Heart Failure

Heart Failure

An Essential Clinical Guide

Edited by

Andreas P. Kalogeropoulos, MD, MPH, PhD, FACC, FHFSA, FASE
Associate Professor of Medicine (Cardiology), Director of Cardiovascular Research,
and Associate Director of the Cardiovascular Fellowship Program
Stony Brook University Medical Center and Renaissance School of Medicine, Stony Brook, NY

Hal A. Skopicki, MD, PhD, FACC, FAHA, FACP
Ambassador Charles A. Gargano Chair of Cardiology, Co-Director of the
Heart Institute, Director of the Heart Failure and Cardiomyopathy Center,
and Co-Director of the Ventricular Assist Device Program
Stony Brook University Medical Center and Renaissance School of Medicine, Stony Brook, NY

Javed Butler, MD, MPH, MBA, FACC, FAHA
Patrick H. Lehan Chair in Cardiovascular Research and
Professor and Chairman of the Department of Medicine
University of Mississippi, Jackson, MS

CRC Press
Taylor & Francis Group
Boca Raton London New York

CRC Press is an imprint of the
Taylor & Francis Group, an **informa** business

First edition published 2023
by CRC Press
6000 Broken Sound Parkway NW, Suite 300, Boca Raton, FL 33487-2742

and by CRC Press
4 Park Square, Milton Park, Abingdon, Oxon, OX14 4RN

CRC Press is an imprint of Taylor & Francis Group, LLC

Library of Congress Cataloging-in-Publication Data

Names: Kalogeropoulos, Andreas, editor. | Skopicki, Hal, editor. | Butler, Javed, editor.
Title: Heart failure : an essential clinical guide / edited by Andreas Kalogeropoulos, Hal Skopicki, Javed Butler.
Other titles: Heart failure (Kalogeropoulos)
Description: First edition. | Boca Raton, FL : CRC Press, 2022. | Includes bibliographical references and index. | Summary: "This "patient-oriented" book provides a practical reference tool for the contemporary assessment and management of patients with heart failure. It evolves around broad patient scenarios to deploy diagnostic and management strategies. It focusses on the areas of current controversies, research needs, and ongoing research for each clinical scenario"-- Provided by publisher.
Identifiers: LCCN 2022002553 (print) | LCCN 2022002554 (ebook) | ISBN 9780367199845 (hardback) | ISBN 9781032278971 (paperback) | ISBN 9780429244544 (ebook)
Subjects: MESH: Heart Failure
Classification: LCC RC685.C53 (print) | LCC RC685.C53 (ebook) | NLM WG 370 | DDC 616.1/29--dc23/eng/20220412
LC record available at https://lccn.loc.gov/2022002553
LC ebook record available at https://lccn.loc.gov/2022002554

ISBN: 9780367199845 (hbk)
ISBN: 9781032278971 (pbk)
ISBN: 9780429244544 (ebk)

DOI: 10.1201/9780429244544

Typeset in Warnock Pro
by Deanta Global Publishing Services, Chennai, India

To my parents, Panagiotis and Angeliki, for their lifelong unconditional support. To my wife, Vicki, who was patient enough to share with me a 20-year journey. And to my beloved children Panagiotis (Takis) and Angeliki (Kiki), my cosmic sources of energy.

—A.P.K.

To my muse and love, Debra. To Hannah, Natalie, and Maddie, whose journey of life-long learning I am fortunate to share. And to my parents, who continue to inspire.

—H.A.S.

To my wife Asma, and children Sophia and Zara.

—J.B.

CONTENTS

PREFACE

No other field of cardiovascular medicine interfaces with as many subspecialties and other medical disciplines as heart failure. A disease of biological aging, heart failure is destined to increase in prevalence as the global population ages and as we get better at treating acute and subacute cardiovascular conditions. The past few decades have seen dramatic progress in the treatment of heart failure and our evidence basis has expanded vastly. Yet, it is amazing how much of our daily heart failure practice is still based on empirical approaches, which sometimes tend to be almost religious in nature.

With improving diagnostics, novel pharmacotherapy targets, and an ever-expanding armamentarium of devices, there are certainly many reasons to be optimistic about the future of heart failure prevention, diagnosis, and management. Yet, there is still a lot of room for improvement in the awareness of heart failure as a preventable and treatable entity among non-specialist practicing internists and cardiologists.

In this spirit, we are excited to present the inaugural edition of *Heart Failure: An Essential Clinical Guide*, a textbook that aspires to be a trigger for further learning and clinical investigation in the field of heart failure. The intended audience is general practitioners and internists with an interest in heart failure, non-heart failure cardiologists, and heart failure specialists—keeping both the practicing clinicians and the clinical investigators in mind. The book is arranged with clinical presentations in mind, but open questions for further investigation are highlighted throughout each chapter to provide the necessary impetus for the next research steps in the field. As there are a number of comprehensive textbooks on heart failure, our goal was to provide an all-around practical overview for a broad clinical audience, while simultaneously intriguing the clinical researcher.

The 36 chapters of the book have been authored by world-class heart failure specialists and clinical investigators in the field of heart failure. We enjoyed every moment working with these accomplished authors to provide the best possible yet compact content to our readers. We learned a great deal during this process—and we hope that you do, too.

Finally, we are fully cognizant of the fact that the field of heart failure is changing at a pace that is not conducive to printed updates. For this purpose, we are planning to provide an online version with live updates for key changes in knowledge and practice.

EDITORS

Andreas P. Kalogeropoulos, MD, MPH, PhD, FACC, FHFSA, FASE, is Associate Professor of Medicine (Cardiology), Director of Cardiovascular Research at Stony Brook University, and Associate Director of the Cardiovascular Fellowship Program, Stony Brook, NY. He is a clinical and outcomes researcher in cardiovascular medicine with expertise in heart failure, echocardiography, and research methodology. Dr. Kalogeropoulos graduated from the University of Patras, Greece (MD, 1994), where he completed his training in internal and cardiovascular medicine (2004) and research methodology (PhD, 2012). He trained in echocardiography, heart failure, and outcomes research (MPH, 2013) at Emory University, Atlanta, GA. Dr. Kalogeropoulos has authored over 180 peer-reviewed articles and five book chapters and has received support for his research from the National Institutes of Health, the American Heart Association, the American Society of Echocardiography, and the Atlanta Clinical and Translational Science Institute. He has chaired the Research Committee of the Heart Failure Society of America (2019–2020) and served on the research committees of the American Society of Echocardiography and the National Cardiovascular Data Registry. Dr. Kalogeropoulos serves on the Editorial Boards of the *Journal of Cardiac Failure* and the *American Heart Journal*, among other cardiovascular journals. His research focuses on (1) risk factors, outcomes, and clinical prediction models for patients with advanced heart failure, with the goal of optimizing management of heart failure patients; (2) risk factors for heart failure; and (3) applications of echocardiography for patients with advanced heart failure and congenital heart disease.

Hal A. Skopicki, MD, PhD, FACC, FAHA, FACP, is the Ambassador Charles A. Gargano Chair of Cardiology, Co-Director of the Heart Institute, Director of the Heart Failure and Cardiomyopathy Center, and Co-Director of the Ventricular Assist Device Program at Stony Brook University Medical Center, Stony Brook, NY. An internationally renowned heart failure scholar and researcher, Dr. Skopicki completed his internship and residency at the Yale-New Haven Hospital and was a clinical and research fellow in Cardiology at the Massachusetts General Hospital and Harvard Medical School. He joined the Heart Failure program at New York–Presbyterian Hospital in New York before being recruited to the Stony Brook University Medical Center. Dr. Skopicki is a fellow of the American Heart Association, the American College of Cardiology, and the American College of Physicians. He is a member of the Heart Failure Society of America and the International Society of Heart and Lung Transplantation. Dr. Skopicki has been rated as a Castle Connolly Top Cardiologist in the New York Metro Area since 2008 and was also honored as a Newsday Top Cardiologist during this time.

Javed Butler, MD, MPH, MBA, FACC, FAHA, is the Patrick H. Lehan Chair in Cardiovascular Research and Professor and Chairman of the Department of Medicine at the University of Mississippi, Jackson, MS. He earned his medical degree from Aga Khan University in Karachi, Pakistan. He completed residency training at Yale University, New Haven, CT, cardiology and advanced heart failure and transplant fellowships at Vanderbilt University, Nashville, TN, and cardiac imaging fellowship at the Massachusetts General Hospital, Harvard Medical School in Boston, MA. He has completed a Master of Public Health degree from Harvard University, Cambridge, MA, and a Master of Business Administration degree from Emory University, Atlanta, GA. Dr. Butler is board certified in cardiology and in advanced heart failure and transplant medicine. His research focuses on clinical trials in patients with heart failure. He serves on several national committees for the American College of Cardiology, the American Heart Association, the National Institutes of Health, and the Heart Failure Society of America Board of Directors. He is a recipient of the Simon Dack Award by the American College of Cardiology as well as the Time, Feeling, and Focus Award by the American Heart Association. Dr. Butler has authored more than 800 peer-reviewed publications. He serves on the editorial board of several peer-reviewed cardiovascular journals.

CONTRIBUTORS

Antonio Abbate
VCU Pauley Heart Center
Virginia Commonwealth University
Richmond, VA

Constantina Aggeli, MD, PhD
Hippokrateio University Hospital
University of Athens Medical School
Athens, Greece

Paulino Alvarez, MD
Division of Cardiovascular Diseases
Section of Heart Failure and Transplant
University of Iowa Hospitals and Clinics
Iowa City, IA

Konstantinos Aznaouridis, MD, PhD
1st Department of Cardiology
Hippokration Hospital
Medical School of National and Kapodistrian University of Athens
Athens, Greece

Georgios Bakosis
Heart Failure Unit
Department of Cardiology
Attikon University Hospital
National and Kapodistrian University of Athens
Athens, Greece

Ana Barradas-Pires
Adult Congenital Heart Centre and National Centre for Pulmonary Hypertension
National Heart and Lung Institute
Imperial College School of Medicine
London, UK

Maria-Anna Bazmpani
1st Department of Cardiology
AHEPA Hospital
Aristotle University
Thessaloniki, Greece

Aris Bechlioulis, MD, PhD
2nd Department of Cardiology
School of Medicine
Faculty of Health Sciences
University of Ioannina
Ioannina, Greece

Kunal Bhatt, MD
Department of Internal Medicine
Division of Cardiology
Emory University School of Medicine
Atlanta, GA

Vasiliki Bistola, MD
Heart Failure Unit
Department of Cardiology
Attikon University Hospital
National and Kapodistrian University of Athens
Athens, Greece

Michelle E. Bloom, MD
Stony Brook University
Renaissance School of Medicine
Stony Brook, NY

Audrey Borghi-Silva
Cardiopulmonary Physical Therapy
Physical Therapy Department
Federal University of São Carlos
São Carlos, Brazil

Alexandros Briasoulis, MD, PhD
Division of Cardiovascular Diseases
Section of Heart Failure and Transplant
University of Iowa Hospitals and Clinics
Iowa City, IA

Rachel A. Bright, BS
Stony Brook University
Renaissance School of Medicine
Stony Brook, NY

Jacob Cao, MD
University of Sydney and Royal Prince Alfred Hospital
Sydney, Australia

Juan Guido Chiabrando
VCU Pauley Heart Center
Virginia Commonwealth University
Richmond, VA

and

Department of Cardiology
Hospital Italiano
Buenos Aires, Argentina

Andrew Constantine
Adult Congenital Heart Centre and National Centre for Pulmonary Hypertension
National Heart and Lung Institute
Imperial College School of Medicine
London, UK

Giulia De Angelis
Cardiovascular Department
Azienda Sanitaria Universitaria Giuliano Isontina (ASUGI)
University of Trieste
Trieste, Italy

Marco Giuseppe Del Buono
VCU Pauley Heart Center
Virginia Commonwealth University
Richmond, VA

and

Department of Cardiovascular and Thoracic Sciences
Catholic University of the Sacred Heart
Rome, Italy

Robert J. DiDomenico, PharmD
Department of Pharmacy Practice
University of Illinois Chicago College of Pharmacy
Chicago, IL

Konstantinos Dimopoulos
Adult Congenital Heart Centre and National Centre for Pulmonary Hypertension
National Heart and Lung Institute
Imperial College School of Medicine
London, UK

Tiffany Dong, MD
Division of Cardiology
Cleveland Clinic Foundation
Cleveland, OH

and

Department of Internal Medicine
Emory University
Atlanta, GA

Stephanie Dwyer Kaluzna, PharmD
Department of Pharmacy Practice
University of Illinois Chicago College of Pharmacy
Chicago, IL

Maxwell Eyram Afari, MD
Cardiac Service Line
Maine Medical Center/Tufts University School of Medicine
Portland, ME

Michael A. Gatzoulis, MD
Adult Congenital Heart Centre and National Centre for Pulmonary Hypertension
National Heart and Lung Institute
Imperial College School of Medicine
London, UK

Philippe Gaudard, MD
Department of Anesthesiology and Critical Care Medicine
Arnaud de Villeneuve Hospital
CHU de Montpellier
Montpellier, France

George Giannakoulas, MD, PhD
1st Department of Cardiology
AHEPA University Hospital of Thessaloniki
Aristotle University of Thessaloniki
Thessaloniki, Greece

Katherine Godfrey, BA
Stony Brook University
Renaissance School of Medicine
Stony Brook, NY

Clive Goulbourne, MD
Stony Brook University
Renaissance School of Medicine
Stony Brook, NY

Prabhjot Grewal, MD
Stony Brook University
Renaissance School of Medicine
Stony Brook, NY

Debbie A. Gunter, RN, MN, FNP-BC, ACHPN
Nell Hodgson Woodruff School of Nursing
Emory University
Atlanta, GA

Salim S. Hayek, MD
Department of Internal Medicine
Division of Cardiology
University of Michigan
Ann Arbor, MI

Stephen B. Heitner, MD
Hypertrophic Cardiomyopathy Center
Knight Cardiovascular Institute
Oregon Health & Science University
Portland, OR

Erika L. Hellenbart, PharmD
Department of Pharmacy Practice
University of Illinois Chicago College of Pharmacy
Chicago, IL

Jenine E. John, MD
Noninvasive Cardiovascular Imaging Program
Departments of Medicine and Radiology
Brigham and Women's Hospital
Boston, MA

Grigorios Kalaitzidis, MD
Department of Neurology
Johns Hopkins University School of Medicine
Baltimore, MD

Eran Kalmanovich, MD
Department of Cardiology
CHU de Montpellier
Montpellier, France

Jesse Kane, MD
Stony Brook University
Renaissance School of Medicine
Stony Brook, NY

and

Montefiore Medical Center
Albert Einstein College of Medicine
Bronx, NY

Theodoros D. Karamitsos
First Department of Cardiology
AHEPA Hospital
Aristotle University
Thessaloniki, Greece

Jodie L. Kenes, MD
Cardiovascular Medicine Section
Wake Forest School of Medicine
Winston–Salem, NC

Panagiotis Korantzopoulos, MD, PhD
First Department of Cardiology
University of Ioannina Faculty of Medicine
Ioannina, Greece

Sean Lal, MD, PhD
University of Sydney and Royal Prince Alfred Hospital
Sydney, Australia

George Lazaros, MD, PhD
First Cardiology Department
Hippokration General Hospital
National and Kapodistrian University of Athens
Athens, Greece

Emilia Lazarou, MD
First Cardiology Department
Hippokration General Hospital
National and Kapodistrian University of Athens
Athens, Greece

Melissa Lyle, MD
Department of Cardiovascular Disease
Mayo Clinic
Jacksonville, FL

and

Department of Internal Medicine
Division of Cardiology
Emory University School of Medicine
Atlanta, GA

Antonis S. Manolis, MD
First Department of Cardiology
Athens University School of Medicine
Athens, Greece

Antonis A. Manolis, DPT, MS
Patras University School of Medicine
Patras, Greece

Theodora A. Manolis, MD
Red Cross Hospital
Athens, Greece

Catherine Marti
Medical College of Georgia
Athens, GA

Constantina Masoura, MD, PhD
Department of Cardiology
Laiko General Hospital
Athens, Greece

Ahmad Masri, MD, MS
Hypertrophic Cardiomyopathy Center
Knight Cardiovascular Institute
Oregon Health & Science University
Portland, OR

Renata Gonçalves Mendes
Cardiopulmonary Physical Therapy
Physical Therapy Department
Federal University of São Carlos
São Carlos, Brazil

Marco Merlo
Cardiovascular Department
Azienda Sanitaria Universitaria Giuliano Isontina (ASUGI)
University of Trieste

Alanna Morris, MD, MSc, FHFSA, FACC, FAHA
Division of Cardiology
Emory University School of Medicine
Atlanta, GA

Sophia Anastasia Mouratoglou, MD, MSc, PhD
Department of Intensive Care and Anesthesiology
AHEPA University Hospital of Thessaloniki
Aristotle University of Thessaloniki
Thessaloniki, Greece

Jonathan Murrow, MD, MSc
Medical College of Georgia
Athens, GA

Evangelos Pavlos Myserlis, MD
Department of Neurology
Harvard Medical School
Boston, MA

Katerina K. Naka, MD
2nd Department of Cardiology
School of Medicine
Faculty of Health Sciences
University of Ioannina
Ioannina, Greece

Aditi Nayak, MD
Division of Cardiology
Emory University School of Medicine
Atlanta, GA

Kent Nilsson
Medical College of Georgia
Athens, GA

Quynh Nguyen, BSc
Division of Cardiology
Department of Medicine
Mazankowski Alberta Heart Institute
Faculty of Medicine and Dentistry
University of Alberta
Edmonton, Canada

John O'Sullivan, MD, PhD
University of Sydney and Royal Prince Alfred Hospital
Sydney, Australia

Gavin Y. Oudit, MD, PhD
Division of Cardiology
Department of Medicine
Mazankowski Alberta Heart Institute
Faculty of Medicine and Dentistry
University of Alberta
Edmonton, Canada

Melissa I. Owen, PhD, RN, FHFSA, CNE
Nell Hodgson Woodruff School of Nursing
Emory University
Atlanta, GA

Alessia Paldino
Cardiovascular Department
Azienda Sanitaria Universitaria Giuliano Isontina (ASUGI)
University of Trieste
Trieste, Italy

Lampros Papadimitriou, MD, PhD
Department of Medicine
University of Mississippi Medical Center
Jackson, MS

Kishan S. Parikh, MD
Duke University Medical Center and Duke Clinical Research Institute
Durham, NC

John Parissis
Heart Failure Unit
Department of Cardiology
and
Emergency Medicine Department
Attikon University Hospital
National and Kapodistrian University of Athens

Kali Polytarchou, MD
Henry Dunnant Hospital Center
Athens, Greece

Eftyhia Polyzogopoulou
Emergency Medicine Department
Attikon University Hospital
National and Kapodistrian University of Athens
Athens, Greece

Arthur Qi, BSc
Division of Cardiology
Department of Medicine
Mazankowski Alberta Heart Institute
Faculty of Medicine and Dentistry
University of Alberta
Edmonton, Canada

Isma Rafiq
Adult Congenital Heart Centre and National Centre for Pulmonary Hypertension
National Heart and Lung Institute
Imperial College School of Medicine
London, UK

Vishal N. Rao, MD, MPH
Duke University Medical Center and Duke Clinical Research Institute
Durham, NC

Krishna Ravindra
VCU Pauley Heart Center
Virginia Commonwealth University
Richmond, VA

Leah Reid, MD
Whitfield Regional Hospital
Demopolis, AL

Jonathan D. Rich
Department of Medicine
Division of Cardiology
Northwestern University Feinberg School of Medicine
Chicago, IL

Fred H. Rodriguez III, MD
Division of Cardiology
Emory University School of Medicine
and
Sibley Heart Center Cardiology
Atlanta, GA

Flávia Rossi Caruso
Cardiopulmonary Physical Therapy
Physical Therapy Department
Federal University of São Carlos
São Carlos, Brazil

François Roubille, MD
Université de Montpellier
Department of Cardiology
CHU de Montpellier
Montpellier, France

Justyna Rybicka
Adult Congenital Heart Centre and National Centre for Pulmonary Hypertension
National Heart and Lung Institute
Imperial College School of Medicine
London, UK

Anita Saraf, MD, PhD
Department of Medicine and Pediatrics and McGowan Regenerative Institute
University of Pittsburgh
Pittsburgh, PA

Victoria Shklar, MD, MS
Mather Hospital
Northwell Health
Port Jefferson, NY

Amil M. Shah, MD, MPH
Cardiovascular Division
Brigham and Women's Hospital
Boston, MA

Gianfranco Sinagra
Cardiovascular Department
Azienda Sanitaria Universitaria Giuliano Isontina (ASUGI)
University of Trieste
Trieste, Italy

Richard B. Stacey, MD
Cardiovascular Medicine Section
Wake Forest School of Medicine
Winston–Salem, NC

Getu Teressa, MD, PhD
Stony Brook University
Renaissance School of Medicine
Stony Brook, NY

Anjan Tibrewala
Department of Medicine
Division of Cardiology
Northwestern University Feinberg School of Medicine
Chicago, IL

Dimitris Tousoulis, MD, PhD
First Cardiology Department
Hippokration General Hospital
National and Kapodistrian University of Athens
Athens, Greece

Lana Tsao, MD
Mass General Heart Center
Boston, MA

Bharathi Upadhya, MD
Cardiovascular Medicine Section
Wake Forest School of Medicine
Winston–Salem, NC

Peter van der Meer, MD, PhD
University of Groningen
University Medical Center Groningen
Groningen, The Netherlands

Haye H. van der Wal, MD
University of Groningen
University Medical Center Groningen
Groningen, The Netherlands

Charalambos Vlachopoulos, MD, PhD
1st Department of Cardiology
Hippokration Hospital
Medical School of National and Kapodistrian University of Athens
Athens, Greece

Haran Yogasundaram, MD
Division of Cardiology
Department of Medicine
Mazankowski Alberta Heart Institute
Faculty of Medicine and Dentistry
University of Alberta
Edmonton, Canada

Ily Kristine T. Yumul-Non, MD
Division of Cardiovascular Diseases
Section of Heart Failure and Transplant
University of Iowa Hospitals and Clinics
Iowa City, IA

Section I
Basic Concepts in Heart Failure

DOI: 10.1201/9780429244544-1

Chapter 1
DEFINITIONS AND CLINICAL DIAGNOSIS OF HEART FAILURE

Katerina K. Naka and Aris Bechlioulis

The Heart Failure Syndrome

Heart failure (HF) is a leading cause of morbidity and mortality worldwide, with increasing prevalence. HF is a common clinical syndrome that can result from any abnormality of cardiac structure or function that may impair the ability of the ventricle to eject blood or to fill with blood, leading to reduced cardiac output which is insufficient to meet the body requirements at rest or on exertion, or sufficient only at the expense of elevated cardiac filling pressures.

HF can arise as a result of almost any abnormality of the structure, mechanical function, or electrical activity of the heart (myocardial disease, systolic or diastolic ventricular dysfunction, abnormalities of the valves, pericardium, endocardium, heart rhythm, and conduction), although more than one abnormality may be present. Each of these abnormalities may require quite different treatments, emphasizing the need to identify the underlying cardiac problem. Most patients with HF have symptoms resulting from impaired left ventricular (LV) myocardial function.

Clinically, HF is a complex clinical syndrome, characterized by typical symptoms (e.g., breathlessness, ankle swelling, fatigue, and limited exercise tolerance), which may be accompanied by typical signs (e.g., elevated jugular venous pressure, pulmonary crackles, and peripheral edema). The term "syndrome" merely describes a constellation of symptoms and signs and, therefore, HF is not a diagnosis per se. Moreover, typical symptoms and signs of HF are non-specific, making clinical confirmation of the syndrome difficult.

Although it has proved difficult to agree on a simple definition of HF, the most pragmatic and concise clinical approach has been advocated by the European Society of Cardiology (ESC) (Table 1.1).[1] This definition of HF is limited to symptomatic stages. However, before symptoms become evident, patients may have asymptomatic structural or functional cardiac abnormalities (e.g., cardiomyopathy or any LV systolic or diastolic dysfunction), that usually precede overt HF. Recognition of these asymptomatic, preclinical stages is important, as these are related to worse outcomes, and early initiation of treatment may reduce mortality in patients with asymptomatic systolic LV dysfunction.[2]

Based on symptom onset and time course, HF may be chronic or acute (*de novo* or acute decompensation of chronic HF). Chronic HF can be further classified based on different aspects of the syndrome:

- Symptomatic severity and functional limitation; the New York Heart Association (NYHA) and Interagency Registry for Mechanically Assisted Circulatory Support (INTERMACS) classifications.
- Risk factors for and stages of development of cardiac dysfunction and HF; the American College of Cardiology (ACC) / American Heart Association (AHA) stage-specific approach.
- Left ventricular ejection fraction (LVEF); HF with reduced ejection fraction (HFrEF) vs midrange ejection fraction (HFmrEF) vs preserved (HFpEF) LVEF phenotypes.
- Ventricle(s) affected; left ventricular vs right ventricular vs bi-ventricular.

New York Heart Association Classification and INTERMACS

The most widely used classification of the functional limitation related to HF is the NYHA functional classification that describes and categorizes the severity of HF symptoms and exercise intolerance. Patients with HF are divided into four categories:

- *NYHA class I*: No limitations in physical activity. Ordinary activity does not cause unusual dyspnea, fatigue, or palpitations.
- *NYHA class II*: Slight limitation in physical activity. Comfortable at rest, but ordinary activity results in unusual dyspnea, fatigue, or palpitations.
- *NYHA class III*: Marked limitation in physical activity. Less than ordinary activity results in unusual dyspnea, fatigue, or palpitations.
- *NYHA class IV*: Unable to participate in any physical activity. Symptoms at rest can be present. Increased discomfort if any activity is undertaken.

There is significant direct correlation between NYHA class and measures of maximal or submaximal exercise capacity in HF patients.[3,4] Although symptomatic severity often correlates poorly with objective measures of LV function, there is a clear relationship between symptoms and prognosis; even mild symptoms are associated with increased risk of hospitalization and death.[3,5] Although reproducibility and validity may be problematic, the NYHA classification independently predicts mortality and it is widely used in research and clinical practice to determine the eligibility of patients for various treatment modalities and health care services.[5]

Patients with advanced HF are those who are still severely symptomatic despite optimal guideline-directed management regardless of LVEF. For patients with advanced HFrEF, further differential classification is recommended to guide advanced therapeutic options. The INTERMACS registry has identified seven distinct profiles (Table 1.2) at different stages of disease progression with variable indications for advanced therapies (i.e., mechanical circulatory support and transplantation) and variable prognoses.[6–8] Furthermore, three modifiers of these profiles indicate worsening of HF, i.e., the need for temporary circulatory support (modifies profiles 1, 2, and 3 in hospital), the presence of arrhythmias (modifies any profile), and the need for frequent emergency visits or hospitalizations (modifies profiles 3 at home, 4, 5,

DOI: 10.1201/9780429244544-2

TABLE 1.1: Definition of Heart Failure as a Clinical Syndrome

1. Symptoms	Typical: breathlessness at rest or on exercise, fatigue, tiredness, ankle swelling	May be atypical or may have been reduced with treatment
AND		
2. Signs	Typical: tachycardia, tachypnea, pulmonary rales, raised jugular venous pressure, pleural effusion, peripheral edema, hepatomegaly	May be more or less specific or may become less evident following treatment
AND		
3. Objective evidence of cardiac structural or functional abnormality at rest	Physical examination: 3rd heart sound, cardiac murmurs Chest X-Ray: cardiomegaly Raised natriuretic peptide levels Echocardiographic abnormalities	Echocardiography is the method most widely used

Source: Modified with permission from: McMurray, Adamopoulos, Anker, et al. ESC Guidelines for the diagnosis and treatment of acute and chronic heart failure 2012: The Task Force for the Diagnosis and Treatment of Acute and Chronic Heart Failure of the European Society of Cardiology. Developed in collaboration with the Heart Failure Association (HFA) of the ESC. *Eur J Heart Fail* 2012;14:803–69.

TABLE 1.2: INTERMACS Classification and Relation to New York Heart Association (NYHA) Classification

INTERMACS	Description	NYHA class
1. Cardiogenic shock: "Crash and burn"	Hemodynamic instability in spite of increasing doses of catecholamines and/or mechanical circulatory support with critical hypoperfusion of target organs	IV
2. Progressive decline despite inotrope support: "Sliding on inotropes"	Intravenous inotrope support with acceptable blood pressure but rapid deterioration of renal function, nutritional state or signs of congestion	IV
3. Stable but inotrope dependent: "Dependent stability"	Hemodynamic stability with low or intermediate doses of inotropes, but necessary due to hypotension, worsening of symptoms or progressive renal failure	IV
4. Resting symptoms	Temporary cessation of inotrope treatment is possible, but patients present with frequent symptom recurrences and typically with fluid overload	IV (ambulatory)
5. Exertion intolerant: "Housebound"	Complete cessation of physical activity, stable at rest, but frequently with moderate fluid retention and some level of renal dysfunction	IV (ambulatory)
6. Exertion limited: "Walking wounded"	Absence of congestion while at rest, easily fatigued by slight activity	III
7. Advanced NYHA III	NYHA III with no current or recent fluid retention	III

Source: Modified with permission from: Stevenson, Pagani, Young, et al. INTERMACS profiles of advanced heart failure: the current picture. *J Heart Lung Transplant* 2009;28:535–41.

and 6).[9] The INTERMACS was developed as an extension of the NYHA classification for classes III–IV, specifically for patients with HFrEF, with the aim of identifying early on the turning point that demands escalation of therapy (mainly long-term mechanical circulatory support and device implantation). A recent statement from ESC further refines the criteria for advanced HF to classify both patients with HFrEF and HFpEF.[9]

Stage-Specific Approach to Heart Failure

The ACC/AHA stage classification aligns with epidemiological principles of prevention and emphasizes the development and progression of HF.[10] This approach recognizes four different stages of HF, starting early in the development of the disease in the presence of risk factors without abnormalities of cardiac function (Stage A), progressing to subclinical asymptomatic disease (Stage B), and finally to clinical symptomatic disease (Stages C and D) (Table 1.3).

The stages are progressive and, once a patient moves to a higher stage, regression to an earlier stage of HF cannot occur. Progression in HF stages is associated with worsening prognosis and different therapeutic interventions at each stage are needed. The focus of this approach is prevention (Stage A) to avoid or delay progression to structural heart disease (Stage B) and to aggressively treat patients with Stage B HF to delay progression to symptomatic HF (Stages C and D). Whether adopting this classification could decrease the incidence of clinical HF and improve outcomes is not known. Both the stage-specific approach and NYHA classification provide useful and complementary information about the presence and severity of HF (Table 1.3).[5] Differentiating Stage C and D HF patients may be challenging, although the early identification of Stage D status is important to proceed with advanced treatment modalities. Although a clear Stage D definition is lacking, INTERMACS profiles provide a practical approach to identifying Stage D HF patients more efficiently than do other sets of criteria or simply the physician's opinion.[11]

The Heart Failure Diagnostic Armamentarium

Diagnostic Algorithm

Although there is no consensus on the criteria required to establish a diagnosis of HF (either acute or chronic), the most comprehensive algorithm for the diagnosis of chronic HF in patients presenting with symptoms or signs of HF for the first time in a non-acute setting, is shown in Figure 1.1 and is based

TABLE 1.3: Stages of Heart Failure (HF) and Relation to New York Heart Association (NYHA) Classification

	ACC/AHA Stages of HF	NYHA Class
A	High risk of HF but no structural heart disease or HF symptoms	–
B	Structural heart disease but no signs or symptoms of HF	I
C	Structural heart disease with prior or current symptoms if HF	I–IV
D	Refractory HF requiring specialized interventions	IV

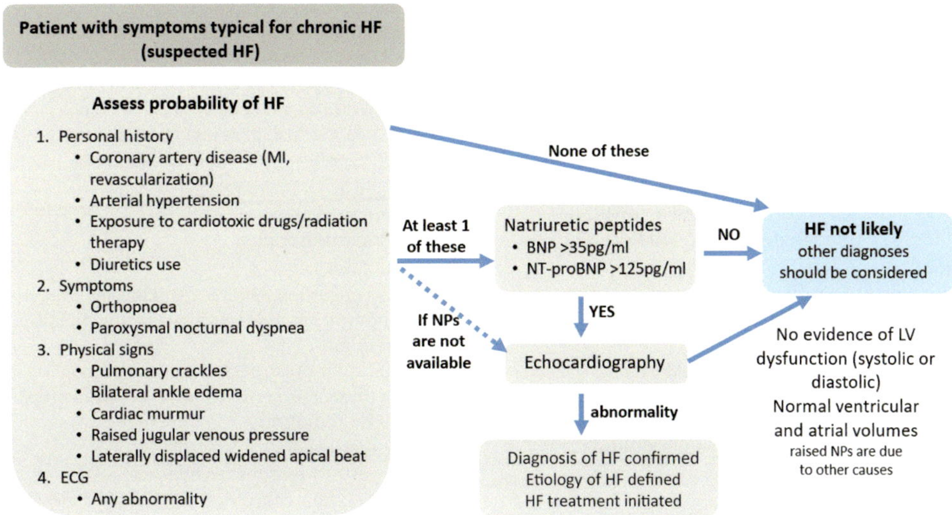

FIGURE 1.1 Diagnostic algorithm for the diagnosis of chronic heart failure. *Abbreviations*: BNP, B-type natriuretic peptide; ECG, electrocardiogram; HF, heart failure; LV, left ventricular; MI, myocardial infarction; NPs, natriuretic peptides; NT-proBNP, N-terminal pro-BNP. (Modified from: Ponikowski, Voors, Anker, et al. 2016 ESC guidelines for the diagnosis and treatment of acute and chronic heart failure: The Task Force for the diagnosis and treatment of acute and chronic heart failure of the European Society of Cardiology (ESC). Developed with the special contribution of the Heart Failure Association (HFA) of the ESC. *Eur J Heart Fail* 2016;18:891–975.)

upon the 2016 ESC guidelines.[2] First, the probability of HF should be assessed based on:

- *Personal history* (coronary artery disease, arterial hypertension, exposure to cardiotoxic medications or radiation therapy, diuretic use)
- *Presenting symptoms* (orthopnea or paroxysmal nocturnal dyspnea)
- *Physical examination* (bilateral ankle edema, increased jugular venous pressure, displaced apical beat)
- *Resting electrocardiogram*

If there is no abnormality in any of the four categories above, HF is considered highly unlikely and other diagnoses should be assessed. If an abnormality is found in ≥1 category then plasma natriuretic peptides should be measured, if available, to identify those who need echocardiography. In cases where natriuretic peptide measurement is not available or where plasma levels are above the proposed cut-offs, echocardiography is indicated.

History and Physical Examination

Symptoms and signs of HF are due to lung congestion, fluid retention, and peripheral hypoperfusion (Table 1.4). Typical symptoms may be present, but often symptoms are nonspecific and presentation is complicated by multiple comorbidities, especially in older adults, in whom HF predominantly occurs.[2] As most patients with HF present with symptoms related to congestion, the most common presentation is dyspnea, a symptom that is neither specific nor sensitive for HF. Furthermore, symptoms and signs of HF due to fluid retention may resolve quickly with diuretic therapy and may be particularly difficult to detect and interpret in older adults, patients with obesity, and those with chronic lung disease.[2]

Some physical signs of HF, such as elevated jugular venous pressure, lateral displacement of the apical impulse, bilateral basal pulmonary end-inspiratory rales, and leg edema may be more specific for HF, but are harder to detect, have poor reproducibility, and sensitivity is ~50–60%. Thus, diagnostic uncertainty often remains high, even after clinical assessment.[12]

Biomarkers: Old and New

Natriuretic Peptides

B-type natriuretic peptide (BNP) and N-terminal pro-BNP (NT-proBNP) are considered the gold standard biomarkers in the diagnosis and prognosis of HF and may play a role in HF management.[12] Natriuretic peptides should be measured in all patients with symptoms suggestive of HF, to facilitate early diagnosis and risk stratification. For chronic HF, natriuretic peptides are recommended as an initial diagnostic test, especially when echocardiography is not immediately available. Natriuretic peptides are reasonable surrogates for intracardiac volumes and filling pressures but should always be used in conjunction with clinical information. A normal value has an excellent negative predictive value to exclude HF, whereas an abnormal value does not confirm the diagnosis of HF but underlines the need for cardiac imaging. Patients with normal

TABLE 1.4: Symptoms and Signs of HF and Main Proposed Pathophysiological Explanations

Symptoms—Typical	Breathlessness	Lung congestion due to raised left atrial pressure, respiratory muscle
	Orthopnea	and chemoreceptor abnormalities
	Paroxysmal nocturnal dyspnea	Increased venous return and lung congestion in the supine position
	Reduced exercise tolerance, fatigue, tiredness	As above and respiratory center depression
	Ankle swelling	Skeletal muscle hypoperfusion and metabolic abnormalities
		Fluid retention
Symptoms—Less Typical	Nocturnal cough	Increased venous return and lung congestion
	Wheezing	Lung congestion
	Bloated feeling	Fluid retention, raised right atrial pressure
	Loss of appetite	Fluid retention
	Confusion (especially in the elderly)	Cerebral hypoperfusion
	Depression	Cerebral hypoperfusion, impaired quality of life
	Palpitations	Tachyarrhythmias, reduced exercise tolerance
	Dizziness and/or syncope	Cerebral hypoperfusion, brady- or tachyarrhythmias
	Bendopnea	Increased venous return and lung congestion when bending
Signs—More Specific	Elevated jugular venous pressure	Raised right atrial pressure
	Third heart sound (gallop rhythm)	Raised left atrial pressure
	Laterally displaced apical impulse	Left ventricular dilatation
Signs—Less Specific	Weight gain (>2 kg/week)	Fluid retention
	Weight loss (in advanced HF), Tissue	Intestinal congestion, chronic cytokine and inflammatory activation
	wasting, cachexia	Mitral and/or tricuspid regurgitation (functional)
	Cardiac murmur	Fluid retention
	Peripheral edema (ankle, sacral, scrotal)	Raised left atrial pressure and lung congestion
	Pulmonary crepitations	Fluid retention, raised right and/or left atrial pressure
	Reduced air entry and dullness to percussion	Sympathetic activation
	at lung bases (pleural effusion)	Atrial or ventricular arrhythmias
	Tachycardia	Lung congestion, response to hypoxia
	Irregular pulse	Respiratory center depression due to lung congestion
	Tachypnoea	Raised right atrial pressure, venous congestion
	Cheyne-Stokes respiration	Raised right atrial pressure, fluid retention
	Hepatomegaly	Peripheral hypoperfusion, reduced cardiac output
	Ascites	Renal hypoperfusion and/or venous congestion
	Cold extremities	Reduced cardiac output
	Oliguria	
	Narrow pulse pressure	

Source: Modified from: Ponikowski, Voors, Anker, et al. 2016 ESC Guidelines for the diagnosis and treatment of acute and chronic heart failure: The Task Force for the diagnosis and treatment of acute and chronic heart failure of the European Society of Cardiology (ESC). Developed with the special contribution of the Heart Failure Association (HFA) of the ESC. *Eur J Heart Fail* 2016;18:891–975.

natriuretic peptide concentrations are unlikely to have HF and do not need echocardiography. Natriuretic peptides accurately discriminate HF from other causes of dyspnea: the higher the level, the greater the likelihood that dyspnea is caused by HF. However, natriuretic peptides cannot identify the underlying cause of HF and therefore, if elevated, must always be used in conjunction with cardiac imaging.[12]

The upper limit of normal in non-acute settings is 35 pg/mL for BNP and 125 pg/mL for NT-proBNP, although higher cut-offs have been suggested for the acute setting. Cut-offs do not differ for HFrEF and HFpEF, although values are lower for HFpEF vs HFrEF patients.[13] The negative predictive value of levels below the cut-offs is high (0.94–0.98) in both acute and chronic settings. However, the positive predictive value is lower, both in the chronic setting (0.44–0.57) and in the acute setting (0.66–0.67).[2] These data suggest that BNP and NT-proBNP are powerful, not only in ruling out HF, but also in confirming a diagnosis of HF, supplementing (but not replacing) clinical judgment. Patients with very high levels (NT-proBNP >2,000 pg/mL) should be referred to a cardiologist (preferably a HF specialist) within two weeks and those with levels between 400 and 2000 pg/mL within six weeks.[14] Several point-of-care devices have been developed to measure natriuretic peptides levels in clinical practice; in addition to blood, the use of saliva is also currently being investigated.[15]

The diagnostic utility of natriuretic peptides in HF is compromised by the various cardiovascular and non-cardiovascular causes that are associated with high natriuretic peptide levels. In the acute setting, these causes include acute coronary syndromes, atrial or ventricular arrhythmias, pulmonary embolism, and severe chronic obstructive pulmonary disease with elevated right heart pressures, renal failure, and sepsis.[1] Other causes in the non-acute setting are age >75 years, atrial arrhythmias, left ventricular hypertrophy, chronic obstructive pulmonary disease, and chronic kidney disease.[1] The most important factors confounding the interpretation of natriuretic peptide levels are atrial fibrillation (AF), age, and renal failure, all causing an increase in natriuretic peptide levels. Obese patients have lower concentrations, mandating lower cut-off levels (about 50% lower). Despite the presence of HF with potentially severe symptoms, natriuretic peptide levels may also be lower in patients already treated for HF, right ventricular failure, pulmonary hypertension, and pericardial causes, as well as HF due to causes upstream of the LV, such as mitral stenosis, acute mitral regurgitation, and flash pulmonary edema. Finally, treatment with neprilysin inhibitors (sacubitril/valsartan) leads to higher BNP levels, which complicates the use of this biomarker in patients treated with this class of agents. In addition to diagnostic use, natriuretic peptides also have a high prognostic value and can identify high-risk patients who should be offered more immediate and aggressive treatment to improve outcomes.[12] Also, natriuretic peptides and troponins are recommended to monitor the use and dosing of cardiotoxic antineoplastic therapy and to identify patients at higher risk of cardiotoxicity.[16]

Another natriuretic peptide, mid-regional pro-ANP, has been studied in the diagnosis of acute HF, with a diagnostic and prognostic profile comparable to that of other natriuretic peptides.[17] This natriuretic peptide has potentially greater stability and higher diagnostic and prognostic value, especially in HFpEF patients. Mid-regional pro-ANP has shown a greater sensitivity for the diagnosis of HFpEF, a stronger, positive correlation with echocardiographic markers, and better discrimination of disease severity than NT-proBNP.[18]

Other Biomarkers

In addition to NPs, newer biomarkers, such as soluble suppression of tumorigenicity 2 (sST2), high-sensitivity troponin, and renal biomarkers, may be useful in risk stratification and patient management. In the context of the pro-inflammatory state associated with HFpEF, an increasing body of evidence suggests that non-natriuretic-peptide biomarkers are better diagnostic tools for HFpEF. Emerging markers reflecting myocardial fibrosis, such as sST2, growth differentiation factor-15, galectin 3, and interleukins 1 and 6, are showing promise, correlating to different degrees with transthoracic echocardiographic parameters of diastolic dysfunction.[19] The utility of these biomarkers in comparison to natriuretic peptides remains to be evaluated. Finally, high levels of serological markers of collagen turnover (collagen type I carboxy-terminal telopeptide and procollagen type III N-terminal propeptide) in subjects free of overt cardiovascular disease have been associated with increased risk of HF, especially HFpEF.[20] Despite extensive research on these newer biomarkers in HF, there is currently no definite evidence to support the use of such biomarkers in clinical practice.

Non-Invasive Imaging and Assessment

Cardiac imaging plays a central role in the diagnosis and management of HF. Assessment of myocardial structure and function using non-invasive imaging is recommended in patients presenting with new or worsening HF symptoms or patients with established HF who have received evidence-based therapy before the decision to escalate treatment. Echocardiography remains the method of choice in suspected HF due to its favorable profile (high availability, low cost, safety, and reasonable accuracy).[2]

Electrocardiography

A resting 12-lead electrocardiogram is recommended in all patients with suspected HF to determine heart rate and rhythm, QRS morphology and duration, as well as to detect other abnormalities. An abnormal electrocardiogram is common in patients with HF but has low specificity. A completely normal electrocardiogram excludes HF diagnosis (high sensitivity). Specific abnormalities on an electrocardiogram may be informative on the etiology of HF (i.e., ischemic heart disease), whereas others are suggestive of specific treatments in a relevant clinical setting (i.e., thromboprophylaxis in atrial fibrillation, pacing for bradycardia, cardiac resynchronization therapy in left bundle branch block, etc.).[2,5]

Chest X-Ray

A chest X-ray is recommended as a first line investigation in patients with a potential HF diagnosis, especially in the acute setting, to identify pulmonary congestion, and can be useful to diagnose or exclude alternative non-cardiac causes (e.g., pulmonary disease) of symptoms. However, there is often discordance between hemodynamics and radiological findings, i.e., absence of pulmonary venous congestion in the presence of high pulmonary capillary pressures.[2,5] Although a chest X-ray is important for the evaluation of patients presenting with symptoms and signs of HF, it should not be the sole determinant of the presence and specific cause of HF because of its low sensitivity and specificity.

Echocardiography

Doppler transthoracic echocardiography (TTE) is the most useful, widely available test in the initial evaluation of patients with suspected HF to establish the diagnosis. It is the method of choice for the assessment of myocardial systolic and diastolic function, wall thickness, wall motion, and valve function. This information is crucial in order to establish the diagnosis and often the cause of HF, to determine the phenotype of HF, and to choose the appropriate treatment accordingly.[2,5] Repeat assessment of LVEF and severity of remodeling is useful in patients with HF who have had a significant change in clinical status, experienced or recovered from a clinical event, received treatment that might have affected cardiac function, or who may be candidates for device therapy.[5] TTE is recommended for the assessment of valve disease in order to identify those suitable for interventions.[2,5]

For LVEF, the modified biplane Simpson's method is recommended, although reporting regional wall motion abnormalities might be particularly relevant for patients with suspected coronary artery disease (CAD) or myocarditis. Three-dimensional echocardiography of adequate quality improves the quantification of LV volumes and LVEF and provides values closest to those obtained with cardiac magnetic resonance (CMR). Although LVEF is still the cornerstone of diagnosis, choice of treatment, and prognosis in HF, the calculation of LVEF has important pitfalls, due to its high load dependence. Thus, true myocardial function often remains underestimated or overestimated under different conditions.[21] Other components of LV geometry and function as well as loading conditions should be considered when assessing cardiac function. The stroke volume index, with a cut-off of $\leq$22 mL/m$^{2.04}$ derived from aortic stenosis studies, corresponding to the previously reported cut-off of 35 mL/m^2 when normalized for body surface area,[22] has been reported to be important, particularly in HFpEF.[23] Recently, tissue Doppler parameters (S′ wave) and myocardial deformation imaging (to assess strain and strain rate) have been shown to be reproducible and feasible for clinical use, especially in detecting subclinical abnormalities in systolic function.[2,5] However, measurements may vary among vendors and software versions.

LV diastolic dysfunction is thought to be the underlying pathophysiological abnormality in patients with HFpEF and HFmrEF, and thus its assessment plays a key role in diagnosis. Echocardiography is currently the only imaging technique that allows for the diagnosis of diastolic dysfunction, but no single variable is sufficiently accurate to be used in isolation to diagnose diastolic dysfunction. Therefore, a comprehensive echocardiograph examination, incorporating all relevant two-dimensional and Doppler data, is recommended.[2,5]

The right ventricle (RV) structure and function should be assessed in all patients with suspected or established HF. The RV systolic function can be assessed by the tricuspid annular plane systolic excursion (TAPSE, abnormal <17 mm) and tissue Doppler-derived tricuspid lateral annular systolic velocity (S′, abnormal <9.5 cm/s). Systolic pulmonary artery pressure is derived from an estimation of the tricuspid systolic gradient, adding an estimate of right atrial (RA) pressure based on inferior vena cava (IVC) size and collapsibility with respiration. Three-dimensional assessment of RV is recommended in experienced laboratories, whereas three-dimensional speckle tracking may be an additional quantitative method to assess RV function in specialized centers.[2,5]

Transesophageal echocardiography (TEE) is not needed in the routine assessment of HF; however, it may be valuable in some patients with valve disease, suspected aortic dissection, suspected endocarditis, or congenital heart disease, and for ruling out intracavitary thrombi in patients with AF requiring cardioversion. When the severity of mitral or aortic valve disease on TTE does not match the severity of symptoms, a TEE should be performed.[2,5] Exercise or pharmacological stress echocardiography may be used to evaluate the patient for inducible ischemia and/or myocardial viability and to assess the severity of valve disease in some scenarios (e.g., dynamic mitral regurgitation, low-flow, low-gradient aortic stenosis).[2,5] If echocardiography is not available or image quality is poor, alternative methods of cardiac imaging can be considered.

Cardiac Magnetic Resonance (CMR) Imaging

CMR is a key imaging technique in patients with suspected HF and plays a key role in cardiac phenotyping, with several clinical advantages over other techniques. CMR is considered the gold standard for comprehensive and reproducible measurements of cardiac anatomy and function, including volumes, mass assessment, wall thickening, and motion of both LV and RV.[2,5,24] Established techniques, e.g., use of gadolinium as a contrast agent, are now widely used in practice, providing information on myocardial perfusion and viability, while late gadolinium enhancement is the preferred method to assess the extent of myocardial fibrosis and to differentiate between ischemic scar and non-ischemic fibrosis.[2,5] Furthermore, CMR enables myocardial tissue characterization and can assist in the etiological diagnosis of myocarditis, amyloidosis, sarcoidosis, arrhythmogenic cardiomyopathy, and other specific cardiomyopathies. Novel techniques, such as myocardial mapping (T1, T2, T2*, and the extracellular volume) may further enhance the diagnostic and prognostic role of CMR.[2,5,24] Advances in CMR may fill gaps in our knowledge, with the potential to change thinking, disease classifications, and definitions, as well as patient management.[24] Limitations include availability and cost, the presence of metallic implants (including rhythm devices in HF patients), and claustrophobia. Gadolinium is contraindicated in patients with glomerular filtration rate<30 mL/min/1.73 m^2 because of the risk of nephrogenic systemic fibrosis.[2,5,24]

Cardiac Computerized Tomography (CCT)

CCT provides an accurate assessment of cardiac structure and function with an excellent correlation between CMR and CCT-derived volumes, mass, and function. Nevertheless, its use over echocardiography and CMR is limited to cases where other methods are suboptimal or contraindicated.[25] Compared to echocardiography, CCT may offer an advantage to characterize the myocardium, although this has not been proven in clinical studies.[26] The main indication of CCT in HF, as suggested by current guidelines, remains the visualization of the coronary anatomy in patients with angina or evidence of myocardial ischemia and low-to-intermediate pre-test probability of CAD (or those with ambiguous non-invasive stress tests) in order to rule out coronary artery stenosis. Functional studies with CCT require electrocardiogram (ECG)-gated acquisition to reconstruct end-diastolic and end-systolic images, whereas radiation, the need for intravenous contrast, and high heart rate are the main limitations to CCT use in practice.[2,5,26]

Nuclear Imaging

Single-photon emission computerized tomography (SPECT) may be useful in assessing coronary ischemia and myocardial viability in HF patients when revascularization is under discussion, while gated SPECT can also provide information on ventricular volumes and function. Positron emission tomography (PET), alone or with computerized tomography (CT), may be used to assess ischemia and viability in HF patients but the availability of tracers is currently limited by excessive cost.[2,5] Radionuclide ventriculography is still the gold standard method for assessment of LVEF. This method is highly reproducible and may be used for the evaluation of cardiac function when other imaging modalities are unavailable or inadequate, although it cannot assess valvular structure/function or myocardial wall thickness and motion. Radionuclide ventriculography is considered to be more accurate than echocardiography, especially for measuring RV function, and its reproducibility is better than that of echocardiography.[27] Myocardial perfusion imaging has an excellent negative predictive value for the detection of significant CAD as the cause of new-onset HF. SPECT has also been used in clinical practice to assess LV dyssynchrony in patients with HF, using commercially available software. Cardiac imaging with radioactive ^{123}I-metaiodobenzyl-guanidine (mIBG) can identify areas of myocardium with impaired sympathetic innervation because of injury or ischemia. In HFrEF, ^{123}I-mIBG imaging improves risk stratification over natriuretic peptides and LVEF.[27] Nuclear imaging modalities may also provide diagnostic and prognostic information in specific cardiomyopathies. PET is routinely used in the management of patients with cardiac sarcoidosis, allowing for identification of inflammation (both cardiac and extracardiac) and management of immunosuppression. Scintigraphy with bone tracers is used to detect cardiac transthyretin amyloidosis, an increasingly important and common disease in older adults, presenting as HFpEF (see also Chapter 35).[27]

Invasive Imaging and Assessment

The indications for invasive diagnostic procedures in patients with HF have been narrowing in the past several years, as these procedures are not necessary to confirm the presence of HF. However, invasive diagnostic procedures may be helpful on an individual basis to determine the etiology of HF and to guide therapy, especially in acute or difficult situations.

Coronary Angiography

Coronary angiography is recommended in patients with HF and known CAD who suffer from angina refractory to medical therapy, provided the patient is suitable for revascularization, as well as in patients with a history of symptomatic ventricular arrhythmia or aborted cardiac arrest.[2] Coronary angiography should be considered in patients with HF and intermediate to high pre-test probability of CAD and/or ischemia in non-invasive stress tests, with the goal of establishing the etiology of HF and assessing the severity of CAD.[2] In practice, coronary angiography is also used as a diagnostic test in patients with HF or LV systolic dysfunction of unknown origin and may also be considered in patients with acute HF with shock not responding to initial therapy.[5]

Right Heart Catheterization (RHC)

Right heart catheterization (RHC) for invasive assessment of hemodynamics is not routinely used in patients with HF and is considered mainly in acute or emergency situations with respiratory distress or impaired perfusion. RHC can be considered in cases where a specific clinical or therapeutic question needs to be addressed or where non-invasive assessment of filling pressures is inconclusive.[5] RHC is part of the initial evaluation of patients with HF who are candidates for heart transplantation or mechanical circulatory support.[2,5] RHC should also be considered in patients with echocardiographic evidence of pulmonary hypertension in order to confirm the presence of pulmonary hypertension and to assess pulmonary vascular resistance for baseline reference.[2,5] RHC can be useful for patients with acute HF who remain severely symptomatic despite initial standard therapies and whose hemodynamic status is unclear.[2,5] Patients with clinically significant hypotension and/or worsening renal function, despite initial therapy that may lead to the use of inotropes/vasoactive medications or mechanical circulatory support, might also benefit from invasive hemodynamic measurements. On the other hand, routine RHC is not recommended in normotensive patients with acute HF who have an adequate response to diuretics and vasodilators.[5]

Myocardial Biopsy

Myocardial biopsy should be considered in patients with rapidly progressive HF despite standard therapy, in whom a specific diagnosis that would influence treatment is suspected.[2,5] These cases include the probable presence of a specific myocarditis or myocardial disease in newly diagnosed HF. Furthermore, myocardial biopsy is routinely used in heart transplant recipients to detect graft rejection. Routine myocardial biopsy is not recommended in HF, given the limited diagnostic yield and the risk of procedure-related complications.[2,5]

Pitfalls in the Diagnosis of Heart Failure

Symptoms and signs usually alert the patient and the physician to the probable presence of a cardiac disorder and may suggest the presence of HF, but are not specific for this syndrome.[28] Comorbidities, such as obesity, chronic pulmonary obstructive disease, chronic kidney disease, anemia, depression, aging, and deconditioning, may present with similar symptoms, making the differential diagnosis difficult, especially in the presence of preserved LVEF. In these cases, natriuretic peptides play a key role, provided that interpretation considers the limitations of these biomarkers.

Pitfalls of Natriuretic Peptides

The cut-off concentrations of natriuretic peptides used for the exclusion of HF differ among scientific societies, potentially causing confusion. For example, the ESC recommends BNP <30 pg/mL or NT-proBNP <125 pg/mL, whereas the National Institute for Health and Care Excellence of England suggests that a NT-proBNP <400 pg/mL in an untreated person makes a diagnosis of HF less likely.[2,14] However, it was recently shown that the NT-proBNP cut-off of 400 pg/mL, albeit cost-effective, was probably too high, as about 20% of patients with HF were not appropriately referred for further investigation and diagnosis.[29] The cut-off levels currently recommended by the ESC focus on a strong rule-out strategy that favors minimizing false-negative results.[17] For NT-proBNP, a stratified approach of 50/75/250 pg/mL for ages <50/50–75/>75 years has been suggested;[17] these age-adjusted cut-off levels address the issue of age-dependent normal values of NT-proBNP as a result of gradual impairment of renal function with age.

In patients with HFpEF, natriuretic peptide levels are often low despite high LV filling pressures, thereby making diagnosis of HF challenging. Low natriuretic peptide levels are also seen with obesity (a common comorbidity in HFpEF), patients of African American origin, and patients on diuretics and HF treatment.[11] In these ambiguous cases, echocardiography can be useful, although a high level of expertise may be needed in difficult-to-diagnose patients. Detailed guidance on the objective assessment and staging of LV diastolic dysfunction and filling pressures has recently been reported.[30]

Pitfalls with Atrial Fibrillation

The presence of AF is another important problem complicating the diagnostic process in HF and especially HFpEF. AF is the most common arrhythmia in persons over age 60 and is common in patients with HF, whereas AF frequently precedes HFpEF.[31] Cardiac structural alterations, such as increased left atrial volume index (LAVI), are common in AF, irrespective of HF, although parameters of LV diastolic dysfunction are more difficult to assess in the presence of AF.[2] Moreover, AF is associated with higher natriuretic peptide values and lower exercise tolerance compared to non-AF patients, irrespective of HF diagnosis.[32] It is unclear whether standard or higher cut-off values of natriuretic peptides should be used for the diagnosis of HF in the presence of AF.[31] Although the use of higher levels is recommended, guidelines have not provided a clear alternative cut-off value for patients with AF.[2] In patients with dyspnea and concurrent AF, HF is present in at least 65% of cases and, thus, these patients should be considered to have HF until proven otherwise.[17]

Heart Failure Symptoms with Normal Cardiac Function

There are clinical situations in which overt HF may occur despite normal or near-normal cardiac structure and function. In these situations, HF may be due to abnormal loading conditions associated with either (1) volume overload (e.g., renal failure or iatrogenic fluid overload) or (2) high-output states (e.g., severe anemia, sepsis, thyrotoxicosis, Paget's disease, arteriovenous fistula, or pregnancy). In the "high-output state" case, HF has been described as "high-output HF," implying that the heart cannot deliver sufficient oxygen to the metabolizing tissues, because of either increased tissue demand or reduced oxygen-carrying content of the blood, despite intact pumping function. In the case of a pre-existing cardiac structural or functional abnormality, the exact etiology may be difficult to distinguish. These causes need to be considered in the differential diagnosis for every patient with newly diagnosed HF.

Diagnosing HFrEF vs HFmrEF vs HFpEF

The terminology that has been historically used to classify HF is based on LVEF measurement. HF may be associated with a wide spectrum of LV structural and functional abnormalities, ranging from normal LV size and preserved LVEF to severe LV dilatation and/or markedly reduced LVEF. In most patients, abnormalities of systolic and diastolic function usually coexist, irrespective of LVEF. In contemporary practice, although the assessment of systolic function is less dependent on LVEF measurement, LVEF is still important in the classification of HF because of prognostic and therapeutic implications, as most clinical trials selected patients based on LVEF.[2,5]

According to current guidelines, HFrEF is defined as the clinical diagnosis of HF and LVEF<40% (Table 1.5); the definition of HFrEF has varied in the past, including LVEF values ≤35%, <40%, and/or ≤40%. In randomized, controlled trials of HFrEF patients that showed beneficial effects of various therapies, patients with LVEF ≤35% or ≤40% were included. Despite heterogeneous etiologies of LV dysfunction in HFrEF, LV volumes and particularly LVEF are still mostly used as robust diagnostic and prognostic variables. Of note, despite individual differences in subsets of patients with certain therapies, the response to therapies targeting reduced LVEF is homogeneous, regardless of the etiology of reduced LVEF, justifying the HFrEF designation.

The prevalence of HF with preserved LVEF (HFpEF) has varied in various clinical studies and registries mainly because of the different EF cut-off diagnostic criteria used: HFpEF has been classified as LVEF >40%, >45%, >50%, and ≥55%. According to current guidelines, HFpEF is defined as the clinical diagnosis of HF and LVEF ≥50%.[2,5] These patients do not have entirely normal LVEF, but there is no major reduction in LV systolic function either and hence the term preserved LVEF has been proposed. In addition to clinical findings and the evidence of preserved or normal LVEF, the diagnosis of HFpEF needs further evidence, including elevated natriuretic peptide levels and other cardiac structural or functional alterations pointing to LV diastolic dysfunction.[2,5] Relevant structural findings include increased LAVI (>34 mL/m^2) or LV mass index (≥115 g/m^2 for males and ≥95 g/m^2 for females). In patients with preserved LVEF, LV geometry has been shown to be a predictor of adverse cardiovascular outcomes.[21] The main echocardiographic parameters related to LV diastolic function and increased filling pressures are considered to be tricuspid regurgitation velocity, mitral annular and mitral inflow velocities, and left atrial size.[33] The currently used algorithm for grading of LV diastolic dysfunction and elevated filling pressures in patients with myocardial disease and preserved or reduced LVEF focuses firstly on mitral inflow velocities and secondly on peak tricuspid regurgitation velocity (abnormal >2.8 m/s), an increased E/E' ratio (i.e., >14), and increased LAVI (Table 1.5).[33] Other parameters derived from myocardial strain analysis may be helpful in the assessment of LV diastolic function (i.e., SR_{IVR}, SR_E, E/SR_{IVR}, LV untwisting rate, etc.), albeit not widely used in clinical practice. All these parameters share various limitations, and their usefulness is dependent on the presence of underlying conditions, such as AF, mitral valve disease, cardiomyopathies, paced rhythm, etc.[33] The effect of exercise on LV function may also be used to reveal LV diastolic dysfunction; various dynamic exercise protocols are available designed to reveal exercise-induced changes in echocardiographic parameters or invasive hemodynamics.[2] A diastolic stress test can be performed using echocardiography with assessment of E/e′ and tricuspid regurgitation velocity, systolic dysfunction (longitudinal strain), and stroke volume and cardiac output changes with exercise.

Currently, there is still no consensus on the definition of HFpEF. The diagnosis of HFpEF is more challenging than the diagnosis of HFrEF, as it is one of excluding other non-cardiac causes of symptoms suggestive of HF. The variety of HFpEF definitions used over time and the significant heterogeneity in patient profiles, exercise capacity, and clinical outcomes highlight the complexity of HFpEF.[34] Patients with HFpEF are usually older, more often women, with a history of hypertension and multiple other comorbidities, such as obesity, CAD, diabetes mellitus, AF, and hyperlipidemia. Hypertension is considered the most important cause of HFpEF, with a prevalence of 60–89% in large, controlled trials, registries, and epidemiological studies. However, comorbidities also play a significant role because they may mimic HF symptoms, and they may lead to either increased (AF) or decreased (obesity) NP levels, further

TABLE 1.5: Definitions of HFrEF, HFmrEF, HFpEF, Left Ventricular Diastolic Dysfunction, and Increased Filling Pressures

HFrEF	Symptoms ± Signs LVEF <40%
HFmrEF	Symptoms ± Signs LVEF 40–49% a) Elevated NP levels (BNP >35 pg/mL and/or NT-proBNP >125 pg/mL) b) At least one additional criterion: • Relevant structural heart disease (LVH and/or LAE) • LV diastolic dysfunction
HFpEF	1. Symptoms ± Signs 2. LVEF ≥50% 3. a) Elevated NP levels (BNP >35 pg/mL and/or NT-proBNP >125 pg/mL) b) At least one additional criterion: • Relevant structural heart disease (LVH and/or LAE) • LV diastolic dysfunction
Diagnosing LV diastolic dysfunction in patients with normal LV ejection fraction	
1. Average E/E' >14	
2. Septal E' <7 cm/s or Lateral E' <10 cm/s	<2 positive → normal diastolic function
3. TR Vmax >2.8 m/s	2 positive → indeterminate diastolic function
4. LAVI >34 mL/m^2	>2 positive → diastolic dysfunction
Estimating LV filling pressures in depressed or normal LV ejection fraction	
E/A ≤0.8 and E ≤0.5 m/s	Normal LV filling pressures
E/A ≥2	Increased LV filling pressures
E/A ≤0.8 and E >0.5 m/s or E/A >0.8 and <2	
Average E/E' >14	0–1 positive → normal LV filling pressures
TR Vmax >2.8 m/s	2–3 positive → increased LV filling pressures
LAVI >34 mL/m^2	

Note: Signs may not be present in early stages of HF (especially in HFpEF) and in patients on diuretics.
Abbreviations: BNP, B-type natriuretic peptide; ECG, electrocardiogram; HFmrEF, heart failure with midrange left ventricular ejection fraction; HFpEF, heart failure with preserved left ventricular ejection fraction; HFrEF, heart failure with reduced left ventricular ejection fraction; LAE, left atrial enlargement; LAVI, left atrial volume index; LV, left ventricular; LVEF, left ventricular ejection fraction; LVH, left ventricular hypertrophy; NP, natriuretic peptides; NT-proBNP, N-terminal pro-BNP; TR Vmax, maximal tricuspid regurgitation velocity.
Source: Modified with permission from: Nagueh. Left ventricular diastolic function: Understanding pathophysiology, diagnosis, and prognosis with echocardiography. *JACC Cardiovasc Imaging* 2020;13:228–44.

confusing the diagnostic process. Comprehensive hemodynamic phenotyping of HFpEF patients may prove to be pivotal in refining HFpEF subgrouping and assessing the differential effect of therapeutic interventions; currently, however, no efficacious treatment for HFpEF exists.[5] Beyond establishing the diagnosis, echocardiography is essential in clinical phenotyping and risk stratification of these patients.[35] The H2FPEF score, based on simple clinical and echocardiographic characteristics, enables discrimination of HFpEF from non-cardiac causes of dyspnea and can assist in determination of the need for further diagnostic testing in the evaluation of patients with suspected HFpEF (Figure 1.2).[36] For additional information on HFpEF, please see Chapters 4 and 15.

Patients with a LVEF in the range of 40–49% represent an intermediate (HFmrEF) group (Table 1.5). These patients are often treated for underlying risk factors and comorbidities and with treatment modalities similar to HFrEF.[37] Patients with HFmrEF most probably have primarily mild LV systolic dysfunction, but with features of LV diastolic dysfunction.[2,5] Of note, similarly poor 5-year survival rates have been reported among patients hospitalized with HF across the spectrum of LVEF, although HF readmission risk was higher in HFrEF and HFmrEF patients than in HFpEF patients.[38] The high variability of LVEF measurements, even more pronounced when assessed by different imaging modalities, raises concern about the need for further subclassification of the HF population based on LVEF, particularly with such narrow boundaries.[21] Nevertheless, the recent HFmrEF designation provides an opportunity to further investigate the characteristics, treatments, and outcomes of these patients, as, until now, patients with midrange LVEF were either excluded from HF studies or were mixed in with other groups. For additional information, see Chapter 16.

Another subset of patients with HFpEF, who previously had had HFrEF, is currently recognized. These patients with improved or recovered LVEF may be clinically distinct from those with persistently preserved or reduced LVEF and further research is needed to better characterize these patients. Evidence suggests that the underlying myocardial abnormalities may not have completely resolved in those patients with improved or recovered LVEF. There are often ongoing HF symptoms and these patients may continue to have neurohormonal activation, abnormal biomarker profile, and detectable functional abnormalities. Furthermore, these patients are still at risk of deterioration of LV function, HF hospitalization, and death, and management remains challenging. There are several reasons to recommend continuation of HF therapies, including device therapies, to prevent clinical deterioration.[39] For more information, see Chapter 16.

Controversies and Research Opportunities

Several areas in the diagnosis and classification of HF remain controversial or unexplored, and thus offer opportunities for further research. We outline several of these areas below:

- Strategies aiming at screening, risk prediction, and early diagnosis of HF; evaluation of the comparative clinical effectiveness and cost effectiveness of the various strategies.
- Refining the HF diagnosis process using machine-learning techniques or big data analysis; evaluation of an integrated approach using echocardiographic indices of cardiac structure and function, clinical parameters and/or biomarkers.
- Use of biomarkers to facilitate screening for earlier diagnosis and treatment initiation in HF.
- Investigation of novel biomarkers for HF diagnosis with greater diagnostic accuracy or for screening at-risk populations.

	Clinical Variable	Values	Points
H_2	Heavy	Body mass index > 30 kg/m^2	2
	Hypertensive	2 or more antihypertensive medicines	1
F	Atrial Fibrillation	Paroxysmal or Persistent	3
P	Pulmonary Hypertension	Doppler Echocardiographic estimated Pulmonary Artery Systolic Pressure > 35 mmHg	1
E	Elder	Age > 60 years	1
F	Filling Pressure	Doppler Echocardiographic E/e' > 9	1
	H_2FPEF score		Sum (0-9)

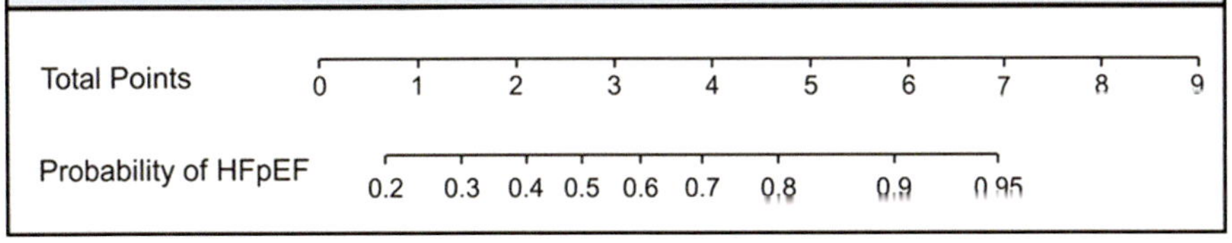

FIGURE 1.2 The H_2FPEF score. (Reproduced with permission from: Reddy, Carter, Obokata M, Redfield, Borlaug. A simple, evidence-based approach to help guide diagnosis of heart failure with preserved ejection fraction. *Circulation.* 2018;138:861–870.)

- Improving classification of HF, based on indexed stroke volume rather than ejection fraction.
- Integration of novel echocardiographic techniques to better understand and define the underlying pathophysiological mechanisms in HfpEF.
- Role of advanced imaging modalities (late-gadolinium enhancement CMR, echocardiographic strain measurements) in groups at risk of HF (patients receiving cardiotoxic drugs, relatives of cardiomyopathy patients, etc.).
- Discrimination of HFmrEF *versus* HFpEF; research into the underlying characteristics, pathophysiology, and diagnosis, using new imaging modalities.
- Description of HfpEF phenotypes based either on comorbidities or specific etiology of cardiac dysfunction.
- Objective assessment of functional capacity to stage and risk stratify HF.
- Addressing complex issues in the primary care setting, e.g., pitfalls in clinical assessment, natriuretic peptide interpretation, echocardiographic assessment, multiple confounders, etc.

References

1. McMurray JJ, Adamopoulos S, Anker SD, et al. ESC guidelines for the diagnosis and treatment of acute and chronic heart failure 2012: the task force for the diagnosis and treatment of acute and chronic heart failure 2012 of the European Society of Cardiology. Developed in collaboration with the Heart Failure Association (HFA) of the ESC. *Eur Heart J.* 2012;33:1787–847.
2. Ponikowski P, Voors AA, Anker SD, et al. 2016 ESC guidelines for the diagnosis and treatment of acute and chronic heart failure: the task force for the diagnosis and treatment of acute and chronic heart failure of the European Society of Cardiology (ESC) developed with the special contribution of the Heart Failure Association (HFA) of the ESC. *Eur J Heart Fail.* 2016;18:891–975.
3. Yap J, Lim FY, Gao F, et al. Correlation of the New York Heart Association classification and the 6-minute walk distance: a systematic review. *Clin Cardiol.* 2015;38:621–8.
4. Lim FY, Yap J, Gao F, et al. Correlation of the New York Heart Association classification and the cardiopulmonary exercise test: a systematic review. *Int J Cardiol.* 2018;263:88–93.
5. Yancy CW, Jessup M, Bozkurt B, et al. 2013 ACCF/AHA guideline for the management of heart failure: executive summary: a report of the American College of Cardiology Foundation/American Heart Association Task Force on practice guidelines. *Circulation.* 2013;128:1810–52.
6. Stevenson LW, Pagani FD, Young JB, et al. INTERMACS profiles of advanced heart failure: the current picture. *J Heart Lung Transplant.* 2009;28:535–41.
7. Stewart GC, Kittleson MM, Patel PC, et al. INTERMACS (Interagency Registry for Mechanically Assisted Circulatory Support) profiling identifies ambulatory patients at high risk on medical therapy after hospitalizations for heart failure. *Circ Heart Fail.* 2016;9:e003032.
8. Samman-Tahhan A, Hedley JS, McCue AA, et al. INTERMACS profiles and outcomes among non-inotrope-dependent outpatients with heart failure and reduced ejection fraction. *JACC Heart Fail.* 2018;6:743–53.
9. Crespo-Leiro MG, Metra M, Lund LH, et al. Advanced heart failure: a position statement of the Heart Failure Association of the European Society of Cardiology. *Eur J Heart Fail.* 2018;20:1505–35.
10. Hunt SA, Abraham WT, Chin MH, et al. 2009 focused update incorporated into the ACC/AHA 2005 guidelines for the diagnosis and management of heart failure in adults: a report of the American College of Cardiology Foundation/American Heart Association Task Force on Practice Guidelines: developed in collaboration with the International Society for Heart and Lung Transplantation. *Circulation.* 2009;119:e391–479.
11. Hedley JS, Samman-Tahhan A, McCue AA, et al. Definitions of Stage D heart failure and outcomes among outpatients with heart failure and reduced ejection fraction. *Int J Cardiol.* 2018;272:250–4.
12. Mueller C, McDonald K, de Boer RA, et al. Heart Failure Association of the European Society of Cardiology practical guidance on the use of natriuretic peptide concentrations. *Eur J Heart Fail.* 2019;21:715–31.
13. Roberts E, Ludman AJ, Dworzynski K, et al. The diagnostic accuracy of the natriuretic peptides in heart failure: systematic review and diagnostic meta-analysis in the acute care setting. *BMJ.* 2015;350:h910.
14. Taylor CJ, Moore J, O'Flynn N. Diagnosis and management of chronic heart failure: NICE guideline update 2018. *Br J Gen Pract.* 2019;69:265–6.
15. Tripoliti EE, Ioannidou P, Toumpaniaris P, et al. Point-of-care testing devices for heart failure analyzing blood and saliva samples. *IEEE Rev Biomed Eng.* 2020;13:17–31.
16. Zamorano JL, Lancellotti P, Rodriguez Munoz D, et al. 2016 ESC position paper on cancer treatments and cardiovascular toxicity developed under the auspices of the ESC Committee for Practice Guidelines: the task force for cancer treatments and cardiovascular toxicity of the European Society of Cardiology (ESC). *Eur J Heart Fail.* 2017;19:9–42.
17. Seferovic PM, Ponikowski P, Anker SD, et al. Clinical practice update on heart failure 2019: pharmacotherapy, procedures, devices and patient management. An expert consensus meeting report of the Heart Failure Association of the European Society of Cardiology. *Eur J Heart Fail.* 2019;21:1169–86.
18. Cui K, Huang W, Fan J, Lei H. Midregional pro-atrial natriuretic peptide is a superior biomarker to N-terminal pro-B-type natriuretic peptide in the diagnosis of heart failure patients with preserved ejection fraction. *Medicine (Baltimore).* 2018;97:e12277.
19. Zakeri R, Cowie MR. Heart failure with preserved ejection fraction: controversies, challenges and future directions. *Heart.* 2018;104:377–84.
20. Kosmala W, Marwick TH. Asymptomatic left ventricular diastolic dysfunction: predicting progression to symptomatic heart failure. *JACC Cardiovasc Imaging.* 2020;13:215–27.
21. Fabijanovic D, Milicic D, Cikes M. Left ventricular size and ejection fraction: are they still relevant? *Heart Fail Clin.* 2019;15:147–58.
22. Dumesnil JG, Pibarot P, Carabello B. Paradoxical low flow and/or low gradient severe aortic stenosis despite preserved left ventricular ejection fraction: implications for diagnosis and treatment. *Eur Heart J.* 2010;31:281–9.
23. De Marco M, Gerdts E, Mancusi C, et al. Influence of left ventricular stroke volume on incident heart failure in a population with preserved ejection fraction (from the strong heart study). *Am J Cardiol.* 2017;119:1047–52.
24. Captur G, Manisty C, Moon JC. Cardiac MRI evaluation of myocardial disease. *Heart.* 2016;102:1429–35.
25. Pickett CA, Cheezum MK, Kassop D, Villines TC, Hulten EA. Accuracy of cardiac CT, radionucleotide and invasive ventriculography, two- and three-dimensional echocardiography, and SPECT for left and right ventricular ejection fraction compared with cardiac MRI: a meta-analysis. *Eur Heart J Cardiovasc Imaging.* 2015;16:848–52.
26. Chahal H, Levsky JM, Garcia MJ. Cardiac CT: present and future applications. *Heart.* 2016;102:1840–50.
27. Sabharwal NK. State of the art in nuclear cardiology. *Heart.* 2017;103:790–9.
28. McMurray JKM, Anker S, Gardner R. Heart failure: epidemiology, pathophysiology and diagnosis. In: Camm AJ, Serruys PW, ed. *The ESC textbook of cardiovascular medicine.* Malden, MA: Blackwell Publishing; 2006: 685–719.
29. Taylor CJ, Roalfe AK, Iles R, et al. Primary care REFerral for EchocaRdiogram (REFER) in heart failure: a diagnostic accuracy study. *Br J Gen Pract.* 2017;67:e94–e102.
30. Nagueh SF, Smiseth OA, Appleton CP, et al. Recommendations for the evaluation of left ventricular diastolic function by echocardiography: an update from the American Society of Echocardiography and the European Association of Cardiovascular Imaging. *Eur Heart J Cardiovasc Imaging.* 2016;17:1321–60.
31. Lam CSP, Santema BT, Voors AA. Atrial fibrillation in heart failure: a common and deadly combination. *JACC Heart Fail.* 2017;5:575–7.
32. Kristensen SL, Jhund PS, Mogensen UM, et al. Prognostic value of N-terminal pro-B-type natriuretic peptide levels in heart failure patients with and without atrial fibrillation. *Circ Heart Fail.* 2017;10:e004409.
33. Nagueh SF. Left ventricular diastolic function: understanding pathophysiology, diagnosis, and prognosis with echocardiography. *JACC Cardiovasc Imaging.* 2020;13:228–44.
34. Ho JE, Zern EK, Wooster L, et al. Differential clinical profiles, exercise responses, and outcomes associated with existing HFpEF definitions. *Circulation.* 2019;140:353–65.
35. Obokata M, Reddy YNV, Borlaug BA. The role of echocardiography in heart failure with preserved ejection fraction: what do we want from imaging? *Heart Fail Clin.* 2019;15:241–56.
36. Reddy YNV, Carter RE, Obokata M, Redfield MM, Borlaug BA. A simple, evidence-based approach to help guide diagnosis of heart failure with preserved ejection fraction. *Circulation.* 2018;138:861–70.
37. Rickenbacher P, Kaufmann BA, Maeder MT, et al. Heart failure with mid-range ejection fraction: a distinct clinical entity? Insights from the Trial of Intensified versus standard Medical therapy in Elderly patients with Congestive Heart Failure (TIME-CHF). *Eur J Heart Fail.* 2017;19:1586–96.
38. Shah KS, Xu H, Matsouaka RA, et al. Heart failure with preserved, borderline, and reduced ejection fraction: 5-year outcomes. *J Am Coll Cardiol.* 2017;70:2476–86.
39. Gulati G, Udelson JE. Heart failure with improved ejection fraction: is it possible to escape one's past? *JACC Heart Fail.* 2018;6:725–33.

Chapter 2
EPIDEMIOLOGY OF HEART FAILURE

Lampros Papadimitriou, Prabhjot Grewal, and Andreas P. Kalogeropoulos

Introduction

Heart failure (HF) encompasses a wide spectrum of clinical scenarios. In the past, attention was drawn almost exclusively to systolic dysfunction of the left ventricle leading to HF with reduced left ventricular ejection fraction (HFrEF). However, recognition that HF can develop in the presence of preserved (≥50%) or midrange (borderline, 40–49%) ejection fraction (HFpEF or HFmrEF, respectively) has expanded the number of cases included in the definition of HF. Additionally, population aging, the increasing ubiquity of risk factors, and improved survival rates as a consequence of both, a better understanding of the underlying mechanism as well as advancement in treatment, have all led to an ever-increasing prevalence of HF. In the United States between 2012 and 2030, it is projected that HF prevalence will increase by 46%, and the total population affected will increase from 2.42% to 2.97%.[1]

Despite significant advances in therapy, HF still carries a high mortality. Depending on the demographic and regional characteristics, one-year mortality after a hospitalization for HF ranges between 20% and 36%.[2–4] It is striking that, among 40,000 hospitalized HF patients included in the Get With The Guidelines HF registry between 2005 and 2009, three out of four patients died within five years regardless of their ejection fraction.[5] These survival rates are lower than with several forms of cancer.[6] HF also affects quality of life, significantly increases morbidity rates, and leads to substantial healthcare costs; in 2014, the cost was estimated at approximately 11 billion dollars in the United States.[7]

Prevalence and Incidence

Estimates and Trends

Most contemporary population-based cohorts in developed countries suggest that the age-standardized incidence of HF is declining.[8–14] In a comprehensive epidemiologic study from the United Kingdom,[15] the population-based incidence of HF for women and men were 3.53 and 8.00 per 10,000 person-years, respectively.

In a large European study of 80,000 subjects between the ages of 25 and 98 years, the rates of incident HF were found to be higher beyond the age of 60 years, and lower in women.[16] In the United States, a report investigating the changes in HF incidence between 1990 and 2009, from both the Framingham Heart Study and the Cardiovascular Health Study, showed that, although HFrEF and HFpEF incidence declined and increased, respectively, overall HF incidence remained unchanged.[17]

As the population ages and HF therapies continue to improve, the prevalence of HF is expected to increase. Based on the National Health and Nutrition Examination Survey (NHANES) 2013–2016 data, the prevalence of HF in the United States overall is 2%, and as expected, increases significantly after the age of 60. The highest prevalence was observed after the age of 80, where 12.8% and 12.0% of males and females, respectively, had a diagnosis of HF.[18] Table 2.1 summarizes the prevalence of HF around the world.

Prevalence of Preclinical (Stage A and B) Heart Failure

The diagnosis of HF is a continuum. Subjects with risk factors such as hypertension, diabetes, coronary artery disease, and obesity are at greater risk of developing HF. To emphasize the importance of prevention, the American Heart Association (AHA) and the American College of Cardiology (ACC) proposed a classification that divides HF into four stages (Table 2.2).[19]

Because of the need for systematic screening to detect subclinical disease, limited data exist on the prevalence of HF Stages A and B. In the Framingham study,[20] the prevalence of Stage A and B was 36.5% and 24.2%, respectively. The prevalence of subclinical disease (Stage B) increased with age. The importance of detecting HF in earlier stages was highlighted by the 2-fold higher mortality of participants with Stage B HF compared with healthy subjects.[20]

The CARDIA study collected clinical, laboratory, and imaging data at two timepoints, 1990 and 2015, on 2189 participants. The prevalence of stage A HF increased from 16% to 42% and that of stage B from 5% to 26%, with African American males affected disproportionately.[21]

Prevalence of Heart Failure with Reduced, Midrange, and Preserved Ejection Fraction

Left ventricular (LV) systolic function, most quantified by the LV ejection fraction (LVEF), has been an established approach to classify HF. Traditionally, HF has been categorized into reduced and preserved ejection fraction HF, with 40% being the most common LVEF cutoff. However, the recognition that there is a significant overlap of phenotypes on both sides of the LVEF cutoff led to the introduction of the midrange LVEF category by the European Society of Cardiology (ESC) in 2016 for patients with LVEF between 41% and 49%.[22] Thus, HF is currently categorized according to LVEF into HF with reduced (≤40%—HFrEF), midrange (41% to 49%—HFmrEF), and preserved (≥50%—HFpEF) ejection fraction.[22] The term HF with recovered ejection fraction (HFrecEF) is reserved for patients initially presenting with HFrEF who later demonstrate improved LVEF (>40% or ≥50% depending on the definition) following guideline-directed therapy,[23] although there is currently no consensus on the appropriate definition of this entity. Table 2.3 summarizes the distribution of LVEF ranges in recent HF registries and cohorts.

Regardless of the exact LVEF cutoff used, literature in recent years points towards an increasing prevalence and incidence of HFpEF relative to HFrEF.[24] This is a result of population aging and increasing prevalence of lifestyle-associated cardiometabolic risk factors in both developing and developed countries. For example, among 894 Framingham Study participants with new-onset HF (mean age 75, 52% women), HFpEF (EF ≥50%) increased from 11.0% between 1985 and 1994 to 56.2% between 2005 and 2014, while HFrEF (EF <40%) decreased from 44.1% to 31.06% during this time.[10]

DOI: 10.1201/9780429244544-3

TABLE 2.1: Population Prevalence of HF in Registries and Surveys across the World

Country	Population Sample	Study Period	Ascertainment of Heart Failure Cases	Total (%)	Men (%)	Women (%)
Sweden (Zarrinkoub, Wettermark et al. 2013)	2.1 million	2010	Primary or secondary diagnosis of HF (ICD-10 code I50) in primary care (2003 to 2010), secondary care (1997 to 2010), or during hospitalization (1997 to 2010)	2.2*	2.2	2.2
Spain (Farre, Vela et al. 2017)	7.5 million	2012	Hospital diagnosis of HF (ICD-9-CM codes 402.X1, 404.X1, 404.X3, 428.X) or outpatient diagnosis followed by loop diuretic prescription between 2011 and 2012	1.2 (among age >15)		
United States (Streng, Nauta et al. 2018)	5,761	2013–2014	National Health and Nutrition Examination Survey, multi-stage probability sampling, self-reported HF*	1.9*	1.8	2.0
United Kingdom (Conrad, Judge et al. 2018)	4.0 million	2002–2014	ICD-10 codes (I50.X, I42.0, I42.9, I11.0, I13.0, I13.2, I25.5) for in-hospital and NHS Read codes for primary care diagnosis of HF in any diagnostic position	1.6	1.8	1.2
South Korea (Lee, Oh et al. 2016)	1.4 million	2014	Adult patients with any outpatient or inpatient services with a primary or secondary diagnosis of HF (ICD-10 codes I50.X, I11.0, I13.0, I13.2, I42.0, I42.5, I25.5) in 2014	1.2 (among age >18)		

* Estimated prevalence in the national population.
Abbreviations: HF: heart failure.
Source: ICD-9-CM: International Classification of Diseases, Ninth Revision, Clinical Modification; ICD-10: International Classification of Diseases, Version 10; NHS: National Health Service.

TABLE 2.2: American Heart Association (AHA) and American College of Cardiology (ACC) Classifications of Heart Failure

Stage	Definition	Treatment
A	At risk of developing heart failure	Lifestyle modifications: Exercise, smoking cessation, and alcohol cessation Management of comorbidities (diabetes, hyperlipidemia, hypertension)
B	Structural heart disease without symptoms of heart failure	Medical therapy: ACEi or ARB; beta-blocker if post MI
C	Structural heart disease with previous or current symptoms of heart failure	Fluid restriction, dietary sodium restriction, diuretics, GDMT ICD or CRT in appropriate cases
D	Heart failure refractory to treatment	Advanced therapies: Ventricular assist devices, clinical trials, continuous IV inotropes, heart transplant Palliative care/hospice referral

Abbreviations: ACEi: angiotensin converting enzyme inhibitor; ARB: angiotensin receptor blocker; MI: myocardial infarction; GDMT: guideline directed medical therapy; ICD: implantable cardioverter defibrillator; CRT: cardiac resynchronization therapy.

TABLE 2.3: Distribution of Ejection Fraction in Recent Heart Failure Registries and Cohorts

Region	HFrEF	HFmrEF	HFpEF	Midrange EF Definition	Setting	Study Design	Age, Years (mean±SD)	Female, %
Europe, Turkey, Israel, Egypt (Chioncel, Lainscak et al. 2017)	60	24	16	40–50%	Outpatient	Registry	64.8±13.3	28.2
Switzerland, Germany (Rickenbacher, Kaufmann et al. 2017)	65	17	18	40–49%	Outpatient	Clinical Trial	76.6±7.7	36.9
Sweden (Koh, Tay et al. 2017)	56	21	23	40–49%	Mixed	Registry	74±12	29–55
Europe Latin America, Australia (Farmakis, Simitsis et al. 2017)	52	25	23	40–49%	Inpatient	Registry	28.3% >75 years	36.2
Spain (Gomez-Otero, Ferrero-Gregori et al. 2017)	41	16	43	40–49%	Inpatient	Registry	71.8±12.1	37.7
United States (Shah, Claggett et al. 2017)	46	8	46	41–49%	Inpatient	Registry	80 (74–86)	54.0

Abbreviations: EF: ejection fraction; HFmrEF: heart failure with midrange ejection fraction; HFpEF: heart failure with preserved ejection fraction; HFrEF: heart failure with reduced ejection fraction.

Lifetime Risk of Heart Failure

In combined data from two large prospective cohorts, the Cardiovascular Heart Study (CHS) and the Multiethnic Study of Atherosclerosis (MESA), with over 12,400 participants (22.2% Black, 45.2% female), the lifetime risk for HF at the index age of 45 years through 90 years of age was higher in men than women (27.4% versus 23.8%).[25] Among HF subtypes, the lifetime risk for HFrEF was higher in men than women (10.6% versus 5.8%), whereas the lifetime risk for HFpEF was similar in men and women. Among participants with antecedent myocardial infarction before HF diagnosis, the remaining lifetime risks for HFpEF and HFrEF were up to 2.5-fold and 4-fold higher, respectively, compared with those without myocardial infarction.[25]

Patient Characteristics

Impact of Demographics and Socioeconomic Status

Age

Age is a major contributor to the development of HF. The incidence and prevalence of HF is considerably higher among middle-aged and older adults. In a recent population-based report from the United Kingdom, mean±SD age at diagnosis was 76.7±12.6 years.[9] A similar median age of 76 to 78 years at HF diagnosis was reported in the inpatient setting in Denmark from 1995 until 2012, stratified by 3-year periods, with most patients diagnosed between age 66 and 85.[8]

Men and women are equally affected by HF. However, sex predominance is affected by age at onset and type of HF.[26] In the United Kingdom, women accounted for 49.0% of new HF cases.[9] A similar 1:1 sex ratio for new cases has been reported elsewhere.[26–28] However, although higher rates of coronary artery disease in men lead to male predominance at younger ages, susceptibility to diastolic dysfunction leads to more women affected by HF at older ages. Men are more likely to develop HFrEF, whereas women are more prone to HFpEF.[29] In the United Kingdom, age at diagnosis was 74±13 years in men vs 79±12 years in women.[9] Similar data have been reported from Sweden.[27] Finally, large studies show that HF affects all races equally.[30,31]

In a meta-analysis of community-based studies, the median prevalence of HF among persons aged ≥60 years was 11.8% (4.7–13.3%).[32] Among Danish adults, the annual incidence of new in-hospital HF diagnosis in 2012 was <0.01% in ages 18-35 years but >1% in ages >74 years (Figure 2.1).[8] In the United States, the annual incidence of HF ranges between 1% and 2% among older adults (age ≥65 years), depending on age, group, and race.[2,33]

Sex

Age-standardized incidence and prevalence of HF is higher in men,[9,27,34] but more women develop HF later in life, therefore contributing almost equally to new HF cases. Therefore the crude prevalence is either only slightly higher in men or comparable between men and women.[9,27,34,35] In the United Kingdom, although the age-standardized incidence was higher in men than in women (incidence rate ratio 1.52, 95% confidence interval [CI] 1.50–1.54), the total number of cases was only 9% higher in men, because of more women being present in older age groups.[9] In the Atherosclerosis Risk in Communities cohort, incidence of HF was higher in men vs women for both Black people and white people and across age groups, but these differences diminished in the >75 age group.[2] Similarly, in Denmark, men had a higher HF incidence than women overall, except in the >74 age group.[8]

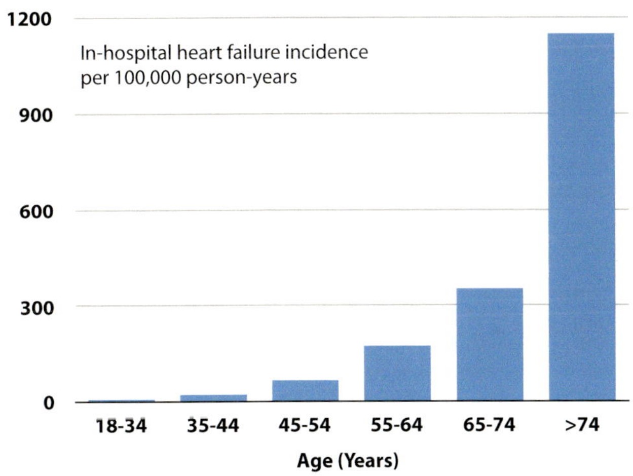

FIGURE 2.1 Incidence of in-hospital heart failure diagnosis among adults in Denmark, 2012. (Data from Christiansen et al., *Circulation* 2017;135:1214–23.)

Socioeconomic Status

Socioeconomic status is a key determinant of HF risk. In the United Kingdom, among persons of the same age and sex, those in the most deprived socioeconomic quintile were more likely to experience HF (incidence rate ratio 1.61, 95% CI 1.58–1.64) than their affluent counterparts. This distinction was more pronounced in the younger age groups.[9] Patients from the most deprived quintile were about 3.5 years younger at diagnosis vs those from the least deprived (74.5±13 vs 78±12 years).[9] Among 27,000 relatively young (age 55.5±10.4 years), low-income white and Black men and women in the United States who were receiving Centers for Medicare and Medicaid Services in years 2002 to 2009, HF incidence was 328 per 100,000 person-years, considerably higher for age compared to other cohorts, with little variation across race or sex.[31]

Patient Characteristics According to Ejection Fraction

There is an age and sex distribution gradient across LVEF categories. In the European Society of Cardiology Heart Failure Long-Term Registry (ESC-HF-LT) registry in Europe, outpatients with HFrEF were younger (64 vs 69 years), more commonly male (78% vs 52%), had an ischemic etiology (49% vs 24%), and a left bundle branch block (24% vs 9%), but they were less likely to have hypertension (56% vs 67%) or atrial fibrillation (18% vs 32%) compared to HFpEF. Patients with HFmrEF mirrored those with HFrEF in terms of age, sex, and ischemic etiology, but had a lower rate of left ventricular and atrial dilation.[29]

Etiology of Heart Failure

Ischemic Cardiomyopathy

Coronary artery disease is a major driving force of HF. Previous longitudinal studies have shown that reductions in short- and long-term mortality after acute myocardial infarction (AMI) in past decades have been translated into increasing rates of HF. In recent registries, post-AMI HF is declining, because of increased use of early interventional strategies. However, HF continues to be a major problem in patients recovering from AMI or acute coronary syndrome (ACS). Estimates of HF after AMI vary because of varying definitions of both AMI and post-AMI HF.

In a Swedish national registry, primary percutaneous coronary intervention increased from 6.0% to 91.5% between 1996 and 2008, accompanied by a decrease in the incidence of HF (defined as presence of crackles or the use of IV diuretics or inotropes) during index admission from 46% to 28%.[36] The decrease was more pronounced for ST-segment elevation AMI. Notably, reduction in post-AMI HF rates has been reported for HFrEF but not HFpEF.[37] In a study from Norway, 18.7% of patients developed new HF during index admission for a first AMI between 2001 and 2009, depending on age and gender (Figure 2.2A).[38] Among patients discharged without HF, 12.6% were admitted or died because of HF after a median of 3.2 years and the risk of HF was highest during the first six months post-AMI (Figure 2.2B).[38] The annual incidence of HF per 1000 person-years was 31% in men and 46% in women (P <0.01).

Comorbidities

As a disease of older adults, HF is rarely an isolated finding. Over 80% of patients have ≥2 concomitant chronic conditions.[9,39,40] The most common comorbidities are hypertension, ischemic heart disease, diabetes mellitus, cerebral and peripheral vascular disease, atrial fibrillation, chronic kidney disease,

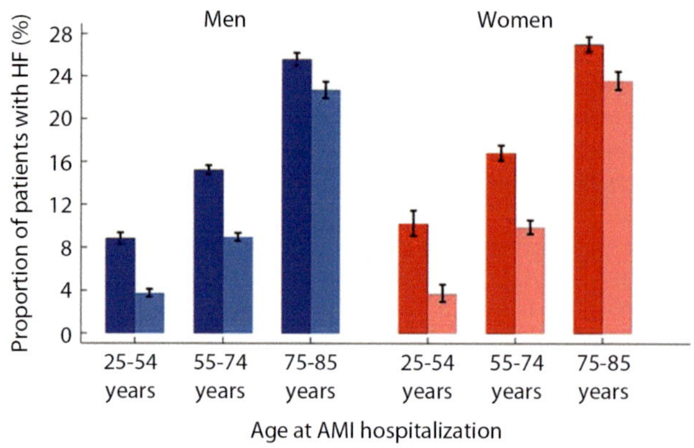

FIGURE 2.2A Proportion of patients with acute myocardial infarction (AMI) complicated with in-hospital (fully colored bars) and post-AMI discharge (light-colored bars) heart failure (HF) by sex and age group in the Cardiovascular Disease in Norway (CVDNOR) project, 2001–2009.

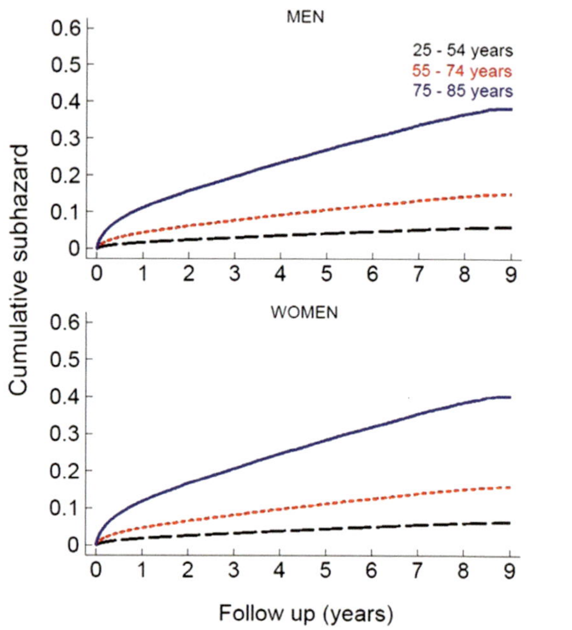

FIGURE 2.2B Sex-specific cumulative incidence of post-AMI discharge heart failure by age group in CVDNOR. (Reproduced under the terms of the Creative Commons Attribution – Non-Commercial (CC BY-NC) License from Sulo et al., *J Am Heart Assoc* 2016;5:e002667.)

chronic obstructive lung disease, anemia, and depression. As the average age at HF diagnosis increases over time,[9] the number of comorbidities and use of medications in patients with HF increases as well.[8,9] In the United Kingdom, the number of comorbidities in patients with HF increased from 3.4±1.9 in 2002 to 5.4±2.5 in 2014 and the percent of patients with ≥3 additional conditions increased from 68% to 87%.[9] Overall, there has been a shift from a model where HF was mainly a consequence of coronary artery disease with male predominance toward a disease of older adults equally affecting both sexes and accompanied by a complex medical profile.

Hypertension

Along with coronary artery disease, hypertension has the highest population-attributable risk for HF.[41] In the Health Aging and Body Composition (ABC) Study, there was a direct association between systolic blood pressure (SBP) and HF risk for levels of SBP as low as <115 mmHg.[42] The 10-year incidence of HF with SBP <120, 120–139, 140–159, and ≥160 mmHg at baseline was 5.9%, 10.5%, 14.8%, and 22.8%, respectively, and over half of cases occurred in individuals with SBP <140 mmHg.[42] The impact of SBP control on HF risk was impressively demonstrated in the landmark Systolic Blood Pressure Intervention Trial (SPRINT), which compared intensive (<120 mmHg) with conventional (<140 mmHg) target SBP; intensive SBP target reduced the risk of HF by 37% (hazard ratio [HR] 0.63; 95% CI, 0.46–0.85; P=0.003) consistently across all subgroups.[43]

Diabetes

Several studies have highlighted the impact of increasingly prevalent metabolic risk factors, including diabetes, glucose intolerance, and insulin resistance, on HF risk. In a nationwide study from Scotland, the incidence of hospitalization for HF among residents ≥30 years old between 2004 to 2013 was 2.4, 5.6, and 12.4 per 1,000 person-years for residents without diabetes, with type 2, and type 1 diabetes, respectively.[44] Despite falling incidence over time, particularly with respect to type 1 diabetes, HF was approximately 2-fold higher among residents with diabetes (type 1 or type 2) vs those without, with higher short-term (30-day) case-fatality in those with type 1 diabetes mellitus.[44]

Atrial Fibrillation

Atrial fibrillation (AF) is common among patients with HF and is a negative prognostic factor. Conversely, AF confers increased risk of HF, especially HFpEF. In the Framingham Heart Study, among 1,737 individuals with new AF (mean age, 75±12 years; 48% women), more than one-third (37%) had HF. Conversely, among 1,166 individuals with new HF (mean age, 79±11 years; 53% women), more than half (57%) had AF. Prevalent AF was more strongly associated with incident HFpEF than HFrEF.[45] In Olmsted County, Minnesota, among ~3,500 patients with new AF (age 71±15 years, 45.5% women), a substantial excess risk of HF was observed after AF diagnosis, with a standardized morbidity ratio of 9.60, 2.13, and 1.70 at 90 days, one year, and three years, respectively.[46] In the community-based Outcomes Registry for Better Informed Treatment of Atrial Fibrillation (ORBIT-AF), among approximately 6,500 outpatients with AF in the United States (median age 74 years, 43.6% female), annualized HF incidence was 1.58% over a two-year follow-up period, with a higher proportion of HFpEF than HFrEF.[47] Of note, in contrast to general HF cases, the incidence of HF after AF does not seem to be declining.[48]

Renal Disease

Renal impairment is common in HF and portends a worse prognosis. Conversely, HF commonly follows renal dysfunction. Even moderate renal impairment, in the absence of diabetes and hypertension, was associated with a higher risk of HF. In pooled data from three community cohorts in the United States, comprising ~14,500 participants (age, 63±12 years; 59% women; 44% African American), chronic kidney disease (CKD; defined as estimated glomerular filtration rate (eGFR) <60 mL/min/1.73 m^2) was present in 10% of participants.[49] The annualized incidence of HF was 2.2% among those with CKD vs 0.62% without. Risk of HF was higher in African Americans and Hispanics.[49] Acute kidney injury also carries an increased risk of HF. In a cohort of 300,000 hospitalized U.S. veterans without HF, a 0.3-mg/dL or 50% increase in serum creatinine from the baseline was associated with a 23% increased two-year risk for

HF.[49] Of note, in a cohort of over 3,500 patients with CKD, cystatin C-based eGFR and albuminuria predicted risk of HF better than creatinine-based eGFR; anemia, insulin resistance, inflammation, and poor glycemic control were additional risk factors.[50]

Outcomes

Despite advances in HF therapy in the past 20 years, HF-related mortality and rehospitalization rates at the population level have proven difficult to curb. This is secondary to (1) increasing patient age and comorbidity burden;[9] (2) negative results of trials with pharmaceuticals/devices targeting non-neurohormonal pathways; and (3) lack of effective treatments for patients with acute HF and HFpEF.

Mortality Causes and Trends

In the large PARADIGM-HF study, a landmark trial in HFrEF, 81% of deaths were attributed to cardiovascular (CV) causes. Of these, 45% were due to sudden cardiac death and 26% due to HF.[51] Even in earlier stages of HF, patients are at a higher risk of sudden cardiac death, making the proper management of Stage B and of mildly symptomatic Stage C HF extremely important.

Mortality appears to be decreasing in long-term trend analyses for both outpatients and inpatients with HF, albeit at different rates for various subgroups. Currently, one-year mortality for outpatients with HF in observational studies in developed countries ranges between 5% and 10%;[29,52,53] however, it is considerably higher (between 10% and 20%) in national registries,[54] developing regions,[4] and in older adults.[12] For hospitalized patients, one-year mortality is generally >20% and exceeds 30% in several national registries.[3,12,52–55]

Hospitalizations for HF and In-Hospital Mortality Trends

Hospitalization for decompensated or *de novo* HF represents a critical point in the natural history of HF, with a marked worsening in outcomes afterward. In the United States, in 2014, there were approximately 2 million emergency department (ED) visits and hospitalizations with a primary diagnosis of HF, costing over 11 billion dollars.[7] In the same study, in 2014, the median length of hospital stay was three days, and the crude number of ED visits and admissions with a primary diagnosis of HF decreased by 3.2% and 20%, respectively, compared with 2006

In France, the overall age-standardized rate of primary HF hospitalizations was 250 per 100,000 people in 2012, only a small change from 2002.[56] Of note, although the age-standardized rate was higher in men (320 vs 200 per 100,000 people), the crude rate was comparable between men and women. In Germany, primary HF-related hospitalizations increased by 65.4% between 2000 and 2013, and by 28.4% after age adjustment (from 261 to 335 per 100,000). HF was the leading cause of hospitalizations and in-hospital deaths in 2013.[57]

In-hospital mortality rates are currently below 10% in developed countries. In the United States, in-hospital mortality among HF patients from the Get With The Guidelines-Heart Failure (GWTG-HF) registry declined from 3.9 % in 2001–2003 to 2.8% in 2011–2016.[58] In Italy, in-hospital mortality remained unchanged at 9.4% in Lombardy between 2000 and 2012; this estimate included patients with HF as secondary diagnosis (13%), who have higher mortality rates.[59] In the same study, mortality decreased among patients <75 years of age; however, the % of older patients increased in the same period.[59] A similar in-hospital mortality of 8% has been reported for years 2014 to 2018 in France.[60] In a Japanese cohort, in-hospital mortality was 7% and was no different among patients with HFrEF, HFmrEF, and HFpEF with rates of 8%, 7%, and 7%, respectively.[61] Of note, length of stay (and therefore, time at risk) is considerably shorter in the United States compared with Europe or Asia.[57,62,63]

Readmission Challenges and Controversy

Readmission rates after a hospitalization for HF remain high, with 20–30% of patients in the United States readmitted within 30 days[55,64,65] and between one-half and two-thirds readmitted within one year.[55,66,67] Concerted efforts to reduce readmissions in the United Stated have been associated with unfavorable mortality trends,[66] highlighting the challenges of improving outcomes in an ever-aging and medically complex HF population.

Rehospitalization rates and trends vary widely across healthcare systems. In the multi-national Acute Study of Clinical Effectiveness of Nesiritide in Decompensated Heart Failure (ASCEND-HF) trial, the mean country-level all-cause 30-day readmission rate ranged from 2.5% to 25.0% and countries with longer length of stay had significantly lower readmission rates.[68]

Readmissions after hospitalization for HF have been a remarkably resistant outcome to curb. In a recent systematic review spanning four decades of acute HF studies, despite continuous improvements in mortality, 30-day and one-year all-cause readmission rates remained roughly unchanged.[69] Between 2005 and 2015, mean length of stay declined marginally from 7.5 days to 7.3 days in Canadian hospitals and remained stable in US hospitals (4.9 days).[70] During the same period, 30-day readmission rates declined only slightly both in Canada (from 19.7% to 17.6% for all-cause and from 8.4% to 6.9% for HF-specific readmissions) and in the United States (from 21.2% to 18.5% for all-cause and from 7.6% to 5.7% for HF-specific readmissions).[70] Interestingly, the Hospital Readmissions Reduction Program that was implemented in the United States did not appear to have an impact on these trends.

Impact of Acute Heart Failure on Mortality

HF hospitalization has a dramatic impact on both short- and long-term mortality. Among 160,000 HF hospitalizations of Medicare beneficiaries from the GWTG-HF registry, 30-day and one-year mortality post HF admission were 12% and 40.5%, respectively.[58] Similarly, in the Italian HF registry, one-year mortality was 24% among patients admitted for HF (19.2% for *de novo* HF and 27.7% for worsening HF) and 5.9% among outpatients.[52] In the European Society of Cardiology Heart Failure Long-Term (ESC-HF-LT) registry, all-cause one-year mortality rate was 23.6% for inpatient vs 6.4% for outpatient enrollees. The composite endpoint of mortality or HF hospitalization within one year was 36.0% and 14.5% for inpatients and outpatients, respectively.[53] Despite a decrease over the past few decades, one-year mortality after hospitalization for HF remains high and exceeds 30% in several healthcare systems (Table 2.4).

Despite decreasing mortality trends,[3,6,28] five-year survival after HF diagnosis in population studies does not exceed 50% in most systems, regardless of setting (outpatient vs inpatient),[27,71] and is as low as 25% in older inpatients regardless of left ventricular EF.[28]

Outcomes in Chronic Heart Failure

Mortality

In contrast to hospitalized patients, data for ambulatory patients with HF are less abundant. In the ESC-HF-LT registry, mortality at 1 year was 8.8% among ~5,500 outpatients with

TABLE 2.4: Mortality Rates after Hospitalization for Heart Failure

	Source	Mortality Estimates	Notes
In-hospital			
United States	National Inpatient Sample (Akintoye, Briasoulis et al. 2017)	4.5% (2001) to 2.9% (2014)	ICD-9-CM codes, primary diagnosis
Italy	Lombardy region, administrative data (Frigerio, Mazzali et al. 2017)	9.4% without temporal trend (2000-2012) Acute HF episodes: 9.1% Cardiomyopathies without acute HF: 5.6% with HF as 2nd diagnosis: 15.9%	ICD-9-CM codes
Germany	German Federal Health Monitoring System (Christ, Stork et al. 2016)	14.8% (2000) to 9.3% (2013)	ICD10-GM codes, primary diagnosis
France	French National Hospitalization Database (Gabet, Juilliere et al. 2015)	7.8% (2012)	ICD-10 codes, primary diagnosis
30-day			
United States	Medicare enrollees from the GWTG-HF program (Gupta, Allen et al. 2018)	7.2% (2006–2010) 8.6% (2012–2014)	Risk-adjusted estimates
International	ALARM-HF Registry (Farmakis, Simitsis et al. 2017)	9.4% (2006–2007)	Patients with documented EF
One-year			
USA	Medicare enrollees from the GWTG-HF program (Gupta, Allen et al. 2018)	31.3% (2006–2010); 36.3% (2012–2014)	Risk-adjusted estimates
Europe	Multicenter registry (Crespo-Leiro, Anker et al. 2016)	23.6% (2011–2013)	Prospective study, only consenting patients included
International	INTER-CHF cohort (Dokainish, Teo et al. 2017)	30.6% (unadjusted)	Middle- or low-income countries
Italy	Italian Network Registry (Xia, Qu et al. 2017)	24.0% (2007–2009) *de novo* HF: 19.2%; Worsening HF: 27.7%	Prospective study, only consenting patients included
Germany	Administrative (Ohlmeier, Mikolajczyk et al. 2015)	23% (2006)	Primary diagnosis, new cases only
Denmark	Registry (Schmidt, Ulrichsen et al. 2016)	34.6% (2003–2007) 32.7% (2008–2012)	ICD codes, primary or secondary diagnosis, new cases only
Five-year			
USA	GWTG-HF (Shah, Claggett et al. 2017)	HFrEF: 75.3%; HFpEF: 75.7%; HFmrEF: 75.7%	Quality improvement initiative
Denmark	Registry (Schmidt, Ulrichsen et al. 2016)	64.1% (2003–2007); 61.3% (2008–2012)	ICD codes, primary or secondary diagnosis, new cases only

Abbreviations: ALARM-HF: Acute Heart Failure Global Registry of Standard Treatment; EF: ejection fraction; GWTG-HF: Get With The Guidelines – Heart Failure; HF: heart failure; HFmrEF: heart failure with midrange ejection fraction; HFpEF: heart failure with preserved ejection fraction; HFrEF: heart failure with reduced ejection fraction.
Source: ICD-9-CM: International Classification of Diseases, 9th Revision, Clinical Modification; ICD-10-GM: International Classification of Diseases, 10th revision, German Modification; INTER-CHF: International Congestive Heart Failure Study.

HFrEF (EF ≤40%, age 64±13 years, 21.6% women), 7.6% among ~2,200 patients with borderline or midrange EF (EF 40%–50%, age 64±14 years, 31.5% women), and 6.3% among approximately 1,500 patients with HFpEF (EF >50%, age 69±14 years, 47.9% women) (Figure 2.3).[29]

Mortality is higher in national registries, which encompass older and sicker patients. Among 11,600 patients with HFrEF in the United States IMPROVE HF registry (EF ≤35%, median age 71 years), mortality at two years was 22.1%.[72] On a positive note, mortality in outpatients is declining. In a study using administrative data from Ontario, Canada, one-year risk-adjusted mortality decreased from 17.7% in 1997 to 16.2% in 2007 (P=0.02).[54]

Quality of care, especially adherence to evidence-based practices, critically affects outcomes in HFrEF. In IMPROVE HF, each 10% improvement in a composite care metric was associated with 13% lower odds of 24-month mortality (adjusted odds ratio, 0.87; 95% CI, 0.84–0.90).[72] In the international, quality improvement-oriented QUALIFY registry, mortality at six months was generally below 7% among outpatients with HFrEF but was highly dependent on adherence to guideline-recommended practices.[73]

Among ~23,500 patients with HF in the United Kingdom who were seen in primary care and had no HF hospitalization record (median age 79, 51.3% women), five-year survival was 43.9% compared with 88.1% in the age- and sex-matched general population.[74] In a primary care cohort in Scotland, five-year survival among about 10,300 men with HF (mean age at diagnosis, 70.5±12.2 years) and about 9,100 women with HF (mean age at diagnosis, 76.4±15.5 years) was 55.8% and 49.5%, respectively, and was comparable to or worse than several forms of cancer.[6]

In a retrospective study from Finland of 8,833 patients with a known diagnosis of HF,[75] compared to an age- and sex-matched control population without a diagnosis of HF, patients with HF had a higher rate of health care resource utilization (with 3.7 more days in the hospital per year) and a higher five-year mortality (62.6% in HF patients vs 28.3% in controls). Further analysis revealed a 13% (95% CI, 2.7% to 25%) higher five-year mortality in patients with HFrEF (defined as LVEF <40%) compared with those with HFpEF (defined as LVEF ≥40%).[75]

In a registry of 10,312 ambulatory patients with HF from Norway, Germany, and the United Kingdom, 68.7% had

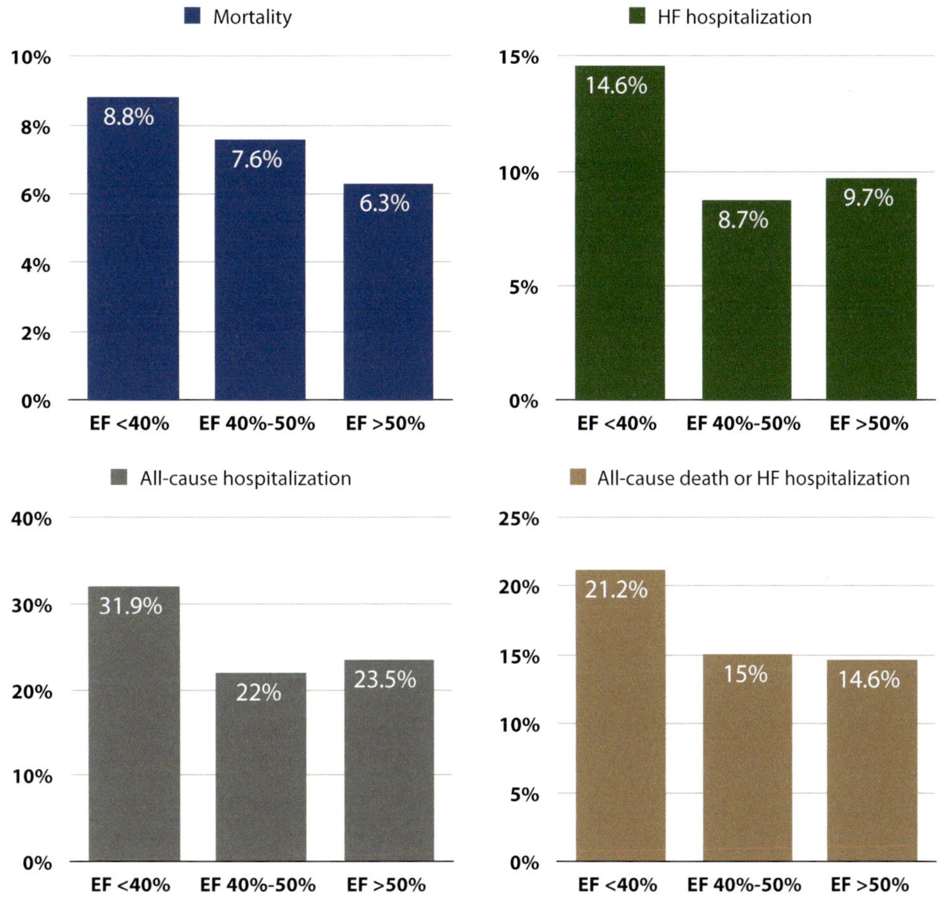

FIGURE 2.3 Outcomes at one year in outpatients with heart failure in the ESC Heart Failure Long-Term Registry. *Abbreviations*: EF: ejection fraction; HF: heart failure. (Data from Chioncel et al., *Eur J Heart Fail* 2017;19:1574–85.)

HFrEF, 20.2% had HFmrEF, and 11.1% had HFpEF.[76] After a median follow up of 66 months, 51.4% of the participants died. Multivariable analysis revealed that mortality was independent of LVEF, and was mainly influenced by age, functional class, levels of natriuretic peptides, and the use of loop diuretics.[76]

Outcomes in Chronic Heart Failure with Improved or Recovered Ejection Fraction

Patients who initially present with HFrEF but subsequently demonstrate improved or recovered EF (HFrecEF) have a distinct clinical course and, as a rule, better outcomes than patients with persistent HFpEF or HFrEF. In a single-center outpatient cohort from the United States, preserved EF (>40%) at inception was present in 37.7% of 2,166 outpatients.[23] Of these, over 40% had previously reduced EF (≤40%). Mortality significantly decelerated among patients with HFrecEF after one year. Age- and sex-adjusted three-year mortality was 16.3%, 13.2%, and 4.8% in patients with HFrEF, HFpEF, and HFrecEF, respectively. Compared with HFpEF or HFrEF, patients with HFrecEF had fewer all-cause and HF-related hospitalizations.[23] In a Spanish cohort of over 1,000 referral outpatients, one in four HFrEF patients showed recovery of EF from <45% to ≥45% within one year.[77] Patients with HFrecEF had lower all-cause, cardiovascular, and HF-related mortality as well as lower sudden death rates, and experienced fewer hospitalizations.[77]

In a prospective cohort of 5,103 Korean patients with HF who were evaluated one year after hospitalization for HF, of the 1,509 patients who initially had HFrEF (defined as an LVEF ≤40% in this study), 720 patients demonstrated improved LVEF on follow-up echocardiography. Positive predictors of LVEF recovery included female sex, a younger age, hypertension, atrial fibrillation, and *de novo* HF. Negative predictors included a diagnosis of diabetes mellitus and ischemic heart disease. Patients with HFrecEF had lower four-year mortality, whereas beta-blocker use was associated with reduced all-cause mortality in these patients (HR: 0.59; 95% CI, 0.40 to 0.87; P= 0.007); this benefit was irrespective of beta-blocker dose.[78]

Sex Differences in Heart Failure Mortality

In the Swedish Heart Failure Registry of approximately 43,000 subjects with ambulatory HF, women presented with higher crude mortality and hospitalization rates in the HFpEF and HFmrEF categories and lower rates in the HFrEF category, compared with men.[79]

In a study from the Netherlands, patients hospitalized for new-onset HF between 2000–2002 and 2008–2010 were stratified by age and sex, with 40,230 men and 41,582 women.[80] In both cohorts, the men (average, 74–75 years) were younger than the women (average, 78–79 years). Men had more comorbidities than women, 37% vs 30%, respectively. In the 2008–2010 cohort, mortality at 30 days, one year, and five years was similar in both sexes: 13%, 32%, and 64% in men vs 14%, 33%, and 66% in women, respectively. Between the two periods, mortality dropped across all ages and equally for men and women, with a one-year absolute risk of death declining by 4% in men and

3.2% in women.[80] Overall, HF-related mortality appears to be comparable in men vs women.

Conclusion

Preventive efforts at the population level, especially those related to hypertension, appear to have curbed the incidence of HF in the more developed countries. However, the overall prevalence of HF continues to increase because of population aging. Mortality after a diagnosis of HF is still high despite advances in pharmacotherapy and device therapy. Therefore, intensification of preventive efforts, with better control of cardiometabolic risk factors, is warranted.

References

1. Heidenreich PA, Albert NM, Allen LA, et al. Forecasting the impact of heart failure in the United States: a policy statement from the American Heart Association. *Circ Heart Fail.* 2013;6:606–19.
2. Chang PP, Chambless LE, Shahar E, et al. Incidence and survival of hospitalized acute decompensated heart failure in four US communities (from the Atherosclerosis Risk in Communities Study). *Am J Cardiol.* 2014;113:504–10.
3. Schmidt M, Ulrichsen SP, Pedersen L, Botker HE, Sorensen HT. Thirty-year trends in heart failure hospitalization and mortality rates and the prognostic impact of co-morbidity: a Danish nationwide cohort study. *Eur J Heart Fail.* 2016;18:490–9.
4. Dokainish H, Teo K, Zhu J, et al. Global mortality variations in patients with heart failure: results from the International Congestive Heart Failure (INTER-CHF) prospective cohort study. *Lancet Glob Health.* 2017;5:e665–72.
5. Shah KS, Xu H, Matsouaka RA, et al. Heart failure with preserved, borderline, and reduced ejection fraction: 5-year outcomes. *J Am Coll Cardiol.* 2017;70:2476–86.
6. Mamas MA, Sperrin M, Watson MC, et al. Do patients have worse outcomes in heart failure than in cancer? A primary care-based cohort study with 10-year follow-up in Scotland. *Eur J Heart Fail.* 2017;19:1095–104.
7. Jackson SL, Tong X, King RJ, et al. National burden of heart failure events in the United States, 2006 to 2014. *Circ Heart Fail.* 2018;11:e004873.
8. Christiansen MN, Kober L, Weeke P, et al. Age-specific trends in incidence, mortality, and comorbidities of heart failure in Denmark, 1995 to 2012. *Circulation.* 2017;135:1214–23.
9. Conrad N, Judge A, Tran J, et al. Temporal trends and patterns in heart failure incidence: a population-based study of 4 million individuals. *Lancet.* 2018;391:572–80.
10. Vasan RS, Xanthakis V, Lyass A, et al. Epidemiology of left ventricular systolic dysfunction and heart failure in the Framingham Study: an echocardiographic study over 3 decades. *JACC Cardiovasc Imaging.* 2018;11:1–11.
11. Sun LY, Tu JV, Sherrard H, et al. Sex-specific trends in incidence and mortality for urban and rural ambulatory patients with heart failure in Eastern Ontario from 1994 to 2013. *J Card Fail.* 2018;24:568–74.
12. Khera R, Pandey A, Ayers CR, et al. Contemporary epidemiology of heart failure in fee-for-service medicare beneficiaries across healthcare settings. *Circ Heart Fail.* 2017;10:e004402.
13. Chang PP, Wruck LM, Shahar E, et al. Trends in hospitalizations and survival of acute decompensated heart failure in four US communities (2005–2014): ARIC study community surveillance. *Circulation.* 2018;138:12–24.
14. Lindmark K, Boman K, Olofsson M, et al. Epidemiology of heart failure and trends in diagnostic work-up: a retrospective, population-based cohort study in Sweden. *Clin Epidemiol.* 2019;11:231–44.
15. Sillars A, Ho FK, Pell GP, et al. Sex differences in the association of risk factors for heart failure incidence and mortality. *Heart.* 2020;106:203–12.
16. Magnussen C, Niiranen TJ, Ojeda FM, et al. Sex-specific epidemiology of heart failure risk and mortality in Europe: results from the BiomarCaRE Consortium. *JACC Heart Fail.* 2019;7:204–13.
17. Tsao CW, Lyass A, Enserro D, et al. Temporal trends in the incidence of and mortality associated with heart failure with preserved and reduced ejection fraction. *JACC Heart Fail.* 2018;6:678–85.
18. Virani SS, Alonso A, Benjamin EJ, et al. Heart disease and stroke statistics-2020 update: a report from the American Heart Association. *Circulation.* 2020;141:e139–596.
19. Hunt SA, American College of C, American Heart Association Task Force on Practice G. ACC/AHA 2005 guideline update for the diagnosis and management of chronic heart failure in the adult: a report of the American College of Cardiology/American Heart Association Task Force on Practice Guidelines (Writing Committee to update the 2001 guidelines for the evaluation and management of heart failure). *J Am Coll Cardiol.* 2005;46:e1–82.
20. Xanthakis V, Enserro DM, Larson MG, et al. Prevalence, neurohormonal correlates, and prognosis of heart failure stages in the community. *JACC Heart Fail.* 2016;4:808–15.
21. Gidding SS, Lloyd-Jones D, Lima J, et al. Prevalence of American Heart Association heart failure stages in Black and White young and middle-aged adults: the CARDIA study. *Circ Heart Fail.* 2019;12:e005730.
22. Ponikowski P, Voors AA, Anker SD, et al. 2016 ESC guidelines for the diagnosis and treatment of acute and chronic heart failure: the task force for the diagnosis and treatment of acute and chronic heart failure of the European Society of Cardiology (ESC)Developed with the special contribution of the Heart Failure Association (HFA) of the ESC. *Eur Heart J.* 2016;37:2129–200.
23. Kalogeropoulos AP, Fonarow GC, Georgiopoulou V, et al. Characteristics and outcomes of adult outpatients with heart failure and improved or recovered ejection fraction. *JAMA Cardiol.* 2016;1:510–8.
24. Honma M, Tanaka F, Sato K, et al. Sex-specific temporal trends in the incidence and prevalence of hospitalized patients with preserved versus reduced left ventricular ejection fraction heart failure: a Japanese community-wide study. *Int J Cardiol Heart Vasc.* 2015;9:15–21.
25. Pandey A, Omar W, Ayers C, et al. Sex and race differences in lifetime risk of heart failure with preserved ejection fraction and heart failure with reduced ejection fraction. *Circulation.* 2018;137:1814–23.
26. Farre N, Vela E, Cleries M, et al. Real world heart failure epidemiology and outcome: a population-based analysis of 88,195 patients. *PLoS One.* 2017;12:e0172745.
27. Zarrinkoub R, Wettermark B, Wandell P, et al. The epidemiology of heart failure, based on data for 2.1 million inhabitants in Sweden. *Eur J Heart Fail.* 2013;15:995–1002.
28. Shah AM, Claggett B, Loehr LR, et al. Heart failure stages among older adults in the community: the atherosclerosis risk in communities study. *Circulation.* 2017;135:224–40.
29. Chioncel O, Lainscak M, Seferovic PM, et al. Epidemiology and one-year outcomes in patients with chronic heart failure and preserved, mid-range and reduced ejection fraction: an analysis of the ESC Heart Failure Long-Term Registry. *Eur J Heart Fail.* 2017;19:1574–85.
30. Silverman MG, Patel B, Blankstein R, et al. Impact of race, ethnicity, and multimodality biomarkers on the incidence of new-onset heart failure with preserved ejection fraction (from the multi-ethnic study of atherosclerosis). *Am J Cardiol.* 2016;117:1474–81.
31. Akwo EA, Kabagambe EK, Wang TJ, et al. Heart failure incidence and mortality in the Southern community cohort study. *Circ Heart Fail.* 2017;10:e003553.
32. van Riet EE, Hoes AW, Wagenaar KP, et al. Epidemiology of heart failure: the prevalence of heart failure and ventricular dysfunction in older adults over time. A systematic review. *Eur J Heart Fail.* 2016;18:242–52.
33. Khan H, Kalogeropoulos AP, Zannad F, et al. Incident heart failure in relation to vascular disease: insights from the Health, Aging, and Body Composition Study. *Eur J Heart Fail.* 2014;16:526–34.
34. Danielsen R, Thorgeirsson G, Einarsson H, et al. Prevalence of heart failure in the elderly and future projections: the AGES-Reykjavik study. *Scand Cardiovasc J.* 2017;51:183–9.
35. Lee H, Oh SH, Cho H, Cho HJ, Kang HY. Prevalence and socio-economic burden of heart failure in an aging society of South Korea. *BMC Cardiovasc Disord.* 2016;16:215.
36. Desta L, Jernberg T, Lofman I, et al. Incidence, temporal trends, and prognostic impact of heart failure complicating acute myocardial infarction. The SWEDEHEART Registry (Swedish web-system for enhancement and development of evidence-based care in heart disease evaluated according to recommended therapies): a study of 199,851 patients admitted with index acute myocardial infarctions, 1996 to 2008. *JACC Heart Fail.* 2015;3:234–42.
37. Desta L, Jernberg T, Spaak J, Hofman-Bang C, Persson H. Heart failure with normal ejection fraction is uncommon in acute myocardial infarction settings but associated with poor outcomes: a study of 91,360 patients admitted with index myocardial infarction between 1998 and 2010. *Eur J Heart Fail.* 2016;18:46–53.
38. Sulo G, Igland J, Vollset SE, et al. Heart failure complicating acute myocardial infarction; burden and timing of occurrence: a nation-wide analysis including 86 771 patients from the cardiovascular disease in Norway (CVDNOR) project. *J Am Heart Assoc.* 2016;5:e002667.
39. Chamberlain AM, St Sauver JL, Gerber Y, et al. Multimorbidity in heart failure: a community perspective. *Am J Med.* 2015;128:38–45.
40. Murad K, Goff DC, Jr., Morgan TM, et al. Burden of comorbidities and functional and cognitive impairments in elderly patients at the initial diagnosis of heart failure and their impact on total mortality: the cardiovascular health study. *JACC Heart Fail.* 2015;3:542–50.
41. Kalogeropoulos A, Georgiopoulou V, Kritchevsky SB, et al. Epidemiology of incident heart failure in a contemporary elderly cohort: the health, aging, and body composition study. *Arch Intern Med.* 2009;169:708–15.

42. Butler J, Kalogeropoulos AP, Georgiopoulou VV, et al. Systolic blood pressure and incident heart failure in the elderly. The Cardiovascular Health Study and the Health, Ageing and Body Composition Study. *Heart.* 2011;97:1304–11.
43. Upadhya B, Rocco M, Lewis CE, et al. Effect of intensive blood pressure treatment on heart failure events in the systolic blood pressure reduction intervention trial. *Circ Heart Fail.* 2017;10:e003613.
44. McAllister DA, Read SH, Kerssens J, et al. Incidence of hospitalization for heart failure and case-fatality among 3.25 million people with and without diabetes mellitus. *Circulation.* 2018;138:2774–86.
45. Santhanakrishnan R, Wang N, Larson MG, et al. Atrial fibrillation begets heart failure and vice versa: temporal associations and differences in preserved versus reduced ejection fraction. *Circulation.* 2016;133:484–92.
46. Chamberlain AM, Gersh BJ, Alonso A, et al. No decline in the risk of heart failure after incident atrial fibrillation: a community study assessing trends overall and by ejection fraction. *Heart Rhythm.* 2017;14:791–98.
47. Pandey A, Kim S, Moore C, et al. Predictors and prognostic implications of incident heart failure in patients with prevalent atrial fibrillation. *JACC Heart Fail.* 2017;5:44–52.
48. Schmidt M, Ulrichsen SP, Pedersen L, et al. 30-year nationwide trends in incidence of atrial fibrillation in Denmark and associated 5-year risk of heart failure, stroke, and death. *Int J Cardiol.* 2016;225:30–6.
49. Bansal N, Katz R, Robinson-Cohen C, et al. Absolute rates of heart failure, coronary heart disease, and stroke in chronic kidney disease: an analysis of 3 community-based cohort studies. *JAMA Cardiol.* 2017;2:314–8.
50. He J, Shlipak M, Anderson A, et al. Risk factors for heart failure in patients with chronic kidney disease: the CRIC (Chronic Renal Insufficiency Cohort) study. *J Am Heart Assoc.* 2017;6:e005336.
51. Desai AS, McMurray JJ, Packer M, et al. Effect of the angiotensin-receptor-neprilysin inhibitor LCZ696 compared with enalapril on mode of death in heart failure patients. *Eur Heart J.* 2015;36:1990–7.
52. Xia J, Qu Y, Yin C, Xu D. Preliminary study of beta-blocker therapy on modulation of interleukin-33/ST2 signaling during ventricular remodeling after acute myocardial infarction. *Cardiol J.* 2017;24:188–94.
53. Crespo-Leiro MG, Anker SD, Maggioni AP, et al. European Society of Cardiology Heart Failure Long-Term Registry (ESC-HF-LT): 1-year follow-up outcomes and differences across regions. *Eur J Heart Fail.* 2016;18:613–25.
54. Yeung DF, Boom NK, Guo H, et al. Trends in the incidence and outcomes of heart failure in Ontario, Canada: 1997 to 2007. *CMAJ.* 2012;184:E765–73.
55. Vivo RP, Krim SR, Liang L, et al. Short- and long-term rehospitalization and mortality for heart failure in 4 racial/ethnic populations. *J Am Heart Assoc.* 2014;3:e001134.
56. Gabet A, Juilliere Y, Lamarche-Vadel A, Vernay M, Olie V. National trends in rate of patients hospitalized for heart failure and heart failure mortality in France, 2000–2012. *Eur J Heart Fail.* 2015;17:583–90.
57. Christ M, Stork S, Dorr M, et al. Heart failure epidemiology 2000–2013: insights from the German Federal Health Monitoring System. *Eur J Heart Fail.* 2016;18:1009–18.
58. Parikh KS, Sheng S, Hammill BG, et al. Characteristics of acute heart failure hospitalizations based on presenting severity. *Circ Heart Fail.* 2019;12:e005171.
59. Frigerio M, Mazzali C, Paganoni AM, et al. Trends in heart failure hospitalizations, patient characteristics, in-hospital and 1-year mortality: a population study, from 2000 to 2012 in Lombardy. *Int J Cardiol.* 2017;236:310–4.
60. Gorlicki J, Boubaya M, Cottin Y, et al. Patient care pathways in acute heart failure and their impact on in-hospital mortality, a French national prospective survey. *Int J Cardiol Heart Vasc.* 2020;26:100448.
61. Shiga T, Suzuki A, Haruta S, et al. Clinical characteristics of hospitalized heart failure patients with preserved, mid-range, and reduced ejection fractions in Japan. *ESC Heart Fail.* 2019;6:475–86.
62. Zhang Y, Zhang J, Butler J, et al. Contemporary epidemiology, management, and outcomes of patients hospitalized for heart failure in China: results from the China Heart Failure (China-HF) Registry. *J Card Fail.* 2017;23:868–75.
63. Akintoye E, Briasoulis A, Egbe A, et al. Regional variation in mortality, length of stay, cost, and discharge disposition among patients admitted for heart failure in the United States. *Am J Cardiol.* 2017;120:817–24.
64. Bergethon KE, Ju C, DeVore AD, et al. Trends in 30-day readmission rates for patients hospitalized with heart failure: findings from the get with the guidelines-heart failure registry. *Circ Heart Fail.* 2016;9:10.
65. Durstenfeld MS, Ogedegbe O, Katz SD, Park H, Blecker S. Racial and ethnic differences in heart failure readmissions and mortality in a large municipal healthcare system. *JACC Heart Fail.* 2016;4:885–93.
66. Gupta A, Allen LA, Bhatt DL, et al. Association of the hospital readmissions reduction program implementation with readmission and mortality outcomes in heart failure. *JAMA Cardiol.* 2018;3:44–53.
67. Pandey A, Golwala H, Xu H, et al. Association of 30-day readmission metric for heart failure under the hospital readmissions reduction program with quality of care and outcomes. *JACC Heart Fail.* 2016;4:935–46.
68. Eapen ZJ, Reed SD, Li Y, et al. Do countries or hospitals with longer hospital stays for acute heart failure have lower readmission rates?: findings from ASCEND-HF. *Circ Heart Fail.* 2013;6:727–32.
69. Kimmoun A, Takagi K, Gall E, et al. Temporal trends in mortality and readmission after acute heart failure: a systematic review and meta-regression in the past four decades. *Eur J Heart Fail.* 2021.
70. Samsky MD, Ambrosy AP, Youngson E, et al. Trends in readmissions and length of stay for patients hospitalized with heart failure in Canada and the United States. *JAMA Cardiol.* 2019;4:444–53.
71. Gerber Y, Weston SA, Redfield MM, et al. A contemporary appraisal of the heart failure epidemic in Olmsted County, Minnesota, 2000 to 2010. *JAMA Intern Med.* 2015;175:996–1004.
72. van Boxtel W, Bulten BF, Mavinkurve-Groothuis AM, et al. New biomarkers for early detection of cardiotoxicity after treatment with docetaxel, doxorubicin and cyclophosphamide. *Biomarkers.* 2015;20:143–8.
73. Komajda M, Cowie MR, Tavazzi L, et al. Physicians' guideline adherence is associated with better prognosis in outpatients with heart failure with reduced ejection fraction: the QUALIFY international registry. *Eur J Heart Fail.* 2017;19:1414–23.
74. Koudstaal S, Pujades-Rodriguez M, Denaxas S, et al. Prognostic burden of heart failure recorded in primary care, acute hospital admissions, or both: a population-based linked electronic health record cohort study in 2.1 million people. *Eur J Heart Fail.* 2017;19:1119–27.
75. Huusko J, Kurki S, Toppila I, et al. Heart failure in Finland: clinical characteristics, mortality, and healthcare resource use. *ESC Heart Fail.* 2019;6:603–12.
76. Frohlich H, Rosenfeld N, Tager T, et al. Epidemiology and long-term outcome in outpatients with chronic heart failure in Northwestern Europe. *Heart.* 2019;105:1252–59.
77. Lupon J, Diez-Lopez C, de Antonio M, et al. Recovered heart failure with reduced ejection fraction and outcomes: a prospective study. *Eur J Heart Fail.* 2017;19:1615–23.
78. Park CS, Park JJ, Mebazaa A, et al. Characteristics, outcomes, and treatment of heart failure with improved ejection fraction. *J Am Heart Assoc.* 2019;8:e011077.
79. Stolfo D, Uijl A, Vedin O, et al. Sex-based differences in heart failure across the ejection fraction spectrum: phenotyping, and prognostic and therapeutic implications. *JACC Heart Fail.* 2019;7:505–15.
80. Buddeke J, Valstar GB, van Dis I, et al. Mortality after hospital admission for heart failure: improvement over time, equally strong in women as in men. *BMC Public Health.* 2020;20:36.

Chapter 3
PATHOPHYSIOLOGY OF HEART FAILURE WITH REDUCED EJECTION FRACTION

Jacob Cao, John O'Sullivan, and Sean Lal

Heart failure with reduced ejection fraction (HFrEF) is a complex collection of disease entities, all resulting in impairment of myocardial contraction such that cardiac output can no longer meet peripheral tissue demands. The list of etiologies is extensive but can all be conceptualized as occurring after one or more index event(s) either directly damaging the myocardium or preventing cardiomyocytes from contracting normally. The index event can be acute, as in the case of a myocardial infarction, chronic, as in the case of hemodynamic overload relating to valvular dysfunction or a progressive dilated cardiomyopathy, or a combination thereof. Cardiomyocytes, unlike other cell types (e.g., hepatocytes), are in a terminally differentiated state, implying limited regenerative capabilities. Although this dogma has been challenged in recent years, significant regenerative capacity has not been proven in human trials and it is still an active area of research. Rather, the damaged cardiomyocytes are typically replaced by fibrous tissues, resulting in global or regional biomechanical inefficiencies. To maintain cardiac output, cascades of neurohormonal, structural (remodeling), and energetic changes are simultaneously triggered, perpetuating the vicious cycle that characterizes the progression of HFrEF. These mechanisms form the basis of our current understanding of heart failure (HF) pathophysiology and serve as targets for established and novel therapies.

Neurohormonal Activation

The neurohormonal hypothesis of HF, first formalized by Milton Packer in 1992, posits that activation of neurohormones helps to maintain circulatory homeostasis in the short term, but causes damage to the heart and circulation when sustained (Figure 3.1).[1] Extensive literature has reported significant positive associations between concentrations of circulating neurohormones and adverse HF outcomes, and conversely benefits associated with inhibition of these neurohormonal systems.

Sympathetic Nervous System

The sympathetic nervous system (SNS) is the first to be involved.[2] Circulatory insufficiencies secondary to the initial myocardial insult are sensed by the high-pressure baroreceptors in the carotid sinus and aortic arch, and the low-pressure mechanoreceptors in the cardiopulmonary system. Stimulation of these receptors disinhibit the sympathetic efferents to the heart with secondary improvement in contractility (inotropy), rate (chronotropy), and relaxation (lusitropy), all designed to restore peripheral perfusion. However, with chronic hemodynamic disturbances, as in the case of HF, there are progressive pathological alterations to the autonomic nervous system, which can be summarized as attenuation of the parasympathetic and augmentation of the sympathetic system. The mechanisms of these changes are multi-factorial. Earlier studies have alluded to blunting of the arterial and cardiopulmonary receptor reflexes, whereas more recent studies have shown significant modulation of the sympathetic nervous system (SNS) by central neural mechanisms and peripheral chemoreceptors. Animal models have shown that central infusion of angiotensin II (AT II) modulates the arterial baroreceptor reflex to increase sympathetic outflow and dampen vagal discharges, whilst aldosterone increases hypothalamic production of angiotensin receptor 1, angiotensin-converting enzyme (ACE), and plasma norepinephrine levels. Conversely, intracerebral administration of the AT II receptor blocker (ARB) losartan and the aldosterone antagonist spironolactone has been shown to reduce or abolish the increased sympathetic outflow. Irrespective of the underlying mechanisms, sustained sympathetic overdrive results in pathological remodeling, as well as secondary damage through stimulation of the renin-angiotensin-aldosterone system (RAAS). This mutual activation of the SNS and RAAS effectively sets up a positive feedback loop, which, if not interrupted by targeted neurohormonal blockade, commonly spirals towards HF exacerbations, hospitalization, and increased mortality.

Renin-Angiotensin-Aldosterone System

Activation of the RAAS occurs late, relative to the SNS.[3] In healthy individuals, RAAS contributes toward salt and fluid homeostasis by modulating the glomerular filtration rate and the degree of sodium and water reabsorption. In HF, the increased SNS activity results in systemic vasoconstriction, including that of the renovascular system, which, in conjunction with low cardiac output, leads to decreased renal perfusion and reduced solute delivery to the macula densa. This triggers the release of renin from the granular cells within the juxtaglomerular apparatus. Hyperreninemia is further promoted by the overactive SNS directly stimulating renin release via the beta-1 adrenergic receptors (β1-ARs) within the juxtaglomerular apparatus. Plasma renin subsequently cleaves angiotensinogen produced by the liver to angiotensin I, which is then converted to AT II by ACE within the pulmonary vasculature. AT II is a potent vasoconstrictor, thereby increasing total peripheral resistance and elevating mean arterial pressure. Additionally, AT II stimulates aldosterone release from the zona glomerulosa of the adrenal glands. Aldosterone, an endogenous mineralocorticoid, acts on the distal collecting duct of the nephron to facilitate salt and water reabsorption. Other mechanisms by which AT II results in volume expansion include directly acting on the proximal tubules to promote sodium reabsorption; stimulating the hypothalamic thirst center; and inducing non-osmotic release of anti-diuretic hormone (ADH) from the posterior pituitary to retain free water in the renal collecting ducts. Altogether, expansion of the effective circulatory volume, in combination with venous constriction, increases cardiac preload, which, by the Frank-Starling relationship, increases stroke volume and cardiac output in the short term. However, in the long term, like SNS activation, sustained RAAS activation also results in pathological remodeling (see below).

Natriuretic Peptides

Various intrinsic counter-regulatory pathways are upregulated in HF to offset the effects of sustained neurohormonal activation. Natriuretic peptides, most prominently the B-type

DOI: 10.1201/9780429244544-4

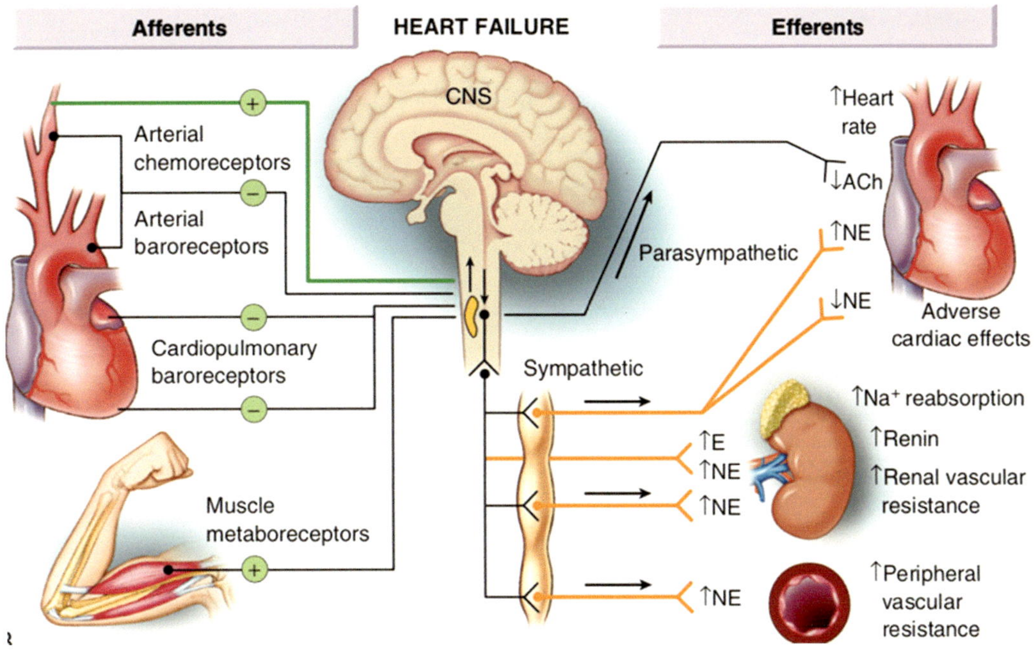

FIGURE 3.1 Sympathetic nervous system and renin-angiotensin-aldosterone system maintain circulatory homeostasis in the short term following the index myocardial insult. However, sustained neurohormonal activation directly results in pathological remodeling and further damage to the heart. (Reproduced with permission from: Hartupee and Mann, *Nat Rev Cardiol* 2017;14:30–8.)

natriuretic peptide (BNP), have been an active area of research in recent years due to their role in diagnosis of HF, in predicting HF outcomes, and as drug targets for therapy. BNP is released in response to ventricular myocardial stretch and serves to offload the heart by sodium and water excretion, peripheral vasodilation, inhibition of renin release, and antagonism of AT II effects (opposite effects of RAAS). Atrial natriuretic peptide (ANP) is released from atrial cells under similar volume overload stress, and it has the same actions as BNP. The C-type natriuretic peptide is primarily derived from endothelial cells and may prevent pathological remodeling after myocardial infarction but is found in only low concentrations in circulating blood.

Based on their physiological mechanisms, multiple natriuretic peptide analogues and endopeptidase inhibitors have progressed through preclinical studies to human trials. Nesiritide, a recombinant BNP, although showing hemodynamic benefits in earlier studies, did not reduce death or rehospitalization compared to placebo in a large long-term trial. Neprilysin is a membrane-bound metalloproteinase that cleaves and inactivates various peptide hormones, including natriuretic peptides, bradykinin, substance P, and beta amyloids. Early neprilysin inhibitors were shown to promote natriuresis, but the effect was not sustained, likely because AT II breakdown was also inhibited. Consequently, dual blockade of neprilysin and ACE was thought to be the solution. The neprilysin-ACE inhibitor omapatrilat was compared with ACE inhibitor alone in the phase III trial OVERTURE,[4] showing no reduction in the composite primary endpoint of all-cause mortality and HF hospitalization, but causing a reduction in the secondary endpoint of all-cause mortality and cardiovascular hospitalization. However, on account of the unacceptable rise in the angioedema rate in the treatment group, related to omapatrilat inhibition of bradykinin breakdown, further development of this agent was ceased. The more recently developed agent sacubitril-valsartan carries the dual advantage that sacubitrilat (active metabolite of sacubitril) does not inhibit aminopeptidase P, which breaks down bradykinin, and that valsartan does not inhibit ACE, which also contributes to bradykinin inactivation (Figure 3.2). Accordingly, sacubitril-valsartan was compared with enalapril for HFrEF patients in the recent phase III trial PARADIGM-HF,[5] demonstrating the marked superiority of sacubitril-valsartan in terms of all-cause mortality, cardiovascular mortality, and HF hospitalization, with a non-significant rise in non-serious angioedema. Replacing ACE inhibitor or ARB with sacubitril-valsartan now holds a level I class of recommendation in all major international guidelines for HFrEF.[6,7]

Negative Remodeling

Negative remodeling refers to alterations in the structure of the heart on a cellular, anatomical, and functional level to accommodate injury or changes in hemodynamic load. The initial injury, such as myocardial infarction and associated regional hemodynamic changes, often sets in motion the process of pathological remodeling, which is perpetuated by sustained neurohormonal overactivity. Whereas activation of RAAS and SNS is beneficial in maintaining peripheral perfusion in the short term, chronic overactivity is associated with deleterious changes to cardiomyocyte biology, extracellular matrix, and ventricular geometry. Under sustained hemodynamic stress, cardiomyocytes have been shown to alter their structure (cellular hypertrophy), metabolism, and excitation-contraction coupling, while simultaneously exhibiting progressive cell loss through necrosis and apoptosis, with their replacement by non-contractile fibrous tissues (increase in extracellular volume).

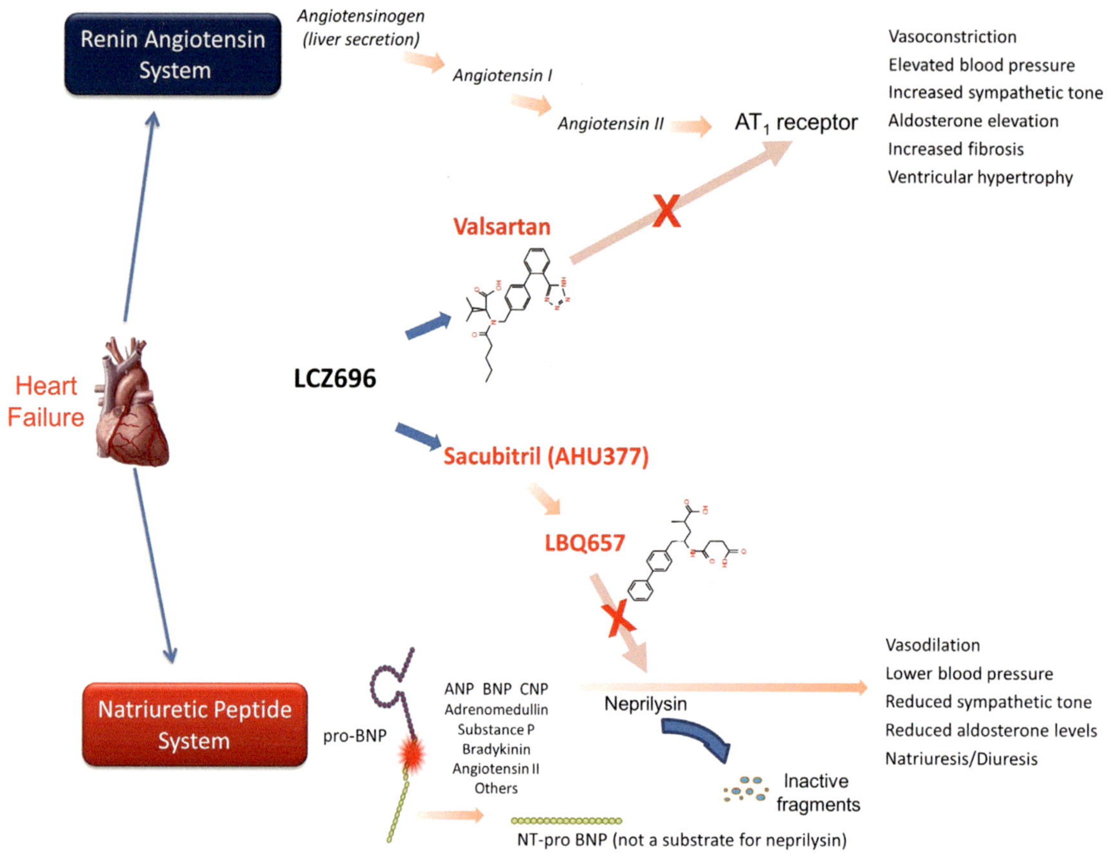

FIGURE 3.2 Sacubitril-valsartan mechanism of action in heart failure. (Reproduced with permission from: Vardeny, Miller, and Solomon, *JACC Heart Fail* 2014;2:663–70.)

Adrenergic Stimulation Desensitization

In the healthy heart, norepinephrine released from the SNS efferent varicosities increase cardiac output through improved inotropy, chronotropy, and lusitropy. On the other hand, innervation from the parasympathetic system (vagus nerves) only decreases inotropy. In cardiomyocytes, norepinephrine acts predominantly on the β1- and β2-adrenergic receptors, although the effect is modulated by coactivation of the α1-adrenergic receptors. β1 accounts for 70–80% of β-adrenergic receptors in the heart. It is linked to the G_s protein-adenylyl cyclase system, such that activation of the β1-receptor triggers a cascade, resulting in the increased production of the secondary messenger, cyclic adenosine monophosphate (cAMP). In contrast, β2 accounts for the remaining 20–30% of β-adrenergic receptors. It is coupled with both G_s and G_i, the latter inhibiting adenylyl cyclase thus reducing cardiac output (Figure 3.3). cAMP subsequently acts on a tertiary messenger, protein kinase A (PKA), which proceeds to phosphorylate various important intracellular targets responsible for the pleiotropic effects of β1 in increasing cardiac output. Key targets include 1) L-type calcium channel, which allows more calcium to enter the cell with every action potential (inotropy) and decreases the action potential threshold (chronotropy); 2) phospholamban, a transmembrane protein that typically inhibits the sarco-endoplasmic reticulum Ca-ATPase 2a (SERCA-2a), which in turn transports calcium from the cytosol into the sarcoplasmic reticulum. Phosphorylation of phospholamban leads to disinhibition of SERCA-2a, thereby allowing faster and greater sarcoplasmic reticulum accumulation of calcium to be released in the next cycle (lusitropy and inotropy); and 3) troponin I and myosin-binding protein C. Phosphorylation of troponin I promotes dissociation of calcium from myofilaments (lusitropy), whereas phosphorylation of myosin-binding protein C accelerates cross-bridge turnover (inotropy and chronotropy).

Sustained β-adrenergic stimulation, as seen in HF, results in desensitization of the receptors thereby impairing augmentation of cardiac output during increased physiological demand.[8] This is mediated through the induction of β-receptor kinase 1 (βARK1), a member of the G-coupled protein kinase family, which increases the affinity of the β-adrenergic receptor for β-arrestin. Activation of the β-adrenergic receptor by β-arrestin subsequently uncouples the G_s protein from adenylyl cyclase, switches coupling from G_s to G_i, and causes internalization and degradation of β-adrenergic receptors. Indeed, the failing heart has been shown to express fewer of the stimulatory β1 receptors relative to the β2 receptors. Experimental HF models have demonstrated improved contractility and survival with βARK1 inhibition, and restoration of normal β-adrenergic signaling with cardiac resynchronization therapy.[9,10]

Excitation Contraction Coupling

Excitation contraction coupling refers to the coordinated process that starts when the action potential arrives at the sarcolemmal membrane and ends with sarcomere contraction and relaxation (Figure 3.4). Calcium plays a pivotal role in this entire process. Upon activation of the voltage-gated L-type calcium channels on the T tubules by the action potential, there is an initial small inward current of calcium. This small current

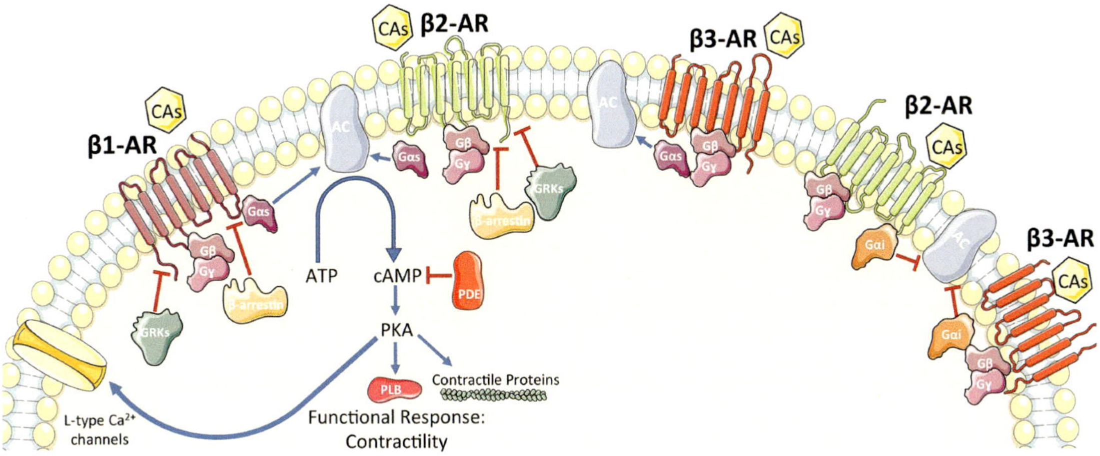

FIGURE 3.3 Normal beta-adrenergic signaling in the heart is mediated through the secondary messenger cyclic adenosine monophosphate (cAMP), and protein kinase A (PKA). PKA has pleotropic downstream effects to modulate lusitropy, inotropy, and chronotropy of the myocardial contractile cells. *Abbreviations*: AR, adrenergic receptor; AC, adenylyl cyclase; CA, catecholamines; GRK: G protein-coupled receptor kinases. (Reproduced under the terms of the Creative Commons Attribution License (CC BY) from: de Lucia, Eguchi, and Koch, *Front Pharmacol* 2018;9:904.)

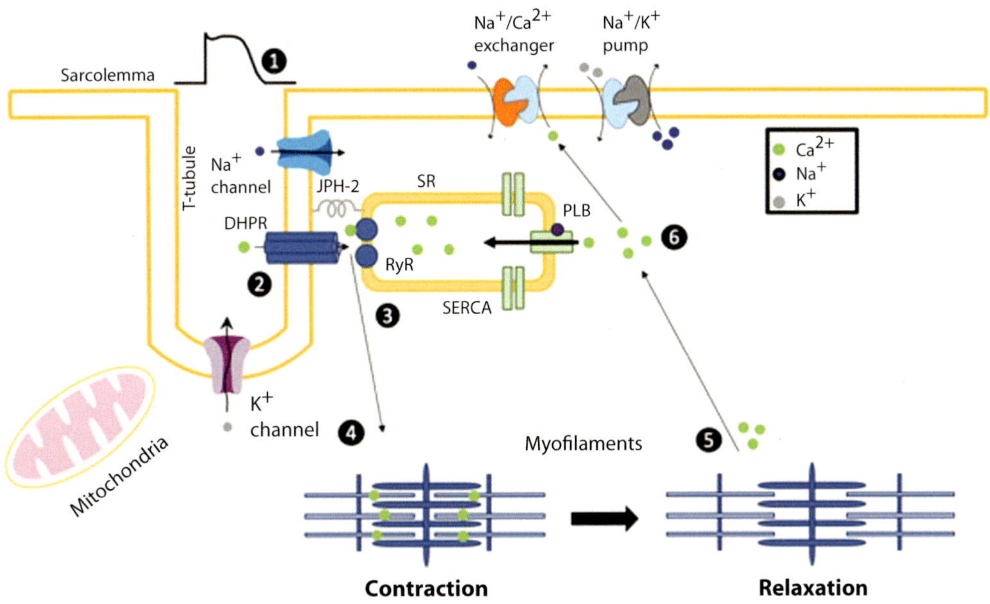

FIGURE 3.4 Excitation contraction coupling in the cardiomyocyte. The cardiac action potential [1] is initiated by influx of Na^+ ions via Na^+ channels, which brings the net cellular potential from negative to positive. This triggers Ca^{2+} release from LTCC [2] found within the invagination of the T-tubule. The localized elevation of Ca^{2+} concentration induces CICR from the closely opposed SR via RyR receptors [3]. Contraction [4] and relaxation [5] of myofilaments are dependent on binding and dissociation of Ca^{2+} from troponin. Diastole is therefore dependent on efflux of Ca^{2+} to either the SR via SERCA or extracellularly via NCX. Return to net negative cellular potential occurs during repolarization and involves efflux of K^+ ions via K^+ channels and NKX. *Abbreviations*: LTCC, L-type Ca^{2+} channels; CICR, calcium induced calcium release; SR, sarcoplasmic reticulum; RyR, ryanodine receptor; SERCA, sarcoplasmic reticulum Ca^{2+} ATPase; NCX, sodium-calcium exchanger; NKX, sodium-potassium exchanger. (Reproduced with permission from: Ge et al., *Heart Fail Rev* 2019;24:743–58.)

acts on the closely apposed ryanodine receptors 2 and triggers a large release of calcium from the sarcoplasmic reticulum (calcium-induced calcium release). The cytosolic calcium subsequently binds to the cardiac troponin C. This induces conformational changes of the contractile proteins, leading to cross-bridge formation and sarcomeric contraction. The peak cytosolic calcium concentration is a major determinant of contractility. Relaxation occurs when the calcium is transported from the cytosol to either the sarcoplasmic reticulum via the SERCA-2a transporter (major mechanism) or out of the cells via the sodium-calcium exchanger (minor mechanism).

In HF, excitation contraction coupling is impaired through three intracellular changes: (1) decreased expression and function of SERCA-2a; (2) increased calcium leak through ryanodine receptors; and (3) increased transport of calcium out of the cell through enhanced expression and function of the sodium-calcium exchanger. Together, these processes impair inotropy through depletion of intracellular calcium and reduced calcium-induced calcium release from the sarcoplasmic reticulum, and lusitropy should be impaired or decreased in heart failure due to slow removal of calcium from the cytosol after completion of an action potential-contraction cycle.[11]

As described previously, the sustained hyperadrenergic state that characterizes HF results in desensitization of cardiomyocytes to further adrenergic stimulation. As a result, there is increased phospholamban-dependent inhibition of SERCA-2a. Indeed, both phospholamban ablation and β blockade have been shown to improve excitation-contraction coupling and calcium handling in both animal and human studies. Upregulation of SERCA-2a function and expression have been trialed with varying success. Istaroxime, a direct SERCA-2a stimulator, has been shown to increase sarcoplasmic reticulum calcium reuptake during diastole and release during systole. In a randomized placebo-controlled trial of 120 patients with acute decompensated HF, istaroxime infusion was shown to improve left heart hemodynamics without any increase in adverse events.[12] There are currently no studies examining istaroxime in chronic HFrEF. Post-translational protein modification has recently emerged as another area of research into improving SERCA-2a function. The conjugation of small ubiquitin-like modifiers (SUMO) to SERCA-2a has been shown to be essential in preserving SERCA-2a ATPase activity, and that HF is associated with a reduction in the extent of conjugation. Additionally, animal studies have demonstrated that restoration of SUMO1 via gene therapy improves cardiac function, with evidence in humans still pending.

Furthermore, numerous animal and human studies have confirmed reduced expression of SERCA-2a at the mRNA and protein levels, and, as such, replenishment of SERCA-2a is theoretically sound. Gene therapy with SERCA-2a-carrying adenovirus has shown promise in pre-clinical and early clinical studies. In the pilot human study, CUPID, intra-coronary delivery of SERCA-2a via the adeno-associated virus vector 1 (SERCA-2a/AAV1) for treatment of moderate-to-severe HFrEF produced an impressive 82% reduction in HF events over three years follow-up.[13] Despite this, in the subsequent randomized controlled trial CUPID II, SERCA-2a/AAV1 treatment failed to achieve significance in its primary endpoint of recurrent HF events.[14] Such discrepancy between the pilot and the randomized trial was possibly a product of inconsistent ventricular transduction of SERCA-2a, and, as such, there is research ongoing into improving transfection techniques prior to further trials.

Inappropriate Cardiac Hypertrophy

Pathological hypertrophy is a key component of remodeling. In HFrEF, eccentric hypertrophy in response to chronic volume overload leads to progressive ventricular dilatation with secondary loss of contractility. Maladaptive hypertrophy is also characterized by genetic changes, possibly driven by neurohormones and inflammatory cytokines.[15] Such changes include increased expression of a set of genes commonly seen in fetal cardiomyocytes, and conversely decreased expression of those typical of adult cardiomyocytes. Specifically, there is reduced production of the V1 isoform of the myosin heavy chain, which contains fast myofibrillar ATPase activity, and conversely increased production of the V3 isoform with slow ATPase activity, combining to impair contractility. Restoration of the normal ratio of V1 to V3 isoform is seen in those with an effective beta blockade. Pathological changes have been additionally described in myosin light chains, the troponin-tropomyosin complex, and titin, and, in advanced HF, biopsies have revealed proteolysis of the contractile proteins and sarcomeres. The myofibrillar ultrastructure is also affected in advanced remodeling, with disruption of the intercellular linkage and loss of the parallel arrangement of sarcomeres required for effective excitation-contraction coupling.

Necrosis and Apoptosis

Necrosis and apoptosis occur at an increased rate in HF and serve as important contributors towards worsening cardiac function, especially in the context of minimal innate cardiomyocyte regeneration. Cardiomyocyte necrosis is stimulated by norepinephrine and AT II at concentrations that are not uncommonly seen in HFrEF patients. Cellular rupture releases intracellular molecules, which incite a sterile inflammatory process, driving further necrosis. In comparison, apoptosis is a more regulated process, but is also driven by neurohormonal activation, resulting in loss of contractile cardiac cells. In murine models, over-expression of caspase 8, an intracellular messenger on the apoptosis pathway, is associated with development of dilated cardiomyopathy, whereas knockout of the pro-apoptotic protein Bnip3 delays development of HF post-myocardial infarction. One study of explanted hearts from patients undergoing transplantation demonstrated an increase in the rate of apoptosis of more than 200-fold.[16] Further support for the pathophysiological role of low-grade apoptosis/necrosis stems from cardiac troponin studies. Elevated troponin levels have been documented in significant proportions of stable, chronic HF patients even in the absence of coronary artery disease. Higher baseline troponin concentration and trends in troponin level over time have been shown to predict greater tendencies to negative remodeling, hospitalization, and death.[17]

Extracellular Matrix

The extracellular matrix of the heart serves as a scaffold for both the resting structure and the contractile coordination of the heart. Excessive matrix increases ventricular stiffness and reduces filling, whereas reduced matrix is associated with progressive ventricular dilatation. A homeostasis between matrix production and destruction is maintained by a balance of fibroblasts and matrix metalloproteinases (MMP). This homeostasis, however, can be disturbed by neurohormonal activation. AT II and aldosterone drive fibroblast differentiation into myofibroblasts which have enhanced collagen production capacity, whereas RAAS blockade with ACE inhibitors and ARBs has been consistently shown to reduce cardiac fibrosis. Neurohormonal activation also drives MMP activity, leading to ventricular wall thinning and pathological remodeling. Human ischemic and dilated cardiomyopathy have been shown to exhibit increased expression of MMP-9 and decreased expression of TIMP-1 and -3, inhibitors of MMP. Accordingly, levels of serum N-terminal type II collagen peptide, a marker of collagen turnover, have been noted to be increased in dilated cardiomyopathy, and serve as predictors of mortality in HF.

Left Ventricular Geometry

The net sum of the previously described cellular and extracellular processes is pathological alterations to the left ventricular (LV) geometry (Figure 3.5).[18] At an anatomical level, the structure of the failing heart undergoes numerous changes, including wall thinning, progressive dilatation, and transformation into a more spherical shape from the normal prolate ellipse. Such changes create new biomechanical burdens, which in themselves can drive further worsening of HF. Firstly, the concurrent increase in ventricular radius and decrease in wall thickness confers greater wall stress (as per Laplace's law of the

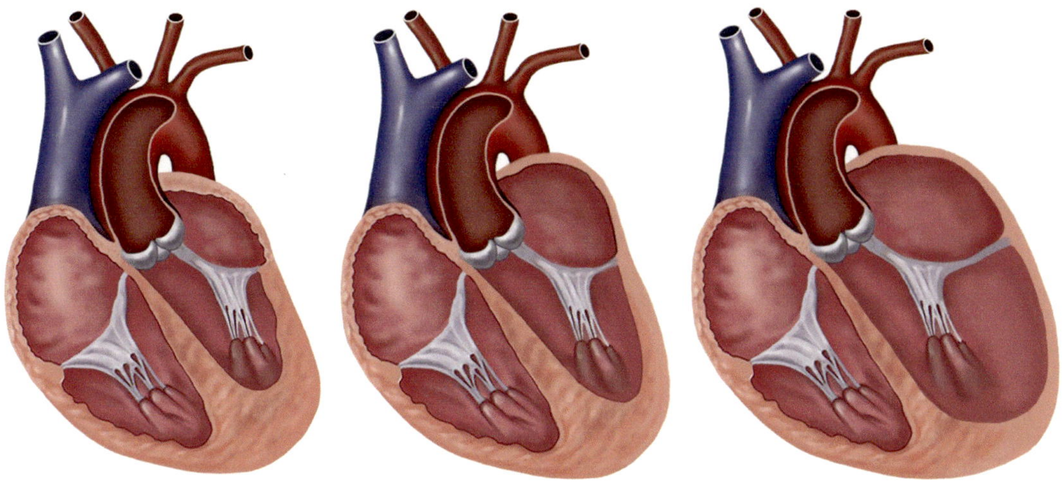

FIGURE 3.5 Negative remodeling in HFrEF is characterized by increased sphericity, ventricular wall thinning, and functional mitral incompetence. (Reproduced with permission from: Fatkin et al., *J Am Coll Cardiol* 2019;74:2921–38.)

heart) and thus greater myocardial oxygen requirement. This is further exacerbated by high end-diastolic pressures leading to intermittent subendocardial ischemia. Secondly, increased LV sphericity results in separation of papillary muscles and distortion of the mitral annulus, resulting in functional mitral regurgitation. In turn, this places the LV under increased volume-related stress, forming a cycle of worsening regurgitation and LV dilatation. Breaking this cycle, as shown by the COAPT trial using percutaneous mitral repair devices, significantly reduces hospitalization for HF at two-year follow-up.[19] However, the concurrently conducted MITRA-FR trial did not demonstrate a reduction in combined all-cause mortality and HF hospitalization at one year.[20] Such discrepancy might have been related to lower severity of HF, smaller effective regurgitant orifice area, fewer patients receiving more than a single clip, and shorter duration of follow-up in the MITRA-FR, compared with the COAPT trial.

Energetics

The healthy heart derives two-thirds of its energy supply from β-oxidation of fatty acids, and the remainder from oxidation of pyruvate, which is generated from lactate and glucose metabolism.[21] The exact proportions vary under physiological conditions, such as during states of hypoglycemia (e.g., fasting), when fatty acid oxidation is favored. The end-product, adenosine triphosphate (ATP), is predominantly used for one of two purposes—myofibrillar contraction and calcium flux. As such, any disturbances in the myocyte energy reserve can precipitate cardiac dysfunction. Under stress, such as in the early stages of HF, an adaptive shift in energy utilization from fatty acid oxidation to glycolysis has been described. Fatty acid oxidation, although able to generate four times as much ATP for every mole of substrate utilized than glycolysis, does require 10–12% more oxygen for the same amount of ATP production. Therefore, under oxygen-restricted circumstances, the metabolic shift to glycolysis maximizes ATP production efficiency. This switch in substrate utilization may be in part driven by upregulation of the fetal gene program and chronic hyperadrenergic states.[21]

As HF progresses, key components of the cardiac energetic system, including metabolites (adenine nucleotides, creatine phosphate) and enzymes (creatine kinase, creatine phosphokinase), are downregulated, with the loss of cardiac energy reserve in HFrEF being predictive of mortality. The etiology of this energy depletion is likely multifactorial, including substrate and oxygen unavailability, mitochondrial dysfunction, and disruption of energy transfer.[22]

Energetic Changes in Heart Failure

Substrate and Oxygen Availability

Coronary delivery of oxygen and substrates may be significantly diminished during HF. Despite the early switch from fatty acid oxidation to carbohydrate metabolism to improve mitochondrial efficiency, there is a concurrent reduction in glucose influx through downregulation of the glucose transporters, GLUT-1 and GLUT-4. GLUT-4 knockout mice exhibit worse cardiac hypertrophy and fibrosis, as well as reduced expression of ryanodine receptors and SERCA-2. Additionally, although glycolytic enzyme activity is increased in HF, the rate of glucose oxidation is reduced, leading to further energy depletion in advanced HF, and accumulation of lactic acid, with secondary regional acidosis and ventricular dysfunction.

Mitochondrial Function

Mitochondrial dysfunction may also contribute toward energetic depletion and generation of cytotoxic reactive oxygen species. Decreased mitochondrial complexes and compromised mitochondrial structural integrity have been noted in both human and animal HF and restored with effective treatment, including resynchronization and neprilysin inhibition. Observational studies have variably noted a correlation between low coenzyme Q10, a key component of the electron transport chain, and poorer HF outcomes. A randomized trial of Q10 supplementation demonstrated significant benefit for HFrEF in terms of long-term cardiovascular death, HF hospitalization, or mechanical support or transplant. However, results need to be interpreted with caution considering the small cohort size and the lack of improvement in biochemical, echocardiographic, and functional correlates with Q10 supplementation. Various other agents, such as flavonoids and melatonin, have been shown to improve mitochondrial function in animal models of HF, but translation to humans is still lacking.

Energy Transfer

Precise transfer of the high-energy phosphate moiety from ATP-producing to ATP-consuming sites is fundamental to cardiac bioenergetics. Numerous enzymatic networks exist to facilitate this process, the most important of which is the creatine kinase system. Multiple alterations to this system, including reduction in total enzyme activity and changes in isoenzyme pattern, are partially responsible for decreased energy utilization in HF.

Metabolic Substrate Modification as a Therapeutic Target

On account of the increased efficiency of carbohydrate metabolism compared with fatty acid metabolism, various agents targeted at modifying substrate utilization have been tested, including etomoxir, perhexiline, trimetazidine, and ranolazine.[23]

Etomoxir is an inhibitor of carnitine palmitoyl transferase 1 (CPT-1), which normally transports fatty acids across the mitochondrial membrane for oxidation. *In vitro* studies of etomoxir have demonstrated improved cardiomyocyte calcium handling via upregulation of SERCA expression. An initial trial of etomoxir in moderate-severity HF patients demonstrated up to 27% increase in ejection fraction after three months of treatment.[24] The subsequent randomized trial was ceased prematurely due to associated liver function derangement, and, at time of cessation, there was no echocardiographic improvement in the treatment groups, although the power was limited.[25]

Perhexilline is an inhibitor of CPT-1 and -2. In small-scale trials with HF patients, one month of treatment was shown to be associated with increased phosphocreatine-to-ATP ratio,[26] a marker of energy reserve, while longer treatment was associated with improvement in peak oxygen consumption, ejection fraction, and HF-related quality of life.[27]

Trimetazidine is a partial inhibitor of 3-ketoacyl CoA thiolase, a key enzyme involved in fatty acid oxidation. Numerous small-scale trials have been conducted, showing variable changes in cardiac function. A meta-analysis of nearly one thousand patients demonstrated improvements in ventricular hemodynamic and clinical outcomes, including exercise capacity, all-cause mortality, and combined cardiovascular events and hospitalization. Although most studies have been limited to ischemic cardiomyopathy, a more recent trial noted improvements in hemodynamic and functional status in non-ischemic cardiomyopathy patients.[28]

Ranolazine is a novel anti-anginal drug. Its main effect is mediated through inhibition of the late sodium channel current but it may also have effects on glucose and fatty acid metabolism. Experimental models of cardiac ischemia-reperfusion injury have shown that ranolazine treatment reduced fatty acid and enhanced glucose metabolism with associated increase in ATP generation. However, human trials of ranolazine in heart failure are lacking.

Sodium-Glucose Transporter 2 (SGLT2) Inhibitors

Sodium-glucose transporter 2 (SGLT2) is a transmembrane protein located in the proximal convoluted tubules of nephrons for reabsorption of filtered glucose. Three large, randomized, placebo-controlled trials (EMPA-REG OUTCOME, CANVAS Program, DECLARE-TIMI 58) have demonstrated impressive reductions of ~30% in HF hospitalization following treatment with the SGLT2 inhibitors empagliflozin, canagliflozin, and dapagliflozin in type 2 diabetes patients (Figure 3.6 and Table 3.1).[29–33] Similar results have been noted in the post-marketing study CVD-REAL of more than 300,000 patients, demonstrating a 39% lower risk of HF hospitalization in those taking SGLT2 inhibitors versus other glucose-lowering agents.[34]

The cardioprotective benefits of SGLT2 inhibitors may not be limited to type 2 diabetes patients alone. In 2019, dapagliflozin was shown in a large, placebo-controlled, randomized trial (DAPA-HF) to reduce composite worsening HF and cardiovascular death by 26% over median 18 months follow-up.[35] Notably, pre-specified subgroup analysis by type 2 diabetes status (nearly half of the patients in the dapagliflozin and placebo arms) demonstrated benefits in both those with and without type 2 diabetes. This has subsequently been confirmed by the EMPEROR-Reduced trial demonstrating a 31% reduction in heart failure hospitalization with empagliflozin compared to placebo regardless of diabetes status.[36]

Various mechanisms have been proposed for the cardioprotective effects of SGLT2 inhibitors. Notably, the reduction in HF hospitalization occurred as early as three months after treatment, meaning that cardiovascular benefits are unlikely to be related to atherosclerosis. Furthermore, the cardioprotective effects are unlikely related to HbA1c lowering or weight loss, both of which are modest at best with SGLT2 inhibitors. To date, three main mechanisms have been proposed to underpin the SGLT2 inhibitors' benefits—substrate utilization modification, hemodynamic unloading, and inhibition of sodium/hydrogen exchangers (NHE) (Figure 3.7).[37]

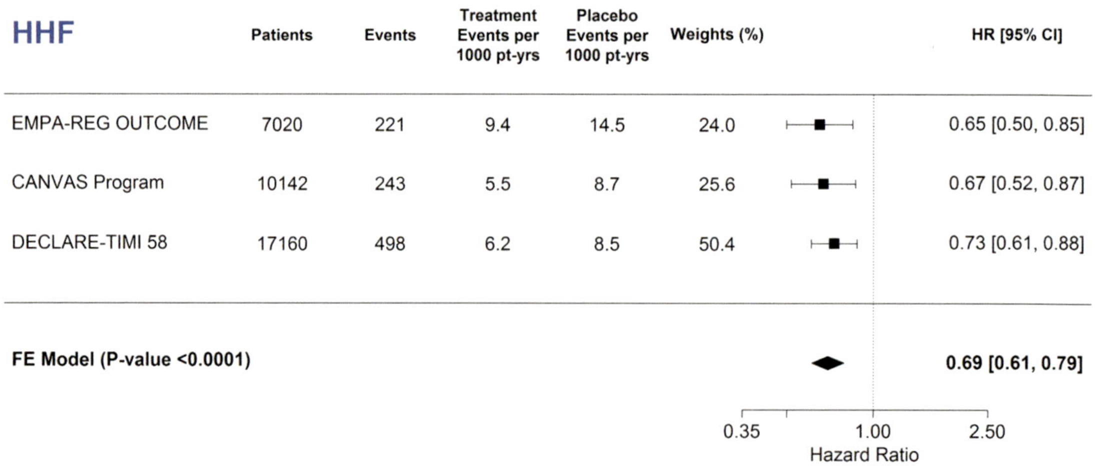

FIGURE 3.6 The rate of heart failure (HF) hospitalization with sodium-glucose transporter 2 (SGLT2) inhibitor treatment. Meta-analysis of all three major trials showing significant homogenous reductions in rate of HF hospitalization. (Reproduced with permission from: Zelniker et al., *Lancet* 2019;393:31–9.)

TABLE 3.1: Completed Human Trials of SGLT2 Inhibitors in Patients with Established HFrEF or at Risk of HFrEF

Trial Name	Population	Intervention	Heart Failure Outcome
EMPA-REG OUTCOME	T2D with established CV disease	Empagliflozin	Reduced heart failure hospitalization (HR 0.65, 95% CI 0.50–0.85)
CANVAS Program	T2D with established ASCVD or high risk of CVD	Canagliflozin	Reduced heart failure hospitalization (HR 0.67, 95% CI 0.52–0.87)
DECLARE-TIMI 58	T2D with established ASCVD or high risk of CVD	Dapagliflozin	Reduced heart failure hospitalization (HR 0.73, 95% CI 0.61–0.88)
CREDENCE	T2D with moderate CKD	Canagliflozin	Reduced heart failure hospitalization (HR 0.61, 95% CI 0.47–0.80)
DAPA-HF	HFrEF	Dapagliflozin	Reduced heart failure hospitalization (HR 0.70, 95% CI 0.59–0.83)
EMPEROR-Reduced	HFrEF	Empagliflozin	Reduced heart failure hospitalization (HR 0.69, 95% CI 0.59–0.81)
VERTIS CV	T2D with established ASCVD	Ertugliflozin	Reduced heart failure hospitalization (HR 0.70, 95% CI 0.54–0.90)
SCORED	T2D with CKD and high risk of CVD	Sotagliflozin	Reduced heart failure hospitalization (HR 0.67, 95% CI 0.55–0.82)
DAPA-CKD	Moderate CKD (eGFR 25–75 mL/min/1.73 m^2)	Dapagliflozin	Reduced heart failure hospitalization or CV death (HR 0.71, 95% CI 0.55–0.92)

Abbreviations: ASCVD = atherosclerotic cardiovascular disease; CKD = chronic kidney disease; CVD = cardiovascular disease; CI = confidence interval; HR = hazard ratio; T2D = type 2 diabetes.

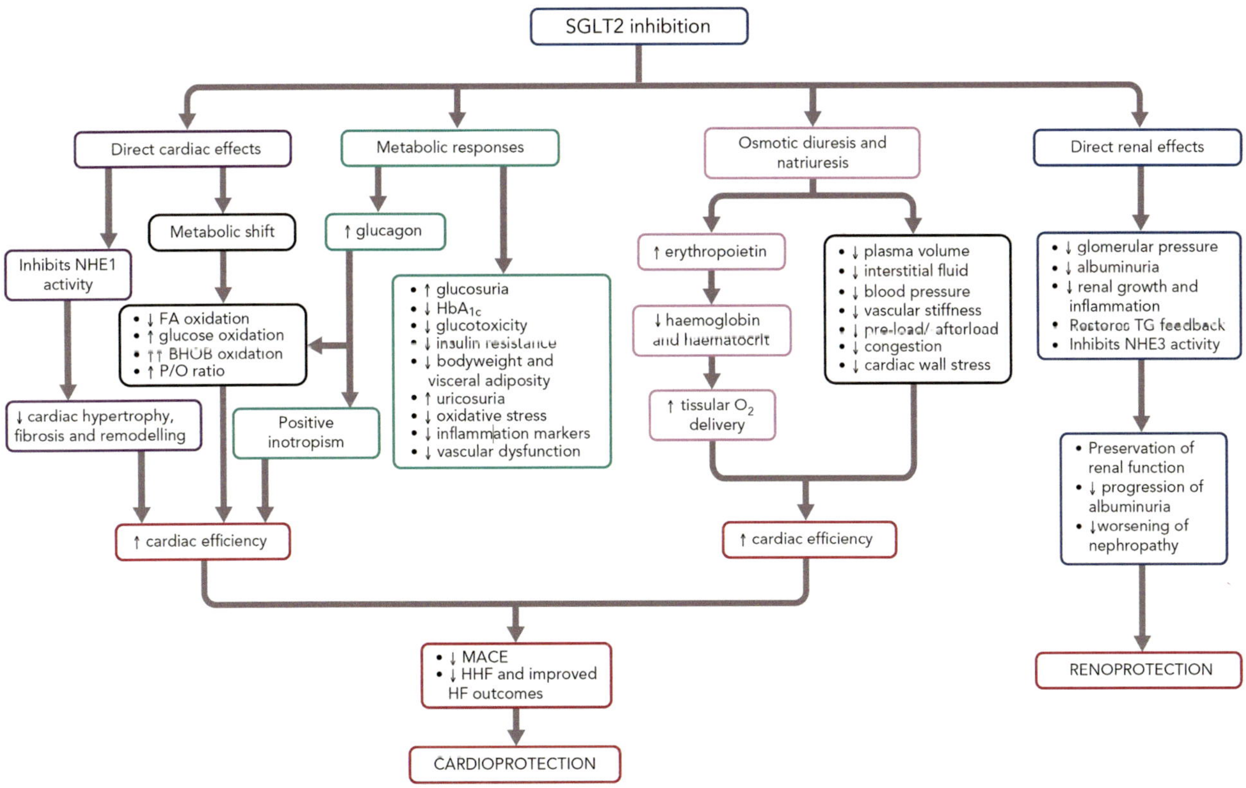

FIGURE 3.7 Multiple mechanisms may underlie the cardioprotective effects of SGLT2 inhibition. *Abbreviations*: BHOB = 3-beta-hydroxybutyrate; FA = fatty acid; HHF = hospitalizations for HF; MACE = major adverse cardiovascular events; NHE = Na$^+$-H$^+$ exchanger; P/O = ATP yield per oxygen atom consumed in oxidative phosphorylation; SGLT2 = sodium-glucose cotransporter 2; TG = tubuloglomerular. (Reproduced under the CC-BY-NC 4.0 License from: Tamargo, *Eur Cardiol* 2019;14:23–32.)

Substrate Utilization Modification

A shift from glucose and fatty acid oxidation to an even more efficient fuel, ketones, may contribute to improved cardiac bioenergetics. The increased lipolysis seen in an insulin-resistant state is enhanced by SGLT2 inhibition due to glucose depletion, insulin suppression, and increased glucagon release. There is also reduced renal ketone excretion, which altogether leads to a mild but persistent state of hyperketonemia. Ketones are preferentially taken up by cardiomyocytes over fatty acids and glucose, as shown by myocardial accumulation of ketone bodies in pigs treated with empagliflozin. The substrate efficiency is enhanced by the hemoconcentrating effects of SGLT2 inhibitors, facilitating better oxygen delivery to the endangered myocardium. Notably, similar metabolic changes have been seen in non-diabetic patients, raising the question of SGLT2 inhibitor efficacy as an HF treatment. This is being explored in ongoing trials.

Hemodynamics

Both cardiac preload and afterload are reduced. Preload lowering is achieved through natriuresis and osmotic diuresis, with magnetic resonance imaging studies showing significant reduction in skin sodium concentration after a brief treatment with dapagliflozin. Afterload lowering is due to reductions in systolic and diastolic blood pressures, which is mediated through total fluid loss, in addition to reduced arterial stiffness and improvement in endothelial health. Although classical diuresis also offers offloading of the heart, SGLT2 inhibitors may offer the additional benefit of maintaining intravascular volume, thereby minimizing risks of renal injury.

NHE

Both sodium-hydrogen exchanger isoform 1 (NHE-1, the cardiac and vasculature isoform) and NHE-3 (the renal isoform) are activated by neurohormones, as well as certain adipokines associated with diabetes. NHE-3 plays an important role in sodium reabsorption, and, as such, excessive activation has been linked to peripheral edema. NHE-1 activation results in a rise in intracellular sodium, with a secondary rise in intracellular calcium. This has been implicated in exacerbating cellular death and cardiac fibrosis. The deleterious effects of prolonged AT II and aldosterone stimulation in HF appear to be at least in part mediated by their action on cardiac NHE-1. Experimental models of HF have demonstrated improvements in response to NHE-1 inhibition in cardiac hypertrophy, fibrosis, and systolic and diastolic function. The direct and indirect actions of SGLT2 inhibitors on myocardium have proven difficult to elucidate due to the absence of SGLT2 receptors in cardiomyocytes. Nonetheless, empagliflozin has been shown in animal studies to inhibit NHE-1 on the myocyte cell membrane, with secondary reductions in intracellular sodium and accumulation of intra-mitochondrial calcium, the latter activating antioxidant pathways to prevent cell death and HF.

It is unclear if the above processes can promote reverse remodeling with SGLT2 inhibition. Myocardial fibrosis and ventricular hypertrophy have been shown to be reduced in small animal models, mediated in part by inhibition of myofibroblast differentiation. Several small series have demonstrated reductions in ventricular mass after three to six months of empagliflozin and dapagliflozin treatment. Larger mechanistic trials are underway to shed further light on structural alterations in humans as a result of SGLT2 inhibition.

Conclusion

The pathophysiology of HFrEF is a complex interplay of neurohormonal, structural, and energetic derangements. As our understanding of each contributing part evolves, so will therapeutics. Model systems have replicated human HF pathophysiology well. Recently, clinical trials pointing towards energetic and substrate-based improvements in HF outcomes have provided the motivation to re-examine the molecular pathophysiology of HF. Enabling technologies, such as "omics" and sophisticated imaging techniques, generate hope for significant advances in the understanding of HF[38] and, ultimately, for novel treatment strategies.

References

1. Packer M. The neurohormonal hypothesis: a theory to explain the mechanism of disease progression in heart failure. *J Am Coll Cardiol.* 1992;20:248–54.
2. Floras JS, Ponikowski P. The sympathetic/parasympathetic imbalance in heart failure with reduced ejection fraction. *Eur Heart J.* 2015;36:1974–82b.
3. Hartupee J, Mann DL. Neurohormonal activation in heart failure with reduced ejection fraction. *Nat Rev Cardiol.* 2017;14:30–38.
4. Packer M, Califf RM, Konstam MA, et al. Comparison of omapatrilat and enalapril in patients with chronic heart failure: the Omapatrilat Versus Enalapril Randomized Trial of Utility in Reducing Events (OVERTURE). *Circulation.* 2002;106:920–6.
5. McMurray JJ, Packer M, Desai AS, et al. Angiotensin-neprilysin inhibition versus enalapril in heart failure. *N Engl J Med.* 2014;371:993–1004.
6. Ponikowski P, Voors AA, Anker SD, et al. 2016 ESC guidelines for the diagnosis and treatment of acute and chronic heart failure: the task force for the diagnosis and treatment of acute and chronic heart failure of the European Society of Cardiology (ESC)Developed with the special contribution of the Heart Failure Association (HFA) of the ESC. *Eur Heart J.* 2016;37:2129–200.
7. Yancy CW, Jessup M, Bozkurt B, et al. 2016 ACC/AHA/HFSA focused update on new pharmacological therapy for heart failure: an update of the 2013 ACCF/AHA guideline for the management of heart failure: a report of the American College of Cardiology/American Heart Association Task Force on Clinical Practice Guidelines and the Heart Failure Society of America. *J Am Coll Cardiol.* 2016;68:1476–88.
8. Penela P, Murga C, Ribas C, et al. Mechanisms of regulation of G protein-coupled receptor kinases (GRKs) and cardiovascular disease. *Cardiovasc Res.* 2006;69:46–56.
9. Rockman HA, Chien KR, Choi DJ, et al. Expression of a beta-adrenergic receptor kinase 1 inhibitor prevents the development of myocardial failure in gene-targeted mice. *Proc Natl Acad Sci U S A.* 1998;95:7000–5.
10. Chakir K, Daya SK, Aiba T, et al. Mechanisms of enhanced beta-adrenergic reserve from cardiac resynchronization therapy. *Circulation.* 2009;119:1231–40.
11. Ge Z, Li A, McNamara J, Dos Remedios C, Lal S. Pathogenesis and pathophysiology of heart failure with reduced ejection fraction: translation to human studies. *Heart Fail Rev.* 2019;24:743–58.
12. Shah SJ, Blair JE, Filippatos GS, et al. Effects of istaroxime on diastolic stiffness in acute heart failure syndromes: results from the hemodynamic, echocardiographic, and neurohormonal effects of istaroxime, a novel intravenous inotropic and lusitropic agent: a randomized controlled trial in patients hospitalized with heart failure (HORIZON-HF) trial. *Am Heart J.* 2009;157:1035–41.
13. Zsebo K, Yaroshinsky A, Rudy JJ, et al. Long-term effects of AAV1/SERCA2a gene transfer in patients with severe heart failure: analysis of recurrent cardiovascular events and mortality. *Circ Res.* 2014;114:101–8.
14. Greenberg B, Butler J, Felker GM, et al. Calcium upregulation by percutaneous administration of gene therapy in patients with cardiac disease (CUPID 2): a randomised, multinational, double-blind, placebo-controlled, phase 2b trial. *Lancet.* 2016;387:1178–86.
15. Lowes BD, Minobe W, Abraham WT, et al. Changes in gene expression in the intact human heart. Downregulation of alpha-myosin heavy chain in hypertrophied, failing ventricular myocardium. *J Clin Invest.* 1997;100:2315–24.
16. Olivetti G, Abbi R, Quaini F, et al. Apoptosis in the failing human heart. *N Engl J Med.* 1997;336:1131–41.

17. Januzzi JL, Jr., Filippatos G, Nieminen M, Gheorghiade M. Troponin elevation in patients with heart failure: on behalf of the third universal definition of myocardial infarction global task force: heart failure section. *Eur Heart J.* 2012;33:2265–71.
18. Mann DL, Bristow MR. Mechanisms and models in heart failure: the biomechanical model and beyond. *Circulation.* 2005;111:2837–49.
19. Stone GW, Lindenfeld J, Abraham WT, et al. Transcatheter mitral-valve repair in patients with heart failure. *N Engl J Med.* 2018;379:2307–18.
20. Obadia JF, Messika-Zeitoun D, Leurent G, et al. Percutaneous repair or medical treatment for secondary mitral regurgitation. *N Engl J Med.* 2018;379:2297–306.
21. Stanley WC, Recchia FA, Lopaschuk GD. Myocardial substrate metabolism in the normal and failing heart. *Physiol Rev.* 2005;85:1093–129.
22. Ventura-Clapier R, Garnier A, Veksler V. Energy metabolism in heart failure. *J Physiol.* 2004;555:1–13.
23. Abozguia K, Clarke K, Lee L, Frenneaux M. Modification of myocardial substrate use as a therapy for heart failure. *Nat Clin Pract Cardiovasc Med.* 2006;3:490–8.
24. Schmidt-Schweda S, Holubarsch C. First clinical trial with etomoxir in patients with chronic congestive heart failure. *Clin Sci (Lond).* 2000;99:27–35.
25. Holubarsch CJ, Rohrbach M, Karrasch M, et al. A double-blind randomized multicentre clinical trial to evaluate the efficacy and safety of two doses of etomoxir in comparison with placebo in patients with moderate congestive heart failure: the ERGO (etomoxir for the recovery of glucose oxidation) study. *Clin Sci (Lond).* 2007;113:205–12.
26. Beadle RM, Williams LK, Kuehl M, et al. Improvement in cardiac energetics by perhexiline in heart failure due to dilated cardiomyopathy. *JACC Heart Fail.* 2015;3:202–11.
27. Lee L, Campbell R, Scheuermann-Freestone M, et al. Metabolic modulation with perhexiline in chronic heart failure: a randomized, controlled trial of short-term use of a novel treatment. *Circulation.* 2005;112:3280–8.
28. Fragasso G, Palloshi A, Puccetti P, et al. A randomized clinical trial of trimetazidine, a partial free fatty acid oxidation inhibitor, in patients with heart failure. *J Am Coll Cardiol.* 2006;48:992–8.
29. Zinman B, Wanner C, Lachin JM, et al. Empagliflozin, cardiovascular outcomes, and mortality in type 2 diabetes. *N Engl J Med.* 2015;373:2117–28.
30. Neal B, Perkovic V, Mahaffey KW, et al. Canagliflozin and cardiovascular and renal events in type 2 diabetes. *N Engl J Med.* 2017;377: 644–57.
31. Wiviott SD, Raz I, Bonaca MP, et al. Dapagliflozin and cardiovascular outcomes in type 2 diabetes. *N Engl J Med.* 2019;380:347–57.
32. Perkovic V, Jardine MJ, Neal B, et al. Canagliflozin and renal outcomes in type 2 diabetes and nephropathy. *N Engl J Med.* 2019;380:2295–306.
33. McMurray JJV, DeMets DL, Inzucchi SE, et al. A trial to evaluate the effect of the sodium-glucose co-transporter 2 inhibitor dapagliflozin on morbidity and mortality in patients with heart failure and reduced left ventricular ejection fraction (DAPA-HF). *European Journal of Heart Failure.* 2019;21:665–75.
34. Kosiborod M, Cavender MA, Fu AZ, et al. Response by Kosiborod et al. to letters regarding article, "lower risk of heart failure and death in patients initiated on sodium-glucose cotransporter-2 inhibitors versus other glucose-lowering drugs: the CVD-REAL study (comparative effectiveness of cardiovascular outcomes in new users of sodium-glucose cotransporter-2 inhibitors)." *Circulation.* 2018;137:989–91.
35. McMurray JJV, Solomon SD, Inzucchi SE, et al. Dapagliflozin in patients with heart failure and reduced ejection fraction. *N Engl J Med.* 2019;381:1995–2008.
36. Packer M, Anker SD, Butler J, et al. EMPEROR-Reduced Trial Investigators. Cardiovascular and renal outcomes with empagliflozin in heart failure. *N Engl J Med.* 2020;383:1413–24.
37. Lytvyn Y, Bjornstad P, Udell JA, Lovshin JA, Cherney DZI. Sodium glucose cotransporter-2 inhibition in heart failure: potential mechanisms, clinical applications, and summary of clinical trials. *Circulation.* 2017;136:1643–58.
38. Cao J, Koay YC, Quek LE, et al. Myocardial substrate changes in advanced ischaemic and advanced dilated human heart failure. *Eur J Heart Fail.* 2019;21:1042–5.

Chapter 4
THE PATHOPHYSIOLOGY OF HEART FAILURE WITH PRESERVED EJECTION FRACTION

Vishal N. Rao and Kishan S. Parikh

Introduction

Heart failure (HF) affects over 6.5 million adults in the United States, and its prevalence is projected to increase to over 8 million adults by the end of 2020.[1] The hallmark clinical syndrome of HF includes symptoms of breathlessness and poor cardiac pump reserve.[2] HF with preserved ejection fraction (HFpEF) is a subtype of HF that accounts for approximately 50% of all cases of HF.[1] HFpEF is a heterogeneous syndrome characterized by reduced left ventricular (LV) relaxation, increased LV filling pressures, and impaired LV systolic function despite having an LV ejection fraction (LVEF) of ≥50%.[3] As HFpEF is associated with aging, hypertension, and obesity, it is becoming one of the most common cardiac conditions.[4]

There exist multiple distinct "phenotypes" in HFpEF, marked by diastolic dysfunction, impaired exercise reserve, abnormal ventricular-arterial coupling, inflammation and endothelial dysfunction, chronotropic incompetence, altered myocardial energetics, altered peripheral skeletal muscle metabolism, and renal insufficiency.[2,5] Biological HFpEF phenotypes may be categorized by their comorbidities, including obesity, hypertensive and aortic disease, skeletal muscle disease, infiltrative cardiomyopathy, pulmonary vascular disease, and lung disease.[6] This heterogeneous syndrome presents several challenges: (1) HFpEF prevalence continues to rise alongside varying comorbid conditions, which contribute to its morbidity and mortality; (2) the multiple pathophysiologic mechanisms make it particularly difficult to study in clinical trials; (3) no well-established human and animal experimental models are available to facilitate better understanding of the distinct phenotypes; and 4) despite the complexity of HFpEF, only vascular decongestion has formed the basis of HFpEF therapy, and further evidence-based effective therapies are limited.[2] In this chapter, we discuss the pathophysiologic mechanisms of HFpEF and describe important implications for the existing HFpEF treatments.

Definition and Epidemiology

What Is HFpEF?

Diagnostic criteria for HFpEF have evolved over the past three decades alongside the increased attention being paid to this complex syndrome. In the 1990s, investigators described HFpEF as "diastolic heart failure," described as observed diastolic dysfunction during exercise—having normal LV function (LVEF >45%) with impaired LV relaxation, filling, and diastolic distensibility with exercise.[7] However, with increasing recognition and diagnosis of HF, the LVEF cutoffs for HFpEF varied across studies between LVEF ≥45 or 50%.[8–11] Among these, the Framingham Heart Study incorporated imaging assessment of ventricular function with LVEF ≥50% alongside other clinical factors.[12] As interest in pathologic analysis of myocardial tissue in HFpEF increased over time, investigators added that alterations in cardiomyocyte structure and function likely contributed to the observed LV diastolic dysfunction and concentric hypertrophy.[13,14] However, a wide variety of definitions persisted until the past decade, when professional organizations provided consensus guidelines on diagnosis of HFpEF: the American College of Cardiology and American Heart Association consensus statement in 2013 stated that HFpEF may be diagnosed based on symptoms and signs of clinical HF with preserved LVEF,[15] whereas the European Society of Cardiology further added that there must be additional objective findings of impaired LV relaxation, filling, diastolic stiffness, and diastolic distensibility.[4]

Prevalence

The proportion of HFpEF has varied over time. Since the 1990s, several studies reported a proportion of HFpEF of between 22.3 and 55%.[16] Over time, studies more consistently classified HFpEF by using ejection fraction cutoffs ≥50% by non-invasive, imaging tools.[16] In the past two decades, the proportion of HFpEF has been reported to be approximately 50% or greater in large cohorts, including the Framingham Heart Study[8] and the Cardiovascular Health Study,[9] findings consistent with reports from other large registries.[1,2,17] Prevalence of HFpEF increases with age, and, at any given age group, it appears that women are more likely to have HFpEF than men.[18] This trend contrasts with that of HFrEF, in which men are more likely to have HFrEF than women across age groups (Figure 4.1).[18]

Incidence

HFpEF accounts for approximately 50% of all incident HF cases and incident HF-related hospitalizations across community studies.[19–21] In the Atherosclerosis Risk in Communities (ARIC) community study, hospitalizations for acute, decompensated HF increased from 2005 to 2014, and these were primarily driven by HFpEF.[21] In the Multi-Ethnic Study of Atherosclerosis (MESA) community study, HFpEF accounted for approximately 51% of all incident hospitalized HF over 11 years.[22] In the community study from Olmstead County, MN, USA, incident HFpEF was approximately 53%.[11] These rates are higher than older population studies, including the Prevention of Renal and Vascular End-Stage Disease (PREVEND) study, the Framingham Heart Study, and Cardiovascular Health Study.[23] It is important to note that, in most of these studies, HFpEF was diagnosed at the time of hospitalization and that the incidence of HFpEF may be underestimated among people who are seen with primary presentation to the outpatient clinics.

Risk Factors

HFpEF is associated with multiple comorbid conditions. Common risk factors for HFpEF include older patients, hypertension, diabetes, kidney disease, and obesity.[5,24–26] Among these risk factors, age beyond 50 years appears to increase the risk of HFpEF for both men and women.[18] However, the risk of HFpEF increases slightly higher in women than men beyond 70 years of age, a trend not apparent in HFrEF.[18] Among the

 DOI: 10.1201/9780429244544-5

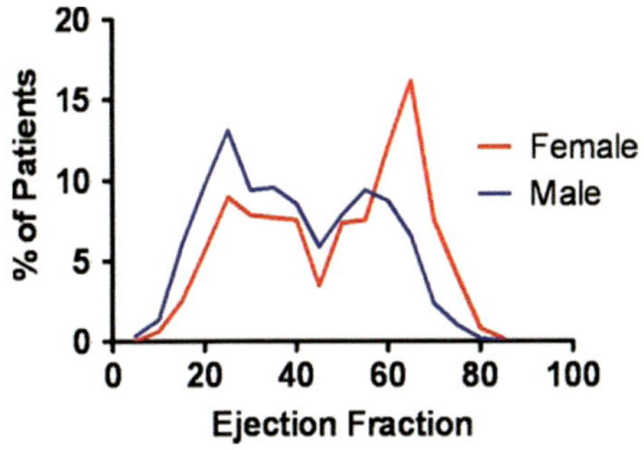

FIGURE 4.1 Distribution of ejection fraction (EF) at baseline in the 1,233 patients diagnosed with incident heart failure in the Olmsted County cohort. (Reproduced with permission from: Dunlay et al., *Circ Heart Fail* 2012;5(6):720–6.)

cardiovascular risk factors, both hypertension and diabetes strongly predict incident HFpEF, yet their effect on the risk of HFpEF and HFrEF appear similar.[23] As for non-cardiovascular risk factors, chronic kidney disease, especially end-stage renal disease, increases the development of HFpEF.[5,24] Obesity, as determined by measure of body mass index (BMI), appears to predict HFpEF, but not HFrEF.[20] The distribution of fat, particularly in central obesity, where there is higher quantity of visceral adiposity, also predicts incident hospitalized HFpEF.[19,27] Targeting these cardiovascular and non-cardiovascular risk factors has drawn attention to future potential therapies to prevent HFpEF, such as weight reduction surgery.[28]

Proposed Pathophysiologic Mechanisms

Diastolic Dysfunction and Delayed Myocardial Relaxation

Prolonged myocardial relaxation, along with passive stiffness, is believed to serve as one physiological component of HFpEF (Figure 4.2).[13] Delayed or impaired diastolic relaxation results in elevations in ventricular end-diastolic pressures with incremental changes in cardiac filling.[13,29–32] The ventricular relaxation delay becomes physiologically apparent under certain vascular loading states[30] or at faster heart rates with reduced total diastolic filling time.[33] Various mechanisms that prolong myocardial relaxation have been proposed.[34] In normal ventricles, calcium removal from the cardiomyocyte cytosol is integral to active relaxation via phospholamban (PLB)-modulated uptake of calcium into the sarcoplasmic reticulum by a calcium-ATPase, calcium extrusion via a sodium-calcium exchanger, mitochondrial calcium uniport, and sarcolemmal calcium-ATPase.[34,35] In HFpEF, cytosolic calcium is incompletely removed and the sarcoplasmic reticulum stores of calcium for the next systolic cycle are reduced due to calcium-ATPase inactivity (SERCA2a), likely due to reduced protein expression and by reduced phosphorylation of its inhibitory modulating protein. Active relaxation is further reduced in HFpEF due to downregulation of beta-adrenergic receptor expression[36] and depressed responsiveness,[37] contributing to signaling irregularities and downstream myocardial changes. Furthermore, the myofilament titin and other elastic elements and their restoring forces facilitate sarcomere movement toward resting length in diastole as well as in the regulation of calcium activation/deactivation during the cardiac cycle, so that reduced levels of titin may contribute to the diastolic dysfunction and reduced myocardial efficiency in HFpEF.[38]

Ventricular Stiffening and Endothelial Dysfunction

In 2013, Paulus and Tschope proposed a novel paradigm which suggests that a systemic pro-inflammatory state, caused by HFpEF-associated comorbidities, including obesity, chronic kidney disease, diabetes, and chronic obstructive pulmonary disease, induces coronary microvascular endothelial inflammation. This microvascular inflammation mediates cardiomyocyte hypertrophy, myocardial stiffening, and replacement fibrosis that contribute to ventricular dysfunction and myocardial remodeling in HFpEF.[39]

Unlike in HFrEF, where exposure to reactive oxygen species (ROS) directly triggers cardiomyocyte autophagy, apoptosis, and necrosis, which is then replaced with fibrosis of the dead cardiomyocytes, HFpEF ventricular remodeling and stiffening is driven by endothelial dysfunction and oxidative stress,[39] as discussed below.

Systemic inflammation affects coronary microvascular endothelial function and induces expression of endothelial adhesion molecules, including E-selectin and vascular cell adhesion molecule-1 (VCAM-1), as confirmed by myocardial biopsy samples of HFpEF patients.[40] These adhesion molecules further attract migrating leukocytes, which, when activated, secrete pro-inflammatory cytokines which trigger production of ROS by the local endothelial cells through activation of reduced nicotinamide adenine dinucleotide phosphate (NADPH) oxidases of the Nox family.[40,41] Higher ROS concentrations limit nitric oxide (NO) bioavailability for adjacent cardiomyocytes, as NO is diverted to peroxynitrite by the superoxide anion. With reduced NO bioavailability, there is reduced vasodilatory response of the coronary microvasculature in HFpEF, which contributes to LV diastolic dysfunction.[42]

When cardiomyocytes adjacent to dysfunctional endothelium are exposed to lower NO and higher peroxynitrite levels, there is downregulation of cyclic guanosine monophosphate (cGMP) production by soluble guanylate cyclase.[43] In HFpEF myocardium, there are lower levels of cGMP and lower protein kinase G (PKG) activity than in normal ventricular myocardium.[44] This change in cGMP and PKG levels is important, since one of the functions of PKG is to stall cardiomyocyte hypertrophy, with reduced PKG activity leading to accelerated cardiomyocyte hypertrophy, which increases resting tension in HFpEF.[44] This mechanism is largely mediated by myocardial titin hypophosphorylation due to low PKG activity in rat models,[45] and the degree of diastolic distensibility improves when suppression of cGMP and PKG functions are reversed in dog models.[46] Inflammation also contributes to changes in the extracellular matrix within the myocardium, as pro-inflammatory cytokines trigger monocyte migration and release transforming growth factor (TGF)-beta to differentiate fibroblasts into myofibroblasts, depositing collagen at sites of microvascular endothelial dysfunction.[40,47] The result is stiffer cardiomyocytes and adjacent interstitial fibrosis, which contribute to higher diastolic LV stiffness and LV mass in HFpEF.[48]

HFpEF-associated comorbidities, including obesity and diabetes, are associated with left ventricular hypertrophy, increased left ventricular stiffness, reduced diastolic relaxation, and coronary microvascular disease.[49–51] These conditions may further potentiate the effects on systemic and local inflammation, production of ROS, endothelial dysfunction, reduced NO bioavailability, reduced cGMP/PKG activity, worsening of arterial smooth muscle relaxation, and augmentation of further myocardial stiffening.[2,40]

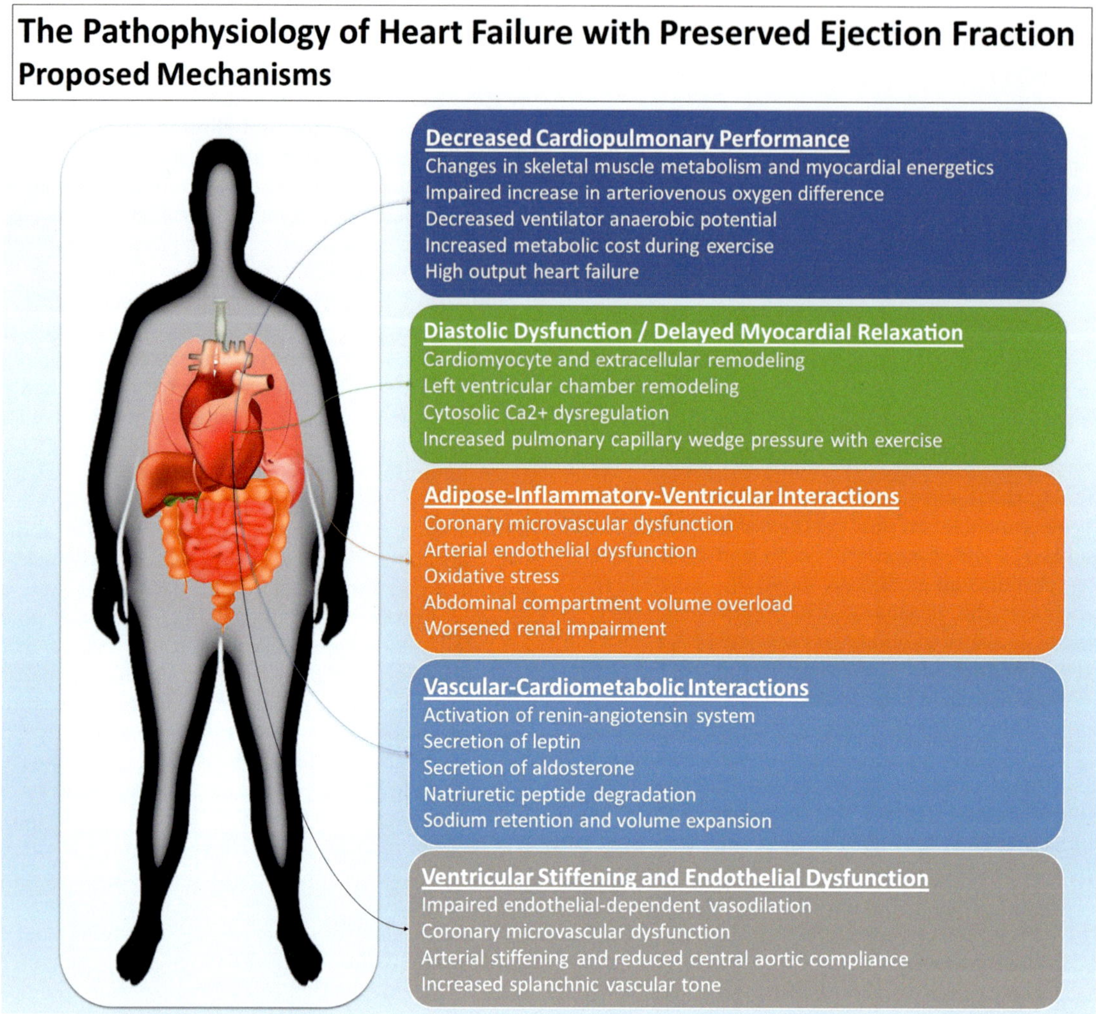

FIGURE 4.2 Current leading proposed mechanisms that contribute to the development of heart failure with preserved ejection fraction.

Ventricular-Arterial Coupling

Stroke volume and systolic ejection time relies on an interaction between the LV and vascular impedance. In normal ventricular and arterial function, arterial resistance decreases during systole to allow for increased stroke volume and augmented blood flow without significant fluctuations in pressure.[52] Patients with HFpEF, however, have abnormal endothelial function compared to those without HFpEF,[53] and rest to exercise peripheral arterial elastance change is blunted in HFpEF.[54] This ventricular-arterial coupling contributes to an inability to augment stroke volume and increases end-diastolic volume in HFpEF (Figure 4.3).[55]

To preserve adequate coupling, a combined ventricular-vascular stiffening occurs in HFpEF that may further contribute to abnormal LV distensibility.[31,52] The result can be blood pressure lability and increased cardiac workload without effective changes in stroke volume at different hemodynamic loading states.[30]

Inflammatory Mechanisms

There are several non-cardiac conditions that are comorbid with HFpEF, which include obesity, hypertension, diabetes, chronic kidney disease, anemia, and chronic obstructive pulmonary disease.[56] Investigators have proposed that comorbid conditions contribute to increased oxidative stress and depressed nitric oxide-signaling which results in upregulation of local and systemic inflammation.[39,57] Obesity, particularly visceral adipose tissue hypertrophy, provides an environment in which macrophages infiltrate adipose tissue, resulting in cell damage and secretion of pro-inflammatory cytokines.[57,58] Chronic kidney disease and salt-sensitive hypertension also contribute to oxidative stress and systemic inflammation upregulation.[59,60]

The upregulation in inflammatory pathways mediate microvascular injury, myocardial fibrosis, and cardiac dysregulation in HFpEF, as described above.[61–63] The pro-inflammatory biomarkers interleukin-6 and tumor necrosis factor-α have been shown to predict HFpEF but not HFrEF in a community population.[64] Additionally, high-sensitivity C-reactive protein is elevated in comorbid obesity-HFpEF but not in normal weight or overweight HFpEF.[65] Inflammation may serve several mechanisms in myocardial dysfunction in HFpEF (Figure 4.4).

As described, systemic inflammation results in endothelial dysfunction from expression of VCAM-1 and E-selectin and the accumulation of ROS.[40] As ROS concentration increases, there is less available nitric oxide to activate cGMP/PKG, having a detrimental effect on arterial smooth muscle, and causing

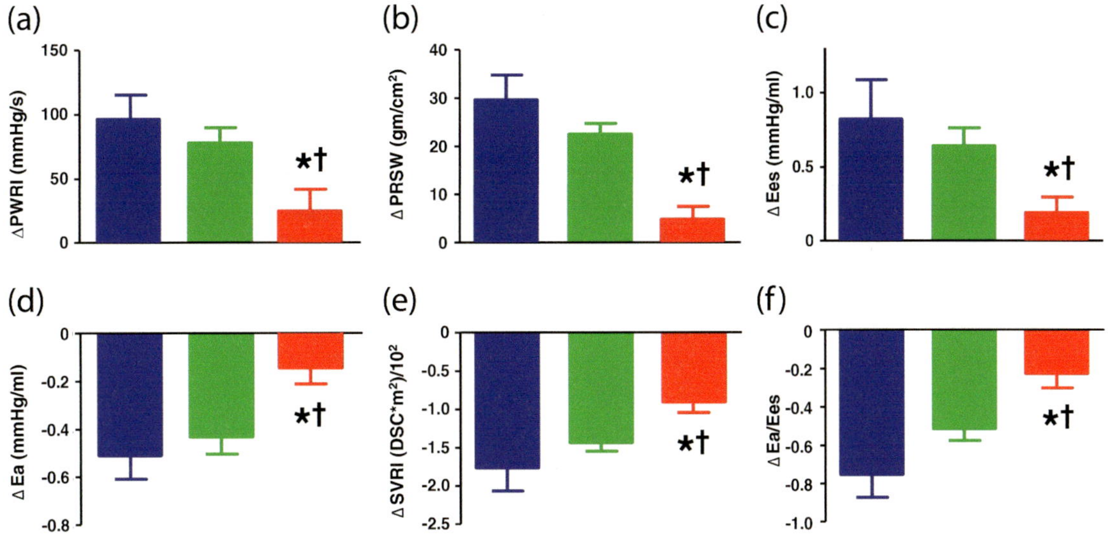

FIGURE 4.3 Contractile, vascular and coupling reserve with low-level exercise (20W). (a–c) Compared with both controls (blue) and hypertensives (green), the contractile reserve was blunted in HFpEF (red) at 20W, as evidenced by blunted increases end-systolic elastance (Ees), preload recruitable stroke work (PRSW), and peak power index (PWRI). (d, e) Vasodilation (reduction in arterial elastance, Ea, and systemic vascular resistance index, SVRI) was also impaired in HFpEF. (f) These deficits led to abnormal ventricular-arterial coupling responses (i.e., less reduction in Ea/Ees ratio) in HFpEF compared with controls and hypertensives. (Reproduced with permission from: Borlaug et al., *J Am Coll Cardiol.* 2010;56(11):845–54.)

myocardial stiffening.[40] Some have also proposed that excess local adiposity may further potentiate this relationship, that, by producing pro-inflammatory cytokines, upregulated metabolic cascades lead to cardiomyocyte hypertrophy, LV remodeling, and subsequent LV diastolic dysfunction.[39] Among patients with visceral adiposity, the secreted cytokines are thought to directly cause microvascular endothelial dysfunction and reduced vascular compliance among obese-HFpEF; however, studies confirming this relationship are lacking.[66–68] Additionally, plasma volume increase occurs more markedly in comorbid obese-HFpEF. The upregulation of systemic inflammation contributes to plasma volume expansion which uniquely and adversely impairs decongestive diuretic therapies in obese-HFpEF.[69] Thus, future studies are needed to investigate whether targeting systemic inflammatory dysregulation may prevent or mitigate progression of HFpEF.

HFpEF-Adiposity Interactions

Adiposity and HFpEF Risk

Among the risk factors for HFpEF, the prevalence of obesity has increased worldwide,[70] and this increase has occurred alongside the rise in HF.[71] Recent HFpEF clinical trials describe obesity and HFpEF conditions presenting comorbidly,[72–75] suggesting the emergence of an obese-HFpEF phenotype.[76] Higher BMI predicts HFpEF, but not HFrEF, and this effect varies by sex.[17,19,20,77] Obesity contributes to HFpEF risk, yet the role which adipose tissue plays in HFpEF pathophysiology is not well understood. Additionally, the harmful effect of obesity on cardiovascular heath may be driven more by the distribution of adipose tissue within the body itself than by obesity-related cardiometabolic risk factors alone,[58] and that regional adiposity may function differently within HFpEF groups with normal, overweight, and high BMI values.

Regional adiposity can be characterized by fat accumulation in different body areas. Visceral adipose tissue (VAT) refers to the intra-abdominal adipose accumulation of fat, whereas subcutaneous adipose tissue (SAT) refers to fat outside the abdominal cavity and intramuscular space.[78] Epicardial adipose tissue (EAT) is fat that surrounds the heart. VAT and EAT exhibit detrimental functions on the heart, including pro-inflammatory and cardiomechanical effects that together worsen diastolic dysfunction (Figure 4.5). VAT and EAT accelerate coronary atherosclerosis, insulin resistance, and hypertension, both in obese and non-obese individuals.[63,79–81] SAT, however, does not appear to be associated with cardiovascular disease.[82,83] Among a multiethnic cohort, VAT accumulation disproportionately increased risk of developing HFpEF and HFpEF-related hospitalizations, whereas SAT had no effect on HFpEF.[19]

Adiposity-Ventricular Interaction

A primary determinant of cardiac dysfunction in HFpEF is decreased left ventricular distensibility.[32,63,84] Change in BMI throughout adulthood contributes to LV diastolic dysfunction.[85] Regional adiposity worsens ventricular compliance of obese-HFpEF. As BMI increases, pulmonary and pulmonary capillary wedge pressures increase compared to those without HFpEF.[32] One hypothesized mechanism focuses on the external mechanical force inflicted by accumulation of fat around the heart. EAT thickness may result in an external pericardial constrictive pathophysiology, as demonstrated in a study comparing non-obese with HFpEF and healthy controls to obese-HFpEF patients, which showed higher right-sided to left-sided filling pressures and septal flattening on echocardiography at rest and with exercise.[32] Epicardial fat may play a key mechanistic role within obese-HF through decreased LV compliance within a fixed pericardial space.

Adiposity and Cardiopulmonary Performance

People with higher BMI have reduced exercise performance compared to those with normal BMI.[86] People with obesity

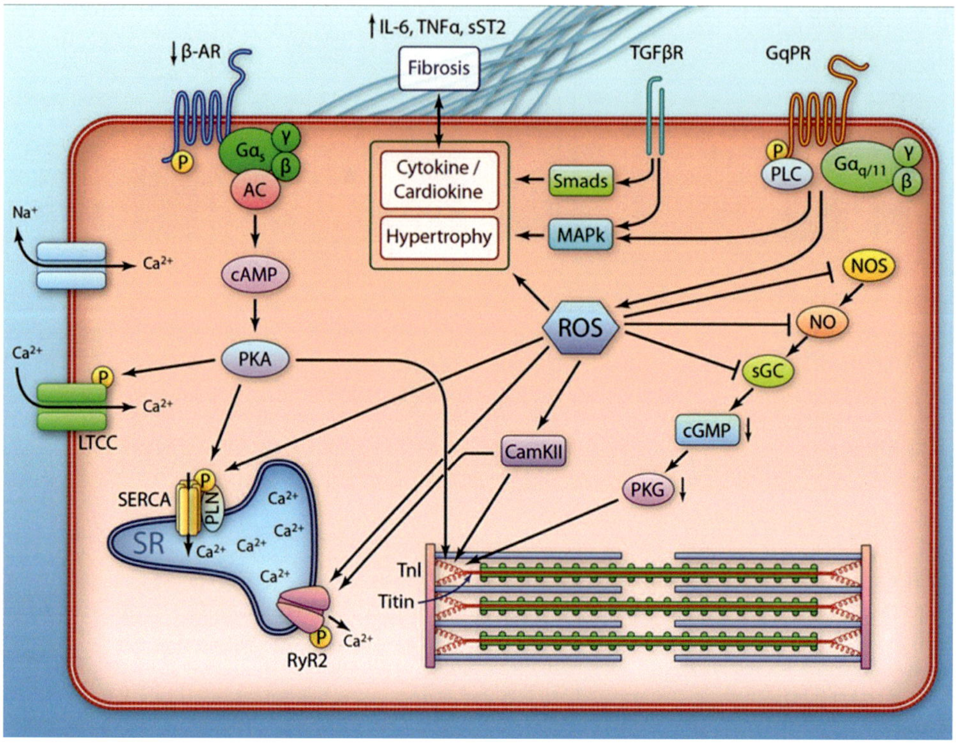

FIGURE 4.4 Schematic of myocardial abnormalities revealed in human HFpEF. The left side shows components of the beta-adrenergic (b-AR) pathway from the receptor to adenyl cyclase (AC), and from generation of cyclic AMP (cAMP) to activation of protein kinase A (PKA). The latter is involved with modification of L-type calcium channels, phospholamban (PLN), titin, and other regulatory thin filament proteins (e.g., troponin I, TnI), which influence myofilament stiffness and contractile activation. Evidence suggests a deficiency in this signaling pathway in HFpEF, with increased titin stiffness and depressed β-AR responsiveness. The middle section shows transforming growth factor b (TGFb) and Gq-protein coupled receptor (GqPR) signaling involving transcription factors (Smad), phospholipase C (PLC) and mitogen-activated kinases (MAPK), which are involved with activation of pro-fibrotic and hypertrophic cascades. At the right is the nitric oxide synthase (NOS) pathway resulting in NO activation of soluble guanylate cyclase (sGC), generation of cyclic GMP (cGMP), and activation of protein kinase G (PKG). In the middle is reactive oxygen species (ROS) activated by TGFb, β-AR, and GqPR-coupled signaling—which inhibits the NOS-cGMP generation and thereby PKG activity, stimulates CamKII which can render sarcoplasmic reticular (SR) calcium release by the ryanodine receptor (RyR2) more promiscuous. ROS and CamKII also impact titin to influence stiffening. Lastly, the upper right side depicts the role of matrix modulation by cytokines/inflammation, and the bI-directional interaction of these factors with the myocyte. (Reproduced with permission from: Sharma and Kass, *Circ Res* 2014;115(1):79–96.) (Illustration credit: Ben Smith.)

and HFpEF may behave differently from a pathophysiologic perspective. Despite having normal LVEF, people with obese-HFpEF have higher left ventricular (LV) mass, demonstrate high-output heart failure, and an inability to augment cardiac output with activity.[87] Additionally, peak exercise oxygen consumption (VO_2) drops as obesity severity worsens,[32,62,67] and these patients have higher right- and left-sided cardiac filling pressures compared with non-obese HFpEF patients and healthy individuals.[32] Relative distribution of adiposity may also impair cardiac function—higher intra-abdominal and visceral fat, but not epicardial fat, worsens peak VO_2, ventilator anaerobic threshold, and 6-minute walk test outcomes in obese-HFpEF individuals.[68]

Neurohormonal Effects

Obesity also affects the neurohormonal axis that impacts cardiac function, LV distensibility, and volume overload.[88,89] Abnormal regulation of adipose tissue stimulates leptin secretion, which is produced by adipocytes, that regulates energy balance and modulates hunger and also regulates the secretion of angiotensin II and aldosterone.[90,91] Excess adiposity can also increase neprilysin activity, which reduces the anti-aldosterone effect by degrading natriuretic peptide hormones.[89] With a direct effect on neurohormonal axis, the renin-angiotensin system activates aldosterone synthesis with subsequent sodium retention, volume expansion, and dysregulated ventricular relaxation in HFpEF.[88]

Skeletal Muscle Metabolism and Myocardial Energetics

A primary chronic symptom in HFpEF is severe exercise intolerance. Changes in cardiac and skeletal muscle metabolism may play a significant role in reduced cardiopulmonary performance in HFpEF. One study described exercise-related changes in LV relaxation and contractile function in HFpEF using ^{31}P-magnetic resonance spectroscopy. Compared with controls, patients with HFpEF when had reduced cardiac phosphate/adenosine triphosphate ratio (indicating reduced cardiac energy reserves) and increased time to peak LV filling, alongside impaired peak maximal oxygen uptake, peak heart

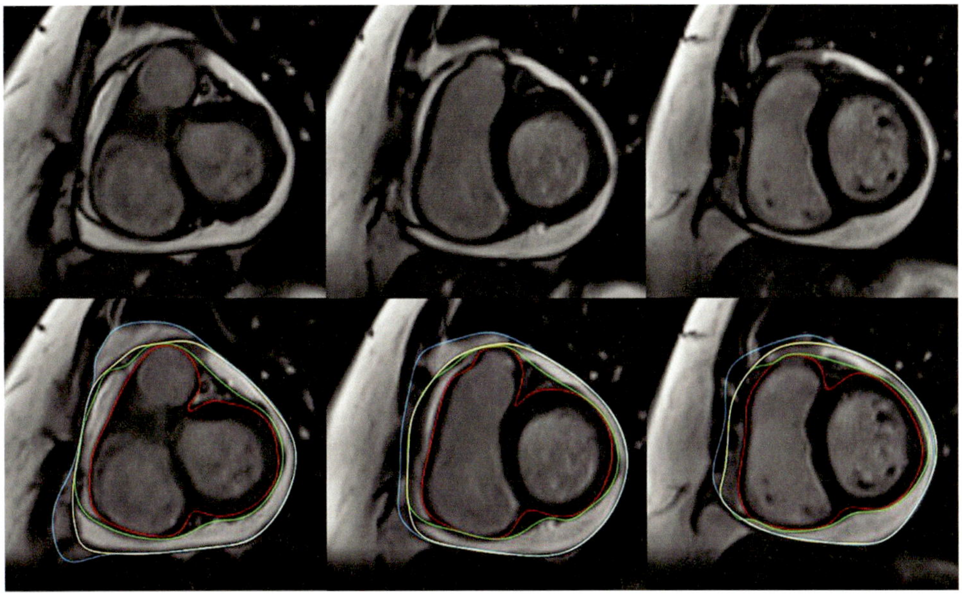

FIGURE 4.5 Upper figure shows a short-axis series, moving from basal to apical slices. The myocardium is shown in red, the visceral layer of the pericardium in green, the parietal layer of the pericardium in yellow, the pericardial fat border in blue. (Reproduced with permission from: van Woerden et al., *Eur J Heart Fail* 2018;20(11):1559–66.)

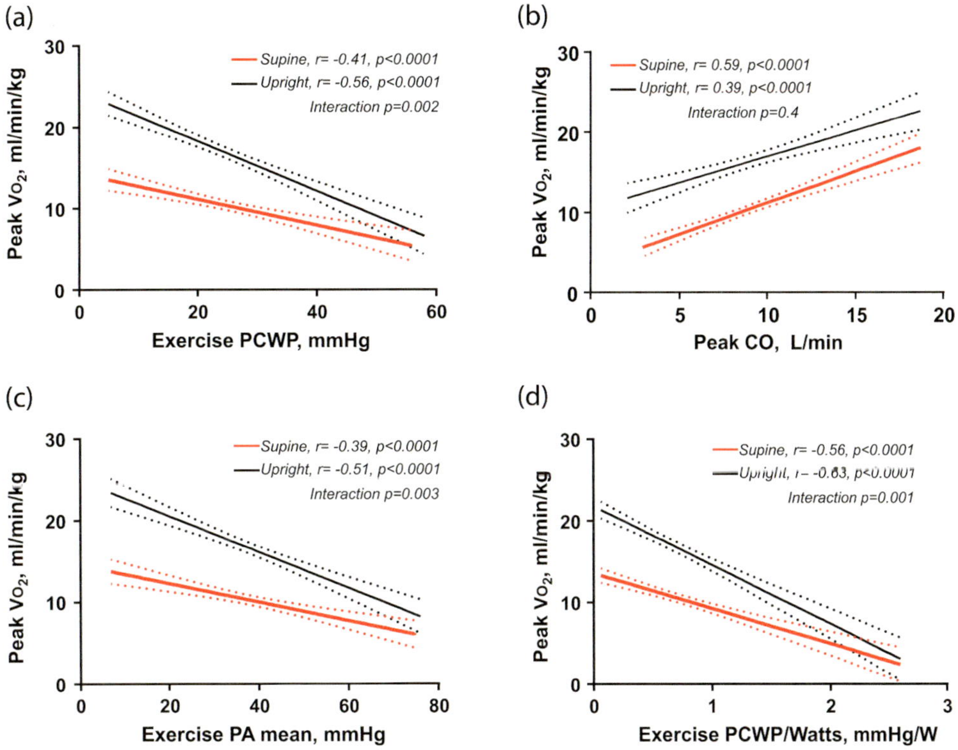

FIGURE 4.6 Correlation between peak VO_2 in both upright (black) and supine (red) positions and exercise pulmonary capillary wedge pressure (PCWP), pulmonary artery (PA) pressure, cardiac output (CO) and PCWP indexed to work performed in watts (W). (Reproduced with permission from: Reddy et al., *JACC Heart Fail* 2018;6(8):665–75.)

rates, stroke volumes, and cardiac output.[54] Skeletal muscle abnormalities additionally contribute to reduced peak exercise oxygen consumption (VO_2) in HFpEF. When compared with controls, HFpEF patients had reduced peak VO_2 and 6-minute walk distance (Figure 4.6).[92]

Furthermore, the percentage of type I fibers and type I-to-type II fiber ratio are markedly reduced, whereas the percentage of type II fibers is elevated in HFpEF, compared with healthy controls.[92] The observed muscle fiber type distribution plays a role in exercise intolerance in the HFpEF syndrome.

Obesity and regional adiposity may further contribute to impaired cardiopulmonary performance. Peak VO_2 drops with higher BMI among obese-HFpEF.[32,67] Additionally, obese HFpEF patients have higher cardiac filling pressures with exercise,[32] worse HF symptoms, and higher metabolic cost of exertion than do non-obese HFpEF.[65] Changes in skeletal muscle composition, particularly higher intramuscular fat-to-skeletal muscle ratios, correlate with reduced peak VO_2 in older HFpEF.[93] Visceral adiposity is also associated with reduced myocardial glucose uptake,[94] impaired efficiency of fatty acid metabolism,[95] impaired myocardial energetics, myocardial steatosis, and concentric LV hypertrophy that mediates LV diastolic dysfunction.[96] These mechanisms may augment the effect observed in that higher visceral fat predicts worse peak VO_2, ventilator anaerobic threshold, and 6-minute walk test outcomes among obese-HFpEF compared with healthy controls, and intra-abdominal adiposity predicts poorer cardiopulmonary performance than epicardial fat.[68]

Restrictive Cardiomyopathies

Among the primary diseases of the heart, restrictive cardiomyopathies are less common than HFpEF syndromes and are characterized as discrete infiltrative and non-infiltrative disorders. Primary restrictive cardiomyopathies include endomyocardial fibrosis and idiopathic restrictive cardiomyopathy, whereas secondary restrictive cardiomyopathy disorders include infiltrative cardiomyopathies (i.e., amyloidosis, sarcoidosis, hemochromatosis), storage disorders (i.e., Fabry disease), and endomyocardial disorders secondary to cancer, cardiotoxic drugs, and radiation exposure. These etiologies of restrictive cardiomyopathy, including their pathophysiology, diagnostic approaches, and treatments, are described elsewhere.[97,98]

Conclusion

The prevalence of HFpEF has grown significantly across the world, partly due to increasing prevalence of comorbid conditions, such as obesity, hypertension, chronic kidney disease, and diabetes. Varying comorbidities contribute to the lack of universal mechanisms within this syndrome, and these distinct HFpEF phenotypes have led to a poor understanding of the onset and disease progression.

Thus, no universal therapies have been effective in preventing or mitigating the morbidity and mortality related to HFpEF. Moving forward, future studies may further our understanding of HFpEF phenotypes and their associated local and systemic interactions with comorbidities, as well as identifying therapeutic targets for the HFpEF syndrome.

Disclosures

Both authors report no relevant conflicts of interest related to the content of this chapter.

References

1. Benjamin EJ, Blaha MJ, Chiuve SE, et al. Heart disease and stroke statistics-2017 update: a report from the American Heart Association. *Circulation.* 2017;135:e146–603.
2. Sharma K, Kass DA. Heart failure with preserved ejection fraction: mechanisms, clinical features, and therapies. *Circ Res.* 2014;115:79–96.
3. Borlaug BA. The pathophysiology of heart failure with preserved ejection fraction. *Nat Rev Cardiol.* 2014;11:507–15.
4. McMurray JJ, Adamopoulos S, Anker SD, et al. ESC guidelines for the diagnosis and treatment of acute and chronic heart failure 2012: the task force for the diagnosis and treatment of acute and chronic heart failure 2012 of the European Society of Cardiology. Developed in collaboration with the Heart Failure Association (HFA) of the ESC. *Eur Heart J.* 2012;33:1787–847.
5. Gladden JD, Linke WA, Redfield MM. Heart failure with preserved ejection fraction. *Pflugers Arch.* 2014;466:1037–53.
6. Lewis GA, Schelbert EB, Williams SG, et al. Biological phenotypes of heart failure with preserved ejection fraction. *J Am Coll Cardiol.* 2017;70:2186–200.
7. How to diagnose diastolic heart failure. European Study Group on Diastolic Heart Failure. *Eur Heart J.* 1998;19:990–1003.
8. Vasan RS, Larson MG, Benjamin EJ, et al. Congestive heart failure in subjects with normal versus reduced left ventricular ejection fraction: prevalence and mortality in a population-based cohort. *J Am Coll Cardiol.* 1999;33:1948–55.
9. Kitzman DW, Gardin JM, Gottdiener JS, et al. Importance of heart failure with preserved systolic function in patients > or = 65 years of age. CHS Research Group. Cardiovascular Health Study. *Am J Cardiol.* 2001;87:413–9.
10. Lam CS, Lyass A, Kraigher-Krainer E, et al. Cardiac dysfunction and noncardiac dysfunction as precursors of heart failure with reduced and preserved ejection fraction in the community. *Circulation.* 2011;124:24–30.
11. Gerber Y, Weston SA, Redfield MM, et al. A contemporary appraisal of the heart failure epidemic in Olmsted County, Minnesota, 2000 to 2010. *JAMA Intern Med.* 2015;175:996–1004.
12. Pfeffer MA, Shah AM, Borlaug BA. Heart failure with preserved ejection fraction in perspective. *Circ Res.* 2019;124:1598–617.
13. Zile MR, Baicu CF, Gaasch WH. Diastolic heart failure--abnormalities in active relaxation and passive stiffness of the left ventricle. *N Engl J Med.* 2004;350:1953–9.
14. Zile MR, Gottdiener JS, Hetzel SJ, et al. Prevalence and significance of alterations in cardiac structure and function in patients with heart failure and a preserved ejection fraction. *Circulation.* 2011;124:2491–501.
15. Yancy CW, Jessup M, Bozkurt B, et al. ACCF/AHA guideline for the management of heart failure: a report of the American College of Cardiology Foundation/American Heart Association Task Force on Practice Guidelines. *J Am Coll Cardiol.* 2013;62:e147–239.
16. Dunlay SM, Roger VL, Redfield MM. Epidemiology of heart failure with preserved ejection fraction. *Nat Rev Cardiol.* 2017;14:591–602.
17. Ho JE, Lyass A, Lee DS, et al. Predictors of new-onset heart failure: differences in preserved versus reduced ejection fraction. *Circ Heart Fail.* 2013;6:279–86.
18. Ceia F, Fonseca C, Mota T, et al. Prevalence of chronic heart failure in Southwestern Europe: the EPICA study. *Eur J Heart Fail.* 2002;4:531–9.
19. Rao VN, Zhao D, Allison MA, et al. Adiposity and incident heart failure and its subtypes: MESA (Multi-Ethnic Study of Atherosclerosis). *JACC Heart Fail.* 2018;6:999–1007.
20. Savji N, Meijers WC, Bartz TM, et al. The association of obesity and cardiometabolic traits with incident HFpEF and HFrEF. *JACC Heart Fail.* 2018;6:701–9.
21. Chang PP, Wruck LM, Shahar E, et al. Trends in hospitalizations and survival of acute decompensated heart failure in four US communities (2005–2014): ARIC study community surveillance. *Circulation.* 2018;138:12–24.
22. Silverman MG, Patel B, Blankstein R, et al. Impact of race, ethnicity, and multimodality biomarkers on the incidence of new-onset heart failure with preserved ejection fraction (from the multi-ethnic study of atherosclerosis). *Am J Cardiol.* 2016;117:1474–81.
23. Ho JE, Enserro D, Brouwers FP, et al. Predicting heart failure with preserved and reduced ejection fraction: the international collaboration on heart failure subtypes. *Circ Heart Fail.* 2016;9:e003116.
24. Steinberg BA, Zhao X, Heidenreich PA, et al. Trends in patients hospitalized with heart failure and preserved left ventricular ejection fraction: prevalence, therapies, and outcomes. *Circulation.* 2012;126:65–75.
25. Morkedal B, Vatten LJ, Romundstad PR, Laugsand LE, Janszky I. Risk of myocardial infarction and heart failure among metabolically healthy but obese individuals: HUNT (Nord-Trondelag Health Study), Norway. *J Am Coll Cardiol.* 2014;63:1071–8.
26. Kenchaiah S, Evans JC, Levy D, et al. Obesity and the risk of heart failure. *N Engl J Med.* 2002;347:305–13.
27. Rao VN, Fudim M, Mentz RJ, Michos ED, Felker GM. Regional adiposity and heart failure with preserved ejection fraction. *Eur J Heart Fail.* 2020;22:1540–50.
28. Jamaly S, Carlsson L, Peltonen M, Jacobson P, Karason K. Surgical obesity treatment and the risk of heart failure. *Eur Heart J.* 2019;40:2131–8.

29. Abudiab MM, Redfield MM, Melenovsky V, et al. Cardiac output response to exercise in relation to metabolic demand in heart failure with preserved ejection fraction. *Eur J Heart Fail.* 2013;15:776–85.
30. Kawaguchi M, Hay I, Fetics B, Kass DA. Combined ventricular systolic and arterial stiffening in patients with heart failure and preserved ejection fraction: implications for systolic and diastolic reserve limitations. *Circulation.* 2003;107:714–20.
31. Lam CS, Roger VL, Rodeheffer RJ, et al. Cardiac structure and ventricular-vascular function in persons with heart failure and preserved ejection fraction from Olmsted County, Minnesota. *Circulation.* 2007;115:1982–90.
32. Obokata M, Reddy YNV, Pislaru SV, Melenovsky V, Borlaug BA. Evidence supporting the existence of a distinct obese phenotype of heart failure with preserved ejection fraction. *Circulation.* 2017;136:6–19.
33. Wachter R, Schmidt-Schweda S, Westermann D, et al. Blunted frequency-dependent upregulation of cardiac output is related to impaired relaxation in diastolic heart failure. *Eur Heart J.* 2009;30:3027–36.
34. ElGuindy A, Yacoub MH. Heart failure with preserved ejection fraction. *Glob Cardiol Sci Pract.* 2012;2012:10.
35. Garcia EH, Perna ER, Farias EF, et al. Reduced systolic performance by tissue Doppler in patients with preserved and abnormal ejection fraction: new insights in chronic heart failure. *Int J Cardiol.* 2006;108:181–8.
36. Hamdani N, Paulus WJ, van Heerebeek L, et al. Distinct myocardial effects of beta-blocker therapy in heart failure with normal and reduced left ventricular ejection fraction. *Eur Heart J.* 2009;30:1863–72.
37. Norman HS, Oujiri J, Larue SJ, et al. Decreased cardiac functional reserve in heart failure with preserved systolic function. *J Card Fail.* 2011;17:301–8.
38. Helmes M, Lim CC, Liao R, et al. Titin determines the Frank-Starling relation in early diastole. *J Gen Physiol.* 2003;121:97–110.
39. Paulus WJ, Tschope C. A novel paradigm for heart failure with preserved ejection fraction: comorbidities drive myocardial dysfunction and remodeling through coronary microvascular endothelial inflammation. *J Am Coll Cardiol.* 2013;62:263–71.
40. Westermann D, Lindner D, Kasner M, et al. Cardiac inflammation contributes to changes in the extracellular matrix in patients with heart failure and normal ejection fraction. *Circ Heart Fail.* 2011;4:44–52.
41. Griendling KK, Sorescu D, Ushio-Fukai M. NAD(P)H oxidase: role in cardiovascular biology and disease. *Circ Res.* 2000;86:494–501.
42. Tschope C, Bock CT, Kasner M, et al. High prevalence of cardiac parvovirus B19 infection in patients with isolated left ventricular diastolic dysfunction. *Circulation.* 2005;111:879–86.
43. Schulz E, Jansen T, Wenzel P, Daiber A, Munzel T. Nitric oxide, tetrahydrobiopterin, oxidative stress, and endothelial dysfunction in hypertension. *Antioxid Redox Signal.* 2008;10:1115–26.
44. van Heerebeek L, Hamdani N, Falcao-Pires I, et al. Low myocardial protein kinase G activity in heart failure with preserved ejection fraction. *Circulation.* 2012;126:830–9.
45. Hamdani N, Franssen C, Lourenco A, et al. Myocardial titin hypophosphorylation importantly contributes to heart failure with preserved ejection fraction in a rat metabolic risk model. *Circ Heart Fail.* 2013;6:1239–49.
46. Bishu K, Hamdani N, Mohammed SF, et al. Sildenafil and B-type natriuretic peptide acutely phosphorylate titin and improve diastolic distensibility in vivo. *Circulation.* 2011;124:2882–91.
47. Kasner M, Westermann D, Lopez B, et al. Diastolic tissue Doppler indexes correlate with the degree of collagen expression and cross-linking in heart failure and normal ejection fraction. *J Am Coll Cardiol.* 2011;57:977–85.
48. Selby DE, Palmer BM, LeWinter MM, Meyer M. Tachycardia-induced diastolic dysfunction and resting tone in myocardium from patients with a normal ejection fraction. *J Am Coll Cardiol.* 2011;58:147–54.
49. Bello NA, Cheng S, Claggett B, et al. Association of Weight and body composition on cardiac structure and function in the ARIC study (atherosclerosis risk in communities). *Circ Heart Fail.* 2016;9:e002978.
50. Wohlfahrt P, Redfield MM, Lopez-Jimenez F, et al. Impact of general and central adiposity on ventricular-arterial aging in women and men. *JACC Heart Fail.* 2014;2:489–99.
51. Tromp J, Lim SL, Tay WT, et al. Microvascular disease in patients with diabetes with heart failure and reduced ejection versus preserved ejection fraction. *Diabetes Care.* 2019;42:1792–9.
52. Borlaug BA, Kass DA. Ventricular-vascular interaction in heart failure. *Heart Fail Clin.* 2008;4:23–36.
53. Borlaug BA, Olson TP, Lam CS, et al. Global cardiovascular reserve dysfunction in heart failure with preserved ejection fraction. *J Am Coll Cardiol.* 2010;56:845–54.
54. Phan TT, Abozguia K, Nallur Shivu G, et al. Heart failure with preserved ejection fraction is characterized by dynamic impairment of active relaxation and contraction of the left ventricle on exercise and associated with myocardial energy deficiency. *J Am Coll Cardiol.* 2009;54:402–9.
55. Reddy YNV, Olson TP, Obokata M, Melenovsky V, Borlaug BA. Hemodynamic correlates and diagnostic role of cardiopulmonary exercise testing in heart failure with preserved ejection fraction. *JACC Heart Fail.* 2018;6:665–75.
56. Ather S, Chan W, Bozkurt B, et al. Impact of noncardiac comorbidities on morbidity and mortality in a predominantly male population with heart failure and preserved versus reduced ejection fraction. *J Am Coll Cardiol.* 2012;59:998–1005.
57. Glezeva N, Baugh JA. Role of inflammation in the pathogenesis of heart failure with preserved ejection fraction and its potential as a therapeutic target. *Heart Fail Rev.* 2014;19:681–94.
58. Bays HE, Gonzalez-Campoy JM, Bray GA, et al. Pathogenic potential of adipose tissue and metabolic consequences of adipocyte hypertrophy and increased visceral adiposity. *Expert Rev Cardiovasc Ther.* 2008;6:343–68.
59. Tian N, Moore RS, Braddy S, et al. Interactions between oxidative stress and inflammation in salt-sensitive hypertension. *Am J Physiol Heart Circ Physiol.* 2007;293:H3388–95.
60. Haass M, Kitzman DW, Anand IS, et al. Body mass index and adverse cardiovascular outcomes in heart failure patients with preserved ejection fraction: results from the Irbesartan in Heart Failure with Preserved Ejection Fraction (I-PRESERVE) trial. *Circ Heart Fail.* 2011;4:324–31.
61. Gomberg-Maitland M, Shah SJ, Guazzi M. Inflammation in heart failure with preserved ejection fraction: time to put out the fire. *JACC Heart Fail.* 2016;4:325–8.
62. Kitzman DW, Nicklas BJ. Pivotal role of excess intra-abdominal adipose in the pathogenesis of metabolic/obese HFpEF. *JACC Heart Fail.* 2018;6:1008–10.
63. Packer M. Epicardial adipose tissue may mediate deleterious effects of obesity and inflammation on the myocardium. *J Am Coll Cardiol.* 2018;71:2360–72.
64. Kalogeropoulos A, Georgiopoulou V, Psaty BM, et al. Inflammatory markers and incident heart failure risk in older adults: the health ABC (health, aging, and body composition) study. *J Am Coll Cardiol.* 2010;55:2129–37.
65. Reddy YNV, Lewis GD, Shah SJ, et al. Characterization of the obese phenotype of heart failure with preserved ejection fraction: a RELAX trial ancillary study. *Mayo Clin Proc.* 2019;94:1199–209.
66. Kitzman DW, Lam CSP. Obese heart failure with preserved ejection fraction phenotype: from pariah to central player. *Circulation.* 2017;136:20–23.
67. Kitzman DW, Brubaker P, Morgan T, et al. Effect of caloric restriction or aerobic exercise training on peak oxygen consumption and quality of life in obese older patients with heart failure with preserved ejection fraction: a randomized clinical trial. *JAMA.* 2016;315:36–46.
68. Haykowsky MJ, Nicklas BJ, Brubaker PH, et al. Regional adipose distribution and its relationship to exercise intolerance in older obese patients who have heart failure with preserved ejection fraction. *JACC Heart Fail.* 2018;6:640–49.
69. Reddy YNV, Obokata M, Testani JM, et al. Adverse renal response to decongestion in the obese phenotype of heart failure with preserved ejection fraction. *J Card Fail.* 2020;26:101–107.
70. Heymsfield SB, Wadden TA. Mechanisms, pathophysiology, and management of obesity. *N Engl J Med.* 2017;376:1492.
71. Bozkurt B, Aguilar D, Deswal A, et al. Contributory risk and management of comorbidities of hypertension, obesity, diabetes mellitus, hyperlipidemia, and metabolic syndrome in chronic heart failure: a scientific statement from the American Heart Association. *Circulation.* 2016;134:e535–78.
72. Borlaug BA, Anstrom KJ, Lewis GD, et al. Effect of inorganic nitrite vs Placebo on exercise capacity among patients with heart failure with preserved ejection fraction: the INDIE-HFpEF randomized clinical trial. *JAMA.* 2018;320:1764–73.
73. Pitt B, Pfeffer MA, Assmann SF, et al. Spironolactone for heart failure with preserved ejection fraction. *N Engl J Med.* 2014;370:1383–92.
74. Redfield MM, Chen HH, Borlaug BA, et al. Effect of phosphodiesterase-5 inhibition on exercise capacity and clinical status in heart failure with preserved ejection fraction: a randomized clinical trial. *JAMA.* 2013;309:1268–77.
75. Redfield MM, Anstrom KJ, Levine JA, et al. Isosorbide mononitrate in heart failure with preserved ejection fraction. *N Engl J Med.* 2015;373:2314–24.
76. Kitzman DW, Shah SJ. The HFpEF obesity phenotype: the elephant in the room. *J Am Coll Cardiol.* 2016;68:200–3.
77. Pandey A, LaMonte M, Klein L, et al. Relationship between physical activity, body mass index, and risk of heart failure. *J Am Coll Cardiol.* 2017;69:1129–42.
78. Tchernof A, Despres JP. Pathophysiology of human visceral obesity: an update. *Physiol Rev.* 2013;93:359–404.
79. Yerramasu A, Dey D, Venuraju S, et al. Increased volume of epicardial fat is an independent risk factor for accelerated progression of sub-clinical coronary atherosclerosis. *Atherosclerosis.* 2012;220:223–30.

80. Okada K, Ohshima S, Isobe S, et al. Epicardial fat volume correlates with severity of coronary artery disease in nonobese patients. *J Cardiovasc Med (Hagerstown).* 2014;15:384–90.
81. Ibrahim MM. Subcutaneous and visceral adipose tissue: structural and functional differences. *Obes Rev.* 2010;11:11–8.
82. Narumi H, Yoshida K, Hashimoto N, et al. Increased subcutaneous fat accumulation has a protective role against subclinical atherosclerosis in asymptomatic subjects undergoing general health screening. *Int J Cardiol.* 2009;135:150–5.
83. Neeland IJ, Ayers CR, Rohatgi AK, et al. Associations of visceral and abdominal subcutaneous adipose tissue with markers of cardiac and metabolic risk in obese adults. *Obesity (Silver Spring).* 2013;21:E439–47.
84. Patel VG, Gupta DK, Terry JG, et al. Left ventricular function across the spectrum of body mass index in African Americans: the Jackson Heart Study. *JACC Heart Fail.* 2017;5:182–90.
85. Khan SS, Shah SJ, Colangelo LA, et al. Association of patterns of change in adiposity with diastolic function and systolic myocardial mechanics from early adulthood to middle age: the coronary artery risk development in young adults study. *J Am Soc Echocardiogr.* 2018;31:1261–9e8.
86. Sharma A, Lavie CJ, Borer JS, et al. Meta-analysis of the relation of body mass index to all-cause and cardiovascular mortality and hospitalization in patients with chronic heart failure. *Am J Cardiol.* 2015;115:1428–34.
87. Mohammed SF, Borlaug BA, Roger VL, et al. Comorbidity and ventricular and vascular structure and function in heart failure with preserved ejection fraction: a community-based study. *Circ Heart Fail.* 2012;5:710–9.
88. Packer M. Derangements in adrenergic-adipokine signalling establish a neurohormonal basis for obesity-related heart failure with a preserved ejection fraction. *Eur J Heart Fail.* 2018;20:873–78.
89. Packer M. Leptin-aldosterone-neprilysin axis: identification of its distinctive role in the pathogenesis of the three phenotypes of heart failure in people with obesity. *Circulation.* 2018;137:1614–31.
90. Xue B, Yu Y, Zhang Z, et al. Leptin mediates high-fat diet sensitization of angiotensin II-elicited hypertension by upregulating the brain renin-angiotensin system and inflammation. *Hypertension.* 2016;67:970–6.
91. Huby AC, Antonova G, Groenendyk J, et al. Adipocyte-derived hormone leptin is a direct regulator of aldosterone secretion, which promotes endothelial dysfunction and cardiac fibrosis. *Circulation.* 2015;132:2134–45.
92. Kitzman DW, Nicklas B, Kraus WE, et al. Skeletal muscle abnormalities and exercise intolerance in older patients with heart failure and preserved ejection fraction. *Am J Physiol Heart Circ Physiol.* 2014;306:H1364–70.
93. Haykowsky MJ, Kouba EJ, Brubaker PH, et al. Skeletal muscle composition and its relation to exercise intolerance in older patients with heart failure and preserved ejection fraction. *Am J Cardiol.* 2014;113:1211–6.
94. Kim G, Jo K, Kim KJ, et al. Visceral adiposity is associated with altered myocardial glucose uptake measured by (18)FDG-PET in 346 subjects with normal glucose tolerance, prediabetes, and type 2 diabetes. *Cardiovasc Diabetol.* 2015;14:148.
95. Peterson LR, Herrero P, Schechtman KB, et al. Effect of obesity and insulin resistance on myocardial substrate metabolism and efficiency in young women. *Circulation.* 2004;109:2191–6.
96. Rayner JJ, Banerjee R, Holloway CJ, et al. The relative contribution of metabolic and structural abnormalities to diastolic dysfunction in obesity. *Int J Obes (Lond).* 2018;42:441–7.
97. Pereira NL, Grogan M, Dec GW. Spectrum of restrictive and infiltrative cardiomyopathies: part 1 of a 2-part series. *J Am Coll Cardiol.* 2018;71:1130–48.
98. Pereira NL, Grogan M, Dec GW. Spectrum of restrictive and infiltrative cardiomyopathies: part 2 of a 2-part series. *J Am Coll Cardiol.* 2018;71:1149–66.

Chapter 5
PRINCIPLES OF HEART FAILURE PHARMACOTHERAPY

Erika L. Hellenbart, Stephanie Dwyer Kaluzna, and Robert J. DiDomenico

Introduction

Heart failure (HF) encompasses both heart failure with reduced ejection fraction (HFrEF) and heart failure with preserved ejection fraction (HFpEF), both of which cause inadequate perfusion to vital organs, dyspnea, and symptoms of volume overload, placing patients at higher risk of complications such as arrhythmias and death. Several of the medications used to treat HF attenuate the adverse neurohormonal activation that occurs and lower mortality risk, ameliorate symptoms, or both. Although most HF therapies are administered orally, patients with acute decompensated heart failure (ADHF) requiring hospitalization are typically treated with parenteral therapies. This chapter reviews the pharmacology of each of the medications used to treat patients with HF.

Neurohormonal Blockers

Neurohormonal Modulation in Heart Failure

Reductions in stroke volume, arterial pressure, and renal perfusion that occur in patients with HF cause baroreceptor dysfunction, leading to stimulation of the sympathetic nervous system (SNS), the renin-angiotensin-aldosterone system (RAAS), and release of vasopressin.[1,2] Mediators of these neurohormonal systems cause adverse hemodynamic changes and promote cardiac remodeling that further impairs cardiac function.[1,3,4] The natriuretic peptides, the atrial natriuretic peptide (ANP) and the B-type natriuretic peptide (BNP), are hormones that are released to counteract the deleterious effects of the SNS, RAAS, and vasopressin.[5] These neurohormonal systems serve as targets for several HF therapies (Figure 5.1).

Unless otherwise contraindicated, all patients with HFrEF should be prescribed an angiotensin-converting enzyme inhibitor (ACEI), an angiotensin receptor blocker (ARB), or an angiotensin receptor-neprilysin inhibitor (ARNI) in combination with a beta-blocker based on proven reductions in HF progression, morbidity, and mortality.[6–10] Adjunctive guideline-directed medical therapies (GDMTs), such as mineralocorticoid receptor antagonists (MRAs) and the combination of hydralazine/isosorbide dinitrate (Hyd/ISDN), should be added for patients with persistent symptoms.[6–10] In the absence of dose-limiting adverse effects, upward titration of the dose should be considered every two weeks until doses achieved in clinical trials (e.g., target doses) are reached (Table 5.1).[6–10]

Anti-RAAS Therapies

Angiotensin-Converting Enzyme Inhibitors (ACEIs)

ACEIs prevent the conversion of angiotensin I to angiotensin II through inhibition of angiotensin-converting enzyme (ACE) (Figure 5.1).[11] Additionally, ACEIs inhibit plasma kininase, the enzyme responsible for inactivation of bradykinin, which is a potent vasodilator that stimulates nitric oxide and improves endothelial function.[4,11] Together, inactivation of these enzymes by ACEIs causes vasodilation, decreasing blood pressure and peripheral vascular resistance.[11] By decreasing circulating levels of angiotensin II, ACEIs also reverse myocardial remodeling and reduce norepinephrine and aldosterone release.[4,12]

Except for captopril and lisinopril, all ACEIs are prodrugs. ACEIs are primarily eliminated by the kidneys, except for fosinopril and moexepril, which are excreted mostly in feces. The half-lives and durations of action of most ACEIs are sufficiently long to allow for once or twice daily dosing, with the exception of captopril (Table 5.1).[12,13] Although enalapril is available in both oral and intravenous (IV, as enalaprilat) formulations, only the oral formulation is recommended for use in patients with HF.[9]

Whereas several adverse effects are common to anti-RAAS therapies (see below), one unique side effect of ACEIs is a dry cough due to increased levels of bradykinin and substance P.[11,12,14] Up to 44% of patients who take an ACEI will develop a dry cough, which can occur within the first few months of therapy and typically resolves within 1–2 weeks of discontinuation.[12,15] Due to the overwhelming benefit of ACEI use in HF treatment, attempts to rule out alternative causes (e.g., increased left ventricular end-diastolic pressure) of the cough should be exhausted prior to discontinuation of therapy.[12,15]

Extensive research and clinical trials have shown that, compared with a placebo in patients with HFrEF, ACEIs slow progression of HF, reduce HF hospitalizations, and increase survival by 20–30%.[16] Available evidence suggests that these benefits exhibit a class effect. However, it is prudent to use agents that have been clinically proven to reduce morbidity and mortality.

Angiotensin II Receptor Blockers (ARBs)

Chronic use of ACEIs can result in "ACE escape," whereby circulating angiotensin II and aldosterone increase despite treatment with an ACEI.[12] Instead of inhibiting the production of angiotensin II, angiotensin II receptor blockers (ARBs) selectively block the angiotensin II type 1 (AT_1) receptor (Figure 5.1). Therefore, ARBs provide a more complete inhibition of angiotensin II-mediated effects than do ACEIs.[11]

Although there are many ARBs available for the treatment of hypertension, only candesartan, valsartan, and losartan have been proven to reduce morbidity and mortality in HFrEF patients and are recommended by treatment guidelines.[6–9] Since ARBs block the AT_1 receptor directly, they do not affect ACE, increase bradykinin levels, nor cause dry cough. Therefore, ARBs are recommended in HFrEF as alternatives in patients intolerant to ACEI due to dry cough.[6–9]

Candesartan is a prodrug that is primarily eliminated renally.[13] Losartan undergoes hepatic metabolism and has an active metabolite, E3174, that is more potent and has a longer half-life than losartan.[13] Valsartan is cleared predominantly in the feces as unchanged drug.[13] Candesartan and losartan are dosed once daily, whereas valsartan is dosed twice daily when used for the treatment of HF.

Angiotensin Receptor-Neprilysin Inhibitor (ARNI)

BNP promotes natriuresis and vasodilation but is cleaved and inactivated by the endopeptidase, neprilysin, which is found in high concentrations in the kidney. Inhibition of neprilysin is

DOI: 10.1201/9780429244544-6

TABLE 5.1: Dosing of Select Guideline-Directed Medical Therapies for Heart Failure

Medication	Starting Dose	Maximum Dose	Mean Daily Dose Achieved in Studies
ACE Inhibitors			
Captopril	6.25 mg TID	50 mg TID	123 mg
Enalapril	2.5 mg BID	10–20 mg BID	17 mg
Fosinopril	5–10 mg daily	40 mg daily	N/A
Lisinopril	2.5–5 mg daily	20–40 mg daily	32–35 mg
Perindopril	2 mg daily	8–16 mg daily	N/A
Quinapril	5 mg BID	20 mg BID	N/A
Ramipril	1.25–2.5 mg daily	10 mg daily	N/A
Trandolapril	1 mg daily	4 mg daily	N/A
Angiotensin Receptor Blockers			
Candesartan	4–8 mg daily	32 mg daily	24 mg
Losartan	25–50 mg daily	50–150 mg daily	129 mg
Valsartan	20–40 mg BID	160 mg BID	254 mg
Angiotensin Receptor-Neprilysin Inhibitor			
Sacubitril/valsartan[a]	24/26 mg BID[b]–49/51 mg BID	97/103 mg BID	375 mg
Mineralocorticoid Receptor Antagonists			
Eplerenone	25 mg daily	50 mg daily	43 mg
Spironolactone	12.5–25 mg daily	25–50 mg daily	26 mg
Beta-Blockers			
Metoprolol succinate	12.5–25 mg daily	200 mg daily	159 mg
Carvedilol	3.125 mg BID	25–50mg BID	37 mg
Carvdilol CR	10 mg daily	80 mg daily	N/A
Bisoprolol	1.25 mg daily	10 mg daily	8.6 mg
Nebivolol	1.25 mg daily	10 mg daily	7.7 mg
Hydralazine/Isosorbide Dinitrate (ISDN) Combination			
Hydralazine	25 mg TID	100 mg TID	N/A
ISDN	20 mg TID	40 mg TID	N/A
BiDil (37.5 mg hydralazine + 20 mg ISDN)	1 tablet TID	2 tablets TID	~175 mg hydralazine + ~90 mg ISDN

[a] Allow a washout period of 36 hours when switching from an ACE inhibitor to sacubitril/valsartan.

[b] The initial dose of sacubitril/valsartan should be 24/26 mg twice daily in the following patients: ACE inhibitor or ARB naive, treated with low doses of an ACE inhibitor (≤enalapril 10 mg/day or equivalent dose of another ACE inhibitor) or ARB (≤valsartan 160 mg/day or equivalent dose of another ACE inhibitor, eGFR <30 mL/min/1.73 m², moderate hepatic impairment, or age ≥75 years.

Abbreviations: ACE = angiotensin converting enzyme, ARB = angiotensin receptor blocker, TID = three times daily, BID = twice daily, N/A = not applicable, eGFR = estimated glomerular filtration rate, CR = controlled release formulation.

now a drug therapy target for HF to prevent the breakdown of natriuretic peptides. Inhibition of neprilysin alone, however, increases levels of angiotensin II which can counteract the benefits of the natriuretic peptides.[17] Therefore, combination with an ARB was designed to mitigate increases in angioedema.

Sacubitril/valsartan is the first approved ARNI. This formulation combines sacubitril, a prodrug which is cleaved into the active neprilysin inhibitor, sacubitrilat (LBQ657), with valsartan, an ARB (Figure 5.1). Sacubitrilat is renally eliminated and has a half-life comparable to valsartan, requiring twice daily dosing.[18]

Two precautions are unique to sacubitril/valsartan compared with other anti-RAAS therapies. Elevations in BNP and N-terminal-pro-BNP (NT-proBNP) concentrations are indicative of volume overload in patients with HF. However, inhibiting neprilysin also prevents the breakdown of BNP, falsely elevating BNP in patients taking an ARNI. NT-proBNP is not a substrate of neprilysin and may be a more appropriate biomarker for patients taking an ARNI. If NT-proBNP is not available at an institution, it is recommended to establish a new "baseline" BNP once a patient is started on an ARNI.[8] Unlike other anti-RAAS therapies, sacubitril/valsartan is contraindicated in patients with severe hepatic impairment (Child-Pugh C) and initial dose reductions are recommended in patients with moderate hepatic impairment (Child-Pugh B) (Table 5.2).[10]

While either an ACEI, ARB, or sacubitril/valsartan are recommended as initial treatment in patients with HFrEF, sacubitril/valsartan is preferred.[6–8,10] Initiation of sacubitril/valsartan in patients with HFrEF hospitalized for acute decompensated heart failure appears to be safe and effective.[19] For patients switching from an ACEI to sacubitril/valsartan, a 36-hour washout period is required to minimize the risk of adverse effects (Table 5.2).[6–8,10]

Common Adverse Effects and Monitoring of ACEIs, ARBs, and ARNI

Due to their effects on the RAAS, ACEI, ARBs, and ARNIs share many of the same adverse effects. Hypotension can occur throughout treatment but is more common early in therapy or following dose adjustments.[9] Risk factors for hypotension include hypovolemia and hyponatremia, often from excessive diuresis.[15] In order to minimize hypotension and worsening

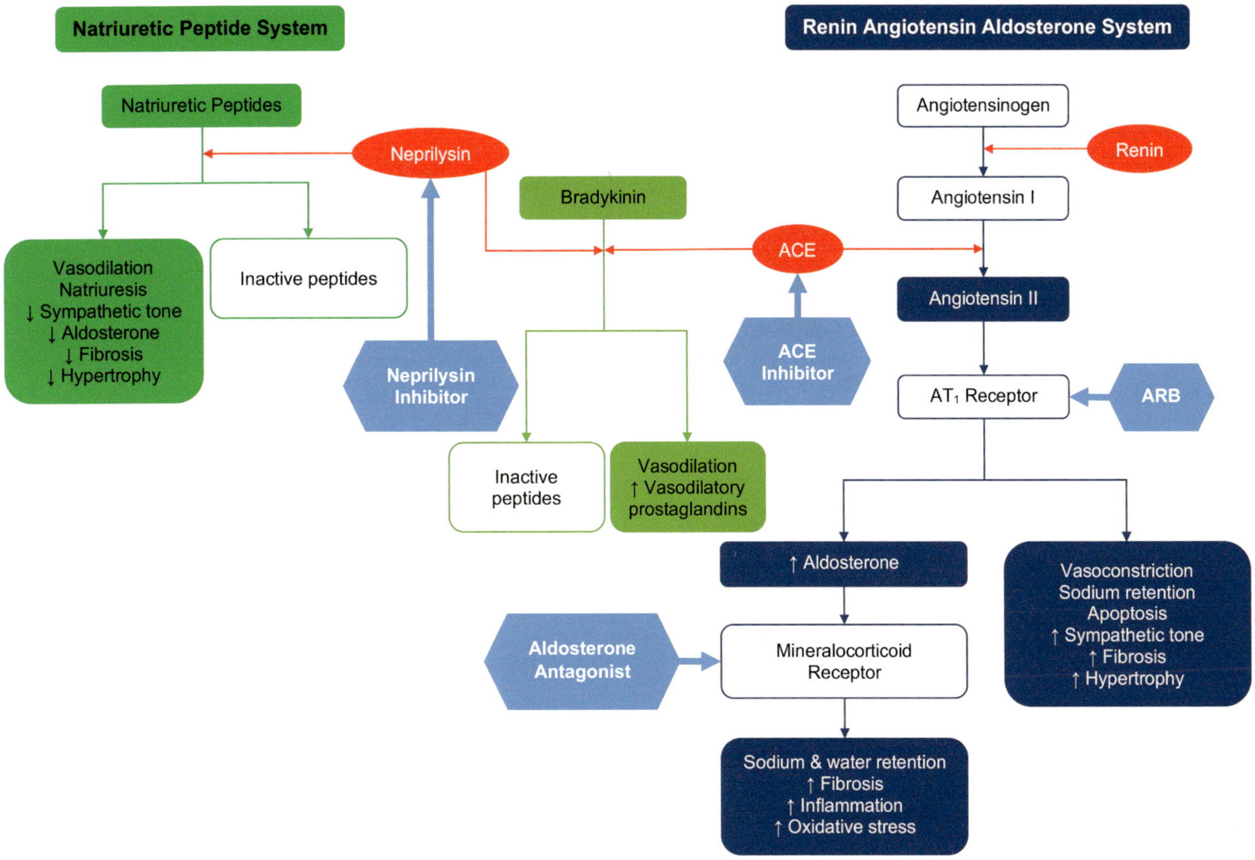

FIGURE 5.1 Renin-angiotensin-aldosterone, natriuretic peptide systems, and drug therapy targets for heart failure. Green rectangles depict neurohormonal systems that are beneficial in treatment of heart failure. Dark blue rectangles depict deleterious neurohormonal systems in heart failure. Red ovals represent enzyme systems catalyzing production and/or degradation of key neurohormones. Light blue shapes depict drug therapy targets for heart failure. *Abbreviations*: ACE = angiotensin converting enzyme, AT_1 = angiotensin II type 1 receptor, ARB = angiotensin receptor blocker.

TABLE 5.2: Pharmacology and Dosing of Beta-Blockers Approved to Treat Heart Failure

	Metoprolol Succinate	Carvedilol	Bisoprolol	Nebivolol
Receptor activity	$\beta_1 >>> \beta_2{}^a$	$\beta_1 = \beta 2 \geq \alpha_1 > \alpha_2$	$\beta_1 >>> \beta_2{}^a$	$\beta_1 >>> \beta_2{}^a$
Pharmacokinetics				
Bioavailability (%)	50–77	25–35	80	12–96
Hepatic metabolism	CYP2D6	CYP2D6	N- and O-dealkylation	CYP2D6
Renal elimination as unchanged drug (%)	<5	<2	50	<1
Half-life (h)	3–7	6–10	9–12	10–30

[a] β_1 Selectivity is observed at lower doses but diminishes at higher doses.
Abbreviation: CYP2D6 = cytochrome P450 isoenzyme 2D6.

renal function (WRF, see below), ACEIs, ARBs, and ARNIs should be initiated at low doses and titrated gradually (e.g., every two weeks) as tolerated (Table 5.2). Hypotension may be minimized by separating administration with other vasoactive agents, such as diuretics and beta-blockers. Asymptomatic hypotension should not be considered a contraindication to initiation or titration.[9]

ACEIs, ARBs, and ARNIs can reduce glomerular capillary hydrostatic pressure secondary to greater vasodilation of efferent than afferent arteriolar flow, leading to WRF which typically manifests as a modest increase in serum creatinine (SCr) and blood urea nitrogen.[2] A SCr increase of up to 20% from the baseline can be anticipated and often returns to baseline without a dose reduction.[2] WRF is more likely in patients with severe HF, hypotension, hyponatremia, volume depletion, bilateral renal artery stenosis (absolute contraindication), and concurrent non-steroidal anti-inflammatory drug (NSAID) use.[12,15] An increase in SCr of 0.5 mg/dL or more for patients with a baseline SCr less than 2.0 mg/dL, (1.0 mg/dL or more if baseline SCr is 2.0 mg/dL or higher) warrants consideration for dose reduction or discontinuation.[2]

The reduction of plasma aldosterone levels by ACEIs, ARBs, and ARNIs reduce urinary potassium excretion, which cause hyperkalemia.[2] Risk of hyperkalemia is higher in patients with chronic kidney disease (CKD), diabetes, concurrent NSAID use, or use of potassium-sparing diuretics or potassium supplements.[2,15] Vital signs, renal function, and serum potassium should be assessed within 1–2 weeks of initiation and following dose titrations.[9] Once stable, monitoring should occur periodically depending on concomitant medications and risk factors for WRF and potassium, typically every 3–12 months.[9]

Angioedema, swelling of the lips, tongue, nose, or throat, can occur in 0.1–0.7% of patients taking an ACEI at any time during a course of therapy.[14] Although rare, angioedema can cause life-threatening asphyxia. Therefore, the offending agent should be discontinued immediately. Risk of ACEI-induced angioedema is five times higher in Black patients.[20] Other risk factors for ACEI-induced angioedema include female gender, age greater than 65 years, drug hypersensitivity, seasonal allergies, and NSAID use.[14] Since ARBs do not affect bradykinin levels, they have a lower risk of angioedema than ACEIs. ARBs can be considered in patients with a history of angioedema on ACEI but angioedema has been reported in 2–17% of patients upon rechallenge with an ARB.[21,22] Therefore, ARBs should be used cautiously in patients with a history of ACEI-induced angioedema and should be avoided in those with a history of life-threatening angioedema from an ACEI.[9,15] ARNI use is contraindicated in patients with a history of angioedema, regardless of severity, to either an ACEI or ARB.[10]

Use of ACEI, ARBs, and ARNIs during second and third trimesters of pregnancy is contraindicated since fetal kidney formation occurs during this time.[9,15] Fetal RAAS is interrupted during ACEI, ARB, and ARNI use, and fetal ischemia can occur from maternal hypotension and/or reduction in fetal-placental blood flow.[15] This can cause WRF in the fetus and abnormalities thought to be due to the reduction of amniotic fluid volume (e.g., limb deformities, cranial ossification deficits, and lung hypoplasia).[15]

Aldosterone Receptor Antagonists (MRAs)

MRAs block the target site of aldosterone on mineralocorticoid receptors. Therefore, MRAs inhibit sodium reabsorption and potassium excretion in the renal tubules as well as inhibiting cardiac fibrosis and remodeling (Figure 5.1).[23]

Both eplerenone and spironolactone are renally eliminated and dosed once daily. Eplerenone is a substrate of cytochrome P450 (CYP) 3A4 isoenzymes and is affected by concurrent use with drugs that inhibit or induce CYP3A4. Eplerenone use with strong CYP3A4 inhibitors should be avoided and use with moderate or weak inhibitors should be done cautiously since these combinations increase hyperkalemia risk.[23]

Since MRAs inhibit potassium excretion in the renal distal tubule and collecting ducts, hyperkalemia is a significant adverse effect that must be monitored closely. MRAs should not be initiated when serum potassium is greater than 5.0 mEq/dL or with other potassium-sparing diuretics. Doses should be reduced or the drug discontinued if serum potassium exceeds 5.5 mEq/dL during therapy. Hyperkalemia risk is increased in patients with renal dysfunction, diabetes, high potassium intake (dietary or supplemental), or concomitant use with ACEI, ARBs, ARNI, or NSAIDs.[23] Renal function should also be monitored closely when using MRAs, and use is not recommended if SCr is above 2.5 mg/dL or estimated glomerular filtration rate (eGFR) is less than 30 mL/min/1.73 m^2. Serum potassium concentrations and renal function should be monitored within 3–7 days after initiation or dose titration. For the first three months, these parameters should be monitored every month, then every three months thereafter, especially if patients are also taking an ACEI, ARB, or an ARNI.[9]

MRAs also block androgen and progesterone receptors, which increase the conversion of testosterone to estradiol. Consequently, gynecomastia (breast enlargement and tenderness) can occur, along with impotence and menstrual irregularities. This occurs more frequently with spironolactone, a non-selective MRA structurally like progesterone. Eplerenone is a selective MRA and has a 100- to 1000-fold lower affinity for androgen and progesterone receptors, significantly reducing rates of these adverse effects.[23]

MRAs are recommended in patients with symptomatic HF and a left ventricular ejection fraction (LVEF) less than 35% (less than 40% following acute myocardial infarction) unless otherwise contraindicated, in order to reduce morbidity and mortality.[6–10] MRAs are also recommended in patients with HFpEF to decrease hospitalizations.[8] Table 5.1 includes MRA dosing recommendations.

Beta-Blockers

In the United States, three beta-blockers—metoprolol succinate, carvedilol, and bisoprolol—are recommended to treat patients with HFrEF, whereas, in Europe, nebivolol may also be considered in older adults with HF.[6,9,10] Beta-blockers competitively antagonize the β_1- adrenergic receptors, decreasing heart rate, blood pressure, and contractility.[24,25] At low doses, metoprolol succinate, bisoprolol, and nebivolol are β_1 selective (Table 5.2). However, at higher doses, receptor selectivity declines and blockade of β_2 receptors also occurs.[25] Carvedilol is a non-selective beta-blocker that predominantly antagonizes β_1 and β_2 receptors but also blocks α_1 receptors, resulting in peripheral vasodilation. Additionally, carvedilol has antioxidant and anti-inflammatory effects.[25,26] Nebivolol also activates nitric oxide synthase, in part, due to stimulation of β_3 receptors on the vascular endothelium, resulting in vasodilation.[24,25,27] Although beta-blockers are negative inotropes, they have been shown to improve LVEF through molecular remodeling.[24,28,29] Improved myocardial energy consumption, upregulation of β_1 receptors, antioxidant and anti-inflammatory effects, and prevention of apoptosis have been postulated as mechanisms.[24,25,29] From a neurohormonal perspective, beta-blockers increase vagal tone while reducing levels of catecholamines, renin, and endothelin.[25,29] Collectively, these effects have translated to reduced rates of sudden cardiac death and improved survival in patients with HFrEF treated with beta-blockers.[24,25,30]

All of the beta-blockers used to treat HFrEF have similar pharmacokinetic profiles (Table 5.2). Beta-blockers undergo first-pass metabolism in the liver to varying degrees, leading to a wide range of oral bioavailability.[25,27] Metoprolol, carvedilol, and nebivolol are each hepatically metabolized by CYP2D6 and are minimally eliminated as unchanged drug in the urine.[24,25,27,31] Therefore, given the genetic variability in CYP2D6 function, plasma concentrations of these beta-blockers in patients who are poor metabolizers of CYP2D6 and/or those treated with CYP2D6 inhibitors may be several-fold higher than extensive metabolizers, potentially increasing the risk of adverse effects.[24,25,27,31] In contrast, bisoprolol undergoes dealkylation in the liver and about 50% is eliminated renally as unchanged drug.[27] Therefore, patients with CKD (eGFR <45 mL/min/1.73 m^2) are at greater risk of bisoprolol-related adverse effects.[32] The dissociation of carvedilol from the β_1 receptors is slow, prolonging the duration of action and resulting in twice daily dosing.[24,31] The half-life of metoprolol is relatively short (3–7 hours) but the approved formulation for HFrEF (metoprolol succinate) delivers metoprolol at a constant rate over 20 hours, allowing for once daily dosing.[31]

When used appropriately, most patients (~85%) with HFrEF tolerate beta-blocker therapy well.[9] Hypotension, dizziness, and bradycardia are the most common adverse events associated with beta-blockers in patients with HFrEF.[33] Additionally, fluid retention, fatigue, and worsening HF are possible.[24,25] These adverse effects are more common in patients with decompensated HF and/or when dose titration occurs too rapidly.[9,24,25] Bronchoconstriction can occur, particularly in patients with asthma or chronic obstructive lung disease, due to β_2 receptor blockade. Therefore, β_1-selective beta-blockers are preferred in these patients and close monitoring of their pulmonary function is warranted, especially during dose titration, since β_1 selectivity diminishes at higher doses.[24,25] Abrupt withdrawal of therapy has been associated with clinical deterioration in up to two-thirds of patients with HFrEF and should be avoided.[9,34]

Hydralazine/Isosorbide Dinitrate (Hyd/ISDN)

Hyd/ISDN is recommended in symptomatic, self-identified Black patients to reduce morbidity and mortality.[6,9,10] Additionally, this combination can be used in patients unable to tolerate ACEIs and ARBs.[6,9] Hyd/ISDN exerts its beneficial effects via complementary mechanisms of action.[35] From a hemodynamic perspective, Hyd/ISDN acts as an arterial and venodilator, reducing afterload and preload, respectively. From a neurohormonal perspective, ISDN serves as a nitric oxide (NO) donor, while hydralazine is thought to act as an antioxidant, reducing inactivation of NO.[35] Specifically, hydralazine may reduce the formation of reactive oxygen species, which are thought to inhibit the development of nitrate tolerance (see IV vasodilator section).[36]

Each component of Hyd/ISDN is available as individual formulations as well as a fixed-dose combination, all requiring thrice daily administration (Table 5.1). Hydralazine is extensively metabolized by the liver during first pass, via acetylation, the rate of which is influenced by genetics, which can impact its bioavailability.[37,38] Slow acetylators may have higher plasma levels of and be more sensitive to hydralazine than fast acetylators, who may be less responsive to the drug. ISDN is eliminated hepatically; serum concentrations may be higher in patients with liver dysfunction.[35]

The most common adverse effects of Hyd/ISDN are headache and dizziness.[35,37] Hypotension, orthostasis, and reflex tachycardia are also possible and require close monitoring of vital signs, particularly when initiating or titrating therapy.[35] Because profound hypotension is possible, ISDN is contraindicated with concomitant use of phosphodiesterase (PDE)-5 inhibitors (avanafil use within 12 hours, vardenafil or sildenafil use within 24 hours, and tadalafil use within 48 hours) and soluble guanylate cyclase (sGC) stimulators (e.g., riociguat).[35,39–44] Although rare, hydralazine has been associated with lupus-like symptoms.[35,37]

Clinical data suggest that self-identified Black patients may derive a greater benefit from the combination of Hyd/ISDN. Black patients may have more derangements in NO homeostasis and NO-mediated cardiovascular effects than non-Black.[45] Therefore, the benefits derived in Black patients with Hyd/ISDN may stem from NO-mediated effects rather than hemodynamic changes.[45]

Vasopressin Antagonists

In select patients hospitalized for ADHF with evidence of volume overload, refractory hyponatremia, or presence of risk factors for hyponatremia-related cognitive symptoms, the short-term use of vasopressin antagonists may be considered.[6,9] Conivaptan is a non-selective IV vasopressin antagonist of both V_{1A} and V_2 receptors with greater affinity for the V_2 receptors (10:1).[46,47] Tolvaptan is a selective V_2 receptor antagonist. Through inhibition of V_2 receptors, both drugs prevent water reabsorption via aquaporin 2 channels in the collecting ducts of the kidney, resulting in aquaresis.[46,47] Blockade of peripheral V_{1A} receptors by conivaptan counteracts vasopressin-induced vasoconstriction, improves hemodynamic indices, and may prevent myocardial hypertrophy.[46–48]

Conivaptan is administered as a 20 mg IV loading dose followed by a continuous infusion of 20–40 mg/day (0.83–1.7 mg/hour).[46,49] In contrast, tolvaptan is administered orally (15 mg once daily) and the dose may be increased every 24 hours to a maximum of 60 mg once daily.[48,50] Both drugs are metabolized by CYP3A4, while conivaptan is also a strong inhibitor of CYP3A4.[46,49,50] Therefore, conivaptan and tolvaptan are contraindicated in combination with strong CYP3A4 inhibitors, and conivaptan should be used cautiously in combination with drugs that are major substrates for CYP3A4.[49,50] Although the half-life of conivaptan is ~5 hours, it exhibits nonlinear pharmacokinetics with a variable half-life due, in part, to inhibition of its own metabolism.[46,48,49] The half-life of tolvaptan is longer (12–24 hours), allowing for once daily dosing.[48,50]

Vasopressin antagonists are generally well tolerated. In patients with HF, dry mouth and thirst are common. Although serum sodium can be expected to rise ~3 mEq/L during initial therapy, hypernatremia has been reported in up to 4% of patients.[47,51] Because correcting hyponatremia too rapidly can cause osmotic demyelination, tolvaptan should only be initiated or reinitiated in the hospital setting where serum sodium and neurologic symptoms can be closely monitored.[50]

Non-Neurohormonal Therapies

Diuretics

Loop Diuretics

Loop diuretics are used to reduce pulmonary congestion, peripheral edema, and other signs and symptoms of fluid retention. Loop diuretics bind to the translocation pocket on the extracellular surface of the sodium-potassium-chloride cotransporter-2 (NKCC2) in the ascending limb of the loop of Henle to block sodium, chloride, and water reabsorption.[52] Intravenous bolus administration of loop diuretics reduces preload within 5 to 15 minutes, presumably by venodilation initially, with peak urinary flow by way of sodium and water excretion occurring within 30 minutes.[53]

Torsemide may prevent disease progression and related outcomes. Animal models suggest torsemide exerts anti-aldosterone effects similar to MRAs, which may contribute to the antifibrotic effects observed in patients with HF.[54] Although limited, torsemide has demonstrated improved NYHA functional class, lower rates of HF hospitalizations, and even lower mortality than furosemide.[55,56]

Furosemide, torsemide, and bumetanide are the most used loop diuretics in HF with subtle differences in their pharmacokinetic profiles (Table 5.3). Furosemide has highly variable oral bioavailability, in the range 10–90% with a mean of 50%.[52,57] The rate of gastrointestinal absorption of furosemide is longer than the excretion half-life, creating absorption-limited pharmacokinetic features. HF patients with abdominal congestion can also see a slowed rate of furosemide absorption, which can decrease its efficacy. Oral bioavailability for bumetanide and torsemide are consistently ~90%, resulting in similar doses

TABLE 5.3: Pharmacokinetics and Dosing of Loop Diuretics

	Furosemide	Torsemide	Bumetanide
Pharmacokinetics			
Oral bioavailability (%)	50	90	90
Onset of action (min)	PO: 30–60 IV: 5	PO: 60 IV: N/A[a]	PO: 30–60 IV: 2–3
Peak effect (h)	2	1–2	1–2
Metabolism	Renal	Hepatic (~80%) via CYP2C9	Partially hepatic
Half-Life			
Healthy (h)	1.5	3–4	1
Renal dysfunction (h)	2.6	4–5	1.6
Heart failure (h)	2.7	6	1.3
Duration of action (h)	6–8	12–16	4–6
Oral Dosing			
Dose equivalence	80 mg	20 mg	1 mg
Initial dose	20–40 mg once or twice daily	10–20 mg daily	0.5–1 mg once or twice daily
Maximum daily dose	600 mg	200 mg	10 mg
Intravenous Dosing			
Dose equivalence	40 mg	N/A[a]	1 mg
Usual bolus dose	40–160 mg IV 1–3 times daily	N/A	0.5–4 mg IV 1–3 times daily
Maximum bolus dose	200 mg/dose	N/A	5 mg/dose
Usual infusion rate	5–20 mg/h	N/A	0.5–2 mg/hr
Maximum infusion rate	40 mg/h	N/A	4 mg/h

[a] IV torsemide no longer available.
Abbreviations: PO = oral, IV = intravenous, CYP2C9 = cytochrome P450 isoenzyme 2C9.

between oral and IV formulations.[52,57] Food decreases the bioavailability of furosemide and bumetanide but does not affect that of torsemide.[52,58] All loop diuretics are highly protein bound (>90%) and are not highly filtered by the glomerulus.[52] They are actively transported into the tubule lumen by organic anion transporters (OAT1 and OAT2).[52,59] Although the half-lives and durations of action of both furosemide and bumetanide are comparable, torsemide has a longer half-life which translates into a longer duration of action that may afford once-daily dosing.[9,54,57,58,60]

Loop diuretics are usually initiated at low doses and adjusted based on symptom assessment, body weight, and net fluid balance (hospitalized patients). However, the response to loop diuretics varies and diuretic tolerance or resistance may develop. Although loop diuretics have steep dose-response curves, they also exhibit a "ceiling" effect whereby increased doses do not produce increased efficacy (Figure 5.2).[52,59] Although the duration of diuresis may last for several hours after administration of loop diuretics, this is often followed by a period when minimal diuresis occurs due to "post-diuretic sodium retention," during which the nephron reabsorbs sodium.[52] A "braking phenomenon" may occur in which an acute decrease in response to loop diuretics occurs during repeated dosing.[52,58,61] A rebound effect can also be observed in which chronic dosing of loop diuretics induces increased sodium reabsorption in the distal tubule.[58,61] Hypertrophy and hyperfunction of the distal nephron may also occur in patients treated chronically with loop diuretics resulting in increased distal reabsorption of sodium.[52,58,61]

Several of these phenomena may be influenced by neurohormonal manipulation in response to loop diuretics. SNS and RAAS activation occur following acute and chronic administration of loop diuretics and may contribute to diuretic resistance.[52] Loop diuretics also increase levels of prostaglandins, causing vasodilation in the proximal tubule which can enhance natriuresis. However, co-administration with NSAIDs and cyclooxygenase-2 (COX-2) inhibitors can inhibit the efficacy of loop diuretics.[52,59] To overcome diuretic resistance, several strategies are often utilized, including more frequent dosing of loop diuretics, administration as a continuous infusion, and combining loop and thiazide diuretics (e.g., "sequential nephron blockade").

Patients hospitalized for ADHF often require IV furosemide or bumetanide (IV torsemide is no longer available[62]) due to their rapid onset of action and ability to bypass impaired gut absorption. However, the most effective dose and administration method is somewhat controversial. Compared with low-dose IV furosemide (1:1 ratio of total IV dose to total oral dose prior to hospitalization), high-dose IV furosemide (2.5:1 ratio of total IV dose to total oral dose prior to hospitalization) has been associated with improved dyspnea, weight loss, and total fluid loss but also an increased incidence of transient WRF.[63] Although continuous infusion of loop diuretics theoretically avoids rebound sodium and fluid retention and the development of diuretic tolerance, no differences were found between the bolus dosing or continuous infusions.[63] Recent meta-analyses have demonstrated that continuous infusion of loop diuretics in patients with ADHF produces significantly better urine output and reduction in body weight, but does not influence HF-related outcomes.[64,65] Therefore, current guidelines state either approach is reasonable to consider.[6,9]

The most common adverse reactions associated with loop diuretics include electrolyte and fluid depletion, azotemia, hypotension, and WRF. Hypokalemia is the most common

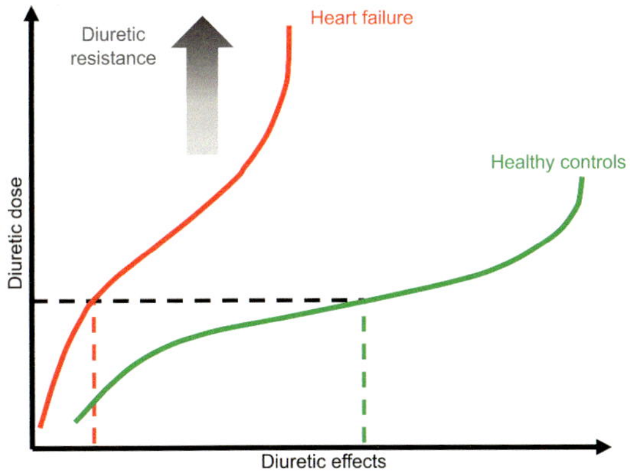

FIGURE 5.2 Relationship between loop diuretic dose and effects. Schematic representation of relationship between administered loop diuretic dose and achieved level of diuresis (water and sodium secretion) in healthy controls (green curve) and heart failure (HF) subjects (red curve). For both cohorts, there is an optimal dose range, depicted by the near-linear ascending middle section of the curves, for which any given dose would conceptually induce predictable amounts of urine production. In HF, markedly higher doses are required for the same absolute amounts of diuresis, and maximum diuretic response is often reduced. In addition, many HF patients show minimal further diuretic response after dose increase in the high-dose portion of the curve, a clinical phenomenon termed diuretic resistance (depicted by shaded gray arrow). (From von Lueder, Atar, Krum; Diuretic use in heart failure and outcomes. *Anesthesiology.* 2013;94(4):490–8. Reprinted with permission from the American Society for Clinical Pharmacology and Therapeutics.)

electrolyte disturbance seen with loop diuretics and has been associated with increased mortality in patients with HF.[66–69] Therefore, serum potassium concentrations should be monitored closely in these patients, with potassium repleted as needed. Because magnesium is required for intracellular potassium transport and hypomagnesemia is also common in patients treated with loop diuretics, serum magnesium levels should also be monitored followed by magnesium supplementation, as necessary. Hypotension, azotemia, and WRF are typically suggestive of intravascular volume depletion due to over-diuresis and typically warrant diuretic dose reduction.[9,59]

A rare but serious side effect of loop diuretics is ototoxicity. Loop diuretics also inhibit NKCC1, another cotransporter located throughout the body, including the ear, which is believed to be the underlying mechanism for ototoxicity.[52] Risk is increased with high-dose IV therapy or at lower doses in patients with CKD or concurrent therapy with other potentially ototoxic medications.

Furosemide, torsemide, and bumetanide all contain a sulfur moiety, are considered sulfonamides, and have the theoretical potential for cross-sensitivity in patients with a sulfonamide allergy. However, there is no convincing evidence of broad cross-reactivity between antimicrobial and non-antimicrobial sulfonamide agents, including loop diuretics.[70] Ethacrynic acid, which does not contain a sulfur moiety, is a potent loop diuretic that is typically reserved for refractory conditions but may be used in patients unable to take other loop diuretics due to a profound sulfonamide allergy.[59]

Thiazide-Like Diuretics

For patients with HF and evidence of volume overload, whose response to optimal doses of loop diuretics (e.g., 160–320 mg/day) is insufficient, sequential nephron blockade, using a combination of loop diuretic and either a thiazide-type diuretic or spironolactone, may be considered.[6,9,71,72] Given that several of the mechanisms contributing to tolerance or resistance to loop diuretics involve sodium and water reabsorption in the distal tubule, adding diuretics that antagonize these renal adaptations can result in synergy and overcome the poor response observed with loop diuretics alone.[48,72]

Several thiazide-like diuretics have been studied as part of sequential nephron blockade and their efficacy is considered a class effect; superiority of a single agent, including IV chlorothiazide, has not been demonstrated.[72–74] Therefore, equipotent doses of any thiazide-like diuretic (Table 5.4) should be effective. Chlorothiazide has the shortest half-life and, along with hydrochlorothiazide, has the shortest duration of action (<24 hours; Table 5.4).[75] In contrast, the half-lives of bendroflumethiazide, indapamide, and metolazone are longer and their effects can persist for 36–48 hours, particularly in patients with CKD.[72,75,76]

The frequency of administration of thiazide-like diuretics as part of sequential nephron blockade often differs by setting. In outpatients, an initial dose of metolazone 2.5 mg two to three times weekly is recommended whereas hospitalized patients may be initiated on 2.5–5 mg once or twice daily.[6,9,71,72,77] Because the peak effect of thiazide-like diuretics is delayed, it is common to administer the thiazide-like diuretic at least 30 minutes before the loop diuretic.[72,75] However, this strategy has not been studied and is largely anecdotal.[72] Because the duration of action of thiazide-like diuretics is longer than that of loop diuretics, the theoretical benefit of this administration strategy is likely negligible after the first dose for patients receiving sequential nephron blockade once or twice daily (e.g., hospitalized patients).

Because sequential nephron blockade can induce a robust diuresis, the most common adverse effects relate to fluid shifts. Electrolyte deficiencies, particularly hypokalemia and

TABLE 5.4: Pharmacokinetics and Dosing of Thiazide-Like Diuretics Used in Sequential Nephron Blockade

Drug	Half-Life (h)	Duration (h)	Equipotent Initial Dose	Maximum Daily Dose
Bendroflumethiazide	9[a]	12–48[a]	2.5 mg	20 mg
Chlorothiazide	1.5–2.5[a]	6–24[a]	250 mg	2,000 mg
Hydrochlorothiazide	6–15[a]	6–24[a]	25 mg	200 mg
Indapamide	16	36	2.5 mg	5 mg
Metolazone	14–20[a]	12–48[a]	2.5 mg	20 mg

[a] Half-life and duration of action may be prolonged in patients with renal insufficiency.

hypomagnesemia, are common despite repletion.[48,72] Although less common, hyponatremia is also possible if sodium excretion exceeds water excretion. Patients may also develop a hypochloremic metabolic alkalosis (e.g., contraction alkalosis). The robust diuresis can also result in hypotension and WRF, the latter leading to prolonged durations of action of the thiazide-like diuretics.[72] Consequently, patients treated with sequential nephron blockade require close monitoring of net urine output, hemodynamics, and frequent (e.g., once or twice daily) monitoring of electrolytes and renal function.[48,72]

Digoxin

Digoxin is a weak positive inotrope and neurohormonal modulator. Inhibition of myocardial sodium-potassium ATPase increases intracellular sodium which promotes an increase in intracellular calcium via the sodium-calcium exchanger leading to increased inotropy.[78–80] Digoxin also increases parasympathetic tone, slowing conduction in the sinoatrial (SA) and atrioventricular (AV) nodes, decreasing heart rate.[78–80] Additionally, digoxin increases baroreceptor sensitivity in patients with HFrEF, leading to decreased neurohormonal activation (e.g., SNS, RAAS).[78–80]

Digoxin exhibits a two-compartment pharmacokinetic model. A 6- to 8-hour distribution phase, during which serum concentrations are often elevated as the drug distributes to the tissues, is followed by a more prolonged elimination phase.[78,80] Therefore, although the onset of action may be less than 2 hours, the peak effect of digoxin is often delayed several hours while it distributes to lean body tissues (e.g., heart, muscle, kidney, liver). Digoxin is largely eliminated renally as unchanged drug (~50–70% of its clearance).[78,80] Digoxin is a substrate for P-glycoprotein, an efflux pump that modulates its absorption, distribution, and excretion. Because several drugs are substrates for and alter the activity of P-glycoprotein, it is a common source for drug interactions with digoxin.[78,79] In adult patients with normal renal function, the half-life of digoxin is ~36 hours but it is prolonged up to 5 days in anuric patients with severe CKD.[78–80]

In HFrEF, digoxin may be considered for patients with symptoms despite treatment with optimal GDMT to decrease hospitalizations for HF.[6,9] The therapeutic range is narrow, requiring precise dosing. Although digoxin has not been shown to lower mortality in HFrEF, an inverse dose-response relationship appears to exist such that patients with serum digoxin concentrations (SDC) <1.0 ng/mL may derive both a reduction in HF hospitalizations and mortality benefit whereas those with SDC above this range derive no benefit and may be at increased risk of mortality.[81–83] Consequently, digoxin dosing should achieve an SDC <1.0 ng/mL, specifically 0.5–0.9 ng/mL.[9,71] Digoxin dosing should be based on a patient's lean body weight (via Devine)[84] and renal function (via Cockcroft Gault).[85] Although several digoxin-dosing methods exist, two have been shown to be effective in achieving the current goal range, one of which is depicted in Figure 5.3.[86–89] Administration of a loading dose is unnecessary in patients with HFrEF. Although several drugs are known to interact with digoxin, notable drug interactions that warrant as much as a 50% reduction in digoxin dose include amiodarone, dronedarone, quinidine, verapamil, and propafenone.[78]

Digoxin is associated with several adverse effects. Digoxin can cause bradycardia and heart block, particularly in elderly patients and in those taking drugs known to interfere with SA or AV nodal conduction (e.g., beta-blockers, calcium channel blockers, or ivabradine) or enhance vagal tone (e.g., cholinesterase inhibitors). The narrow therapeutic range makes patients susceptible to digoxin toxicity, often in the setting of inappropriate dosing or WRF.[78–80] Symptoms of digoxin toxicity may include anorexia, nausea, vomiting, and visual disturbances.[78,79] In more serious cases, digoxin toxicity can cause complete heart block, hyperkalemia, and life-threatening ventricular arrhythmias.[78,79]

Ivabradine

Since bradycardia has been suggested as the major mechanism by which beta-blockers provide benefit, therapies that

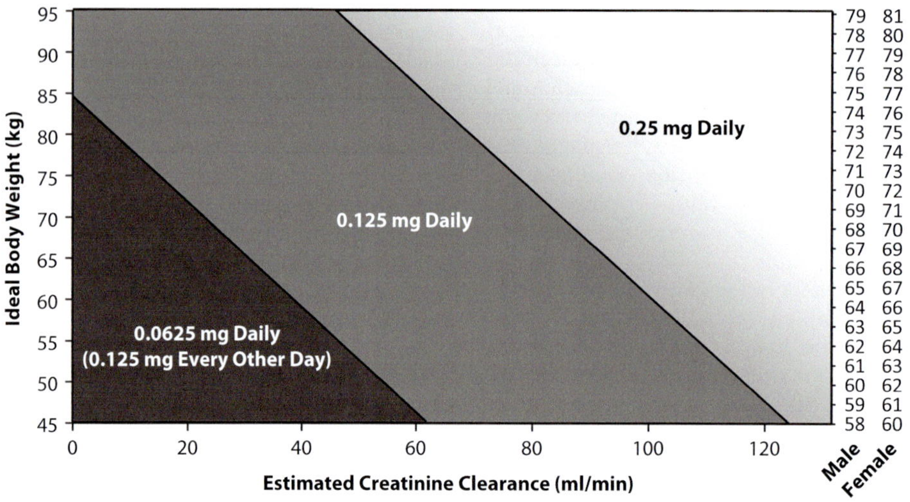

FIGURE 5.3 Dosing nomogram for digoxin in patients with heart failure. To select an appropriate digoxin dose, plot a patient's creatinine clearance[a] (x-axis) (to convert creatinine clearance to mL per second, multiply by 0.01667) against their ideal body weight[b] (y-axis). The shaded area where a patient's creatinine clearance and ideal body weight intersect corresponds to the recommended digoxin dose. If the ideal body weight has not or cannot be calculated, an appropriate digoxin maintenance dose can be determined by plotting a patient's creatinine clearance (x-axis) and their height (z-axis), depending on patient gender. In the 0.25 mg daily area of the nomogram, one may also consider a digoxin maintenance dose of 0.125 mg alternating with 0.25 mg every other day (average daily dose of 0.1875 mg/day) as represented by the gradual shading of this area. [a] Calculated using the Cockcroft and Gault equation utilizing ideal body weight. [b] Calculated using the Devine equation. (Reproduced with permission from Bauman JL, et al., *Arch Intern Med.* 2006;166:2539–45.)

lower heart rate, such as ivabradine, have been developed for the treatment of HFrEF.[90] Ivabradine is a selective and specific inhibitor of hyperpolarization-activated current, I_f, that regulates intrinsic pacemaker activity of the SA node.[91] Inhibition of I_f by ivabradine produces a dose-dependent reduction in heart rate without affecting contractility.[91,92]

The pharmacokinetic profile of ivabradine is linear. The bioavailability of ivabradine is approximately 40% and reaches peak concentrations within 60–90 minutes.[92,93] Food delays absorption but increases bioavailability by 20–40%.[93,94] Metabolism by CYP3A4 accounts for most (80%) of ivabradine's total body clearance.[92-94] Ivabradine has an active N-dealkylated metabolite, S-18982, which exhibits a similar pharmacokinetic profile.[92–94] Whereas the distribution half-life of ivabradine in plasma is two hours, the effective half-life is approximately 6–10 hours, allowing for twice-daily dosing.[93–96]

Ivabradine is recommended for patients with HFrEF and persistent symptoms despite treatment with optimal GDMT to decrease hospitalizations for HF, more specifically in patients who are in sinus rhythm, whose resting heart rate is 70 bpm or higher.[6–8,10] In most patients, ivabradine should be initiated at a dose of 5 mg twice daily with food and titrated to achieve a resting heart rate, in sinus rhythm, between 50–60 bpm.[10,93] In patients who may be susceptible to the heart rate lowering effects (pediatrics, older adults), a starting dose of 2.5 mg twice daily may be considered; the dosage range is 2.5–7.5 mg twice daily.[10,93] Ivabradine is contraindicated in combination with drugs that are strong CYP3A4 inhibitors and should be avoided in combination with other inhibitors and inducers of CYP3A4.[93,94] Although ivabradine has been shown to increase the QT interval by about 20–40 ms, when corrected for heart rate (QTc), no significant differences were observed.[97,98] Nevertheless, ivabradine should be used cautiously in patients with pre-existing QTc interval prolongation and/or patients taking other drugs known to prolong the QTc interval as cases of QTc prolongation and Torsades de Pointes have been reported.[93,99,100]

With the exception of bradycardia, which can occur in up to 10% of patients, ivabradine is well-tolerated.[101] Atrial fibrillation occurs in significantly more patients with HFrEF treated with ivabradine compared to placebo.[101] For this reason, ivabradine is not recommended for patients in atrial fibrillation and should be discontinued if it develops.[93] Ivabradine has also been associated with visual disturbances and phosphenes, a transient enhancement of brightness in a restricted area of the visual field, thought to be due to inhibition of hyperpolarization current, I_h, in the retina.[101,102]

IV Vasoactive Therapies

IV Vasodilators

Consensus guidelines currently recommend the use of three IV vasodilators—nitroglycerin, nitroprusside, and nesiritide—in select patients hospitalized for ADHF to relieve symptoms of congestion.[6,9] In 2018, nesiritide was discontinued by the manufacturer, leaving IV nitroglycerin and nitroprusside as the currently available IV vasodilators to treat ADHF.[103]

Nitroglycerin and nitroprusside are venodilators, decreasing venous return to the heart (preload) and improving dyspnea. These agents also have varying degrees of arterial dilation and afterload reduction, which can further improve cardiac output and symptoms. Nitroglycerin and nitroprusside exert their vasodilatory properties by forming NO.[104,105] Nitroglycerin causes vasodilation of both peripheral veins and arteries, but it has more prominent effects on veins. At higher doses, nitroglycerin also dilates coronary arteries to improve myocardial blood flow, making nitroglycerin a preferred vasodilator in patients with ADHF and ischemic heart disease.[106] Nitroprusside acts as a prodrug that reacts with sulfhydryl groups on various proteins to release NO.[107] Nitroprusside produces equipotent dilation of veins and arteries, resulting in significant decreases in ventricular filling pressures and afterload.

The onset of action for nitroglycerin and nitroprusside is virtually immediate (Table 5.5).[38,104,105] Both drugs are rapidly metabolized, resulting in short half-lives and brief durations of action (less than 10 min). Therefore, both nitroglycerin and nitroprusside are administered as continuous infusions and require titration to the desired hemodynamic response. Each molecule of nitroprusside contains five anions of cyanide which are released when nitroprusside reacts with oxyhemoglobin in vivo.[38,104,105,107] Hepatic detoxification of cyanide, via rhodanese, produces thiocyanate, which is slowly excreted by the kidneys (half-life ~3 days) and may lead to toxicity (Table 5.5).[38,105]

Tachyphylaxis, or tolerance to the hemodynamic effects of IV nitroglycerin, may occur in as many as half of patients.[108] Nitrate tolerance can occur within 3–12 hours of initiation of IV nitroglycerin.[108,109] Although the mechanism of nitrate tolerance is

TABLE 5.5: Dosing and Pharmacokinetics of Intravenous Vasodilators Used to Treat Acute Decompensated Heart Failure

	Nitroglycerin	Nitroprusside
Pharmacokinetics		
Onset	Immediate	Immediate
Metabolism	Hepatic, non-hepatic	Non-hepatic to methemoglobin, nitric oxide, and cyanide; hepatic (cyanide) to thiocyanate
Elimination	Renal (inactive metabolites)	Renal (thiocyanate)
Half-life (min)	1–4	Nitroprusside: 2; thiocyanate: 3 days
Duration of action (min)	3–5	1–10
Dosing		
Initial	10–20 mcg/min	0.3–0.5 mcg/kg/min
Titration	10–20 mcg/min every 5–10 min	0.5 mcg/kg/min every 5 min
Maximum	200–500 mcg/min	10 mcg/kg/min

poorly understood, nitrate-induced supersensitivity to vasoconstrictors, desensitization to sGC, production of reactive oxygen species, NO synthase dysfunction, and increased phosphodiesterase activity have been proposed.[104] A dosing strategy that provides a nitrate-free interval—no or low nitrate exposure—is the generally accepted method to prevent nitrate tolerance but may be impractical when using IV nitroglycerin to treat ADHF.[104] Therefore, monitoring for nitrate tolerance in patients treated with IV nitroglycerin is important and may require more frequent titration, higher doses, or alternative therapies if it occurs.

In addition to hypotension, headache is a common and treatment-limiting adverse effect seen with nitroglycerin. Although rare, cyanide and thiocyanate toxicity are possible with nitroprusside and the risk increases with higher doses (>2 mcg/kg/min), longer infusion durations (>72 hours), and CKD (SCr >3 mg/dL or eGFR <30 mL/min).[105,107] In patients with coronary artery disease, the phenomenon of coronary steal has also been linked to nitroprusside, due to dilation of smaller coronary vessels and a decrease in coronary perfusion pressure in ischemic areas. Coronary steal may explain why nitroprusside has been associated with increased mortality when started early (within nine hours) in patients hospitalized for acute myocardial infarction complicated by left ventricular failure.[107,110]

Because IV nitroglycerin and nitroprusside can cause hypotension, continuous blood pressure monitoring is warranted and both are contraindicated in the setting of cardiogenic shock, low systolic blood pressure (<90 mmHg), and in combination with certain medications.[6,9] Because profound hypotension has been observed when used in combination, both IV nitroglycerin and nitroprusside are contraindicated in patients with recent use of PDE-5 inhibitors (within 12 hours of avanafil use, 24 hours of vardenafil and sildenafil use, or 48 hours of tadalafil use) or chronic use of sGC stimulators (riociguat).[39–42,44]

Because of the risk of hemodynamic compromise, IV nitroglycerin or nitroprusside should be used cautiously in patients with right ventricular (RV) failure, significant mitral or aortic stenosis, HFpEF, and restrictive cardiomyopathies.[104] Nitroprusside has been associated with increases in intracranial pressure (ICP) and should be used cautiously in patients with or at risk of elevated ICP (e.g., intracranial lesions).[107]

Inodilators

Intravenous inotropes are used to treat ADHF in patients with HFrEF and evidence of reduced cardiac output and/or cardiogenic shock.[6,9] Inotropes are categorized as either inodilators or inopressors, depending on their effects on afterload and vascular resistance. Most inotropes are catecholamine derivatives that stimulate adrenergic receptors (Table 5.6). The varying degrees of receptor-mediated and direct vascular effects yield different hemodynamic profiles for both inodilators and inopressors (Table 5.7).

Intravenous inodilators include dobutamine, milrinone, levosimendan, and enoximone. In addition to directly augmenting contractility and heart rate, these agents induce varying degrees of vasodilation, reducing afterload and indirectly increasing stroke volume and cardiac output.[111–115]

Dobutamine

Dobutamine is an adrenergic receptor agonist with affinity for β_1, β_2, and α_1 receptors (Table 5.6).[116] Dobutamine is a racemic mixture, the (+) enantiomer being a strong β_1 and β_2 agonist, responsible for its inotropic properties. Additionally, the (+) enantiomer has weak α_1 antagonism properties. The (-) enantiomer acts as an α_1 receptor agonist, causing vasoconstriction. β_2-induced vasodilation and α_1-induced vasoconstriction offset one another, resulting in net mild vasodilation.[117] Comparatively, dobutamine results in the least amount of vasodilation among inodilators and has little effect on the pulmonary vasculature (Table 5.7).

Because dobutamine has a rapid onset of action (1–2 minutes), bolus dosing is not necessary.[118] Dobutamine is rapidly metabolized in the liver to inactive metabolites.[118] Consequently, it has a short half-life (<2 minutes) and brief duration of action, allowing for frequent titration if necessary.[118]

In some patients, the effects of dobutamine may be diminished. Concurrent use of beta-blockers and dobutamine often

TABLE 5.6: Receptor Activity and Mechanism of Action of Inodilators and Inopressors

	Dosing	α_1	β_1	β_2	Other
Inodilators					
Dobutamine	2–20 mcg/kg/min	+	+++++	+++	N/A
Milrinone	0.25–0.75 mcg/kg/min[a,b]	N/A	N/A	N/A	PDE-3 inhibitor
Levosimendan	0.05–0.2 mcg/kg/min[c]	N/A	N/A	N/A	Calcium sensitizer
Enoximone	5–20 mcg/kg/min[b,d]	N/A	N/A	N/A	PDE-3 inhibitor
Inopressor					
Norepinephrine	0.2–1 mcg/kg/min	+++++	+++	++	N/A
Dopamine	3–20 mcg/kg/min	+++[e]	++++[f]	++[f]	Dopaminergic (D_1, D_2)[g]
Epinephrine	0.05–0.5 mcg/kg/min	+++++[h]	++++[i]	+++[i]	N/A

[a] IV bolus of 25–75 mcg/kg over 10–20 min may be considered if a more rapid response is desired and blood pressure is adequate.
[b] Initial infusion rate should be reduced in patients with renal impairment.
[c] IV bolus of 12 mcg/kg over 10 min may be considered if a more rapid response is desired and blood pressure is adequate.
[d] Accumulation may occur at doses ≥10 mcg/kg/min.
[e] Observed at doses ≥5–10 mcg/kg/min.
[f] Observed at doses ≥3 mcg/kg/min.
[g] Observed at doses <3 mcg/kg/min.
[h] Observed at doses >0.1 mcg/kg/min.
[i] Observed at doses ≤0.1 mcg/kg/min.
Abbreviations: N/A = not applicable; PDE = phosphodiesterase.

TABLE 5.7: **Hemodynamic Effects of Intravenous Inodilators and Inopressors**

	Cardiac Output	Heart Rate	PCWP	SVR	MAP	Cardiac O_2 Consumption
Inodilators						
Dobutamine	↑↑	↑	↔/↓	↔/↓	↓/↔/↑	↑↑
Milrinone	↑↑	↑	↓↓	↓↓	↓/↔	↑
Levosimendan	↑↑	↔/↑	↓↓	↓↓	↓↓	↔
Enoximone	↑↑	↑	↓↓	↓↓	↓	↑
Inopressors						
Norepinephrine	↓/↑	↑	↑	↑↑	↑↑	↑↑
Dopamine	↑	↑↑	↑	↑	↑	↑↑
Epinephrine	↑↑	↑↑	↑	↑	↑↑	↑↑

Abbreviations: PCWP = pulmonary capillary wedge pressure, SVR = systemic vascular resistance, MAP = mean arterial pressure, O_2 = oxygen.

leads to a decreased clinical response to dobutamine due to opposing mechanisms of action. In the setting of concomitant beta-blocker treatment or overdose, PDE-3 inhibitors may be more effective than dobutamine at treating low cardiac output.[119,120] In patients treated with dobutamine for several days, pharmacologic tolerance can occur, perhaps due to downregulation of β_1 receptors.[117,121,122] If tachyphylaxis occurs with dobutamine, higher doses may be required or another inodilator considered if inotropic support remains necessary.

Milrinone and Enoximone

Milrinone and enoximone exert their inotropic effect via inhibition of the PDE-3 enzyme in the cardiac and vascular tissue, which is responsible for the breakdown of intracellular cyclic-AMP (cAMP).[121] Inhibition of cAMP breakdown leads to release of calcium from the sarcoplasmic reticulum into the cytosol, resulting in increased contractility, whereas in the vasculature it produces smooth muscle relaxation and vasodilation. In settings where β_1 receptor downregulation is a concern (e.g., chronic beta-blocker therapy, dobutamine tolerance), the use of either milrinone or enoximone may be more advantageous.[119]

Milrinone has a half-life of 2–4 hours and is almost completely eliminated renally as unchanged drug.[115,122] Enoximone has a half-life of 4–7 hours and is hepatically metabolized to active metabolites, which are eliminated renally and more slowly than enoximone.[123,124] The onset of action for both enoximone and milrinone is often delayed. Consequently, if a more rapid response is desired and blood pressure is adequate, both milrinone and enoximone can be initiated with bolus doses prior to starting continuous infusions.[6] However, the bolus doses of these drugs are often avoided due to the risk of hypotension. Because of their longer half-lives, particularly in the setting of renal dysfunction, the effects of both enoximone and milrinone may be prolonged for hours.

Levosimendan

Levosimendan predominantly augments contractility via binding to cardiac troponin C during systole, increasing sensitivity of the myofilaments to calcium.[124] Levosimendan exerts its inotropic properties, not by increasing intracytosolic calcium like adrenergic agonists and PDE-3 inhibitors, but rather by improving response to the existing calcium. The vasodilatory properties of levosimendan are thought to be secondary to stimulation of the ATP-sensitive potassium channels in small vessels and calcium-activated potassium channels in large vessels.[124] Levosimendan also has PDE-3 inhibitor properties, thought to be synergistic with its calcium sensitizing effects.[121]

Levosimendan has a relatively short half-life (0.6–1 hour).[121] Levosimendan is metabolized in the liver to OR-1896, an active metabolite with both calcium-sensitizing and PDE-3 inhibitory properties.[125] OR-1896 is eliminated renally and has a much longer half-life (80–96 hours) than levosimendan, yielding hemodynamic effects that persist for several days, particularly in the setting of renal dysfunction.[123,124,126]

Inopressors

Inopressors increase vascular resistance in addition to increasing contractility and cardiac output. These agents are indicated specifically in the setting of cardiogenic shock with hypotension, defined as systolic blood pressure <90 mmHg, and persistent hypoperfusion.[6] Each of the inopressors used to treat patients with cardiogenic shock stimulate α_1 receptors, resulting in increased afterload and blood pressure while also increasing cardiac output via β_1-receptor stimulation to varying degrees (Table 5.6).

Norepinephrine

Among the three inopressors, norepinephrine has the greatest α_1 activity but the least activity at the β_1 and β_2 receptors (Table 5.6).[122] Consequently, norepinephrine is among the most potent inopressors in terms of increasing both afterload and mean arterial pressure (MAP) in addition to positive inotropic effects (Table 5.7). Thus, when inopressors are indicated, norepinephrine is recommended initially, occasionally in combination with an inodilator.[6,9]

Dopamine

The receptor activity of dopamine increases with increasing dose (Table 5.6), resulting in dose-related differences in the hemodynamic profile. Unique among the inopressors, lower doses (<3 mcg/kg/min) of dopamine stimulate dopaminergic receptors (D_1 and D_2), which induce vasodilation in the renal, mesenteric, and coronary arteries and inhibit norepinephrine release.[113,122] At medium doses (≥3 mcg/kg/min), increasing heart rate and contractility are observed due to β_1 agonism.[113,122] At higher doses (≥5–10 mcg/kg/min), α_1 stimulation produces vasoconstriction, increasing both vascular resistance and MAP.[113,122]

Historically, "renal dose" dopamine, in which low doses are administered in patients with ADHF and WRF, has been proposed as a strategy to improve diuresis and preserve or improve renal function. However, studies have demonstrated that this approach does not improve outcomes in critically ill patients including those treated for ADHF.[127–129] Additionally, when compared to norepinephrine, dopamine was associated with an increase in tachyarrhythmias in all shock states and increased mortality in patients with cardiogenic shock.[130]

Epinephrine

Like dopamine, the receptor activity of epinephrine increases as the dose is increased, although it tends to have more balanced effects across the β_1, β_2, and α_1 receptors (Table 5.6). At low doses ($\leq$0.1 mcg/kg/min), epinephrine is the most potent β_1 agonist among the inopressors, leading to increases in contractility and heart rate.[113] At higher doses (>0.1 mcg/kg/min), α_1-mediated vasoconstriction increases both vascular resistance and MAP.[113,122]

Epinephrine has a limited role in patients treated for cardiogenic shock. Epinephrine has been associated with an increased rate of refractory shock compared with norepinephrine in patients with cardiogenic shock following myocardial infarction.[131] Consequently, epinephrine is recommended in cardiogenic shock with refractory hypotension despite adequate filling pressures and the use of other IV vasoactive drugs.[6]

Pharmacokinetics and Dosing of Inopressors

Each inopressor has an onset of action of less than 5 minutes.[118] Inopressors have many metabolic fates, rapidly undergoing oxidative deamination via monoamine oxidase to aldehyde intermediates and subsequently to inactive metabolites.[118,132] Inopressors are also metabolized by catechol-*O*-methyltransferase to inactive metabolites.[118] Dopamine is a precursor in the formation of norepinephrine, which accounts for about 25% of dopamine metabolites.[118] Each of the inopressors has short half-lives (<7 minutes) resulting in brief durations of action and allowing for rapid titration to achieve the desired hemodynamic effects.[9,133,134] Although inopressor pharmacokinetics may be altered in critically ill patients, resulting in reduced clearance, their short half-lives make dosage adjustments unnecessary in critically ill patients including those with renal or hepatic dysfunction.[134]

Adverse Effects and Monitoring of Inodilators and Inopressors

All inodilators and inopressors increase the risk of tachyarrhythmias through either direct β_1 stimulation or calcium modulation, which may explain, in part, why long-term use of inodilators has been associated with increased mortality.[6,122] Among inodilators, dobutamine may cause more tachyarrhythmias whereas dopamine has been associated with higher rates compared with other inopressors (e.g., norephinephrine).[121,130] Continuous monitoring of both heart rate and ECG is essential during therapy. Caution is also recommended when considering the use of these agents in patients with recent myocardial infarction as inotropic agents increase myocardial oxygen consumption and may exacerbate ischemia.[6,135]

Because of their vasodilatory properties, hypotension can occur with all inodilators and is often a dose-limiting effect of PDE-3 inhibitors and levosimendan. Inodilators should be avoided or used with caution in patients with concomitant diseases in which vasodilation may worsen the condition or increase the risk of hypotension (e.g., hypovolemia, septic shock, or hypertrophic cardiomyopathy with outflow obstruction). In patients treated with inodilators and/or inopressors, MAP should be measured frequently, perhaps continuously using invasive monitoring, because of their hemodynamic effects. Likewise, volume status and indicators of end-organ perfusion (e.g., mental status, renal function, and urine output) should be monitored closely.

Some adverse effects are unique to inopressors. Epinephrine is known to increase blood glucose and lactate levels, due to increased glycolysis and glycogenolysis in the skeletal muscle.[136] All inopressor agents may cause extravasation and, ideally, should be administered through central catheters. Lastly, peripheral and/or tissue ischemia is possible with inopressors, particularly when used at high doses.[122]

Given that many patients requiring inodilators and most requiring inopressors are critically ill, invasive hemodynamic monitoring using a pulmonary artery catheter may be warranted. In patients with invasive hemodynamic monitoring in place, pulmonary capillary wedge pressure, central venous pressure, cardiac index, systemic vascular resistance, and central venous oxygen saturation are frequently monitored and used to titrate therapies.

Conclusion

Pharmacotherapy of HF typically includes the combination of multiple drugs from several drug classes to improve both symptoms and clinical outcomes. Chronically, the most common and efficacious therapies are those that antagonize neurohormonal systems. In the absence of contraindications, the combination of at least one anti-RAAS drug with a beta-blocker forms the backbone for GDMT for patients with HFrEF. Adjunctive therapies that have less or no neurohormonal manipulation may also be used, particularly for patients hospitalized for ADHF. Drug selection, dosing, drug interactions, and adverse effects are all impacted by pharmacological differences between drugs across and within drug classes. Therefore, clinicians must understand and consider these pharmacological differences to individualize therapy and optimize HF outcomes.

References

1. Schrier RW, Abraham WT. Hormones and hemodynamics in heart failure. *N Engl J Med.* 1999;341:577–85.
2. Schoolwerth AC, Sica DA, Ballermann BJ, et al. Renal considerations in angiotensin converting enzyme inhibitor therapy: a statement for healthcare professionals from the Council on the Kidney in Cardiovascular Disease and the Council for High Blood Pressure Research of the American Heart Association. *Circulation.* 2001;104:1985–91.
3. De Luca L, Orlandi C, Udelson JE, Fedele F, Gheorghiade M. Overview of vasopressin receptor antagonists in heart failure resulting in hospitalization. *Am J Cardiol.* 2005;96:24L–33L.
4. Sayer G, Bhat G. The renin-angiotensin-aldosterone system and heart failure. *Cardiol Clin.* 2014;32:21–32, vii.
5. King JB, Bress AP, Reese AD, Munger MA. Neprilysin inhibition in heart failure with reduced ejection fraction: a clinical review. *Pharmacotherapy.* 2015;35:823–37.
6. Ponikowski P, Voors AA, Anker SD, et al. 2016 ESC guidelines for the diagnosis and treatment of acute and chronic heart failure: the task force for the diagnosis and treatment of acute and chronic heart failure of the European Society of Cardiology (ESC)Developed with the special contribution of the Heart Failure Association (HFA) of the ESC. *Eur Heart J.* 2016;37:2129–200.
7. Yancy CW, Jessup M, Bozkurt B, et al. 2016 ACC/AHA/HFSA focused update on new pharmacological therapy for heart failure: an update of the 2013 ACCF/AHA guideline for the management of heart failure: a report of the American College of Cardiology/American Heart Association Task Force on Clinical Practice Guidelines and the Heart Failure Society of America. *J Am Coll Cardiol.* 2016;68:1476–88.
8. Yancy CW, Jessup M, Bozkurt B, et al. 2017 ACC/AHA/HFSA focused update of the 2013 ACCF/AHA guideline for the management of heart failure: a report of the American College of Cardiology/American Heart Association Task Force on Clinical Practice Guidelines and the Heart Failure Society of America. *J Am Coll Cardiol.* 2017;70:776–803.

9. Yancy CW, Jessup M, Bozkurt B, et al. 2013 ACCF/AHA guideline for the management of heart failure: a report of the American College of Cardiology Foundation/American Heart Association Task Force on Practice Guidelines. *J Am Coll Cardiol.* 2013;62:e147–239.
10. Maddox TM, Januzzi JL Jr., Allen LA, et al. 2021 update to the 2017 ACC expert consensus decision pathway for optimization of heart failure treatment: answers to 10 pivotal issues about heart failure with reduced ejection fraction. *J Am Coll Cardiol.* 2021;77:772–810.
11. Benowitz NL. Antihypertensive agents. In: Katzung BG, ed. *Basic & clinical pharmacology.* 14th ed. New York: McGraw-Hill Education; 2019. http://accesspharmacy.mhmedical.com/content.aspx?bookid=2249&sectionid=175216763. Accessed August 06, 2019.
12. Wong J, Patel RA, Kowey PR. The clinical use of angiotensin-converting enzyme inhibitors. *Prog Cardiovasc Dis.* 2004;47:116–30.
13. Ogawa R, Stachnik JM, Echizen H. Clinical pharmacokinetics of drugs in patients with heart failure: an update (part 2, drugs administered orally). *Clin Pharmacokinet.* 2014;53:1083–114.
14. Campo P, Fernandez TD, Canto G, Mayorga C. Angioedema induced by angiotensin-converting enzyme inhibitors. *Curr Opin Allergy Clin Immunol.* 2013;13:337–44.
15. Sica DA. Angiotensin-converting enzyme inhibitors side effects--physiologic and non-physiologic considerations. *J Clin Hypertens (Greenwich).* 2004;6:410–6.
16. Garg R, Yusuf S. Overview of randomized trials of angiotensin-converting enzyme inhibitors on mortality and morbidity in patients with heart failure. Collaborative group on ACE inhibitor trials. *JAMA.* 1995;273:1450–6.
17. Jhund PS, McMurray JJ. The neprilysin pathway in heart failure: a review and guide on the use of sacubitril/valsartan. *Heart.* 2016;102:1342–7.
18. Nielsen PM, Grimm D, Wehland M, Simonsen U, Kruger M. The combination of valsartan and sacubitril in the treatment of hypertension and heart failure - an update. *Basic Clin Pharmacol Toxicol.* 2018;122:9–18.
19. Velazquez EJ, Morrow DA, DeVore AD, et al. Angiotensin-neprilysin inhibition in acute decompensated heart failure. *N Engl J Med.* 2019;380:539–48.
20. Brown NJ, Ray WA, Snowden M, Griffin MR. Black Americans have an increased rate of angiotensin converting enzyme inhibitor-associated angioedema. *Clin Pharmacol Ther.* 1996;60:8–13.
21. Beavers CJ, Dunn SP, Macaulay TE. The role of angiotensin receptor blockers in patients with angiotensin-converting enzyme inhibitor-induced angioedema. *Ann Pharmacother.* 2011;45:520–4.
22. Haymore BR, Yoon J, Mikita CP, Klote MM, DeZee KJ. Risk of angioedema with angiotensin receptor blockers in patients with prior angioedema associated with angiotensin-converting enzyme inhibitors: a meta-analysis. *Ann Allergy Asthma Immunol.* 2008;101:495–9.
23. Butler J, Ezekowitz JA, Collins SP, et al. Update on aldosterone antagonists use in heart failure with reduced left ventricular ejection fraction. Heart Failure Society of America Guidelines Committee. *J Card Fail.* 2012;18:265–81.
24. Eschenhagen T. Therapy of heart failure. In: Brunton LL, Hilal-Dandan R, Knollmann BC, eds. *Goodman & Gilman's: the pharmacological basis of therapeutics.* 13th ed. New York: McGraw-Hill; 2018. http://accesspharmacy.mhmedical.com/content.aspx?bookid=2189&sectionid=170271080. Accessed November 01, 2019.
25. Robertson D, Biaggioni I. Adrenoreceptor antagonist drugs. In: Katzung BG, ed. *Basic & clinical pharmacology.* 14th ed. New York: McGraw Hill; 2018. http://accesspharmacy.mhmedical.com/content.aspx?bookid=2249&sectionid=175216621. Accessed November 01, 2019.
26. Dandona P, Ghanim H, Brooks DP. Antioxidant activity of carvedilol in cardiovascular disease. *J Hypertens.* 2007;25:731–41.
27. Veverka A, Salinas JL. Nebivolol in the treatment of chronic heart failure. *Vasc Health Risk Manag.* 2007;3:647–54.
28. Lowes BD, Gilbert EM, Abraham WT, et al. Myocardial gene expression in dilated cardiomyopathy treated with beta-blocking agents. *N Engl J Med.* 2002;346:1357–65.
29. Silke B. Beta-blockade in CHF: pathophysiological considerations. *European Heart Journal Supplements.* 2006;8:C13–8.
30. Chatterjee S, Biondi-Zoccai G, Abbate A, et al. Benefits of beta blockers in patients with heart failure and reduced ejection fraction: network meta-analysis. *BMJ.* 2013;346:f55.
31. Talbert RL. Pharmacokinetics and pharmacodynamics of beta blockers in heart failure. *Heart Fail Rev.* 2004;9:131–7.
32. Castagno D, Jhund PS, McMurray JJ, et al. Improved survival with bisoprolol in patients with heart failure and renal impairment: an analysis of the cardiac insufficiency bisoprolol study II (CIBIS-II) trial. *Eur J Heart Fail.* 2010;12:607–16.
33. Ko DT, Hebert PR, Coffey CS, et al. Adverse effects of beta-blocker therapy for patients with heart failure: a quantitative overview of randomized trials. *Arch Intern Med.* 2004;164:1389–94.
34. Waagstein F, Caidahl K, Wallentin I, Bergh CH, Hjalmarson A. Long-term beta-blockade in dilated cardiomyopathy. Effects of short- and long-term metoprolol treatment followed by withdrawal and readministration of metoprolol. *Circulation.* 1989;80:551–63.
35. Cheng JW. A review of isosorbide dinitrate and hydralazine in the management of heart failure in black patients, with a focus on a new fixed-dose combination. *Clin Ther.* 2006;28:666–78.
36. Hare JM. Nitroso-redox balance in the cardiovascular system. *N Engl J Med.* 2004;351:2112–4.
37. Arce C, Segura-Pacheco B, Perez-Cardenas E, et al. Hydralazine target: from blood vessels to the epigenome. *J Transl Med.* 2006;4:10.
38. Eschenhagen T. Treatment of hypertension. In: Brunton LL, Hilal-Dandan R, Knollmann BC, eds. *Goodman & Gilman's: the pharmacological basis of therapeutics.* 13th ed. New York: McGraw-Hill, 2018. http://accesspharmacy.mhmedical.com/content.aspx?bookid=2189&sectionid=170270855. Accessed August 09, 2019.
39. Viagra (sildenafil) [prescribing information]. New York, NY: Pfizer, Inc.; 2017.
40. Stendra (avanafil) [prescribing information]. Freehold, NJ: Metuchen Pharmaceuticals, LLC; 2019.
41. Levitra (vardenafil hydrochloride) [prescribing information]. Whippany, NJ: Bayer HealthCare Pharmaceuticals Inc.; 2018.
42. Cialis (tadalafil) [prescribing information]. Indianapolis, IN: Lilly USA, LLC; 2018.
43. Webb DJ, Freestone S, Allen MJ, Muirhead GJ. Sildenafil citrate and blood-pressure-lowering drugs: results of drug interaction studies with an organic nitrate and a calcium antagonist. *Am J Cardiol.* 1999;83:21C–28C.
44. Adempas (riociguat) [prescribing information]. Whippany, NJ: Bayer HealthCare Pharmaceuticals Inc.; 2021.
45. Cole RT, Kalogeropoulos AP, Georgiopoulou VV, et al. Hydralazine and isosorbide dinitrate in heart failure: historical perspective, mechanisms, and future directions. *Circulation.* 2011;123:2414–22.
46. Ghali JK, Farah JO, Daifallah S, Zabalawi HA, Zmily HD. Conivaptan and its role in the treatment of hyponatremia. *Drug Des Devel Ther.* 2009;3:253–68.
47. Finley JJt, Konstam MA, Udelson JE. Arginine vasopressin antagonists for the treatment of heart failure and hyponatremia. *Circulation.* 2008;118:410–21.
48. Sam R, Ives HE, Pearce D. Diuretic agents. In: B. G. Katzung, ed. *Basic & clinical pharmacology.* 14th ed. New York: McGraw-Hill; 2018. http://accesspharmacy.mhmedical.com/content.aspx?bookid=2249&sectionid=175217531. Accessed November 06, 2019.
49. Vaprisol (conivaptan hydrochloride) [prescribing information]. Nashville, TN: Cumberland Pharmaceuticals Inc.; 2017.
50. Samsca (tolvaptan) [prescribing information]. Rockville, MD: Otsuke America Pharmaceutical, Inc.; 2021.
51. Konstam MA, Kiernan M, Chandler A, et al. Short-term effects of tolvaptan in patients with acute heart failure and volume overload. *J Am Coll Cardiol.* 2017;69:1409–19.
52. Ellison DH, Felker GM. Diuretic treatment in heart failure. *N Engl J Med.* 2017;377:1964–75.
53. Dikshit K, Vyden JK, Forrester JS, et al. Renal and extrarenal hemodynamic effects of furosemide in congestive heart failure after acute myocardial infarction. *N Engl J Med.* 1973;288:1087–90.
54. Buggey J, Mentz RJ, Pitt B, et al. A reappraisal of loop diuretic choice in heart failure patients. *Am Heart J.* 2015;169:323–33.
55. Cosin J, Diez J, TORIC investigators. Torasemide in chronic heart failure: results of the TORIC study. *Eur J Heart Fail.* 2002;4:507–13.
56. Murray MD, Deer MM, Ferguson JA, et al. Open-label randomized trial of torsemide compared with furosemide therapy for patients with heart failure. *Am J Med.* 2001;111:513–20.
57. Vargo DL, Kramer WG, Black PK, et al. Bioavailability, pharmacokinetics, and pharmacodynamics of torsemide and furosemide in patients with congestive heart failure. *Clin Pharmacol Ther.* 1995;57:601–9.
58. Brater DC. Update in diuretic therapy: clinical pharmacology. *Semin Nephrol.* 2011;31:483–94.
59. von Lueder TG, Atar D, Krum H. Diuretic use in heart failure and outcomes. *Clin Pharmacol Ther.* 2013;94:490–8.
60. Brater DC, Day B, Burdette A, Anderson S. Bumetanide and furosemide in heart failure. *Kidney Int.* 1984;26:183–9.
61. Hardin EA, Grodin JL. Diuretic strategies in acute decompensated heart failure. *Curr Heart Fail Rep.* 2017;14:127–33.
62. Wheeler M, Jensen L. Torsemide injection. Current drug shortages. Accessed American Society of Health-System Pharmacists, 2018. https://www.ashp.org/Drug-Shortages/Current-Shortages/Drug-Shortage-Detail.aspx?id=168. Accessed March 23, 2022.
63. Felker GM, Lee KL, Bull DA, et al. Diuretic strategies in patients with acute decompensated heart failure. *N Engl J Med.* 2011;364:797–805.
64. Ng KT, Yap JLL. Continuous infusion vs. intermittent bolus injection of furosemide in acute decompensated heart failure: systematic review and meta-analysis of randomised controlled trials. *Anaesthesia.* 2018;73:238–47.
65. Kuriyama A, Urushidani S. Continuous versus intermittent administration of furosemide in acute decompensated heart failure: systematic review and meta-analysis. *Heart Fail Rev.* 2019;24:31–9.

66. Basnet S, Dhital R, Tharu B, et al. Influence of abnormal potassium levels on mortality among hospitalized heart failure patients in the US: data from National Inpatient Sample. *J Community Hosp Intern Med Perspect.* 2019;9:103–7.
67. Linde C, Qin L, Bakhai A, et al. Serum potassium and clinical outcomes in heart failure patients: results of risk calculations in 21 334 patients in the UK. *ESC Heart Fail.* 2019;6:280–90.
68. Matsushita K, Sang Y, Yang C, et al. Dyskalemia, its patterns, and prognosis among patients with incident heart failure: a nationwide study of US veterans. *PLoS One.* 2019;14:e0219899.
69. Salah K, Pinto YM, Eurlings LW, et al. Serum potassium decline during hospitalization for acute decompensated heart failure is a predictor of 6-month mortality, independent of N-terminal pro-B-type natriuretic peptide levels: an individual patient data analysis. *Am Heart J.* 2015;170:531–42 e1.
70. Wulf NR, Matuszewski KA. Sulfonamide cross-reactivity: is there evidence to support broad cross-allergenicity? *Am J Health Syst Pharm.* 2013;70:1483–94.
71. Hollenberg SM, Warner Stevenson L, Ahmad T, et al. 2019 ACC expert consensus decision pathway on risk assessment, management, and clinical trajectory of patients hospitalized with heart failure: a report of the American College of Cardiology Solution Set Oversight Committee. *J Am Coll Cardiol.* 2019;74:1966–2011.
72. Jentzer JC, DeWald TA, Hernandez AF. Combination of loop diuretics with thiazide-type diuretics in heart failure. *J Am Coll Cardiol.* 2010;56:1527–34.
73. Cardinale M, Altshuler J, Testani JM. Efficacy of intravenous chlorothiazide for refractory acute decompensated heart failure unresponsive to adjunct metolazone. *Pharmacotherapy.* 2016;36:843–51.
74. Shulenberger CE, Jiang A, Devabhakthuni S, et al. Efficacy and safety of intravenous chlorothiazide versus oral metolazone in patients with acute decompensated heart failure and loop diuretic resistance. *Pharmacotherapy.* 2016;36:852–60.
75. Welling PG. Pharmacokinetics of the thiazide diuretics. *Biopharm Drug Dispos.* 1986;7:501–35.
76. Caruso FS, Szabadi RR, Vukovich RA. Pharmacokinetics and clinical pharmacology of indapamide. *Am Heart J.* 1983;106:212–20.
77. Ellison DH. Clinical pharmacology in diuretic use. *Clin J Am Soc Nephrol.* 2019;14:1248–57.
78. DiDomenico R, Page RI. Chapter 13. Digoxin. In: Murphy J, ed. *Clinical pharmacokinetics.* Bethesda, MD: American Society of Health-System Pharmacists; 2017.
79. Bauman JL, Didomenico RJ, Galanter WL. Mechanisms, manifestations, and management of digoxin toxicity in the modern era. *Am J Cardiovasc Drugs.* 2006;6:77–86.
80. Gheorghiade M, Adams KF, Jr., Colucci WS. Digoxin in the management of cardiovascular disorders. *Circulation.* 2004;109:2959–64.
81. Adams KF, Jr., Patterson JH, Gattis WA, et al. Relationship of serum digoxin concentration to mortality and morbidity in women in the digitalis investigation group trial: a retrospective analysis. *J Am Coll Cardiol.* 2005;46:497–504.
82. Ahmed A, Rich MW, Love TE, et al. Digoxin and reduction in mortality and hospitalization in heart failure: a comprehensive post hoc analysis of the DIG trial. *Eur Heart J.* 2006;27:178–86.
83. Rathore SS, Curtis JP, Wang Y, Bristow MR, Krumholz HM. Association of serum digoxin concentration and outcomes in patients with heart failure. *JAMA.* 2003;289:871–8.
84. Devine BJ. Gentamicin therapy. *Drug Intelligence & Clinical Pharmacy.* 1974;8:650–655.
85. Cockcroft DW, Gault MH. Prediction of creatinine clearance from serum creatinine. *Nephron.* 1976;16:31–41.
86. Bauman JL, DiDomenico RJ, Viana M, Fitch M. A method of determining the dose of digoxin for heart failure in the modern era. *Arch Intern Med.* 2006;166:2539–45.
87. DiDomenico RJ, Bress AP, Na-Thalang K, et al. Use of a simplified nomogram to individualize digoxin dosing versus standard dosing practices in patients with heart failure. *Pharmacotherapy.* 2014;34:1121–31.
88. Konishi H, Shimizu S, Chiba M, et al. Predictive performance of serum digoxin concentration in patients with congestive heart failure by a hyperbolic model based on creatinine clearance. *J Clin Pharm Ther.* 2002;27:257–65.
89. Muzzarelli S, Stricker H, Pfister O, et al. Individual dosage of digoxin in patients with heart failure. *QJM.* 2011;104:309–17.
90. Nagatsu M, Spinale FG, Koide M, et al. Bradycardia and the role of beta-blockade in the amelioration of left ventricular dysfunction. *Circulation.* 2000;101:653–9.
91. Manz M, Reuter M, Lauck G, Omran H, Jung W. A single intravenous dose of ivabradine, a novel I(f) inhibitor, lowers heart rate but does not depress left ventricular function in patients with left ventricular dysfunction. *Cardiology.* 2003;100:149–55.
92. Ragueneau I, Laveille C, Jochemsen R, et al. Pharmacokinetic-pharmacodynamic modeling of the effects of ivabradine, a direct sinus node inhibitor, on heart rate in healthy volunteers. *Clin Pharmacol Ther.* 1998;64:192–203.
93. Corlanor (ivabradine) [prescribing information]. Thousand Oaks, CA: Amgen Inc.; 2021.
94. Tse S, Mazzola N. Ivabradine (Corlanor) for heart failure: the first selective and specific I f inhibitor. *P T.* 2015;40:810–4.
95. Portoles A, Calvo A, Terleira A, et al. Lack of pharmacokinetic interaction between omeprazole or lansoprazole and ivabradine in healthy volunteers: an open-label, randomized, crossover, pharmacokinetic interaction clinical trial. *J Clin Pharmacol.* 2006;46:1195–203.
96. Portoles A, Terleira A, Calvo A, Martinez I, Resplandy G. Effects of Hypericum perforatum on ivabradine pharmacokinetics in healthy volunteers: an open-label, pharmacokinetic interaction clinical trial. *J Clin Pharmacol.* 2006;46:1188–94.
97. Camm AJ, Lau CP. Electrophysiological effects of a single intravenous administration of ivabradine (S 16257) in adult patients with normal baseline electrophysiology. *Drugs R D.* 2003;4:83–9.
98. Murat SN, Orcan S, Akdemir R, et al. Arrhythmic effects of ivabradine in patients with coronary artery disease. *Clin Invest Med.* 2009;32:E322–6.
99. Cocco G, Jerie P. Torsades de pointes induced by the concomitant use of ivabradine and azithromycin: an unexpected dangerous interaction. *Cardiovasc Toxicol.* 2015;15:104–6.
100. Mittal SR. Slow junctional rhythm, QTc prolongation and transient torsades de-pointes following combined use of Ivabradine, Diltiazem and Ranolazine. *J Assoc Physicians India.* 2014;62:426–7.
101. Swedberg K, Komajda M, Bohm M, et al. Ivabradine and outcomes in chronic heart failure (SHIFT): a randomised placebo-controlled study. *Lancet.* 2010;376:875–85.
102. Cervetto L, Demontis GC, Gargini C. Cellular mechanisms underlying the pharmacological induction of phosphenes. *Br J Pharmacol.* 2007;150:383–90.
103. Jensen L. Nesiritide injection. Current drug shortages. Accessed American Society of Health-System Pharmacists, 2018. https://www.ashp.org/Drug-Shortages/Current-Shortages/Drug-Shortage-Detail.aspx?id=440 Accessed March 23, 2022.
104. Divakaran S, Loscalzo J. The role of nitroglycerin and other nitrogen oxides in cardiovascular therapeutics. *J Am Coll Cardiol.* 2017;70:2393–410.
105. Elkayam U, Janmohamed M, Habib M, Hatamizadeh P. Vasodilators in the management of acute heart failure. *Crit Care Med.* 2008;36 Supplement:S95–105.
106. Boden WE, Padala SK, Cabral KP, Buschmann IR, Sidhu MS. Role of short-acting nitroglycerin in the management of ischemic heart disease. *Drug Des Devel Ther.* 2015;9:4793–805.
107. Hottinger DG, Beebe DS, Kozhimannil T, Prielipp RC, Belani KG. Sodium nitroprusside in 2014: a clinical concepts review. *J Anaesthesiol Clin Pharmacol.* 2014;30:462–71.
108. Elkayam U, Kulick D, McIntosh N, et al. Incidence of early tolerance to hemodynamic effects of continuous infusion of nitroglycerin in patients with coronary artery disease and heart failure. *Circulation.* 1987;76:577–84.
109. Elkayam U, Akhter MW, Singh H, Khan S, Usman A. Comparison of effects on left ventricular filling pressure of intravenous nesiritide and high-dose nitroglycerin in patients with decompensated heart failure. *Am J Cardiol.* 2004;93:237–40.
110. Cohn JN, Franciosa JA, Francis GS, et al. Effect of short-term infusion of sodium nitroprusside on mortality rate in acute myocardial infarction complicated by left ventricular failure: results of a Veterans Administration cooperative study. *N Engl J Med.* 1982;306:1129–35.
111. Feneck RO, Sherry KM, Withington PS, Oduro-Dominah A, European Milrinone Multicenter Trial G. Comparison of the hemodynamic effects of milrinone with dobutamine in patients after cardiac surgery. *J Cardiothorac Vasc Anesth.* 2001;15:306–15.
112. Janicki JS, Shroff SG, Weber KT. Physiologic response to the inotropic and vasodilator properties of enoximone. *Am J Cardiol.* 1987;60:15C–20C.
113. Jentzer JC, Coons JC, Link CB, Schmidhofer M. Pharmacotherapy update on the use of vasopressors and inotropes in the intensive care unit. *J Cardiovasc Pharmacol Ther.* 2015;20:249–60.
114. Slawsky MT, Colucci WS, Gottlieb SS, et al. Acute hemodynamic and clinical effects of levosimendan in patients with severe heart failure. Study Investigators. *Circulation.* 2000;102:2222–7.
115. Benotti JR, Lesko LJ, McCue JE, Alpert JS. Pharmacokinetics and pharmacodynamics of milrinone in chronic congestive heart failure. *Am J Cardiol.* 1985;56:685–9.
116. Dubin A, Lattanzio B, Gatti L. The spectrum of cardiovascular effects of dobutamine - from healthy subjects to septic shock patients. *Rev Bras Ter Intensiva.* 2017;29:490–8.

117. Majerus TC, Dasta JF, Bauman JL, Danziger LH, Ruffolo RR, Jr. Dobutamine: ten years later. *Pharmacotherapy*. 1989;9:245–59.
118. Miller B, Clements E. Pharmacology of vasopressor agents. In: Tintinalli J, Stapczynski J, Ma O, Cline D, Cydulka R and Meckler G, eds. *Tintianlli's emergency medicine: a comprehensive study guide*. 7th ed. ed. New York: McGraw-Hill; 2011. http://accessmedicine.mhmedical.com/content.aspx?bookid=348&sectionid=40381485. Accessed October 09, 2019.
119. Metra M, Nodari S, D'Aloia A, et al. Beta-blocker therapy influences the hemodynamic response to inotropic agents in patients with heart failure: a randomized comparison of dobutamine and enoximone before and after chronic treatment with metoprolol or carvedilol. *J Am Coll Cardiol*. 2002;40:1248–58.
120. Lowes BD, Tsvetkova T, Eichhorn EJ, Gilbert EM, Bristow MR. Milrinone versus dobutamine in heart failure subjects treated chronically with carvedilol. *Int J Cardiol*. 2001;81:141–9.
121. Maack C, Eschenhagen T, Hamdani N, et al. Treatments targeting inotropy. *Eur Heart J*. 2019;40:3626–44.
122. Overgaard CB, Dzavik V. Inotropes and vasopressors: review of physiology and clinical use in cardiovascular disease. *Circulation*. 2008;118:1047–56.
123. Okerholm RA, Chan KY, Lang JF, Thompson GA, Ruberg SJ. Biotransformation and pharmacokinetic overview of enoximone and its sulfoxide metabolite. *Am J Cardiol*. 1987;60:21C–26C.
124. Toller WG, Stranz C. Levosimendan, a new inotropic and vasodilator agent. *Anesthesiology*. 2006;104:556–69.
125. Takahashi R, Talukder MA, Endoh M. Inotropic effects of OR-1896, an active metabolite of levosimendan, on canine ventricular myocardium. *Eur J Pharmacol*. 2000;400:103–12.
126. Lilleberg J, Laine M, Palkama T, et al. Duration of the haemodynamic action of a 24-h infusion of levosimendan in patients with congestive heart failure. *Eur J Heart Fail*. 2007;9:75–82.
127. Chen HH, Anstrom KJ, Givertz MM, et al. Low-dose dopamine or low-dose nesiritide in acute heart failure with renal dysfunction: the ROSE acute heart failure randomized trial. *JAMA*. 2013;310:2533–43.
128. Triposkiadis FK, Butler J, Karayannis G, et al. Efficacy and safety of high dose versus low dose furosemide with or without dopamine infusion: the Dopamine in Acute Decompensated Heart Failure II (DAD-HF II) trial. *Int J Cardiol*. 2014;172:115–21.
129. Friedrich JO, Adhikari N, Herridge MS, Beyene J. Meta-analysis: low-dose dopamine increases urine output but does not prevent renal dysfunction or death. *Ann Intern Med*. 2005;142:510–24.
130. De Backer D, Biston P, Devriendt J, et al. Comparison of dopamine and norepinephrine in the treatment of shock. *N Engl J Med*. 2010;362:779–89.
131. Levy B, Clere-Jehl R, Legras A, et al. Epinephrine versus norepinephrine for cardiogenic shock after acute myocardial infarction. *J Am Coll Cardiol*. 2018;72:173–82.
132. Eisenhofer G, Kopin IJ, Goldstein DS. Catecholamine metabolism: a contemporary view with implications for physiology and medicine. *Pharmacol Rev*. 2004;56:331–49.
133. Abboud I, Lerolle N, Urien S, et al. Pharmacokinetics of epinephrine in patients with septic shock: modelization and interaction with endogenous neurohormonal status. *Crit Care*. 2009;13:R120.
134. Beloeil H, Mazoit JX, Benhamou D, Duranteau J. Norepinephrine kinetics and dynamics in septic shock and trauma patients. *Br J Anaesth*. 2005;95:782–8.
135. Ruffolo RR, Jr. The pharmacology of dobutamine. *Am J Med Sci*. 1987;294:244–8.
136. Levy B. Bench-to-bedside review: is there a place for epinephrine in septic shock? *Crit Care*. 2005;9:561–5.

Chapter 6
IMPLANTABLE DEVICE THERAPY IN HEART FAILURE

Maxwell Eyram Afari and Lana Tsao

Introduction

Heart failure (HF) therapy has undergone a remarkable evolution over the past four decades. Prior to the 1980s, bedrest and fluid restriction were the hallmarks of the non-pharmacological era of HF therapy. The 1980s and 1990s represent the "pharmacological era," where guideline-directed medical therapy (GDMT) targeting vasodilation and neurohormonal blockade were proven to be effective. In the 2000s, the "device era," we witnessed the remarkable growth of the HF device-based industry.

Device therapy in HF can be categorized into (1) acute and durable circulatory support or (2) ambulatory management of chronic HF. Acute and durable mechanical circulatory support devices are discussed in Chapters 9 and 17, respectively. This chapter reviews implantable devices for treatment and monitoring of ambulatory HF patients, including investigational therapeutic devices (Figure 6.1).

Therapeutic Heart Failure Devices

Therapeutic HF devices target three broad areas: prevention of sudden cardiac death (SCD), improvement of cardiovascular efficiency and/or hemodynamics, and reducing sympathetic activation. As HF portends an increased risk of arrhythmias and SCD,[1] and elimination of arrhythmias with medication (discussed in Chapter 21) has proven problematic, implantable cardioverter-defibrillators (ICDs) to abort malignant arrhythmias are efficacious in this setting. Although several classes of medication improve the contractility of the left ventricle (LV) and improve symptoms and prognosis, medications alone cannot correct mechanical disadvantages, e.g., ventricular dyssynchrony, a result of conduction delays commonly seen in HF that has a deleterious mechanical effect on the failing ventricle.[2] This has led to the development of cardiac resynchronization therapy (CRT), cardiac contractility modulation (CCM), and transcatheter mitral valve repair devices. Finally, sympathetic overdrive and resulting deleterious tachycardia that cannot be mitigated by beta blockade alone have been the target of several investigational devices.

Implantable Cardioverter-Defibrillators (ICDs)

The goal of treating HF is to improve survival. Despite GDMT, patients are still at risk of SCD due to malignant arrhythmias. ICDs were developed more than three decades ago and can terminate ventricular arrhythmias through defibrillation. ICDs are configured similarly to a pacemaker and feature a "shocking coil" in various configurations, including single-chamber (pace and defibrillate from the right ventricle [RV]; Figure 6.2a), dual-chamber (extra pacing lead in the right atrium for atrial synchronized pacing; Figure 6.2b), and biventricular pacing (extra pacing lead in the coronary sinus; Figure 6.2c) configurations.

ICDs can be implanted for primary or secondary prevention of SCD. After resuscitated SCD or syncope likely due to ventricular tachyarrhythmia, ICD is indicated for secondary prevention since those patients have already experienced a life-threatening arrhythmic event and are at an increased risk of recurrence. Implantation is indicated for primary prevention in patients who have not experienced SCD or syncope due to malignant ventricular arrhythmias but are at significant risk based on structural characteristics (severely impaired systolic function), specific genetic background in cases of cardiomyopathies, or ECG or monitoring evidence of malignant arrhythmias.

Table 6.1 summarizes class I indications for ICD placement according to the "2017 AHA/ACC/HRS Guideline for management of patients with ventricular arrhythmias and the prevention of sudden cardiac death"[3] and the "2015 ESC Guidelines for the management of patients with ventricular arrhythmias and the prevention of sudden cardiac death."[4] The DANISH (Defibrillator Implantation in Patients with Non-ischemic Systolic Heart Failure) trial questioned the survival benefits of ICD when used in addition to optimal GDMT in patients with non-ischemic cardiomyopathy with left ventricular ejection fraction (LVEF) ≤35% in comparison to GDMT only.[5] However, a CRT-capable system was implanted in 58% of patients in this trial, thus making it difficult to generalize these findings to all patients requiring ICD. The findings from the DANISH trial are yet to make it to any of the major guidelines. A recent metanalysis, which pooled data from six randomized-control trials, demonstrated 23% reduction by ICD in all causes of mortality in non-ischemic cardiomyopathy.[6]

Subcutaneous defibrillators can be considered when an indication for ICD exists, but vascular access is inadequate or the risk of infection is unacceptably high. The need for standard pacing, an indication for CRT, or a need for anti-tachycardiac capabilities would be contradictions for subcutaneous defibrillators.

Cardiac Resynchronization Therapy (CRT)

The timing and pattern of ventricular conduction can dictate the efficiency of cardiac output in a failing heart. Electrical conduction defects, such as wide QRS complexes, can result in a phasic intraventricular delay resulting in ventricular dyssynchrony. The mechanism of LV dyssynchrony is attributed to temporal delay in electrical activation of different regions of the heart. In left bundle branch block (LBBB), there is a temporal delay between the activation of the septum and the eventual activation of the lateral wall.[2] Ventricular dyssynchrony results in discoordination of myocardial shortening, resulting in suboptimal ventricular filling, prolonged duration of mitral regurgitation, paradoxical septal wall motion, and decreased left ventricular (LV) contractility.[2]

CRT, also known as biventricular pacing, emerged in the 1990s as the therapy of choice for ventricular dyssynchrony. Two pacing leads are placed in both ventricles (epicardial RV lead and LV lead inserted via the coronary sinus). The configurations of CRT devices are CRT-D (with defibrillator) or CRT-P (with pacer), depending on indications for ICD. A CRT-D device has both defibrillation and biventricular pacing options. CRT has been shown to decrease the risk of hospitalization or death from any cause and, when combined with an ICD, significantly improves survival in patients with advanced chronic HF.[7]

DOI: 10.1201/9780429244544-7

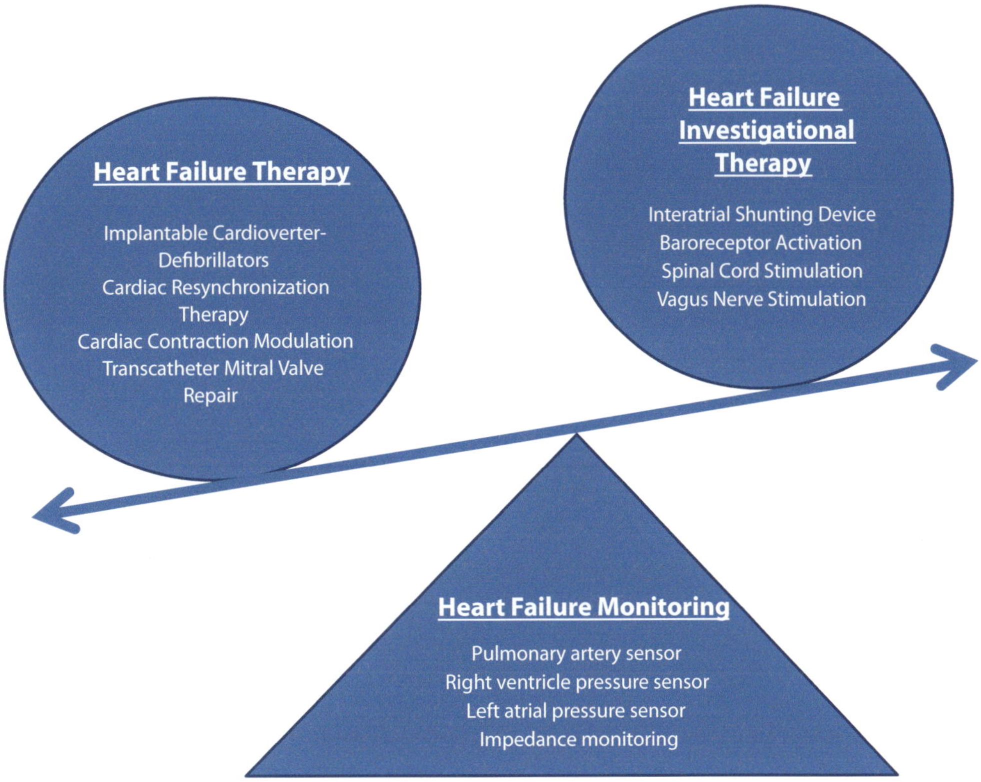

FIGURE 6.1 Summary of HF devices discussed in this chapter.

Table 6.2 summarizes the landmark clinical trials which have demonstrated the clinical utility of CRT. New York Heart Association (NYHA) class III and IV patients were investigated in the Multisite Stimulation in Cardiomyopathy (MUSTIC),[8] Multicenter In Sync Randomized Clinical Evaluation (MIRACLE),[9] MIRACLE ICD,[10] CONTAK CD,[11] Comparison of Medical Therapy, Pacing and Defibrillation in Heart Failure (COMPANION),[7] and CARE-HF (Cardiac Resynchronization in Heart Failure Study).[12] NYHA class I and II patients were investigated in the trials Resynchronization Reverses Remodeling in Systolic Left Ventricular Dysfunction (REVERSE),[13] Multicenter Automatic Defibrillator Implantation Trial with Cardiac Resynchronization Therapy (MADIT-CRT),[14] and Resynchronization/Defibrillation for Ambulatory Heart Failure Trial (RAFT).[15] It is noteworthy that 30–40% of HF patients in clinical trials are non-responders to CRT. This refers to patients who fail to show significant improvement in symptoms, functional capacity, LV reverse modeling (measured via echocardiogram or hemodynamic changes), and clinical outcomes (morbidity °and mortality). The following factors are associated with CRT non-response: non-LBBB, narrow QRS, and suboptimal LV lead position. Comorbidities such as HF disease progression, ventricular scar, and suboptimal atrioventricular or interventricular timing, can also cause CRT non-response.

Table 6.3 summarizes class I indications for CRT from the "2016 ESC Guidelines for the diagnosis and treatment of acute and chronic HF"[16] and the "2013 ACCF/AHA Guideline for the management of HF."[17]

Cardiac Contractility Modulation

Cardiac contractility modulation (CCM), shown in Figure 6.2d, applies non-excitatory electrical signals to the cardiac tissue during the absolute refractory period, when the tissue cannot be activated.[18] It is similar to a pacemaker system, consisting of a generator system connected to three leads (one atrial lead and two RV leads; Figure 6.2d). After delivery of high voltage (≈7.5 V), atrial-sensed biphasic impulse is sent to the RV septum which triggers the release of calcium in the sarcoplasmic reticulum. Calcium release is important in the cardiac excitation–contraction coupling, ultimately improving contractile performance without extra systolic contractions. Fundamentally, it differs from the pacemaker by the fact that it modulates contraction instead of the rhythm.

The Food and Drug Administration (FDA) in 2019 approved the Optimizer Smart System (Impulse Dynamics, Marlton, NJ, USA) in the United States. The device is already available in Europe, China, Brazil, Australia, and India. The indication for CCM according to the European Guidelines would be for patients in sinus rhythm with LVEF in the range 25–45%, NYHA class III disease despite GDMT, and normal QRS (<120 milliseconds), who are not candidates for CRT.[16]

Three studies have been pivotal in establishing the efficacy of CCM. In the FIX-HF-4 trial, three months of CCM were shown to improve exercise tolerance and quality of life (QoL).[19] In the FIX-HF-5 trial, peak VO_2 and QoL improved, but the study failed to achieve the FDA-mandated primary endpoint of anaerobic threshold measured by cardiopulmonary exercise testing.[20] The FIX-HF-5C trial was a prospective multicentric study of 160 patients with NYHA class III/IV symptoms and narrow QRS (<130 ms), LVEF ≥25% and ≤45%, randomized to medical therapy alone or CCM. The treatment arm showed improvement in QoL, NYHA functional class, and 6-min walk test.[21] Based on the results of this trial, the FDA approved CCM for NYHA class III patients, with LVEF 25% to 45% on GDMT, in sinus rhythm, and without an indication for CRT.

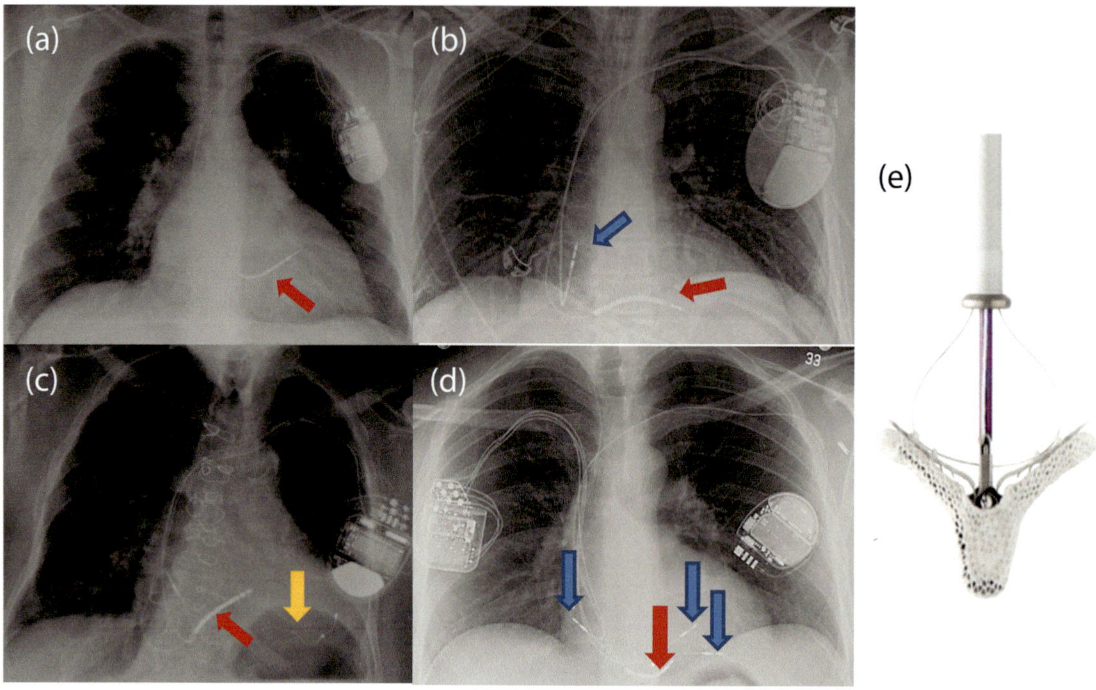

FIGURE 6.2 Therapeutic heart failure devices. (a) Single-chamber implantable cardioverter-defibrillator ICD. On the chest radiograph, the defibrillator coil (red arrow) is seen abutting the right ventricular septum. (b) Dual chamber ICD. The chest radiograph demonstrates a right atrial lead (blue arrow) and a defibrillator coil lead in the right ventricle (red arrow). (c) Biventricular ICD, also known as cardiac resynchronization therapy and defibrillator (CRT-D) device. The chest radiograph shows right ventricular defibrillator coil lead (red arrow), as well as a left ventricular pacing lead placed through the coronary sinus lead (yellow arrow). (d) The posteroanterior chest radiograph shows an ICD on the left upper chest with a defibrillator coil lead (red arrow) and the cardiac contractility modulation (CCM) device on the right upper chest with its leads (blue arrows). (Reproduced with permission from: Al-Ghamdi et al., *HeartRhythm Case Rep.* 2017;3:229–232.) (e) MitraClip NT Clip Delivery System. (Reproduced with permission from Abbott Laboratories, Minneapolis, MN, USA.)

TABLE 6.1: Class I Indications for Implantable Cardioverter-Defibrillator According to American and European Guidelines

Secondary Prevention
Ischemic heart disease which survives SCA due to VT/VF or which experiences hemodynamically unstable VT or stable sustained VT (irreversible).
Ischemic heart disease and unexplained syncope with inducible sustained monomorphic VT on EP study.
NICM which survives SCA due to VT/VF or experiences hemodynamically unstable VT or stable sustained VT (irreversible).
Primary Prevention
LVEF ≤35% due to ischemic heart disease >40 days' post-MI and at least 90 days post- revascularization, with NYHA class II or III HF despite GDMT.
LVEF ≤30% due to ischemic heart disease >40 days' post-MI and >90 days post-revascularization, with NYHA class I HF despite GDMT.
NSVT due to prior MI, LVEF ≤40%, and inducible sustained VT or VF at electrophysiological study.
NICM with NYHA class II–III symptoms and an LVEF ≤35% despite GDMT >3 months with at least 1 year with good functional status.

Abbreviations: EP: electrophysiology, GDMT: guideline-directed medical therapy, HF: heart failure, LVEF: left ventricle ejection fraction, MI: myocardial infarction, NSVT: non-sustained ventricular tachycardia, NYHA: New York Heart Association, SCA: sudden cardiac arrest, VT: ventricular tachycardia, VF: ventricular fibrillation.

Sources: Al-Khatib et al., 2017 AHA/ACC/HRS guideline for management of patients with ventricular arrhythmias and the prevention of sudden cardiac death: executive summary. *Circulation*. 2018;138:e210–e271. Priori et al., 2015 ESC guidelines for the management of patients with ventricular arrhythmias and the prevention of sudden cardiac death: The Task Force for the Management of Patients with Ventricular Arrhythmias and the Prevention of Sudden Cardiac Death of the European Society of Cardiology (ESC). Endorsed by Association for European Paediatric and Congenital Cardiology (AEPC). *Eur Heart J*. 2015;36:2793–867.

Transcatheter Mitral Valve Repair

The dilated LV causes functional mitral regurgitation (MR) through a number of mechanisms, eventually leading to LV volume overload and further decompensation of HF. Patients with functional MR experience higher mortality and increased hospitalization rates.[22] Unlike primary MR, surgery for functional MR does not attenuate this risk. However, functional MR can be corrected percutaneously by the approximation of the anterior and posterior mitral leaflets with the MitraClip System (Abbott Laboratories, Minneapolis, MN, USA), Figure 6.2e. The MitraClip is based on the principle of the Alfieri edge-to-edge repair, which results in a double-orifice MR area.[23]

TABLE 6.2: Landmark Clinical Trials Confirming the Clinical Utility of Cardiac Resynchronization Therapy

Name of Trial	Trial Design	NYHA Class	Patients	Inclusion Criteria	Randomization	Clinical Endpoint	Results	Comments
MUSTIC (Cazeau, Leclercq et al. 2001)	First randomized single-blinded trials	III	58	Normal sinus rhythm, QRS duration >150 msec	Randomized to CRT on and off for 12 weeks, with cross over	$\dot{V}O_2$, 6MHWD test, QOL determined using the MLWHF questionnaire	6MHWD > 23% in CRT, improvement in QoL and NYHA functional class ranking	
MIRACLE (Abraham, Fisher et al. 2002)	Double-blind, parallel-controlled clinical trial	III and IV	453	LVEF ≤35%, QRS >130 msec	CRT (n=228) control group (n=225)	NYHA class, QOL determined using the MLWHF questionnaire, and 6MHWD	Significant improvement in MLWHF, 6MHWD, and NYHA functional class ranking	50% reduction hospitalization
MIRACLE ICD (Young, Abraham et al. 2003)	Randomized, double-blind, parallel-controlled	III and IV	369	LVEF ≤35%; LVEDD ≥55 mm, QRS ≥130 msec, indication for ICD	CRT+ICD 187 ICD 182	NYHA class, QOL determined using the MLWHF questionnaire, and 6MHWD	Improvement in median QoL score and functional class	
CONTAK CD (Higgins, Hummel et al. 2003)	Crossover design changed to parallel design	III and IV	490	LVEF ≤35%, QRS interval ≥120 msec, indications for implant of an ICD	CRT+ICD (n=245) ICD (n=245)	Composite endpoint of HF hospitalization, all-cause mortality, and ventricular arrhythmia requiring defibrillator therapies	Not significant	Improvement in peak VO_2 and quality of life
COMPANION (Bristow, Saxon et al. 2004)	Multicenter, prospective randomized control trial	III and IV	1520	LVEF ≤35%, QRS interval >120 msec, PR interval >150 msec, sinus rhythm	1:2:2 allocation: GDMT (n=308), GDMT+CRT (n=617), GDMT+CRT-D (n=595)	Composite of all-cause mortality and all-cause hospitalization	Reduction of 35% in CRT and 40% of CRT-ICD (both P <0.001).	
CARE HF (Cleland, Daubert et al. 2005)	Unblended randomized control trial	III and IV	813	LVEF ≤35%, QRS duration ≥150 msec or 120-150 msec (with echocardiographic evidence of dyssynchrony)	CRT+GDMT 409 GDMT 404	Risk of death from any cause or unplanned hospitalization for a major cardiac event	37% reduction in CRT+GDMT (hazard ratio [HR], 0.63; 95%CI 0.51 to 0.77; P<0.001)	36% reduction in all-cause mortality with CRT, 46% reduction in all-cause mortality + HF hospitalization
MADIT-CRT (Moss, Hall et al. 2009)	Multicenter RCT	I and II	1820	LVEF ≤30%, QRS ≥130 msec	CRT+ICD or ICD only	Any cause death or nonfatal HF event	CRT+ICD with RRR of 34% (HR, 0.66; 95% CI 0.52 to 0.84; P<0.001)	Significant benefit was driven by a 41% reduction in HF events
REVERSE (Linde, Abraham et al. 2008)	Double blinded RCT	I and II	610	QRS ≥120 msec, LVEF ≤40%, LVEDD ≥55 mm	CRT off (n=191) CRT+GDMT (n=419)	Clinical composite HF score	CRT versus control (16% vs. 21%; P <0.10)	53% RRR in the time to first HF hospitalization
RAFT (Tang, Wells et al. 2010)	Multicenter, double-blind, randomized, controlled study	II or III	1798	LVEF ≤30%, QRS ≥120 msec	CRT+ICD or ICD	All-cause mortality or HF hospitalization	RRR with CRT of 17.5 HR ICD-CRT group, 0.75; 95% CI 0.64 to 0.87; P <0.001	

Abbreviations NYHA; New York Heart Association Heart Failure class, CRT: cardiac resynchronization therapy, VO_2: peak oxygen consumption, 6MHWD: 6-minute hall walk distance, QoL: Quality of Life, MLWHF: Minnesota Living with Heart Failure, LVEF: left ventricular ejection fraction, LVEDD: left ventricle end-diastolic diameter, ICD: implantable cardioverter defibrillator, GDMT: guideline-directed medical therapy, RRR: relative risk reduction, HF: heart failure.

TABLE 6.3: Class I Indications for Cardiac Resynchronization Therapy According to American and European Guidelines

2016 ESC Heart Failure Guidelines CRT Class I Indications
Symptomatic patients with HF in sinus rhythm with a QRS duration ≥150 ms and LBBB QRS morphology with LVEF ≤35% despite GDMT.
Symptomatic patients with HF in sinus rhythm with QRS duration of 130–149 ms and LBBB QRS morphology with LVEF ≤35% despite GDMT.
CRT rather than RV pacing is recommended for patients with HFrEF regardless of NYHA class, who have an indication for ventricular pacing and high-degree AV block.
2012 ACC/AHA/HRS Guidelines CRT Class I Indications
LVEF less than or equal to 35%, sinus rhythm, LBBB with a QRS duration ≥150 ms, and NYHA class II, III, or ambulatory IV symptoms on GDMT.

Abbreviations: ESC: European Society of Cardiology, CRT: cardiac resynchronization therapy, GDMT: guideline-directed medical therapy, HFrEF: heart failure with reduced ejection fraction, NYHA: New York Heart Association, AV: atrioventricular, LVEF: left ventricle ejection fraction, LBBB: left bundle branch block.
Sources: Adapted from Ponikowski et al. ESC guidelines for the diagnosis and treatment of acute and chronic heart failure. *Eur Heart J*. 2016;37(27):2129–200. Yancy et al. ACCF/AHA guideline for the management of heart failure. *Circulation*. 2013;128(16):1810–52.

In the COAPT (Cardiovascular Outcomes Assessment of the MitraClip Percutaneous Therapy for Heart Failure Patients with Functional Mitral Regurgitation) trial,[24] symptomatic patients with HF and moderate to severe MR were randomized to MitraClip in addition to GDMT. Compared to medical therapy only, transcatheter mitral-valve repair resulted in a lower rate of annualized rate of HF hospitalizations (35.8% versus 67.9% per patient-year) and lower all-cause mortality (29.1% versus 46.1%) in the COAPT trial. Prior to the COAPT trial, in the Endovascular Valve Edge-to-Edge Repair Study (EVEREST) II trial, percutaneous repair was less effective in reducing MR compared to surgical repair, albeit safer.[25] The Multicentre Study of Percutaneous Mitral Valve Repair MitraClip Device in Patients With Severe Secondary Mitral Regurgitation (Mitra FR) trial failed to show reduction in death or hospitalization for HF compared to medical therapy.[26]

The discrepancy of results in these trials with COAPT could be attributed to the following factors. First, only a small percentage of EVEREST II patients had functional MR. Second, the procedural success in COAPT was 98% with immediate improvement in MR. In MITRA-FR, there were twice as many procedural complications. Third, MITRA-FR potentially enrolled patients with advanced HF with LV end- systolic dimension>70 mm and LVEF <20%. Fourth, patients with effective regurgitant orifice (ERO) <0.4 cm^2 were excluded from the COAPT study whereas MITRA FR included patients with ERO ~0.2. Finally, some patients with dilated LV with associated annular dilatation have what has been termed "proportionate MR." These patients would benefit from therapies that decrease LV size such as neurohormonal blockade or an LV assist device. In contrast, LV dyssynchrony results in "disproportionate MR." The latter tends to respond to therapies that target the valve (CRT, MitraClip).[27] This concept of "proportionate MR" and "disproportionate MR" is yet to be validated in a prospective study. The population likely to benefit from this therapy are patients with HF and LVEF ≥20% and ≤50%, with moderate-severe or severe MR deemed to be at high surgical risk.

Investigational Therapeutic Devices

Several additional devices not yet approved for clinical practice are currently undergoing rigorous evaluation. Below, we discuss interatrial shunting, baroreceptor activation therapy, spinal cord stimulation, and vagus nerve stimulation.

Interatrial Shunting Device

Elevated LAP with resulting increased pressure in the pulmonary capillaries is the mechanism of exercise intolerance and symptoms in both HFpEF and HF with reduced ejection fraction (HFrEF). Left atrial decompression has emerged as a therapeutic strategy for chronic HF. After a trans-septal puncture, an interatrial shunting device (IASD) is deployed through a sheath, creating a communication between the atria. Blood then flows from the high-pressure left atrium to the right atrium, decompressing the left atrium. The IASD System (Corvia Medical, Tewksbury, MA, USA) shown in Figure 6.3a and subsequently the V-Wave shunt device (V-Wave Ltd, Caesarea, Israel) are at different stages of development. In the REDUCE LAP-HF (The REDUCE Elevated Left Atrial Pressure in Patients with HF) Phase 1 trial, the Corvia IASD was evaluated in 64 patients with NYHA class III–IV symptoms, LVEF >40%, and elevated PCWP (≥15 mmHg at rest or ≥25 mmHg during supine bicycle exercise). The device improved NYHA class and QoL, lowered pulmonary capillary wedge pressure, and increased exercise capacity at six[28] and 12 months.[29] In REDUCE LAP-HF I, a phase 2 trial, where participants were randomized to IASD or sham control procedure, the IASD resulted in greater reduction in PCWP compared with the sham control (P=0.028, accounting for all stages of exercise at one month.[30] At one year, the patency of IASD and safety were confirmed (assessed by major adverse cardiac, cerebrovascular, or renal events).[31] REDUCE LAP-HF II, NCT03088033, is an ongoing multicenter, randomized, controlled pivotal study of the IASD System II in treating HFpEF and HF with midrange ejection fraction (HFmrEF). The first in-man experience of the V-wave interatrial shunt system involved 38 patients [HFpEF (n=8), HFrEF (n=30)]; a 78% and 60% improvement in NYHA class (from III–IV to I–II) was seen at 3 months and 12 months, respectively.[32]

Baroreceptor Activation Therapy (BAT)

Baroreceptors in the carotid artery and the carotid sinus are the physiological means for the body to react to changes in blood flow. The Barostim NEO System (CVRx Inc., Minneapolis, MN, USA) is an investigational device where mechanism of action is based on the stimulation of the baroreceptors in the carotid (Figure 6.3b). The system consists of a pulse generator implanted below the clavicle with an electrode tunneled to the carotid sinus. Programmable impulses are sent to the carotid sinus, and baroreceptors then send signals to the brain. The brain sends feedback signals which augment the parasympathetic system while withdrawing sympathetic activity. Initial trials have demonstrated improvement in NYHA class, quality of life and 6-min walk test.[33,34] Notably, non-CRT patients tend to do better, suggesting that the CRT modulation of sympathetic activity outflow can attenuate its benefit.[35] Baroreflex Activation Therapy for Heart Failure (BeAT-HF) is an ongoing Phase III trial of NYHA class III patients with LVEF of ≤35% not requiring CRT, who were randomized to

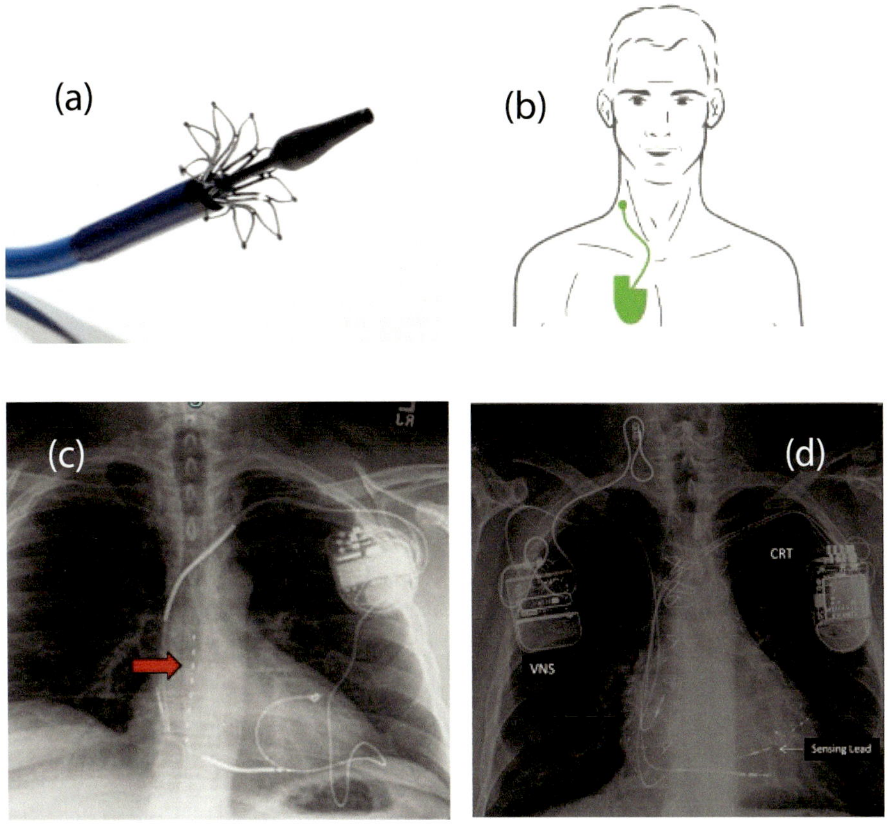

FIGURE 6.3 Mechanism of action of investigational implantable devices for heart failure therapy. (a) Corvia Interatrial shunt device. (Permission from Corvia Medical Inc, Tewksbury, MA, USA.) (b) Baroreceptor Activation Therapy. Pulse generator implanted below the clavicle with an electrode tunneled to the carotid sinus. This is transmitted to the brain which sends message via the efferent pathway for parasympathetic activation and sympathetic inhibition. (Figure obtained from CVRx Inc., Minneapolis, MN, USA.) (c) Spinal Cord Stimulation. Subcutaneous pulse generator transmits impulse to electrode leads inserted percutaneously into the epidural space at the mid-thoracic level. (d) Vagus Nerve Stimulation. Standard right ventricle transmits information to the stimulator, which sends electrical impulses to the vagal nerve. [(c) and (d) Reprinted from Chatterjee and Singh. Novel Interventional Therapies to Modulate the Autonomic Tone in Heart Failure, *JACC Heart Fail* 2015;3(10):786–802. Copyright (2021), with permission from Elsevier.]

BAT+GDMT or GDMT. Preliminary results presented at the Heart Rhythm Society Scientific Meeting in 2019 demonstrated that Barostim NEO improved walk distance and quality of life on the Minnesota Living with Heart Failure questionnaire at 6 months.[36] The Barostim NEO System was approved by the FDA through the Premarket Approval (PMA) pathway in the summer of 2019 for patients with LVEF <35%, who were not candidates for CRT.

Spinal Cord Stimulation

The spinal cord stimulation system relies on electrical stimulations sent directly to nerve fibers in the spinal cord. The system is currently utilized in clinical practice for treating chronic pain and refractory angina. Electrical impulses are generated from a subcutaneous pulse generator to electrode leads inserted percutaneously into the epidural space at the mid-thoracic level (Figure 6.3c). The reduction of catecholamine and increase in blood pressure is hypothesized to be the basis for the treatment of systolic HF in this system. Its efficacy in clinical trials thus far has been equivocal.[37,38] The variance in results from the SCS-HEART (Thoracic Spinal Cord Stimulation for Heart Failure as a Restorative Treatment) and DEFEAT-HF (Determining the Feasibility of Spinal Cord Neuromodulation for the Treatment of Chronic Systolic Heart Failure) trials is likely due to the different techniques used in delivering treatment. Whereas DEFEAT-HF used single 8-electrode stimulation, SCS-HEART used two 8-electrode stimulation at T1-T3 levels. Also, continuous stimulation of impulse was delivered in SCS-HEART, whereas DEFEAT-HF had 12 hours of stimulation per day. Further studies are needed to establish the most effective treatment strategy.

Vagus Nerve Stimulation

The rationale for vagus nerve stimulation (VNS) is based on the principle of parasympathetic stimulation as an HF treatment strategy. The VNS system has a standard RV lead and an electrode tunneled to the vagal nerve near the carotid artery bifurcation (Figure 6.3d). Both components are connected to a subcutaneous stimulator. The RV transmits the sensed heart rate to the stimulator, which sends electrical impulses to the vagal nerve in response. To date, clinical trials have been equivocal in showing improvements in HF endpoints.[39–43] Next-generation VNS devices will focus on patient selection, VNS protocol improvement, and whether the laterality of the vagal nerve affects outcomes. The VNS Therapy System (Cyberonics, Houston, TX, USA) and the CardioFit system (BioControl

Medical, Yehud, Israel) were investigated in the aforementioned trials.

Heart Failure Monitoring Devices

Effective monitoring of HF requires early identification of impending decompensation. Conceptually, it has been shown that up to two weeks before patients develop symptoms of HF, there are already hemodynamic changes suggestive of fluid overload.[44,45] An accurate interpretation of fluid status requires an invasive acquisition of the LV end-diastolic pressure (LVEDP) or pulmonary artery capillary wedge pressure (PCWP), which is impractical for outpatient management. This clinical conundrum has led to the emergence of implantable devices for ambulatory HF monitoring. There are two categories of monitors: (1) *de novo* implantation of an implantable pulmonary artery sensor or left atrial pressure monitor, reserved for patients with severe or recurrent HF symptoms; or (2) "bonus" monitoring system added to a device that a patient qualifies for, such as a pacemaker, CRT (e.g., impedance). The disadvantages of the latter include battery life draining and therefore on/off status may need individualization. Table 6.4 summarizes the currently available HF monitoring devices.

Implantable Pulmonary Artery Sensor

The Cardio-Microelectromechanical system (CardioMEMS; Abbott, Sylmar, CA, USA) is a remote monitoring system, which is effective in the early detection of rising intracardiac filling pressures. CardioMEMS has a sensor which is placed directly into the pulmonary artery through right heart catheterization. This sensor uses the microelectromechanical systems (MEMS) technology to transmit via wireless frequencies to an external measurement system which determines the pulmonary artery pressure (PAP). Patients lie on a special pillow containing an antenna which transmits sensor readings to an electronic unit, which afterwards transmits data to a secure website accessible to health care practitioners. Figure 6.4a shows transmitted pulmonary artery pressures of a patient with fluid overload while Figure 6.4b shows transmitted pressures after taking diuretics.

In the CHAMPION trial, patients treated with the guidance of CardioMEMS had a 37% reduction in hospitalization over a 15-month period, compared with the average of the standard care only.[46] Most pressure-based medication changes were for diuretics and vasodilators. CardioMEMS-guided therapy of patients with HF and preserved ejection fraction (HFpEF) has also been shown to decrease hospitalization.[47] The 2016 European Society of Cardiology (ESC) guidelines recommend CardioMEMS placement (class IIb indication) for patients with NYHA class III symptoms who have been hospitalized for HF in the previous year.[16]

Recently, Abraham et al. retrospectively compared patients implanted with CardioMEMS to a propensity-matched HF cohort who received standard care. The investigators showed a lower rate of mortality in the CardioMEMS cohort (0.23 deaths/year vs 0.30 deaths/ year; hazard ratio [HR], 0.70 [95% confidence interval (CI), 0.59–0.83]; P<0.001) compared with the standard care cohort.[48] As these data come from a claims database, without adjusting for HF severity, caution should be applied in interpreting these data. CardioMEMS is the only FDA (2014) and Conformitè Europëenne (CE) mark (2010) -approved HF monitor shown to reduce hospitalization and improve QoL in patients with NYHA class III symptoms. Other implantable monitors for HF discussed below are in various stages of development and have not attained CE Mark or FDA approval yet.

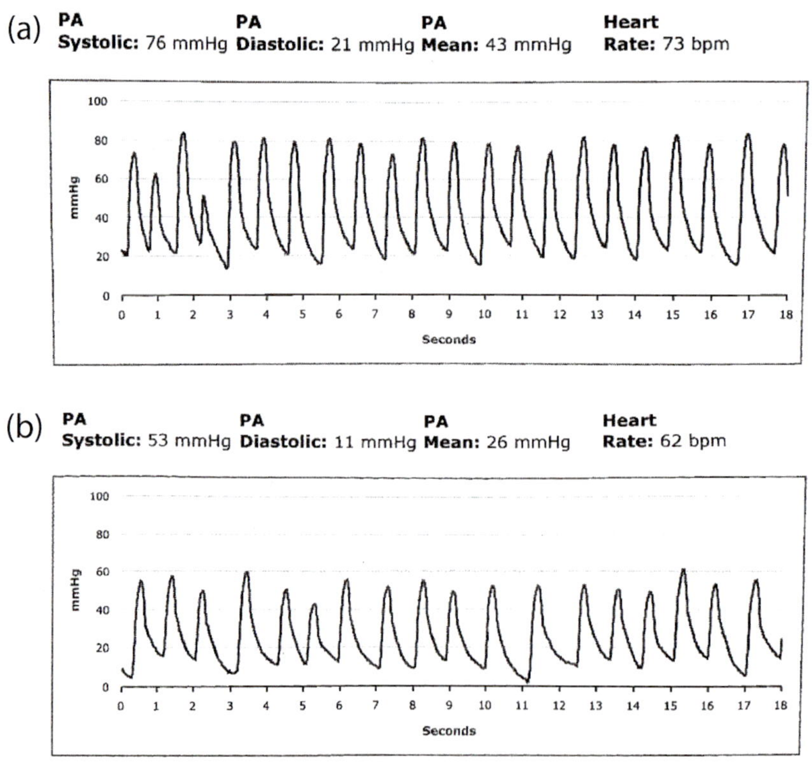

FIGURE 6.4 (a) Transmitted pulmonary artery pressures of a patient with fluid overload. (b) After being treated with diuretics, a significant reduction in filling pressures was observed.

TABLE 6.4: Summary of Heart Failure Monitoring Devices

Device	Clinical Trial	Location	Sensor Type	Transmission	Regulatory Status
De Novo *Implantation*					
CardioMEMs	CHAMPION (Abraham, Stevenson et al. 2016)	Pulmonary artery	Micro-electromechanical systems-pulmonary artery pressure	Wireless frequencies	FDA-approved NYHA III HF admission in past 12 months
HeartPod V-LAP	HOMEOSTASIS (Ritzema, Troughton et al. 2010) LAPTOP-HF (Maurer, Adamson et al. 2015)	Left atrial septum	Left atrial pressure	Miniature, wireless, microcomputer	Newer generation V-LAP is under preclinical and clinical investigation (VECTOR HF Trial)
Bonus Monitoring System					
CHRONICLE	COMPASS (Bourge, Abraham et al. 2008) REDUCEhf (Adamson, Gold et al. 2011)	Part of ICD system (right ventricle septum)	Right ventricular pressure, estimated pulmonary diastolic pressure	Handheld radio frequency wand which transmits data through a telephone line to a secure server	Not approved
OPTIVOL COGNIS CRT-D	FAST (Abraham, Compton et al. 2011) Multi SENSE (Boehmer, Hariharan et al. 2017)	Part of CRT system	Intrathoracic IMPEDANCE	Download during follow-up visit or remote LATITUDE transmissions	FDA approved

Abbreviations: CRT: cardiac resynchronization therapy; FDA: US Food and Drug Administration; HF: heart failure; ICD: implantable cardioverter defibrillator; NYHA: New York Heart Association.

Left Atrial Pressure (LAP) Monitoring

Ongoing efforts have targeted the measuring of left atrial pressure (LAP) as a strategy to get ahead of rising left-sided filling pressures. The HeartPOD (Abbott, Sylmar, CA, USA) is a sensor lead which is implanted in the left atrium using a transseptal technique. In the HOMEOSTASIS (Hemodynamically Guided Home Self-Therapy in Severe Heart Failure Patients) trial,[49] LAP fell by 16% when patients were managed with the guidance of LAP monitoring, compared with usual care. However, the momentum around HeartPOD has slowed down with the early termination of the LAPTOP-HF (Left Atrial Pressure Monitoring to Optimize Heart Failure Therapy) trial[50] due to transseptal technique-related complications. A newer-generation device, V-LAP (Vectorious Medical Technologies, Tel Aviv, Israel), is under preclinical and clinical investigation.[51] Via the transseptal approach, the sensor is implanted in the septum and, in addition to LAP, can also obtain other physiological data, such as heart rate variability and arrhythmias.

Right Ventricle Pressure Monitoring

Prior to the approval of the implantable pulmonary artery sensor, studies focused on the measurement of the RV end-systolic pressure, RV end-diastolic pressure, and the estimated diastolic PAP through systems which had already been implanted for other reasons, like pacemakers or ICDs. The sensors on the RV lead measure pressure during pulmonic valve opening, estimating the diastolic PAP. In the COMPASS-HF (Chronicle Offers Management to Patients with Advanced Signs and Symptoms of Heart Failure) trial, the Chronicle implantable hemodynamic monitor (Medtronic, Inc., Minneapolis, MN, USA) system failed to show significant reduction in HF-related events compared to standard care.[45] However, COMPASS-HF did show that a gradual increase in diastolic PAP preceded the onset of symptoms. The Chronicle ICD system was similarly investigated in the REDUCEhf (Reducing Decompensation Events Utilizing Intracardiac Pressures in Patients with Chronic Heart Failure) trial. However, the incidence of HF-related events (defined as hospitalizations ≥24 hours, hospitalizations <24 hours requiring IV therapy, emergency department visits, or urgent clinic visits requiring IV therapy) was similar between treatment arms.[52] These studies have dampened the excitement around RV pressure monitoring through pacemaker leads.

Impedance Monitoring

Bioimpedance refers to the electrical resistance of tissue to the flow of current. An inverse relationship exists between fluid accumulation in the lungs and intrathoracic impedance (ITI), a measurement built into select pacemaker, ICD, or CRT systems. The Medtronic Optivol is an example of a fluid-monitoring feature built into a CRT device. The Optivol fluid index tracks the variation of ITI, which is transmitted to health care providers when the index exceeds a certain threshold value. Despite ITI monitoring having failed to demonstrate reductions in HF hospitalizations,[53,54] the device has been shown to predict HF hospitalization.[55–57] Lung conditions, such as pneumonia, chronic obstructive lung disease, interstitial lung disease, and pneumothorax, impact on the impedance of the lungs, which challenges the specificity and utility of ITI readings. Furthermore, it is difficult to discriminate between lung impedance and chest wall impedance. Lung impedance is the difference between chest wall and thoracic impedances. Edema Guard (CardioSet Medical, Bnei Brak, Israel), a non-invasive monitoring device currently under investigation, uses a proprietary algorithm to determine lung independence through three electrodes attached to the anterior and posterior chest. Edema Guard has been shown to reduce all-cause hospitalizations and HF hospitalizations by 57% and 39%, respectively, in the IMPEDANCE-HF (Non-Invasive Lung IMPEDANCE-Guided Preemptive Treatment in Chronic Heart Failure Patients) trial.[58]

The HeartLogic multi-sensor HF index and alert algorithm, which is part of the COGNIS CRT-D system (Boston Scientific, St. Paul, MN, USA), uses input from multiple sensors. The data obtained are based on third heart sounds, thoracic impedance, respiration rate, heart rate, and patient activity. In the Multi SENSE (Multisensor Chronic Evaluation in Ambulatory Heart Failure Patients) trial, HeartLogic predicted HF events with 70% sensitivity.[59] A median 34-day advance warning was transmitted prior to an HF event (admission, need for IV diuretic/inotrope or vasodilator), suggesting a role for this device in ambulatory monitoring of HF patients who have a CRT system. The tradeoff would be the impact on the battery life.

Conclusion

This is an exciting time for the treatment of HF. Besides established life-saving therapies, including the ICD and CRT devices, many implantable HF devices are in development as current technologies continue to evolve. These devices will be important in taming the burden of HF.

References

1. Lorvidhaya P, Addo K, Chodosh A, et al. Sudden cardiac death risk stratification in patients with heart failure. *Heart Fail Clin.* 2011;7:157–74, vii.
2. Cheng A, Helm RH, Abraham TP. Pathophysiological mechanisms underlying ventricular dyssynchrony. *Europace.* 2009;11 Suppl 5:v10–14.
3. Al-Khatib SM, Stevenson WG, Ackerman MJ, et al. 2017 AHA/ACC/HRS guideline for management of patients with ventricular arrhythmias and the prevention of sudden cardiac death: executive summary: a report of the American College of Cardiology/American Heart Association Task Force on Clinical Practice Guidelines and the Heart Rhythm Society. *Circulation.* 2018;138:e210–71.
4. Priori SG, Blomstrom-Lundqvist C, Mazzanti A, et al. 2015 ESC guidelines for the management of patients with ventricular arrhythmias and the prevention of sudden cardiac death: the task force for the management of patients with ventricular arrhythmias and the prevention of sudden cardiac death of the European Society of Cardiology (ESC). Endorsed by: Association for European Paediatric and Congenital Cardiology (AEPC). *Eur Heart J.* 2015;36:2793–867.
5. Kober L, Thune JJ, Nielsen JC, et al. Defibrillator implantation in patients with nonischemic systolic heart failure. *N Engl J Med.* 2016;375:1221–30.
6. Golwala H, Bajaj NS, Arora G, Arora P. Implantable cardioverter-defibrillator for nonischemic cardiomyopathy: an updated meta-analysis. *Circulation.* 2017;135:201–3.
7. Bristow MR, Saxon LA, Boehmer J, et al. Cardiac-resynchronization therapy with or without an implantable defibrillator in advanced chronic heart failure. *N Engl J Med.* 2004;350:2140–50.
8. Cazeau S, Leclercq C, Lavergne T, et al. Effects of multisite biventricular pacing in patients with heart failure and intraventricular conduction delay. *N Engl J Med.* 2001;344:873–80.
9. Abraham WT, Fisher WG, Smith AL, et al. Cardiac resynchronization in chronic heart failure. *N Engl J Med.* 2002;346:1845–53.
10. Young JB, Abraham WT, Smith AL, et al. Combined cardiac resynchronization and implantable cardioversion defibrillation in advanced chronic heart failure: the MIRACLE ICD trial. *JAMA.* 2003;289:2685–94.
11. Higgins SL, Hummel JD, Niazi IK, et al. Cardiac resynchronization therapy for the treatment of heart failure in patients with intraventricular conduction delay and malignant ventricular tachyarrhythmias. *J Am Coll Cardiol.* 2003;42:1454–9.
12. Cleland JG, Daubert JC, Erdmann E, et al. The effect of cardiac resynchronization on morbidity and mortality in heart failure. *N Engl J Med.* 2005;352:1539–49.
13. Linde C, Abraham WT, Gold MR, et al. Randomized trial of cardiac resynchronization in mildly symptomatic heart failure patients and in asymptomatic patients with left ventricular dysfunction and previous heart failure symptoms. *J Am Coll Cardiol.* 2008;52:1834–43.
14. Moss AJ, Hall WJ, Cannom DS, et al. Cardiac-resynchronization therapy for the prevention of heart-failure events. *N Engl J Med.* 2009;361:1329–38.
15. Tang AS, Wells GA, Talajic M, et al. Cardiac-resynchronization therapy for mild-to-moderate heart failure. *N Engl J Med.* 2010;363:2385–95.
16. Ponikowski P, Voors AA, Anker SD, et al. 2016 ESC guidelines for the diagnosis and treatment of acute and chronic heart failure: the task force for the diagnosis and treatment of acute and chronic heart failure of the European Society of Cardiology (ESC)Developed with the special contribution of the Heart Failure Association (HFA) of the ESC. *Eur Heart J.* 2016;37:2129–200.
17. Yancy CW, Jessup M, Bozkurt B, et al. 2013 ACCF/AHA guideline for the management of heart failure: executive summary: a report of the American College of Cardiology Foundation/American Heart Association Task Force on practice guidelines. *Circulation.* 2013;128:1810–52.
18. Brunckhorst CB, Shemer I, Mika Y, Ben-Haim SA, Burkhoff D. Cardiac contractility modulation by non-excitatory currents: studies in isolated cardiac muscle. *Eur J Heart Fail.* 2006;8:7–15.
19. Borggrefe MM, Lawo T, Butter C, et al. Randomized, double blind study of non-excitatory, cardiac contractility modulation electrical impulses for symptomatic heart failure. *Eur Heart J.* 2008;29:1019–28.
20. Kadish A, Nademanee K, Volosin K, et al. A randomized controlled trial evaluating the safety and efficacy of cardiac contractility modulation in advanced heart failure. *Am Heart J.* 2011;161:329–37 e1–2.
21. Abraham WT, Kuck KH, Goldsmith RL, et al. A randomized controlled trial to evaluate the safety and efficacy of cardiac contractility modulation. *JACC Heart Fail.* 2018;6:874–83.
22. Sannino A, Smith RL, 2nd, Schiattarella GG, et al. Survival and cardiovascular outcomes of patients with secondary mitral regurgitation: a systematic review and meta-analysis. *JAMA Cardiol.* 2017;2:1130–9.
23. Maisano F, La Canna G, Colombo A, Alfieri O. The evolution from surgery to percutaneous mitral valve interventions: the role of the edge-to-edge technique. *J Am Coll Cardiol.* 2011;58:2174–82.
24. Stone GW, Lindenfeld J, Abraham WT, et al. Transcatheter mitral-valve repair in patients with heart failure. *N Engl J Med.* 2018;379:2307–18.
25. Feldman T, Foster E, Glower DD, et al. Percutaneous repair or surgery for mitral regurgitation. *N Engl J Med.* 2011;364:1395–406.
26. Obadia JF, Messika-Zeitoun D, Leurent G, et al. Percutaneous repair or medical treatment for secondary mitral regurgitation. *N Engl J Med.* 2018;379:2297–306.
27. Packer M, Grayburn PA. Contrasting effects of pharmacological, procedural, and surgical interventions on proportionate and disproportionate functional mitral regurgitation in chronic heart failure. *Circulation.* 2019;140:779–89.
28. Hasenfuss G, Hayward C, Burkhoff D, et al. A transcatheter intracardiac shunt device for heart failure with preserved ejection fraction (REDUCE LAP-HF): a multicentre, open-label, single-arm, phase 1 trial. *Lancet.* 2016;387:1298–304.
29. Kaye DM, Hasenfuss G, Neuzil P, et al. One-year outcomes after transcatheter insertion of an interatrial shunt device for the management of heart failure with preserved ejection fraction. *Circ Heart Fail.* 2016;9:1–6.
30. Feldman T, Mauri L, Kahwash R, et al. Transcatheter interatrial shunt device for the treatment of heart failure with preserved ejection fraction (REDUCE LAP-HF I [Reduce Elevated Left Atrial Pressure in Patients With Heart Failure]): a phase 2, randomized, sham-controlled trial. *Circulation.* 2018;137:364–75.
31. Shah SJ, Feldman T, Ricciardi MJ, et al. One-year safety and clinical outcomes of a transcatheter interatrial shunt device for the treatment of heart failure with preserved ejection fraction in the reduce elevated left atrial pressure in patients with heart failure (REDUCE LAP-HF I) trial: a randomized clinical trial. *JAMA Cardiol.* 2018;3:968–77.
32. Rodes-Cabau J, Bernier M, Amat-Santos IJ, et al. Interatrial shunting for heart failure: early and late results from the first-in-human experience with the V-wave system. *JACC Cardiovasc Interv.* 2018;11:2300–10.
33. Abraham WT, Zile MR, Weaver FA, et al. Baroreflex activation therapy for the treatment of heart failure with a reduced ejection fraction. *JACC Heart Fail.* 2015;3:487–96.
34. Gronda E, Seravalle G, Brambilla G, et al. Chronic baroreflex activation effects on sympathetic nerve traffic, baroreflex function, and cardiac haemodynamics in heart failure: a proof-of-concept study. *Eur J Heart Fail.* 2014;16:977–83.
35. Zile MR, Abraham WT, Weaver FA, et al. Baroreflex activation therapy for the treatment of heart failure with a reduced ejection fraction: afety and efficacy in patients with and without cardiac resynchronization therapy. *Eur J Heart Fail.* 2015;17:1066–74.
36. Zile MR, Lindenfield JW, Zannad F, Gale E, Rogers T, Abraham WT. Baroreflex activation therapy in patients with heart failure with a reduced ejection fraction. Paper presented at Heart Rhythm Society; 2019; San Francisco, CA.
37. Tse HF, Turner S, Sanders P, et al. Thoracic spinal cord stimulation for heart failure as a restorative treatment (SCS HEART study): first-in-man experience. *Heart Rhythm.* 2015;12:588–95.
38. Zipes DP, Neuzil P, Theres H, et al. Determining the feasibility of spinal cord neuromodulation for the treatment of chronic systolic heart failure: the DEFEAT-HF study. *JACC Heart Fail.* 2016;4:129–36.
39. Premchand RK, Sharma K, Mittal S, et al. Autonomic regulation therapy via left or right cervical vagus nerve stimulation in patients with chronic heart failure: results of the ANTHEM-HF trial. *J Card Fail.* 2014;20:808–16.
40. Zannad F, De Ferrari GM, Tuinenburg AE, et al. Chronic vagal stimulation for the treatment of low ejection fraction heart failure: results of the NEural Cardiac TherApy foR Heart Failure (NECTAR-HF) randomized controlled trial. *Eur Heart J.* 2015;36:425–33.
41. Gold MR, Van Veldhuisen DJ, Hauptman PJ, et al. Vagus nerve stimulation for the treatment of heart failure: the INOVATE-HF trial. *J Am Coll Cardiol.* 2016;68:149–58.
42. Premchand RK, Sharma K, Mittal S, et al. Extended follow-up of patients with heart failure receiving autonomic regulation therapy in the ANTHEM-HF study. *J Card Fail.* 2016;22:639–42.
43. Nishizaki A, Sakamoto K, Saku K, et al. Optimal titration is important to maximize the beneficial effects of vagal nerve stimulation in chronic heart failure. *J Card Fail.* 2016;22:631–8.
44. Yu CM, Wang L, Chau E, et al. Intrathoracic impedance monitoring in patients with heart failure: correlation with fluid status and feasibility of early warning preceding hospitalization. *Circulation.* 2005;112:841–8.

45. Bourge RC, Abraham WT, Adamson PB, et al. Randomized controlled trial of an implantable continuous hemodynamic monitor in patients with advanced heart failure: the COMPASS-HF study. *J Am Coll Cardiol.* 2008;51:1073–9.
46. Abraham WT, Stevenson LW, Bourge RC, et al. Sustained efficacy of pulmonary artery pressure to guide adjustment of chronic heart failure therapy: complete follow-up results from the CHAMPION randomised trial. *Lancet.* 2016;387:453–61.
47. Adamson PB, Abraham WT, Bourge RC, et al. Wireless pulmonary artery pressure monitoring guides management to reduce decompensation in heart failure with preserved ejection fraction. *Circ Heart Fail.* 2014;7:935–44.
48. Abraham J, Bharmi R, Jonsson O, et al. Association of ambulatory hemodynamic monitoring of heart failure with clinical outcomes in a concurrent matched cohort analysis. *JAMA Cardiol.* 2019;4:556–63.
49. Ritzema J, Troughton R, Melton I, et al. Physician-directed patient self-management of left atrial pressure in advanced chronic heart failure. *Circulation.* 2010;121:1086–95.
50. Abraham WT. Hemodynamic monitoring in advanced heart failure: results from the LAPTOP-HF trial. Paper presented at: HFSA; 2016; Orlando, FL.
51. Perl L, Soifer E, Bartunek J, et al. A novel wireless left atrial pressure monitoring system for patients with heart failure, first ex-vivo and animal experience. *J Cardiovasc Transl Res.* 2019;12:290–8.
52. Adamson PB, Gold MR, Bennett T, et al. Continuous hemodynamic monitoring in patients with mild to moderate heart failure: results of the Reducing Decompensation Events Utilizing Intracardiac Pressures in Patients with Chronic heart failure (REDUCEhf) trial. *Congest Heart Fail.* 2011;17:248–54.
53. van Veldhuisen DJ, Braunschweig F, Conraads V, et al. Intrathoracic impedance monitoring, audible patient alerts, and outcome in patients with heart failure. *Circulation.* 2011;124:1719–26.
54. Bohm M, Drexler H, Oswald H, et al. Fluid status telemedicine alerts for heart failure: a randomized controlled trial. *Eur Heart J.* 2016;37:3154–63.
55. Small RS, Wickemeyer W, Germany R, et al. Changes in intrathoracic impedance are associated with subsequent risk of hospitalizations for acute decompensated heart failure: clinical utility of implanted device monitoring without a patient alert. *J Card Fail.* 2009;15:475–81.
56. Whellan DJ, Ousdigian KT, Al-Khatib SM, et al. Combined heart failure device diagnostics identify patients at higher risk of subsequent heart failure hospitalizations: results from PARTNERS HF (Program to Access and Review Trending Information and Evaluate Correlation to Symptoms in Patients With Heart Failure) study. *J Am Coll Cardiol.* 2010;55:1803–10.
57. Abraham WT, Compton S, Haas G, et al. Intrathoracic impedance vs daily weight monitoring for predicting worsening heart failure events: results of the fluid accumulation status trial (FAST). *Congest Heart Fail.* 2011;17:51–5.
58. Shochat MK, Shotan A, Blondheim DS, et al. Non-invasive lung IMPEDANCE-guided preemptive treatment in chronic heart failure patients: a randomized controlled trial (IMPEDANCE-HF trial). *J Card Fail.* 2016;22:713–22.
59. Boehmer JP, Hariharan R, Devecchi FG, et al. A multisensor algorithm predicts heart failure events in patients with implanted devices: results from the MultiSENSE study. *JACC Heart Fail.* 2017;5:216–25.

Section II
Acute Decompensated Heart Failure

DOI: 10.1201/9780429244544-8

Chapter 7
PATHOPHYSIOLOGY AND CLINICAL EVALUATION OF THE PATIENT WITH ACUTE HEART FAILURE

Georgios Bakosis, Vasiliki Bistola, Eftyhia Polyzogopoulou, and John Parissis

Introduction

Acute heart failure (AHF) is a potentially life-threatening condition, with sudden and abrupt onset or aggravation of symptoms and/or signs of heart failure (HF), requiring urgent evaluation and escalation of treatment, typically through hospital admission.[1] AHF is a rather heterogeneous clinical syndrome with different clinical presentations.[2,3] Several attempts have been made over the past number of years in order to categorize AHF syndromes, using different criteria each time.

Pathophysiology

Four key pathogenetic mechanisms have been proposed in AHF: volume overload, volume redistribution, myocardial loss and cardiogenic shock, and impaired ventricular filling (Figure 7.1). We discuss these mechanisms briefly below.

Volume Overload

In acutely decompensated chronic HF, which represents ~50% of AHF cases,[4] true fluid overload is the principal pathogenetic mechanism. In this patient subgroup, pre-existing HF leads to activation of several neurohormonal pathways, including the renin-angiotensin-aldosterone system (RAAS), the sympathetic nervous system, and the arginine-vasopressin system, all of which result in sodium and fluid retention by the kidneys.[5–7] The hemodynamic consequence of increased circulating volume, i.e., elevated filling pressures, may be present sub-clinically and can be detected days or even weeks before fluid accumulation, occurring in visceral organs and lungs (with subsequent reductions in intrathoracic impedance), while excessive weight gain and symptoms of congestion become evident just before overt clinical deterioration.[5,8] In this scenario, arterial blood pressure is usually normal but in advanced cases it can be low. Clinical symptoms and signs of pulmonary congestion are usually present but not dramatic and signs and symptoms of systemic congestion (jugular venous distention, peripheral edema) are also evident. A specific trigger of HF decompensation may be identified but, sometimes, it is unprovoked and thus attributable to progressive deterioration of cardiac function and the ineffectiveness of compensatory mechanisms (Table 7.1).

Cardio-renal interactions, also known as cardio-renal syndrome (CRS), appear to play a critical role in the pathogenesis of volume overload in decompensated HF. Although traditionally low cardiac output leading to low perfusion pressure in the afferent arteriole was considered to be the main cause of renal dysfunction in AHF (CRS type 1),[9] recent data highlight the importance of increased central venous pressure (CVP) as the principal mechanism contributing to the reduction of glomerular filtration rate in AHF, through increases in renal interstitial pressure[10] and intra-abdominal pressure (CRS type 2),[11] thereby contributing to exaggeration of maladaptive sodium and water retention. Less frequently, development of AHF may result due to an acute deterioration of kidney function (CRS type 3) through increased fluid retention, intolerance to treatment with RAAS antagonists, and resistance to loop diuretics. Adverse cardio-renal interactions are frequently aggravated by precipitating factors and comorbidities, such as aging, diabetes, hypertension, atherosclerosis, anemia, etc. These factors trigger adverse pathophysiological responses (neurohormonal activation, inflammation, apoptosis, and fibrosis), which in turn compromise the function of both organs.

Recently, the role of cardio-hepatic interactions in the pathogenesis of AHF has been investigated. A similar model to CRS has been proposed, where acutely reduced cardiac output and peripheral hypoperfusion results in acute cardiogenic liver injury (cardio-hepatic syndrome [CHS] type 1), whereas gradually deteriorating systemic congestion, back- transmitted to hepatic and portal circulation, results in cardiac cirrhosis (CHS type 2).[12] Conversely, acute liver failure (CHS type 3), which is characterized by systemic inflammatory response and multiorgan involvement, may result in hyperdynamic circulation and portal hypertension that could lead to AHF development.[13]

Volume Redistribution

Fluid redistribution from systemic to pulmonary circulation, due to excessive and abrupt vasoconstriction without the presence of true volume overload, is considered the primary pathophysiologic mechanism of pulmonary congestion in the so-called "vascular" type or hypertensive AHF. Redistribution appears to be caused by venoconstriction of the systemic venous bed on one hand, which leads to the sudden displacement of plasma volume from the splanchnic and peripheral venous system (preload) to the right heart and pulmonary circulation; under normal circumstances, venous capacitance vessels contain up to 25% of the total blood volume, buffering volume overload.[14,15] On the left side, arterial vasoconstriction increases left ventricular afterload, thus reducing stroke volume and further increasing left ventricular end-diastolic pressure. This in turn can lead to increased pulmonary capillary pressures and interstitial and alveolar fluid extravasation, particularly in cases with severe diastolic dysfunction. Clinically, the primary contribution of fluid redistribution, rather than that of fluid accumulation, in hypertensive AHF is suspected by the minimal body weight increase before hospital admission reported by the majority of patients with vascular AHF (<1 kg).[4,8,16] Although the pathophysiological mechanisms leading to vasoconstriction are not fully elucidated, increased sympathetic drive, inflammation, vascular stiffness, and impaired arterial distensibility are considered to play key roles.[17,18]

Myocardial Loss—Cardiogenic Shock

In a small proportion of patients (4–12%), AHF manifests as cardiogenic shock, the most ominous type of AHF, which is characterized by low cardiac output despite adequate left ventricular filling, resulting in end-organ hypoperfusion.[1,19–21] Acute coronary syndromes (ACS), especially those with severe

DOI: 10.1201/9780429244544-9

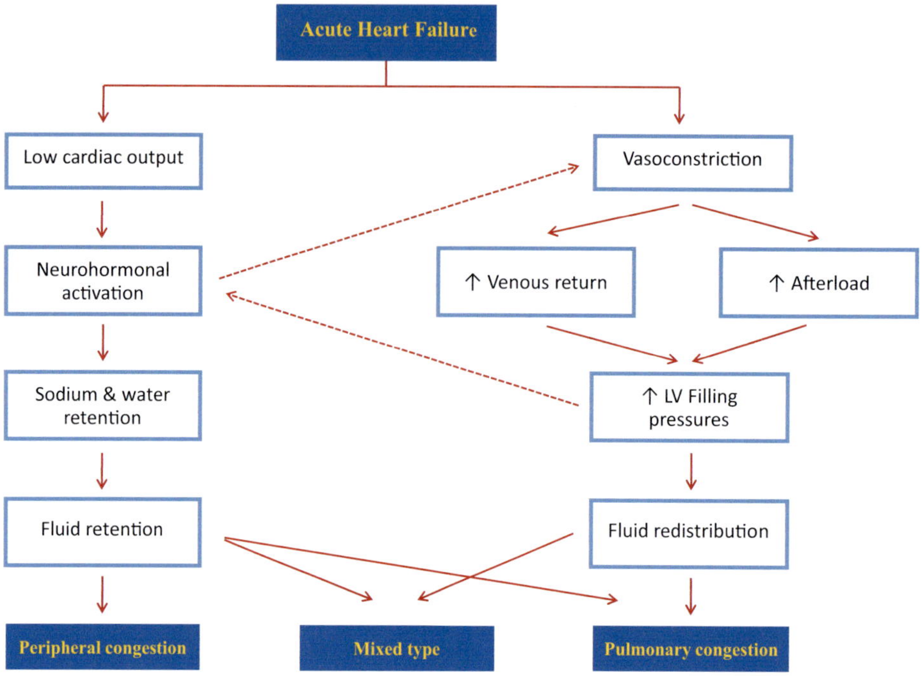

FIGURE 7.1 Pathophysiology of acute heart failure. (Modified from Farmakis et al. *The ESC Textbook of Intensive and Acute Cardiovascular Care. Acute Heart Failure: Epidemiology, Classification, and Pathophysiology.* Oxford University Press, 2018.)

TABLE 7.1: Precipitating Factors of Acute Heart Failure

I. Cardiovascular
Acute coronary syndromes (large myocardial infarction, right ventricular infarction)
Tachyarrhythmias (i.e., atrial fibrillation, ventricular tachycardia)
Bradyarrhythmias or conduction disturbances
Hypertensive crisis
Acute valve incompetence due to endocarditis or thrombosis
Myocarditis
Acute mechanical cause (myocardial rupture or acute mitral regurgitation complicating acute coronary syndromes, aortic dissection, pulmonary embolism, cardiac tamponade)
High output (shunt)
II. Non Cardiovascular
Infection/sepsis
Chronic obstructive pulmonary disease or asthma exacerbation
Renal dysfunction
Metabolic/hormonal derangements (i.e., thyroid and adrenal dysfunction, anemia)
Stress-induced cardiomyopathies (Takotsubo, peripartum)
III. Patient Related
Increased salt/fluid intake
Medication non-adherence
Drugs (e.g., nonsteroidal anti-inflammatory drugs, corticosteroids, cardiotoxic chemotherapeutics)
Alcohol
Surgery and perioperative complications

Source: Modified from Ponikowski et al. 2016 ESC Guidelines for the diagnosis and treatment of acute and chronic heart failure: The Task Force for the diagnosis and treatment of acute and chronic heart failure of the European Society of Cardiology (ESC). *Eur J Heart Fail* 2016;18:891–975.

presentation (e.g., affecting >40% of left ventricular mass, complicated with right ventricular infarction or mechanical complications), are the leading cause of cardiogenic shock (80% of cases) and are associated with the highest mortality rates. Other, less frequent etiologies of cardiogenic shock include end-stage cardiomyopathy, fulminant myocarditis, stress-induced cardiomyopathy, and drug toxicity.[22] At times, cardiac contractility may be preserved in cardiogenic shock, e.g., acute valvular disease, arrhythmias, pericardial effusion, aortic dissection, and pulmonary embolism (Table 7.2).

TABLE 7.2: **Causes of Cardiogenic Shock**

I. Impaired Cardiac Function
Acute coronary syndromes
Large MI (>40% of LV mass)
RV infarction
Acute mechanical complication
Free wall rupture
Interventricular septum rupture
Acute mitral regurgitation due to papillary muscle rupture
End-stage cardiomyopathy
Myocarditis (fulminant myocarditis)
Stress-induced cardiomyopathies (Takotsubo, peripartum)
Drug toxicity (e.g., non-steroidal anti-inflammatory drugs, corticosteroids, cardiotoxic chemotherapeutics)
Septic shock with myocardial depression
Prolonged cardiopulmonary bypass
Myocardial contusion
II. Preserved Cardiac Function
Acute valve incompetence (endocarditis, thrombosis, chordal rupture)
Arrhythmias (tachyarrhythmias, bradyarrhythmias, conduction disturbances)
Aortic dissection
Pulmonary embolism
Cardiac tamponade
Flow obstruction (hypertrophic obstructive cardiomyopathy, cardiac tumors)
Pheochromocytoma

Source: Modified from Topalian et al. Cardiogenic shock. *Crit Care Med* 2008;36:S6674.

There is growing recognition that, whereas myocardial loss and severely deteriorated cardiac function is the primary insult in most cardiogenic shock cases, peripheral vascular dysfunction, along with neurohormonal and cytokine systems activation, also seems to play a role in the perpetuation of hemodynamic derangements. Myocardial injury causes left ventricular systolic and diastolic dysfunction, resulting in increased end-diastolic pressures and wall stress, pulmonary congestion, reduced oxygenation, and impaired cellular metabolism. On the other hand, a decrease in stroke volume and cardiac output reduces coronary and peripheral perfusion, triggering catecholamine release. Compensatory sympathetic activation promotes positive inotropic and chronotropic actions, albeit at the expense of further increases in oxygen demand as well as proarrhythmic and cardiotoxic effects. Sympathetic activation in conjunction with reflex vasoconstriction of peripheral arterioles (stage I of cardiogenic shock) and activation of neurohormonal cascades promote salt and water retention in an attempt to maintain vital organ perfusion in the early stages of shock.[21,23,24] However, as compensatory mechanisms gradually fail to maintain organ function, excess release of inflammatory mediators (e.g., interleukin-6, tumor necrosis factor), due to systemic inflammatory response along with nitric oxide (NO) overproduction, cause inappropriate precapillary vasodilation, whereas venules remain constricted, resulting in microcirculation stasis (stage II/stagnant hypoxia) and severely decreased cardiac preload.[25–27] This vicious circle promotes new myocardial injury and further deterioration of myocardial performance, refractory hypotension, and irreversible end-organ dysfunction (refractory shock stage).

Impaired Ventricular Filling

Several conditions can cause AHF through reducing preload, thereby impairing ventricular filling that, according to the Frank-Starling principle, leads to reduced myocyte contraction. Characteristic examples are tachyarrhythmias that may reduce diastolic period, pericardial effusion, and restrictive cardiomyopathies.

A distinct entity, formerly known as *de novo* or new-onset HF, refers to the first manifestation of heart disease in previously asymptomatic or oligosymptomatic individuals.[28] Data from the European Heart Failure Survey II have indicated that new-onset HF accounts for approximately 20% of all AHF hospital admissions, presents more frequently as acute pulmonary edema (26% of cases), and tends to be more hypertensive on admission, in comparison to acutely decompensated HF.[19] However, *de novo* AHF may also present as cardiogenic shock in a minority of patients (6.8% of cases). Although in-hospital mortality of new-onset AHF appears to be similar or even higher (when complicated with shock), compared with acutely decompensated HF, long-term prognosis is more favorable due to the greater prevalence of reversible causes (ACS, acute myocarditis, hypertension) and lower prevalence of comorbidities.[29]

Although our understanding of AHF has evolved in recent years, not all pathophysiological adaptations leading to abnormal hemodynamic responses are totally understood as yet. To make matters more complicated, in practice, several mechanisms may be simultaneously present in the same patient. For example, whereas an ACS primarily causes myocardial injury leading to pump failure, the development of associated acute mitral insufficiency or ventricular tachyarrhythmias would deteriorate AHF, as acute volume overload and impaired ventricular filling would be superimposed on the initial insult. Therefore, the pathophysiology of AHF can be better understood if it is considered as the result of interactions between triggering factors, patients' underlying cardiac dysfunction, and activation of adaptive compensatory mechanisms, resulting in specific sets of clinical signs and symptoms. Instead, attempts to interpret AHF pathophysiology, using simplistic and unified models, appear to have become irrelevant in the current era.

Clinical Assessment of Acute Heart Failure

Due to its life-threatening nature, AHF requires immediate diagnostic assessment and early management to improve outcomes (Figure 7.2). Diagnostic evaluation of patients presenting with suspected AHF may be challenging due to the complex pathophysiology, overlapping symptoms, multiple precipitating factors, and comorbidities. Therefore, clinical judgment is required for thorough assessment of medical history, physical examination, laboratory data, and diagnostic tests to:

1. Assess the severity of AHF
2. Confirm diagnosis
3. Identify possible precipitants
4. Guide treatment

The primary target in each patient with suspected AHF is to assess hemodynamic and respiratory status and provide appropriate management if hemodynamic instability or respiratory distress are present. In such cases, urgent admission to and management in an intensive care unit is required. Assessment of vital signs (pulse oximetry and systolic blood pressure [SBP]) is the first step in the diagnostic evaluation of AHF. Unfavorable findings include low (<100 mmHg) SBP and high (>25 breaths/min) or disproportionately low (<8 breaths/min) respiratory rate despite evident dyspnea, along with accessory muscles use to augment breathing, indicating the need for supportive ventilation.[30] After initial assessment, an in-depth clinical evaluation should follow to assess the presence of symptoms and signs of HF. Clinical manifestations most frequently reflect volume overload and/or redistribution (peripheral congestion and/or pulmonary edema), and less often low cardiac output with peripheral hypoperfusion. Dyspnea of any kind (breathlessness on exertion, orthopnea, paroxysmal nocturnal dyspnea, bendopnea, nocturnal cough) indicates elevated ventricular filling pressures and is usually the main reason to seek medical help. Physical examination may reveal tachycardia, sometimes with irregular pulse, a displaced apical impulse due to cardiac enlargement and a late (S_4) or early (S_3) diastolic sound. A murmur due to valvular regurgitation may be present. Tachypnea, hypoxia, use of accessory respiratory muscles, and pathological lung auscultation (rales, crackles, dullness of lung bases due to pleural effusion, wheezing) may be present. Right-sided congestion is evident as jugular vein distention, hepatojugular reflux, bilateral peripheral edema, ascites, hepatomegaly with icterus, and increased body weight. Finally, clinical manifestations of hypoperfusion include hypotension (SBP <90 mmHg), narrow pulse pressure, cold extremities, oliguria (<30 mL/h or 0.5 mL/kg/h), dizziness, and confusion.[1]

According to a modification of the Nohria and Stevenson classification for advanced HF, patients with AHF can be classified according to the presence or absence of symptoms/signs of organ congestion ("wet" vs "dry," respectively) and hypoperfusion ("warm" vs "cold," respectively) (Table 7.3).[31] This classification allows clinicians to identify high-risk patients, carries

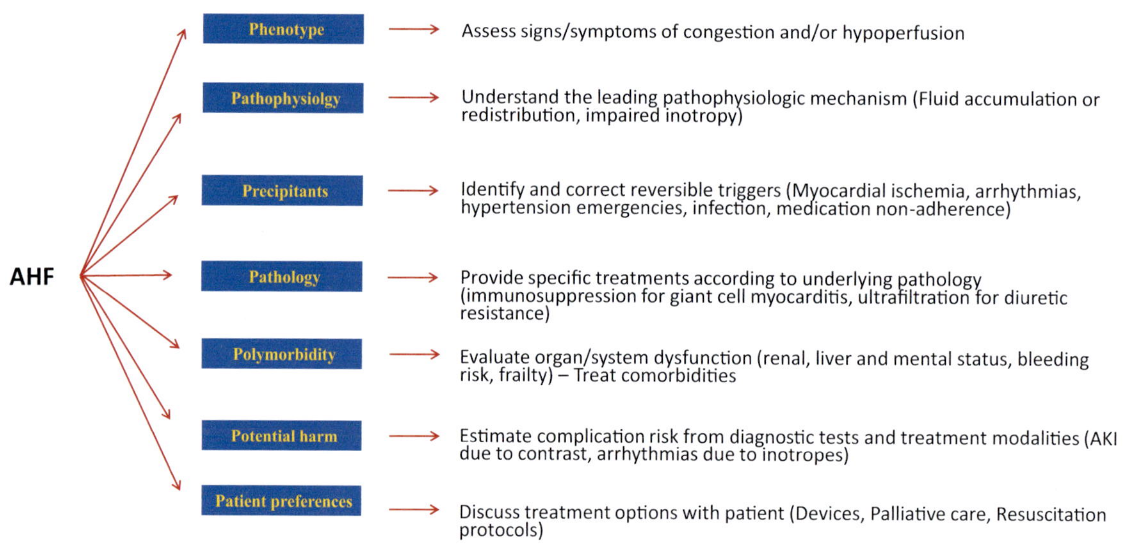

FIGURE 7.2 The seven principles for initial evaluation patients with acute heart failure. (Modified from Arrigo et al. Optimising heart failure therapies in the acute setting. *Card Fail Rev* 2018;4:38–42.)

TABLE 7.3: Clinical Profiles of Acute Heart Failure Patients Based on Volume Status and Peripheral Perfusion

		Volume Status	
		Dry	Wet
Peripheral Circulation	**Warm**	Well perfused—not congested	Well perfused and congested
	Cold	Hypoperfused—not congested	Hypoperfused and congested

Source: Modified from Ponikowski et al. 2016 ESC Guidelines for the diagnosis and treatment of acute and chronic heart failure: The Task Force for the diagnosis and treatment of acute and chronic heart failure of the European Society of Cardiology (ESC). *Eur J Heart Fail* 2016;18:891–975.

TABLE 7.4: **Typical Differences between Cardiac and Vascular Failure**

	"Cardiac" AHF	"Vascular" AHF
Mechanism	↓ Contractility	↑ Afterload and/or LV diastolic dysfunction
Main cause of symptoms	Fluid retention	Fluid redistribution
Heart failure type	Acute decompensated heart failure	*De novo*
Onset	Progressive (days)	Abrupt (hours)
Signs	Peripheral (mostly) and pulmonary congestion	Pulmonary congestion
Blood pressure	Normal or low	Normal or elevated
Left ventricular ejection fraction	Reduced	Preserved
Filling pressures	Reduced	Elevated
Cardiac output	Reduced	Normal
Body weight gain	Significant	Minimal
Type of therapy	Diuretics	Vasodilators ± diuretics
Heart failure rehospitalizations	Frequent	Occasional
Mortality	Higher	Lower

Source: Modified from Farmakis et al. *The ESC Textbook of Intensive and Acute Cardiovascular Care. Acute Heart Failure: Epidemiology, Classification, and Pathophysiology*. Oxford University Press, 2018.

TABLE 7.5: **Diagnostic Modalities for the Assessment of Patients with Acute Heart Failure**

Laboratory	Natriuretic peptides
	Troponins
	Creatinine
	Electrolytes (potassium, sodium)
	Liver function tests (transaminases, γ-glutamyl transferase, alkaline phosphatase, bilirubin, coagulation status)
	Full blood count (hemoglobin, white blood cells, platelets)
	Arterial blood gas (pH, lactate)
	D-dimers
Imaging	Chest X-ray
	Echocardiography
	Lung ultrasound
Catheterization	Pulmonary artery catheter (in selected cases)
Other	Electrocardiogram

prognostic information, and, most importantly, can guide initial treatment.[32,33] Both the American[34] and the European[1] guidelines recommend clinical classification for initial assessment of patients with suspected AHF, especially as routine invasive hemodynamic evaluation has failed to prove its efficacy to guide therapy compared with rigorous clinical assessment.[35] Patients with the "warm" and "wet" profile (50% of patients with AHF) fall into two categories: those with predominant hypertension and fluid redistribution (vascular type), who primarily require vasodilators combined with low doses of diuretics, and the normotensive patients with congestion due to fluid accumulation (cardiac type), who usually represent decompensation of chronic HF and primarily require diuretic therapy (usually at higher dose or a combination of diuretics) and low-dose vasodilators, provided blood pressure is not severely reduced (SBP >90–100 mmHg) (Table 7.4). On the other hand, "cold" and "wet" patients (up to 20% of patients with AHF), especially those with hypotension (SBP <90 mmHg), represent the highest-risk population, who require inotropic support, usually in combination with a vasopressor. In patients with refractory symptoms, despite first-line therapy, mechanical circulatory support remains the final option. Lastly, "dry" and "cold" patients (up to 5% of patients with AHF) commonly present with reduced preload due to dehydration from overdiuresis with resultant reduced cardiac output. Therefore, they initially require a fluid challenge to correct preload and to reassess perfusion status.

Laboratory Tests in the Evaluation of Acute Heart Failure

Given the limited sensitivity and specificity of the symptoms and signs of AHF, clinical evaluation should integrate information from laboratory tests.[33,36] Therefore, upon presentation, assessments shown in Table 7.5 should be performed.

Natriuretic peptides are counter-regulatory hormones with vasodilatory, lusitropic, antifibrotic, and natriuretic effects.[37,38] Circulating natriuretic peptide levels reflect elevated ventricular filling pressures and are associated with adverse outcomes in HF. Natriuretic peptides have high sensitivity but sub-optimal specificity for HF diagnosis, so that elevated levels do not confirm the diagnosis of AHF, as they may be increased under a plethora of cardiac and non-cardiac conditions (Table 7.6). On the contrary, low natriuretic peptide levels (B-type natriuretic peptide [BNP] <100 pg/mL; N-terminal pro-BNP [NT-proBNP] <300 pg/mL; or mid-regional pro-atrial natriuretic peptide [MR-proANP] <120 pg/mL) have a 98% negative predictive value for HF diagnosis. Therefore, natriuretic peptides are recommended as excellent rule-out markers for AHF in patients presenting with acute dyspnea.[39] Limitations include falsely low levels in obese patients, in very early presenters in the emergency room, in right-sided AHF, or in flash pulmonary edema commonly seen in acute mitral regurgitation.

Troponins are frequently elevated in AHF even in the absence of acute coronary syndrome, reflecting ongoing subclinical

TABLE 7.6: Causes of Elevated Levels of Natriuretic Peptides

Cardiac
Heart failure, including right ventricular failure syndromes
Acute coronary syndrome
Heart muscle disease, including left ventricular hypertrophy
Valvular heart disease
Pericardial disease
Atrial fibrillation
Myocarditis
Cardiac surgery
Cardioversion
Non-Cardiac
Advancing age
Anemia
Renal failure
Pulmonary: obstructive sleep apnea, severe pneumonia, pulmonary hypertension
Critical illness
Bacterial sepsis
Severe burns
Toxic-metabolic insults, including cancer chemotherapy and envenomation

Source: Modified from Ponikowski et al. 2016 ESC Guidelines for the diagnosis and treatment of acute and chronic heart failure: The Task Force for the diagnosis and treatment of acute and chronic heart failure of the European Society of Cardiology (ESC). *Eur J Heart Fail* 2016;18:891–975.

myocardial injury caused by elevated myocyte stretch, and neurohormonal, inflammatory and oxidative stress-induced cell death,[40–42] with resultant replacement by fibrotic tissue (remodeling).[43] Troponins are useful risk stratification markers in AHF, as abnormally elevated baseline levels have been associated with increased short- and long-term mortality and an increase of ≥20% over baseline within 24h of presentation nearly doubles mortality risk.[44] Also, evidence of ongoing ischemia may have important implications for the selection of appropriate HF therapies, such as by limiting the use of agents that may promote ischemia through increased myocardial oxygen consumption, e.g., inotropes.[45] On the other hand, other indices of neurohormonal activation, inflammation, oxidative stress, or myocardial remodeling, including adrenomedullin, sST2, and galectin 3, have not yet proven their value in routine clinical practice as prognostic markers in AHF.

Evaluation of renal function is an integral element of clinical profiling in AHF, with important therapeutic and prognostic implications. Moreover, worsening of renal function (usually defined as an increase of serum creatinine of ≥0.3 mg/dL or ≥25% from baseline levels) when associated with persistent symptoms/signs of congestion resistant to diuretic treatment is an ominous sign, portending unfavorable outcomes.[46] Abnormalities in serum electrolytes are frequent in AHF. Potassium abnormalities are associated with increased risk of arrhythmogenesis whereas hyponatremia (<135 mmol/L) may reflect advanced HF syndrome that is associated with increased risk of subsequent rehospitalizations and mortality if persistently present throughout discharge.[47]

Liver function tests may also be impaired in AHF patients due to impaired hemodynamics, resulting in reduced cardiac output and increased venous congestion. Apart from their prognostic value,[12,48] specific patterns of hepatic enzyme elevations are particularly useful in identification of the predominant pathophysiologic mechanism of liver injury. Rapid and marked elevation of transaminases (>10×–20× of the upper reference limit), along with bilirubin increases, indicate shock liver with centrocellular hepatocyte damage and necrosis due to hypoperfusion (CHS I),[49,50] whereas cholestatic liver dysfunction with primarily elevated gamma-glutamyl transferase and alkaline phosphatase activities is mainly related to right-sided congestion (CHS II).[51]

Hematologic parameters (complete blood count) may reveal anemia or underlying infection. Arterial blood gas is particularly helpful to assess respiratory or metabolic acidosis in cases with persistent respiratory distress,[52] although serum lactate is considered to be a good prognosticator of outcome in shock.[53] D-dimer testing is indicated in patients with suspected acute pulmonary embolism.

An electrocardiogram upon admission is rarely normal in AHF.[54] Although sinus tachycardia is the most common and non-specific finding, a 12-lead electrocardiogram can also be diagnostic of specific precipitants of AHF, including myocardial ischemia, rapid atrial fibrillation, ventricular arrhythmias, and conduction disturbances.

Imaging in Acute Heart Failure

Imaging modalities used in the assessment of AHF include chest X-ray, echocardiography, and, recently, lung ultrasound. Chest X-ray is mostly used for the detection of pulmonary congestion (pulmonary vascular redistribution, peri-bronchial cuffing, Kerley's B lines, batwing pattern, pleural effusion, or cardiomegaly). However, interpretation of results is highly subjective, with it being nearly normal in about 20% of cases.[55,56] Chest X-ray may also identify non-cardiac conditions that can cause or contribute to patients' symptoms, such as pneumonia or pneumothorax.

Immediate echocardiography is mandatory for patients with hemodynamic instability or for patients with AHF suspected to be caused by acute mechanical cause (free wall rupture, ventricular septal defect, or acute mitral regurgitation complicating acute coronary syndrome, acute native or prosthetic valve dysfunction, aortic dissection, pulmonary embolism, or cardiac tamponade). Otherwise, comprehensive echocardiography (within 24 h of admission) should be considered in all patients with *de novo* AHF or in cases of altered cardiac structure and function with a particular interest in the evaluation of left ventricular ejection fraction, valvular abnormalities, filling pressures (E/e' ratio) and volume status (inferior vena cava diameter and collapsibility index).

Accumulating evidence highlights the importance of lung ultrasound as a useful method in the evaluation of lung congestion (bilateral b-lines) in AHF.[57,58] Moreover, a rapid cardiothoracic ultrasound protocol, combining sequential assessment of cardiac filling pressures by echocardiography with severity of pulmonary congestion, can monitor volume status and possibly guide decongestive therapy, resulting in faster and more efficient decongestion, with resultant abbreviated hospital stay.[59–61]

Due to advances in non-invasive modalities, routine use of pulmonary artery catheter may be considered currently only in selected patients with refractory symptoms despite initial intravenous therapies, in order to directly assess the patient's hemodynamics.[1,35]

Conclusion

Acute heart failure is a potentially life-threatening clinical syndrome which requires prompt diagnosis and initiation of treatment to prevent dismal outcomes. Understanding its pathophysiology is a key element toward this goal. Congestion is the hallmark of AHF, either due to "cardiac" failure and fluid retention or due to "vascular" failure, resulting in fluid redistribution. Myocardial loss leading to cardiac pump incompetence, hemodynamic compromise, and end-organ dysfunction (cardiogenic shock) is a rarer but much more severe contributing mechanism. Frequently, though, several mechanisms coexist in the same patient, leading to complex clinical manifestations and often making differential diagnosis challenging. An in-depth clinical evaluation is required to confirm the diagnosis, assess its severity, and identify and treat possible precipitants. A detailed medical history, along with physical examination, with specific interest in early detection of signs and/or symptoms of congestion and organ hypoperfusion, is recommended, while natriuretic peptide testing, combined with cardio-thoracic echocardiography, can promote early diagnosis and guide therapy already in the emergency room.

References

1. Ponikowski P, Voors AA, Anker SD, et al. 2016 ESC guidelines for the diagnosis and treatment of acute and chronic heart failure: the task force for the diagnosis and treatment of acute and chronic heart failure of the European Society of Cardiology (ESC) developed with the special contribution of the Heart Failure Association (HFA) of the ESC. *Eur Heart J.* 2016;37:2129–200.
2. Gheorghiade M, Filippatos G, De Luca L, Burnett J. Congestion in acute heart failure syndromes: an essential target of evaluation and treatment. *Am J Med.* 2006;119 Supplement 1:S3–S10.
3. Weintraub NL, Collins SP, Pang PS, et al. Acute heart failure syndromes: emergency department presentation, treatment, and disposition: current approaches and future aims: a scientific statement from the American Heart Association. *Circulation.* 2010;122:1975–96.
4. Chaudhry SI, Wang Y, Concato J, Gill TM, Krumholz HM. Patterns of weight change preceding hospitalization for heart failure. *Circulation.* 2007;116:1549–54.
5. Adamson PB. Pathophysiology of the transition from chronic compensated and acute decompensated heart failure: new insights from continuous monitoring devices. *Curr Heart Fail Rep.* 2009;6:287–92.
6. McKie PM, Schirger JA, Costello-Boerrigter LC, et al. Impaired natriuretic and renal endocrine response to acute volume expansion in pre-clinical systolic and diastolic dysfunction. *J Am Coll Cardiol.* 2011;58:2095–103.
7. Nijst P, Verbrugge FH, Grieten L, et al. The pathophysiological role of interstitial sodium in heart failure. *J Am Coll Cardiol.* 2015;65:378–88.
8. Zile MR, Bennett TD, St John Sutton M, et al. Transition from chronic compensated to acute decompensated heart failure: pathophysiological insights obtained from continuous monitoring of intracardiac pressures. *Circulation.* 2008;118:1433–41.
9. Ljungman S, Laragh JH, Cody RJ. Role of the kidney in congestive heart failure. Relationship of cardiac index to kidney function. *Drugs.* 1990;39 Suppl 4:10–21; discussion 22–4.
10. Mullens W, Abrahams Z, Francis GS, et al. Importance of venous congestion for worsening of renal function in advanced decompensated heart failure. *J Am Coll Cardiol.* 2009;53:589–96.
11. Verbrugge FH, Dupont M, Steels P, et al. Abdominal contributions to cardiorenal dysfunction in congestive heart failure. *J Am Coll Cardiol.* 2013;62:485–95.
12. Poelzl G, Ess M, Mussner-Seeber C, et al. Liver dysfunction in chronic heart failure: prevalence, characteristics and prognostic significance. *Eur J Clin Invest.* 2012;42:153–63.
13. Zamora Nava LE, Aguirre Valadez J, Chavez-Tapia NC, Torre A. Acute-on-chronic liver failure: a review. *Ther Clin Risk Manag.* 2014;10:295–303.
14. Greenway CV. Role of splanchnic venous system in overall cardiovascular homeostasis. *Fed Proc.* 1983;42:1678–84.
15. Arrigo M, Parissis JT, Akiyama E, Mebazaa A. Understanding acute heart failure: pathophysiology and diagnosis. *European Heart Journal Supplements.* 2016;18:G11–8.
16. Yu CM, Chan JY, Zhang Q, et al. Biventricular pacing in patients with bradycardia and normal ejection fraction. *N Engl J Med.* 2009;361:2123–34.
17. Colombo PC, Onat D, Sabbah HN. Acute heart failure as "acute endothelitis"—Interaction of fluid overload and endothelial dysfunction. *Eur J Heart Fail.* 2008;10:170–5.
18. Ponikowski P, Jankowska EA. Pathogenesis and clinical presentation of acute heart failure. *Rev Esp Cardiol (Engl Ed).* 2015;68:331–7.
19. Nieminen MS, Brutsaert D, Dickstein K, et al. EuroHeart failure survey II (EHFS II): a survey on hospitalized acute heart failure patients: description of population. *Eur Heart J.* 2006;27:2725–36.
20. Mebazaa A, Parissis J, Porcher R, et al. Short-term survival by treatment among patients hospitalized with acute heart failure: the global ALARM-HF registry using propensity scoring methods. *Intensive Care Med.* 2011;37:290–301.
21. van Diepen S, Katz JN, Albert NM, et al. Contemporary management of cardiogenic shock: a scientific statement from the American Heart Association. *Circulation.* 2017;136:e232–68.
22. Topalian S, Ginsberg F, Parrillo JE. Cardiogenic shock. *Crit Care Med.* 2008;36 Supplement:S66–74.
23. Reynolds HR, Hochman JS. Cardiogenic shock: current concepts and improving outcomes. *Circulation.* 2008;117:686–97.
24. Thiele H, Allam B, Chatellier G, Schuler G, Lafont A. Shock in acute myocardial infarction: the cape horn for trials? *Eur Heart J.* 2010;31:1828–35.
25. de Werra I, Jaccard C, Corradin SB, et al. Cytokines, nitrite/nitrate, soluble tumor necrosis factor receptors, and procalcitonin concentrations: comparisons in patients with septic shock, cardiogenic shock, and bacterial pneumonia. *Crit Care Med.* 1997;25:607–13.
26. Geppert A, Steiner A, Zorn G, et al. Multiple organ failure in patients with cardiogenic shock is associated with high plasma levels of interleukin-6. *Crit Care Med.* 2002;30:1987–94.
27. Hochman JS. Cardiogenic shock complicating acute myocardial infarction: expanding the paradigm. *Circulation.* 2003;107:2998–3002.
28. Hunt SA, Abraham WT, Chin MH, et al. ACC/AHA 2005 guideline update for the diagnosis and management of chronic heart failure in the adult: a report of the American College of Cardiology/American Heart Association Task Force on Practice Guidelines (Writing Committee to Update the 2001 Guidelines for the Evaluation and Management of Heart Failure): developed in collaboration with the American College of Chest Physicians and the International Society for Heart and Lung Transplantation: endorsed by the Heart Rhythm Society. *Circulation.* 2005;112:e154–235.
29. Tavazzi L, Maggioni AP, Lucci D, et al. Nationwide survey on acute heart failure in cardiology ward services in Italy. *Eur Heart J.* 2006;27:1207–15.
30. Chun S, Tu JV, Wijeysundera HC, et al. Lifetime analysis of hospitalizations and survival of patients newly admitted with heart failure. *Circ Heart Fail.* 2012;5:414–21.
31. Nohria A, Tsang SW, Fang JC, et al. Clinical assessment identifies hemodynamic profiles that predict outcomes in patients admitted with heart failure. *J Am Coll Cardiol.* 2003;41:1797–804.
32. Chioncel O, Mebazaa A, Maggioni AP, et al. Acute heart failure congestion and perfusion status - impact of the clinical classification on in-hospital and long-term outcomes; insights from the ESC-EORP-HFA Heart Failure Long-Term Registry. *Eur J Heart Fail.* 2019;21:1338–52.

33. Drazner MH, Hellkamp AS, Leier CV, et al. Value of clinician assessment of hemodynamics in advanced heart failure: the ESCAPE trial. *Circ Heart Fail.* 2008;1:170–7.
34. Yancy CW, Jessup M, Bozkurt B, et al. ACCF/AHA guideline for the management of heart failure: executive summary: a report of the American College of Cardiology Foundation/American Heart Association Task Force on practice guidelines. *Circulation.* 2013;128:1810–52.
35. Binanay C, Califf RM, Hasselblad V, et al. Evaluation study of congestive heart failure and pulmonary artery catheterization effectiveness: the ESCAPE trial. *JAMA.* 2005;294:1625–33.
36. Stevenson LW, Perloff JK. The limited reliability of physical signs for estimating hemodynamics in chronic heart failure. *JAMA.* 1989;261:884–8.
37. Hobbs RE, Mills RM. Endogenous B-type natriuretic peptide: a limb of the regulatory response to acutely decompensated heart failure. *Clin Cardiol.* 2008;31:407–12.
38. Maisel A, Mueller C, Adams K, Jr., et al. State of the art: using natriuretic peptide levels in clinical practice. *Eur J Heart Fail.* 2008;10:824–39.
39. Peacock WFt, De Marco T, Fonarow GC, et al. Cardiac troponin and outcome in acute heart failure. *N Engl J Med.* 2008;358:2117–26.
40. Bott-Flugel L, Weig HJ, Uhlein H, et al. Quantitative analysis of apoptotic markers in human end-stage heart failure. *Eur J Heart Fail.* 2008;10:129–32.
41. Januzzi JL, Jr., Filippatos G, Nieminen M, Gheorghiade M. Troponin elevation in patients with heart failure: on behalf of the third Universal Definition of Myocardial Infarction Global Task Force: heart failure section. *Eur Heart J.* 2012;33:2265–71.
42. Tsutsui H, Kinugawa S, Matsushima S. Oxidative stress and heart failure. *Am J Physiol Heart Circ Physiol.* 2011;301:H2181–90.
43. Biolo A, Fisch M, Balog J, et al. Episodes of acute heart failure syndrome are associated with increased levels of troponin and extracellular matrix markers. *Circ Heart Fail.* 2010;3:44–50.
44. Metra M, Cotter G, Davison BA, et al. Effect of serelaxin on cardiac, renal, and hepatic biomarkers in the relaxin in acute heart failure (RELAX-AHF) development program: correlation with outcomes. *J Am Coll Cardiol.* 2013;61:196–206.
45. Metra M, Felker GM, Zaca V, et al. Acute heart failure: multiple clinical profiles and mechanisms require tailored therapy. *Int J Cardiol.* 2010;144:175–9.
46. Metra M, Davison B, Bettari L, et al. Is worsening renal function an ominous prognostic sign in patients with acute heart failure? The role of congestion and its interaction with renal function. *Circ Heart Fail.* 2012;5:54–62.
47. Gheorghiade M, Rossi JS, Cotts W, et al. Characterization and prognostic value of persistent hyponatremia in patients with severe heart failure in the ESCAPE Trial. *Arch Intern Med.* 2007;167:1998–2005.
48. Nikolaou M, Parissis J, Yilmaz MB, et al. Liver function abnormalities, clinical profile, and outcome in acute decompensated heart failure. *Eur Heart J.* 2013;34:742–9.
49. Ebert EC. Hypoxic liver injury. *Mayo Clin Proc.* 2006;81:1232–6.
50. Henrion J, Schapira M, Luwaert R, et al. Hypoxic hepatitis: clinical and hemodynamic study in 142 consecutive cases. *Medicine (Baltimore).* 2003;82:392–406.
51. Auer J. What does the liver tell us about the failing heart? *Eur Heart J.* 2013;34:711–4.
52. Masip J, De Mendoza D, Planas K, et al. Peripheral venous blood gases and pulse-oximetry in acute cardiogenic pulmonary oedema. *Eur Heart J Acute Cardiovasc Care.* 2012;1:275–80.
53. Harjola VP, Lassus J, Sionis A, et al. Clinical picture and risk prediction of short-term mortality in cardiogenic shock. *Eur J Heart Fail.* 2015;17:501–9.
54. Wang CS, FitzGerald JM, Schulzer M, Mak E, Ayas NT. Does this dyspneic patient in the emergency department have congestive heart failure? *JAMA.* 2005;294:1944–56.
55. Chakko S, Woska D, Martinez H, et al. Clinical, radiographic, and hemodynamic correlations in chronic congestive heart failure: conflicting results may lead to inappropriate care. *Am J Med.* 1991;90:353–9.
56. Collins SP, Lindsell CJ, Storrow AB, et al. Prevalence of negative chest radiography results in the emergency department patient with decompensated heart failure. *Ann Emerg Med.* 2006;47:13–8.
57. Al Deeb M, Barbic S, Featherstone R, Dankoff J, Barbic D. Point-of-care ultrasonography for the diagnosis of acute cardiogenic pulmonary edema in patients presenting with acute dyspnea: a systematic review and meta-analysis. *Acad Emerg Med.* 2014;21:843–52.
58. Russell FM, Rutz M, Pang PS. Focused ultrasound in the emergency department for patients with acute heart failure. *Card Fail Rev.* 2015;1:83–6.
59. Palazzuoli A, Ruocco G, Beltrami M, Nuti R, Cleland JG. Combined use of lung ultrasound, B-type natriuretic peptide, and echocardiography for outcome prediction in patients with acute HFrEF and HFpEF. *Clin Res Cardiol.* 2018;107:586–96.
60. Ohman J, Harjola VP, Karjalainen P, Lassus J. Focused echocardiography and lung ultrasound protocol for guiding treatment in acute heart failure. *ESC Heart Fail.* 2018;5:120–8.
61. Price S, Platz E, Cullen L, et al. Expert consensus document: echocardiography and lung ultrasonography for the assessment and management of acute heart failure. *Nat Rev Cardiol.* 2017;14:427–40.

Chapter 8
THERAPEUTIC APPROACHES IN ACUTE HEART FAILURE

Getu Teressa, Rachel A. Bright, and Andreas P. Kalogeropoulos

Background and Epidemiology

Although no universal definition of acute heart failure (AHF) exists, it can be defined as new- onset or decompensation of chronic signs and symptoms of heart failure (HF), requiring unscheduled care or hospital admission.[1] Although the word "acute" suggests a sudden onset of symptoms, many patients might have a more subacute course, with gradual worsening of symptoms that ultimately reach a level of severity sufficient to seek acute medical care. Chapter 7 describes in more detail the distribution of the various forms and presentations of AHF.

More than 80% of patients presenting to an emergency department (ED) with AHF in the United States are admitted for inpatient management,[2] leading to ~1 million hospitalizations per year, an incidence which has remained unchanged over the past two to three decades (Figure 8.1).[3] Hospitalization for AHF accounts for the single largest proportion of HF expenditure.[4] Likewise, patients with AHF admitted to the hospital have increasing non-cardiovascular comorbidities.[5] In-hospital mortality for AHF is unacceptably high and is greater than that for acute myocardial infarction, ranging from 2% to 20%.[6] Furthermore, AHF hospitalization is a sentinel event associated with high rates of morbidity, re-hospitalization, and mortality that remain high for more than one year, compared with stable outpatients with chronic HF.[7,8] The rates of mortality and readmission during the first 60–90 days of the post-discharge period, termed the "vulnerable phase," are particularly high, and approaches 15%–30%, respectively.[9–11] Therefore, the care of AHF patients, and their proper transition to the community, plays a crucial role in shaping outcomes among patients with HF.

Initial Management in the Emergency Department

Overview

The most important initial goals of care are early diagnosis, identification of precipitants that need urgent management (e.g., acute coronary syndrome), clinical stabilization, and treatment to improve symptoms. The hemodynamic and respiratory status of patients with AHF should be assessed promptly via history taking and physical examination. The clinical condition is classified based on the findings of bedside physical examination, aiming mainly to detect clinical signs/symptoms of congestion ("wet" or "dry") and tissue perfusion ("warm" or "cold") according to the Forrester classification (Chapter 7).[12]

Symptoms and signs of poor perfusion are present in about 5% of patients with AHF and may require advanced therapy, discussed in Chapter 9. Most patients exhibit congestion and good peripheral perfusion ("warm and wet" clinical profile), representing nearly all patients with HF and preserved ejection fraction (HFpEF) and over 80% of patients with HF and reduced ejection fraction (HFrEF), and the therapeutic approaches are discussed in this chapter. Despite the heterogeneity of patient profiles, the goals for and approaches to AHF management in the ED follow general principles (Table 8.1). Although no single, universal approach exists, Figure 8.2 can provide guidance to frontline care providers in the initial management of AHF patients.

As part of the initial management, coexisting life-threatening triggers of AHF (discussed in detail in Chapter 7) and other clinically comorbid conditions should be identified and managed urgently. Most AHF episodes have identifiable triggers. Data from 256 US hospitals in the OPTIMIZE-HF study revealed that over 60% of AHF patients had one or more triggers.[13] Ascertaining the precipitating factors early in the treatment course may allow for further risk stratification of AHF patients and may provide a guide for both inpatient and immediate post- hospitalization management (Table 8.2).[13,14]

Risk Stratification and Disposition from the Emergency Department

Disposition of AHF patients from the ED is complex and challenging, as a wide spectrum of clinical and non-clinical, social determinants of health must be considered. AHF patients who are discharged from the ED may have substantial risk of early mortality,[15] repeat ED visits, and non-elective hospitalizations[16] compared with hospitalized AHF patients. This is paradoxical, as ED physicians are more likely to discharge low-risk AHF patients. This highlights the complexity of disposition decision making and the need for a risk-stratification tool to assist ED physicians in identifying low-risk AHF patients safe for direct discharge from the ED. Although there are risk scores specifically developed for ED AHF patients,[17–19] robust validation studies are still needed before these tools can be used in practice. Furthermore, there is a paucity of data on outcomes of AHF management in ED Observation Units or specialized outpatient same-day access clinics (SDACs) for IV diuresis, strategies which are being entertained as alternatives to hospitalizations. Given the high proportion of patients currently admitted from the ED and significant post-hospitalization mortality and morbidity rates, an ED-SDAC-Home or ED Observation Unit-Home route is an attractive care strategy and transition pathway for low-risk patients that can potentially address the multiple challenges of AHF management.[20] Until this is realized, patient profiles indicating elevated, immediate, and short-term clinical risk currently dictate hospitalization (Table 8.3). It should be noted, however, that the absence of high-risk features does not necessarily mean the patient is low risk for discharge from the ED.

For admitted patients, ICU/CCU vs general ward admission should be considered. High-risk patients, as well as those who require intubation, have signs/symptoms of hypoperfusion, have persistently low O_2 saturation (<90%), are using accessory muscles to breathe, have heart rate <40 or >130bpm, or systolic BP <90 mmHg should be considered for ICU/CCU admission.

Acute Respiratory Failure: Oxygen Therapy and Ventilatory Support

Acute respiratory failure is defined as hypoxia (SpO_2<90% or PaO_2<60 mmHg), respiratory distress (increased work of breathing, respiratory rate >25 breaths/minute), or hypercapnia

DOI: 10.1201/9780429244544-10

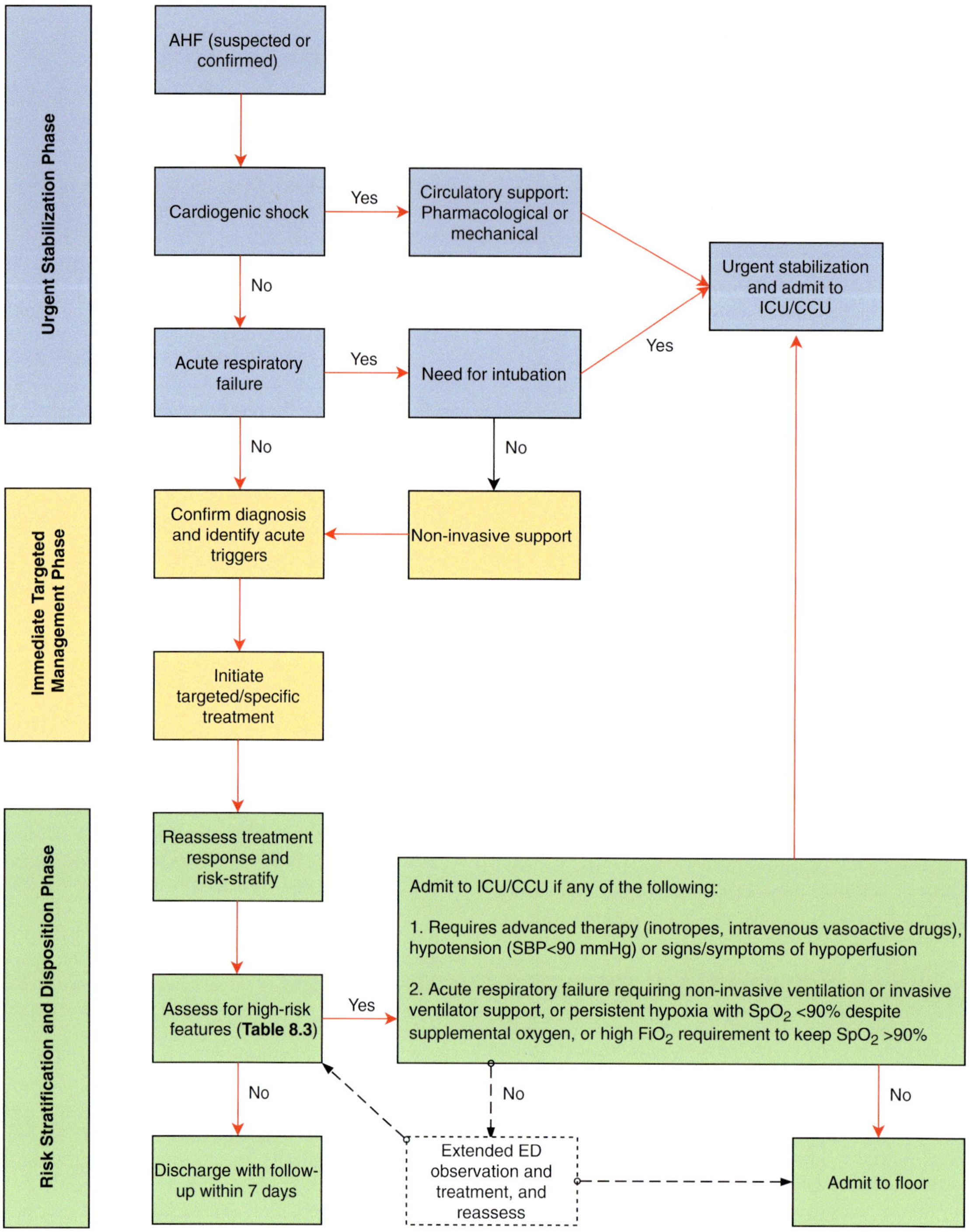

FIGURE 8.1 Proposed algorithm for the initial management of AHF patients in the ED. *Abbreviations*: AHF: acute heart failure; CCU: cardiac care unit; ED: emergency department; FiO_2: fractional inspired O_2 concentration; ICU: intensive care unit; SBP: systolic blood pressure; SpO_2: oxygen saturation.

($PaCO_2$ >50 mmHg and arterial pH <7.35). Signs of increased work of breathing are subjective assessments that include accessory muscle use and retractions, paradoxical abdominal breathing, inability to speak full sentences (or sentences interrupted by labored breath), which may be associated with diaphoresis, restlessness/agitation, or decline in mental status.

Patients presenting with AHF should have transcutaneous measurement of O_2 saturation (SpO_2) (class I, Level C). Measurement of blood gas (to obtain PaO_2, $PaCO_2$, and pH) should be considered, especially in patients with acute pulmonary edema or history of lung disease (class IIa, Level C). Although dyspnea/breathlessness is a chief complaint in 90% of patients with AHF,[21] and some degree of pulmonary and/or alveolar edema may be observed in most patients,[22] less than half of AHF patients present with acute respiratory failure.[23] The latter is observed in the setting of cardiogenic pulmonary edema (CPE) and in the presence of concomitant pulmonary conditions such as chroming lung disease, asthma, pneumonia,

TABLE 8.1: Phases of Initial Management of Patients with Acute Heart Failure in the Emergency Department

Phase	Goal of Emergency Department Management
I. Urgent Stabilization Phase	Ensure stability of Airway, Breathing, and Circulation or resuscitate immediately
II. Immediate Targeted/ Specific Therapy	Ensure diagnosis of acute heart failure and begin treatment.
	Identify acute triggers and treat any other potential life threats (i.e., ST-elevation myocardial dysfunction, dysrhythmias)
	Consider the potential contribution of other co-morbid conditions and whether they require urgent treatment
III. Risk Stratification and Disposition Phase	Re-evaluate improvement in symptoms, hemodynamics, and respiratory status
	Assess for high-risk features (Table 8.3)
	Disposition planning (Discharge, Observation, Admission to ward or ICU/CCU)

Abbreviations: CCU: coronary care unit; ICU: intensive care unit.

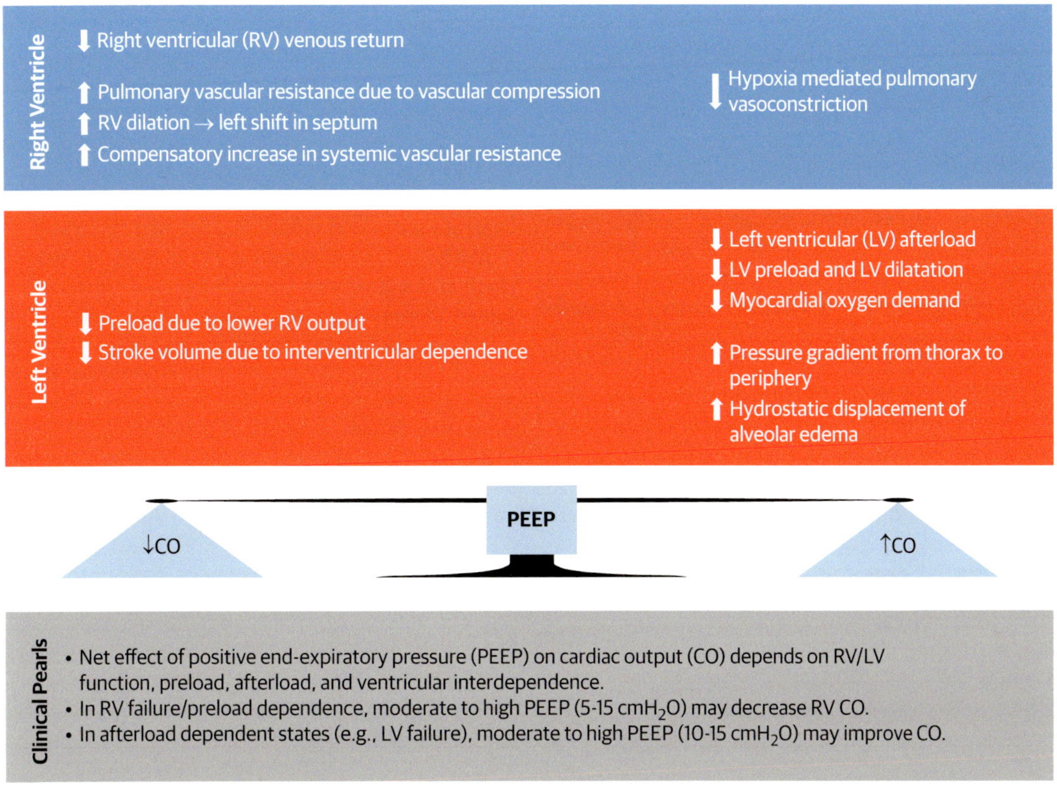

FIGURE 8.2 Potential physiological effects of positive end-expiratory pressure on ventricular function and cardiac output. Positive end-expiratory pressure (PEEP) will have variable effects on cardiac output (CO) depending on left ventricular (LV) and right ventricular (RV) function, preload, and filling pressures. Note that, in patients with noncompliant lungs from causes other than cardiogenic pulmonary edema, the effect of PEEP on pleural pressure and preload might not be as pronounced. (Reproduced with permission from Alviar et al. *J Am Coll Cardiol*. 2018;72(13):1532–53.)

or pulmonary embolism.[22,24] CPE is characterized by accumulation of protein-poor fluid in the pulmonary interstitial and alveolar spaces, impairing gas exchange and resulting in shunt-like physiology. This usually occurs in the setting of an acute rise in pulmonary capillary pressure resulting in transvascular fluid filtration that overwhelms the lymphatic interstitial drainage capacity.[25,26] "Flash" pulmonary edema is used to describe a particularly dramatic progression to severe AHF, often progressing within minutes to a life-threatening condition. The pathophysiology is similar to CPE, but "flash" pulmonary edema is associated with pulmonary capillary stress failure and increased permeability manifesting as high-permeability edema and/or alveolar hemorrhage. The fluid has higher concentration of protein than would be expected in CPE.[27] Nonetheless, the therapeutic goal and management is similar to CPE.[27] The common triggers for pulmonary edema are hypertensive crisis, acute myocardial ischemia/infarction, acute aortic regurgitation, and acute mitral regurgitation.

Oxygen Therapy

Supplemental O_2, which has long been the cornerstone of acute cardiac care, is currently losing traction. Small studies in stable HFrEF[28,29] and AHF with HFrEF[30] indicated that hyperoxia or routine use of supplemental O_2 in normoxemic patients is associated with detrimental physiological effects such as decreased cardiac output[28–30] and increased systemic vascular resistance.[28,29] A more contemporary pilot study in AHF patients randomized to high vs low SpO_2 targets showed

TABLE 8.2: Common Precipitating Factors in Acute Heart Failure

Acute coronary syndrome
Arrhythmia (most commonly, atrial fibrillation)
Uncontrolled blood pressure
Infection (especially pneumonia)
Exacerbation of chronic lung disease
Worsening renal function
Medication non-adherence
Non-adherence to dietary restrictions (debatable)

no observed differences in NT-proBNP or dyspnea changes 72 hours post-randomization, and there were no differences in in-hospital mortality or 30-day HF readmission rates.[31] Further studies with larger sample sizes are warranted to determine the efficacy and safety of O_2 therapy in AHF. Given no demonstrable benefit weighed against a risk of potential harm, supplemental O_2 should be avoided in normoxemic AHF patients. Hyper-oxygenation could also suppress the ventilatory drive and lead to hypercapnia in AHF patients with concomitant chronic lung disease. Therefore, O_2 therapy is recommended only in hypoxic AHF patients (class I, Level C) most commonly by use of standard nasal cannulas (delivers maximum flow of 6 L/min) or high-flow nasal cannulas (deliver warmed, humidified O_2 up to 60 L/min) or low-flow reservoir masks. High-flow nasal cannulas have the added advantage of providing 3–5 cmH_2O of positive end-expiratory pressure in patients with increased work in breathing.

Ventilatory Support

Non-invasive ventilation (NIV) refers to positive pressure ventilation via a non-invasive interface (full facemasks, oronasal masks, nasal mask, or nasal prongs) rather than through an invasive endotracheal tube. In patients with AHF complicated by acute respiratory failure, especially CPE, NIV improves outcomes such as hospital mortality and decreases rate of mechanical/invasive ventilation compared with standard medical care alone,[32–34] although some studies have shown neutral effects on mortality in contrast to series of meta-analyses.[35,36]

NIV can be delivered either through continuous positive airway pressure (CPAP) or bi-level positive airway pressure (BiPAP), with no clear advantage of one technique over the other.[34,37,38] BiPAP delivers both inspiratory and expiratory positive airway pressure and may be more effective in those with hypercapnia; however, there is insufficient data in these subgroups of patients with AHF complicated by ARF.

There is a lack of consensus across HF guidelines regarding the indications for NIV use. The American College of Cardiology Foundation/American Heart Association guidelines do not make any specific statements. The NICE (British) guideline recommends not routinely using NIV in people with AHF and CPE but advises to consider starting NIV without delay if there is CPE associated with severe dyspnea and acidemia. This is different from the recent European Society of Cardiology (ESC) guidelines, which recommend considering NIV as early as possible in patients with respiratory distress (respiratory rate >25 breaths/minute, SpO_2<90%) to alleviate breathlessness and reduce the rate of mechanical intubation.

Mechanical endotracheal intubation is recommended if there is contraindication of NIV (Table 8.4) or if respiratory failure cannot be managed non-invasively (after a 60–90 min NIV trial) as demonstrated by persistent or worsening hypoxia, hypercapnia, acidosis, respiratory distress, or development or worsening of altered mental status, progressive signs of fatigue, or persistent hemodynamic instability.[39]

Despite limited data and consensus on the indication and best strategy for ventilator support in acute respiratory failure complicating AHF, there is an increasing use of NIV in AHF/CPE populations[40] with substantial variation across hospital centers.[41] In practice, management strategies are largely extrapolated from data from acute respiratory failure due to primary pulmonary disorders.[42] Therefore, this poses limitations on any

TABLE 8.3: High-Risk Features Requiring Hospital Admission (i.e., Patients Are Not Candidates for Discharge from the Emergency Department)

*Hypotension (SBP <90 mmHg) with or without signs of hypoperfusion, heart rate >120–130 bmp or <40–50 bpm, or electrical instability
Acute respiratory failure (SpO_2 < 90–92%, PaO_2<60 mmHg, respiratory rate >25 breaths/min)
New-onset heart failure
Presence of concomitant acute or chronic comorbidities
Renal dysfunction, estimated glomerular filtration rate <50 mL/min/1.73 m^2
Liver dysfunction
Sepsis
Stroke
Hemodynamically significant arrythmia
Severe aortic stenosis or other severe valvular disease
Pneumonia
Other predictors of elevated risk
Elevated cardiac troponin with or without acute coronary syndrome
Marked natriuretic peptide elevations or other signs or symptoms of marked congestion
Major electrolyte disturbances
Unclear triggers for decompensation of chronic heart failure or inability to address the trigger in the ED setting
Absence of information about chronic therapies and comorbidities
Inadequate response to initial ED-based therapy or after more prolonged surveillance in the observation unit
Barriers to self-care, limitations of support in the home environment, or inability for post-ED discharge medical follow-up

* Patients with advanced heart failure may have low (<90 mmHg) SBP at baseline. Evaluation should rather be guided by careful assessment of organ perfusion and volume status.

Abbreviations: ED: emergency department; SBP: systolic blood pressure.

TABLE 8.4: Contraindications to Non-Invasive Ventilation and Indications for Mechanical Positive Pressure Ventilation in the Setting of Acute Respiratory Failure Requiring Positive Pressure Ventilation

Cardiac or respiratory arrest, or impending hemodynamic or respiratory collapse
Refractory hypotension
Aspiration risk (vomiting, inability to control secretions, or expectorating copious secretions)
Inability to keep patient airway open (uncontrolled agitation, coma or altered mental status, seizures)
Facial deformities because of pathology, recent surgery, or trauma
Non-respiratory multi-organ failure
Upper gastrointestinal bleeding
Recent upper gastrointestinal or airway surgery
Reduced respiratory drive
Isolated right ventricular failure

untailored application to the AHF population, whose hemodynamics are sensitive to the complex interaction between positive pressure ventilation and cardiopulmonary physiologies. Physicians managing AHF patients complicated by acute respiratory failure should be aware of the cardiopulmonary physiological effects of positive pressure ventilation and its cumulative effect on cardiac output.[43] When positive pressure is used during either non-invasive or endotracheal ventilation, blood pressure, as well as other markers of alterations in cardiac output, should be closely monitored.

Pharmacotherapy

Therapeutic options for chronic HFrEF are well delineated and are grounded in strong clinical trial evidence. In contrast, therapy for AHF has been met with largely negative or neutral clinical trials. The goal of pharmacotherapy in AHF centers on relieving congestion and restoration or maintenance of systemic perfusion, while addressing triggers and concomitant acute as well as contributory chronic illness. Diuretics are the mainstay of decongestive therapy, often combined with vasodilators in non-hypotensive patients. In some refractory cases, ultrafiltration and vasopressin receptor antagonists can be employed. Vasodilator therapy takes a central role in hypertensive AHF patients. Advanced therapies with vasoactive drugs, including inotropic agents and vasopressors, as well as mechanical circulatory support, are discussed in Chapter 9.

Diuretic Strategies

There are no large-scale clinical trials that have examined the use of diuretics for AHF, but loop diuretics are generally considered the preferred first-line therapy, whereas other classes of diuretics are used as adjuncts. Commonly used loop diuretics include furosemide, torsemide, bumetanide, and ethacrynic acid. Ethacrynic acid is a non-sulfonamide-based loop diuretic commonly used in patients with hypersensitivity to sulfonamide. Adjunct non-loop diuretics commonly used are thiazide or thiazide-like diuretics, and sometimes natriuretic doses of mineralocorticoid receptor antagonists (MRAs). A basic understanding of diuretic pharmacology is covered in Chapter 5. Additional major points relevant to AHF are discussed in the current chapter.

Loop Diuretics

Loop diuretics are the preferred diuretic class for patients with HF and should be promptly administered intravenously in patients with AHF.[44,45] When administered intravenously, loop diuretics also have an additional acute vasodilatory effect that precedes their natriuresis effect.[46]

Pharmacology

Loop diuretics inhibit the activity of the Na^+-K^+-$2Cl^-$ symporter (NKCC2) found at the apical surface of the thick ascending limb (TAL) cells of the loop of Henle. Up to 25% of filtered Na^+ and Cl^- is reabsorbed by the activity of this symporter. Although the proximal tubule reabsorbs about 65% of filtered Na^+, diuretics acting only in the proximal tubule have limited efficacy because the TAL has the capacity to reabsorb most of the Na^+ that escapes reabsorption at the proximal tubule. On the other hand, nephron segments beyond the TAL do not possess the resorptive capacity to rescue the Na^+ exiting the TAL. This contributes to the robust diuretic effect of loop diuretics, compared with other diuretics acting at other sites of the nephron.

Other mechanisms also contribute to the robust natriuretic effect: by blocking active NaCl reabsorption in the TAL, NKCC2 inhibitors interfere with a critical step in the mechanism that produces a hypertonic medullary interstitium. Therefore, loop diuretics block the kidney's ability to concentrate urine. Additionally, because TAL is part of the diluting segment, inhibitors of NKCC2 markedly impair the kidney's ability to excrete a dilute urine during water diuresis.

Loop diuretics are organic anions that circulate tightly bound to protein (>90%), limiting their volumes of distribution. Low albumin impairs diuretic delivery to the kidney, promoting diuretic resistance in patients with severe hypoalbuminemia.[47,48] Small-scale studies showed only a transient modest increase in urinary volume and sodium excretion with albumin/loop-diuretic co-administration in hypoalbuminemic patients.[49] The extensive protein-bound state of loop diuretics in plasma largely precludes their glomerular filtration. Instead, loop diuretics gain access to their site of action along the luminal membrane of TAL by secretion across proximal tubular cells, predominantly through organic anion transporters. The efficacy of loop diuretics can thus be diminished by factors limiting loop diuretic binding to the secretory protein (organic anion transporter) or the NKCC2 symporter. These factors include decreased numbers of functioning nephrons as in chronic kidney disease (CKD), drugs (e.g., nonsteroidal anti-inflammatory drugs), and endogenous organic anions (which often accumulate in CKD) that bind to the symporter, resulting in a rightward shift in the natriuretic dose-response curve.[50] The mechanisms of diuretic resistance in CKD patients are complex and beyond the scope of this chapter.

Dose, Routes, and Modes of Administration

Generally, patients with AHF are given intravenous dosing to circumvent decreased rate of drug absorption[51] due to mucosal edema and decreased intestinal perfusion. Chapter 5 discusses relevant findings regarding continuous *versus* bolus doses of IV diuretics;[52] guidelines state that either option is acceptable. For patients receiving oral loop diuretics as outpatients, treatment with an initial IV dose that is at least equivalent to the oral dose as intermittent boluses or as a continuous infusion can be employed.[44] This simple approach should be modified according to specific conditions, such as changes in renal function. For patients naïve to loop diuretics, IV furosemide at an initial dose of 20–40 mg can be used. Patients with congestion from volume redistribution (as in flash pulmonary edema), as opposed to those with worsening total volume overload, may not require aggressive diuretic administration with urgent and adequate blood pressure control with vasodilators. Diuretic dosages should be adjusted based on urine output and symptom improvement. If adequate diuresis is not achieved with higher doses of IV loop diuretics, adjunct treatment strategies, such as sequential nephron blockade, can be employed.

Maximum Safe and Effective Dose

In patients with HF, as is the case in patients with cirrhosis, nephrotic syndrome, or CKD, the natriuretic dose-response curve is shifted to the right and the ceiling is diminished. This response requires that higher doses are administered to achieve a diuresis response comparable with that of normal individuals, and a lower maximal natriuretic response is achieved. Although it is recommended to use an initial dose that is at least their home dose in intravenous form and to titrate upward toward the goal based on clinical response, the maximum safe dose is yet to be well established.

In clinical practice, achieving adequate decongestion safely with loop diuretics in the acute setting can be limited by diuresis-related side effects, such as electrolyte abnormalities, worsening renal function, and hypotension.[53] In addition to these effects, the activation of the renin-angiotensin-aldosterone system (RAAS) by high-dose loop diuretics has been suggested to link observed associations between high doses of loop diuretics and adverse clinical outcomes.[54,55] However, these observational data do not delineate whether higher doses of diuretics are markers of illness severity or triggers of adverse outcomes.

More studies are needed to clarify the impact of diuretic dosing, during either the active decongestion period or at discharge on short- or long-term outcomes. Data from the DOSE trial supports the use of an initial furosemide dose at 2.5 times the home dose, which was not associated with worse secondary clinical outcomes such as in-hospital mortality, or 60-day composite outcomes of death, rehospitalizations, and ED visits compared with home-equivalent furosemide. Since furosemide is renally metabolized, elimination half-life is prolonged and the relative potency compared with bumetanide and torsemide narrows in patients with CKD, and the toxic potential of furosemide is increased in this setting.

Ototoxicity is a rare but serious toxicity that occurs with high dose of diuretic therapy at a dose above 250 mg IV bolus infusion of furosemide or equivalent doses of bumetanide and torsemide. Ototoxicity can occur at lower doses in patients with renal failure, hypoproteinemia, or concurrent therapy with aminoglycoside or other ototoxic drugs. Compared with other loop diuretics, ethacrynic acid may be more toxic at higher doses. Ototoxicity may manifest as tinnitus, temporary hearing loss, or in rare cases, permanent deafness. The mechanism of ototoxicity development is discussed further in Chapter 5.

Door-to-Diuretics

The concept of "door-to-diuretic" in the management of AHF was coined as a possible strategy to improve outcomes with early decongestion, thereby preventing organ dysfunction.[56] Available prospective data are limited to two prospective observational studies that yielded discordant findings. In REALITY-HF, early IV furosemide (administered within <60 minutes of arrival at ED) was associated with decreased in-hospital mortality, but not decreased 30-day mortality, compared with later treatments applied within 24 hours.[57] In contrast, another prospective observational study failed to show any association between door-to-diuretic and outcomes.[58] Ethical considerations may preclude a randomized controlled trial of early vs late diuretic therapy in AHF patients.

Diuretic Resistance

Fluid overload refractory to conventional treatment with escalating loop diuretics, as evidenced by lack of appreciable improvement in urine output and unimproved congestion, can complicate both acute and chronic HF management. Once a loop diuretic is administered, the effect will last hours; however, as the concentration of diuretic decreases over time, "post-diuretic sodium retention" starts to occur, where sodium is reabsorbed, and diuresis slows. This can be mediated somewhat by restricting dietary sodium and by more frequent administration of the loop diuretic. Additionally, when extracellular fluid volume reaches a low point, the natriuretic response to each dose of diuretic administered decreases, leading to the second notable adaptation termed the "braking phenomenon." Both phenomena are discussed in depth in Chapter 5.

Thiazide or Thiazide-Like Diuretics

Thiazide diuretics inhibit the Na-Cl symporter in the apical membrane of the distal convoluted tubule epithelial cells, achieving only 5% of Na^+ excretion, making them less efficacious than loop diuretics. In situations where there is increased delivery of sodium chloride by loop diuretics, the distal nephrons are stimulated to increase their resorptive capacity. Chronic use of loop diuretics leads to distal tubular remodeling; thus, thiazides can be added to achieve a synergistic sequential nephron blockade effect (ACCF/AHA class IIa, Level B). Although the safety and clinical efficacy of such a strategy has not been examined in large-scale clinical trials, it can result in more than doubled daily urine sodium excretion, at the risk of inducing severe hypokalemia in addition to hyponatremia, hypotension, and worsening renal function.[59] This approach is discussed in greater detail in Chapter 5. Most thiazide diuretics, except for metolazone and indapamide, are ineffective when estimated glomerular filtration rate (eGFR) is <30–40 mL/min.

Vasopressin Receptor Antagonist (Aquaretics)

Medications in this class of drugs may be used short-term for inpatients with HF who show signs of volume overload along with severe hypervolemic hyponatremia unresponsive to optimized medical therapy, or who are at risk of having active cognitive symptoms secondary to hyponatremia.[44] In the setting of AHF, hyponatremia indicates water accumulation/retention, which is associated with a poorer prognosis.[60] Chapter 5 addresses details of V_1 and V_2 receptor selectivity and other important pharmacologic characteristics of vasopressin receptor antagonists (VRAs). Tolvaptan and conivaptan are the two

VRAs most used to induce aquaresis in these patients. The Efficacy of Vasopressin Antagonism in Heart Failure: Outcome Study with Tolvaptan (EVEREST) study sought to evaluate patients hospitalized with HF and compare outcomes in those given tolvaptan or a placebo. The study ultimately showed no difference in long-term clinical outcomes between the two groups, although it did show a benefit in the tolvaptan group with regard to symptomatology and volume overload.[61] Other smaller studies have failed to reproduce these results.[62] Both tolvaptan and conivaptan are contraindicated for use in combination with strong CYP450 3A4 inhibitors.

Mineralocorticoid Antagonists

Mineralocorticoid antagonists (MRAs), such as spironolactone and eplerenone, have been shown to decrease morbidity and mortality among HF patients and are therefore recommended for those with symptomatic HF and a left ventricular ejection fraction (LVEF) less than 35%, or less than 40% following acute myocardial infarction (MI), unless otherwise contraindicated.[44] They are also recommended for patients with HFpEF.[45] Renal function should be monitored, and generally low doses are used to avoid hyperkalemia. MRAs should not be used if eGFR is <30 mL/min/1.73 m^2. The pharmacology and dosing of MRAs are discussed in detail in Chapter 5. Though some small studies have suggested that high doses may improve congestion in AHF, the ATHENA-HF study did not reflect improved congestive symptoms with high doses of spironolactone.[63]

Ultrafiltration and Renal Replacement Therapy

Ultrafiltration can be considered for refractory congestion (ACCF/AHA class IIb, Level C), but comparisons with diuresis show inconsistent results, including increased risk of serious adverse events. This topic is discussed further in Chapter 9.

Vasodilators

About 95% of AHF patients present with "warm and wet" clinical profiles. Data from registries, such as the EuroObservational[64] and Get with The Guidelines HF,[65] shows that the mean SBP among these AHF patients is 144 mmHg and 140 mmHg, respectively. These patients may benefit from adjunctive therapy with vasodilators such as nitroglycerin, nitroprusside, or nesiritide if they remain symptomatic despite initial diuretic treatment (ACCF/AHA class IIb, Level A). Although nesiritide may not reduce mortality, rehospitalization, or dyspnea in patients with acute HF and in fact increases risk of hypotension,[66] nitrates for AHF have insufficient evidence for effects on clinical outcomes. However, in patients with congestion resulting from volume redistribution (vascular type "warm and wet" clinical profile) characterized by elevated blood pressure (commonly above 180 mmHg), a dramatic improvement in symptoms can be achieved by use of vasodilators and sublingual nitrates. followed by IV vasodilators, in addition to diuretic therapy as outlined before. The use of these agents is further discussed in Chapter 5 and Chapter 9.

Inotropic Agents and Vasopressors

The use of these agents is discussed in Chapter 5 and Chapter 10.

Additional Therapeutic Considerations

Management of Third Space Fluid (Thoracentesis and Paracentesis)

Peripheral pitting edema, ascites, and large pleural effusions reflect a large extravascular fluid reservoir that may take many days to mobilize. Although there are no specific interventions for pitting edema (besides diuretics), the ESC guidelines suggest that in patients with AHF and large pleural effusions, fluid evacuation through pleurocentesis may be considered to alleviate dyspnea.[67] Similarly, in patients with ascites, paracentesis may be considered to improve symptoms and can also improve renal filtration through reduction in intra-abdominal pressure.[67] However, high-quality data to support the use of these procedures are lacking.

Opiates

Morphine is a venodilator and a weak arterial vasodilator. Data on the utility of morphine in AHF is limited. Retrospective studies suggest morphine may be associated with increased mortality in patients with AHF[68, 69] and may not relieve dyspnea,[70] but the patients who received morphine tend to be severely ill. Therefore, the routine use of opioids is not recommended in patients with AHF,[71] but they may be considered to relieve severe dyspnea and anxiety (ESC class IIB, Level B).[67] Patients should be monitored for nausea and respiratory depression, and naloxone (Narcan) should be available in case of respiratory depression.[72]

Management of Atrial Fibrillation in Acute Heart Failure

Atrial fibrillation (AF) and AHF frequently co-exist and exacerbate each other. AF is present in about 35% of patients with AHF.[67,73] AF can be the only or at least the predominant trigger of AHF, the consequence of AHF, or an innocent bystander; of note, both AHF and AF can be simultaneously triggered by the same pathological process.[74] By inducing a rapid ventricular response and altering diastolic function, AF can cause HF symptoms even in patients with normal left ventricular (LV) systolic function.[67,75]

In a large US-based registry, the presence of AF, particularly newly diagnosed, in patients admitted with AHF, was independently associated with increased in-hospital mortality and longer duration of stay.[76] Higher heart rate (HR) on admission was shown to be independently associated with worse outcomes in patients admitted for HF, both for those in sinus rhythm and in AF.[77]

The management of AF in AHF should first be focused on correcting reversible causes or triggers of AF, such as acute coronary syndrome, thyroid disease, anemia, infection, pulmonary embolism, etc.[67] A lenient initial HR target, e.g., <110 bpm should be adequate in acute settings, followed by a lower target, e.g., <80 bpm, when the patient is stabilized.[78] In non-hypotensive patients with HFpEF, rate control can be attempted first with IV non-dihydropyridine calcium channel blockers or beta-blockers, followed by digoxin if HR control cannot be achieved.[78] Beta-blockers can be used in AHF in non-hypotensive patients with HFrEF, followed by digoxin,[78] although amiodarone is probably the first option in patients with severely depressed LVEF.[74]

For patients who are hypotensive and/or patients with severe HFrEF, the choice of drug includes IV amiodarone if the patient is fully anticoagulated or where AF onset is <48 hours earlier, and digoxin can be added if amiodarone fails to control HR. Patients receiving long-term digoxin therapy should be continued during AHF. Limited retrospective data suggest a role for digoxin therapy in reducing 30-day readmission, 12-month HF readmission, and 12-month all-cause mortality in patients with LVEF<45%.[79] The role of short-term use of digoxin during AHF episode is unknown.

It is unclear if prompt restoration of sinus rhythm would improve outcomes in AHF, as the recurrence rate is very high in the still-decompensated patient. Rhythm control in the acute setting is rarely necessary and should be avoided if the individual is not fully anticoagulated or if the onset of AF is not known to be <48 hours earlier. Cardioversion can be considered when attempts to control rate and relieve congestion are unsuccessful, or if hemodynamic instability is present. In less acute cases, transesophageal echocardiogram should be considered in patients without adequate anticoagulation, followed by maintenance anticoagulation. When pharmacological rhythm control is considered in AHF, antiarrhythmic drugs are contraindicated except for amiodarone.[80] If rhythm control is unsuccessful and the patient remains symptomatic with elevated heart rates, atrioventricular junctional ablation, often with a biventricular pacing system, is an additional option that can be considered.[81]

Management of Evidence-Based Chronic Heart Failure Therapy

Guideline-directed therapy can be continued in the absence of hemodynamic instability or contraindications (ACCF/AHA class I, Level B).[82] Continuation of the usual outpatient beta-blocker regimen during acute decompensation of chronic HF does not worsen symptoms or increase inpatient mortality or length of hospital stay,[83] and in fact it is associated with lower post-discharge mortality at 60–90 days.[84] Beta-blockers can also be initiated in the hospital after optimization of volume status and successful discontinuation of IV diuretics (ACCF/AHA class I, Level B.[84] Likewise, in absence of hemodynamic instability or contraindications, angiotensin-converting enzyme (ACE) inhibitors (or angiotensin receptor blocker [ARB]) can be started or continued in stable patients prior to hospital discharge (ACCF/AHA class I, Level B),[82] and mineralocorticoid receptor antagonists can also be initiated in appropriate patients with NYHA class II–IV HF and LVEF ≤35%, unless contraindicated, to reduce morbidity and mortality (ACCF/AHA class I, Level A).[82]

Venous Thromboembolism Prophylaxis

Patients admitted to the hospital with AHF should receive venous thromboembolism (VTE) prophylaxis with anticoagulant medication if the risk-benefit ratio is favorable (ACCF/AHA class I, Level B).[82] Candidates for VTE prophylaxis can receive unfractionated heparin or related medications such as low-molecular-weight heparin (LMWH), or fondaparinux. In patients with risk factors for VTE who are at high risk of bleeding, intermittent pneumatic compression is preferred over graduated compression stockings for the prevention of VTE.[85] Transition to a pharmacologic agent should occur as soon as the bleeding risk becomes acceptably low.

Monitoring of Clinical Course and Readiness for Discharge

Clinical Status/Treatment Effect/ Trajectory Monitoring

The clinical trajectory of AHF patients should be continuously assessed from admission, during the process of decongestion and medication optimization, to transition to outpatient care. The trajectory could exhibit either a continuously improving trend towards treatment target, no improvement, or stalled improvement after initial response, or worsening.

Clinical trajectory monitoring assesses resolution of signs and symptoms of congestion, adequate perfusion, end-organ function recovery, and maintenance of acceptable vital signs. Assessing improvement in dyspnea, orthopnea, crackles, and jugular venous pressure (JVP) are important indicators of treatment trajectory as they indirectly reflect left-sided filling pressure. The presence of rales or fine crackles usually indicates higher filling pressures than the baseline and can be present before detection of pulmonary edema radiographically. However, these findings can be often absent in chronic HF patients owing to compensation of the pulmonary lymphatic system. JVP measures right-sided filling pressure and can serve as a surrogate for left-sided filling pressures. However, other processes may lead to disproportionately higher right-sided filling pressure than left-sided filling pressure. In the case of uncertainty in assessing intracardiac filling pressures clinically, invasive hemodynamic monitoring can be considered to guide therapy in the setting of respiratory distress or clinical evidence of impaired perfusion (ACCF/AHA class I, Level C). However, pulmonary artery catheterization does not reduce mortality or length of hospitalization, and in fact may increase adverse events.[86] Therefore, routine use of invasive hemodynamic monitoring is not recommended.[82]

Other objective parameters that can be utilized in assessing treatment response include daily weight and daily fluid balance measured at the same time each day.[82] Data on the role of natriuretic peptide (NP)-guided treatment in AHF is limited. A small, randomized trial showed NT-proBNP-guided therapy (goal of >30% reduction) after clinical stabilization may not reduce the composite of all-cause mortality and heart failure readmission in patients with AHF.[87]

If the clinical trajectory of decongestion goal is slow, stalled, or worsening, diuretic therapy can be intensified while assessing other parameters such as blood pressure, electrolytes, and renal function. To achieve the goal of net negative fluid balance, fluid restriction (1.5–2 L/day) can be considered in patients with stage D heart failure, particularly in patients with hyponatremia (ACCF/AHA class IIa, Level C).[82] However, aggressive sodium and fluid restriction was shown not to affect weight loss or clinical stability at three days compared with a standard hospital diet in patients with acute decompensated heart failure.[88]

Renal dysfunction is one of many complex aspects of AHF management, and can have several etiologies: low cardiac output, increased venous pressure, altered intrarenal hemodynamics, and tubuloglomerular feedback. Most recent evidence suggests that elevated central venous pressure imposes an increased "afterload" on the kidney and is the most common dominant factor in renal dysfunction in AHF.[89]

The use of the indwelling urinary catheter facilitates accurate urine output monitoring and thus has theoretical benefits in the management of AHF patients with significant volume overload. However, the routine use of indwelling urethral catheter in AHF has not been shown to improve heart failure outcomes and is associated with increased urinary tract complications.[90]

Criteria for Hospital Discharge

Readiness for discharge during hospitalization for HF remains highly subjective, as the evidence base is limited, and individual practices are highly heterogeneous.[91] Recommended practices include reaching a presumable baseline dry weight, achieving resolution of dyspnea on exertion,[91] and observing patients for at least 24 hours before discharge to ensure effectiveness of maintenance oral diuretic therapy and to prevent early readmission.[92]

The maintenance oral diuretic dose set in the hospital, where patients' diet and fluid intake have been controlled, may fail to achieve the intended fluid balance in the outpatient setting. Therefore, a back-up rescue diuretic plan, triggered by weight gain or symptoms of congestion, can be included in the discharge planning for select patients, in addition to close post-discharge follow-up or access to health care providers via telemedicine to guide the patient. The rescue diuretic dosing may include increasing dose and/or frequency of the loop diuretic or adding a thiazide-type diuretic for sequential nephron blockage.

Patients who require high doses of loop diuretics may also require potassium supplements. The decision to add potassium supplement should consider patients' renal function and concomitant therapies with ACEI, ARB, ARNI, or MRA, all of which increase the risk of hyperkalemia. A stable pattern of serum potassium during hospitalization may provide a clue as to which patients may need potassium supplementation on discharge. In the event of uncertainty, a post-discharge laboratory measurement of electrolytes and renal function is needed soon after discharge.

Post-Discharge Follow-Up

Up to 25% of patients admitted for AHF are readmitted within the first 30 days of discharge. Therefore, discharge follow-up planning is crucial to mitigate this. Practices vary widely across healthcare systems but may comprise of a follow-up phone call or telemedicine encounter within two to three days of discharge. These encounters assess clinical signs and symptoms of congestion or medication side effects (e.g., symptomatic hypotension) and ensure understanding of and adherence to discharge instructions, then followed by a clinic visit.[93] It is reasonable to plan for a follow-up visit within two weeks from hospital discharge (ESC recommendation).[44] In a highly publicized study from Medicare data in the United States, early (within seven days) post-discharge follow-up has been associated with lower 30-day readmission dates, leading to adoption of this practice as a quality metric for HF care in the United States.[94,95] In general, individual patient's risk assessment at time of hospital discharge, consideration for advanced therapy or palliative care, need for outpatient initiation or titration of GDMT, and electrolyte and renal function monitoring (especially after major changes in diuretics, ACEI, ARB, ARNI, or MRA), warrant early post-discharge follow-up. It is also important to engage patients and families in a shared decision when establishing follow-up planning and management after discharge. Unfortunately, clinical risk scores do not perform well in predicting risk of hospital readmission.[82,96]

Conclusion

The management of AHF has been challenging, as most practices are guided by experience and pathophysiology, with few practices being backed up by high-quality evidence. In addition, there is substantial patient and presentation heterogeneity, which hampers systematic evaluation of diagnostic and therapeutic strategies in AHF. Of note, no pharmacotherapy has been shown to date to improve acute-phase outcomes in AHF, although early initiation of evidence-based medications does improve prognosis. Optimal use of agents with hemodynamic effects, diuretic strategies, disease-modifying therapies, appropriate triage, in-hospital management, and discharge strategies are areas of active investigation in AHF.

References

1. Gheorghiade M, Zannad F, Sopko G, et al. Acute heart failure syndromes: current state and framework for future research. *Circulation.* 2005;112:3958–68.
2. Storrow AB, Jenkins CA, Self WH, et al. The burden of acute heart failure on U.S. emergency departments. *JACC Heart Fail.* 2014;2:269–77.
3. Benjamin EJ, Virani SS, Callaway CW, et al. Heart disease and stroke statistics-2018 update: a report from the American Heart Association. *Circulation.* 2018;137:e67–e492.
4. Heidenreich PA, Albert NM, Allen LA, et al. Forecasting the impact of heart failure in the United States: a policy statement from the American Heart Association. *Circ Heart Fail.* 2013;6:606–19.
5. Sharma A, Zhao X, Hammill BG, et al. Trends in noncardiovascular comorbidities among patients hospitalized for heart failure: insights from the get with the guidelines-heart failure registry. *Circ Heart Fail.* 2018;11:e004646.
6. Targher G, Dauriz M, Laroche C, et al. In-hospital and 1-year mortality associated with diabetes in patients with acute heart failure: results from the ESC-HFA heart failure long-term registry. *Eur J Heart Fail.* 2017;19:54–65.
7. Bello NA, Claggett B, Desai AS, et al. Influence of previous heart failure hospitalization on cardiovascular events in patients with reduced and preserved ejection fraction. *Circ Heart Fail.* 2014;7:590–5.
8. Kristensen SL, Jhund PS, Køber L, et al. Comparison of outcomes after hospitalization for worsening heart failure, myocardial infarction, and stroke in patients with heart failure and reduced and preserved ejection fraction. *Eur J Heart Fail.* 2015;17:169–76.
9. Greene SJ, Fonarow GC, Vaduganathan M, et al. The vulnerable phase after hospitalization for heart failure. *Nat Rev Cardiol.* 2015;12:220–9.
10. Cook TD, Greene SJ, Kalogeropoulos AP, et al. Temporal changes in postdischarge mortality risk after hospitalization for heart failure (from the EVEREST trial). *Am J Cardiol.* 2016;117:611–6.
11. Khan H, Greene SJ, Fonarow GC, et al. Length of hospital stay and 30-day readmission following heart failure hospitalization: insights from the EVEREST trial. *Eur J Heart Fail.* 2015;17:1022–31.
12. Forrester JS, Diamond G, Chatterjee K, Swan HJ. Medical therapy of acute myocardial infarction by application of hemodynamic subsets (second of two parts). *N Engl J Med.* 1976;295:1404–13.
13. Fonarow GC, Abraham WT, Albert NM, et al. Factors identified as precipitating hospital admissions for heart failure and clinical outcomes: findings from OPTIMIZE-HF. *Arch Intern Med.* 2008;168:847–54.
14. Arrigo M, Gayat E, Parenica J, et al. Precipitating factors and 90-day outcome of acute heart failure: a report from the intercontinental GREAT registry. *Eur J Heart Fail.* 2017;19:201–8.
15. Lee DS, Schull MJ, Alter DA, et al. Early deaths in patients with heart failure discharged from the emergency department: a population-based analysis. *Circ Heart Fail.* 2010;3:228–35.
16. Brar S, McAlister FA, Youngson E, Rowe BH. Do outcomes for patients with heart failure vary by emergency department volume? *Circ Heart Fail.* 2013;6:1147–54.
17. Lee DS, Stitt A, Austin PC, et al. Prediction of heart failure mortality in emergent care: a cohort study. *Ann Intern Med.* 2012;156:767–75, W-261, W-262.
18. Stiell IG, Clement CM, Brison RJ, et al. A risk scoring system to identify emergency department patients with heart failure at high risk for serious adverse events. *Acad Emerg Med.* 2013;20:17–26.
19. Collins SP, Jenkins CA, Harrell FE, Jr., et al. Identification of emergency department patients with acute heart failure at low risk for 30-day adverse events: the STRATIFY decision tool. *JACC Heart Fail.* 2015;3:737–47.
20. Zsilinszka R, Mentz RJ, DeVore AD, et al. Acute heart failure: alternatives to hospitalization. *JACC Heart Fail.* 2017;5:329–36.
21. Mebazaa A, Pang PS, Tavares M, et al. The impact of early standard therapy on dyspnoea in patients with acute heart failure: the URGENT-dyspnoea study. *Eur Heart J.* 2010;31:832–41.
22. Dickstein K, Cohen-Solal A, Filippatos G, et al. ESC guidelines for the diagnosis and treatment of acute and chronic heart failure 2008: the task force for the diagnosis and treatment of acute and chronic heart failure 2008 of the European Society of Cardiology. Developed in collaboration with the Heart Failure Association of the ESC (HFA) and endorsed by the European Society of Intensive Care Medicine (ESICM). *Eur Heart J.* 2008;29:2388–442.
23. Park JJ, Choi DJ, Yoon CH, et al. The prognostic value of arterial blood gas analysis in high-risk acute heart failure patients: an analysis of the Korean Heart Failure (KorHF) registry. *Eur J Heart Fail.* 2015;17:601–11.
24. Nieminen MS, Bohm M, Cowie MR, et al. Executive summary of the guidelines on the diagnosis and treatment of acute heart failure: the task force on acute heart failure of the European Society of Cardiology. *Eur Heart J.* 2005;26:384–416.

25. Ware LB, Matthay MA. Clinical practice. Acute pulmonary edema. *N Engl J Med.* 2005;353:2788–96.
26. Gropper MA, Wiener-Kronish JP, Hashimoto S. Acute cardiogenic pulmonary edema. *Clin Chest Med.* 1994;15:501–15.
27. Rimoldi SF, Yuzefpolskaya M, Allemann Y, Messerli F. Flash pulmonary edema. *Prog Cardiovasc Dis.* 2009;52:249–59.
28. Mak S, Azevedo ER, Liu PP, Newton GE. Effect of hyperoxia on left ventricular function and filling pressures in patients with and without congestive heart failure. *Chest.* 2001;120:467–73.
29. Park JH, Balmain S, Berry C, Morton JJ, McMurray JJ. Potentially detrimental cardiovascular effects of oxygen in patients with chronic left ventricular systolic dysfunction. *Heart.* 2010;96:533–8.
30. Haque WA, Boehmer J, Clemson BS, et al. Hemodynamic effects of supplemental oxygen administration in congestive heart failure. *J Am Coll Cardiol.* 1996;27:353–7.
31. Sepehrvand N, Alemayehu W, Rowe BH, et al. High vs. low oxygen therapy in patients with acute heart failure: HiLo-HF pilot trial. *ESC Heart Fail.* 2019;6:667–77.
32. Berbenetz N, Wang Y, Brown J, et al. Non-invasive positive pressure ventilation (CPAP or bilevel NPPV) for cardiogenic pulmonary oedema. *Cochrane Database Syst Rev.* 2019;4:CD005351.
33. Mariani J, Macchia A, Belziti C, et al. Noninvasive ventilation in acute cardiogenic pulmonary edema: a meta-analysis of randomized controlled trials. *J Card Fail.* 2011;17:850–9.
34. Weng CL, Zhao YT, Liu QH, et al. Meta-analysis: noninvasive ventilation in acute cardiogenic pulmonary edema. *Ann Intern Med.* 2010;152:590–600.
35. Miro O, Martinez G, Masip J, et al. Effects on short term outcome of non-invasive ventilation use in the emergency department to treat patients with acute heart failure: a propensity score-based analysis of the EAHFE registry. *Eur J Intern Med.* 2018;53:45–51.
36. Gray A, Goodacre S, Newby DE, et al. Noninvasive ventilation in acute cardiogenic pulmonary edema. *N Engl J Med.* 2008;359:142–51.
37. Peter JV, Moran JL, Phillips-Hughes J, Graham P, Bersten AD. Effect of non-invasive positive pressure ventilation (NIPPV) on mortality in patients with acute cardiogenic pulmonary oedema: a meta-analysis. *Lancet.* 2006;367:1155–63.
38. Li H, Hu C, Xia J, et al. A comparison of bilevel and continuous positive airway pressure noninvasive ventilation in acute cardiogenic pulmonary edema. *Am J Emerg Med.* 2013;31:1322–7.
39. Masip J, Peacock WF, Price S, et al. Indications and practical approach to non-invasive ventilation in acute heart failure. *Eur Heart J.* 2018;39:17–25.
40. Demoule A, Chevret S, Carlucci A, et al. Changing use of noninvasive ventilation in critically ill patients: trends over 15 years in francophone countries. *Intensive Care Med.* 2016;42:82–92.
41. Kulkarni VT, Kim N, Dai Y, et al. Hospital variation in noninvasive positive pressure ventilation for acute decompensated heart failure. *Circ Heart Fail.* 2014;7:427–33.
42. Miller PE, van Diepen S, Ahmad T. Acute decompensated heart failure complicated by respiratory failure. *Circ Heart Fail.* 2019;12:e006013.
43. Alviar CL, Miller PE, McAreavey D, et al. Positive pressure ventilation in the cardiac intensive care unit. *J Am Coll Cardiol.* 2018;72:1532–53.
44. Ponikowski P, Voors AA, Anker SD, et al. ESC guidelines for the diagnosis and treatment of acute and chronic heart failure: the task force for the diagnosis and treatment of acute and chronic heart failure of the European Society of Cardiology (ESC)Developed with the special contribution of the Heart Failure Association (HFA) of the ESC. *Eur Heart J.* 2016;37:2129–200.
45. Yancy CW, Jessup M, Bozkurt B, et al. ACC/AHA/HFSA focused update of the 2013 ACCF/AHA guideline for the management of heart failure: a report of the American College of Cardiology/American Heart Association Task Force on Clinical Practice Guidelines and the Heart Failure Society of America. *J Card Fail.* 2017;23:628–51.
46. Oppermann M, Hansen PB, Castrop H, Schnermann J. Vasodilatation of afferent arterioles and paradoxical increase of renal vascular resistance by furosemide in mice. *Am J Physiol Renal Physiol.* 2007;293:F279–87.
47. Inoue M, Okajima K, Itoh K, et al. Mechanism of furosemide resistance in analbuminemic rats and hypoalbuminemic patients. *Kidney Int.* 1987;32:198–203.
48. Pichette V, Geadah D, du Souich P. Role of plasma protein binding on renal metabolism and dynamics of furosemide in the rabbit. *Drug Metab Dispos.* 1999;27:81–5.
49. Kitsios GD, Mascari P, Ettunsi R, Gray AW. Co-administration of furosemide with albumin for overcoming diuretic resistance in patients with hypoalbuminemia: a meta-analysis. *J Crit Care.* 2014;29:253–9.
50. Ellison DH. Clinical pharmacology in diuretic use. *Clin J Am Soc Nephrol.* 2019;14:1248–57.
51. Brater DC, Day B, Burdette A, Anderson S. Bumetanide and furosemide in heart failure. *Kidney Int.* 1984;26:183–9.
52. Felker GM, Lee KL, Bull DA, et al. Diuretic strategies in patients with acute decompensated heart failure. *N Engl J Med.* 2011;364:797–805.
53. Felker GM, O'Connor CM, Braunwald E, Heart failure clinical research network I. Loop diuretics in acute decompensated heart failure: necessary? Evil? A necessary evil? *Circ Heart Fail.* 2009;2:56–62.
54. Peacock WF, Costanzo MR, De Marco T, et al. Impact of intravenous loop diuretics on outcomes of patients hospitalized with acute decompensated heart failure: insights from the ADHERE registry. *Cardiology.* 2009;113:12–9.
55. Okabe T, Yakushiji T, Kido T, et al. The association between high-dose loop diuretic use at discharge and cardiovascular mortality in patients with heart failure. *ESC Heart Fail.* 2018;5:87–94.
56. Maisel AS, Peacock WF, McMullin N, et al. Timing of immunoreactive B-type natriuretic peptide levels and treatment delay in acute decompensated heart failure: an ADHERE (Acute Decompensated Heart Failure National Registry) analysis. *J Am Coll Cardiol.* 2008;52:534–40.
57. Matsue Y, Damman K, Voors AA, et al. Time-to-furosemide treatment and mortality in patients hospitalized with acute heart failure. *J Am Coll Cardiol.* 2017;69:3042–51.
58. Park JJ, Kim SH, Oh IY, et al. The effect of door-to-diuretic time on clinical outcomes in patients with acute heart failure. *JACC Heart Fail.* 2018;6:286–94.
59. Jentzer JC, DeWald TA, Hernandez AF. Combination of loop diuretics with thiazide-type diuretics in heart failure. *J Am Coll Cardiol.* 2010;56:1527–34.
60. Rusinaru D, Tribouilloy C, Berry C, et al. Relationship of serum sodium concentration to mortality in a wide spectrum of heart failure patients with preserved and with reduced ejection fraction: an individual patient data meta-analysis(dagger): meta-analysis global group in chronic heart failure (MAGGIC). *Eur J Heart Fail.* 2012;14:1139–46.
61. Pang PS, Konstam MA, Krasa HB, et al. Effects of tolvaptan on dyspnoea relief from the EVEREST trials. *Eur Heart J.* 2009;30:2233–40.
62. Felker GM, Mentz RJ, Cole RT, et al. Efficacy and safety of tolvaptan in patients hospitalized with acute heart failure. *J Am Coll Cardiol.* 2017;69:1399–406.
63. Butler J, Anstrom KJ, Felker GM, et al. Efficacy and safety of spironolactone in acute heart failure: the ATHENA-HF randomized clinical trial. *JAMA Cardiol.* 2017;2:950–8.
64. Maggioni AP, Dahlstrom U, Filippatos G, et al. EURObservational research programme: regional differences and 1-year follow-up results of the heart failure pilot survey (ESC-HF Pilot). *Eur J Heart Fail.* 2013;15:808–17.
65. DeVore AD, Cox M, Eapen ZJ, et al. Temporal trends and variation in early scheduled follow-up after a hospitalization for heart failure: findings from get with the guidelines-heart failure. *Circ Heart Fail.* 2016;9:e002344.
66. Gong B, Wu Z, Li Z. Efficacy and safety of nesiritide in patients with decompensated heart failure: a meta-analysis of randomised trials. *BMJ Open.* 2016;6:e008545.
67. Ponikowski P, Voors AA, Anker SD, et al. 2016 ESC guidelines for the diagnosis and treatment of acute and chronic heart failure: the task force for the diagnosis and treatment of acute and chronic heart failure of the European Society of Cardiology (ESC) developed with the special contribution of the Heart Failure Association (HFA) of the ESC. *Eur Heart J.* 2016;37:2129–2200.
68. Peacock WF, Hollander JE, Diercks DB, et al. Morphine and outcomes in acute decompensated heart failure: an ADHERE analysis. *Emerg Med J.* 2008;25:205–9.
69. Iakobishvili Z, Cohen E, Garty M, et al. Use of intravenous morphine for acute decompensated heart failure in patients with and without acute coronary syndromes. *Acute Card Care.* 2011;13:76–80.
70. Gray A, Goodacre S, Seah M, Tilley S. Diuretic, opiate and nitrate use in severe acidotic acute cardiogenic pulmonary oedema: analysis from the 3CPO trial. *Qjm.* 2010;103:573–81.
71. National Clinical Guideline C. *National Institute for Health and Care Excellence: clinical guidelines. Acute heart failure: diagnosing and managing acute heart failure in adults.* London: National Institute for Health and Care Excellence (UK). National Clinical Guideline Centre; 2014.
72. McMurray JJ, Adamopoulos S, Anker SD, et al. ESC guidelines for the diagnosis and treatment of acute and chronic heart failure 2012: the task force for the diagnosis and treatment of acute and chronic heart failure 2012 of the European Society of Cardiology. Developed in collaboration with the Heart Failure Association (HFA) of the ESC. *Eur Heart J.* 2012;33:1787–847.
73. Mebazaa A, Yilmaz MB, Levy P, et al. Recommendations on pre-hospital and early hospital management of acute heart failure: a consensus paper from the Heart Failure Association of the European Society of Cardiology, the European Society of Emergency Medicine and the Society of Academic Emergency Medicine – short version. *European Heart Journal.* 2015;36:1958–66.
74. Gorenek B, Halvorsen S, Kudaiberdieva G, et al. Atrial fibrillation in acute heart failure: a position statement from the Acute Cardiovascular Care Association and European Heart Rhythm Association of the European Society of Cardiology. *Eur Heart J Acute Cardiovasc Care.* 2020;9:348–57.

75. Kotecha D, Piccini JP. Atrial fibrillation in heart failure: what should we do? *Eur Heart J.* 2015;36:3250–7.
76. Mountantonakis SE, Grau-Sepulveda MV, Bhatt DL, et al. Presence of atrial fibrillation is independently associated with adverse outcomes in patients hospitalized with heart failure: an analysis of get with the guidelines-heart failure. *Circ Heart Fail.* 2012;5:191–201.
77. Bui AL, Grau-Sepulveda MV, Hernandez AF, et al. Admission heart rate and in-hospital outcomes in patients hospitalized for heart failure in sinus rhythm and in atrial fibrillation. *Am Heart J.* 2013;165:567–574.e6.
78. Hindricks G, Potpara T, Dagres N, et al. 2020 ESC guidelines for the diagnosis and management of atrial fibrillation developed in collaboration with the European Association for Cardio-Thoracic Surgery (EACTS): the task force for the diagnosis and management of atrial fibrillation of the European Society of Cardiology (ESC) Developed with the special contribution of the European Heart Rhythm Association (EHRA) of the ESC. *Eur Heart J.* 2021;42:373–498.
79. Ahmed A, Bourge RC, Fonarow GC, et al. Digoxin use and lower 30-day all-cause readmission for Medicare beneficiaries hospitalized for heart failure. *Am J Med.* 2014;127:61–70.
80. Kirchhof P, Benussi S, Kotecha D, et al. 2016 ESC guidelines for the management of atrial fibrillation developed in collaboration with EACTS. *Eur J Cardiothorac Surg.* 2016;50:e1–e88.
81. DiMarco JP. Atrial fibrillation and acute decompensated heart failure. *Circulation: Heart Failure.* 2009;2:72–3.
82. Yancy C, Jessup M, Bozkurt B, et al. ACCF/AHA guideline for the management of heart failure: a report of the American College of Cardiology Foundation/American Heart Association task force on practice guidelines. *Circulation.* 2013;128:e240–327.
83. Jondeau G, Neuder Y, Eicher JC, et al. B-CONVINCED: Beta-blocker CONtinuation Vs. INterruption in patients with Congestive heart failure hospitalizED for a decompensation episode. *Eur Heart J.* 2009;30:2186–92.
84. Fonarow GC, Abraham WT, Albert NM, et al. Influence of beta-blocker continuation or withdrawal on outcomes in patients hospitalized with heart failure: findings from the OPTIMIZE-HF program. *J Am Coll Cardiol.* 2008;52:190–9.
85. Guyatt GH, Norris SL, Schulman S, et al. Methodology for the development of antithrombotic therapy and prevention of thrombosis guidelines: antithrombotic therapy and prevention of thrombosis, 9th ed: American College of Chest Physicians Evidence-Based Clinical Practice Guidelines. *Chest.* 2012;141:53s–70s.
86. Binanay C, Califf RM, Hasselblad V, et al. Evaluation study of congestive heart failure and pulmonary artery catheterization effectiveness: the ESCAPE trial. *JAMA.* 2005;294:1625–33.
87. Stienen S, Salah K, Moons AH, et al. NT-proBNP (N-Terminal pro-B-Type Natriuretic Peptide)-guided therapy in acute decompensated heart failure: PRIMA II randomized controlled trial (can NT-ProBNP-guided therapy during hospital admission for acute decompensated heart failure reduce mortality and readmissions?). *Circulation.* 2018;137: 1671–83.
88. Aliti GB, Rabelo ER, Clausell N, et al. Aggressive fluid and sodium restriction in acute decompensated heart failure: a randomized clinical trial. *JAMA Intern Med.* 2013;173:1058–64.
89. Husain-Syed F, Gröne HJ, Assmus B, et al. Congestive nephropathy: a neglected entity? Proposal for diagnostic criteria and future perspectives. *ESC Heart Fail.* 2021;8:183–203.
90. Jang AY, O'Brien C, Chung WJ, et al. Routine indwelling urethral catheterization in acute heart failure patients is associated with increased urinary tract complications without improved heart failure outcomes. *Circ J.* 2018;82:1632–9.
91. Bhatt AB, Cheeran DD, Shemisa K, et al. Physician-specific practice patterns about discharge readiness and heart failure utilization outcomes. *Circ Cardiovasc Qual Outcomes.* 2018;11:e004365.
92. Laliberte B, Reed BN, Devabhakthuni S, et al. Observation of patients transitioned to an oral loop diuretic before discharge and risk of readmission for acute decompensated heart failure. *J Card Fail.* 2017;23: 746–52.
93. Hollenberg SM, Warner Stevenson L, Ahmad T, et al. 2019 ACC expert consensus decision pathway on risk assessment, management, and clinical trajectory of patients hospitalized with heart failure: a report of the American College of Cardiology Solution Set Oversight Committee. *J Am Coll Cardiol.* 2019;74:1966–2011.
94. Hernandez AF, Greiner MA, Fonarow GC, et al. Relationship between early physician follow-up and 30-day readmission among Medicare beneficiaries hospitalized for heart failure. *JAMA.* 2010;303:1716–22.
95. Figueroa JF, Wadhera RK, Frakt AB, et al. Quality of care and outcomes among medicare advantage vs fee-for-service medicare patients hospitalized with heart failure. *JAMA Cardiol.* 2020;5:1349–57.
96. Ross JS, Mulvey GK, Stauffer B, et al. Statistical models and patient predictors of readmission for heart failure: a systematic review. *Arch Intern Med.* 2008;168:1371–86.

Chapter 9
ADVANCED THERAPEUTIC OPTIONS IN ACUTE HEART FAILURE

Tiffany Dong, Aditi Nayak, and Alanna Morris

Introduction to Therapies for Acute Heart Failure

Therapy for patients presenting with symptoms of acute decompensated heart failure (ADHF) is largely driven by presentation evidence of congestion and the underlying hemodynamic profile. Those who present as "warm and wet" are defined by symptoms of congestion without evidence of hypoperfusion,[1] for which diuresis remains the cornerstone of therapy. Alternatively, those who present as "cold and wet" are not only congested but also have evidence of hypoperfusion resulting in end-organ dysfunction, while a minority of patients will present as "cold and dry" with no evidence of congestion, but evidence of decreased end-organ perfusion. Treatment for these phenotypes consists of diuretics to relieve congestion when present, as well as chemical and mechanical support to restore end-organ perfusion.

This chapter will first focus on therapies pertaining for those presenting as "warm and wet" followed by the treatment for "cold and wet." Specific treatments for right-sided heart failure (HF) and the role of palliative care conclude the chapter.

Management of Volume Overload

Role of Diuretics

For patients with symptoms of congestion, intravenous diuretics represent the mainstay of therapy. Given their higher potency, loop diuretics, such as furosemide, torsemide, bumetanide, and ethacrynic acid, are preferred over other classes of diuretics. The initial loop diuretic dose for ADHF should be at least 2.5 times the potency of the patient's home dose.[2] The Diuretic Optimization Strategies Evaluation (DOSE) trial allowed for randomized patients with ADHF to receive furosemide administered intravenously at either a low dose (equivalent to the patient's previous oral dose) or a high dose (2.5 times the previous oral dose) by means of either a bolus every 12 hours or continuous infusion.[2] Although there was no difference in the primary endpoints of global assessment in symptoms after 72 hours, the group randomized to higher-dose furosemide showed more rapid improvement in dyspnea, weight change, and fluid balance at the cost of an increase in creatinine of >0.3 mg/dL. There was no difference in those receiving continuous infusions compared to intermittent dosing.[2] According to the 2013 guidelines from the American College of Cardiology (ACC) and the American Heart Association (AHA), the initial IV diuretic dose should equal or exceed the patient's home dose and may be given continuously or as a bolus. Both of these are class I recommendations.[3]

With increasing diuretic use, many patients will develop diuretic resistance, which occurs when congestion persists despite diuretic therapy. The pathophysiology of diuretic resistance includes cell hypertrophy in the connecting tubule and collecting ducts of the kidney that may be driven by the renin-angiotensin and sympathetic systems.[4] In these cases, adding a thiazide diuretic, such as chlorothiazide, or a thiazide-like diuretic, like metolazone, may be beneficial. The combination of a loop with a thiazide for diuresis is termed "dual nephron blockade," as the thiazide blocks the sodium-chloride transporter in the ascending limb and distal tubule while the loop diuretic blocks the sodium, chloride, and potassium cotransporter of the loop of Henle. The combined effect leads to improved natriuresis.[5]

Ultrafiltration

In patients who fail maximal diuretic therapy, ultrafiltration is an option that functions similarly to dialysis, as it removes isotonic fluid from blood. A nephrology consult is warranted when considering ultrafiltration. Data supporting ultrafiltration over diuresis is limited, with two major trials, UNLOAD and CARRESS-HF, having conflicting outcomes. UNLOAD studied 200 patients admitted for ADHF and randomized subjects to ultrafiltration or diuretic therapy. The ultrafiltration group had greater weight and fluid loss after 48 hours without a change in dyspnea compared with the diuretic group. In addition, this group had lower rehospitalization rates at 90 days, but no change in mortality.[6] Despite these promising results, this study had major design flaws, as low doses of diuretics were utilized, limiting reproducibility. Moreover, it did not specify the degree of renal dysfunction, unlike the CARRESS-HF trial. In the latter trial, 188 patients with decompensated heart failure and worsening cardiorenal syndrome, defined by an increase of creatinine >0.3 mg/dL, were randomly assigned to ultrafiltration or tailored diuretic therapy for a goal of 3–5L of daily urine output. CARRESS-HF failed to achieve its primary outcome of weight loss. Furthermore, the ultrafiltration group had worse renal function and higher rates of adverse events, including renal failure, heart failure, anemia, thrombocytopenia, and infection, than the diuretic therapy.[7] Thus, utilizing ultrafiltration for ADHF carries a class IIb recommendation according to the ACC/AHA.[3]

Vasodilators

Vasodilators (Table 9.1) decrease filling pressures while preserving systolic blood pressure. These medications can improve hemodynamic function, increasing oxygenation and perfusion while theoretically relieving congestive symptoms. However, routine use of vasodilators does not improve outcomes for ADHF. A Cochrane review of four randomized trials utilizing isosorbide dinitrate or nitroglycerin failed to demonstrate symptom relief compared with alternative therapies.[8] In a post-hoc analysis from the ESCAPE trial, vasodilators were not associated with mortality benefit.[9]

The type of vasodilator depends on the phenotype of HF. In those with adequate cardiac output but persistently elevated left ventricular (LV) filling pressures, venodilators are a viable option. Among nitroglycerin, nesiritide, and nitroprusside, nitroglycerin offers the greatest venous dilatation compared with arterial dilation. Nitroglycerin provides a source of nitric

DOI: 10.1201/9780429244544-11

TABLE 9.1: Vasodilators Utilized in Acute Decompensated Heart Failure

Vasodilators	Dosages	Mechanism of Action	Venous vs Arterial	Indications	Adverse Effects
Nitroglycerin	10–200 mcg/min	NO donor	V > A dilation	• ADHF (off-label) • Hypertensive emergency • Intractable angina • Acute coronary syndrome (↓ myocardial O_2 demand)	• Headache • Orthostatic hypotension • Tachyphylaxis
Nitroprusside	5–400 mcg/min	NO donor	A = V dilation	• ADHF • Hypertensive emergency • Cardiogenic shock with high systemic, vascular resistance	• Coronary steal syndrome • Cyanide toxicity • Hypotension
Nesiritide	Bolus 2 mcg/kg then continuous infusion at 0.01 mcg/kg/min	Recombinant BNP	A and V dilation	• ADHF with dyspnea at rest	• Hypotension • Kidney injury

Abbreviations: ADHF: acute decompensated heart failure; BNP: B-type natriuretic peptide; NO: nitric oxide.

oxide that leads to smooth vascular muscle relaxation. Doses start at 5–10 mcg/min and are titrated up to 200 mcg/min, with higher doses leading to more arterial dilation.[10] Through venodilation, nitroglycerin lowers LV filling pressure and, at higher doses, decreases systemic vascular resistance and LV afterload. However, tachyphylaxis with nitroglycerin can occur hours after high doses. Alternatively, nitroprusside is another option for elevated LV filling pressures and causes equal amounts of venous and arterial dilation by providing nitric oxide. Nitroprusside can be beneficial for acute mitral regurgitation or aortic regurgitation. Patients with renal dysfunction and those on higher doses (>400 mcg/min) are at higher risk of cyanide toxicity. Because nitroprusside is a more balanced arterial and venous dilator, hypotension occurs more frequently.

Nesiritide is a recombinant form of brain natriuretic peptide (BNP), causing arterial and venous dilation, and has been approved for early relief of dyspnea, as studied in the ASCEND-HF trial. This trial randomized patients with ADHF and dyspnea at rest to nesiritide or placebo and showed improvement in subjective assessment of dyspnea at both 6- and 24-hour time points. There was an increased risk of symptomatic hypotension and no mortality benefit.[11] Current guidelines recommend that IV nitroglycerin, nitroprusside, or nesiritide can be an adjuvant to diuretics for dyspneic patients, in the absence of symptomatic hypotension.[3]

Novel vasodilators include serelaxin and ularitide. Serelaxin is a recombinant form of relaxin, which releases nitric oxide allowing for cardiovascular and renal adaptations during pregnancy. In the RELAX-AHF trial, which enrolled 1,161 patients with ADHF, the serelaxin arm attained the primary endpoint of relief of dyspnea by day five but not day one.[12] A follow-up study with 6,800 patients with ADHF (RELAX-AHF-2), failed to show cardiovascular mortality benefit or improvement in heart failure by day 5.[13] Ularitide is a synthetic form of urodilatin, which is spliced into atrial natriuretic peptide, thus promoting natriuresis by the distal tubules and the collecting duct.[14] In the SIRIUS II trial, patients who were randomized to a 24-h infusion of ularitide had dose-dependent reductions in pulmonary capillary wedge pressure (PCWP) and in dyspnea score at six hours. Patients on higher doses also had lower systemic vascular resistance and increased cardiac index that persisted 24 hours after starting ularitide.[15] Despite these promising results, ularitide failed to improve cardiovascular mortality and clinical outcomes after 48-hours in a study of 2,157 patients.[16]

Management of Low Cardiac Output

While diuretics, ultrafiltration, and vasodilators alleviate congestion, other therapies are warranted for systolic heart failure patients who present with low cardiac output or "cold and wet." These patients often meet criteria for cardiogenic shock with systolic blood pressure <90 mmHg or cardiac index <2.2 L/min/m^2 along with signs of end-organ damage. Treatment for shock encompasses inotropes and mechanical circulatory support (MCS).

Monitoring Hemodynamics

Many patients who qualify for inotropic or mechanical support may require a pulmonary artery catheter (PAC) to assess hemodynamics. The catheter measures filling pressures from which cardiac output and pulmonary and systemic vascular resistance can be derived. While PAC may be useful in certain contexts, data have not shown benefit consistently. In the ESCAPE trial, 433 patients with left ventricular ejection fraction (LVEF) <30% and symptoms of congestion were randomized to PAC or clinical assessment alone with the primary endpoint of 60-day survival after discharge. The trial was discontinued due to PAC complications and futility. However, only 180 patients in the trial required inotropes and thus PACs may still be indicated.[17] The guidelines recommend PAC use in patients with respiratory distress or decreased perfusion when cardiac filling pressures cannot be clinically ascertained (class I, level of evidence C). There is a class IIA indication with level C evidence for ADHF refractory to standard therapy if there is uncertainty regarding hemodynamics, persistently low systolic blood pressure, worsening renal function, use of IV vasoactive medications, or when considering MCS or transplant.[3]

Inotropes

Inotropes (Table 9.2) improve hemodynamics and include dobutamine, milrinone, and dopamine. Despite favorable effects on cardiac output and filling pressures, inotropes are associated with ischemia from higher myocardial consumption, arrhythmias, and higher mortality—though these patients tend to be very ill.[18] The OPTIME-CHF trial demonstrated higher in-hospital and 60-day mortality in patients with ADHF on milrinone compared to placebo. This group had increased incidence of atrial arrhythmias and hypotension, requiring intervention.[19] This association with mortality is noted in the guidelines, as long-term continuous or intermittent use of IV inotropes for reasons other than palliation is harmful.

TABLE 9.2: Inotropes Utilized in Acute Decompensated Heart Failure

Inotrope	Dosages	Mechanism of Action	Indications	Adverse Effects
Dobutamine	2–20 mcg/kg/min	• β-1 > β-2 agonist	• Cardiogenic shock • Palliative	• Arrhythmia • Ischemia
Dopamine	3–10 mcg /kg/min	• Acts as a pressor and inotrope • β-1 and β-2 agonist > α-1 agonist	• Septic shock • Cardiogenic shock • Bradycardia	• Arrhythmia • Ischemia
Milrinone	0.375–0.75 mcg/kg/min	• PDE III inhibitor	• Cardiogenic shock • RV failure • Decreases PVR	• Ischemia • Arrhythmias • Hypotension

Abbreviations: PDE: phosphodiesterase; PVR: pulmonary vascular resistance; RV: right ventricle.

Inotropes are indicated as a temporizing measure in cardiogenic shock or as a bridge to MCS or transplant.[3] Thus, inotropes should be utilized judiciously in patients with systolic dysfunction and low cardiac index with evidence of hypoperfusion and should be discontinued when clinically indicated.

Dobutamine

Dobutamine acts primarily on β_1 receptors and partially on β_2 receptors to increase stroke volume and cardiac output while decreasing systemic, vascular resistance and PCWP to a certain degree. Dobutamine assists in unloading the LV and improving volume status.[20] For heart failure, the recommended starting infusion dose is 2.5–5 mcg/kg/min and doses can be titrated up to 20 mcg/kg/min.[3] Side effects include arrhythmias at higher doses and worsening ischemia in severe coronary artery disease through increased myocardial demand. Dobutamine is contraindicated in sulfite allergy. Tolerance can develop after several days due to downregulation of β receptors.

Milrinone

Milrinone inhibits phosphodiesterase 3, ultimately preventing breakdown of cyclic adenosine monophosphate (cAMP). This increases myocardial inotropy and diastolic compliance, while reducing systemic and pulmonary vascular resistance, and thus improves cardiac index, filling pressures, and afterload.[21] Milrinone can also be used for right ventricular (RV) failure.[22] Doses range from 0.125 to 0.75 mcg/kg/min. There is a synergistic effect with dobutamine as both increase cAMP. Compared with dobutamine, milrinone may be appropriate in patients who have downregulation of their adrenergic receptors. Side effects include hypotension, cardiac ischemia due to increased myocardial demand, and arrhythmias. Caution should be used in patients with renal dysfunction, as milrinone is renally cleared.[3]

Dopamine

Unlike dobutamine and milrinone, dopamine offers both inotropic and vasopressor support. It is useful in patients with bradycardia, septic shock, and/or cardiogenic shock. At doses of 3–10 mcg/kg/min, dopamine acts on the β_1-adrenergic receptors, which leads to increased stroke volume, augmenting cardiac output. Higher doses lead to α–adrenergic stimulation, increasing systemic, vascular resistance. There is theoretical renal dilation at 1–3 mcg/kg/min. However, in the ROSE trial, which investigated whether low-dose dopamine, added to diuretics, would help with decongestion while preserving kidney function in patients with ADHF, dopamine neither increased urine output nor improved renal function and actually led to more arrhythmias.[23]

Novel Inotropes

Omecamtiv is a novel inotrope that activates cardiac myocytes, ultimately prolonging systole in reduced LVEF. In the ATOMIC-AHF study, 606 patients with ADHF were randomized to either three different doses of omecamtiv or placebo for 48 hours. Although the trial failed to reach the primary endpoint of dyspnea improvement, the group on the highest dose had improvement in dyspnea. Moreover, LVEF increased whereas end-systolic dimension decreased with higher plasma concentrations. Unlike other inotropes, omecamtiv was not associated with tachyarrhythmias.[24]

Mechanical Circulatory Support (MCS)

In general, MCS utilizes pump technology to augment cardiac output. Benefits include end-organ perfusion, lowering of intracardiac pressures with improvement in cardiac volumes, ameliorating congestive symptoms, improving wall stress, decreasing myocardial O_2 demand, and augmenting coronary perfusion. The guidelines currently support MCS for stage D heart failure with reduced LVEF with plans for definite management or expected cardiac recovery.[3] Other indications for MCS include cardiogenic shock, refractory malignant arrhythmias, support for percutaneous interventions, or cardiac arrest. There are two types of MCS: nondurable or durable. Nondurable or temporary MCS includes the intra-aortic balloon pump (IABP), the Impella and TandemHeart devices, and extracorporeal membrane oxygenation (ECMO). Durable devices are intended for long-term use and encompass ventricular assist device (VAD) or total artificial heart (TAH) as strategies for destination therapy, bridge to therapy, or bridge to candidacy. The ideal timing for MCS placement remains unknown.[25] Risk factors for mortality despite MCS include RV failure, acuity, and severity of the condition. In this chapter, we focus on temporary MCS; additional information on durable MCS can be found in Chapter 18.

Intra-Aortic Balloon Pump (IABP)

The IABP is the most employed form of MCS, given its cost-effectiveness and easier insertion. The pump consists of a balloon catheter and a pump console controller and, compared with other MCS devices, provides modest hemodynamic support (Figure 9.1). The catheter is a double-lumen 7.5–8.0 French with a balloon attached to the distal end. The pump attaches to one lumen and inflates the balloon with helium, whereas the second lumen allows for guidewire insertion and transduction of aortic pressure. It can be placed through either a femoral or axillary approach and travels retrograde, so that the balloon ends in the aorta. Timing of inflation and deflation depends on electrocardiogram (EKG) or pressure triggers, with inflation occurring at the end of diastole, which is the middle of the T-wave representing repolarization. Deflation begins with systole or the peak of the R-wave.

The IABP improves hemodynamics by increasing coronary perfusion during diastole through inflation in the proximal

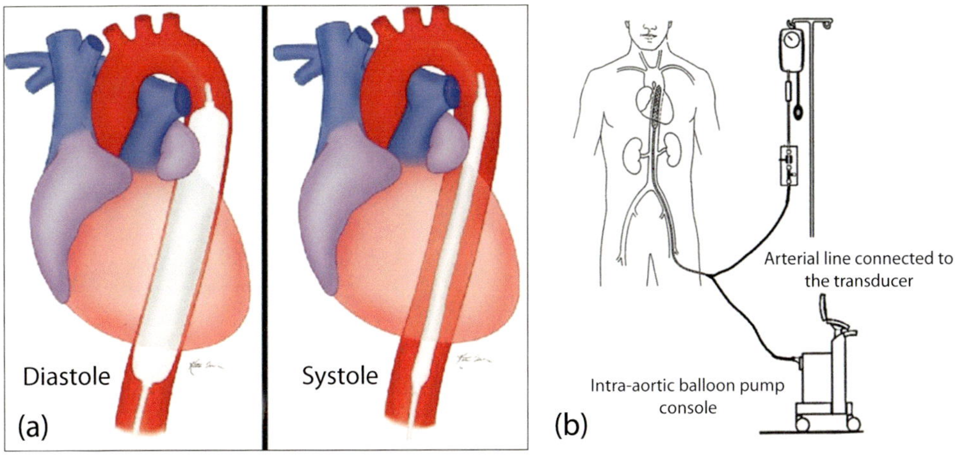

FIGURE 9.1 The intra-aortic balloon pump. (a) Intra-aortic balloon pump inflated within the aorta during diastole and deflated during systole. (Reproduced under a Creative Commons Attribution License from Ginat et al. Imaging of mechanical cardiac-assist devices. *J Clin Imaging Sci.* 2011;1:21.) (b) Mechanical setup of the intra-aortic balloon pump. (Reproduced under a Creative Common CC BY license from Limbert and Amiri. Intra-aortic balloon pump for patients with cardiac conditions: An update on available techniques and clinical applications. *Reports.* 2019;2:19.)

aorta, creating an augmented diastolic flow. By deflating during systole, IABP creates a vacuum effect and decreases LV afterload, which in turn decreases wall tension and reduces myocardial demand. Moderate (as opposed to severe) LV dysfunction and low burden of arrhythmias yield optimal IABP dynamics. Daily assessments of IABP include waveform analysis, heparin monitoring, and correct placement 1–4 cm below the aortic arch.

As IABP depends on EKG, arrhythmias result in incorrect balloon mechanics. Newer IABPs utilize fiber optics that can ameliorate the burden of arrhythmias. Complications are largely vascular and include dissection, pseudoaneurysm, hemorrhage, stroke, and limb ischemia. Other complications include anemia, thrombocytopenia, infection, and those related to incorrect positioning of the pump, e.g., acute kidney injury and bowel ischemia. Balloon rupture rarely occurs, and the device is designed to aspirate helium to prevent gas emboli. Contraindications are moderate to severe aortic valve regurgitation, peripheral arterial disease, and aortic dissection or aneurysm. Sepsis and severe coagulopathy are relative contraindications.

Impella

The Impella is a rotatory, axial-flow pump that propels blood from the LV to the aorta (Figure 9.2). The system includes a flexible pigtail end that sits in the LV and connects to a distal cannula that comes in three different sizes. The cannula houses the pump inlet and outlet, motor, and pump pressure monitor. A proximal 9-Fr catheter contains the motor leads as well as the purge and pressure lumens. This catheter attaches to a console cable and side arms for purge solution and pressure tubing. The device is commonly placed through the femoral artery via a cut-down or in the axillary artery, which allows patients to ambulate, and is advanced retrogradely to cross the aortic valve. The pump rotates at a set speed and draws blood out of the LV into the aorta.

The axial flow unloads the LV, which results in less myocardial O_2 consumption, better mean arterial pressure, and lower PCWP. The larger the distal cannula, the greater the flow, with Impella 2.5 providing the least hemodynamic support and Impella 5.0 providing the most support. The Impella 2.5 generates about 2.5 L/m flow, utilizing a 12-Fr pump motor. Compared to the IABP, Impella 2.5 provides greater cardiac output. The Impella CP provides approximately 3–4 L/m of flow with a 14-Fr pump motor. Compared to IABP, the Impella CP did not improve all-cause mortality at one or six months in patients with myocardial infarction complicated with severe cardiogenic shock requiring immediate percutaneous, coronary intervention.[26] However, this population was very ill with the most common cause of death being anoxic brain injury.[26] The Impella 5.0 generates the greatest flow, using a 21-Fr pump motor, which gives 5.0 L/m cardiac output. A single-center study of 40 patients with stage D heart failure demonstrated efficacy in stabilization as well as safety of the Impella 5.0 device while waiting for transplant or VAD.[27]

Unlike IABP, the Impella does not rely on EKGs for timing and is stable during transient arrhythmias. However, the device is not effective during asystole or ventricular tachycardia, because of RV failure. Other complications include vascular injury similar to IABP, those related to pump migration, and aortic or mitral valve injury. Suction events can occur, especially in low preload states. If hemolysis persists and causes acute kidney injury, then the device should be removed. Contraindications include thrombus either in the LV or left atrium (LA), severe aortic stenosis or insufficiency, mechanical aortic valve, bleeding, ventricular septal defect, and severe peripheral arterial disease.

TandemHeart

Similar to the Impella, TandemHeart can also generate up to 5.0 L/m of flow. The device pumps blood from the LA to the iliofemoral system and thus bypasses the LV (Figure 9.3). TandemHeart consists of four parts: a control console, a centrifugal pump, a femoral arterial cannula, and a transseptal cannula. The cannula contains holes, which aspirate blood from the LA. An electromagnetic motor moves the blood to the femoral system. To place the device, the operator inserts the venous catheter into the femoral vein and advances, ultimately making a transseptal puncture into the LA. The arterial cannula is placed into the iliofemoral system.

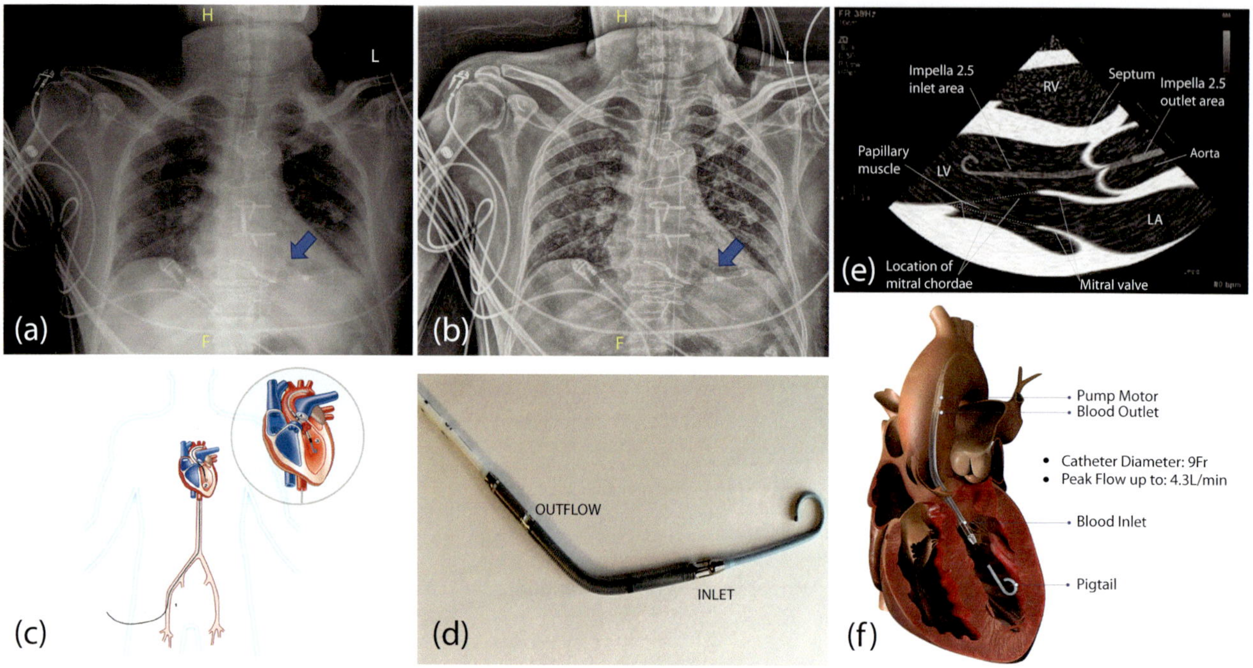

FIGURE 9.2 The Impella device (Abiomed, Inc., Danvers, MA). (a) and (b): Anteroposterior chest radiographs of a patient with an Impella device (arrows). (c) The Impella catheter is inserted percutaneously through the femoral artery and advanced under fluoroscopic or echocardiographic monitoring into the left ventricular cavity. The inlet is within the left ventricle and the outlet is in the ascending aorta. (Reproduced with permission from Glazier and Kaki. The Impella device: Historical background, clinical applications and future directions. *Int J Angiol.* 2019;28:118–23.) (d) The Impella 2.5 device. (Reproduced with permission from Glazier and Kaki. The Impella device: Historical background, clinical applications and future directions. *Int J Angiol.* 2019;28:118–23.) (e) Transthoracic echocardiogram parasternal long-axis view illustrating the correct positioning of an Impella device. LA, left atrium; LV, left ventricle; RV, right ventricle. (Image reproduced with the permission of Abiomed, Inc.). (Reproduced under a Creative Commons Attribution 4.0 International License (CC-BY) from Kaki et al. Impella-induced incessant ventricular tachycardia. *Ochsner J.* 2019;19:248–51.) (f) Impella CP. The Impella is placed retrograde across the aortic valve, with the pigtail and inlet area in the left ventricle and the outlet area in the ascending aorta. Blood is continuously pulled from the left ventricle into the ascending aorta. CP: cardiac power. (© 2018 Abiomed, Inc., image used with permission. Reproduced under a Creative Commons Attribution 4.0 International License from: Primary Angioplasty: A Practical Guide [Internet]. Lo and Ohman. Chapter 19 Mechanical Circulatory Support in ST-Elevation Myocardial Infarction, 2018.) (www.ncbi.nlm.nih.gov/books/NBK543576/.)

Advantages of TandemHeart include decreased LV preload, workload, wall stress, myocardial demand, and filling pressures.[28] The device works in "tandem" with the heart, as the LV still contributes to cardiac output. However, the LV often will cease contracting. As with most MCS studies, the number of subjects is limited. A study with 33 patients with cardiogenic shock due to either acute myocardial infarction or ADHF showed that TandemHeart recipients had greater cardiac indices and reductions in PCWP over the first 16 h, compared with IABP recipients. Safety profiles were similar. However, the study failed to show difference in 30-day mortality.[29] Other studies confirmed this improvement in hemodynamics without significant change in 30-day survival. However, one study did report higher rates of bleeding and limb ischemia with TandemHeart compared with IABP.[30,31]

Procedural complications include tamponade from the transseptal approach, residual atrial septal defect, thromboemboli, and air emboli. Other complications include bleeding, arrhythmias, limb ischemia, and hemolysis. Movement can displace the venous catheter. If retracted into the right atrium, the venous catheter causes a massive right-to-left shunt. If advanced into the pulmonary vein, the device can malfunction. TandemHeart relies on adequate RV function and, thus, RV failure is a contraindication to placement. Other contraindications include right or left atrial thrombus, aortic insufficiency, ventricular septal defect, or significant peripheral arterial disease. In certain patients, a 5–6 Fr sheath can be placed antegrade into the superficial femoral artery and cut into the arterial cannula to provide limb perfusion.

Extracorporeal Membrane Oxygenation (ECMO)

ECMO provides artificial lung and heart support via a membrane oxygenator and a non-pulsatile, centrifugal pump (Figure 9.4). There are two types of ECMO: veno-veno (V-V) or veno-arterial (V-A). As V-V ECMO only provides oxygenation and V-A provides both oxygenation and circulatory support, this chapter will focus only on V-A ECMO. Indications for V-A ECMO include cardiogenic shock requiring cardiac and pulmonary support, inability to wean from cardiogenic bypass, bridge to transplant, and post-cardiac arrest. ECMO consists of a centrifugal blood pump, a membrane oxygenator, an inflow or venous 20-Fr cannula, and an outflow or arterial 17-Fr cannula. The venous cannula removes deoxygenated blood that then moves to the membrane oxygenator for gas exchange. The oxygenated blood is infused back into the patient. This device can be placed also at the bedside under ultrasonographic or fluoroscopic guidance. ECMO can be placed either peripherally or centrally in the operating room with sternotomy. In peripheral

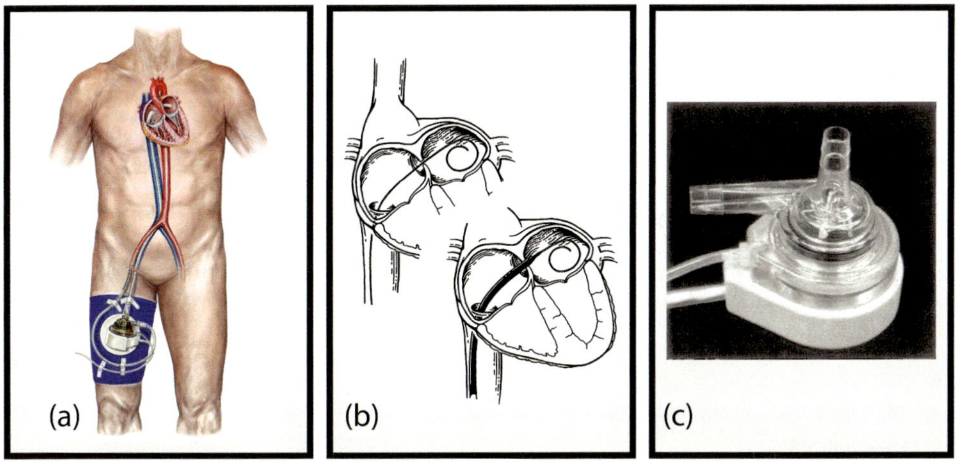

FIGURE 9.3 The TandemHeart device (CardiacAssist, Inc., Pittsburgh, PA). (a) The TandemHeart is a left atrial to arterial extracorporeal device that requires atrial transseptal puncture. A cannula is situated into the left atrium and aspirates oxygenated blood, which is delivered to the body by a femoral artery outflow cannula. (Image used with permission from CardiacAssist. (Reproduced under a Creative Commons Attribution 4.0 International License from: Primary Angioplasty: A Practical Guide [Internet]. Lo and Ohman: Chapter 19 Mechanical Circulatory Support in ST-Elevation Myocardial Infarction, 2018.) (www.ncbi.nlm.nih.gov/books/NBK543576/.) (b) A looped wire is present in the left atrium and a dilator is then advanced over the wire to dilate the septal puncture site. Next, a venous cannula is passed over the wire and positioned in the left atrium. The arterial return cannula is inserted into the common femoral artery, using the Seldinger technique. (Reproduced with permission from Magovern and Lasorda: Implantation of the TandemHeart percutaneous left ventricular assist device. *Operative Techniques in Thoracic and Cardiovascular Surgery*, 2002;7:112–19.) (c) The TandemHeart pump is a small centrifugal pump driven by an electromagnetic motor. On a mock loop, the device can flow up to 10 L/min, but, in the clinical setting, the average flow is 3 to 4 L/min owing to limitations from cannula size. (Reproduced with permission from Magovern and Lasorda. Implantation of the TandemHeart percutaneous left ventricular assist device. *Operative Techniques in Thoracic and Cardiovascular Surgery*, 2002;7:112–19.)

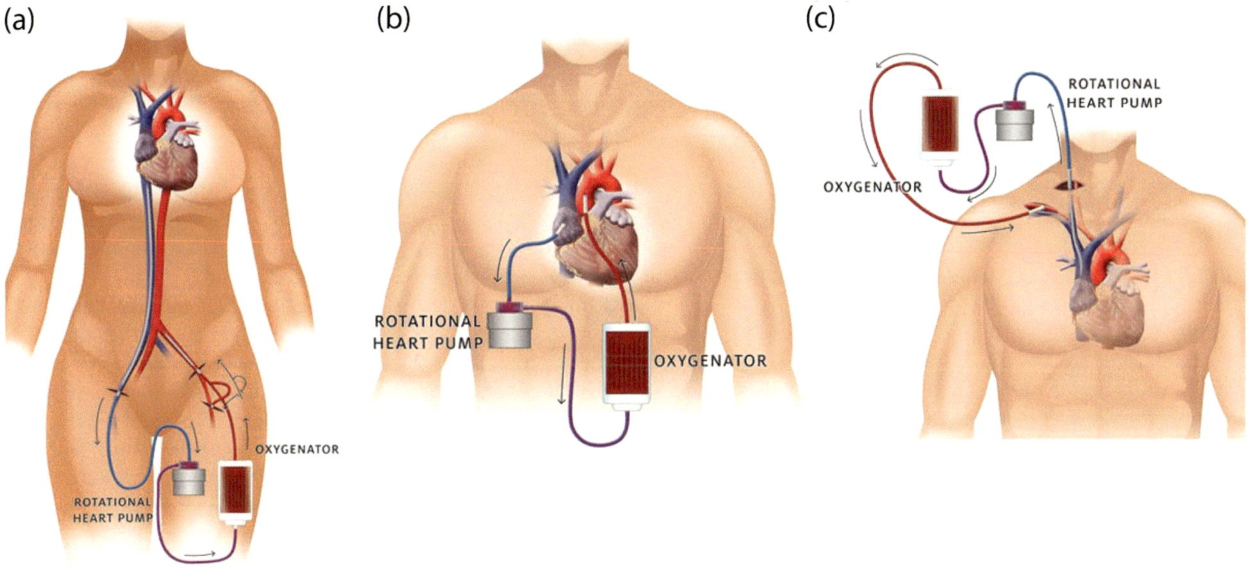

FIGURE 9.4 Extracorporeal membrane oxygenation (ECMO). (a) Peripheral veno-arterial ECMO (femoro-femoral configuration). (b) Central veno-arterial ECMO. (c) Peripheral veno-arterial ECMO ("sport" configuration). (Reproduced with permission from Rao. Circulation: Venoarterial extracorporeal membrane oxygenation for cardiogenic shock and cardiac arrest. *Circ Heart Fail.*, 2018;11:e004905.)

placement, the inflow cannula is usually placed in the RA via the internal jugular or femoral vein as drainage, with the outflow cannula placed in the femoral artery. Centrally placed ECMO has the venous cannula in the RA and the arterial cannula in the ascending aorta.

The management of ECMO consists of fluid flow, sweep gas flow, and anticoagulation. After a patient is connected to ECMO, the fluid flow needs to be adjusted. Initially the operator mixes priming fluid with the patient's blood and then the rate is increased gradually to reach maximum flow as determined by the patient's circulation and resistance within the machine. Once the maximum flow is attained, the rate is then decreased to the lowest level that supports an adequate mean arterial pressure. Another variable in ECMO is the flow of the sweep gas that removes CO_2 while infusing O_2 into the patient's blood. The rate is usually equal to the blood flow but can be increased for CO_2 clearance while not affecting oxygenation. Anticoagulation also needs to be monitored while on ECMO. Heparin is most used with the goal of activated clotting time 1.5 times the upper limit of normal. Advantages of ECMO include a cardiac output of up to 6 L/min depending on cannula size. However, retrograde blood flow from the femoral artery can lead to LV distension along with higher afterload, ultimately causing higher wall stress and decreasing LV outflow. In these cases, the LV may need additional MCS support with an IABP or Impella device.[32]

Complications of ECMO are largely hematologic, including bleeding, thromboemboli, and hemolysis. Clots can occur in the machine and/or the patient. Cannulation itself can lead to thrombosis in veins and arteries. Another complication is North-South syndrome, which occurs in patients with recovering cardiac output. In this syndrome, the recovering heart pumps blood to the pulmonary system but does not attain proper oxygenation. This relatively deoxygenated blood perfuses the upper limbs while ECMO delivers oxygenated blood to the lower limbs. Contraindications to device placement include severe aortic regurgitation, aortic dissection, severe peripheral artery disease, disseminated cancer, bleeding, recent stroke, head trauma, and severe chronic diseases e.g., cirrhosis, renal failure, or emphysema.

Ventricular Assist Device (VAD)

Unlike IABP, Impella and ECMO, VADs are a form of long-term mechanical support that can be placed for RV or LV support. Cardiac surgeons place the inlets in the LV apex and the outflow graft connects the unit to the ascending aorta. The pump placement depends on the model. The types of pumps have evolved over time. The first-generation pumps, including HeartMate I, Thoratec pneumatic, and Novacor, were pulsatile, producing a pulse pressure. Due to issues with durability and complication rates, first-generation models are no longer implanted. Second-generation models rely on a rotatory pump generating axial, continuous flow, and a battery-powered electric motor. The HeartMate II, Jarvik 2000, and DeBakey VADs are examples of second-generation devices. The HeartMate II demonstrated better survival and low rates of malfunction and thromboembolic events,[33,34] and was shown to be a reasonable therapeutic option as a destination therapy, compared with first-generation devices.[35] Third-generation devices use a centrifugal, continuous-flow pump with a levitating rotor or impeller. The magnetic or hydrodynamic levitation reduces the wear and heat production of the system. HeartMate 3, HeartWare, and DuraHeart are examples of third-generation devices. HeartMate 3 demonstrated superiority over HeartMate II, with lower reoperation rates for device malfunction and disabling stroke after two years in the MOMENTUM 3 trial in 366 patients with VAD placed either as bridge-to-transplant or destination therapy. In addition, the HeartMate 3 group had lower rates of pump thrombosis and bleeding. However, the device did not meet the secondary endpoints of reduction in death or disabling stroke.[36]

Complications with VADs include ischemic and hemorrhagic stroke, gastrointestinal bleeding, pump thrombosis, hemolysis, and acquired von Willebrand factor deficiency secondary to shearing of the von Willebrand protein in axial-flow pumps. Patients are also at risk of driveline infection, worsening aortic regurgitation, and RV failure. Risk factors for RV failure include pre-existing RV dysfunction,[37] higher pulmonary vascular resistance, and destination therapy indication.

Total Artificial Heart (TAH)

For those who require biventricular support, a TAH may be a long-term bridge option. Placement requires a body surface area of 1.7–2.5 m^2 or >10 cm between the 10th thoracic vertebra and the sternum. With TAH, the work of the native ventricles and valves is replaced by a pneumatically powered artificial heart. Complications include stroke, bleeding, thrombosis, and infections, e.g., mediastinitis. TAH has been associated with renal failure due to BNP withdrawal.[38] Anemia in TAH recipients is multifactorial, with etiologies including hemolysis, inflammation, and decreased erythropoiesis.[39] A study comparing an implantable biventricular assist device with TAH reported that TAH had lower stroke rates with better 90-day survival.[40] TAH also improved survival to cardiac transplant and post-transplant survival.[41] Durable devices are discussed in more detail in Chapter 18.

Right Heart Failure

Right heart failure is associated with increased morbidity and mortality. Treatment includes addressing the underlying causes, e.g., ischemia, maintaining sufficient preload and afterload, and improving RV contractility. Medical management encompasses either volume or diuretics for preload optimization, pulmonary vasodilators for RV afterload reduction, and inotropes for patients in shock. Similar to LV failure, if RV is refractory to medical management, MCS should be considered. Devices capable of RV support include the Impella RP, the TandemHeart Right Ventricular Assist Device (TH-RVAD), and VA-ECMO. The Impella RP is placed in the femoral vein and advanced across both the tricuspid and pulmonic valves into the pulmonary artery (PA). The device moves blood from the inferior vena cava to the PA, providing up to 5 L/min of flow. Patients after myocardial infarction and cardiac surgery who received an Impella RP had immediate improvement in central venous pressure and cardiac index in the RECOVER RIGHT trial.[42] The device is contraindicated in respiratory failure. Similarly, the TH-RVAD provides flow from the RA to the PA, bypassing the RV. One inflow cannula is placed into the RA while the outflow cannula is placed into the main PA, using either bilateral femoral veins or the internal, jugular vein and femoral vein. The inflow cannula drains blood from the RA, which then travels to the centrifugal pump that returns it to the PA. The TH-RVAD was associated with improvement in hemodynamics in a retrospective, multicenter study.[43] ECMO can also be utilized either as VA or veno-veno-arterial (VVA) in conjunction with a centrifugal pump (TandemHeart, CentriMag, or Rotaflow). In VA-ECMO, the inflow cannula is placed in the RA and returns blood into the arterial system. In VVA-ECMO, two inflow cannulas drain the RA and PA, then deposit blood into the arterial system. Both configurations decrease RV preload and RV output. By increasing arterial flow, however, ECMO can increase afterload and worsen an already impaired LV. VA-ECMO has been shown to help hemodynamics in RV failure of multiple etiologies.[44] Moreover, the Impella RP and TH-RVAD can be combined with the left-sided therapies mentioned above.

Heart Transplant

Patients with Stage D heart failure refractory to medication, MCS, and surgical management should be considered for heart transplant. Candidacy depends on institutional reviews, but absolute contraindications include limited life expectancy regardless of transplant, current substance abuse, medical non-adherence, and severe, symptomatic cerebrovascular disease. Irreversible pulmonary hypertension may be a contraindication, but the degree of hypertension remains institutionally dependent. Other relative contraindications include older patients, diabetes, severe kidney disease, obesity, active infection, cancer, and limited social support.

Palliative Care

Palliative care plays a vital role in advanced heart failure, consistent with the HF guidelines. In the PAL-HF trial, 150 patients received usual care with or without palliative care involvement. The palliative care arm had better quality of life after six months, as measured by the Kansas City Cardiomyopathy Questionnaire and the Functional Assessment of Chronic Illness Therapy–Palliative Care scale. Moreover, this group experienced less depression and anxiety while reporting higher levels of spiritual well-being.[45] Thus, the role of palliative care cannot be overstated in advanced heart failure.

Conclusion

In acute heart failure, treatment depends on hemodynamics. If hemodynamically stable, patients should undergo IV diuresis, although certain individuals may benefit from ultrafiltration. Vasodilators can also be considered to improve filling pressures and perfusion, while aiding with congestion. For cardiogenic shock, inotropes such as dobutamine, milrinone, and dopamine may be utilized. If refractory to medical management, the patient should be evaluated for short-term and/or long-term MCS as well as for heart transplant. Palliative care should be involved early for those with advanced heart failure.

References

1. Nohria A, Tsang SW, Fang JC, et al. Clinical assessment identifies hemodynamic profiles that predict outcomes in patients admitted with heart failure. *J Am Coll Cardiol.* 2003;41:1797–804.
2. Felker GM, Lee KL, Bull DA, et al. Diuretic strategies in patients with acute decompensated heart failure. *N Engl J Med.* 2011;364:797–805.
3. Yancy CW, Jessup M, Bozkurt B, et al. ACCF/AHA guideline for the management of heart failure: A report of the American College of Cardiology Foundation/American Heart Association Task Force on practice guidelines. *J Am Coll Cardiol.* 2013;62:e147–239.
4. Casu G, Merella P. Diuretic therapy in heart failure - Current approaches. *Eur Cardiol.* 2015;10:42–47.
5. Brater DC. Diuretic therapy. *N Engl J Med.* 1998;339:387–95.
6. Costanzo MR, Guglin ME, Saltzberg MT, et al. Ultrafiltration versus intravenous diuretics for patients hospitalized for acute decompensated heart failure. *J Am Coll Cardiol.* 2007;49:675–83.
7. Bart BA, Goldsmith SR, Lee KL, et al. Ultrafiltration in decompensated heart failure with cardiorenal syndrome. *N Engl J Med.* 2012;367:2296–304.
8. Wakai A, McCabe A, Kidney R, et al. Nitrates for acute heart failure syndromes. *Cochrane Database Syst Rev.* 2013:CD005151.
9. Elkayam U, Tasissa G, Binanay C, et al. Use and impact of inotropes and vasodilator therapy in hospitalized patients with severe heart failure. *Am Heart J.* 2007;153:98–104.
10. Imhof PR, Ott B, Frankhauser P, Chu LC, Hodler J. Difference in nitroglycerin dose-response in the venous and arterial beds. *Eur J Clin Pharmacol.* 1980;18:455–60.
11. O'Connor CM, Starling RC, Hernandez AF, et al. Effect of nesiritide in patients with acute decompensated heart failure. *N Engl J Med.* 2011;365:32–43.
12. Teerlink JR, Cotter G, Davison BA, et al. Serelaxin, recombinant human relaxin-2, for treatment of acute heart failure (RELAX-AHF): A randomised, placebo-controlled trial. *Lancet.* 2013;381:29–39.
13. Teerlink JR, Voors AA, Ponikowski P, et al. Serelaxin in addition to standard therapy in acute heart failure: Rationale and design of the RELAX-AHF-2 study. *Eur J Heart Fail.* 2017;19:800–9.
14. Singh A, Laribi S, Teerlink JR, Mebazaa A. Agents with vasodilator properties in acute heart failure. *Eur Heart J.* 2017;38:317–25.
15. Mitrovic V, Seferovic PM, Simeunovic D, et al. Haemodynamic and clinical effects of ularitide in decompensated heart failure. *Eur Heart J.* 2006;27:2823–32.
16. Packer M, O'Connor C, McMurray JJV, et al. Effect of ularitide on cardiovascular mortality in acute heart failure. *N Engl J Med.* 2017;376:1956–64.
17. Binanay C, Califf RM, Hasselblad V, et al. Evaluation study of congestive heart failure and pulmonary artery catheterization effectiveness: The ESCAPE trial. *JAMA.* 2005;294:1625–33.
18. Abraham WT, Adams KF, Fonarow GC, et al. In-hospital mortality in patients with acute decompensated heart failure requiring intravenous vasoactive medications: An analysis from the Acute Decompensated Heart Failure National Registry (ADHERE). *J Am Coll Cardiol.* 2005;46:57–64.
19. Cuffe MS, Califf RM, Adams KF, Jr., et al. Short-term intravenous milrinone for acute exacerbation of chronic heart failure: A randomized controlled trial. *JAMA.* 2002;287:1541–7.
20. Liang CS, Sherman LG, Doherty JU, Wellington K, Lee VW, Hood WB, Jr. Sustained improvement of cardiac function in patients with congestive heart failure after short-term infusion of dobutamine. *Circulation.* 1984;69:113–9.
21. Simonton CA, Chatterjee K, Cody RJ, et al. Milrinone in congestive heart failure: Acute and chronic hemodynamic and clinical evaluation. *J Am Coll Cardiol.* 1985;6:453–9.
22. Chen EP, Bittner HB, Davis RD, Jr., Van Trigt P, 3rd. Milrinone improves pulmonary hemodynamics and right ventricular function in chronic pulmonary hypertension. *Ann Thorac Surg.* 1997;63:814–21.
23. Chen HH, Anstrom KJ, Givertz MM, et al. Low-dose dopamine or low-dose nesiritide in acute heart failure with renal dysfunction: The ROSE acute heart failure randomized trial. *JAMA.* 2013;310:2533–43.
24. Teerlink JR, Felker GM, McMurray JJV, et al. Acute treatment with omecamtiv mecarbil to increase contractility in acute heart failure: The ATOMIC-AHF study. *J Am Coll Cardiol.* 2016;67:1444–55.
25. Rihal CS, Naidu SS, Givertz MM, et al. 2015 SCAI/ACC/HFSA/STS clinical expert consensus statement on the use of percutaneous mechanical circulatory support devices in cardiovascular care: Endorsed by the American Heart Association, the Cardiological Society of India, and Sociedad Latino Americana de Cardiologia Intervencion; Affirmation of Value by the Canadian Association of Interventional Cardiology-Association Canadienne de Cardiologie d'intervention. *J Am Coll Cardiol.* 2015;65:e7–e26.
26. Ouweneel DM, Eriksen E, Sjauw KD, et al. Percutaneous mechanical circulatory support versus intra-aortic balloon pump in cardiogenic shock after acute myocardial infarction. *J Am Coll Cardiol.* 2017;69:278–87.
27. Lima B, Kale P, Gonzalez-Stawinski GV, Kuiper JJ, Carey S, Hall SA. Effectiveness and safety of the Impella 5.0 as a bridge to cardiac transplantation or durable left ventricular assist device. *Am J Cardiol.* 2016;117:1622–8.
28. Kapur NK, Paruchuri V, Urbano-Morales JA, et al. Mechanically unloading the left ventricle before coronary reperfusion reduces left ventricular wall stress and myocardial infarct size. *Circulation.* 2013;128:328–36.
29. Burkhoff D, Cohen H, Brunckhorst C, O'Neill WW, TandemHeart Investigators G. A randomized multicenter clinical study to evaluate the safety and efficacy of the TandemHeart percutaneous ventricular assist device versus conventional therapy with intraaortic balloon pumping for treatment of cardiogenic shock. *Am Heart J.* 2006;152:469 e461–468.
30. Thiele H, Sick P, Boudriot E, et al. Randomized comparison of intra-aortic balloon support with a percutaneous left ventricular assist device in patients with revascularized acute myocardial infarction complicated by cardiogenic shock. *Eur Heart J.* 2005;26:1276–83.
31. Kar B, Gregoric ID, Basra SS, Idelchik GM, Loyalka P. The percutaneous ventricular assist device in severe refractory cardiogenic shock. *J Am Coll Cardiol.* 2011;57:688–96.
32. Koeckert MS, Jorde UP, Naka Y, Moses JW, Takayama H. Impella LP 2.5 for left ventricular unloading during venoarterial extracorporeal membrane oxygenation support. *J Card Surg.* 2011;26:666–8.
33. John R, Kamdar F, Liao K, Colvin-Adams M, Boyle A, Joyce L. Improved survival and decreasing incidence of adverse events with the HeartMate II left ventricular assist device as bridge-to-transplant therapy. *Ann Thorac Surg.* 2008;86:1227–34; discussion 1234–25.
34. John R, Kamdar F, Liao K, et al. Low thromboembolic risk for patients with the Heartmate II left ventricular assist device. *J Thorac Cardiovasc Surg.* 2008;136:1318–23.

35. Slaughter MS, Rogers JG, Milano CA, et al. Advanced heart failure treated with continuous-flow left ventricular assist device. *N Engl J Med.* 2009;361:2241–51.
36. Mehra MR, Goldstein DJ, Uriel N, et al. Two-year outcomes with a magnetically levitated cardiac pump in heart failure. *N Engl J Med.* 2018;378:1386–95.
37. Hayek S, Sims DB, Markham DW, Butler J, Kalogeropoulos AP. Assessment of right ventricular function in left ventricular assist device candidates. *Circ Cardiovasc Imaging.* 2014;7:379–89.
38. Delgado R, 3rd, Wadia Y, Kar B, et al. Role of B-type natriuretic peptide and effect of nesiritide after total cardiac replacement with the AbioCor total artificial heart. *J Heart Lung Transplant.* 2005;24:1166–70.
39. Mankad AK, Tang DG, Clark WB, et al. Persistent anemia after implantation of the total artificial heart. *J Card Fail.* 2012;18:433–8.
40. Kirsch M, Mazzucotelli JP, Roussel JC, et al. Survival after biventricular mechanical circulatory support: Does the type of device matter? *J Heart Lung Transplant.* 2012;31:501–8.
41. Copeland JG, Smith RG, Arabia FA, et al. Cardiac replacement with a total artificial heart as a bridge to transplantation. *N Engl J Med.* 2004;351:859–67.
42. Anderson MB, Goldstein J, Milano C, et al. Benefits of a novel percutaneous ventricular assist device for right heart failure: The prospective RECOVER RIGHT study of the Impella RP device. *J Heart Lung Transplant.* 2015;34:1549–60.
43. Kapur NK, Paruchuri V, Jagannathan A, et al. Mechanical circulatory support for right ventricular failure. *JACC Heart Fail.* 2013;1: 127–34.
44. Truby L, Mundy L, Kalesan B, et al. Contemporary outcomes of venoarterial extracorporeal membrane oxygenation for refractory cardiogenic shock at a large tertiary care center. *ASAIO J.* 2015;61:403–9.
45. Rogers JG, Patel CB, Mentz RJ, et al. Palliative care in heart failure: The PAL-HF randomized, controlled clinical trial. *J Am Coll Cardiol.* 2017;70:331–41.

Section III
Managing Chronic Heart Failure

DOI: 10.1201/9780429244544-12

Chapter 10
OUTPATIENT MANAGEMENT OF STABLE HEART FAILURE WITH REDUCED EJECTION FRACTION

Leah Reid, Jonathan Murrow, Kent Nilsson, and Catherine Marti

Introduction

Although therapies for HF with preserved ejection fraction (HFpEF) are lacking, there are many therapies available to patients with HF with reduced ejection fraction (HFrEF), regardless of symptomatology.[1] Careful consideration should be taken at every encounter to evaluate not only volume status but also to optimize guideline-directed medical therapy as well as device therapy. In this chapter, we outline the current therapy available for outpatient management of HFrEF (Table 10.1).

Beta-Blockers

Maladaptive activation of the sympathetic nervous system in HFrEF can lead to worsening congestion, malperfusion, and arrhythmias.[2] Blockade of β-adrenergic receptors has proven in multiple clinical trials to reduce morbidity and mortality—specifically with metoprolol succinate and bisoprolol, which selectively block β-1-receptors, and with carvedilol, which selectively blocks α-1, β-1 and β-2 receptors.[3]

In the landmark Cardiac Insufficiency Bisoprolol Study II (CIBIS-II), patients with HFrEF (ejection fraction [EF] ≤35%) and New York Heart Association (NYHA) class II–IV symptoms had a 34% relative risk reduction in all-cause mortality with bisoprolol therapy vs placebo.[4] The Metoprolol CR/XL Randomized Intervention Trial in Congestive Heart Failure (MERIT-HF) and carvedilol trials likewise demonstrated reduced risk of death or HF hospitalization (Figure 10.1).[5–7] To reduce morbidity and mortality, the 2013 American College of Cardiology/American Heart Association (ACC/AHA) Heart Failure Guidelines thus recommend using either bisoprolol, carvedilol, or sustained-release metoprolol succinate for all patients with current or prior symptoms of HFrEF unless contraindicated (class I, level of evidence [LOE]: A). Importantly, the benefit of β blockers is dose dependent, with lower achieved heart rates associated with improved outcomes, albeit this effect is mostly relevant to patients in sinus rhythm and not among those with atrial fibrillation.[8] A network meta-analysis of 21 trials found a mortality benefit of β blockers vs placebo at 12 months (odds ratio [OR] 0.69, confidence interval [CI] 0.56 to 0.80); no obvious differences in clinical outcomes were observed between differing β blockers, nor did one dominate others in terms of improvements in left ventricular EF.[9] An individual patient data meta-analysis of 11 trials demonstrated reduction of mortality in HFrEF across the age distribution (40–85 years old), reporting an absolute reduction for the cohort of 13,833 patients of 4.3% over a median follow-up of 1.3 years. Heart failure readmission was reduced by β blockers, but less so in older patients. Drug discontinuation for side effects was similar across the age distribution and between men and women. Notably, rates of discontinuation for dizziness or lethargy were not different from rates reported in placebo-treated cohorts.[10]

The overall clinical goal is to achieve the highest tolerated dose, best done by starting with a low dose and increasing the dose over time while being mindful of precipitating fluid retention among those without concurrent diuretic therapy. MERIT-HF[11] showed a mortality reduction of over 30% when targeting 200 mg/day. This dose was achieved in 64% of patients; the mean dose was 159 mg/day.[5] In the Carvedilol Prospective Randomized Cumulative Survival Study (COPERNICUS) trial, four out of five patients reached the target dose of 50 mg daily.[12] Furthermore, side effects reported with carvedilol were actually less than those reported with placebo. Importantly, reactive airways disease or asymptomatic bradycardia should not necessarily constrain the use of beta-blockers.[13] In most health systems, beta-blocker prescription costs are low, yielding an Incremental Cost Effectiveness Ratio of only $34/quality-adjusted life years in one analysis.[14]

Angiotensin-Converting Enzyme Inhibitors

Angiotensin-converting enzyme inhibitors (ACEI) are well established in HF therapy, with overwhelming evidence in symptomatic and asymptomatic HFrEF (left ventricular EF<40%).[15–17] ACEIs interfere with the renin angiotensin system, inhibiting the enzyme that is responsible for converting angiotensin I to angiotensin II (Figure 10.2). Because of inhibition of kininase II, ACEIs may also lead to the upregulation of bradykinin, further enhancing effects of angiotensin suppression. These agents have been shown to reduce mortality, reduce hospitalization for HF, result in left ventricular remodeling, and improve quality of life.[18] As such, the ACC/AHA HF Guidelines have given the use of ACEI a class I, LOE: A recommendation.[1]

ACEIs should be initiated at the lowest dose and titrated quickly, every 3–5 days, to the highest tolerated dose that has been shown to be effective in clinical trials. Higher doses have been shown to be more effective than lower doses in preventing hospitalization, although even low doses are effective in reducing mortality and HF hospitalization.[19] ACEIs can reduce blood pressure, increase potassium, and increase creatinine. In the Studies of Left Ventricular Dysfunction (SOLVD) treatment trial, side effects were reported in 87% of the patients with enalapril, but high rates of side effects were also reported with placebo (82%).[18] Blood pressure, renal function, and potassium should be checked 1–2 weeks after initiation of ACEI use. Extra caution should be taken in patients with diabetes mellitus, preexisting renal dysfunction, azotemia, hyponatremia, or previous allergy to ACEI. Importantly, most patients tolerate mild hypotension related to suppression of the renin angiotensin system, although, if hypotension is accompanied by dizziness or syncope, the dose of ACEI can be decreased and/or diuretics decreased before ACEIs are considered to be poorly tolerated.

Importantly, more attention needs to be paid to achieving target doses of medications in practice. In the Registry to

DOI: 10.1201/9780429244544-13

TABLE 10.1: Starting and Target Doses of Select Established and Novel Therapies for Heart Failure

	Starting Dose (mg)	Target Dose (mg)
Beta-Blockers		
Bisoprolol	1.25 daily	10 daily
Carvedilol	3.125 b.i.d.	25 b.i.d. for weight <85 kg and 50 b.i.d. for weight ≥85 kg
Metoprolol succinate	12.5–25 daily	200 daily
Angiotensin Receptor Neprilysin Inhibitors		
Sacubitril/valsartan	24/26–49/51 b.i.d.	97/103 b.i.d.
Angiotensin-Converting Enzyme Inhibitors		
Captopril	6.25 t.i.d.	50 t.i.d.
Enalapril	2.5 b.i.d.	10–20 b.i.d.
Lisinopril	2.5–5.0 daily	20–40 daily
Ramipril	1.25 daily	10 daily
Angiotensin II Receptor Blockers		
Candesartan	4–8 daily	32 daily
Losartan	25–50 daily	150 daily
Valsartan	40 b.i.d.	160 b.i.d.
Aldosterone Antagonists		
Eplerenone	25 daily	50 daily
Spironolactone	12.5–25 daily	25–50 daily
Sodium-Glucose Cotransporter-2 Inhibitors		
Dapagliflozin	10 daily	10 daily
Empagliflozin	10 daily	10 daily
Vasodilators		
Hydralazine	25 t.i.d.	75 t.i.d.
Isosorbide dinitrate	20 t.i.d.	40 t.i.d.
Fixed-dose combination isosorbide dinitrate/hydralazine	20/37.5 (1 tab) t.i.d.	2 tabs t.i.d.
Ivabradine		
Ivabradine	2.5–5 b.i.d.	Titrate to heart rate 50–60 beats/min. Maximum dose 7.5 b.i.d.

Notes: Isosorbide mononitrate is not recommended by current guidelines, which consider either the fixed-dose combination or the separate combination of isosorbide dinitrate and hydralazine as appropriate guideline-directed therapies for heart failure.
Abbreviations: b.i.d. = bis in die (twice daily); t.i.d. = ter in die (three times daily).
Source: Reproduced with permission from: Maddox et al., *J Am Coll Cardiol* 2021;77:772–810.

Improve the Use of Evidence-Based Heart Failure Therapies in the Outpatient Setting (IMPROVE HF), only one-third of the patients were treated at target dose of ACEIs.[20] In addition, ACEI therapy should be carried out in conjunction with other HF therapies, even if lower doses of either medication are necessary. The mortality benefit of combined beta-blocker and ACEI therapy is apparent, regardless of ACEI dose.[21]

A certain proportion of patients taking ACEI will develop a non-productive cough (10–15% of patients) or angioedema (1% of patients). In patients that cannot tolerate ACEIs because of a cough or angioedema, angiotensin receptor blockers can be substituted.[18]

Angiotensin Receptor Blockers

Angiotensin receptor blockers (ARBs) are well tolerated in most patients and should be used to reduce mortality, prevent rehospitalization, and improve quality of life in symptomatic and asymptomatic patients with HF (left ventricular EF <40%). ARBs inhibit the renin-angiotensin system, but by a different mechanism than ACEIs. ARBs block the effects of angiotensin II on the angiotensin type I receptor, the subtype which is responsible for the adverse effects relevant to angiotensin II as it relates to cardiac remodeling in HF. Clinical trials have demonstrated that ARBs are as effective as ACEIs in decreasing mortality, reducing hospitalization, reversing the process of left ventricular remodeling, and improving quality of life.[22] Similar to ACEI, the ACC/AHA HF Guidelines have given the use of ARB in HF patients a class I, LOE: A recommendation.[1]

ARBs should be initiated at the doses listed and titrated to the highest tolerated dose that was effective in clinical trials as quickly as possible. Similar to ACEIs, renal function, potassium, and blood pressure should be checked 1–2 weeks after initiation of ARB usage to monitor for significant dysfunction, as well as with changes in dosage.

Angiotensin Receptor Neprilysin Inhibitor

The combination of the ARB valsartan with the neprilysin inhibitor sacubitril has proven to offer better outcomes in HFrEF

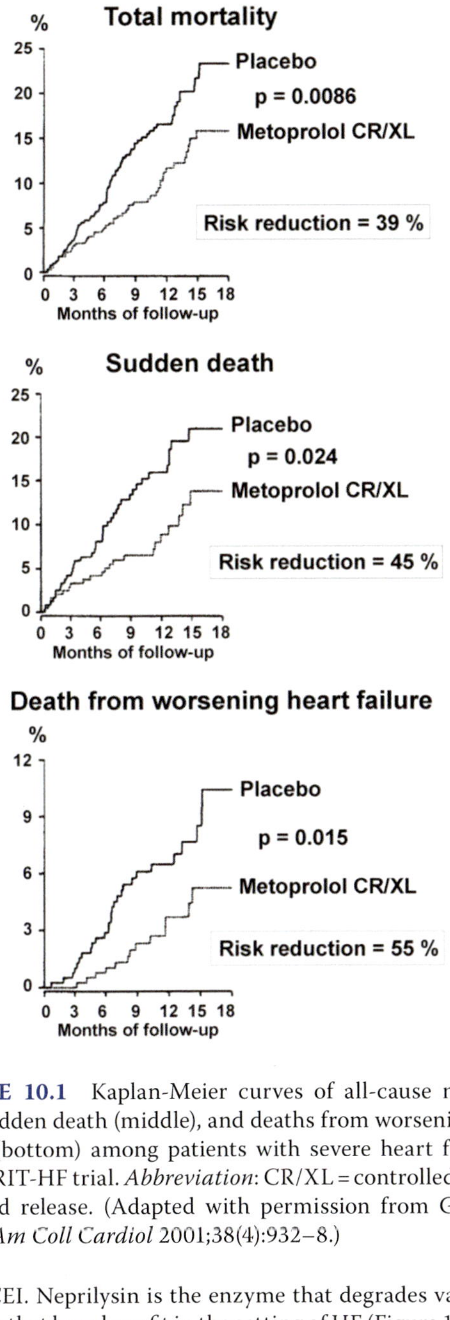

FIGURE 10.1 Kaplan-Meier curves of all-cause mortality (top), sudden death (middle), and deaths from worsening heart failure (bottom) among patients with severe heart failure in the MERIT-HF trial. *Abbreviation*: CR/XL = controlled release/extended release. (Adapted with permission from Goldstein et al., *J Am Coll Cardiol* 2001;38(4):932–8.)

over ACEI. Neprilysin is the enzyme that degrades vasoactive peptides that have benefit in the setting of HF (Figure 10.3). The Prospective comparison of Angiotensin Receptor-neprilysin inhibitor (ARNI) with ACEI to Determine Impact on Global Mortality and morbidity in Heart Failure (PARADIGM-HF trial) was the largest HF trial to date, demonstrating improved outcomes with ARNI among patients with symptomatic HF and left ventricular EF ≤40%, in conjunction with one additional risk marker (elevated B-type natriuretic peptide [BNP] or HF hospitalization).[23] The primary outcome (cardiovascular death or HF hospitalization) was more common in those receiving enalapril than those receiving valsartan-sacubitril (hazard ratio [HR] 0.80 [CI: 0.73, 0.87]).[23] A subsequent meta analysis of neprilysin inhibitors demonstrated that, as compared with a strategy of ACE inhibition, neprilysin inhibition led to a consistent reduction in mortality.[24] In the Comparison of Sacubitril-Valsartan vs Enalapril on Effect on N terminal proBNP in Patients Stabilized from an Acute Heart Failure Episode trial (PIONEER-HF), patients hospitalized with HFrEF were randomly assigned to enalapril or sacubitril-valsartan while still in hospital. A larger reduction in N terminal proBNP was noted in patients who received sacubitril-valsartan than in those that received enalapril. These findings bolster the use of sacubitril-valsartan in the acute HF setting in stabilized patients. Because of the robust data supporting a significant benefit in HF, the ACC/AHA HF Guidelines have given the use of ARNI a class I, LOE: B-R recommendation as either initial therapy, or as replacement for ACEI/ARB.[1]

In PARADIGM-HF, patients receiving sacubitril-valsartan experienced more hypotension than those receiving enalapril; typically this did not necessitate cessation of medication. However, there was less severe hyperkalemia and cough among those receiving sacubitril-valsartan than those receiving enalapril. Treatment-naïve patients should be started at the lowest dose of sacubitril-valsartan and rapidly titrated up to the maximum tolerated dose. Importantly, the magnitude of benefit with low-, moderate-, or high-dose valsartan-sacubitril, relative to corresponding enalapril doses, was similar.[25]

Hydralazine and Nitrates

Endothelial dysfunction, impaired nitric oxide bioavailability, and increased oxidative stress occur with structural remodeling of the left ventricle seen in HFrEF.[26] Isosorbide mononitrate augments nitric oxide and hydralazine reduces oxidative stress. The combination of both has been posited to slow the progression of left ventricular dysfunction. Clinical trials of hydralazine and nitrates for HFrEF have in fact shown some clinical benefit; a systematic review of seven trials including 2,626 patients found a reduction in all-cause mortality and cardiovascular mortality associated with hydralazine/nitrate therapy vs placebo, but less clinical efficacy when compared to ACEI.[27]

Subgroup analysis of a large clinical trial observed a significant benefit in African American subjects treated with hydralazine and nitrates.[28] The follow-up randomized clinical trial enrolling self-identified African Americans demonstrated improved outcomes in HF with hydralazine/isosorbide treatment in addition to ACEI or ARB therapy, aldosterone antagonism, and beta-blockers.[26] Thus, the ACC/AHA HF guidelines confer a class I indication for the combination of hydralazine and isosorbide dinitrate for patients self-described as African Americans with NYHA class III–IV HFrEF receiving optimal therapy with ACE inhibitors and beta-blockers (LOE A).[1,13] For patients unable to tolerate other vasodilators, hydralazine/isosorbide may be helpful (class IIA, LOE B).[1,13]

While the high pill burden in hydralazine/isosorbide dosing, in addition to drug side effects, may limit adherence, an analysis of African American Veterans Affairs patients eligible for this therapy observed significant underutilization—and most concerningly a higher mortality rate among untreated patients after controlling for patient selection.[29]

Ivabradine

Lowering myocardial oxygen demand (MVO_2) in patients with HFrEF remains a therapeutic goal to mitigate the high-energy phosphate depletion associated with impaired contractility.[30] Historically, pharmacologic means of reducing MVO_2 have been limited to beta-adrenergic blockers. Though beta-blockers exert a pronounced salutary effect in HFrEF, optimal dosing to reduce heart rate is constrained by their concomitant

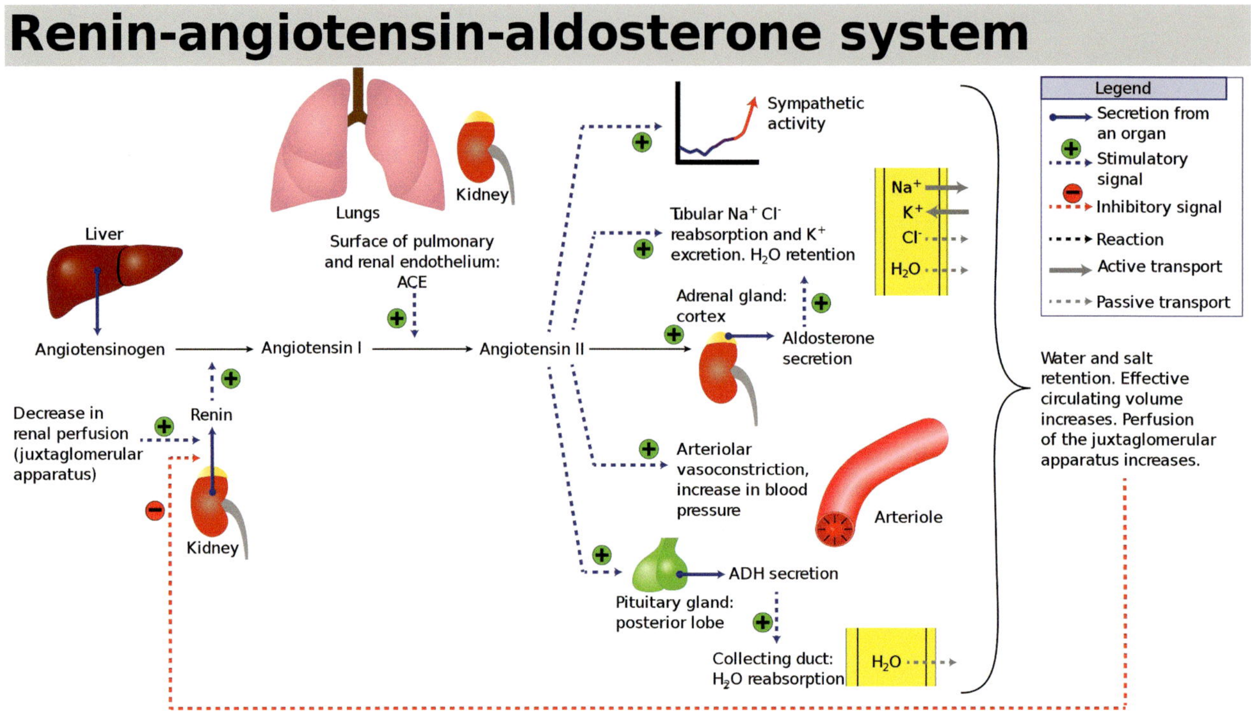

FIGURE 10.2 The renin-angiotensin-aldosterone system (RAAS). (Figure obtained from Wikipedia Commons, reproduced under the Creative Commons Attribution-Share Alike 4.0 International license. https://commons.wikimedia.org/w/index.php?curid=66583851.)

impact on systemic arterial pressure. Ivabradine is a comparatively novel pharmacologic agent that reduces heart rate without affecting blood pressure, inotropy, and vascular resistance.[31] Ivabradine works at the sinoatrial node where it inhibits the inward "funny" current (I_f), which is critical in determining the automaticity (spontaneous pacemaker activity) rate of the pacemaker cells. Selective inhibition of I_f leads to an increase in diastole duration without alteration of other phases of the action potential, and thus lowers heart rate.[31]

The Systolic Heart Failure Treatment with the I_f Inhibitor Ivabradine Trial (SHIFT) tested ivabradine in a randomized, double-blind, placebo-controlled, parallel-group study of 6,558 patients with symptomatic (NYHA class II–IV) HFrEF (left ventricular EF ≤35%), sinus rhythm heart rates ≥70 beats per minute with hospital admission for HF within the previous year and on optimal medical therapy.[32] The primary endpoint, a composite of cardiovascular death or hospital admission for worsening HF, was reduced by 18% in the ivabradine group (HR 0.82; CI: 0.75, 0.90) and was driven by a 26% reduction in hospitalizations for HF over 23 months. Although there was no difference in all-cause mortality, there was a 26% reduction in HF deaths, an 11% reduction in all-cause hospitalizations, and a 15% reduction in any cardiovascular hospitalization. Subsequently, ivabradine was given a class IIA (LOE B-R) recommendation by 2016 ACC/AHA/Heart Failure Society of America (HFSA) Focused Update on New Pharmacological Therapy for HF.[33] Ivabradine is best viewed as a second-line therapy and can be beneficial to reduce HF hospitalization for patients with symptomatic (NYHA class II–III) stable chronic HFrEF (left ventricular EF ≤35%), who are receiving goal-directed therapy including a beta-blocker at maximum tolerated dose, and who are in sinus rhythm with resting heart rate of ≥70 beats per minute.

Constraints to use of ivabradine include cost, with a recent cost-effectiveness analysis determining its incremental cost effectiveness ratio of $24920 per quality-adjusted life year.[34] In addition, ivabradine is not indicated for patients with atrial fibrillation as it acts on the sinus node.

Digoxin

Digoxin is the most prescribed cardiac glycoside due to its pharmacokinetics, alternative routes of administration, and availability to measure serum drug level measurements. Digoxin has been shown to be effective in relieving HF symptoms associated with atrial fibrillation with a rapid ventricular rate. However, in HF patients with normal sinus rhythm, its efficacy has been questioned.

The effect of digoxin on survival among patients with HF was assessed in the Digitalis Investigator Group (DIG) trial.[35] Almost 6,800 patients, with symptomatic HF on baseline therapy with ACE inhibitors and diuretics as clinically indicated, were studied. After an average of 37 months follow-up, there was no difference in terms of survival between patients on digoxin or placebo. However, use of digoxin was associated with a trend toward lower mortality related to worsening HF (11.6% vs 13.2% for placebo, P=0.06). More recent meta-analyses have shown that digoxin use in HF is associated with a neutral to increased risk of mortality compared to placebo, further constraining its widespread use in HFrEF.[36,37] Likewise, the ACC/AHA HF Guidelines suggest that the use of digoxin to minimize symptoms of HF is not well established (class IIb, LOE: C).[1]

Digoxin poisoning can be a life-threatening event. Among patients with HF, significant toxicity most commonly emerges at serum concentrations greater than 2.0 ng/mL. Frequently,

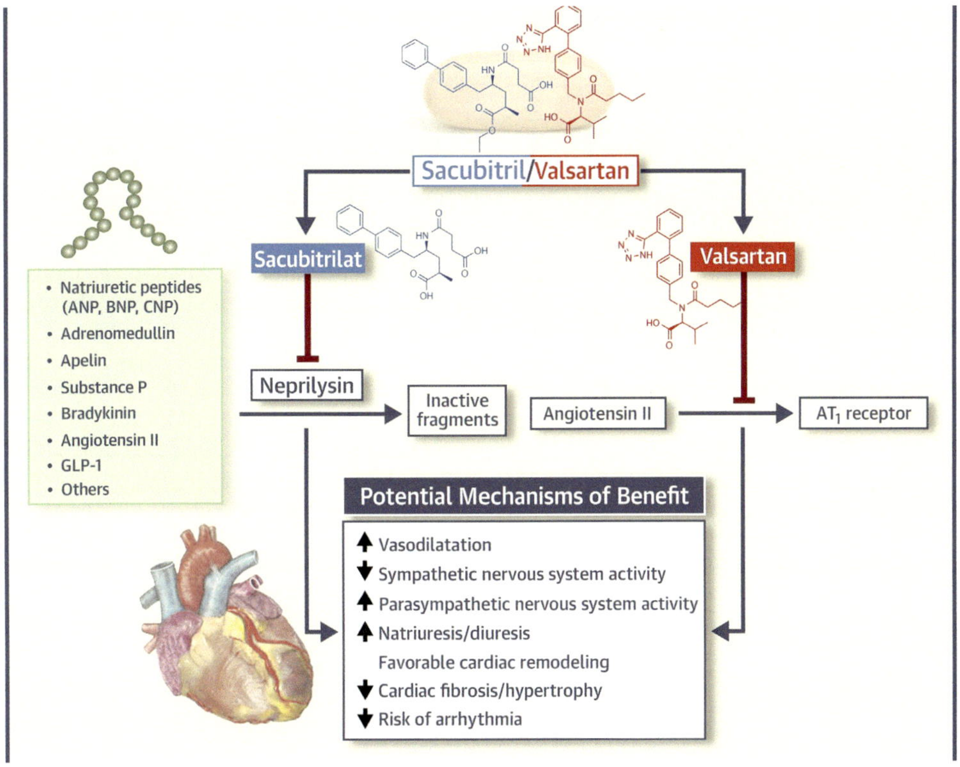

FIGURE 10.3 Mechanism of action of sacubitril/valsartan. Sacubitril/valsartan is a combination of an angiotensin receptor blocker (valsartan) and a neprilysin inhibitor pro-drug (sacubitril). In binding to the AT1 receptor, valsartan attenuates the vasoconstrictive, sodium-retaining, and pro-fibrotic and pro-mitotic effects of angiotensin II. Neprilysin is responsible for the breakdown of a variety of vasoactive peptides. Sacubitrilat inhibits neprilysin activity, thereby increasing endogenous levels of these peptides, resulting in increased vasodilation, natriuresis, and diuresis, along with a reduction in cardiac fibrosis and hypertrophy. Red lines denote inhibitory actions. *Abbreviations*: ANP: atrial natriuretic peptide; BNP: B-type natriuretic peptide; CNP: C-type natriuretic peptide. (Reproduced with permission from Docherty et al., *J Am Coll Cardiol HF* 2020;8:800–10.)

neurological or gastrointestinal symptoms are the first symptoms. Disturbances in cardiac conduction are also commonly seen with toxicity, including ectopic beats of atrioventricular, junctional, or ventricular origin; atrioventricular block; a slow ventricular rate response to atrial fibrillation; or an accelerated atrioventricular junctional rhythm.[38] Life-threatening digoxin toxicity can be reversed with anti-digoxin immunotherapy.[39]

Diuretics

Diuretics are used to remove excess fluid from patients with HF (Table 10.2). They are important not only in patients with decompensated HF but also in those with stable, chronic HF to maintain euvolemia. There have been no randomized, controlled trials addressing the use of non-potassium sparing diuretics in patients with HF. As volume regulation is at the center of HF therapy, it would be unethical to withhold therapy and any trial with a placebo control would result in substantial crossover. Thus, most of the recommendations regarding diuretics in HF are based on clinical experience. Despite the lack of randomized data, the ACC/AHA HF Guidelines support the use of diuretics to control pulmonary congestion and peripheral edema with a class I, LOE: C recommendation.[1]

TABLE 10.2: Commonly Used Diuretics in the Management of Outpatient Heart Failure

Diuretic	Category	Dose Range (mg per day)	Starting Dose (mg)
Furosemide	Loop	20–600	20
Bumetanide	Loop	0.5–10	0.5
Torsemide	Loop	20–200	20
Metolazone	Thiazide	2.5–10	2.5

Loop diuretics are the most potent of all diuretic agents. The four most used drugs in this class are furosemide, bumetanide, torsemide, and ethacrynic acid. Loop diuretics are protein-bound and not freely filtered by the glomerulus; they are secreted into the tubular lumen. Importantly, this secretion is impaired by and the action of these drugs limited by the concurrent presence of organic acids, which occurs in renal failure or in the presence of probenecid, salicylates, or nonsteroidal anti-inflammatory drugs.[40] Once secreted into the tubule, loop diuretics compete with chloride molecules to bind to the $Na^+/K^+/2Cl^-$ cotransporter, thereby inhibiting reabsorption of sodium and chloride. Urinary diuretic concentration correlates with the natriuretic response following administration of a diuretic.[41]

Furosemide is the most widely used loop diuretic with an oral bioavailability of about 50% in patients with normal renal function. The onset of action after an oral dose is within 30–60 min and has a duration of action of six hours.[42] In renal insufficiency, the elimination half-life can be prolonged and there is reduced drug delivery to the main site of action within the tubule.[43] In HF patients, the absorption of oral furosemide can be delayed, which prolongs the time to peak concentration as well as efficacy. Bumetanide is 40 times more potent than furosemide with a bioavailability of 80%. The duration of action is between three and six hours for most patients. Torsemide differs from other loop diuretics as 80% of the drug is metabolized in the liver, so that its half-life is less altered by renal dysfunction. It is absorbed rapidly and has a bioavailability of 80%. The natriuretic response following dosing of torsemide is not affected by route of administration.[44] The onset of action is one to two hours after administration with a half-life of 3.3 hours, but this can be prolonged in the setting of cirrhosis.[41, 45] When selecting an oral agent for patients with HF, torsemide may be advantageous as its absorption is unimpaired and more consistent than that of furosemide.[41]

Fluid and electrolyte abnormalities can be a result of diuresis—hypokalemia and metabolic alkalosis, hyperuricemia, hyponatremia, and hypotension. Therefore, careful monitoring is required, especially in patients with chronic kidney disease or hypotension at baseline. Hypersensitivity reactions can also occur, typically manifested with a rash or less commonly as acute interstitial nephritis. Loop diuretics can also cause an allergic reaction in patients with a known sulfonamide allergy.[46]

There are limited data on dosing of diuretics in HF. Many factors can result in persistent fluid retention among patients with HF. Most commonly, this is related to inadequate diuretic dose and excess sodium intake. However, delayed intestinal absorption of oral drugs, decreased diuretic excretion, and increased sodium reabsorption in the nephron are also potential causes of fluid retention.[47–49] Importantly, non-steroidal anti-inflammatory drugs should be discontinued. Diminished synthesis of both vasodilator and natriuretic prostaglandins can significantly impair diuretic responsiveness.[50,51]

Sodium-Glucose Co-Transporter 2 Inhibitors

Sodium-glucose co-transporter 2 inhibitors (SGLT2i) were initially developed as glucose-lowering agents, as these drugs block the sodium-glucose cotransporter protein 2 in the proximal convoluted tubule of the kidney, therefore increasing urinary glucose and sodium excretion. In cardiovascular safety trials, these agents led to a reduction of HF events in patients with diabetes regardless of baseline-prevalent HF.[52,53] These favorable effects of SGLT2i led to the hypothesis that SGLT2i have favorable disease- modifying effects in HF. [54] The pivotal DAPA-HF trial evaluated the effect of 10 mg of dapagliflozin vs placebo in HF patients with LVEF ≤40% and NYHA II–IV HF symptoms who were on guideline-directed medical therapy.[55] Patients on dapagliflozin had a 26% reduction in the composite of hospitalization or urgent visit for HF (resulting in intravenous diuretic therapy) or death from cardiovascular (CV) causes (HR 0.74, 95%CI 0.65–0.85, P<0.001).[55] The effect was consistent across all the components of the primary endpoint and independent of the presence of diabetes.

Similar to the cardioprotective effects of SGLT2i, data suggest that the beneficial effects of SGLT2i in patients with prevalent HFrEF are a class effect. In the EMPEROR-Reduced trial, 3,730 patients with HFrEF with or without diabetes were randomized to receive either 10 mg of empagliflozin or placebo.[56] Empagliflozin achieved a 25% reduction in the primary composite endpoint of CV death or hospitalization for worsening HF (HR 0.75, 0.65–0.86, P<0.001).[56] The total number of hospitalizations for HF was 30% lower in the empagliflozin arm (HR 0.70, 95%CI 0.58–0.85; P <0.001). Importantly, the annual rate of decline in the estimated glomerular filtration rate (a prespecified endpoint in the study) was slower in the empagliflozin arm (–0.55 vs –2.28 mL per minute per 1.73 m^2 per year, P <0.001), and empagliflozin-treated patients had a lower risk of serious renal outcomes.[56]

Initial findings from the CANVAS trial fueled concerns about a direct association between SGLT2i use and a higher rate of amputations.[53] This association was not confirmed as a class effect in other studies or meta-analyses, in which a favorable safety profile was seen. However, in patients on canagliflozin, a close monitoring for ulcers, sores, and signs of infections should be strongly advised, and, if any of the above occur, canagliflozin should be discontinued.[57] The main side effects are mycotic genital infections, as well as urinary tract infections, dehydration, and hypotension.[58] Additional details on the action of these agents are provided in Chapter 22.

Based on the overwhelmingly positive results, a recent ACC expert consensus decision pathway document recommends that after initiation of use of beta-blockers and renin-angiotensin-aldosterone system antagonists, with close monitoring of electrolytes, SGLT2i should be considered for patients with HFrEF and NYHA class II–IV symptoms (Figure 10.4).[59]

Device Therapy in Chronic Heart Failure

Multiple epidemiologic studies have identified reduced left ventricular EF as a significant risk factor for sudden cardiac death (SCD).[60,61] In addition to the increased risk of SCD with a decreased EF, the pathology underlying the cardiomyopathy influences the risk of SCD: patients with infiltrative/ischemic cardiomyopathies have a significantly higher risk of SCD than do patients with a non-ischemic cardiomyopathy.[60] For patients with reduced left ventricular EF, implantable cardioverter defibrillators (ICD) have been shown to reduce both cardiovascular and all-cause mortality.[62–65] In patients with HFrEF exacerbated by dyssynchrony (e.g., left bundle branch block, right ventricular pacing), cardiac resynchronization therapy (CRT) has been demonstrated to not only decrease mortality, but also to improve EF, quality of life, and exercise capacity.[61,66,67] The benefits of ICD implantation, however, need to be weighed against the acute (pneumothorax, cardiac tamponade) and chronic (infection, inappropriate therapies, lead fracture) risks of device placement. Use of both ICD and CRT devices in HF is highly recommended by the ACC/AHA HF Guidelines in the appropriate patient (class I, LOA: A).[1,13] Additional details on ICD and CRT options for patients with HF are provided in Chapters 6 and 21.

Heart Failure Self-Care

Lifestyle modifications are an important aspect of HF care in Stage C HFrEF, with particular emphasis on physical activity and dietary prescriptions.[68] The Heart Failure: A Controlled Trial Investigating Outcomes of Exercise Training (HF-ACTION) study randomized 2,331 medically stable outpatients with HFrEF to usual care plus aerobic exercise training in both supervised and home-based training or usual care alone.[69] Over the median 30-month follow-up, exercise training resulted in no significant reductions in the primary end point of all-cause mortality or hospitalization. A subsequent meta-analysis of 44 cardiac rehabilitation trials that included 5,783 patients for a median of six months observed reduced hospitalization (RR: 0.70; 95% CI: 0.60, 0.80) but not mortality.[70]

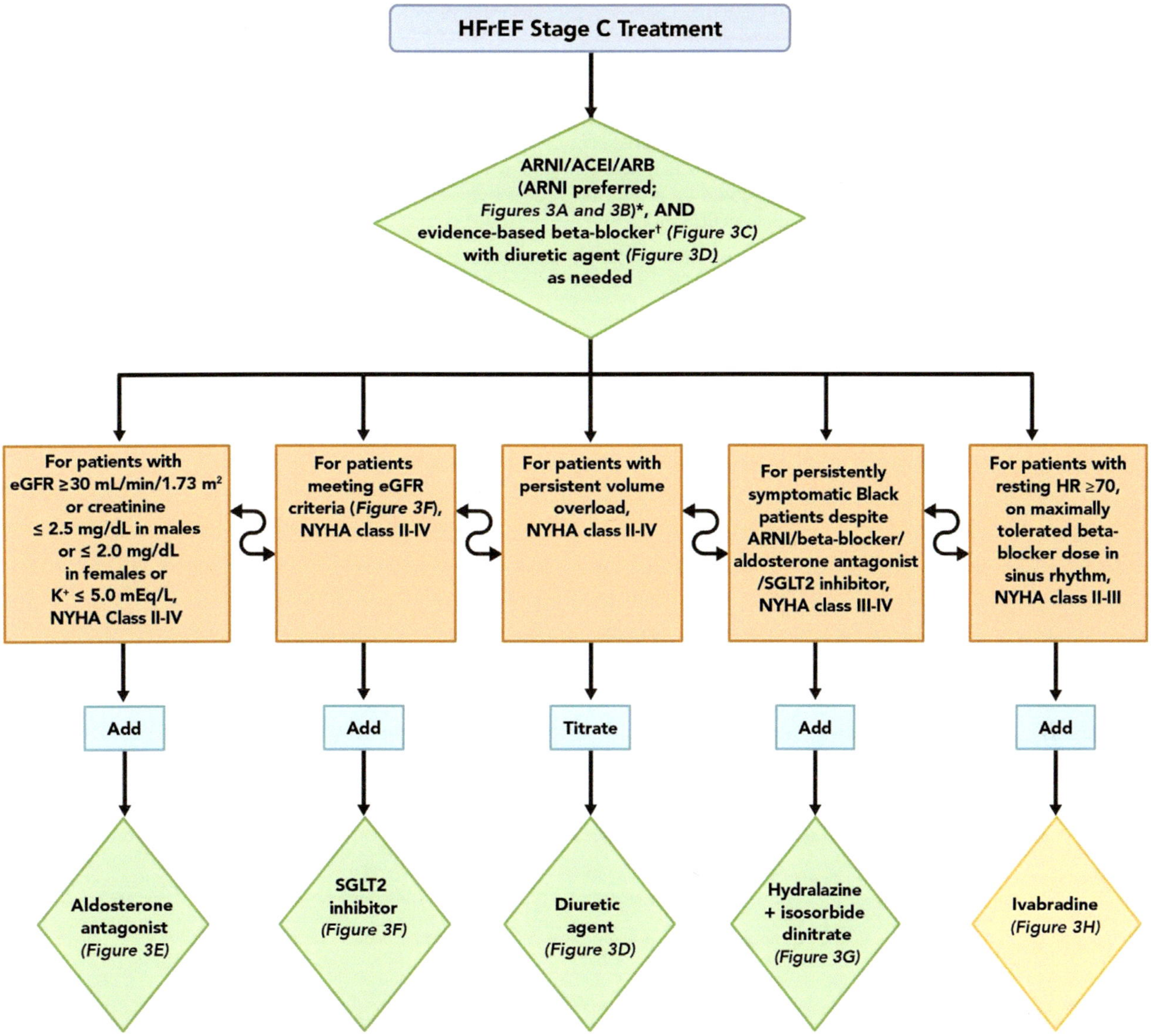

*ACEI/ARB should only be considered in patients with contraindications, intolerance or inaccessibility to ARNI. In those instances, please consult Figure 3 and text for guidance on initiation.

†Carvedilol, metoprolol succinate, or bisoprolol.

ACEI = angiotensin-converting enzyme inhibitors; ARNI = angiotensin receptor-neprilysin inhibitors; ARB = angiotensin receptor blocker; eGFR = estimated glomerular filtration rate; HFrEF = heart failure with reduced ejection fraction; HR = heart rate; K^+ = potassium; NYHA = New York Heart Association; SGLT2 = sodium-glucose cotransporter-2.

FIGURE 10.4 Treatment algorithm for guideline-directed medical therapy, including novel therapies. Green color identifies a class I therapy from clinical practice guidelines, whereas a yellow color indicates a class II therapy. (Reproduced with permission from Maddox et al., *J Am Coll Cardiol* 2021;77:772–810.)

Accordingly, the 2013 ACC/AHA heart failure guidelines recommend physical activity to improve symptoms (class I, LOE: A), and supervised exercise through cardiac rehabilitation to reduce morbidity and mortality (class IIA, LOE: B).[13]

Dietary modification—primarily through advice for sodium restriction—remains a key focus in self-management of HFrEF.[71] There remains a dearth of evidence, however, to support recommending specific sodium intake levels—made complicated by several studies showing worse outcomes in patients randomized to lower sodium intake. The 2013 ACCF/AHA HF Guideline recommends sodium restriction of <3 g/day in patients with stage C HF to avoid congestion.[13]

There is increasing interest in leveraging the widespread use of new technologies that may easily provide reminders, track dietary intake and physical activity, and motivational tools for people attempting to adopt healthy habits.[72] Exergaming (games to improve physical exercise) was studied as a potential alternative approach to increasing exercise capacity in elderly, chronically ill cardiac patients in a small study.[73] Fear of physical activity is also one potential psychological barrier to physical activity in patients with HF.[74] Significant barriers to recruiting and enrolling patients with HFrEF into cardiac rehabilitation exist and recruitment strategies and factors that improve adherence are potential areas for research in this area.[75]

Conclusion

Heart failure is a common and deadly condition. However, there are many therapies available to patients with HFrEF that can dramatically change the course of the disease process.[1, 13] Every effort should be made to initiate all therapies available to patients and titrate to the highest tolerated dose as quickly as possible. When titrating therapies, care should be given to prioritizing therapies with the most proven benefit.

References

1. Yancy CW, Jessup M, Bozkurt B, et al. 2017 ACC/AHA/HFSA focused update of the 2013 ACCF/AHA guideline for the management of heart failure: A report of the American College of Cardiology/American Heart Association Task Force on Clinical Practice Guidelines and the Heart Failure Society of America. *J Am Coll Cardiol.* 2017;70:776–803.
2. Lechat P, Hulot JS, Escolano S, et al. Heart rate and cardiac rhythm relationships with bisoprolol benefit in chronic heart failure in CIBIS II trial. *Circulation.* 2001;103:1428–33.
3. Yancy CW, Jessup M, Bozkurt B, et al. 2013 ACCF/AHA guideline for the management of heart failure: A report of the American College of Cardiology Foundation/American Heart Association Task Force on Practice Guidelines. *J Am Coll Cardiol.* 2013;62:e147–239.
4. CIBIS-II Investigators and Committees. The Cardiac Insufficiency Bisoprolol Study II (CIBIS-II): A randomised trial. *Lancet.* 1999;353:9–13.
5. MERIT-HF Study Group. Effect of metoprolol CR/XL in chronic heart failure: Metoprolol CR/XL Randomised Intervention Trial in Congestive Heart Failure (MERIT-HF). *Lancet.* 1999;353:2001–7.
6. Investigators C. Effect of carvedilol on outcome after myocardial infarction in patients with left-ventricular dysfunction: The CAPRICORN randomised trial. *The Lancet.* 2001;357:1385–90.
7. Goldstein S, Fagerberg B, Hjalmarson A, et al. Metoprolol controlled release/extended release in patients with severe heart failure: Analysis of the experience in the MERIT-HF study. *J Am Coll Cardiol.* 2001;38:932–8.
8. Kotecha D, Flather MD, Altman DG, et al. Heart rate and rhythm and the benefit of beta-blockers in patients with heart failure. *J Am Coll Cardiol.* 2017;69:2885–96.
9. Chatterjee S, Biondi-Zoccai G, Abbate A, et al. Benefits of beta blockers in patients with heart failure and reduced ejection fraction: Network meta-analysis. *BMJ.* 2013;346:f55.
10. Kotecha D, Manzano L, Krum H, et al. Effect of age and sex on efficacy and tolerability of beta blockers in patients with heart failure with reduced ejection fraction: Individual patient data meta-analysis. *Bmj.* 2016;353:i1855.
11. Hjalmarson A, Goldstein S, Fagerberg B, et al. Effects of controlled-release metoprolol on total mortality, hospitalizations, and well-being in patients with heart failure: The Metoprolol CR/XL Randomized Intervention Trial in congestive heart failure (MERIT-HF). MERIT-HF Study Group. *JAMA.* 2000;283:1295–302.
12. Packer M, Coats AJ, Fowler MB, et al. Effect of carvedilol on survival in severe chronic heart failure. *N Engl J Med.* 2001;344:1651–8.
13. Yancy CW, Jessup M, Bozkurt B, et al. ACCF/AHA guideline for the management of heart failure: Executive summary: A report of the American College of Cardiology Foundation/American Heart Association Task Force on practice guidelines. *Circulation.* 2013;128:1810–52.
14. Banka G, Heidenreich PA, Fonarow GC. Incremental cost-effectiveness of guideline-directed medical therapies for heart failure. *J Am Coll Cardiol.* 2013;61:1440–6.
15. Group CTS. Effects of enalapril on mortality in severe congestive heart failure. Results of the Cooperative North Scandinavian Enalapril Survival Study (CONSENSUS). *N Engl J Med.* 1987;316:1429–35.
16. SOLVD Investigators, Yusuf S, Pitt B, et al. Effect of enalapril on mortality and the development of heart failure in asymptomatic patients with reduced left ventricular ejection fractions. *N Engl J Med.* 1992;327:685–91.
17. Pfeffer MA, Braunwald E, Moye LA, et al. Effect of captopril on mortality and morbidity in patients with left ventricular dysfunction after myocardial infarction. Results of the survival and ventricular enlargement trial. The SAVE Investigators. *N Engl J Med.* 1992;327:669–77.
18. SOLVD Investigators, Yusuf S, Pitt B, et al. Effect of enalapril on survival in patients with reduced left ventricular ejection fractions and congestive heart failure. *N Engl J Med.* 1991;325:293–302.
19. Packer M, Poole-Wilson PA, Armstrong PW, et al. Comparative effects of low and high doses of the angiotensin-converting enzyme inhibitor, lisinopril, on morbidity and mortality in chronic heart failure. ATLAS Study Group. *Circulation.* 1999;100:2312–8.
20. Heywood JT, Fonarow GC, Yancy CW, et al. Comparison of medical therapy dosing in outpatients cared for in cardiology practices with heart failure and reduced ejection fraction with and without device therapy: Report from IMPROVE HF. *Circ Heart Fail.* 2010;3:596–605.
21. Ghali JK, Dunselman P, Waagstein F, et al. Consistency of the beneficial effect of metoprolol succinate extended release across a wide range dose of angiotensin-converting enzyme inhibitors and digitalis. *J Card Fail.* 2004;10:452–9.
22. Heran BS, Musini VM, Bassett K, Taylor RS, Wright JM. Angiotensin receptor blockers for heart failure. *Cochrane Database Syst Rev.* 2012:CD003040.
23. McMurray JJ, Packer M, Desai AS, et al. Angiotensin-neprilysin inhibition versus enalapril in heart failure. *N Engl J Med.* 2014;371:993–1004.
24. Solomon SD, Claggett B, McMurray JJ, Hernandez AF, Fonarow GC. Combined neprilysin and renin-angiotensin system inhibition in heart failure with reduced ejection fraction: A meta-analysis. *Eur J Heart Fail.* 2016;18:1238–43.
25. Vardeny O, Claggett B, Packer M, et al. Efficacy of sacubitril/valsartan vs. enalapril at lower than target doses in heart failure with reduced ejection fraction: The PARADIGM-HF trial. *Eur J Heart Fail.* 2016;18:1228–34.
26. Taylor AL, Ziesche S, Yancy C, et al. Combination of isosorbide dinitrate and hydralazine in blacks with heart failure. *N Engl J Med.* 2004;351:2049–57.
27. Farag M, Mabote T, Shoaib A, et al. Hydralazine and nitrates alone or combined for the management of chronic heart failure: A systematic review. *Int J Cardiol.* 2015;196:61–9.
28. Cohn JN, Archibald DG, Ziesche S, et al. Effect of vasodilator therapy on mortality in chronic congestive heart failure. Results of a Veterans Administration Cooperative Study. *N Engl J Med.* 1986;314:1547–52.
29. Ziaeian B, Fonarow GC, Heidenreich PA. Clinical effectiveness of hydralazine-isosorbide dinitrate in African-American patients with heart failure. *JACC Heart Fail.* 2017;5:632–9.
30. Neubauer S. The failing heart--an engine out of fuel. *N Engl J Med.* 2007;356:1140–51.
31. Koruth JS, Lala A, Pinney S, Reddy VY, Dukkipati SR. The clinical use of ivabradine. *J Am Coll Cardiol.* 2017;70:1777–84.
32. Swedberg K, Komajda M, Bohm M, et al. Ivabradine and outcomes in chronic heart failure (SHIFT): A randomised placebo-controlled study. *Lancet.* 2010;376:875–85.
33. Yancy CW, Jessup M, Bozkurt B, et al. 2017 ACC/AHA/HFSA focused update of the 2013 ACCF/AHA guideline for the management of heart failure: A report of the American College of Cardiology/American Heart Association Task Force on Clinical Practice Guidelines and the Heart Failure Society of America. *Circulation.* 2017;136(6):e137–e161.
34. Kansal AR, Cowie MR, Kielhorn A, et al. Cost-effectiveness of ivabradine for heart failure in the United States. *J Am Heart Assoc.* 2016;5:e003221.
35. Digitalis Investigation Group. The effect of digoxin on mortality and morbidity in patients with heart failure. *N Engl J Med.* 1997;336:525–33.
36. Vamos M, Erath JW, Benz AP, Lopes RD, Hohnloser SH. Meta-analysis of effects of digoxin on survival in patients with atrial fibrillation or heart failure: An update. *Am J Cardiol.* 2019;123:69–74.
37. Ziff OJ, Lane DA, Samra M, et al. Safety and efficacy of digoxin: Systematic review and meta-analysis of observational and controlled trial data. *BMJ.* 2015;351:h4451.
38. Hauptman PJ, Kelly RA. Digitalis. *Circulation.* 1999;99:1265–70.
39. Bosse GM, Pope TM. Recurrent digoxin overdose and treatment with digoxin-specific Fab antibody fragments. *J Emerg Med.* 1994;12:179–85.
40. Valette H, Apoil E. Interaction between salicylate and two loop diuretics. *Br J Clin Pharmacol.* 1979;8:592–4.
41. Brater DC. Clinical pharmacology of loop diuretics in health and disease. *Eur Heart J.* 1992;13 Suppl G:10–4.
42. Knoben J. *Clinical drug data.* 6th ed. Illinois: Drug Intelligence Publications; 1988.
43. Voelker JR, Cartwright-Brown D, Anderson S, et al. Comparison of loop diuretics in patients with chronic renal insufficiency. *Kidney Int.* 1987;32:572–8.
44. Rudy DW, Gehr TW, Matzke GR, et al. The pharmacodynamics of intravenous and oral torsemide in patients with chronic renal insufficiency. *Clin Pharmacol Ther.* 1994;56:39–47.
45. Schwartz S, Brater DC, Pound D, et al. Bioavailability, pharmacokinetics, and pharmacodynamics of torsemide in patients with cirrhosis. *Clin Pharmacol Ther.* 1993;54:90–7.
46. Strom BL, Schinnar R, Apter AJ, et al. Absence of cross-reactivity between sulfonamide antibiotics and sulfonamide nonantibiotics. *N Engl J Med.* 2003;349:1628–35.
47. Rose BD. Diuretics. *Kidney Int.* 1991;39:336–52.
48. Brater DC. Contemporary issues in nephrology pharmacology of renal disease and hypertension. In: Bennet W (ed.), *Use of diuretics in patients with renal disease.* New York, NY: Churchill Livingstone.
49. Ellison DH. Diuretic drugs and the treatment of edema: From clinic to bench and back again. *Am J Kidney Dis.* 1994;23:623–43.

50. Brater DC. Analysis of the effect of indomethacin on the response to furosemide in man: Effect of dose of furosemide. *J Pharmacol Exp Ther.* 1979;210:386–90.
51. Brater DC, Day B, Burdette A, Anderson S. Bumetanide and furosemide in heart failure. *Kidney Int.* 1984;26:183–9.
52. Zinman B, Wanner C, Lachin JM, et al. Empagliflozin, cardiovascular outcomes, and mortality in type 2 diabetes. *N Engl J Med.* 2015;373:2117–28.
53. Neal B, Perkovic V, Mahaffey KW, et al. Canagliflozin and cardiovascular and renal events in type 2 diabetes. *N Engl J Med.* 2017;377:644–57.
54. McMurray JJV, DeMets DL, Inzucchi SE, et al. A trial to evaluate the effect of the sodium-glucose co-transporter 2 inhibitor dapagliflozin on morbidity and mortality in patients with heart failure and reduced left ventricular ejection fraction (DAPA-HF). *Eur J Heart Fail.* 2019;21:665–75.
55. McMurray JJV, Solomon SD, Inzucchi SE, et al. Dapagliflozin in patients with heart failure and reduced ejection fraction. *N Engl J Med.* 2019;381:1995–2008.
56. Packer M, Anker SD, Butler J, et al. Cardiovascular and renal outcomes with empagliflozin in heart failure. *N Engl J Med.* 2020;383: 1413–1424.
57. Katsiki N, Dimitriadis G, Hahalis G, et al. Sodium-glucose co-transporter-2 inhibitors (SGLT2i) use and risk of amputation: An expert panel overview of the evidence. *Metabolism.* 2019;96:92–100.
58. McGill JB, Subramanian S. Safety of sodium-glucose co-transporter 2 inhibitors. *Am J Cardiol.* 2019;124 Supplement 1:S45–S52.
59. Maddox TM, Januzzi JL, Jr., et al. Update to the 2017 ACC expert consensus decision pathway for optimization of heart failure treatment: Answers to 10 pivotal issues about heart failure with reduced ejection fraction: A report of the American College of Cardiology Solution Set Oversight Committee. *J Am Coll Cardiol.* 2021;77:772–810.
60. Al-Khatib SM, Stevenson WG, Ackerman MJ, et al. 2017 AHA/ACC/HRS guideline for management of patients with ventricular arrhythmias and the prevention of sudden cardiac death: Executive summary: A report of the American College of Cardiology/American Heart Association Task Force on Clinical Practice Guidelines and the Heart Rhythm Society. *Heart Rhythm.* 2018;15:e190–e252.
61. Al-Khatib SM, Hellkamp AS, Fonarow GC, et al. Association between prophylactic implantable cardioverter-defibrillators and survival in patients with left ventricular ejection fraction between 30% and 35%. *JAMA.* 2014;311:2209–15.
62. Bardy GH, Lee KL, Mark DB, et al. Amiodarone or an implantable cardioverter-defibrillator for congestive heart failure. *N Engl J Med.* 2005;352:225–37.
63. Buxton AE, Lee KL, Fisher JD, et al. A randomized study of the prevention of sudden death in patients with coronary artery disease. Multicenter Unsustained Tachycardia Trial Investigators. *N Engl J Med.* 1999;341:1882–90.
64. Greenberg H, Case RB, Moss AJ, et al. Analysis of mortality events in the Multicenter Automatic Defibrillator Implantation Trial (MADIT-II). *J Am Coll Cardiol.* 2004;43:1459–65.
65. Kadish A, Dyer A, Daubert JP, et al. Prophylactic defibrillator implantation in patients with nonischemic dilated cardiomyopathy. *N Engl J Med.* 2004;350:2151–8.
66. Cleland JG, Daubert JC, Erdmann E, et al. The effect of cardiac resynchronization on morbidity and mortality in heart failure. *N Engl J Med.* 2005;352:1539–49.
67. Curtis AB, Worley SJ, Adamson PB, et al. Biventricular pacing for atrioventricular block and systolic dysfunction. *N Engl J Med.* 2013;368:1585–93.
68. Aggarwal M, Bozkurt B, Panjrath G, et al. Lifestyle modifications for preventing and treating heart failure. *J Am Coll Cardiol.* 2018;72:2391–2405.
69. Whellan DJ, O'Connor CM, Lee KL, et al. Heart failure and a controlled trial investigating outcomes of exercise training (HF-ACTION): Design and rationale. *Am Heart J.* 2007;153:201–11.
70. Long L, Mordi IR, Bridges C, et al. Exercise-based cardiac rehabilitation for adults with heart failure. *Cochrane Database Syst Rev.* 2019;1:CD003331.
71. Gupta D, Georgiopoulou VV, Kalogeropoulos AP, et al. Dietary sodium intake in heart failure. *Circulation.* 2012;126:479–85.
72. Zhang L, Babu SV, Jindal M, Williams JE, Gimbel RW. A patient-centered mobile phone app (iHeartU) with a virtual human assistant for self-management of heart failure: Protocol for a usability assessment study. *JMIR Res Protoc.* 2019;8:e13502.
73. Klompstra L, Jaarsma T, Stromberg A. Exergaming to increase the exercise capacity and daily physical activity in heart failure patients: A pilot study. *BMC Geriatr.* 2014;14:119.
74. Hoffmann JM, Hellwig S, Brandenburg VM, Spaderna H. Measuring fear of physical activity in patients with heart failure. *Int J Behav Med.* 2018;25:294–303.
75. Rengo JL, Savage PD, Barrett T, Ades PA. Cardiac rehabilitation participation rates and outcomes for patients with heart failure. *J Cardiopulm Rehabil Prev.* 2018;38:38–42.

Chapter 11
EXERCISE AND REHABILITATION IN HEART FAILURE

Audrey Borghi-Silva, Flávia Rossi Caruso, and Renata Gonçalves Mendes

Introduction

Heart failure (HF) has a marked negative impact on exercise capacity, inducing progressive impairment in the performance of daily life tasks and quality of life.[1] Although HF has multiple etiologies and thus can affect people of all ages, it is mostly a disease of older adults. A major concern is that the prevalence of IC continues to rise over time with the aging population. An estimated 5.7 million of American adults had HF between 2009 and 2012 contrasted with 6.2 million between 2013 and 2016, according NHANES data.[2] Exercise intolerance is a prominent manifestation in patients with HF, especially those with New York Heart Association functional classes III and IV.[1]

Pronounced fatigue and dyspnea are key symptoms reported by patients with HF, causing a progressive reduction in exercise capacity and consequently an increasingly sedentary lifestyle which has a major impact on quality of life.[3] Recent guidelines for the diagnosis and treatment of chronic HF have incorporated recommendations for regular exercise training programs as part of a multifaceted cardiac rehabilitation approach. Table 11.1 shows the goals of these programs: improved functional capacity, minimized symptoms, and reduced risk of exacerbations that culminate in hospitalizations, with associated increases in morbidity, mortality, and health care costs.[4–6]

This chapter aims to (1) address the importance of exercise as a core component of rehabilitation programs in patients with HF and preserved or reduced ejection fraction (HFpEF or HFrEF) and review recent scientific evidence; (2) present innovative non-pharmacological approaches as adjuncts to physical exercise in order to optimize performance and outcomes; and (3) discuss early mobilization and initiation of rehabilitation for HF patients in the hospital environment through intravenous, pharmacological interventions.

Pathophysiological Responses during Exercise in HF with Preserved and Reduced Ejection Fraction (HFpEF and HFrEF)

Exercise intolerance is a clinical hallmark of HF, characterized by dyspnea and fatigue during exertion[7]. It can be objectively measured as decreased oxygen uptake (VO_2) and is associated with adverse outcomes, including poor health-related quality of life (HRQoL), increased risk OF hospital admission, elevated mortality risk, and higher health care costs.[8,9]

Physical exercise requires the coordinated function of the interdependent systems (Wasserman's gears); however, in HF, the integrated machinery is impaired at multiple levels. Up-to-date evidence suggests that there are several determinants linked to the pathophysiology of exercise intolerance in patients with HF, including decreased cardiac output, chronotropic incompetence, abnormal lung mechanics, impaired convective and diffusive oxygen transport, skeletal muscle dysfunction (muscle fibers, oxidative enzymes, capillary density, autonomic dysfunction, mitochondrial volume), exaggerated ventilatory responses (ergoreflex activation), and impaired vasoreactivity,[7,8,10–12] (Figure 11.1).

Although HF with preserved and reduced ejection fraction (HFpEF and HFrEF) are phenotypically different, with significant phenotypic variations within each type, peak VO_2 is decreased in both HFrEF and HFpEF patients compared with healthy controls. However, different factors are involved in peak VO_2 impairment according to HF phenotype.[8,12] In patients with HFrEF, both central and peripheral factors have been associated with the exercise intolerance, whereas, in those with HFpEF, the peripheral factors have been postulated to play a relatively greater role in limiting exercise performance.[8,12] Regarding central and peripheral hemodynamic responses to exercise, Tucker et al.[11] and Haykowsky et al.[12] have demonstrated evidence involving both large and small muscle mass groups (cycle or treadmill and unilateral knee extension, respectively) for different HF phenotypes (Table 11.2).

Distinct determinants of VO_2, including heart rate, arterio-mixed venous oxygen content difference (C[a-v] O_2) and stroke volume, should be considered when assessing the capacity to augment VO_2. Normal exercise-related responses include greater increase in heart rate and C(a-v) O_2 (≈2.5×) and lower increase in stroke volume (≈1.3×). Dhakal et al. demonstrated that relative augmentation of C(a-v) O_2 exceeded that of heart rate and stroke volume during maximum incremental exercise in both HFpEF and HFrEF.[13] Furthermore, specifically for patients with HFpEF, 75% presented with impaired C(a-v) O_2, demonstrating that peripheral O_2 extraction was a major determinant of exercise capacity.[13]

The Role of Exercise and Rehabilitation in HFpEF and HFrEF

A combination of medical and lifestyle management is recommended for all patients with HF. Exercise intolerance has been an important therapeutic target in HF and an exercise-based cardiac rehabilitation (EXCR) should be considered for all patients. The Cochrane review (2019) included 5,783 participants with HF and reported that EXCR may confer a clinical improvement in HRQoL, reducing risk of all-cause and HF-specific hospital admissions, as well as a possible reduction in mortality over the long-term, albeit it appears to have no impact on short-term (<12-month) mortality.[9]

Taylor et al. have undertaken an individual participant data meta-analysis to assess the impact of EXCR on exercise capacity and HRQoL in patients with HF.[14] Using data from 3,990 randomized patients (97% with HFrEF), the investigators have shown evidence in favor of exercise for both exercise capacity and HRQoL in a 12-month follow-up. In another meta-analysis, benefits on resting left ventricular ejection fraction, end-diastolic, end-systolic volumes, and peak VO_2 were observed with moderate-intensity continuous aerobic exercise in patients with HFrEF compared with the control group, with the greatest benefits occurring with long-term (≥6 months) training.[15]

Focusing on abnormalities in peripheral muscle tissue in patients with HF, Giuliano and colleagues conducted a meta-analysis, examining the effects of resistance training on muscle

DOI: 10.1201/9780429244544-14

TABLE 11.1: Current Guidelines for the Recommendations for Regular Exercise Training Programs for Chronic HF

	Australia Position Statement, 2010[16]	ECPR, 2011[17]	Canadian Cardiovascular Society Guidelines, 2017[18]	ACC/AHA Guidelines, 2019[19]
Exercise training intervention	AE, NYHA I–II	AE	AE	AE
	AE, NYHA III–IV RE, NYHA I–II Flexibility, NYHA I–IV	RE IMT	RE ISO	RE
Type of exercise	Walking/running, cycling and swimming Circuit weight training, theraband exercise, body weight exercise	Endurance, AE (continuous and interval) IET (CE, treadmill) Three types of RE IMT-RE	Walk, treadmill, CE and swimming ISO/RE	AE, RE
Intensity	↓ Myocardial ischemic threshold RPE 11–14 (Borg 6–20), or 0% to 75% of HRp, higher intensities (up to 80% – VO_2peak)—applied in hospitals/ exercise centers	Endurance, AE 40–50% at the starting point, increasing to 70–80% of the percentage VO_2peak	AE Moderate intensity: RPE 3-5, or 65%-85% maximum HR, or 50%–75% VO_2peak Moderate-intensity Intervals 15–30 min, RPE of 3–5, Rest intervals of 15–30 min	Moderate to vigorous intensity
	AE, NYHA III–IV RPE ≤13, or 40–65% of HRp, or 40–60% of VO_2peak RE RPE 11–15	10–30 s moderate to high intensity (50–100% p), recovery (80–60 s)—low or no workload 3 Types: 1) <30% 1RM, RPE <12 2) 30–40% 1RM, RPE 12–13 3) 40–60% 1RM, RPE <15	ISO/RE 10–20 rep of 5- to 10-pound free weights	
	RE, NYHA III–IV 6–15 rep/set Start one set/exercise, progressing to three sets of 4–8 different exercises RPE 10–13 4–10 rep/set Start one set/exercise, progressing to two sets 3–4 major muscle groups	IMT RE 30% of MIP (PImax) and to readjust the intensity every 7–10 days up to a maximum of 60%		
Time intervention	AE, NYHA I-II 10–15 min progressing according to tolerance to 45–60 min	↑ 45–60 min duration	20–30 min	150 min/week of moderate intensity AE or 75 min/week of vigorous intensity
	RE, NYHA I–II 20 min at target exercise intensities, progressing according to patient's tolerance – 45–60 min	30 and 60 s – hard segments are accomplished at 50%: power output achieved during incremental test	Starting with 10–15 min Goal: 30 min	
	RE, NYHA III–IV 20 min at target exercise intensities, progressing gradually according to tolerance to 45–60 min	Types 1. 5–10 rep 2. 12–25 rep 3. 8–15 rep		
	Flexibility, NYHA I–IV 5–10 min	IMT 20–30 min		
Intervention, frequency and duration	AE, NYHA I-IV and RE NYHA III–IV 2 X/week	AE 3–5×/week	IMT 3–5×/week: minimum of 8 weeks	-
		RE 2–3×/week	2–3×/week	
	Flexibility, NYHA I–IV 2–3×/week	IMT 3–5×/week—minimum 8 weeks		

Abbreviations: AE: aerobic exercise; CE: cycle ergometer; HR: heart rate, HRR: heart rate reserve, IET: interval exercise training; NYHA: New York Heart Association; VO_2peak, peak oxygen uptake; ISO: isometric; PPO: peak power output; RE: resistance exercise; RPE: rate of perceived exertion scale; IMT: inspiratory muscle training; MIP: maximum inspiratory pressure; p: peak.

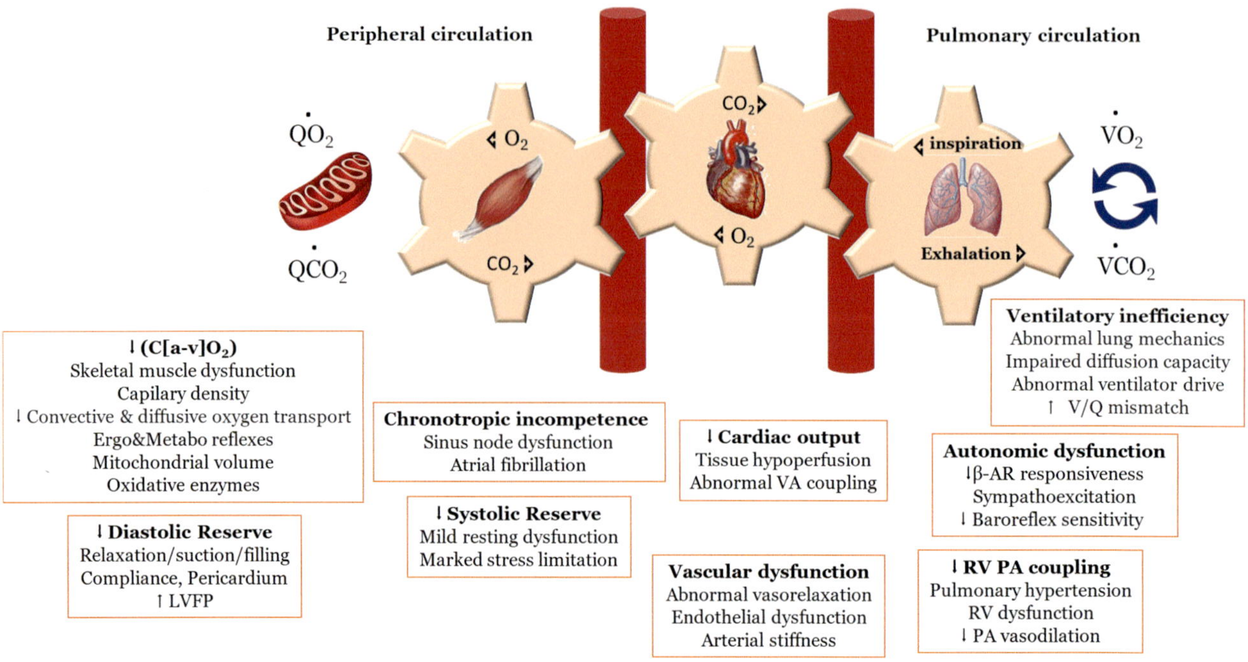

FIGURE 11.1 Adapted illustration of possible pathophysiological mechanisms governing exercise intolerance in heart failure patients. *Abbreviations*: (C[a-v] O_2), arterio-mixed venous oxygen content differences; β-AR, beta-adrenoreceptor; LVFP, left ventricular filling pressures; PA, pulmonary artery; RV, right ventricle; VA, ventricular arterial.

TABLE 11.2: Hemodynamic Responses in Patients with Reduced or Preserved Ejection Fraction Compared with Healthy Controls during Maximal Large and Small Muscle Mass Exercise in Heart Failure

Variable	HFREF vs control	HFPEF vs control
Large Muscle Mass Exercise		
Cardiac output	↓	↓
Heart rate	↓	↓
Stroke volume end-diastolic volume	↓	↓
End-systolic volume	↓	↓
Ejection fraction	↓	↓
Mean arterial blood pressure	↓	↔
Systemic vascular resistance	↑	↑↔
Pulmonary capillary wedge pressure	↑	↑
Arterial-mixed venous oxygen difference	↔	↔
Small Muscle Mass Exercise		
Leg oxygen uptake	↓	Not studied
Leg blood flow	↓	Not studied
Leg oxygen delivery	↓	Not studied
Leg vascular resistance	↑	Not studied
Leg arterial-venous oxygen difference	↔	Not studied
Muscle oxygen diffusional conductance	↓	Not studied

Sources: Adapted from Tucker et al.[11] and Haykowsky et al.[12]

strength, considering the one-repetition maximum test (1RM) and Peak Torque, aerobic capacity (VO_2peak and 6- min walk), and HRQoL.[20] The results demonstrated that resistance training as a single intervention can increase muscle strength, aerobic capacity, and HRQoL in patients with HF.

Inspiratory muscle training also offers an alternative to exercise training. Previous meta-analyses indicated that inspiratory muscle training (IMT) can improve cardio-respiratory fitness (VO_2peak, 6-min walk distance, V_E/VCO_2 slope, maximal inspiratory pressure (MIP) and HRQoL), and may provide an initial alternative to the more severely de-conditioned patients with HF.[21–23] Another meta-analysis was conducted to assess the benefits and harms of EXCR to people with implantable ventricular assist devices.[24] A total of 40 participants were included, and aerobic and/or resistance training modalities (50% of VO_2 reserve or ranging from 60% to 80% of heart rate reserve) for six to eight weeks were considered. Scores from the 36-item Short Form Health Survey (SF-36) and the Kansas City Cardiomyopathy Questionnaire (KCCQ) were used to measure HRQoL. A large difference in HRQoL was observed between groups (exercise vs usual care group) at the end of the follow-up. However, the authors of this meta-analysis pointed out that the evidence was of rather low quality and should be interpreted with caution.[25]

Designing the Optimal Exercise and Rehabilitation Regimen for Your HF Patient

Currently, it is recommended to introduce aerobic and resistance (combined) training programs with moderate to high intensities (40–80% of maximum HR) for aerobic exercise. For resistance training, an intensity between 60% and 65% of 1-repetition maximum and two to three times a week is recommended. The total period of the training program is recommended from six to 26 weeks. Tables 11.3 and 11.4 summarize randomized, controlled studies involving exercise interventions in HF patients with reduced and preserved ejection fraction.

For ventilatory muscle training programs, a recent meta-analysis by Wu et al. demonstrated that a 6-week minimum of inspiratory muscle training led to improvements in HRQoL, maximum inspiratory pressure, and perceived dyspnea.[17] The intervention group that received 40–60% of inspiratory pressure load showed improvement in maximal inspiratory pressure when compared with patients that received 10–15% of maximum inspiratory pressure.[17] In this sense, a moderate training load of 40–60% of maximum inspiratory pressure may be ideal for patients with HFpEF. However, limited evidence exists regarding the optimal protocol for ventilatory muscle training. Thus, current recommendations of muscle training are based on the few studies that have been performed to date, especially in patients who have ventilatory muscle weakness.

Exercise training recommendations and guidelines for HFpEF are still under development. Which exercise and protocols should be used and what is the appropriate intensity, volume, and type of exercise that should be introduced to patients with HFpEF are still open questions.

Although not always evident from the existing literature, careful design of the training program for this population is key to successful training and requires cautious and careful handling, especially in patients with HFrEF. According to recommendations and guidelines,[21] patients with HFpEF and HFrEF have increased need for monitoring of physical exercise tolerance that is usually accompanied by hemodynamic changes with altered blood pressure and symptoms. Table 11.5 illustrates a number of important points that must be taken into account when conducting a training program for patients with HF.

Non-Pharmacological Adjunct Therapies to Improve Functional Capacity in HF

Dyspnea is a cardinal symptom of advanced HF, resulting in exercise intolerance, sedentarism, and reduced HRQoL. Dyspnea and respiratory and locomotor muscle fatigue of lower limbs is often reported during physical exertion by these patients, negatively impacting functional capacity and ability to carry out activities of daily living. These symptoms reduce the ability of these patients to increase their physical efforts, leading to limited gains during the rehabilitation process.

In this context, some strategies that promote unloading of respiratory muscles and improve peripheral muscle fatigue could help these patients exercise at higher intensity and thus benefit more from a rehabilitation program. In hospitalized patients, Oliveira et al. showed that a short exercise training program combined with non-invasive ventilation can be safely applied to patients with acute HF, leading to improvements in walking distance, amelioration of dyspnea, and reduced length of stay.[22] Other studies have shown the potential effects of various modalities of non-invasive ventilation, e.g., proportional assisted ventilation,[23,24] continuous or bilevel positive airway pressure,[24] reducing the overload of respiratory muscles, reducing dyspnea, and improving exercise tolerance in chronic HF.[24–26] However, larger studies are needed to confirm these results.

Another strategy recently used to improve functional capacity and reduce muscle fatigue in advanced HF is the neuromuscular electrical stimulation (NMES) that can be applied in hospitalized, ambulatory, or at-home patients. NMES has been considered as a safe tool that may increase muscle strength and exercise tolerance, positively impacting HRQoL of these patients. Other potential effects observed by NMES include beneficial effects on pro-inflammatory cytokines, oxidative activity, protein anabolic and catabolic metabolism, and on endothelial dysfunction, reducing muscle wasting in HF.

Early Rehabilitation during Hospitalization in Exacerbated HF

Patients with HF experience frequent rehospitalizations, which compromise mobility and result in muscle atrophy, leading to deconditioning and functional disability. Previous studies demonstrated that hospital admission is an important marker for increased risk of mortality in these patients.[27] Decompensations of HF are often accompanied by signs and symptoms of congestion and fluid retention, electrical instability with potential arrhythmogenic responses, and hemodynamic instability,[28] hampering but not hindering early mobilization.

In general, in decompensated patients with congestion but who are well perfused, it is important to optimize diuretics, beta-blockers and vasodilatory drugs, whereas in patients with congestion who are hypoperfused, it is recommended to introduce IV inotropic support and vasopressors.[28] IV pharmacological therapy may limit some movements and exercises out of bed such as walking. In this sense, early mobilization is also dependent on the medical conduct and experience of the care team.

Regarding scientific evidence, a study showed that an exercise-based protocol composed of deep breathing exercises, sedestation, orthostatic exercises, and walking in a corridor during the hospitalization period was safe and promoted beneficial effects of cardiac autonomic modulation in patients hospitalized for HF[29] Other studies have suggested that early moderate exercise after an episode of decompensation is safe and effective in improving exercise tolerance in selected patients after achievement of clinical stability[30] and may prevent important functional decline, muscle deconditioning, and atrophy[31] resulting in better outcomes of functionality.[32] Evidence of beneficial autonomic adaptations was shown after implementation of a short-term (≅5 days) inpatient progressive physiotherapy program (active exercises of lower and upper limbs plus walking with maximal estimated energy

TABLE 11.3: Summary of Randomized, Controlled Studies Involving Exercise Interventions in Heart Failure Patients with Reduced Ejection Fraction from 2009 to 2019

Study, Year	Study Sample and Size	Exercise Training Intervention	Intervention Frequency, Duration, Setting	Outcomes
Jolly et al., 2009 (24)	***NYHA***: I:6%, II: 74%, III 20% ***LVEF***: ≤40% ***Total***: 169 (EG: 84, CG: 85)	***Modality***: *AE* and RE ***Intensity***: 70% VO_{2p} or Borg 12–13 ***CG***: Specialist HF nurse care	***Frequency***: 5×/week ***Duration***: 20 to 30 min ***Total duration***: 6/month ***Setting***: center and home-based	HRQoL: ↔ MLWHF ↑ EQ-5D at 6 months ↓ Hospital Anxiety and Depression Scale
HF ACTION, 2009 (25)	***NYHA***: II 63%, III 35%, IV 1% ***LVEF***: 25% ***Total***: 2331 (EG: 1159, CG: 1172)	***Modality***: AE ***Intensity***: 60% to 70% HRR ***CG***: Usual care	***Frequency***: 3–5×/week ***Duration***: 15 to 35 min/session ***Total duration***: 30 months ***Setting***: supervised and home-based	Modest reduction: Mortality and hospitalization: HRQoL: ↑ KCCQ
Gary et al., 2010 (26)	***NYHA***: II 43.3%; III 56.7% ***LVEF***: ≥5% ***Total***: 65	***Modality***: walking */AE* ***Intensity***: org <15 ("moderate") ***Other***: ET + CBT group: weekly 1-hour sessions of CBT for 12 weeks ***CG***: Usual care	***Frequency***: 3×/week ***Duration***: 30 to 45 min/session ***Total duration***: 12 weeks ***Setting***: home-based	↑ HRQoL: MLWHF ↓ HAM-D (depression) ↑ 6MWT distance (CBT+ exercise)
Davidson et al., 2010 (27)	***NYHA***: I: EG 2%; II: EG 38%, CG 33%; III: EG 60%, CG 67%; ***LVEF***: not reported ***Total***: 105 (EG: 53, CG: 52)	***Modality***: gymnasium: treadmills, stationary and recumbent cycles/AE ***Intensity***: not reported	***Frequency***: 1×/week ***Duration***: 30 to 50 min ***Total duration***: 12 weeks ***Setting***: gymnasium, home-based	↑HRQoL: MLWHF; ↓ all-cause and cardiovascular-related hospital admission; ↑ 6MWT
Wall et al., 2010 (28)	***NYHA***: mean of 2 (SE: 0.13) ***LVEF***: ≤60% ***Total***: 19 (EG: 9, CG: 10)	***Modality***: treadmill/AE ***Intensity***: not reported ***CG***: Comprehensive disease management.	***Frequency***: 3×/week ***Duration***: >15 min ***Total duration***: 12 months ***Setting***: hospital-based and home	Disease-specific HRQoL (Chronic Heart Failure Questionnaire), mortality
Yeh et al., 2011 (29)	***NYHA***: I: 20%, II: 63%, III: 17% ***LVEF***: 29% (SD 8%) ***Total***: 100 (EG:50, CG: 50)	***Modality***: Tai Chi /AE ***Intensity***: not reported ***CG***: Educational group	***Frequency***: 2×/week ***Duration***: 1-h (30 min warm-up) ***Total duration***: 12 weeks ***Setting***: center and home	↑ HRQoL (MLWHF questionnaire)
Belardinelli et al., 2012 (30)	***NYHA***: II: 59%, III: 41% ***LVEF***: 37% (SD 8) ***Total N***: 123 (EG: 63, CG: 60)	***Modality***: cycling/AE ***Intensity***: 60% to 70% max VO_2 ***CG***: Standard medical care	***Frequency***: 2–3×/week ***Duration***: 40 min/session ***Total duration***: 10 years; 8-week supervised, 12 months' maintenance ***Settings***: hospital and home	↑ HRQoL (MLWHF questionnaire); ↓ mortality; ↓ morbidity (including hospitalization) cost-effectiveness
Norman et al., 2012 (31)	***NYHA***: II: EG: 64%, CG:45%; III: EG36%, CG: 55% ***LVEF***: *m*ean 33% (SD 7) ***Total***: 42 (EG: 22, CG:20)	***Modality***: *AE*: not reported; RE: weight machines, free-weights, or elastic bands ***Intensity***: AE: 40–70% HRR, or Borg 11–14; resistance: not reported ***CG***: Usual care	***Frequency***: AE 3×/week, RE 2 /week ***Duration***: AE: 30 min; RE: 8-10 exercises, 1 set of 10–15 rep ***Total duration***: 24 weeks ***Setting***: *s*upervised, hospital's wellness or home	↑ HRQoL (KCCQ); ↑ 6MWT ↔ BNP
Witham et al., 2012 (32)	***NYHA***: II 79%, III 21% ***LVEF***: not reported ***Total***: 107 (EG:53, CG:54)	***Modality***: home, walking/mix ***Intensity***: not reported ***CG***: Usual care	***Frequency***: 2×/week ***Duration***: ≤60 min ***Total duration***: 24 weeks ***Setting***: hospital and home	Disease-specific ↔ HRQoL (MLWHF questionnaire); ↔ HRQoL (EuroQoL-5D); mortality; ↔ cost
Mehani, 2013 (33)	***NYHA***: I to III ***LVEF***: EG*:* 33.09±4.77%, CG: 35.8 ± 6.87% ***Total***: 40 (EG:20, CG:20)	***Modality***: AE: circuit training (Stairmaster, bicycle, treadmill) ***Intensity***: AE: 80% of HRR ***CG***: Usual care	***Frequency***: 3×/week ***Duration***: AE; 45 min/session ***Total duration***: 28 weeks ***Setting***: hospital (supervised)	↓ diastolic and systolic dysfunction ↑ peak VO_2 ↓ resting HR

(*Continued*)

TABLE 11.3 (Continued): Summary of Randomized, Controlled Studies Involving Exercise Interventions in Heart Failure Patients with Reduced Ejection Fraction from 2009 to 2019

Study, Year	Study Sample and Size	Exercise Training Intervention	Intervention Frequency, Duration, Setting	Outcomes
Cowie et al., 2014 (34)	***NYHA***: II: 56.3%, III: 40% ***LVEF***: not reported ***Total***: 46 (EG: 30; CG:16)	***Modality***: circuit training-AE ***Intensity***: not specified ***CG***: Usual care	***Frequency***: 2×/week ***Duration***: 60 min ***Total duration***: 8 weeks ***Setting***: hospital and home-based	Similar hospitalizations, costs
Kaltsatou et al., 2014 (35)	***NYHA***: not reported ***LVEF***: dance 49.3 ± 3.4%, formal exercise 49.1 ± 2.4%, CG: 49.6 ± 3.5% ***Total***: 57 (dance 19, exercise 19, CG: 19)	***Modality***: dancing, cycling, or treadmill (RE to EG) ***Intensity***: moderate: exercise perceived exertion 13–14 on the Borg 6 to 20 scale ***CG***: Usual care	***Frequency***: 3×/week ***Duration***: 60 min ***Total duration***: 32 weeks ***Setting***: home setting (supervised training at a public gym)	↑ HRQoL (Greek version of SF-36) ↑ peak VO_2 ↓ (VE/VCO_2) slope ↑ Intrinsic Motivation Inventory
Hassanpour et al., 2015 (36)	***NYHA***: I: 0; II: EG:20%, CG: 19.33%; III: EG:83%, CG:81%; ***LVEF***: EG: 32±4%; CG: 33±5% ***Total***: 61 (EG: 30, CG: 31)	***Modality***: walking/AE ***Intensity***: 60% to 70% of HRR ***Control group***: Usual care	***Frequency***: 3×/week ***Duration***: 40 min ***Total duration***: 24 weeks ***Setting***: hospital sport facility or gymnasium (supervised)	↑ HRQoL (MacNew Questionnaire) ↑ EF
Antonicelli et al., 2016 (37)	***NYHA***: not reported. ***LVEF***: total 48.4±13.4% ***Total***: 343 (EG: 170, CG: 173)	***Modality***: AE (cycling) ***Intensity***: 20 min (60 rpm, 60–70% maximum HR) ***CG***: Usual care	***Frequency***: 3×/week ***Duration***: 50 min ***Total duration***: 24 weeks ***Settings***: hospital and home	↑ HRQoL (MLWHF) ↑ 6MWT distance ↑ activities of daily living scores ↓ risk of rehospitalization
Reeves et al., 2017 (38)	***NYHA***: not reported ***LVEF***: EG: 40±13%, CG: 34±18% ***Total***: 27 (EG: 15, CG: 12)	***Modality***: AE and RE/ mix ***Intensity***: individually: low intensity on self-reported score ***CG***: Usual care	***Frequency***: 3×/week ***Duration***: 60 min ***Total duration***: 12 weeks ***Setting***: hospital and home	↓ All-cause hospital admissions ↑ physical function (Short Physical Performance Battery [SPPB])
Chen et al., 2018 (39)	***NYHA***: II to IV ***LVEF***: mean 43.5%, SD 13.8 ***Total N***: 62 (EG: 31, CG: 31)	***Modality***: walking/mix ***Intensity***: as tolerated ***CG***: Standard of care	***Frequency***: up 3×/week ***Duration***: 20–40 min/ session ***Total duration***: 26 weeks ***Setting***: hospital	↑ HRQoL (MLWHF questionnaire), ↓ depressive symptoms
Du et al., 2018 (40)	***NYHA***: II: total 92 (70%), III: total 40 (30%) ***LVEF***: EG: 32, CG: 33 ***Total N***: 132 (EG: 67, CG: 65)	***Modality***: walking/AE ***Intensity***: tailored to individual ***Other***: usual care ***CG***: Usual care	***Frequency***: 1×/week ***Duration***: 6 min/session ***Total duration***: 24 weeks ***Setting***: home-based	HRQoL (SF-36 and MLWHF questionnaire) ↑ self-care behavior ↑ physical activity level
Dalal et al., 2019 (41)	***NYHA***: II: EG 59%, CG: 58%; III: EG: 19%, CG: 24% ***LVEF***: mean 34% ***Total***: 216 (EG: 107; CG: 109)	***Modality***: not reported/ AE ***Intensity***: not reported ***CG***: Usual care	***Frequency***: 2–3×/week ***Duration***: 12 weeks ***Total duration***: 12 weeks ***Setting***: home-based	↑ HRQoL (MLWHF questionnaire) ↔ HeartQoL, EQ-5D-3L

Abbreviations: AE: aerobic exercise, BNP: brain natriuretic peptide, CBT: cognitive behavioral therapy; CG: control group; EG: exercise group; ET: exercise training, HFpEF: heart failure preserved ejection fraction, HFrEF: heart failure reduced ejection fraction, HRQoL: health-related quality of life; HR: heart rate, HRR: heart rate reserve; KCCQ: Kansas City Cardiomyopathy Questionnaire, LVEF: left ventricular ejection fraction, MLWHF: Minnesota Living With Heart Failure; 6MWT: 6-minute walking test, NYHA: New York Heart Association, RE: resistance exercise, SPPB: short physical performance battery, VO_2: oxygen uptake.

cost 3–4 metabolic equivalents [METS]) in hospitalized but stable patients. Superior, autonomic outcomes were observed in patients with reduced ventricular function compared with patients with preserved ejection fraction.[33] These findings have particular relevance since the improvement of cardiac autonomic modulation could be associated with a lower risk of arrhythmias and sudden death.[34]

Considering the implementation of early exercise rehabilitation therapy in intravenous drug use, a case study demonstrated that when an aerobic exercise program consisting of motor driver, stationary rowing machines, treadmills, arm ergometers, and stairs steps with intensity using HR reserve and Borg scale was introduced in a patient using continuous infusion of dobutamine for 10 months prior, improvements in oxygen uptake, exercise duration, and a discontinuation of the dobutamine therapy were observed[35] Another case study showed safety and efficacy of aerobic exercise training in a patient awaiting heart transplant while on intravenous milrinone use. The study indicated that the patient showed a 38% increase in aerobic exercise time and a 34% increase in sustainable exercise workload with no other adverse events reported.[36] Utilizing other non-pharmacological strategies, a recent study of a randomized, controlled trial by Forestieri et al. demonstrated that NMES introduced earlier in hospitalized HF improved exercise tolerance and reduced the need for intravenous inotropics.[37]

TABLE 11.4: **Summary of Main Studies with Exercise Training Programs in Patients with HfpEF**

Study, Year	Study Sample	Exercise Training Intervention	Intervention Frequency, Duration	Outcomes
Alves et al., 2002 (42)	***Total***: 98 Moderate–severe 34, *LVEF*: 37.3 ± 7.9 mild: 33, *LVEF*: 49.3 ± 1.9, and preserved: 31, *LVEF*: 56.3 ± 2.5	***Modality***: AE first month: ***Frequency***: treadmill or CE, 5 sets of 3 min ***Intensity***: 70–75% HRmax Following 5 months	***Duration***: 15 min and ↑ up to 35 min by increasing the number and duration of exercise (7×5 min) ***Total duration***: 6 months	Modify left ventricular dimensions
Gary et al., 2004 (26)	***Total***: 32 women (LVEF > 45%), (NYHA) class II or III	***Modality***: AE. Walking program self-monitoring of symptom severity, and self-monitoring of exertion level ***Intensity***: Low-moderate: 40–60% of HR	***Duration***: 20 min ***Total duration***: 12 weeks	↑ functional capacity and quality of life
Kitzmann et al., 2013 (43)	***Total***: 63 HFpEF Exercise n: 32 and control: 31	***Modality***: ET (walking, arm, and leg ergometry) ***Intensity***: Initially at 40–50% HR: 5–10 min of walking and ergometry:70% HR	***Total duration***: 16 weeks, Control: every 2 weeks	↑ VO_2 without altering endothelial function
Endelmann et al., 2011 (44)	***Total***: 64 patients. Training n: 44 and control n: 20	***Modality***: AE ***Intensity***: 1–4 weeks: 2 sessions, 50–60% of VO_2, 5 weeks: 3 sessions,70% of VO_2 ***Modality***: RE: 15 rep 60–65% 1RM	***Duration***: 2×/week. ***Total duration***: 32 sessions	↑ quality of life, exercise capacity and left ventricular diastolic function
Karavidas et al., 2013 (45)	***Total***: 30 HFpEF patients, 18 female and 12 male NYHA II or III and EF 63±6%	***Modality***: FES in (quadriceps and gastrocnemius muscles) ***Intensity***: 25 Hz for 5 s followed by 5-s rest ***Intensity***: 5 Hz in placebo group	***Duration***: 30 min/day, 5×/week ***Total duration***: 6 weeks	↑ exercise capacity, quality of life, emotional status, and endothelial function
Palau et al., 2014 (46)	***Total***: 26 HFpEF patients IMT n: 14 and control n: 12	***Modality***: IMT and usual care. ***Intensity***: 25–30% of MIP for 1 week – resistance was modified each session (25–30%) of MIP	***Duration***: 2×/day, 20 min ***Total duration***: 12 weeks	↑ MIP, VO_2 p, ventilatory efficiency, metabolic equivalents, 6MWT and quality of life
Angadi et al., 2015 (47)	***Total***: 19 HFpEF patients, NYHA II–III. Randomized, clinical trial (pilot study)	***Modality***: HIIT ***Intensity***: 85–90% HRp interspersed by 3 min active recovery at 50% HRp ***Modality***: MCT: 15 min at 60% HRp, increasing to 30 min, at 70% HRp, start of 2nd week	***Duration***: 3×/week ***Total duration***: 12–24 weeks	FMD remained unchanged after HIIT and no changes on FMD were observed after MCT
Pandey et al., 2015 (48)	***Total***: 48 HF patients. HFrEF n: 24 and HFpEF n: 24	***Modality***: ET ***Intensity***: increased 40 to 50% of HR in the first 2 weeks to 60–70% over	***Duration***: 15 to 20 min each of walking and CE, 3×/week ***Total duration***: 16 weeks	↑ VO_2
Fukuta et al., 2016 (49)	***Total***: 245 HFpEF patients and controls 5 trials NYHA II–III	***Modality***: AE (walking/cycling) ***Duration***: 30 min–1 h, 3×/week ***Modality***: AE, RE ***Control***: Education program, and usual care	***Duration***: 20–40 min, 2–3×/week ***Total duration***: 12–24 weeks	↑ Emotional status, physical capacity, quality of life and symptoms of depression
Fu et al., 2016 (50)	***Total***: 120 HF patients, divided into HFpEF and HFrEF NYHA II–III supervised hospital-based	***Modality***: AIT ***Intensity***: 40–80%, 30 min and general health care	***Duration***: 3 weekly sessions ***Total duration***: 12 weeks	↑ in exercise capacity, quality of life and diastolic function. Increased cerebral blood distribution and extraction of O_2 muscular
Chan et al., 2016 (51)	***Total***: 317 patients. Exercise n: 174 and controls n: 143	***Modality***: Walking, CE, FES and IMT	***Duration***: 2–5×/week ***Total duration***: 6–26 weeks	↑ in quality of life
Palau et al., 2016 (52)	***Total***: 60 patients with HFpEF. NYHA II–III/IV	***Modality***: IMT, FES, IMT and FES (IMT + FES) and standard treatment ***Intensity***: 25% to 30% of their MIP	***Duration***: 2×/day, 20 min/session ***Total duration***: 12 weeks	↑ in quality of life and autonomy

(Continued)

TABLE 11.4 (Continued): Summary of Main Studies with Exercise Training Programs in Patients with HfpEF

Study, Year	Study Sample	Exercise Training Intervention	Intervention Frequency, Duration	Outcomes
Klempfner et al., 2018 (53)	*Total*: 216 HFrEF n: 170 and HFrEF n: 46	***Modality***: AE ***Intensity***: moderate to high, 40–50% of HR with increment up to 70–80% of HR ***Modality***: RE ***Intensity***: Initially 10–12 rep and later 15–18, according to Borg scale	***Duration***: up to 45 min (AE) ***Duration***: 15 minutes (RE) ***Total duration***: 6 months	↑ exercise capacity
Tanaka et al., 2018 (54)	*Total*: 78 patients. HFpEF n: 40 and HFrEF n: 38	***Modality***: AE/RE	***Duration***: 2–3×/week ***Total duration***: 20 weeks	HFpEF not received benefits on endothelium function

Abbreviations: AE: aerobic exercise, AIT: aerobic interval training, CE: cycle ergometer, ET: exercise training, HFpEF: heart failure preserved ejection fraction, HFrEF: heart failure reduced ejection fraction, HR: heart rate, IMT: inspiratory muscle training, FMD: flow mediated dilation, FES: functional electrical stimulation, HIIT: high-intensity interval training, HRR: heart rate reserve, MCT: moderate continuous training, 6MWT: 6-minute walking test, MIP: maximum inspiratory pressure, NYHA: New York Heart Association, RE: resistance exercise, p: peak.

TABLE 11.5: Summary of Recommendations of Exercise Training (ET) Programs in Heart Failure Patients

Recommendations of Program Training in HF Patients

1. To have maximum or symptom-limited exercise testing before ET
2. To evaluate 1 Repetition Maximum(1RM) testing before ET
3. Measurement before, during, and after training of arterial blood pressure, heart rate, oxygen saturation, respiratory rate, and lungs auscultation
4. Observe the symptoms/signs such as:
   - Hypoperfusion, confusion, cold sweated extremities
   - Presence of pulmonary crackles in base
   - Headache, dizziness, palpitations, chest pains, motion sickness
   - Increased edema of lower limbs
   - Exacerbation of dyspnea
   - Arrhythmias such as atrial fibrillation and ventricular tachycardia
   - Weight alterations after 24 h of ET

Abbreviations: HF: heart failure, ET: exercise training.

Therefore, the introduction of inotropic drugs during an acute HF episode associated with early mobilization, to initiate the physical rehabilitation of these patients as early as possible, may contribute to the amelioration of muscle mass losses and to increased functional capacity. Despite these interesting preliminary results, there is still limited evidence to recommend early rehabilitation in patients undergoing IV inotropic support, and future studies should be carried out on this line of research.[38]

Conclusion

Exercise training is an essential tool for rehabilitation in HFpEF and HFrEF. Moderate-intensity exercise programs are recommended, whereas HIIT may be applied under more stable clinical conditions. Non-pharmacological therapies as an adjunct to ET, such as ventilatory muscle training, non-invasive ventilation, and neuromuscular electrical stimulation have gained prominence and scientific relevance. Future studies should be performed to confirm the effects of these adjunct therapies on larger samples. Although the evidence base is less robust during the hospitalization period, studies have demonstrated that exercise implemented early after an episode of decompensation is safe and beneficial in several clinical and functional outcomes in selected patients after achievement of clinical stability.

References

1. Del Buono MG, Arena R, Borlaug BA, et al. Exercise intolerance in patients with heart failure. *J Am Coll Cardiol.* 2019;73(17):2209–25. doi:10.1016/j.jacc.2019.01.072
2. Benjamin EJ, Muntner P, Alonso A, et al. Heart disease and stroke statistics-2019 update: a report from the American Heart Association. *Circulation.* 2019;139:e56–e528.
3. Borghi-Silva A, Trimer R, Mendes RG, Arena RA, Schwartzmann P V. Rehabilitation practice patterns for patients with heart failure. *Heart Fail Clin.* 2015;11(1):73–82. doi:10.1016/j.hfc.2014.08.004
4. Haykowsky MJ, Daniel KM, Bhella PS, Sarma S, Kitzman DW. Heart failure: Exercise-based cardiac rehabilitation: Who, when, and how intense? *Can J Cardiol.* 2016;32(10) Supplement 2:S382–7. doi:10.1016/j.cjca.2016.06.001
5. Miller S, Mandrusiak A, Adsett J. Getting to the heart of the matter: What is the landscape of exercise rehabilitation for people with heart failure in Australia? *Hear Lung Circ.* 2018;27(11):1350–6. doi:10.1016/j.hlc.2017.08.016
6. Ezekowitz JA, O'Meara E, McDonald MA, et al. 2017 comprehensive update of the Canadian cardiovascular society guidelines for the management of heart failure. *Can J Cardiol.* 2017;33(11):1342–433. doi:10.1016/j.cjca.2017.08.022
7. Piepoli MF, Guazzi M, Boriani G, et al. Exercise intolerance in chronic heart failure: Mechanisms and therapies. Part I. *Eur J Cardiovasc Prev Rehabil.* 2010;17(6):637–42. doi:10.1097/HJR.0b013e3283361dc5
8. Poole DC, Richardson RS, Haykowsky MJ, Hirai DM, Musch TI. Exercise limitations in heart failure with reduced and preserved ejection fraction. *J Appl Physiol.* 2018;124(1):208–24. doi:10.1152/japplphysiol.00747.2017
9. Long L, Mordi IR, Bridges C, et al. Exercise-based cardiac rehabilitation for adults with heart failure. *Cochrane Database Syst Rev.* January 2019. doi:10.1002/14651858.CD003331.pub5
10. Esposito F, Mathieu-Costello O, Shabetai R, Wagner PD, Richardson RS. Limited maximal exercise capacity in patients with chronic heart failure. *J Am Coll Cardiol.* 2010;55(18):1945–54. doi:10.1016/j.jacc.2009.11.086
11. Tucker WJ, Lijauco CC, Hearon CM, et al. Mechanisms of the improvement in peak VO 2 with exercise training in heart failure with reduced or preserved ejection fraction. *Hear Lung Circ.* 2018;27(1):9–21. doi:10.1016/j.hlc.2017.07.002
12. Haykowsky MJ, Tomczak CR, Scott JM, Paterson DI, Kitzman DW. Determinants of exercise intolerance in patients with heart failure and reduced or preserved ejection fraction. *J Appl Physiol.* 2015;119(6):739–44. doi:10.1152/japplphysiol.00049.2015
13. Dhakal BP, Malhotra R, Murphy RM, et al. Mechanisms of exercise intolerance in heart failure with preserved ejection fraction. *Circ Hear Fail.* 2015;8(2):286–94. doi:10.1161/CIRCHEARTFAILURE.114.001825
14. Taylor RS, Walker S, Smart NA, et al. Impact of exercise rehabilitation on exercise capacity and quality-of-life in heart failure. *J Am Coll Cardiol.* 2019;73(12):1430–43. doi:10.1016/j.jacc.2018.12.072

15. Tucker WJ, Beaudry RI, Liang Y, et al. Meta-analysis of exercise training on left ventricular ejection fraction in heart failure with reduced ejection fraction: A 10-year update. *Prog Cardiovasc Dis.* 2019;62(2):163–71. doi:10.1016/j.pcad.2018.08.006
16. Australia Position Statement, 2010.
17. ECPR, 2011.
18. Canadian Cardiovascular Society Guidelines, 2017.
19. ACC/AHA Guidelines, 2019.
20. Giuliano C, Karahalios A, Neil C, Allen J, Levinger I. The effects of resistance training on muscle strength, quality of life and aerobic capacity in patients with chronic heart failure — A meta-analysis. *Int J Cardiol.* 2017;227:413–23. doi:10.1016/j.ijcard.2016.11.023
21. Wu J, Kuang L, Fu L. Effects of inspiratory muscle training in chronic heart failure patients: A systematic review and meta-analysis. *Congenit Heart Dis.* 2018;13(2):194–202. doi:10.1111/chd.12586
22. Smart NA, Giallauria F, Dieberg G. Efficacy of inspiratory muscle training in chronic heart failure patients: A systematic review and meta-analysis. *Int J Cardiol.* 2013;167(4):1502–7. doi:10.1016/j.ijcard.2012.04.029
23. Montemezzo D, Fregonezi GA, Pereira DA, Britto RR, Reid WD. Influence of inspiratory muscle weakness on inspiratory muscle training responses in chronic heart failure patients: A systematic review and meta-analysis. *Arch Phys Med Rehabil.* 2014;95(7):1398–407. doi:10.1016/j.apmr.2014.02.022
24. Yamamoto S, Hotta K, Ota E, Matsunaga A, Mori R. Exercise-based cardiac rehabilitation for people with implantable ventricular assist devices. *Cochrane Database Syst Rev.* September 2018. doi:10.1002/14651858.CD012222.pub2
25. Ponikowski P, Voors AA, Anker SD, et al. ESC guidelines for the diagnosis and treatment of acute and chronic heart failure. *Rev Española Cardiol (English Ed).* 2016;69(12):1167. doi:10.1016/j.rec.2016.11.005
26. Oliveira MF, Santos RC, Artz SA, et al. Safety and efficacy of aerobic exercise training associated to non-invasive ventilation in patients with acute heart failure. *Arq Bras Cardiol.* 2018. doi:10.5935/abc.20180039
27. Borghi-Silva A, Carrascosa C, Oliveira CC, et al. Effects of respiratory muscle unloading on leg muscle oxygenation and blood volume during high-intensity exercise in chronic heart failure. *Am J Physiol Circ Physiol.* 2008;294(6):H2465–72. doi:10.1152/ajpheart.91520.2007
28. Chermont S, Quintão MMP, Mesquita ET, Rocha NN, Nóbrega ACL. Noninvasive ventilation with continuous positive airway pressure acutely improves 6-minute walk distance in chronic heart failure. *J Cardiopulm Rehabil Prev.* 2009;29(1):44–48. doi:10.1097/HCR.0b013e3181927858
29. Wittmer VL, Simoes GMS, Sogame LCM, Vasquez EC. Effects of continuous positive airway pressure on pulmonary function and exercise tolerance in patients with congestive heart failure. *Chest.* 2006;130(1):157–63. doi:10.1378/chest.130.1.157
30. Gomes Neto M, Duarte LFG, Rodrigues E de S, et al. Effects of non-invasive ventilation with bilevel positive airway pressure on exercise tolerance and dyspnea in heart failure patients. *Hell J Cardiol.* 2018;59(6):317–20. doi:10.1016/j.hjc.2017.11.005
31. Heidenreich PA, Albert NM, Allen LA, et al. Forecasting the impact of heart failure in the United States. *Circ Hear Fail.* 2013;6(3):606–19. doi:10.1161/HHF.0b013e318291329a
32. Kurmani S, Squire I. Acute heart failure: Definition, classification and epidemiology. *Curr Heart Fail Rep.* 2017;14(5):385–92. doi:10.1007/s11897-017-0351-y
33. Rossi Caruso FC, Arena R, Mendes RG, Reis MS, Papa V, Borghi-Silva A. Heart rate autonomic responses during deep breathing and walking in hospitalised patients with chronic heart failure. *Disabil Rehabil.* 2011;33(9):751–7. doi:10.3109/09638288.2010.511420
34. Doletsky A, Andreev D, Giverts I, et al. Interval training early after heart failure decompensation is safe and improves exercise tolerance and quality of life in selected patients. *Eur J Prev Cardiol.* 2018;25(1):9–18. doi:10.1177/2047487317724575
35. Acanfora D, Scicchitano P, Casucci G, et al. Exercise training effects on elderly and middle-age patients with chronic heart failure after acute decompensation: A randomized, controlled trial. *Int J Cardiol.* 2016;225:313–23. doi:10.1016/j.ijcard.2016.10.026
36. Piepoli MF, Conraads V, Corrà U, et al. Exercise training in heart failure: From theory to practice. A consensus document of the Heart Failure Association and the European Association for Cardiovascular Prevention and Rehabilitation. *Eur J Heart Fail.* 2011;13(4):347–57. doi:10.1093/eurjhf/hfr017
37. Borghi-Silva A, Mendes R, Simões R, et al. Left-ventricular function and autonomic cardiac adaptations after short-term inpatient cardiac rehabilitation: A prospective clinical trial. *J Rehabil Med.* 2011;43(8):720–7. doi:10.2340/16501977-0843
38. Kudaiberdieva G, Görenek B, Timuralp B. Heart rate variability as a predictor of sudden cardiac death. *Anadolu Kardiyol Derg.* 2007;7 Suppl 1:68–70.
39. Kataoka T, Keteyian SJ, Marks CR, Fedel FJ, Levine AB, Levine TB. Exercise training in a patient with congestive heart failure on continuous dobutamine. *Med Sci Sports Exerc.* 1994;26(6):678–81.
40. Arena R, Humphrey R, Peberdy MA. Safety and efficacy of exercise training in a patient awaiting heart transplantation while on positive intravenous inotropic support. *J Cardiopulm Rehabil.* 20(4):259–61.
41. Forestieri P, Bolzan DW, Santos VB, et al. Neuromuscular electrical stimulation improves exercise tolerance in patients with advanced heart failure on continuous intravenous inotropic support use—randomized controlled trial. *Clin Rehabil.* 2018;32(1):66–74. doi:10.1177/0269215517715762
42. Amiya E, Taya M. Is exercise training appropriate for patients with advanced heart failure receiving continuous inotropic infusion? A review. *Clin Med Insights Cardiol.* 2018;12:117954681775143. doi:10.1177/1179546817751438

Chapter 12
THE PATIENT WITH ISCHEMIC HEART FAILURE

Konstantinos Aznaouridis, Constantina Masoura, and Charalambos Vlachopoulos

Introduction

Coronary artery disease (CAD) comprises one of the major causes of death worldwide and is the most common etiology of heart failure in modern western societies. Patients with heart failure due to CAD have a higher rate of adverse cardiac events and a worse prognosis compared with patients with non-ischemic heart failure. The prevalence of ischemic heart failure has increased during the recent decades, which reflects the improved overall survival of patients with CAD. This is due to the benefit conferred mainly by emergency revascularization with percutaneous coronary intervention in subjects with acute coronary syndromes and by optimal medical therapy for patients with chronic CAD. Although these recent advances have led to improved survival of patients across the spectrum of CAD, they are also associated with an increasing incidence of left ventricular remodeling and dysfunction, and thus with a higher incidence of ischemic heart failure.[1–4]

Ischemic heart failure can be defined as presence of symptoms and signs of heart failure with preserved or—more frequently—impaired systolic function of the left ventricle (usually ejection fraction <40%), with one of the following: presence of angina or history of prior myocardial infarction, history of prior myocardial revascularization, or presence of significant (>70%) left main or proximal left anterior descending (LAD) stenosis, or significant (>70%) 2-vessel stenosis. There are several pathological, pathophysiological, neurohormonal, and humoral factors that contribute to the development of ischemic heart failure. The principal mechanisms include the presence of necrotic (scarred and non-viable) myocardium and hibernated (dysfunctional, but non-necrotic and thus viable) myocardium, and usually a combination of both. Irreversible necrosis of myocardial tissue in a particular left ventricular segment secondary to prior myocardial infarction prevents recovery of myocardial function after coronary revascularization, as the infarcted tissue is not viable (Figure 12.1). Alternatively, hibernation is an adaptive process of the ischemic myocardium due to reduced myocardial blood flow usually secondary to significant epicardial coronary artery stenosis.[1–6] Hibernated myocardium adapts itself to a lower level of energy demands to preserve its viability. This results in (1) a hypocontractile status and systolic dysfunction, the degree of which depends on the extent of ischemia, and (2) recovery of contractile ability after appropriate revascularization. Myocardial stunning is a transient myocardial dysfunction following an acute ischemic insult; repetitive episodes of stunning may induce functional and structural adaptive mechanisms in the myocardium and eventually lead to hibernation. The previously commonly used term "ischemic cardiomyopathy" now tends to be abandoned, as an impaired left ventricle due to coronary artery disease does not represent a true cardiomyopathy.[3–5]

The treatment of ischemic heart failure is based on two main axes:

1) Medical therapy for heart failure, a regimen which is similar to that of heart failure secondary to other causes, and particularly evidence-based medications to downregulate the sympathetic nervous system, inhibits the renin-angiotensin-aldosterone system and modifies left ventricular remodeling such as β-adrenergic receptor blockers, angiotensin converting enzyme inhibitors, or angiotensin receptor blockers, and aldosterone receptor blocker, neprilysin inhibitors and ivabradine to decrease heart rate.
2) Percutaneous or surgical revascularization in patients with a straightforward indication, such as angina, large area of ischemia, or acute coronary syndrome.

The role of revascularization in patients with ischemic heart failure without one of the above indications for revascularization is rather unclear, as the only large, randomized relevant STICH Trial (Surgical Treatment of Ischemic Heart Failure) has provided rather contradictory results (described in detail below). In this chapter, we will present current evidence and practice regarding the role of coronary revascularization in subjects with ischemic heart failure. Evidence regarding the role of modern imaging techniques to characterize hibernated (and thus viable) myocardium with a potential to recover after revascularization, will also be presented.

Myocardial Stunning, Hibernation, and Viability: Pathophysiological and Clinical Considerations

Ischemic heart failure comprises a wide spectrum of pathological, pathophysiological, and clinical states, which depend on the severity and distribution of the coronary stenoses, the extent of myocardial hypoperfusion and ischemia, and the extent of normal, hibernated, and scarred myocardium. The mechanisms underlying those processes are rather complex. Interestingly, there is evidence suggesting that, in patients with coronary disease and chronic angina, even myocardial segments supplied by unobstructed coronaries may have impaired flow reserve and metabolic changes, suggesting that ischemia may be associated with adaptations of remote myocardial segments which are apparently unaffected by ischemia. It has been shown that these remote "unaffected by ischemia" myocardial segments may even have an impaired, reversible contractile function, which likely serves as an energy-preserving mechanism.[4-7]

Myocardial stunning is a condition of reversible contractile dysfunction of the myocardium due to an acute single or recurrent ischemic event (i.e., during acute coronary syndrome) that may persist much longer than the duration of the ischemia. During an acute coronary syndrome, a stunned myocardial segment may remain hypocontractile for some period even after normal blood flow has been restored. Depletion of ATP in the myocardial fibers, reduced responsiveness to calcium, and increased intracellular levels of free oxygen radicals comprise the principal pathophysiological mechanisms leading to stunning. In contrast, hibernation is a condition related to a more sustained hypoperfusion of the myocardium, which is usually

DOI: 10.1201/9780429244544-15

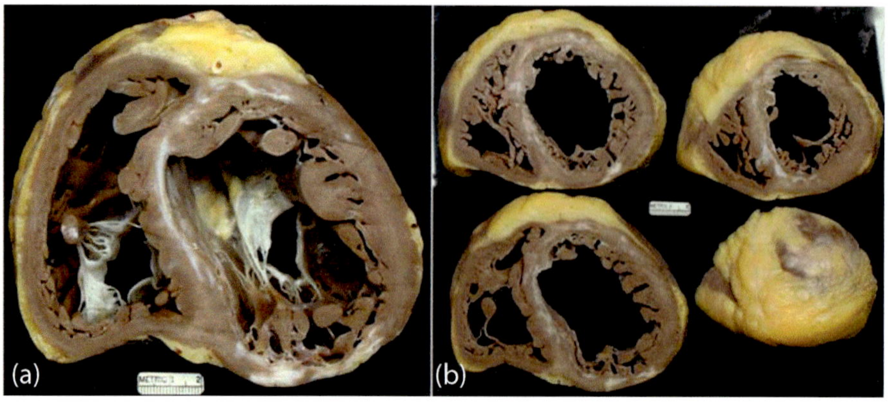

FIGURE 12.1 Gross pathology of ischemic heart failure. Heart of a middle-aged man with a history of two acute myocardial infarctions (of the anterior and posterior walls), with severe dilation and remodeling of the left ventricle. The healed myocardial tissue in the anteroseptal and posterior walls of the left ventricle appears white. (a) View of the heart showing both tricuspid and mitral valves. Both ventricles are greatly dilated. The two healed myocardial infarcts are clearly seen, and they are opposite one another. The left ventricular cavity measures up to 8 cm. (b) Views of the cardiac ventricles caudal to the picture shown on the left. (Reproduced with permission from Roberts et al., *Medicine* 2014;93:211–35.)

accompanied by structural myocardial adaptations. These may include a significant decrease or even complete loss of sarcomeres and sarcoplasmic reticulum, which comprise the main contractile apparatus of the cardiomyocytes. Depending on the severity and duration of hypoperfusion, the structural changes in hibernated myocardial areas may be reversible or irreversible. Irreversibility is usually due to fibrosis and myocardial scarring. In most patients with hibernated myocardium, a variable mixture of reversible (viable) and scarred (non-viable) areas is usually found, which is determined by a complex interplay of several molecular, pathophysiological, and structural adaptations.

Remodeling of the left ventricle is an adaptive structural process secondary to acute or chronic ischemic or non-ischemic insults (i.e., valvular regurgitations). In early stages, remodeling is associated with thinning of the wall and dilation of the ventricle, whereas, in later stages, remodeling is due to irreversible fibrosis and scarring of the myocardium. In general, remodeling due to coronary disease is mostly secondary to necrosis and presence of scar tissue following an acute myocardial infarction. However, even hibernated, predominantly non-necrotic myocardium with minimal scar due to chronic obstructive coronary artery disease may also lead to LV remodeling. From a clinical point of view, it is crucial to identify the patients with predominantly hibernating myocardium, and the patients who have scarred myocardium. In patients with heart failure and hibernated, viable myocardium due to coronary artery disease, it is expected that their symptoms and overall prognoses improve after appropriate revascularization.[6–9] On the other hand, patients with heart failure and scarred, non-viable myocardium are mainly treated with heart failure medications and devices (biventricular pacemakers and/or implantable cardioverter defibrillators [ICDs]). Therefore, the presence and the extent of viability is important in the management of patients with ischemic heart failure. Several imaging modalities have been developed to detect hibernated/viable myocardium and are briefly described herein.

Assessment of Myocardial Viability

Several imaging tools have been used to characterize and detect myocardial viability. The detection of hibernated—and thus, viable—myocardium is considered to play a major role in selecting patients for coronary revascularization. The principle is that the greater the degree of viability in a dysfunctional myocardial segment, the more likely this segment will recover after revascularization. Different imaging modalities use different pathophysiological aspects to define viability.

Echocardiography

Echocardiography allows a thorough assessment of left ventricular systolic and diastolic function, perfusion, and contractile reserve. At rest, transthoracic 2-D echocardiography enables the quantification of LV systolic function, assessment of regional wall motion abnormalities, and estimation of the ejection fraction. In patients with ischemic heart failure, dysfunctional myocardial segments of the left ventricle with an end-diastolic thickness of less than 6 mm are considered to be predominantly non-viable, having a rather low possibility of recovery after revascularization. The infusion of low-dose dobutamine during stress echocardiography allows the evaluation of contractile reserve, which is the cornerstone of viability and a predictor of myocardial recovery after revascularization. Finally, intravenous infusion of microbubbles allows the characterization of myocardial blood flow with contrast echocardiography. The greater the contrast enhancement, the higher the possibility of improvement of myocardial contractility following revascularization.[5–8]

Cardiac Magnetic Resonance (CMR) Imaging

CMR is a very delicate and accurate modality that provides an estimation of the amount of non-viable scar in infarcted myocardial territories with the use of gadolinium. Scarred myocardium appears bright after administration of gadolinium (late gadolinium enhancement), allowing quantification of infarct transmurality (Figure 12.2). The absence of gadolinium uptake from a dysfunctional myocardial segment is a strong predictor of functional recovery after revascularization. In general, a scar transmurality >50% is a predictor of poor or no recovery after revascularization. However, a transmurality <50% is not necessarily a prognosticator of significant functional recovery. In those cases where late gadolinium enhancement offers equivocal results, additional assessment of the contractile reserve with

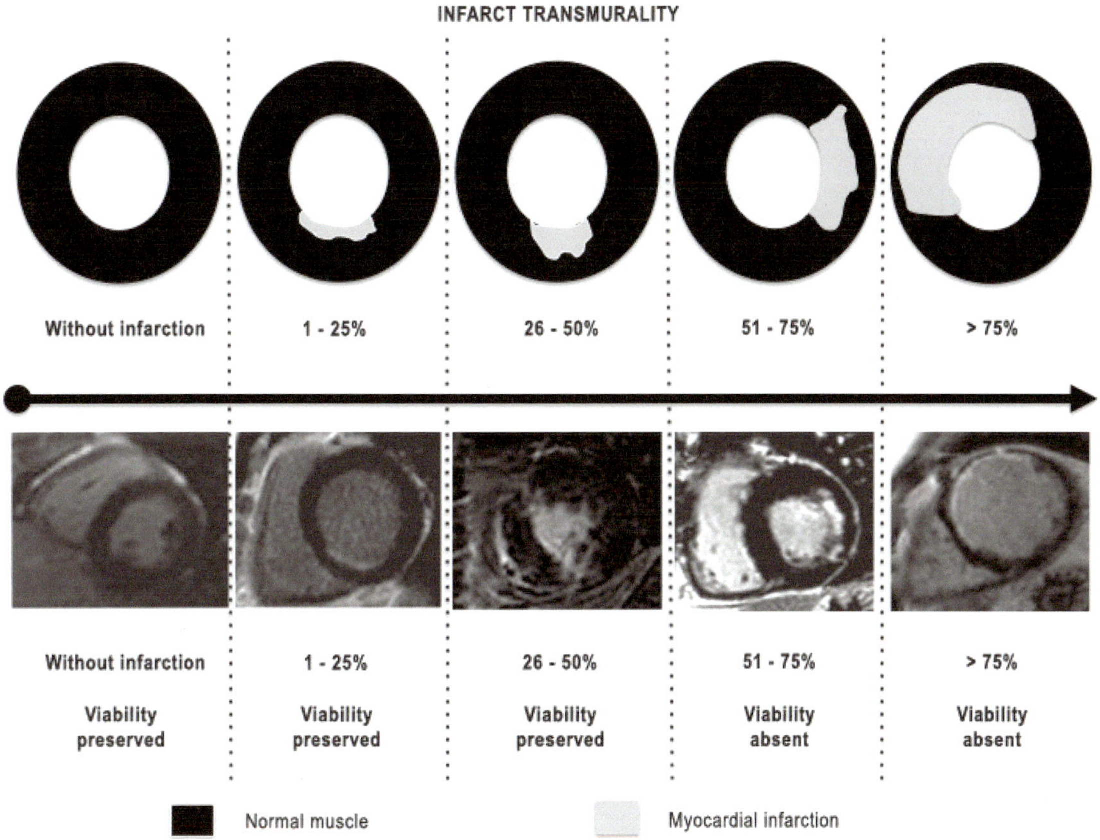

FIGURE 12.2 Ischemic myocardium visualized via gadolinium enhancement. Schematic drawings (top) and cardiac magnetic resonance (CMR) imaging with gadolinium enhancement (bottom) in a patient without infarction (left panel) and in four different patients with histories of myocardial infarction and varying amounts of infarcted myocardium (the other four panels). Scarred/infarcted myocardium appears bright with gadolinium, allowing quantification of infarct transmurality. Scar transmurality >50% (the two right-hand panels) is a predictor of poor recovery of the corresponding myocardial segments after revascularization. (Reproduced under the terms of the Creative Commons Attribution License from Souto et al., *Arq Bras Cardiol* 2017;108:458–69.)

stress cardiac magnetic resonance during dobutamine infusion allows a more comprehensive assessment of viability.[6–11]

Single Photon Emission Computerized Tomography (SPECT) and Positron Emission Tomography (PET)

These modalities are based on nuclear imaging and evaluate myocardial viability by assessing the functional integrity of the cardiomyocyte's membrane. SPECT and PET can differentiate hibernated (viable) from scarred (nonviable) myocardial tissue by demonstrating the presence or absence of cellular metabolism. SPECT uses radioactive tracers such as thallium and technetium compounds during resting and stress conditions. The distribution of the radioactive tracers immediately post-injection is indicative of blood flow (ischemia), whereas images taken several hours later demonstrate the integrity of the cellular membrane (viability) (Figure 12.3). PET is a more sophisticated imaging modality which simultaneously assesses myocardial perfusion and metabolism. It is limited, however, by its rather limited availability and its high cost. Rubidium-82 and N-13 ammonia are the most widely employed tracers used to assess ischemia by way of capturing perfusion.[18] Fluorodeoxyglucose is the radiotracer used to assess metabolism, and thus represents a marker of viability. Dual assessment of perfusion and metabolism allows an accurate characterization of myocardial segments as normal (with normal perfusion and metabolism), hibernated/viable (with impaired perfusion but preserved metabolism: perfusion-metabolism mismatch), or infarcted/non-viable (with impaired perfusion and metabolism) (Figure 12.4).[12–15]

Treatment of Ischemic Heart Failure

The cornerstones of treatment in patients with ischemic heart failure are (1) optimal medical therapy along with lifestyle modifications in all patients, (2) implantable devices (implantable cardioverter-defibrillators and cardiac resynchronization therapy) in appropriately selected patients, and (3) coronary revascularization in appropriately selected patients.

Medical Therapy

The medical treatment of patients with ischemic heart failure comprises a combination of (1) medical treatment of heart failure, plus (2) secondary prevention of coronary artery disease, as well as anti-ischemic/anti-anginal therapy, if needed. In brief, treatment includes a beta-blocker, an angiotensin-converting enzyme inhibitor (ACEi), a statin at high dose (at least 40 mg of atorvastatin or 20 mg of rosuvastatin daily), and antiplatelet therapy (low-dose aspirin at 75 to 160 mg daily). An angiotensin receptor blocker is given to patients who do not tolerate ACEi

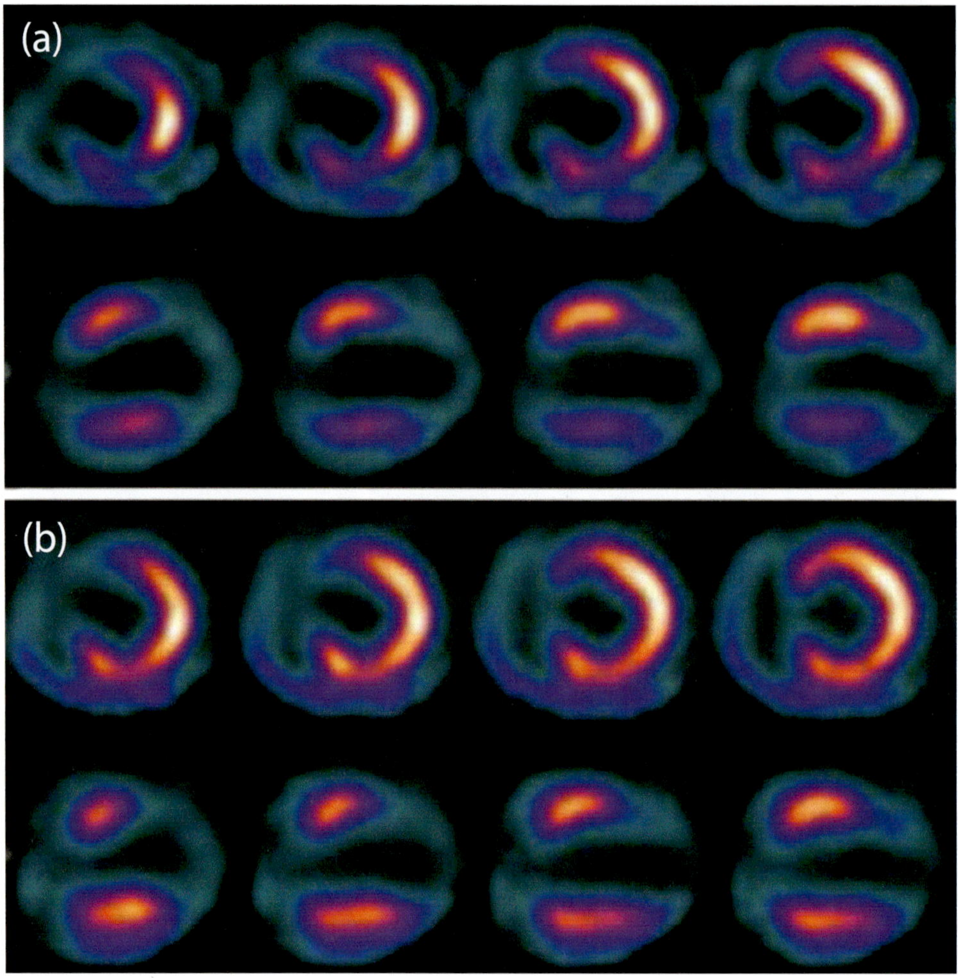

FIGURE 12.3 Technetium Tc-99m tetrofosmin gated SPECT in a patient with ischemic heart failure. Panel (a) shows lack of perfusion in the apical segments and the interventricular septum and severely reduced perfusion in the inferior wall. Panel (b) (delayed images) shows improved tracer uptake in the inferior wall, indicating viability. (Reproduced with permission from Raja et al., *J Nucl Cardiol* 2012;19:1176–81.)

(due to hypersensitivity or non-productive cough). Loop diuretics are given to patients with volume overload for symptomatic relief. Other medications, such as mineralocorticoid receptor antagonists (spironolactone or eplerenone), ivabradine, and neprilysin inhibitors (i.e., sacubitril-valsartan), are considered for particular patients.[16,17]

Lifestyle modifications, including smoking cessation, regular exercise, and weight loss, are of paramount importance in all patients with ischemic heart failure. Medications which have been shown to exert adverse effects on patients with severe LV systolic dysfunction, such as non-steroidal anti-inflammatory medications, some antiarrhythmic medications, and the non-dihydropyridine calcium channel blockers (diltiazem and verapamil), should be avoided.[16–21]

Device Therapy

Patients with severely impaired left ventricular systolic function and symptoms of heart failure, despite optimal medical therapy, are considered for cardiac resynchronization therapy with a biventricular pacemaker or a biventricular ICD. The patients who are considered for ICD for primary prevention of sudden cardiac death should be assessed no less than 40 days after myocardial infarction and more than three months after revascularization. Patients on sinus rhythm with prolonged QRS duration (≥120 ms) and severely depressed LV systolic function with ejection fraction <35%, who remain symptomatic despite maximally tolerated medical therapy, are good candidates for cardiac resynchronization therapy with biventricular pacing to improve symptoms and survival. Most of the patients who fulfill the above criteria are candidates for ICD as well, and therefore receive a biventricular pacemaker-ICD.[16–21]

Revascularization in the Ischemic Patient with Heart Failure

Evidence from Observational, Non-Randomized Studies

The initial evidence that coronary revascularization improves LV systolic dysfunction and benefits prognosis comes from the early studies of coronary artery bypass grafting (CABG). The Coronary Artery Surgery Study (CASS) registry showed that CABG is more likely to improve prognosis in patients with multivessel disease and LV systolic dysfunction.[22] There is no doubt that, compared with the current era, CASS and similar early studies are limited as none of the current evidence-based heart failure and anti-atherosclerotic medical therapy were

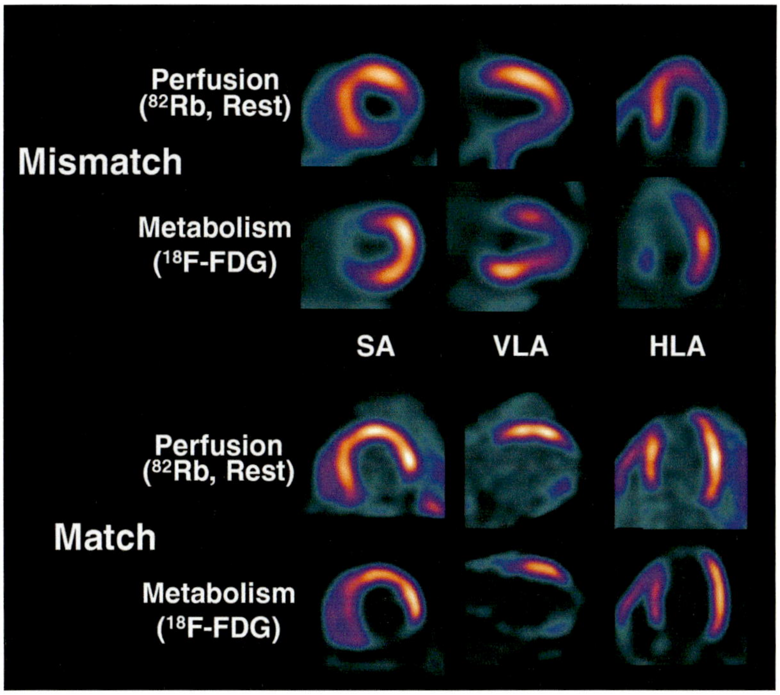

FIGURE 12.4 Positron emission tomography (PET) perfusion/metabolism imaging for assessment of myocardial viability. Top: A mismatch study with reduced rest perfusion (measured by ^{82}Rb) and preserved or increased metabolism (measured by ^{18}F-FDG) is shown in the inferolateral wall, indicating compromised but viable "hibernating" myocardium. Bottom: A matched perfusion/metabolism defect in the inferior wall, indicating a non-viable scar. reduced rest perfusion (measured by ^{82}Rb) and preserved or increased metabolism. *Abbreviations*: FDG = fluorodeoxyglucose; HLA = horizontal long axis; SA=short axis; VLA = vertical long axis. (Reproduced with permission from Bengel et al., *J Am Coll Cardiol* 2009;54:1–15.)

used concurrently with data collection. Despite these apparent limitations, however, these studies provide strong evidence that surgical revascularization is likely to be an effective and beneficial treatment in patients with ischemic heart failure.

The above findings were further confirmed by a large meta-analysis of 24 observational studies that showed a strong mortality benefit with revascularization in patients with coronary artery disease and LV systolic dysfunction. In total, 3,088 patients with ischemic heart failure with an ejection fraction of 32±8% were included in this meta-analysis, and myocardial viability was evaluated using dobutamine stress echocardiography, SPECT, or PET. Patients with viability who were revascularized had a clear mortality benefit, as their annual mortality was 3.2%, compared with an annual mortality of 16% in the subgroup of patients who were treated with medications only. Despite the apparent limitations of such a meta-analysis (heterogeneity among studies, observational, non-randomized data, selection and possible publication bias, variability in methods and thresholds used to define viability, and, most importantly, lack of robust, evidence-based, current medical and device therapy), this analysis delineates the beneficial role of revascularization in select patients with ischemic heart failure.[3,20–27]

Evidence from Randomized Trials

Few randomized studies have investigated the role of coronary revascularization on major outcomes in patients with ischemic heart failure. The early Heart Failure Revascularization Trial (HEART) trial did not show any benefit from revascularization. Furthermore, its findings can be regarded as inconclusive at best, as this study was terminated early due to slow recruitment, with only 138 patients ultimately being enrolled out of the planned 800 patients.[28]

The F-18-Fluorodeoxyglucose Positron Emission Tomography Imaging-Assisted Management of Patients with Severe Left Ventricular Dysfunction and Suspected Coronary Disease (PPAR-2) trial was designed to determine the role of F-18-fluorodeoxyglucose-based PET in the management of patients with ischemic heart failure. The PET-guided management was not associated with improved mortality in intention to treat analysis.[29] However, almost one in four patients did not receive the recommended PET-guided management in this study. In an analysis confined to the patients who eventually received the recommended therapy, PET-guided therapy was associated with a significant reduction in mortality in those patients (relative risk reduction of 38%).

The Surgical Treatment for Ischemic Heart Failure (STICH) trial published in 2011 is the largest and most important study in this field. STICH randomized 1,212 patients with ischemic heart failure and addressed the impact of surgical revascularization with CABG.[30] The patients were randomly allocated to optimal medical therapy alone vs coronary artery bypass grafting (CABG) in addition to optimal medical therapy (OMT). All-cause mortality was the primary outcome of the trial. The trial also assessed two additional secondary outcomes: cardiovascular mortality, and a combined endpoint of all-cause mortality and hospitalization for cardiac causes. The enrolled patients had severe LV systolic dysfunction with an ejection fraction <35% and were followed for a mean period of 4.7 years. Patients who had significant left main stenosis or acute coronary syndromes were excluded. The intention to treat analysis showed a trend toward a benefit of revascularization in terms of the primary endpoint of all-cause mortality (36% with CABG plus OMT compared to 41% with OMT alone), which was not statistically significant (p=0.12). There was, however, a significant benefit of CABG in terms of the secondary endpoints of cardiovascular death and the combined endpoint of all-cause mortality and hospitalization for cardiac causes in the CABG group. The effect of revascularization on all-cause mortality may have been underestimated by a significant cross-over rate in the trial's population. Importantly, a considerable 17% of the patients who had initially been randomized to medical therapy only were eventually offered CABG. Additionally, 9% of the patients who had initially been randomized to CABG did not undergo revascularization. The "as treated" analysis showed a significant reduction of all-cause mortality with CABG, with a number needed to treat of 9.1 to prevent one death.

The STICH trial is a landmark study in the field of ischemic heart failure but has also been the subject of intense criticism. A formal assessment of myocardial viability was not a prerequisite for enrollment, and almost half of the patients had no viability prestudy. Therefore, patients with predominantly non-viable myocardium may have been randomized. Patients who were offered CABG had a relatively high peri-CABG mortality in STICH, which may have influenced the results. Furthermore, some patients had non-severe coronary artery disease and therefore a potential alternative cause of their severe LV systolic dysfunction, and those patients could not benefit from revascularization.

As reported above, only half of the enrolled patients (601 subjects) had a viability assessment in STICH (with dobutamine stress echo or SPECT). Separate analysis of the subgroup of patients with viable myocardium (487 patients) did not show any benefit of revascularization in terms of survival. The presence of myocardial viability was related to improved overall survival independent of treatment compared to the absence of viability in STICH. However, the presence of viability did not predict a mortality benefit with revascularization compared with patients without myocardial viability. These data have questioned the role of viability testing before surgical revascularization in patients with ischemic heart failure. This important viability sub-analysis was limited by its non-randomized and non-blinded nature. Furthermore, statistical power issues may have ensued, as only 60 patients with no demonstrable viability were subjected to CABG.

The extended follow-up from STICH (STICH Extension Study -STICHES), published in 2016,[31] supports a significant overall survival benefit of CABG combined with medical therapy vs medical therapy alone in a median observation period of almost ten years. The primary outcome of all-cause mortality was significantly lower in the CABG plus medical therapy group compared with patients treated only with optimal medical therapy, resulting in an absolute reduction of 7% in all-cause death (59% vs 66%, hazard ratio 0.84, 95% confidence interval 0.73–0.97). CABG was also associated with a significant ~9% absolute reduction in cardiovascular mortality (40.5% vs 49.3%, hazard ratio 0.79, 95% confidence interval 0.66–0.93), as well as in the combined endpoint of all-cause mortality plus hospitalization for cardiac causes (76.6% vs 87.0%, hazard ratio 0.72, 95% confidence interval 0.64–0.82).

PCI or CABG in Patients with Ischemic Heart Failure?

Evidence regarding the role of percutaneous coronary intervention (PCI) in patients with ischemic heart failure is limited.[32–41] The currently performed Percutaneous Revascularization for Ischemic Ventricular Dysfunction (REVIVED-BCIS2 Trial) is a prospective, multi-center, randomized, controlled trial which will evaluate whether PCI, in combination with optimal medical therapy, reduces all-cause death and hospitalization for HF compared with a strategy of optimal medical therapy alone in patients with ischemic heart failure (EF ≤35%), extensive coronary disease, and/or demonstrable myocardial viability.[36]

Evidence from observational studies suggests that PCI and CABG are equivalent in terms of survival in patients with ischemic heart failure. The large New York State registry followed 4,616 patients with coronary artery disease and impaired LV systolic function (EF ≤35%) who underwent PCI (mostly with everolimus drug-eluting stents) or CABG, without randomization.[42] Of them, 2,126 matched patients were assessed after a follow-up of 2.9 years, and no difference in survival was found (hazard ratio 1.01; 95% confidence interval 0.81–1.28) (Figure 12.5). The patients on the CABG arm had a lower need for repeat revascularization. As expected, CABG was associated with a higher risk of stroke. Furthermore, PCI was associated with a higher risk of myocardial infarction in patients with incomplete revascularization. The findings of this study support that multivessel PCI is a potential strategy in patients with ischemic heart failure if complete revascularization can be achieved.

Similarly, analysis of the small subgroup of patients in the Angina with Extremely Serious Operative Mortality Evaluation (AWESOME) trial who had low ejection fraction <35% did not show any mortality difference between the randomly assigned PCI and CABG.[35] However, the design of AWESOME and the small number of patients with severe LV systolic dysfunction included in this study is not conducive to drawing definitive conclusions.

Guidelines for Revascularization in Ischemic Heart Failure

The most recent 2018 European Society of Cardiology guidelines on myocardial revascularization recommend coronary revascularization in patients with severe LV systolic dysfunction and/or coronary artery disease suitable for intervention for benefit in prognosis (recommendation IB). Surgical revascularization (CABG) is recommended as the preferred strategy

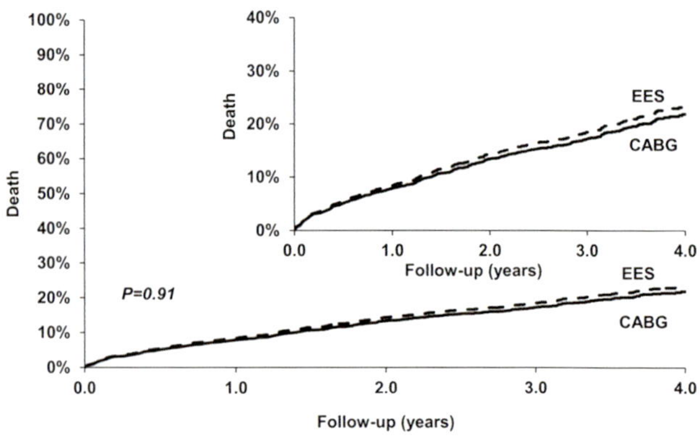

FIGURE 12.5 Long-term outcome assessment of PCI with everolimus-eluting stents (EES) vs CABG. No difference in terms of survival in patients with ischemic heart failure was detected between percutaneous coronary intervention with EES or CABG. (Data for the New York State registry (observational study). Reproduced with permission from Bangalore et al., *Circulation* 2016;133:2132–40.)

in patients with multivessel disease and acceptable surgical risk (IB).[43] In subjects with one- or two-vessel disease, PCI should be considered as an alternative to CABG when complete revascularization can be achieved (IIaC). In patients with three-vessel disease, the choice between CABG or PCI should be made after evaluation of the coronary anatomy, estimation of the potential completeness of revascularization, and consideration of the comorbidities (diabetes, valvular disease, functional status, etc.) by the Heart Team (IIaC).

Conclusion

Ischemic heart failure describes a common phenotype of severely impaired left ventricular function (ejection fraction ≤35–40%) secondary to coronary artery disease. This can result from either a permanent, irreversible loss of myocardial tissue because of a previous myocardial infarction, or from a transient and reversible hypocontractile state due to severe chronic ischemia in a viable myocardial territory.

All patients with ischemic heart failure should receive optimal medical therapy and engage with lifestyle modifications. Coronary revascularization and device therapy (implantable cardioverter-defibrillators and cardiac resynchronization therapy with biventricular pacemaker) should be considered in patients with appropriate indications.

Considering the findings of STICH and STICHES and the evidence they provide for reduction in long-term overall and cardiovascular mortality, it is recommended to offer CABG surgery in addition to optimal medical therapy to patients with severe coronary artery disease amenable to surgery and/or severe LV systolic dysfunction. In patients with comorbidities and a high surgical risk or with a coronary anatomy which is unfavorable for CABG, PCI can be offered.

Although myocardial viability is an important pathophysiological concept, its role in predicting the outcomes after myocardial revascularization has been a subject of debate. It seems that routine assessment of myocardial viability prior to CABG is not a universal need. There are, however, some subsets of patients who merit more sophisticated assessment, such as in extremely remodeled and dilated left ventricles, in the case of uncertainty regarding the possibility of complete revascularization, or in the presence of comorbidities that increase the risk of CABG significantly. In those patients, evaluation of viability may enable the clinicians to tailor the risk/benefit balance of CABG and drive decisions for revascularization.

References

1. Roberts W, et al. Morphologic features of the recipient heart in patients having cardiac transplantation and analysis of the congruence or incongruence between the clinical and morphologic diagnoses. *Medicine.* 2014;93:211–35.
2. Morbach C, et al. Heart failure in patients with coronary heart disease: Prevalence, characteristics and guideline implementation - Results from the German EuroAspire IV cohort. *BMC Cardiovasc Disord.* 2017;17:108.
3. Albakri A. Ischemic cardiomyopathy: A review of literature on clinical status and meta-analysis of diagnostic and clinical management. *Biol Eng Med.* 2018;3:1–13.
4. Remme W. Overview of the relationship between ischemica and congestive heart failure. *Clin Cardiol.* 2000;23:4–8.
5. Underwood S, et al. Imaging techniques for the assessment of myocardial hibernation: Report of a study group of the European Society of Cardiology. *Eur Heart J* 2004;25:815.
6. Cleland J, et al. Myocardial viability as a determinant of the ejection fraction response to carvedilol in patients with heart failure (CHRISTMAS trial): Randomised controlled trial. *Lancet.* 2003;362:14.
7. Desideri A, et al. The extent of perfusion-F18-fluorodeoxyglucose positron emission tomography mismatch determines mortality in medically treated patients with chronic ischemic left ventricular dysfunction. *J Am Coll Cardiol.* 2005;46:1264–9.
8. Allman K, et al. Myocardial viability testing and impact of revascularization on prognosis in patients with coronary artery disease and left ventricular dysfunction: A meta-analysis. *J Am Coll Cardiol.* 2002;39:1151.
9. Bonow R. The hibernating myocardium: Implications for management of congestive heart failure. *Am J Cardiol.* 1995;75:17A.
10. Souto A, et al. Myocardial viability on cardiac magnetic resonance. *Arq Bras Cardiol.* 2017;108:458–69.
11. Al-Sabeq B, et al. Assessment of myocardial viability by cardiac MRI. *Curr Opin Cardiol.* 2019;34:502–9.
12. Auerbach M, et al. Prevalence of myocardial viability as detected by positron emission tomography in patients with ischemic cardiomyopathy. *Circulation.* 1999;99:2921.
13. Madsen S, et al. Myocardial viability testing by positron emission tomography: Basic concepts, mini-review of the literature and experience from a tertiary PET center. *Semin Nucl Med.* 2020;50:248–59.
14. Raja S, et al. Comparison of nitrate augmented Tc-99m tetrofosmin gated SPECT imaging with FDG PET imaging for the assessment of myocardial viability in patients with severe left ventricular dysfunction. *J Nucl Cardiol.* 2012;19:1176–81.
15. Khalaf S, et al. Assessment of myocardial viability by PET. *Curr Opin Cardiol.* 2019;34:466–72.
16. Panza J, et al. Myocardial viability and long-term outcomes in ischemic cardiomyopathy. *N Engl J Med.* 2019;381:739–48.
17. Schinkel A, et al. Assessment of myocardial viability in patients with heart failure. *J Nucl Med.* 2007;48:1135–46.
18. Bock A and Estep J. Myocardial viability: Heart failure perspective. *Curr Opin Cardiol.* 2019;34:459–65.
19. Ghaffar YA, et al. Low dose wall motion score predicts the short and long-term benefit of surgical revascularization in patients with ischemic left ventricular dysfunction. *Int J Cardiovasc Imaging.* 2019;35:1651–9.
20. Arora Y, et al. Impact of hibernating and viable myocardium on improvement in perfusion and left ventricular ejection fraction after coronary artery bypass graft. *Nucl Med Commun.* 2019;40:325–32.
21. Brundage B, et al. Improved regional ventricular function after successful surgical revascularization. *J Am Coll Cardiol.* 1984;3:902.
22. Passamani E, et al. A randomized trial of coronary artery bypass surgery: Survival of patients with low ejection fraction. *N Engl J Med.* 1985;312:1665–71.
23. Lee K, et al. Prognosis of patients with left ventricular dysfunction, with and without viable myocardium after myocardial infarction: Relative efficacy of medical therapy and revascularization. *Circulation.* 1994;90:2687.
24. Kwon D, et al. Survival in patients with severe ischemic cardiomyopathy undergoing revascularization versus medical therapy: Association with end-systolic volume and viability. *Circulation.* 2012;126 Supplement 1:S3–8.
25. Pagley P, et al. Improved outcome after coronary bypass surgery in patients with ischemic cardiomyopathy and residual myocardial viability. *Circulation.* 1997;96:793.
26. Bax J, et al. Improvement of left ventricular ejection fraction, heart failure symptoms and prognosis after revascularization in patients with chronic coronary artery disease and viable myocardium detected by dobutamine stress echocardiography. *J Am Coll Cardiol.* 1999;34:163.
27. Gerber B, et al. Prognostic value of myocardial viability by delayed-enhanced magnetic resonance in patients with coronary artery disease and low ejection fraction: Impact of revascularization therapy. *J Am Coll Cardiol.* 2012;59:825.
28. Cleland J, et al. The Heart Failure Revascularization Trial (HEART). *Eur Heart J.* 2011;13:227–33.
29. Beanlands R, et al. F-18 fluorodeoxyglucose positron emission tomography imaging-assisted management of patients with severe left ventricular dysfunction and suspected coronary disease: A randomized, controlled trial (PARR-2). *J Am Coll Cardiol.* 2007;50:2002–12.
30. Velazquez E, et al. Coronary-artery bypass surgery in patients with left ventricular dysfunction. *N Engl J Med.* 2011;28:1607–16.
31. Velazquez E, et al. Coronary-artery bypass surgery in patients with ischemic cardiomyopathy. *N Engl J Med.* 2016;374:1511–20.
32. Bax J, et al. Radionuclide techniques for the assessment of myocardial viability and hibernation. *Heart.* 2004;90 Supplement 5 v26.
33. Bonow R, et al. Myocardial viability and survival in ischemic left ventricular dysfunction. *N Engl J Med.* 2011;364:1617.
34. Schinkel A, et al. Why do patients with ischemic cardiomyopathy and a substantial amount of viable myocardium not always recover in function after revascularization? *J Thorac Cardiovasc Surg.* 2004;127:385.
35. Sedlis S, et al. Outcome of percutaneous coronary intervention versus coronary bypass grafting for patients with low left ventricular ejection fractions, unstable angina pectoris, and risk factors for adverse outcomes with bypass (the AWESOME Randomized Trial and Registry). *Am J Cardiol.* 2004;94:118.

36. Perera D, et al. Percutaneous revascularization for ischemic ventricular dysfunction: Rationale and design of the REVIVED-BCIS2 trial: Percutaneous coronary intervention for ischemic cardiomyopathy. *JACC Heart Fail.* 2018;6:517–26.
37. Chareonthaitawee P, et al. Revascularization in severe left ventricular dysfunction: The role of viability testing. *J Am Coll Cardiol.* 2005;46:567.
38. Velazquez E, Bonow R. Revascularization in severe left ventricular dysfunction. *J Am Coll Cardiol.* 2015;65:615.
39. Vedin O, et al. Significance of ischemic heart disease in patients with heart failure and preserved, midrange, and reduced ejection fraction: A nationwide cohort study. *Circ Heart Fail.* 2017;10:pii: e003875.
40. Guyton R, Smith A. Coronary bypass—Survival benefit in heart failure *N Engl J Med.* 2016;374:1576–7.
41. Lamblin N, et al. First hospitalization for heart failure in outpatients with stable coronary artery disease: Determinants, role of incident myocardial infarction, and prognosis. *J Card Fail.* 2018;24:815–22.
42. Bangalore S, et al. Revascularization in patients with multivessel coronary artery disease and severe left ventricular systolic dysfunction: Everolimus-eluting stents versus coronary artery bypass graft surgery. *Circulation.* 2016;133:2132–40.
43. Neumann F, et al. 2018 ESC/EACTS guidelines on myocardial revascularization. *EuroIntervention.* 2019;14:1435–534.

Chapter 13
THE NON-ISCHEMIC HEART FAILURE PATIENT

Maria-Anna Bazmpani and Theodoros D. Karamitsos

Epidemiology

Although ischemic heart disease remains the most common cause of heart failure (HF), 30–40% of patients with HF have non-ischemic cardiomyopathy (NICM), according to large-scale registries.[1–4] In clinical practice and multicenter HF clinical trials, the term dilated cardiomyopathy (DCM) has been used as an equivalent to NICM. However, NICM incorporates a diverse group of cardiac abnormalities, including hypertension, valvular heart disease, genetic abnormalities, pericardial and endomyocardial pathologies, immune-mediated and inflammatory damage, infiltration, and toxic damage.[5] Contemporary data from developed countries demonstrate a shift in NICM epidemiology with an increase in idiopathic NICM as opposed to hypertensive cardiomyopathy.[6,7] NICM manifests either with preserved left ventricular (LV) systolic function or, more commonly, with reduced LV systolic function. According to HF guidelines, there is no significant management differentiation between ischemic and non-ischemic cardiomyopathy.[5] However, identification of NICM etiology is important, as some causes are reversible (hypertension, valvular heart disease, tachycardia-induced cardio myopathy, substance abuse) and some types may require specific treatments. In addition, pathophysiology may differ and consequently the prognosis may vary as well.[7] An integrated approach, targeting etiological characterization and early diagnosis, can help improve outcomes. The classification of NICM is presented in Figure 13.1.

Dilated Physiology

LV dilatation and gradual systolic impairment in the absence of significant coronary artery disease and abnormal loading conditions (hypertension and valvular heart disease) define DCM.[8,9] The etiology of DCM is quite heterogenous and causes can be classified as genetic or familial and non-genetic or acquired. In some cases, environmental factors interact with genetic predisposition, resulting in manifestation of DCM.[8]

Recently, the European Society of Cardiology (ESC) working group on myocardial and pericardial diseases has proposed a revised definition of DCM in an effort to better identify and ultimately treat patients with DCM. The newly proposed definition requires that systolic dysfunction is defined by abnormal LV ejection fraction (LVEF) measured using any modality, preferably echocardiography or cardiac magnetic resonance (CMR), and shown either by two separate imaging modalities or on two different occasions by the same technique.[10] LV or biventricular global systolic dysfunction without dilatation (defined as LVEF $<45\%$), not explained by abnormal loading conditions or coronary artery disease, has been defined as hypokinetic non-dilated cardiomyopathy. Hypokinetic non-dilated cardiomyopathy could be the result of an early DCM diagnosis. See also Chapter 31.

The DCM phenotype is common in various heart disorders, rendering identification of etiology challenging. Phenotypic overlap between DCM and other cardiomyopathies, such as arrhythmogenic cardiomyopathy or end-stage hypertrophic cardiomyopathy (HCM), highlight the need for diagnostic methods to differentiate DCM from other conditions. The differential diagnosis of DCM from conditions with overlap is presented in Table 13.1. Innovative imaging methods, modern genetics, biomarkers, and endomyocardial biopsy (EMB) allow for exclusion of other causes that, up until recently, fell under the umbrella of DCM.

After exclusion of prominent acquired factors, a genetic basis for DCM should be sought. Several gene mutations have been implicated in the manifestation of DCM.[11,12] See also Chapter 31 for a detailed discussion of genetic causes of DCM. The etiology and characteristics of DCM are presented in Table 13.2.

Although the causes of DCM are various, myocardial injury leading to worsening LV function and clinical manifestation of HF is a common pathway as disease progresses. Evolution of acute myocarditis to DCM and systolic dysfunction has been reported with an incidence between 14% and 52%.[13] Hence, the establishment of an accurate and complete diagnosis and the timely initiation of evidence-based treatment are pivotal.

Non-Dilated Physiology and Progression to HF

Hypertrophic Cardiomyopathy

The pathophysiology of HF in HCM is heterogenous. Some patients develop symptoms due to LV systolic dysfunction and LV outflow tract obstruction,[14] whereas others have preserved LVEF with a small LV cavity but impaired diastolic function. Reverse remodeling is a lifelong process in HCM that is characterized by structural and functional modifications, including increasing LV fibrosis and function, wall thinning, moderate to severe diastolic dysfunction, atrial dilatation, and LV apical aneurysms.[15,16] LV remodeling and evolution to HF is the outcome of microvascular ischemia, energy depletion, and eventually apoptosis of myocytes, which lead to fibrosis of the myocardium.[17,18] Genetic background, characteristics and diagnostic work-up in patients with HCM phenotypes are discussed in Table 13.2.

Arrhythmogenic Right Ventricular Cardiomyopathy-Dysplasia

Arrhythmogenic right ventricular cardiomyopathy-dysplasia (ARVC/D) may present with a wide range of clinical manifestations. Less favorable long-term outcomes include sudden cardiac death and HF.[19] Although arrhythmogenic cardiomyopathy was considered a disease of the right ventricle, it is not infrequent to involve the LV and result in biventricular failure.[20] In a cohort of 130 patients with ARVC/D, almost one-third died of sudden death while the remaining two-thirds died of progressive HF.[21] In the same study, LV systolic dysfunction was strongly associated with cardiovascular death. See also Table 13.2.

Left Ventricular Non-Compaction

The pathophysiologic background of HF in LV non-compaction is not entirely clear. Systolic dysfunction is thought to be a result of hypoperfusion of the subendocardium in the presence of normal coronary arteries.[22] Diastolic dysfunction with abnormal

DOI: 10.1201/9780429244544-16

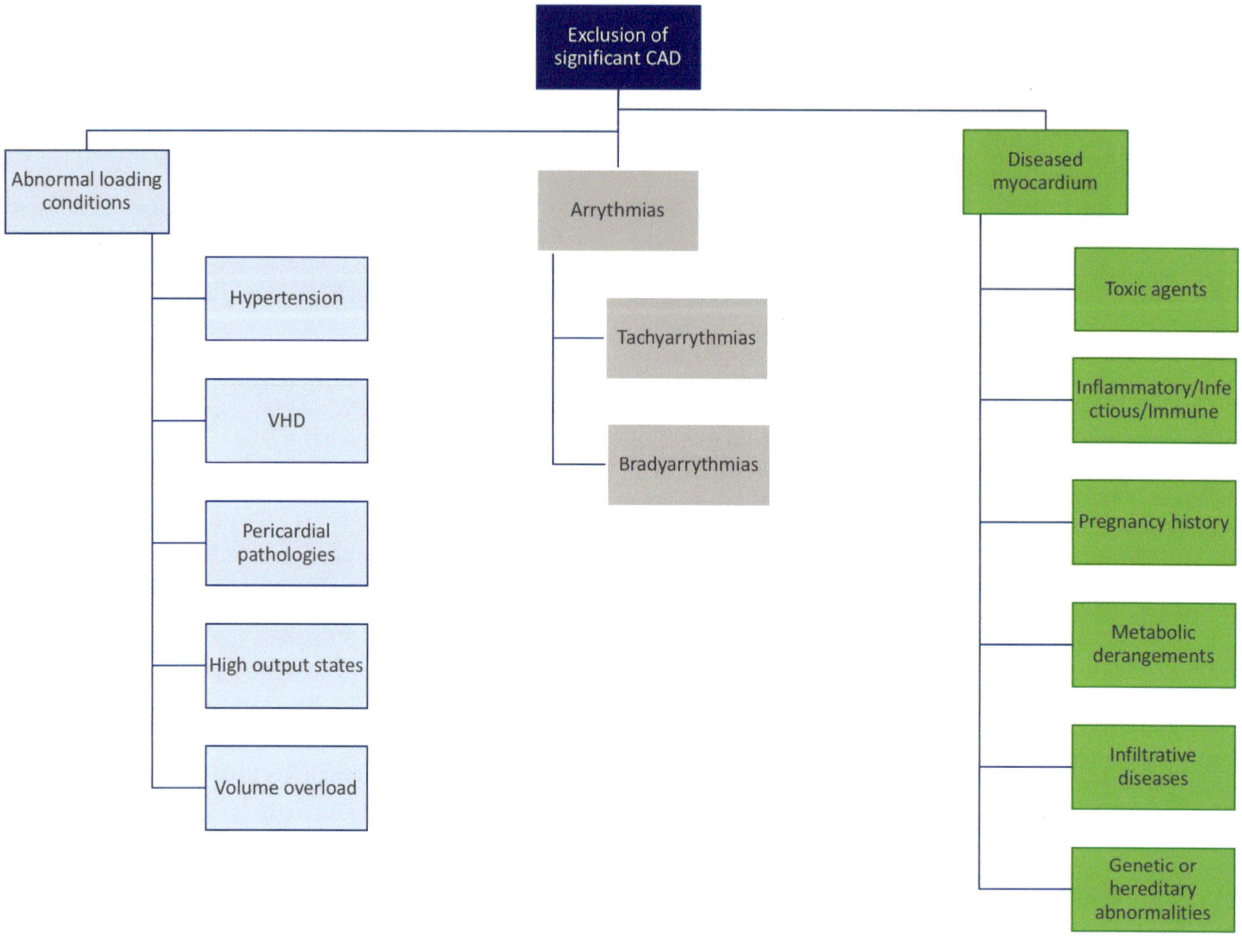

FIGURE 13.1 Differential diagnosis of non-ischemic heart failure patient.

relaxation and restrictive filling pattern may be attributed to ventricular hypertrabeculation.[23] See also Table 13.2.

Restrictive Cardiomyopathy

Restrictive cardiomyopathy is a rare type of cardiomyopathy. It is defined as restrictive ventricular physiology in the presence of normal or reduced diastolic volumes, normal or reduced systolic volumes, and normal ventricular wall thickness.[8] As disease progresses, patients present with systemic and pulmonary venous congestion, and atrial fibrillation, and have a poor prognosis.[24] See also Table 13.2.

Valvular Heart Disease (see also Chapter 14)

Valvular heart disease (VHD) and HF often coexist. VHD may cause HF or cause deterioration of pre-existing HF symptoms. In a prospective cohort study of community patients with suspected HF in the UK, 14% of patients were diagnosed with at least moderate VHD [25] whereas 69.8% of patients with moderate and severe native VHD included in the Euro Heart Survey presented with HF symptoms.[26] When evaluating a patient with HF and VHD, it is important to determine the presence of symptoms, particularly dyspnea, which is of prognostic value. Although echocardiography remains the cornerstone of imaging in VHD, CMR and computed tomography play a supplementary role in the quantification of the severity of valvular disease and accurate assessment of LV size and function.

A multidisciplinary heart team is necessary for determining the best treatment strategy. It has been well established that patients with HF and VHD are at increased risk. Without intervention, these patients have a poor prognosis, and late intervention leads to worse post-operative outcomes.[27] Timely and optimal intervention in patients with VHD and HF depends on determining whether LV dysfunction is due to disease of the valve or the ventricle.[28] For a complete approach on assessment of VHD in HF, please see Chapter 14.

Diagnostic Work-Up in Patients with HF and Suspected NICM

The diagnostic work-up of patients with HF and suspected NICM is summarized in Figure 13.2. Tables 13.2 and 13.3 summarize the differential and proposed work-up for patients with dilated and nondilated physiology, respectively.

History, Clinical Examination, ECG, and Laboratory Work-Up

Upon initial assessment of a patient with HF and suspected NICM, a detailed clinical and family history should be obtained. Clinical history should include potential causes of systolic dysfunction, e.g., hypertension, known VHD, exposure to toxins, drugs, or alcohol, prior myocarditis, or arrhythmias. A detailed family history aims to identify other family members with known or suspected myocardial disease. Questions should include history of sudden cardiac death, HF, skeletal muscle disease, or stroke at a young age.[29] A family pedigree

TABLE 13.1: Differential Diagnosis of Non-Ischemic Cardiomyopathy from Conditions with Overlap

Condition	Characteristics in Favor of Alternative Diagnosis	Comments
Hypertensive heart disease	• Chronic hypertension, poorly controlled • Increased LV wall thickness	• May be challenging to differentiate from HCM[57] • Regression of LV hypertrophy with treatment of hypertension argues against HCM • Majority of patients with hypertensive LV hypertrophy have maximal interventricular septal thickness less than 15 mm[58]
Hypertrophic cardiomyopathy	• Long-standing history of HCM • Extensive myocardial fibrosis with a patchy pattern on LGE-CMR • Increased LV wall thickness	• Burn-out HCM (hypokinetic dilated phase of HCM) may be misdiagnosed as DCM[58] • Differentiation from Anderson-Fabry disease and amyloidosis[40,59]
ARVC	• ARVC task force criteria[32] • Disproportionate RV remodeling and dysfunction • RV regional wall motion abnormalities or localized dyssynchrony ("accordion sign") in subtricuspid region • Strong arrhythmic propensity exceeding severity of LV impairment • Characteristic LGE patterns (e.g., LGE in RV free wall and/or LV inferolateral subepicardium or circumferential LV mid-wall LGE extending to right side of septum)	• LV involvement ranging from scars on CMR to severe LV dilation and systolic impairment, which has been reported in up to 76% of patients[10,60] • Causation overlap (desmosomal gene mutations in both DCM and ARVC) • Myocarditis with or without a DCM phenotype can mimic ARVC. Endomyocardial biopsy has a role in differential diagnosis[61]

Left ventricular non-compaction	• Intertrabecular recesses on color Doppler[62,63]
	• CMR diagnostic criteria for non-compaction[64,65]
	  • Ratio of non-compacted to compacted myocardium > 2.3 at end-diastole
	  • Trabeculation in basal segments 4–6
	  • Non-compacted myocardial mass > 25%/ mass index > 15 g/m²
	  • Trabeculated LV mass > 20% of total LV mass
		• No unified CMR and echocardiographic criteria for diagnosis
		• Left ventricular non-compaction may be isolated or associated with other cardiomyopathies (HCM, DCM, ARVC)[66]

Athlete's heart [67,68]	• Asymptomatic • Negative family history • Training-related ECG changes • Normal BNP and NT-proBNP levels • Negative genetic testing • Dilatation of all cardiac chambers with mildly increased wall thickness • High peak VO_2 on cardiopulmonary exercise testing • No late gadolinium enhancement in CMR • Regression of findings with deconditioning	• Athlete's heart should be distinguished from cardiomyopathies (HCM, DCM, left ventricular non-compaction) • 12-lead electrocardiogram, echo parameters, cardiopulmonary exercise testing, Holter monitoring, CMR aid in the differentiation of athlete's heart from cardiomyopathies
Cirrhotic cardiomyopathy	• Advanced chronic liver disease • QT prolongation > 440 ms • Reduced contractile response to stress, and/or altered diastolic relaxation and/or electrophysiological abnormalities[69]	• High suspicion in patients with cirrhotic liver who develop heart failure and hemodynamic deterioration

Abbreviations: ARVC: arrhythmogenic right ventricular cardiomyopathy; BNP: B-type natriuretic peptide; CMR: cardiac magnetic resonance; DCM: dilated cardiomyopathy; HCM: hypertrophic cardiomyopathy; LGE: late gadolinium enhancement; LV: left ventricular; NT-proBNP: N-terminal pro-B-type natriuretic peptide; RV: right ventricular.
Source: Adapted from Japp et al. *J Am Coll Cardiol*. 2016;67:2996–3010.[56]

facilitates determination of genetic transmission mode of several cardiomyopathies.

Physical examination for signs typical of HF should follow. Bilateral leg edema, hepatojugular reflex, or laterally displaced apical impulse are common HF signs. Auscultation may reveal cardiac murmur in cases of significant VHD. As several genetically determined cardiomyopathies are a manifestation of multisystem diseases, phenotypic expressions typical of specific cardiomyopathies should be sought.

A standard electrocardiogram (ECG) may suggest specific myocardial disease or morphological variants. In early stages of cardiomyopathies, ECG abnormalities often precede manifestation of symptoms. In patients with HF, apart from pointing towards a specific diagnosis, ECG findings provide indications for interventions, e.g., cardiac resynchronization therapy (CRT) device implantation if QRS prolongation is present. Patients with HCM may have normal 12-lead ECG or LV hypertrophy, ST and T-wave abnormalities as well as pathological Q-waves.[30] Short P-R interval/preexcitation is a characteristic of storage diseases (Pompe, Danon, PRKAG2) and mitochondrial disorders. Atrioventricular block may be found in mitochondrial diseases, Anderson-Fabry, amyloidosis, and Danon disease,[31] and may be present in desmin-related RCM. In patients with DCM phenotype, atrioventricular block may be suggestive of laminopathy, Emery Dreifuss 1, acute myocarditis (*Trypanosoma cruzi*, diphtheria, and Lyme disease in particular), sarcoidosis, myotonic dystrophy, and desminopathy. Extreme LV hypertrophy (Sokolow >50) should raise suspicion of storage diseases (Pompe or Danon), while extreme superior QRS axis is a typical finding of Noonan syndrome. ECG findings in ARVC/D with biventricular involvement include low QRS voltage, atypical RBBB, inverted T-waves in inferolateral leads, and epsilon waves.[32] Low QRS voltage despite increased LV wall thickness is found in amyloidosis. Pseudo-infarction pattern despite non-obstructive coronary arteries may be present in HCM or amyloidosis.[33] Posterior or posterolateral infarct pattern in DCM patients hints at dystrophin-related diseases such as Duchenne's or Becker's muscular

TABLE 13.2: Etiology, Characteristics, and Proposed Diagnostic Work-Up for Cardiomyopathies with Dilated Physiology

Causes[8,10]	Characteristics	Diagnostic Work-Up[56]

Familial/Genetic
• Main genes associated with cardiac phenotype: TTN, LMNA, MYH7, TNNT2, MYBPC3, RBM20, MYPN, SCN5A, BAG3, PLN
• Neuromuscular disorders
  • Duchenne muscular dystrophy
  • Becker muscular dystrophy
  • Myotonic dystrophy or Steinert
• Syndromic diseases
  • Mitochondrial
  • Tafazzin
Nonfamilial
• Infectious (viral, bacterial, fungal, protozoal, spirochetal)
• Inflammatory/Infiltrative/Autoimmune (hemosiderosis, sarcoidosis, connective tissue disorders, vasculitis, hypersensitivity myocarditis)
• Drugs and alcohol
• Nutritional deficiency – thiamine, carnitine, selenium, hypocalcemia, hypophosphatemia
• Electrolyte disorders
• Endocrinology
• Tachycardiomyopathy
• Peripartum cardiomyopathy
	• Left ventricular dilatation and left ventricular systolic dysfunction.
	• Absence of hypertension, valvular heart disease, or significant coronary artery disease
	• Dilation and dysfunction of the right ventricle might be present
		1. Family history
		2. Clinical examination
		3. Electrocardiogram
		4. Ferritin and transferrin saturation
		5. History of toxin exposure (liver function tests and γ-glutamyl transferase, mean corpuscular volume on complete blood count)
		6. Urea, creatinine, electrolytes, thyroid function tests, plasma glucose, urinary metanephrines, creatine kinase
		7. Specific serum antibodies
		8. Urinary/plasma catecholamines
		9. Echocardiography
		10. Cardiac magnetic resonance
		11. Endomyocardial biopsy

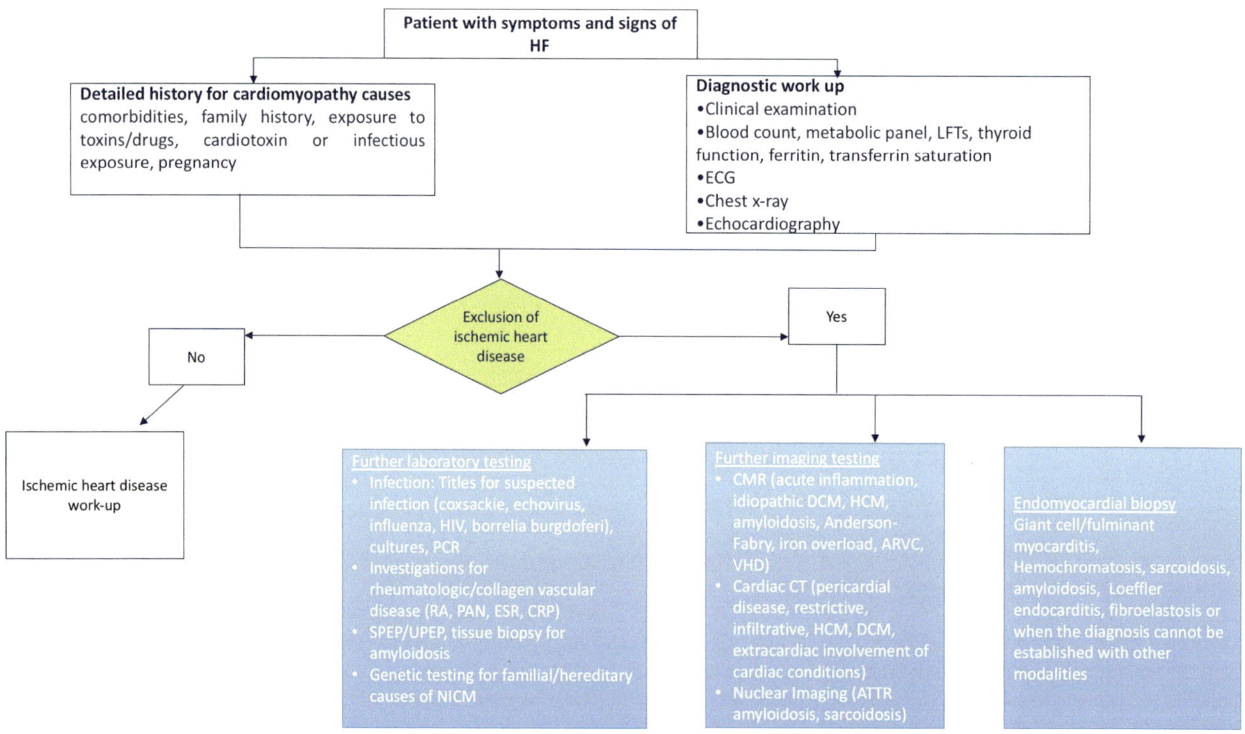

FIGURE 13.2 Algorithm for evaluation and diagnosis of non-ischemic heart failure. (Adapted from Bozkurt, Colvin, Cook, et al. Current diagnostic and treatment strategies for specific dilated cardiomyopathies. A scientific statement from the American Heart Association. *Circulation*. 2016;134:e579–e64.)

dystrophy.[34] Persistent tachyarrhythmia may be suggestive of tachycardia-induced cardiomyopathy. Diagnosis is confirmed if LV systolic dysfunction resides with rate control.

Laboratory work-up in patients with HF should include natriuretic peptides for diagnosis and prognosis,[35,36] cardiac troponin, creatinine, urea or blood urea nitrogen, electrolytes (sodium and potassium), liver function tests, thyroid-stimulating hormone, glucose, full blood count, and ferritin. The value of routine laboratory tests is the detection of secondary organ dysfunction. For patients with suspected cardiomyopathy, serum creatine phosphokinase (CK) should be measured. In patients with DCM, elevated CK may suggest dystrophin-related disorders, a laminopathy, desminopathies, or myofibrillar myopathies. CK in patients with a HCM phenotype is linked to mitochondrial diseases and Danon disease.[37,38] CK is often elevated in desminopathies causing RCM. Proteinuria

TABLE 13.3: Etiology, Characteristics, and Proposed Diagnostic Work-Up for Cardiomyopathies with Non-Dilated Physiology

Type	Etiology	Characteristics	Diagnostic Workup
Hypokinetic non-dilated cardiomyopathy	Same causes as dilated cardiomyopathy	Left ventricular or biventricular global systolic dysfunction without dilatation (defined as LVEF $\leq$45%), not explained by abnormal loading conditions or coronary artery disease.	
Hypertrophic cardiomyopathy[58]	Sarcomere protein gene mutations • MYH7 • MYBPC3 • TNNI3 • TMMT2 • TPM1 • MYL3 Metabolic disorders • Anderson-Fabry • PRKAG2 • Danon Mitochondrial cardiomyopathies Neuromuscular diseases Malformation syndromes Infiltrative disease • AL amyloidosis • ATTR amyloidosis Endocrine disorders Drugs	Wall thickness $\geq$15 mm in one or more LV myocardial segments—as measured by any imaging technique	1. History and clinical examination 2. Resting and ambulatory echocardiography 3. Echocardiography • Assessment of left ventricular wall thickness • Abnormalities of mitral valve and LVOT • Assessment of latent obstruction • Left atrial enlargement • Diastolic function • Systolic function 4. CMR • Ventricular morphology and function • Myocardial fibrosis • Differential diagnosis 5. Nuclear imaging (for ATTR amyloidosis) and computerized tomography 6. Laboratory tests including NT-proBNP 7. Genetic testing and family screening
ARVC[70]	Genetic variations in the desmosomes Identified gene mutations • JUP • DSP • PKP2 • DSG2 • DSC2 • TGFβ3 • TMEM43	• Global or regional dysfunction and structural alterations of right ventricle • Fibrofatty replacement of myocytes • Repolarization abnormalities • Arrhythmias • Family history *Definite diagnosis*: two major, or one major and two minor, or four minor criteria from different diagnostic categories *Borderline diagnosis*: one major and one minor, or three minor criteria from different diagnostic categories *Possible diagnosis*: one major or two minor criteria from different diagnostic categories.	1. Clinical and family history 2. ECG 3. SAECG 4. Holter 5. Echocardiography 6. CMR 7. Genetic testing
LV non-compaction[71]	Heart with normal size and function • Individual variability Genetic LV non-compaction • Chromosomal anomalies • Monogenic syndromes • Cardiomyopathies • CHD Non-genetic LVNC reported in athletes, sickle cell anemia, pregnancy, CKD, polycystic kidney	Trabecular morphology of LV wall May be part of other cardiomyopathies or CHD	1. Medical history 2. Family history 3. Clinical examination 4. Electrocardiogram 5. Cardiac imaging (2D echocardiography and when indicated LGE-CMR) • Non- compacted>>compacted layer • LV size/systolic dysfunction 6. Family screening 7. Genetic testing
Restrictive cardiomyopathy[8,24,29]	**Familial** Familial, unknown gene Sarcomeric protein mutations • Troponin I • Light chain of myosin Familial amyloidosis Desminopathy Pseuxanthoma elasticum Hemochromatosis Anderson-Fabry disease Glycogen storage disease **Nonfamilial** Amyloid Scleroderma Endomyocardial fibrosis • Hypereosinophilic syndrome • Idiopathic • Drugs Carcinoid Metastatic cancer Radiation	Biatrial enlargement Thrombi often present in atrial appendages Normal cavity size of ventricles Normal myocardial mass Normal or reduced systolic dysfunction Impaired diastolic function	1. Medical history 2. Clinical examination 3. Electrocardiogram 4. 2-D Echocardiography 5. CMR/CT 6. Cardiac catheterization 7. Endomyocardial biopsy

Abbreviations: AL: light chain amyloidosis; ARVC: arrhythmogenic right ventricular cardiomyopathy; ATTR; transthyretin amyloidosis; CMR: cardiac magnetic resonance; CT: computed tomography; LV: left ventricular; LVEF: left ventricular ejection fraction; LVOT: left ventricular outflow tract; RV: right ventricular; SAECG: signal-averaged electrocardiogram.

with or without glomerular filtration rate, when other causes of proteinuria are excluded, raises suspicion of Anderson-Fabry disease or amyloidosis. If amyloidosis is suspected, serum immunoglobulin free light chains, serum and urine immunofixation, and electrophoresis of urine should be performed. Finally, in patients with high transferrin saturation or ferritin, hemochromatosis is likely. Genetic testing in suspected cardiomyopathy is discussed in detail in Chapter 31.

Imaging Methods

Advances in cardiac imaging have offered a new understanding of cardiac function, pathophysiology, and mechanisms leading to HF. Diagnostic and prognostic utility of novel imaging techniques guide treatment for patients with HF, and novel imaging biomarkers are being introduced.[39] For example, the ESC HF guidelines recommend the use of myocardial strain in subjects at risk of developing HF in order to identify myocardial dysfunction at the preclinical stage. Also, CMR with late gadolinium enhancement (LGE) should be considered in patients with DCM to distinguish from ischemic and non-ischemic myocardial damage, and also for tissue characterization and etiologic differentiation of non-ischemic HF damage.[5]

Echocardiography

The frontline investigation for assessment of cardiac morphology and function in patients with HF of non-ischemic etiology is two-dimensional (2D) and Doppler echocardiography. Although it is challenging to establish diagnosis only with echocardiography, there are some clues which, when present, will identify specific diseases to be considered. When HCM phenotype with increased interatrial septum thickness is present, amyloidosis should be considered.[40] Increased atrioventricular valve thickness and RV free wall thickness are features of both amyloidosis and Anderson-Fabry disease. A sparkling appearance of the myocardium is found in amyloidosis, whereas concentric hypertrophy is usual in glycogenosis, Anderson-Fabry, Danon and Pompe diseases. DCM following acute myocarditis may present with wall motion abnormalities not related to coronary artery territories, whereas, in fulminant cases, wall thickness may be increased due to edema, accompanied by LV systolic dysfunction and mild dilatation.[41] Increased early diastolic filling velocity, decreased atrial filling velocity, decreased deceleration time and isovolumic relaxation time on Doppler are hallmarks of RCM. Inspiratory augmentation of hepatic vein diastolic reversal is often present.[42]

Three-dimensional echocardiography has entered everyday clinical practice and can help discriminate HF etiology. In a small study, 3D speckle tracking echocardiography was useful in differentiating cardiac amyloidosis from HCM; gradual increase of radial strain from base to apex in amyloidosis correlated with LGE CMR. Global longitudinal strain has the ability to detect subtle alterations in cardiac function and thus it is superior to EF in the diagnosis of chemotherapy-induced cardiotoxicity and LV dysfunction due to VHD.[43,44]

Cardiac Magnetic Resonance

CMR has an established and rapidly expanding role in the HF population. Late gadolinium enhancement provides both diagnostic and prognostic information in a substantial proportion of HF patients. In recent years, novel CMR techniques, such as T1 mapping, extracellular volume, T2 mapping and T2* mapping, allow more extensive tissue characterization, developments which have revolutionized the role of CMR in the evaluation of the non-ischemic HF patient.

Proposed indications for CMR in patients with HF of non-ischemic etiology are: [45]

1. Assessment of ventricular size and function particularly in patients with technically limited images from echo
2. Evaluation of myocarditis
3. Evaluation of specific cardiomyopathies:
   a. DCM
   b. HCM
   c. ARVC
   d. RCM
   e. Cardiac amyloidosis
   f. Cardiac sarcoidosis
   g. Anderson-Fabry disease
   h. Iron-overload cardiomyopathy
   i. LV non-compaction
4. Assessment of dyssynchrony prior to CRT
5. Evaluation of native and prosthetic heart valves
6. Evaluation of cardiac masses

The role of CMR in the diagnosis of the non-ischemic HF patient is summarized in Table 13.4. Although EMB is still considered the gold standard and has a distinct role to play in patients with giant cell myocarditis or eosinophilic myocarditis,[46] CMR is an excellent non-invasive diagnostic tool in assessment of acute myocarditis.[47] Novel CMR techniques, such as T1 and T2 mapping, have superior diagnostic accuracy compared with conventional CMR tools to detect edema for the diagnosis of acute myocarditis.[48]

Computed Tomography

Contemporary multidetector computed tomography (MDCT) scanners allow non-invasive imaging of cardiac structures and coronary arteries.[49] According to the 2019 Appropriate Use Criteria for Multimodality Imaging in the Assessment of Cardiac Structure and Function in Nonvalvular Heart Disease,[50] coronary MDCT is useful in excluding coronary artery disease in patients with HF and LV systolic dysfunction without angina. MDCT has a high negative predictive value for coronary artery disease, particularly in patients with new onset of symptoms.[51,52] Although CMR is considered the gold standard for assessment of cardiac function and structure, MDCT can be considered to be an alternative in specific situations, including patients with non-MRI compatible devices. It may also be of aid for the diagnosis of suspected inherited or acquired cardiomyopathy (restrictive, infiltrative, hypertrophic, or dilated) as well as for the initial evaluation of LV function in patients who are scheduled for or have received chemotherapy.[50] Other uses include suspected pericardial disease, anatomic description of cardiac valves, and assessment of cardiac dyssynchrony.

Nuclear Imaging

Single photon emission computed tomography (SPECT) with thallium-201 or technetium-99m plays an indisputable role in differentiating ischemic from non-ischemic etiology of HF (see Chapter 12). SPECT with ^{123}I-MIBG tracer has been utilized to detect hyperactivity of the autonomic nervous system, offering valuable information about the neurohormonal activation taking place in a failing heart.[53] Imaging with ^{123}I-MIBG has been used to detect myocardial involvement in amyloid transthyretin (ATTR) amyloidosis, although its use in patients with AL-type amyloidosis has not been extensively studied.[54] Imaging with diphosphonate ^{99m}Tc agents, originally

TABLE 13.4: Role of Cardiac Magnetic Resonance in the Diagnostic Work-Up of the Patient with Non-Ischemic HF

Condition	LGE	T1 Mapping	Extracellular Volume	T2 Mapping	T2*
Acute myocarditis	Sub-epicardial or mid-myocardial enhancement suggestive of fibrosis[74] Large areas of scarring may still be visible after healing[75]	Increased native T1	Increased in presence of edema/myocardial free water content/ necrosis/scar	Increased T2	—
DCM	Mid-wall fibrosis in approximately 30–40% of patients[76]	Increased T1 associated with increased risk for events and heart failure[77]	Increased[78,79]	—	—
HCM	Patchy/diffuse pattern or focal Common in anterior and posterior RV insertion points[80,81] Transmural scarring of apical aneurysms	Increased T1 in both areas with and without LGE[77]	Increased even in the absence of left ventricular hypertrophy[82]	Increased in areas of edema due to acute microvascular ischemia[83]	—
Amyloidosis	Global subendocardial/ transmural LGE with a dark blood pool typical of AL amyloidosis[84]	Increased native T1	Moderate or severe increase	—	—
Anderson-Fabry	LGE typically spares subendocardium Mid-wall LGE pattern in inferolateral segments[45]	Low native T1 (highly characteristic and diagnostic of Anderson-Fabry)	—	—	—
Iron overload		Decreased in iron overload[85]	May be increased in patients with thalassemia major and iron overload[86]	—	Decreased in cardiac iron overload[87] Monitoring of disease progression and therapy[88,89]
ARVC	LGE and fibrofatty replacement of myocardium in RV and LV[90,91]	May be increased in hot phases of disease (edema)	May be increased in hot phases of disease (edema)	—	—
Valvular heart disease	No specific pattern May be associated with worse outcomes if present[92]	Shorter post- contrast T1 time in chronic aortic regurgitation[93]	Higher in patients with aortic stenosis[94,95]	—	—

Abbreviations: AL: light chain amyloidosis; ARVC: arrhythmogenic right ventricular cardiomyopathy; CMR: cardiac magnetic resonance; DCM: dilated cardiomyopathy; HCM: hypertrophic cardiomyopathy; LGE: late gadolinium enhancement; LV: left ventricular; RV: right ventricular.
Sources: Adapted from (72) and (73).

designed for bone imaging, are critical in differentiating ATTR from AL-type amyloidosis. This information is crucial for determining management of patients with cardiac amyloidosis.[55] For a complete discussion, see Chapter 35. Finally, positron-emission tomography plays an established role in the identification of cardiac sarcoidosis as a cause of HF.[43]

Treatment

Etiological characterization and early treatment initiation are the cornerstones of management of DCM. Every effort should be made to administer optimal medical treatment for systolic HF. After three to nine months of optimal medical treatment, patients should be reassessed for reverse remodeling. Improvements in left and right ventricular systolic function, mitral regurgitation, and diastolic function are favorable findings during follow-up. Persistently symptomatic patients with severely reduced LVEF (<35%) should be evaluated for CRT or implantable cardioverter defibrillator (ICD) implantation. Patients with DCM, especially in the presence of cardiovascular risk factors, should often be re-assessed for the onset of new comorbidities and negative prognostic factors, such as atrial fibrillation, right ventricular dysfunction, left bundle brunch block, mitral regurgitation, or even coronary atherosclerosis. See Chapter 31 for ICD indications in DCM. Details on the management of stable patients with systolic HF are provided in Chapter 10. The management of patients with preserved and midrange LVEF is discussed in Chapters 15 and 16, respectively. Finally, advanced therapeutic options for patients with refractory symptoms are discussed in Chapter 17.

Conclusion

NICM incorporates a wide spectrum of heterogeneous myocardial conditions that result in LV dysfunction and progression to HF. Almost 30–40% of patients with HF have NICM as the primary cause. Rapid growth in molecular genetics and biomarkers, and advances in cardiac imaging have facilitated timely diagnosis of non-ischemic HF and have significantly improved the quality of management. Targeted treatment of certain causes of non-ischemic HF, on top of evidence-based HF therapies, may induce reverse remodeling and restoration of normal cardiac function. Integrating innovative imaging methods into daily practice is expected to revolutionize diagnosis, prognosis, and management of non-ischemic HF population.

References

1. Crespo-Leiro MG, Anker SD, Maggioni AP, et al. European Society of Cardiology Heart Failure Long-Term Registry (ESC-HF-LT): 1-year follow-up outcomes and differences across regions. *Eur J Heart Fail.* 2016;18:613–25.
2. Rajadurai J, Tse HF, Wang CH, et al. Understanding the epidemiology of heart failure to improve management practices: An Asia-Pacific perspective. *J Card Fail.* 2017;23:327–39.

3. Adams KF, Fonarow GC, Emerman CL, et al. Characteristics and outcomes of patients hospitalized for heart failure in the United States: Rationale, design, and preliminary observations from the first 100,000 cases in the Acute Decompensated Heart Failure National Registry (ADHERE). *Am Heart J.* 2005;149:209–16.
4. Maggioni AP, Dahlström U, Filippatos G, et al. EURObservational Research Programme: Regional differences and 1-year follow-up results of the Heart Failure Pilot Survey (ESC-HF Pilot). *Eur J Heart Fail.* 2013;15:808–17.
5. Ponikowski P, Voors AA, Anker SD, et al. 2016 ESC guidelines for the diagnosis and treatment of acute and chronic heart failure. *Eur J Heart Fail.* 2016;18:891–975.
6. Shore S, Grau-Sepulveda M V., Bhatt DL, et al. Characteristics, treatments, and outcomes of hospitalized heart failure patients stratified by etiologies of cardiomyopathy. *JACC Heart Fail.* 2015;3:906–16.
7. Follath F. Nonischemic heart failure: Epidemiology, pathophysiology and progression of disease. *J Cardiovasc Pharmacol.* 1999;33 Supplement 3: S31–5.
8. Elliott P, Andersson B, Arbustini E, et al. Classification of the cardiomyopathies: A position statement from the European Society of Cardiology Working Group on Myocardial and Pericardial Diseases. *Eur Heart J.* 2008;29:270–6.
9. Mcmurray JJV, Adamopoulos S, Anker SD, et al. ESC guidelines for the diagnosis and treatment of acute and chronic heart failure 2012. *Eur J Heart Fail.* 2012;14:803–69.
10. Pinto YM, Elliott PM, Arbustini E, et al. Proposal for a revised definition of dilated cardiomyopathy, hypokinetic non-dilated cardiomyopathy, and its implications for clinical practice: A position statement of the ESC working group on myocardial and pericardial diseases. *Eur Heart J.* 2016;37:1850–8.
11. Dellefave L, McNally EM. The genetics of dilated cardiomyopathy. *Curr Opin Cardiol.* 2010;25:198–204.
12. Mestroni L, Rocco C, Gregori D, et al. Familial dilated cardiomyopathy: Evidence for genetic and phenotypic heterogeneity. Heart Muscle Disease Study Group. *J Am Coll Cardiol.* 1999;34:181–90.
13. D'Ambrosio A, Patti G, Manzoli A, et al. The fate of acute myocarditis between spontaneous improvement and evolution to dilated cardiomyopathy: A review. *Heart.* 2001;85:499–504.
14. Melacini P, Basso C, Angelini A, et al. Clinicopathological profiles of progressive heart failure in hypertrophic cardiomyopathy. *Eur Heart J.* 2010;31:2111–23.
15. Maron MS, Appelbaum E, Harrigan CJ, et al. Clinical profile and significance of delayed enhancement in hypertrophic cardiomyopathy. *Circ Heart Fail.* 2008;1:184–91.
16. Olivotto I, Maron BJ, Appelbaum E, et al. Spectrum and clinical significance of systolic function and myocardial fibrosis assessed by cardiovascular magnetic resonance in hypertrophic cardiomyopathy. *Am J Cardiol.* 2010;106:261–7.
17. Yacoub MH, Olivotto I, Cecchi F. "End-stage" hypertrophic cardiomyopathy: From mystery to model. *Nat Clin Pract Cardiovasc Med.* 2007;4:232–3.
18. Maron MS, Olivotto I, Maron BJ, et al. The case for myocardial ischemia in hypertrophic cardiomyopathy. *J Am Coll Cardiol.* 2009;54:866–75.
19. Corrado D. CARDIOMYOPATHY: Arrhythmogenic right ventricular cardiomyopathy: Diagnosis, prognosis, and treatment. *Heart.* 2000;83:588–95.
20. Awad MM, Calkins H, Judge DP. Mechanisms of disease: Molecular genetics of arrhythmogenic right ventricular dysplasia/cardiomyopathy. *Nat Clin Pract Cardiovasc Med.* 2008;5:258–67.
21. Hulot JS, Jouven X, Empana JP, Frank R, Fontaine G. Natural history and risk stratification of arrhythmogenic right ventricular dysplasia/cardiomyopathy. *Circulation.* 2004;110:1879–84.
22. Sato Y, Matsumoto N, Matsuo S, et al. Subendomyocardial perfusion abnormality and necrosis detected by magnetic resonance imaging in a patient with isolated noncompaction of the ventricular myocardium associated with ventricular tachycardia. *Cardiovasc Revascul Med.* 2009;10:66–8.
23. Agmon Y, Connolly HM, Olson LJ, Khandheria BK, Seward JB. Noncompaction of the ventricular myocardium. *J Am Soc Echocardiogr.* 1999;12:859–63.
24. Ammash NM, Seward JB, Bailey KR, Edwards WD, Tajik AJ. Clinical profile and outcome of idiopathic restrictive cardiomyopathy. *Circulation.* 2000;101:2490–6.
25. Marciniak A, Glover K, Sharma R. Cohort profile: Prevalence of valvular heart disease in community patients with suspected heart failure in UK. *BMJ Open.* 2017;7:e012240.
26. Iung B. A prospective survey of patients with valvular heart disease in Europe: The Euro heart survey on valvular heart disease. *Eur Heart J.* 2003;24:1231–43.
27. Roques F, Nashef SAM, Michel P, et al. Risk factors and outcome in European cardiac surgery: Analysis of the EuroSCORE multinational database of 19030 patients. *Eur J Cardio-thoracic Surg.* 1999;15:816–23.
28. Mrsic Z, Hopkins SP, Antevil JL, Mullenix PS. Valvular heart disease. *Prim Care Clin Off Pract.* 2018;45:81–94.
29. Chan K, Harper AR, Ashrafian H, Yavari A. Cardiomyopathies. *Medicine (Baltimore).* 2018;46:606–17.
30. McLeod CJ, Ackerman MJ, Nishimura RA, et al. Outcome of patients with hypertrophic cardiomyopathy and a normal electrocardiogram. *J Am Coll Cardiol.* 2009;54:229–33.
31. Rapezzi C, Arbustini E, Caforio ALP, et al. Diagnostic work-up in cardiomyopathies: Bridging the gap between clinical phenotypes and final diagnosis. A position statement from the ESC Working Group on Myocardial and Pericardial Diseases. *Eur Heart J.* 2013;34:1448–58.
32. Marcus FI, McKenna WJ, Sherrill D, et al. Diagnosis of arrhythmogenic right ventricular cardiomyopathy/Dysplasia: Proposed modification of the task force criteria. *Circulation.* 2010;121:1533–41.
33. Veselka J, Anavekar NS, Charron P. Hypertrophic obstructive cardiomyopathy. *Lancet.* 2017;389:1253–67.
34. Sanyal SK, Johnson WW. Cardiac conduction abnormalities in children with Duchenne's progressive muscular dystrophy: Electrocardiographic features and morphologic correlates. *Circulation.* 1982;66:853–63.
35. Krishnaswamy P, Lubien E, Clopton P, et al. Utility of B-natriuretic peptide levels in identifying patients with left ventricular systolic or diastolic dysfunction. *Am J Med.* 2001;111:274–9.
36. Kelder JC, Cramer MJ, Verweij WM, Grobbee DE, Hoes AW. Clinical utility of three B-type natriuretic peptide assays for the initial diagnostic assessment of new slow-onset heart failure. *J Card Fail.* 2011;17: 729–34.
37. Brancaccio P, Lippi G, Maffulli N. Biochemical markers of muscular damage. *Clin Chem Lab Med.* 2010;48:757–67.
38. Tesi Rocha C, Hoffman EP. Limb–girdle and congenital muscular dystrophies: Current diagnostics, management, and emerging technologies. *Curr Neurol Neurosci Rep.* 2010;10:267–76.
39. Čelutkienė J, Plymen CM, Flachskampf FA, et al. Innovative imaging methods in heart failure: A shifting paradigm in cardiac assessment. Position statement on behalf of the Heart Failure Association of the European Society of Cardiology. *Eur J Heart Fail.* 2018;20:1615–33.
40. Rapezzi C, Merlini G, Quarta CC, et al. Systemic cardiac amyloidoses: Disease profiles and clinical courses of the 3 main types. *Circulation.* 2009;120:1203–12.
41. Felker GM, Boehmer JP, Hruban RH, et al. Echocardiographic findings in fulminant and acute myocarditis. *J Am Coll Cardiol.* 2000;36:227–32.
42. Ha JW, Ommen SR, Tajik AJ, et al. Differentiation of constrictive pericarditis from restrictive cardiomyopathy using mitral annular velocity by tissue Doppler echocardiography. *Am J Cardiol.* 2004;94:316–9.
43. Plana JC, Galderisi M, Barac A, et al. Expert consensus for multimodality imaging evaluation of adult patients during and after cancer therapy: A report from the American Society of Echocardiography and the European Association of Cardiovascular Imaging. *Eur Heart J Cardiovasc Imaging.* 2014;15:1063–93.
44. Smiseth OA, Torp H, Opdahl A, Haugaa KH, Urheim S. Myocardial strain imaging: How useful is it in clinical decision making? *Eur Heart J.* 2016;37:1196–207.
45. Karamitsos TD, Francis JM, Myerson S, Selvanayagam JB, Neubauer S. The role of cardiovascular magnetic resonance imaging in heart failure. *J Am Coll Cardiol.* 2009;54:1407–24.
46. Leone O, Veinot JP, Angelini A, et al. 2011 consensus statement on endomyocardial biopsy from the Association for European Cardiovascular Pathology and the Society for Cardiovascular Pathology. *Cardiovasc Pathol.* 2012;21:245–74.
47. Friedrich MG, Sechtem U, Schulz-Menger J, et al. Cardiovascular magnetic resonance in myocarditis: A JACC white paper. *J Am Coll Cardiol.* 2009;53:1475–87.
48. Kotanidis CP, Bazmpani MA, Haidich AB, et al. Diagnostic accuracy of cardiovascular magnetic resonance in acute myocarditis: A systematic review and meta-analysis. *JACC Cardiovasc Imaging.* 2018;11:1583–90.
49. Mangalat D, Kalogeropoulos A, Georgiopoulou V, Stillman A, Butler J. Value of cardiac CT in patients with heart failure. *Curr Cardiovasc Imaging Rep.* 2009;2:410–7.
50. Doherty JU, Kort S, Mehran R, et al. ACC/AATS/AHA/ASE/ASNC/HRS /SCAI/SCCT/SCMR/STS 2019 appropriate use criteria for multimodality imaging in the assessment of cardiac structure and function in nonvalvular heart disease: A report of the American College of Cardiology Appropriate Use Criteria. *J Am Soc Echocardiogr.* 2019;32:553–79.
51. Nielsen LH, Olsen J, Markenvard J, Jensen JM, Nørgaard BL. Effects on costs of frontline diagnostic evaluation in patients suspected of angina: Coronary computed tomography angiography vs. conventional ischaemia testing. *Eur Heart J Cardiovasc Imaging.* 2013;14:449–55.

52. Andreini D, Pontone G, Pepi M, et al. Diagnostic accuracy of multidetector computed tomography coronary angiography in patients with dilated cardiomyopathy. *J Am Coll Cardiol.* 2007;49:2044–50.
53. Perrone-Filardi P, Paolillo S, Dellegrottaglie S, et al. Assessment of cardiac sympathetic activity by MIBG imaging in patients with heart failure: A clinical appraisal. *Heart.* 2011;97:1828–33.
54. Noordzij W, Glaudemans AWJM, Longhi S, et al. Nuclear imaging for cardiac amyloidosis. *Heart Fail Rev.* 2015;20:145–54.
55. Vrana JA, Gamez JD, Madden BJ, et al. Classification of amyloidosis by laser microdissection and mass spectrometry-based proteomic analysis in clinical biopsy specimens. *Blood.* 2009;114:4957–9.
56. Japp AG, Gulati A, Cook SA, Cowie MR, Prasad SK. The diagnosis and evaluation of dilated cardiomyopathy. *J Am Coll Cardiol.* 2016;67:2996–3010.
57. D'Andrea A, D'Andrea L, Caso P, et al. The usefulness of Doppler myocardial imaging in the study of the athlete's heart and in the differential diagnosis between physiological and pathological ventricular hypertrophy. *Echocardiography.* 2006;23:149–57.
58. Zamorano JL, Anastasakis A, Borger MA, et al. 2014 ESC guidelines on diagnosis and management of hypertrophic cardiomyopathy. *Eur Heart J.* 2014;35:2733–79.
59. Falk RH. Diagnosis and management of the cardiac amyloidoses. *Circulation.* 2005;112:2047–60.
60. Sen-Chowdhry S, Morgan RD, Chambers JC, McKenna WJ. Arrhythmogenic cardiomyopathy: Etiology, diagnosis, and treatment. *Annu Rev Med.* 2010;61:233–53.
61. Mahon NG, Madden BP, Caforio ALP, et al. Immunohistologic evidence of myocardial disease in apparently healthy relatives of patients with dilated cardiomyopathy. *J Am Coll Cardiol.* 2002;39:455–62.
62. Oechslin E, Jenni R. Left ventricular non-compaction revisited: A distinct phenotype with genetic heterogeneity? *Eur Heart J.* 2011;32:1446–56.
63. Jenni R, Oechslin E, Schneider J, Attenhofer Jost C, Kaufmann PA. Echocardiographic and pathoanatomical characteristics of isolated left ventricular non-compaction: A step towards classification as a distinct cardiomyopathy. *Heart.* 2001;86:666–71.
64. Jacquier A, Thuny F, Jop B, et al. Measurement of trabeculated left ventricular mass using cardiac magnetic resonance imaging in the diagnosis of left ventricular non-compaction. *Eur Heart J.* 2010;31:1098–104.
65. Petersen SE, Selvanayagam JB, Wiesmann F, et al. Left ventricular non-compaction: Insights from cardiovascular magnetic resonance imaging. *J Am Coll Cardiol.* 2005;46:101–5.
66. Arbustini E, Weidemann F, Hall JL. Left ventricular noncompaction: A distinct cardiomyopathy or a trait shared by different cardiac diseases? *J Am Coll Cardiol.* 2014;64:1840–50.
67. Brosnan MJ, Rakhit D. Differentiating athlete's heart from cardiomyopathies—The left side. *Hear Lung Circ.* 2018;27:1052–62.
68. Maron BJ. Distinguishing hypertrophic cardiomyopathy from athlete's heart: A clinical problem of increasing magnitude and significance. *Heart.* 2005;91:1380–2.
69. Moller S, Henriksen JH. Cardiovascular complications of cirrhosis. *Gut.* 2008;57:268–78.
70. Marcus FI, McKenna WJ, Sherrill D, et al. Diagnosis of arrhythmogenic right ventricular cardiomyopathy/dysplasia. *Eur Heart J.* 2010;31:806–14.
71. Arbustini E, Favalli V, Narula N, Serio A, Grasso M. Left ventricular noncompaction. *J Am Coll Cardiol.* 2016;68:949–66.
72. Captur G, Manisty C, Moon JC. Cardiac MRI evaluation of myocardial disease. *Heart.* 2016;102:1429–35.
73. Messroghli DR, Moon JC, Ferreira VM, et al. Clinical recommendations for cardiovascular magnetic resonance mapping of T1, T2, T2* and extracellular volume: A consensus statement by the Society for Cardiovascular Magnetic Resonance (SCMR) endorsed by the European Association for Cardiovascular Imaging. *J Cardiovasc Magn Reson.* 2017;19:75.
74. Mahrholdt H, Goedecke C, Wagner A, et al. Cardiovascular magnetic resonance assessment of human myocarditis. *Circulation.* 2004;109:1250–8.
75. Mahrholdt H, Wagner A, Deluigi CC, et al. Presentation, patterns of myocardial damage, and clinical course of viral myocarditis. *Circulation.* 2006;114:1581–90.
76. Assomull RG, Prasad SK, Lyne J, et al. Cardiovascular magnetic resonance, fibrosis, and prognosis in dilated cardiomyopathy. *J Am Coll Cardiol.* 2006;48:1977–85.
77. Puntmann VO, Carr-White G, Jabbour A, et al. T1-mapping and outcome in nonischemic cardiomyopathy all-cause mortality and heart failure. *JACC Cardiovasc Imaging.* 2016;9:40–50.
78. aus dem Siepen F, Buss SJ, Messroghli D, et al. T1 mapping in dilated cardiomyopathy with cardiac magnetic resonance: Quantification of diffuse myocardial fibrosis and comparison with endomyocardial biopsy. *Eur Heart J Cardiovasc Imaging.* 2015;16:210–6.
79. Sibley CT, Noureldin RA, Gai N, et al. T1 mapping in cardiomyopathy at cardiac MR: Comparison with endomyocardial biopsy. *Radiology.* 2012;265:724–32.
80. Moon JCC, McKenna WJ, McCrohon JA, et al. Toward clinical risk assessment in hypertrophic cardiomyopathy with gadolinium cardiovascular magnetic resonance. *J Am Coll Cardiol.* 2003;41:1561–7.
81. To ACY, Dhillon A, Desai MY. Cardiac magnetic resonance in hypertrophic cardiomyopathy. *JACC Cardiovasc Imaging.* 2011;4:1123–37.
82. Ho CY, Abbasi SA, Neilan TG, et al. T1 measurements identify extracellular volume expansion in hypertrophic cardiomyopathy sarcomere mutation carriers with and without left ventricular hypertrophy. *Circ Cardiovasc Imaging.* 2013;6:415–22.
83. Gastl M, Gotschy A, von Spiczak J, et al. Cardiovascular magnetic resonance T2* mapping for structural alterations in hypertrophic cardiomyopathy. *Eur J Radiol Open.* 2019;6:78–84.
84. Dungu JN, Valencia O, Pinney JH, et al. CMR-based differentiation of AL and ATTR cardiac amyloidosis. *JACC Cardiovasc Imaging.* 2014;7:133–42.
85. Sado DM, Maestrini V, Piechnik SK, et al. Noncontrast myocardial T 1 mapping using cardiovascular magnetic resonance for iron overload. *J Magn Reson Imaging.* 2015;41:1505–11.
86. Hanneman K, Nguyen ET, Thavendiranathan P, et al. Quantification of myocardial extracellular volume fraction with cardiac MR imaging in Thalassemia Major. *Radiology.* 2015;279:720–30.
87. Kirk P, Roughton M, Porter JB, et al. Cardiac T2* magnetic resonance for prediction of cardiac complications in Thalassemia Major. *Circulation.* 2009;120:1961–8.
88. Pennell DJ, Porter JB, Piga A, et al. Sustained improvements in myocardial T2* over 2 years in severely iron-overloaded patients with beta thalassemia major treated with deferasirox or deferoxamine. *Am J Hematol.* 2015;90:91–6.
89. Tanner MA, Galanello R, Dessi C, et al. A randomized, placebo-controlled, double-blind trial of the effect of combined therapy with deferoxamine and deferiprone on myocardial iron in thalassemia major using cardiovascular magnetic resonance. *Circulation.* 2007;115:1876–84.
90. Tandri H, Saranathan M, Rodriguez ER, et al. Noninvasive detection of myocardial fibrosis in arrhythmogenic right ventricular cardiomyopathy using delayed-enhancement magnetic resonance imaging. *J Am Coll Cardiol.* 2005;45:98–103.
91. Pfluger HB, Phrommintikul A, Mariani JA, Cherayath JG, Taylor AJ. Utility of myocardial fibrosis and fatty infiltration detected by cardiac magnetic resonance imaging in the diagnosis of arrhythmogenic right ventricular dysplasia-A single centre experience. *Hear Lung Circ.* 2008;17:478–83.
92. Dweck MR, Joshi S, Murigu T, et al. Midwall fibrosis is an independent predictor of mortality in patients with aortic stenosis. *J Am Coll Cardiol.* 2011;58:1271–9.
93. Sparrow P, Messroghli DR, Reid S, et al. Myocardial T1 mapping for detection of left ventricular myocardial fibrosis in chronic aortic regurgitation: Pilot study. *AJR Am J Roentgenol.* 2006;187:W630–5.
94. Flett AS, Hayward MP, Ashworth MT, et al. Equilibrium contrast cardiovascular magnetic resonance for the measurement of diffuse myocardial fibrosis: Preliminary validation in humans. *Circulation.* 2010;122:138–44.
95. White SK, Sado DM, Fontana M, et al. T1 mapping for myocardial extracellular volume measurement by CMR: Bolus only versus primed infusion technique. *JACC Cardiovasc Imaging.* 2013;6:955–62.

Chapter 14
VALVULAR HEART DISEASE AND HEART FAILURE

Kali Polytarchou and Constantina Aggeli

Introduction

Valvular heart disease (VHD) is a common cause of heart failure (HF).[1] Conversely, HF with reduced and even preserved left ventricular ejection fraction (LVEF) can result in secondary VHD, due to remodeling of cardiac chambers.[2] In many cases, causality is unclear when HF and VHD coexist. Careful evaluation of patients with HF and VHD should provide answers on the mechanism of HF and the etiology of valvulopathy.[3] The presence of VHD aggravates prognosis of HF and treatment strategies in this context are not always well established. In this chapter, we focus on forms of VHD most encountered in adults with HF.

Aortic Stenosis

Epidemiology and Etiology

Aortic stenosis (AS) is the most common VHD that causes HF and needs hospitalization. Degenerative aortic valve disease affects 25% of patients over 65 years old[4] and this increases to 48% over age 75. The prevalence of significant AS is 4–6% among patients over the age of 65 years old.[5] Degenerative AS, i.e., calcification of a normal tricuspid or dysplastic (bicuspid, monocuspid) valve, accounts for about 80% of cases. Rheumatic disease is the second most common cause and is characterized by fibrosis and fusion of commissures.[6] In contrast, degenerative disease insults the basis of the cusps first, while commissures remain unaffected. Other rare causes are familial hypercholesterolemia, hyperparathyroidism, hyperuricemia, Fabry disease, Paget disease, lupus, and drugs. Congenital AS is the most common cause in very young patients.

Pathophysiology

AS results in left ventricular (LV) pressure overload, leading to concentric LV hypertrophy. Myocardial hypertrophy leads to fibrosis and reduced LV compliance, preload reduction, and increase in end-diastolic pressure. Consequently, coronary flow is reduced. In conjunction with increased oxygen demands due to LV hypertrophy, this results in myocardial ischemia and impaired LV function. Initially, LVEF remains normal or increased. As LV dysfunction progresses, LV systolic function and cardiac output decline and the patient decompensates.[7]

Clinical Presentation

Degenerative AS usually becomes symptomatic in the 7th decade of life, bicuspid valve disease in the 4th to 5th,[8] and rheumatic disease in the 2nd to 4th. Symptoms include dyspnea or angina on exertion, fatigue, and syncope during exercise. When angina occurs, median survival is five years; with syncope, three years; and with occurrence of HF symptoms, two years.[9]

Diagnostic Evaluation and Assessment of Severity

In a patient with severe AS, aortic valve calcification, ascending aorta dilation, and boot-shaped cardiac silhouette are typical findings on chest radiographs.[10] On ECG, left ventricular and atrial enlargement, repolarization disturbances, left axis deviation, left bundle branch block, and AF are common findings.[11]

Echocardiography is the main tool for the evaluation of AS. Normal aortic valve area (AVA) is 3–4 cm^2. Table 14.1 summarizes the classification of AS severity. Maximum velocity through the aortic valve (AoV_{max}) ≥4 m/s and AVA ≤1 cm^2 is considered to be severe AS (Figure 14.1). However, the anatomy of the aortic valve and the cardiac chambers, LVEF, and the LV contractile reserve should also all be considered. Stroke volume (SV) is an important parameter that should always be evaluated and indexed to body surface area to classify AS. The patient should be stable, and blood pressure and heart rate well controlled. Conditions with high cardiac output, such as anemia or fever, should be avoided or treated beforehand.

AS can be classified into four hemodynamic types: (1) the typical "high-gradient" AS with AVA ≤1 cm^2 and mean transaortic pressure gradient (PG) ≥40 mmHg; (2) the "low-flow, low-gradient" AS with reduced or preserved LVEF and, finally (3) the "normal-flow, low-gradient" and preserved LVEF ≥50% with AVA ≤1 cm^2, mean PG <40 mmHg, and SV index ≥35 mL/m^2 (Table 14.1). Difficulty in differential diagnosis of true severe AS from pseudosevere AS exists in patients with the low-flow state (Figure 14.2).[12]

Low-dose dobutamine stress echocardiography (DSE) is an important diagnostic and prognostic tool for the evaluation of patients with low-flow, low-gradient AS and reduced LVEF (Figure 14.2). Aortic valve area projected (AVA_{proj}) can be calculated in cases with disagreement between changes in AVA and mean PG or when SV index does not adequately increase. True severe is the AS with AVA_{proj} <1 cm^2. Little evidence exists regarding patients with low-flow, low-gradient AS and preserved LVEF. These patients are elderly, mostly women with small left ventricular chamber size and left ventricular hypertrophy or arterial hypertension.[13] Multidetector computed tomography and exercise SE may be useful tools for these patients. Considering the clinical and imaging characteristics in combination with the information derived from exercise SE and calcium score, one can give an accurate answer about the severity of valvulopathy (Table 14.1).

Importantly, patients with AS may have mitral regurgitation. Careful evaluation is needed, especially before interventional treatment, as mitral regurgitation is overestimated due to increased LV end-diastolic pressure. If there are no morphological abnormalities in the mitral valve (such as flail, prolapse, or endocarditis), then mitral regurgitation will probably improve after aortic valve replacement.[14]

Exercise stress test or exercise SE are used for asymptomatic patients with severe AS in order to unmask symptoms.[15, 16] The occurrence of symptoms, the drop in blood pressure, and the increase in mean PG by more than 18 mmHg and the increase in systolic pulmonary artery pressure (SPAP) >60 mmHg constitute negative prognostic markers for these patients.

The assessment of peak-to-peak PG with retrograde LV catheterization is rarely useful for the estimation of AS. Aortic valve

DOI: 10.1201/9780429244544-17

TABLE 14.1: Echocardiographic Severity Stratification of Aortic Stenosis and Criteria That Increase the Likelihood of Severe Aortic Stenosis in a Patient with Low-Flow, Low-Gradient, and Preserved Ejection Fraction Aortic Stenosis

Severity of Aortic Stenosis

	AoVmax	Mean PG	AVA (or AVAi)
Mild	2–3 m/s	<25 mmHg	>1.5 cm^2
Moderate	3–4 m/s	25–39 mmHg	1–1.5 cm^2
Severe	≥4 m/s	≥40 mmHg	≤1 cm^2 (or ≤0.6 cm^2/m^2)
Very severe	≥5 m/s	≥60 mmHg	≤1 cm^2 (or ≤0.6 cm^2/m^2)
Low-flow, low-gradient with reduced EF <50% (SVi <35 mL/m^2)	<4 m/s	<40 mmHg	≤1 cm^2 (or ≤0.6 cm^2/m^2)
Low-flow, low-gradient with preserved EF >50% (SVi <35 mL/m^2)	<4 m/s	<40 mmHg	≤1 cm^2 (or ≤0.6 cm^2/m^2)

Criteria that increase the likelihood of severe aortic stenosis in a patient with low-flow, low-gradient and preserved ejection fraction aortic stenosis

Clinical criteria	Typical symptoms without other explanation Elderly patients over 70 years old
Qualitative imaging data	Left ventricular hypertrophy (additional history of hypertension to be considered) Reduced left ventricular longitudinal function without other explanation
Quantitative imaging data	MeanPG between 30 and 40 mmHg AVA <0.8 cm^2 Low flow (with SVi <35 mL/m^2) confirmed by techniques other than standard Doppler techniques (MDCT, cardiac magnetic resonance, or invasively) Calcium score by MDCT. Severe aortic stenosis is • Very likely if calcium score is ≥3,000 for men and 1,600 for women • Likely if calcium score is ≥2,000 for men and 1,200 for women • Unlikely if calcium score is <1,600 for men and 800 for women

Abbreviations: AVA: aortic valve area (calculated with continuity equation AVA= $CSA_{LVOT}XVTI_{LVOT}/VTI_{AV,}$ where CSA_{LVOT} is the cross sectional area and VTI_{LVOT} is the velocity-time integral of left ventricular outflow tract, and VTI_{AV} is the velocity-time integral of aortic valve, AVAi: aortic valve area indexed, AoVmax: maximum aortic velocity, LVEF: left ventricular ejection fraction, SVi: stroke volume index, MDCT: multidetector computed tomography, mean PG: mean transaortic pressure gradient.

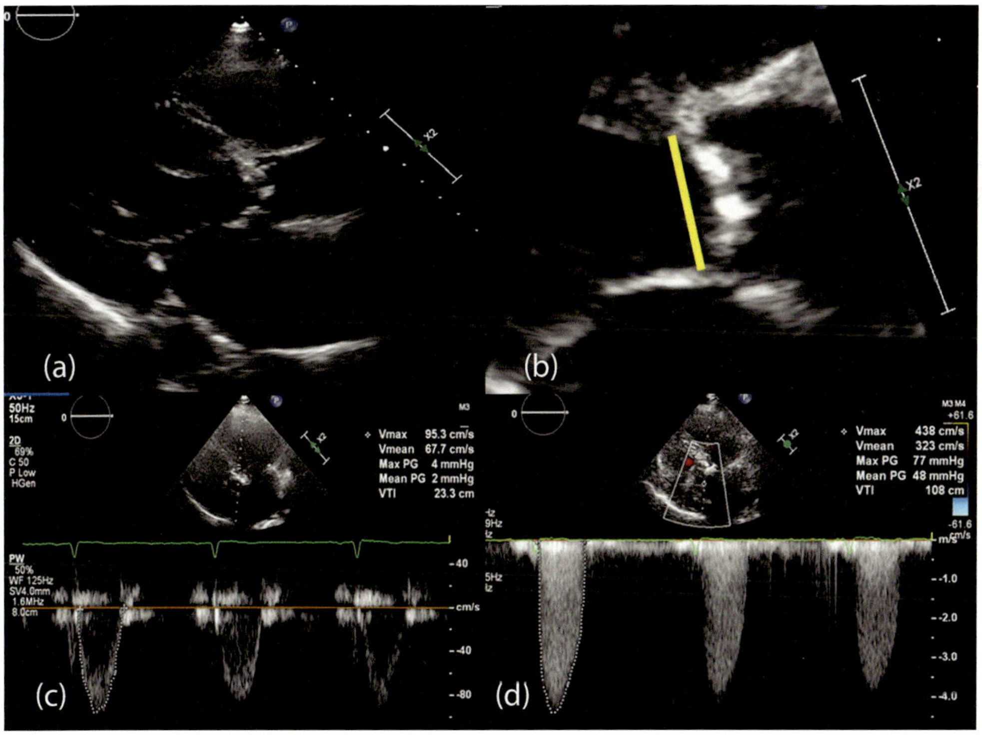

FIGURE 14.1 True high gradient severe aortic stenosis. (a) On 2-D echocardiography, concentric left ventricular hypertrophy is typical. (b) Left ventricular outflow tract diameter is measured at end-systole from edge to edge. (c) Pulse wave velocity is used for measurement of left ventricular outflow tract time-velocity interval. (d) Continuous wave Doppler is used for aortic valve time-velocity interval, maximum velocity, and mean pressure gradient. From these parameters, aortic valve area can be calculated with the continuity equation.

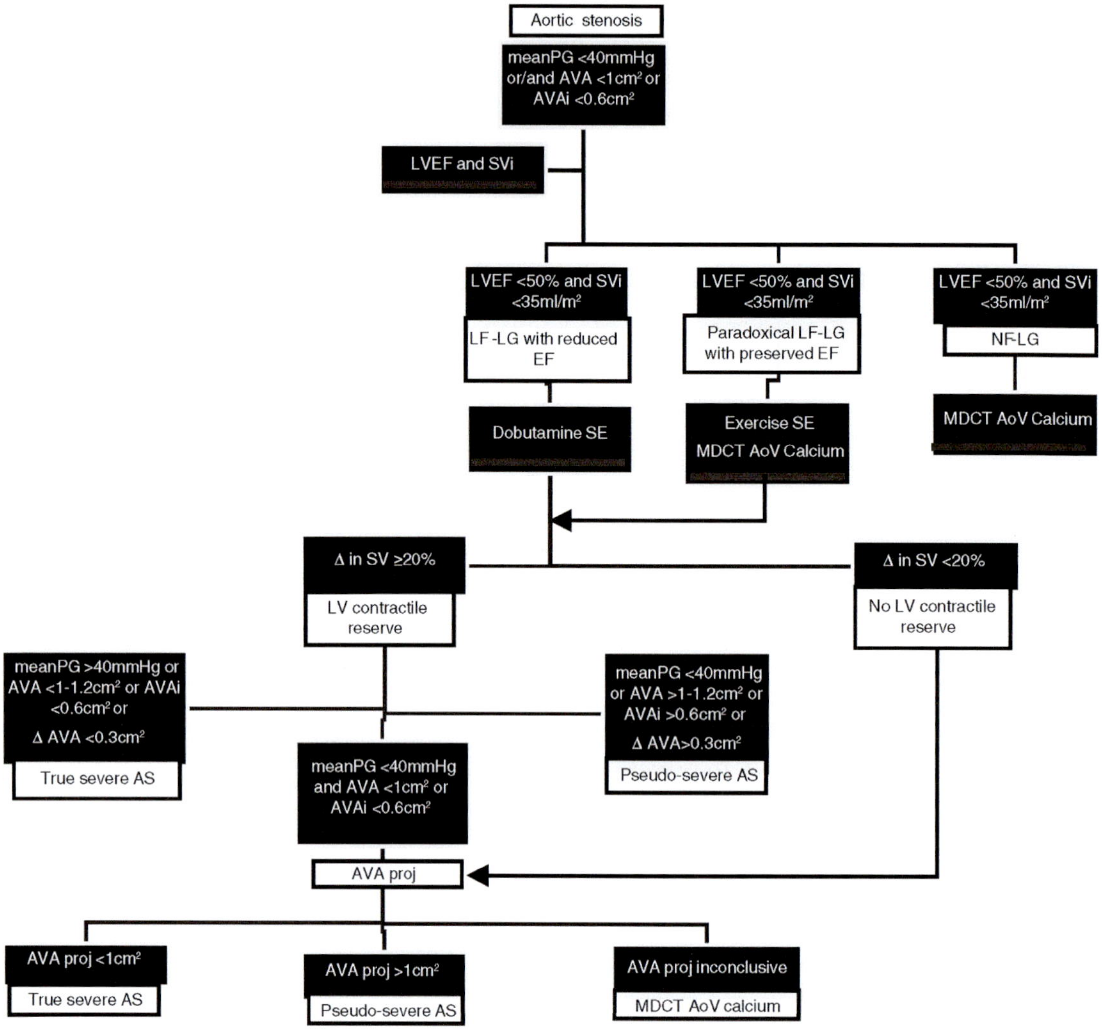

FIGURE 14.2 Algorithm for the diagnostic evaluation and management of patients with low transaortic pressure gradient aortic stenosis. *Abbreviations*: AoV: aortic valve; AVA: aortic valve area; AVAi: AVA indexed; AVAproj: AVA projected; LF-LG: low-flow, low-gradient; LVEF: left ventricular ejection fraction; MDCT: multidetector computed tomography; NF-LG: normal-flow, low-gradient; PG: pressure gradient; SE: stress echocardiography; SVi: stroke volume indexed; Δ: absolute difference. (Reproduced from Aggeli et al., *Clin Cardiol*. 2018;41(12):1600–10.)

area is calculated with the Gorlin formula (AVA = cardiac output/44.3 × heart rate × systolic ejection period × square root (mean transaortic PG). This formula estimates the anatomical AVA, whereas the continuity equation using echocardiography estimates the physiological AVA, which is smaller than the anatomical measured by Gorlin.[17]

Treatment and Recommendations

Treatment of AS includes surgical aortic valve replacement (SAVR), transcatheter aortic valve implantation (TAVI), balloon angioplasty, and medical therapy. The latter includes treatment of risk factors for atherosclerosis. When symptoms of HF occur, treatment with angiotensin-converting enzyme inhibitors, angiotensin-receptor blockers, diuretics, or digoxin is indicated. Statins are not recommended, as there is no clear evidence of benefit in AS.[18,19]

TAVI has been established as an effective alternative to SAVR for patients with severe AS and intermediate or high surgical risk, with very high success rates and about 85–95% one-year survival rates (Figure 14.3). Accumulating evidence supports use of TAVI even in low surgical-risk patients, although to date this is not recommended by current European or American guidelines.[20, 21] TAVI complications include cerebrovascular events (1–5%), atrioventricular block and need for permanent pacemaker (8–13% with balloon-expanded valves and 25–40% with self-expanding valves), vascular complications (20%), paravalvular leaks (commonly mild or trace, 3–4% moderate to severe) (Figure 14.4). Less common but severe complications include aortic or left ventricular rupture, coronary artery occlusion, or "suicidal LV" with LV outflow tract obstruction after TAVI in patients with hypertrophic LV wall segments. When compared with SAVR, post-interventional AVA and mean PG are better. SAVR results in higher rates of acute renal failure and AF. However, the technical improvement of new generation transcatheter valves tends to minimize these complications.

Factors that favor transcatheter implantation are surgical risk >4% as projected by the Society of Thoracic Surgeons (STS) score or Euroscore II, the presence of comorbidities, age >75 years, prior cardiac surgery, frailty or restricted mobility, suitable transfemoral access, prior chest radiotherapy, porcelain aorta, chest deformation, and expected patient–prosthesis mismatch (mostly when the annulus size is 18–29 mm). Factors that favor surgical aortic valve replacement are STS or

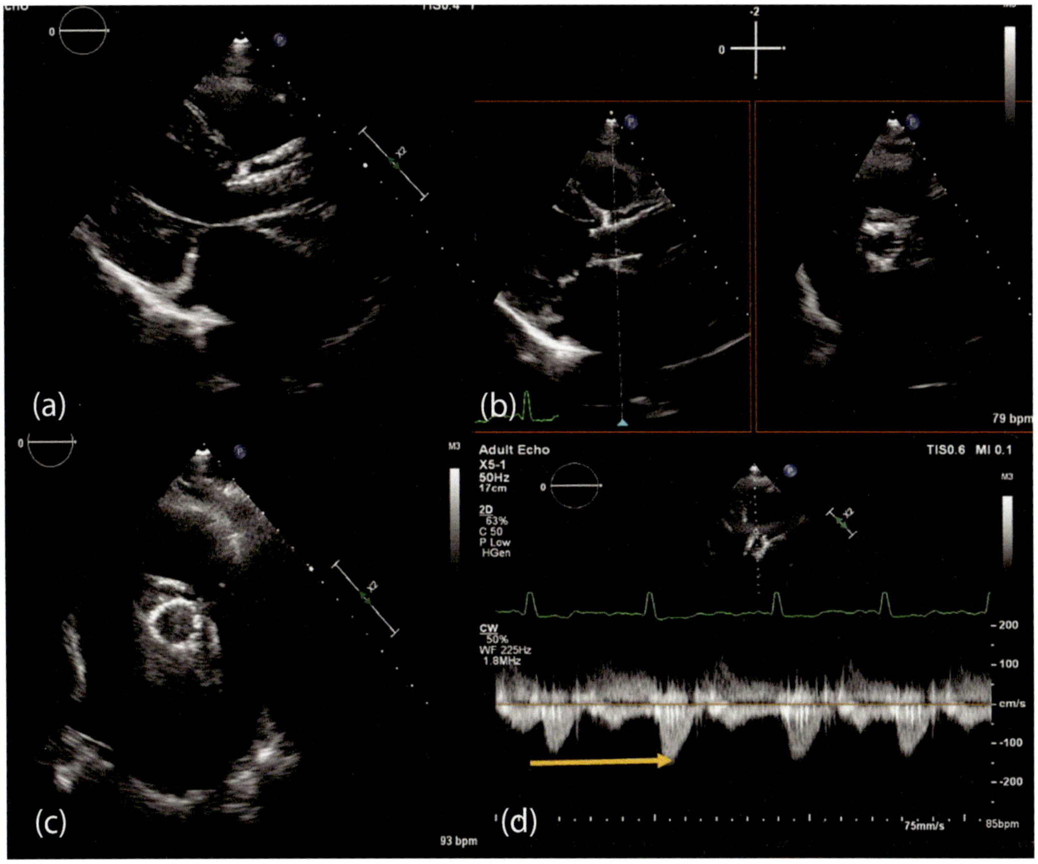

FIGURE 14.3 Successful transcatheter aortic valve implantation. (a) Parasternal long axis view, (b) biplane view, (c) parasternal short axis view, and (d) normal transaortic mean pressure gradient (yellow arrow).

Euroscore II risk <4%, infective endocarditis, short distance between coronary ostia and aortic annulus, dysplastic aortic valve, presence of LV thrombus, and need for cardiac surgery due to severe coronary artery disease, aortic aneurysm or other severe concomitant VHD. However, Heart Team plays an important role in the decision of treatment strategy in patients with severe symptomatic AS.[22]

Patients with symptomatic severe AS, either high-gradient or low-flow, low-gradient, are recommended for surgical replacement or TAVI. The presence of LV contractile reserve in a patient with true severe AS and reduced LVEF constitutes a positive prognostic impact factor, although intervention is recommended even in the absence of contractile reserve. As mentioned before, the choice between transcatheter and surgical intervention is taken from Heart Team based on surgical risk and clinical characteristics. Balloon valvotomy is only reserved as a bridge for hemodynamically unstable patients scheduled for intervention, for patients with severe symptomatic AS scheduled for urgent non-cardiac surgery, and for diagnostic purposes in patients with renal or other organ failure planed for TAVI.

Asymptomatic severe AS should be managed with surgical aortic valve replacement if LVEF falls below 50% and exercise stress test reveals symptoms or drop in blood pressure. For patients with severe asymptomatic AS and LVEF ≥50%, surgery is recommended for low surgical-risk patients and at least one of: AoV_{max} >5.5 m/s, annual increase of AoV_{max} by ≥0.3 m/s and severe aortic calcification, severe increase of brain natriuretic peptide (>3 times the normal range for age- and sex-matched individuals), or SPAP ≥60 mmHg measured ideally with catheterization. To date, TAVI is not recommended for asymptomatic patients.[21]

Finally, aortic valve replacement is recommended for patients with severe or moderate AS scheduled for another cardiac surgery or surgery for the ascending aorta.

Regular follow-up every six months is recommended for patients with asymptomatic severe aortic stenosis. For patients with mild or moderate disease, follow-up is recommended every one to two years.

Aortic Regurgitation

Epidemiology and Etiology

Aortic regurgitation (AR) rarely causes symptoms of HF, as this valvular disease progresses slowly. However, early referral for treatment before the occurrence of LV dysfunction is crucial and decisions should not be based only on LVEF, as HF with reduced LVEF usually manifests postoperatively. Acute AR can manifest with acute cardiogenic shock.

AR can result from abnormalities of the aortic valve or ascending aorta. In general, three phenotypes have been recognized: presence of aortic root aneurysm (defined as sinuses of Valsalva dimensions >45 mm), presence of ascending aorta aneurysm (defined as sinuses of Valsalva dimensions between 40 mm and 45 mm), and lone aortic regurgitation due to aortic valve abnormalities (when all dimensions of the aorta are <40 mm). According to the underlying mechanism, AR can be categorized as type 1, when there is aortic dilation and the aortic cusps are normal, or type 2, when there is aortic cusp prolapse, or type 3 with aortic cusp retraction (Figure 14.5).

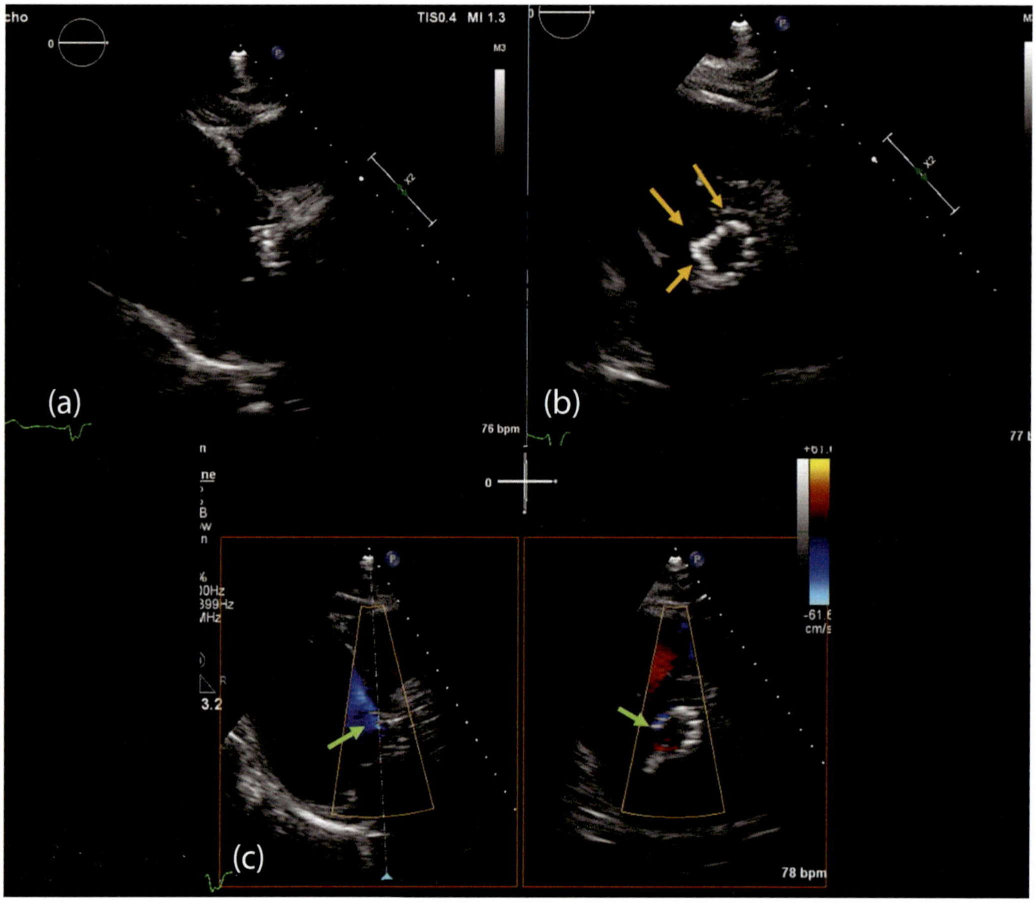

FIGURE 14.4 Echocardiographic imaging of transcatheter valve. (a) Parasternal long-axis view and (b) short-axis view of a transcatheter valve implantation with malposition and inadequate expansion (yellow arrows); (c) color Doppler reveals paravalvular regurgitation (green arrows).

About two out of three cases of aortic regurgitation are caused by degenerative bicuspid or dysplastic aortic valves.[21] Other causes are infective endocarditis, rheumatic disease, ventricular septal defect, post TAVI or balloon valvulotomy, radiation, drugs, or collagenic autoimmune disease, such as rheumatoid arthritis, systemic lupus erythematosus, ankylosing spondylitis, and Adamantiades-Behcet syndrome, which can affect both the aortic valve and the ascending aorta. Arterial hypertension, Marfan syndrome, annuloaortic ectasia, Loeys–Dietz syndrome, Ehler-Danlos syndrome, Turner syndrome, syphilis, psoriasis, Takayasu arteritis, and giant cell arteritis are diseases that cause aortic dilatation and aortic regurgitation. Trauma, infective endocarditis, or acute aortic dissection are causes of acute aortic regurgitation.

Pathophysiology

In chronic AR, left ventricular SV regurgitates to the left ventricle during diastole, resulting in an increase in LV end-diastolic volume and wall tension. The left ventricle responds to this with eccentric wall hypertrophy in order to keep end-diastolic pressure and SV within normal ranges. However, this leads to LV fibrosis, decrease in LV compliance, and an increase in LV end-diastolic pressure. This constitutes the chronic decompensated stage with LV dilation and drop in LVEF and SV (Table 14.2). Moreover, diastolic pressure of the aorta decreases and there is an increase in pulse pressure.

Acute AR leads to an acute increase in LV end-diastolic pressure and pulmonary capillary wedge pressure, resulting in acute pulmonary edema, since the left ventricle cannot compensate for the acute end-diastolic volume overload. Moreover, coronary flow decreases significantly, resulting in myocardial ischemia. Diastolic mitral regurgitation is typical of acute AR due to the premature mitral valve closure at the beginning of diastole. Tachycardia is common in AR, as the body attempts to decrease the regurgitant volume (Rvol).

Clinical Presentation

Chronic regurgitation is asymptomatic for a very long time. The typical symptom is angina, especially during sleep, when heart rate decreases and Rvol increases. Palpitation, dyspnea, orthopnea, and nocturnal paroxysmal dyspnea may exist. Several typical signs of increased pulse have been traditionally described in severe AR but are rarely met nowadays.[23]

First heart sound (S1) may be reduced or even silent in cases of LV dysfunction or premature mitral valve closure. Second heart sound may be paradoxically split due to prolonged ejection time. Fourth heart sound is a usual clinical finding in patients with AR, while S3 is heard when LVEF is reduced. A diastolic decrescendo blowing murmur following the aortic component of S2 and heard at the left third or fourth intercostal space parasternal, with radiation to the apex, is typical for AR. The murmur increases in duration when AR becomes more severe. However, at the end stage of the disease the murmur decreases because of increase in LV end-diastolic pressure. The Austin-Flint murmur is a mid-to-end diastolic low-pitched rumble that results from the direction of the regurgitant jet

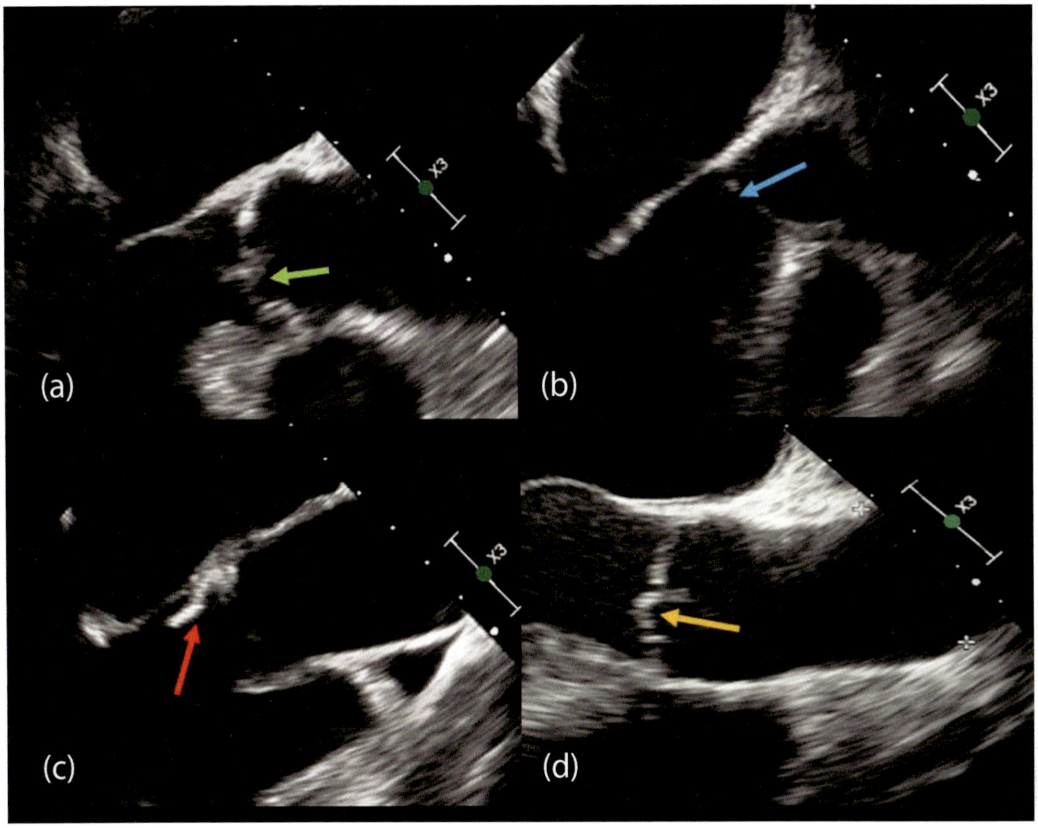

FIGURE 14.5 Echocardiographic imaging of different etiologies of aortic regurgitation. (a) Aortic cusp proptosis, (b) Aortic valve puncture, (c) flail aortic valve, (d) partial aortic cusp proptosis.

TABLE 14.2: Hemodynamics in Various Stages of Aortic Regurgitation

Normal	Acute AR	Chronic Compensated AR	Chronic Decompensated AR	Post Aortic Valve Replacement
AoP=120/80 mmHg	AoP=130/70 mmHg	AoP=190/60 mmHg	AoP=170/60 mmHg	AoP=120/80 mmHg
LVEDP=10 mmHg	LVEDP=50 mmHg	LVEDP=12 mmHg	LVEDP=25 mmHg	LVEDP=15 mmHg
EDV=150 cc	EDV=170 cc	EDV=250 cc	EDV=300 cc	EDV=230 cc
ESV=50 cc	ESV=50 cc	ESV=50 cc	ESV=150 cc	ESV=130 cc
—	Total SV=120cc	Total SV=200 cc	Total SV=150 cc	Total SV=100 cc
Forward SV=100cc	Forward SV=60cc	Forward SV=100 cc	Forward SV=75 cc	Forward SV=100 cc
—	RF=50%	RF=50%	RF=50%	—
LVEF=67%	LVEF=71%	LVEF=80%	LVEF=50%	LVEF=43%

Abbreviations: AoP: aortic pressure, EDV: end-diastolic volume, ESV: end-systolic volume, LVEDP: left ventricular end-diastolic pressure, LVEF: left ventricular ejection fraction, RF: regurgitant fraction, SV: stroke volume.

toward the anterior mitral leaflet. A mid-systolic ejection murmur may be heard at the base of the heart with radiation to the neck, due to an increased SV.[10]

In acute AR, all the above-mentioned signs are absent. First heart sound is diminished due to premature mitral valve closure and the diastolic murmur is light and short in duration or absent when LV end-diastolic pressure equals aortic diastolic pressure.

Diagnostic Evaluation and Severity Stratification

Chest Radiograph

Possible findings may be cardiomegaly or ascending aorta dilatation.

ECG

In chronic AR, LV hypertrophy, left axis deviation, and LA abnormalities may be present. A sign of LV volume overload constitutes the presence of Q-waves in I, aVL, V4–V6 leads and R-wave in V1 lead. In acute AR, non-specific ST and T segment abnormalities may be present.[11]

Echocardiography

Echocardiography is the best method for the evaluation of the etiology and severity of aortic regurgitation. Stages of AR are demonstrated in Table 14.3. With 2-D echocardiography, one can obtain measurements of LV, aortic root, and ascending aorta dimensions (best measured on parasternal long-axis view at end-diastole from leading edge to leading edge). Severe AR is considered the valvular disease with flail or coaptation defect. Diastolic "flutter" and reverse doming of the anterior mitral leaflet are signs of severe AR, whereas the premature mitral valve closure and diastolic mitral regurgitation are signs of acute valvular disease. Color Doppler demonstrates large central or eccentric regurgitant jet (estimated at Nyquist limit 50–60 cm/s), dense signal of regurgitant jet and holodiastolic flow reversal in the descending aorta with end-diastolic velocity>20 cm/s (Figure 14.6).[24]

TABLE 14.3: Echocardiographic Severity Stratification of Aortic Regurgitation

Stages of Aortic Regurgitation	Mild	Moderate	Severe
Jet width (% of LVOT)	<25%	25–64%	≥65%
Vena contracta (cm)	<0.3	0.3–0.6	0.3–0.59
EROA (cm^2)	<0.1	0.1–0.29	≥0.3
RVol (mL/beat)	<30	>60	≥60
RF (%)	<30	30–49	≥50
PHT (msec)	>500	200–500	<200
LVESD (or LVESDi)	Normal	≤50 mm	>50 mm (or >25 mm/m^2)
Other			Holodiastolic flow reversal in the descending aorta with end-diastolic velocity>20 cm/s

Abbreviations: EROA: effective regurgitant orifice area (estimated as 2π×(PISA radius)2×aliasing velocity/maximum velocity of regurgitant jet), LVESD: left ventricular end-systolic dimension, LVESDi: LVESD indexed, LVOT: left ventricular outflow tract, RF: regurgitant fraction, Rvol: regurgitant volume (estimated as EROA × velocity time interval [VTI] of the regurgitant jet), PHT: pressure half-time.

Transesophageal echocardiography is helpful for cases of congenital valve disease or infective endocarditis. Stress echocardiography may be useful to assess contractile reserve and possible latent LV dysfunction. LVEF is load-dependent and preserved despite severity of AR and LV remodeling, as is demonstrated in Table 14.2.[25] Post-operatively, LVEF decreases. Therefore, patients should be referred for aortic valve replacement or repair before the occurrence of irreversible LV dysfunction. The presence of LV contractile reserve and global longitudinal strain during dobutamine echocardiography constitutes a prognostic parameter that may predict the recovery of LV systolic function post-operatively.

Cardiac catheterization is rarely needed. Aortography can stage AR severity.

Treatment

Aortic valve replacement or Bentall procedure, with aortic valve and graft replacement, are the indicated methods of treatment. However, aortic valve repair is preferable where feasible, in the hands of experienced surgeons. Optimal candidates for aortic valve repair are younger patients with tricuspid aortic valve, without any calcification, and type I (aortic root dilation) or II (aortic cusp prolapse) mechanism of AR. Repair usually consists of re-implantation or remodeling of the native aortic valve with annuloplasty.[21] Although transcatheter aortic valve implantation is promising, limited evidence exists for AR.

Medical therapy includes angiotensin-converting enzyme inhibitors, angiotensin receptor blockers, and beta-blockers, especially for patients with collagen disease. Losartan in combination with beta-blocker is indicated for patients with Marfan syndrome. Vasodilators and inotropes are used only as bridges to surgery.

Guideline Recommendations

Surgery is recommended for patients with severe symptomatic AR or asymptomatic patients with LVEF ≤50%. Patients with severe AR undergoing cardiac surgery for another reason should proceed to aortic valve repair or replacement, irrespective of symptoms. Finally, asymptomatic patients with severe AR and preserved LVEF should be managed surgically when LV end-diastolic dimension is >70 mm or when end-systolic dimension is >50 mm (or >25 mm/m^2 indexed to body surface area for small people).[21]

Patients with aortic root or ascending aorta aneurysm should undergo aortic valve repair or replacement, irrespective of the severity of valvular disease. In general, surgery is recommended for patients with aortic dimension ≥55 mm. In Marfan syndrome, surgery is recommended when the ascending aorta dimension is ≥50 mm or ≥45 mm with concomitant risk factors (such as personal or family history of aortic or other vascular dissection, severe aortic or mitral regurgitation, desire for pregnancy, arterial hypertension, or annual increase of aortic diameter ≥3 mm/year). Patients with Loeyz–Dietz syndrome or *TGFBR1* or *TGFBR2* gene mutations should undergo surgery when aortic dimension is ≥45 mm. Patients with bicuspid aortic valve or coarctation of the aorta and presence of the above risk factors should procced to surgery when aortic dimension is ≥50 mm. For patients with an indication for aortic valve replacement or repair, aortic root and ascending aorta replacement is indicated when dimension is ≥45 mm.[21]

Follow-up of patients with mild or moderate AR is recommended every one to two years. Asymptomatic patients with severe AR should be evaluated clinically every six months. Measurement of brain natriuretic peptide might be helpful for those patients.[21]

Mitral Regurgitation

Etiology and Epidemiology

Mitral regurgitation (MR) can be the result of mitral valve abnormalities (primary) or LV or LA remodeling (secondary). According to the Carpentier classification of MR, Type I is characterized by normal mitral leaflet motion and MR is due to annular dilatation or leaflet perforation, such as ischemia of the inferolateral myocardial wall or papillary muscle, dilated cardiomyopathy, infective endocarditis, or cleft mitral valve. Type II is characterized by leaflet prolapse or chordal elongation or rupture (degenerative, Barlow or Marfan disease, trauma, or rheumatic). Type III is due to leaflet motion restriction and is further categorized into type IIIa, where leaflet motion is restricted due to chordal or papillary muscle retraction, and type IIIb, where leaflets are tented as a consequence of annular or LV dilation.[26]

MR is the most common valvular disease in the general population and the 2nd most common one following AS in patients hospitalized with HF. Degenerative MR is the most common form and can manifest as leaflet prolapse or myxomatous degeneration with valve thickening, tissue proliferation, and calcification. Mitral valve prolapse is common in patients with Marfan or Ehler-Dahnlos disease.[27] Rheumatic valvulopathy often presents as combined stenosis and regurgitation and is characterized by commissural fusion and leaflet retraction.

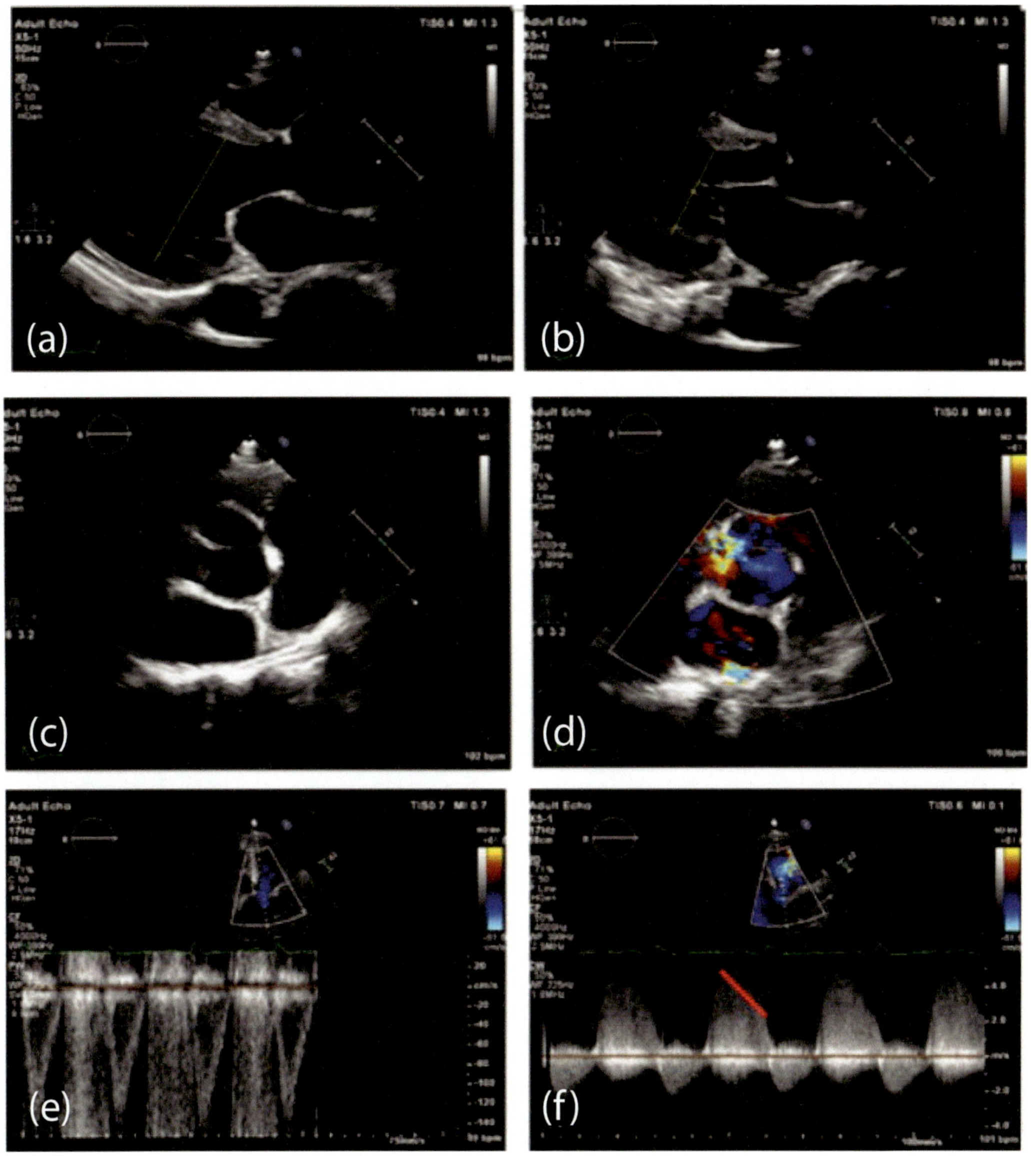

FIGURE 14.6 Severe aortic regurgitation in a patient with dysplastic aortic valve. (a) Left ventricular dilation with end-diastolic diameter 58 mm, (b) end-systolic diameter 45 mm, and (c) hypoplastic non coronary aortic cusp. (d) Color Doppler reveals eccentric regurgitant jet. (e) Pulse wave Doppler in left ventricular outflow tract reveals increase in stroke volume. (f) Continuous wave Doppler signal of aortic regurgitation has the same density as forward flow, and pressure half-time is <200 msec.

Radiation therapy typically affects the anterior mitral leaflet and the aorto-mitral continuity, resulting in excessive calcification. In contrast, degenerative disease is characterized by calcification of the posterior mitral annulus.

Pathophysiology and Clinical Presentation

MR is characterized by volume regurgitation from LV to LA during systole. In chronic MR, there is LV volume overload with increase in total LV output and ejection fraction, in order to maintain adequate forward cardiac output. This results in eccentric LV hypertrophy with LV dilation, while diastolic function is supra-normal. With disease progression, LVEF and cardiac output decrease, leading to elevated LA pressures and HF symptoms (Table 14.4).

In acute MR, there is abrupt decrease in LV afterload and acute LA and LV volume overload. Subsequently, the acute decrease in cardiac output and increase in LA pressure results in acute pulmonary edema and cardiogenic shock. Tachycardia and high LVEF are typical findings in acute MR. Chronic decompensated MR results in dyspnea on exertion, fatigue, or palpitation. Atrial fibrillation (AF) is common in severe MR. Secondary MR is a dynamic clinical condition and symptoms may worsen with exercise or arterial hypertension.[2] Flash pulmonary edema is typical of secondary MR due to acute coronary artery syndromes.

On clinical examination the apical impulse is displaced to the left. On auscultation, S1 is reduced and S2 is widely split. An S3 is usually present due to increased transmitral diastolic inflow during LV early diastolic filling. Fourth heart sound (S4) is often present in acute MR. Typically, a holosystolic blowing murmur is best heard in the apex and usually radiates to the axilla. The murmur begins after the onset of S1, is continuous after S2, and does not change with an extrasystole or AF. However, in severe MR with increased LA pressure,

TABLE 14.4: Hemodynamics in Various Stages of Mitral Regurgitation

Normal	Acute MR	Chronic Compensated MR	Chronic Decompensated MR
LAP= 10 mmHg	LAP= 25 mmHg	LAP= 15 mmHg	LAP= 25 mmHg
EDV=120 cc	EDV=120 cc	EDV=200 cc	EDV=220 cc
ESV=50 cc	ESV=30 cc	ESV=60 cc	ESV=100 cc
Total SV=70 cc	Total SV=90 cc	Total SV=140 cc	Total SV=120 cc
Forward SV=70 cc	Forward SV=45 cc	Forward SV=70 cc	Forward SV=60 cc
Rvol= 0	Rvol= 45 cc	Rvol= 70 cc	Rvol= 60 cc
LVEF=58%	LVEF=75%	LVEF=70%	LVEF=55%

Abbreviations: EDV: left ventricular end-diastolic volume, ESV: left ventricular end-systolic volume, LAP: left atrial pressure, LVEF: left ventricular ejection fraction, Rvol: regurgitant volume, SV: stroke volume.

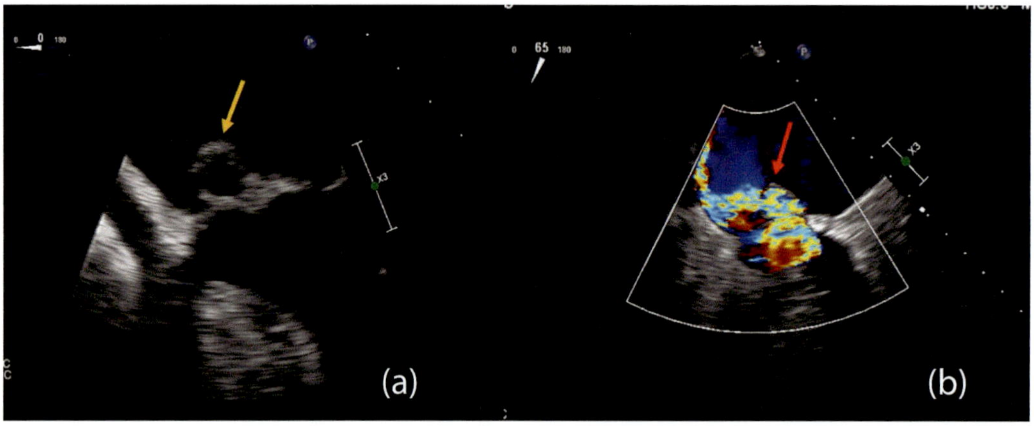

FIGURE 14.7 Echocardiographic imaging of mitral regurgitation. (a) Transesophageal echocardiography in a patient with acute dyspnea reveals the presence of an aneurysm of the anterior leaflet of the mitral valve due to endocarditis. (b) Color Doppler demonstrates a large eccentric regurgitant jet indicating severe mitral regurgitation.

the murmur may be not heard. In mitral valve prolapse, the murmur is usually mid-to-late systolic crescendo with a mid-systolic click. Maneuvers that increase venous return and decrease contractility, such as squatting, decrease the duration of the murmur and the click is moved to late systole.

Diagnostic Evaluation and Severity Stratification

Chest radiography may reveal cardiomegaly or interstitial pulmonary edema. The ECG may reveal LA enlargement, LV hypertrophy, or AF. In acute MR, there is a hypercontractile LV with high LVEF on echocardiography, whereas LA and LV dimensions are normal. Presence of vegetation or a ruptured papillary muscle can reveal the etiology of acute MR. In chronic MR, if the effective regurgitant orifice area (EROA) is small, regurgitation occurs in early systole, whereas, in mitral valve prolapse, regurgitation takes place during mid and late systole, and, in ischemic heart disease, the regurgitation occurs in early and end-systolic period and typically depends on LV contractility and volume. In addition, in mitral leaflet prolapse, the regurgitant jet is oriented opposite to the prolapsing leaflet, whereas, in mitral leaflet tension or retraction, the regurgitant jet is oriented at the same site to the affected leaflet. Severe MR is considered to occur with a valve with anatomic abnormalities, such as a flail valve, papillary muscle rupture, or large coaptation defect, with a large central or eccentric regurgitant jet that swirls and reaches the posterior LA wall (Figure 14.7). Table 14.5 summarizes the stages of primary MR. MR should be evaluated without anesthetic medication, as anesthesia reduces systematic vascular resistance and afterload, and thus MR is underestimated. The anatomy of the mitral valve and the etiology of MR is best evaluated with 3-D echocardiography (Figures 14.8 and 14.9).[28] Moreover, it seems that regurgitant volume can be accurately estimated with 3-D echocardiography. Transesophageal echocardiography is essential before intervention, for planning the surgical strategy, and during surgical or transcatheter interventional procedure.

Treatment and Recommendations

Treatment includes mitral valve replacement (MVR), surgical or percutaneous repair, and medical therapy. Surgical repair includes quadrangular or triangular mitral leaflet resection in A2 or P2 scallop prolapse or chordal rupture, edge-to-edge repair, which is rarely preferred, annuloplasty ring, which is almost always performed in addition to valve repair, and the use of polytetrafluoroethylene neochordae.[29,30]

Transcatheter edge-to-edge mitral valve repair (MitraClip) is a technique based on the placement of a clip between the A2 and P2 scallops of the mitral valve. Subsequently, two mitral valve areas are formed, while there is usually a residual mild to moderate MR. Echocardiographic criteria help assess patient eligibility for MitraClip (A2 or P2 prolapse, coaptation length >2 mm and depth <11 mm, flail gap <10 mm and width <15 mm, mobile leaflet length >1 cm and mitral valve area (MVA) >4 cm^2). It is recommended for symptomatic patients with severe MR, who are ineligible for cardiac surgery due to prohibitive surgical risk.[31]

Transcatheter MVR may be a promising treatment option. The implantation of a transcatheter aortic valve in a bioprosthetic mitral valve with severe calcification ("valve-in-valve" technique) in high surgical-risk patients is under investigation.

TABLE 14.5: Echocardiographic Severity Stratification of Primary and Secondary Mitral Regurgitation

Stages of Primary MR	Mild	Moderate	Severe	Severe Secondary MR
Jet width (% of LA)	<20%	20–40%	>40%	≥20%
Vena contracta (cm)	<0.3	<0.7	≥0.7 (or eight biplane)	>0.3
EROA (cm²)		<0.4	≥0.4	≥0.3
RVol (mL/beat)		<60	≥60	≥45
RF (%)		<50	≥50	≥50
LVESD (mm)	normal	>40	≥40	
Other			• Dense and triangular transmitral continuous wave Doppler • Reversal of the systolic wave in pulmonary vein flow • E-wave ≥1.5 m/s • Mitral to aortic VTI ratio >1.4	

Abbreviations: E: transmitral early diastolic inflow wave, EROA: effective regurgitant orifice area (estimated as $2\pi r^2$ × aliasing velocity / maximum velocity of regurgitant jet, where r is the proximal isovelocity surface area radius), LA: left atrium, LVESD: left ventricular end-systolic dimension, RF: regurgitant fraction, Rvol: regurgitant volume (equals EROA × VTI of the regurgitant jet, where VTI is time-velocity interval). Vena contracta is estimated at Nyquist limit 50–60 cm/s.

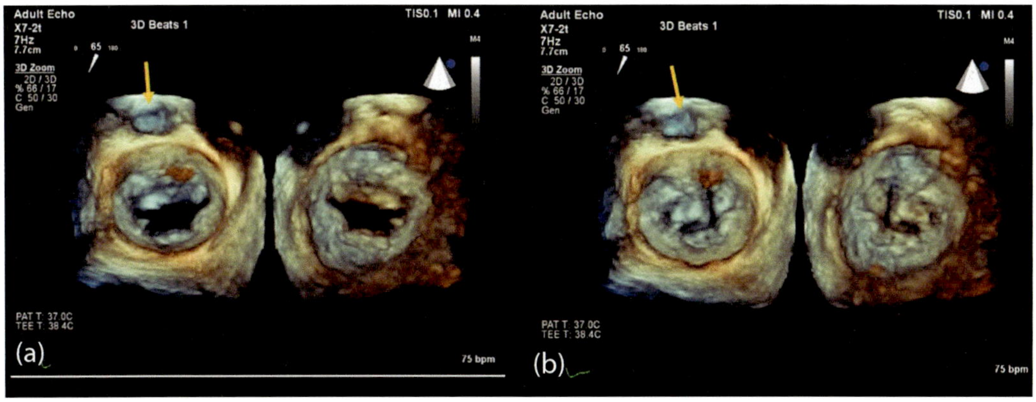

FIGURE 14.8 Three-dimensional echocardiography of mitral regurgitation. 3D-reconstruction of degenerative mitral regurgitation and cleft of A2-A3 scallops of the anterior mitral leaflet. Aortic valve is in the 12th hour (yellow arrow).

The technique poses challenges, as the valve has not adequate support from the mitral apparatus and may cause left ventricular outflow tract obstruction or valve emboli.[32]

Medical treatment is indicated only for patients with chronic MR with HF who are ineligible for surgery and includes angiotensin-converting enzyme inhibitors, beta-blockers, mineralocorticoid receptor antagonists, or diuretics. In acute MR, nitrates, diuretics, sodium nitroprusside, inotropes, and intra-aortic balloon pump are used as a bridge to acute surgery repair or replacement.[21]

Surgery is indicated for symptomatic patients with severe MR and LVEF >30% and asymptomatic patients with documented LV dysfunction, defined as LVEF ≤60% and LV end-systolic dimension ≥45 mm. Mitral valve repair is preferred over replacement. Moreover, asymptomatic patients with severe MR and normal LV can proceed to surgical treatment if AF or increase in SPAP >50 mmHg occurs, measured invasively. If the patient is eligible for mitral valve repair and is on sinus rhythm, the threshold for surgery is lower. These patients can proceed to surgery in the case of flail valve and LV end-systolic dimensions between 40 and 45 mm or LA volume index ≥60 mL/m².[21] Mitral valve repair may be considered for patients with LVEF <30% and LV end-systolic dimension >55 mm, who are symptomatic despite optimal HF treatment. Asymptomatic patients with severe MR and LVEF >60% should be followed up every six months and those with moderate valvulopathy every one to two years.

Functional (Secondary) Mitral Regurgitation

Functional mitral regurgitation (FMR) is the result of annular dilation, ventricular remodeling, or reduced closing forces, while the valve anatomy is normal.

Etiology and Pathophysiology

Ischemic, dilated, restrictive, or hypertrophic cardiomyopathy are characterized by structural remodeling, with increased tethering and reduced closing forces of atrioventricular valves, leading to FMR. LA enlargement can also lead to FMR (Table 14.6).

In ischemic heart disease, FMR can be the result of scar or reduced contractility of LV mid-myocardial segments or posteromedial papillary muscle, which leads to asymmetric tethering and reduced closing forces of mitral leaflets resulting in eccentric regurgitant jet.[21] Contrary to mitral valve prolapse, the jet is directed toward the tethered valve (Figure 14.10).

In patients with ischemic or non-ischemic cardiomyopathy with reduced LVEF and LV dilation, FMR can result from mitral annulus dilation and papillary muscle displacement. The regurgitant jet is early and end-systolic or holosystolic with semilunar EROA parallel to the leaflet coaptation zone. Typically, there is tethering of both leaflets. The regurgitant

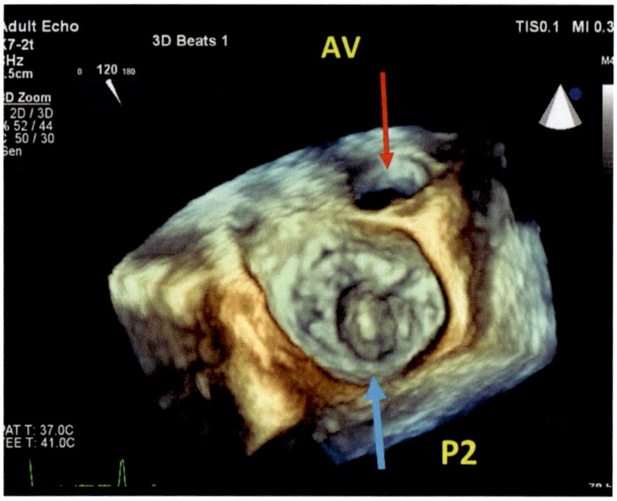

FIGURE 14.9 Transesophageal 3D echo from atrial perspective. 3D-zoom of the mitral valve in a patient with prolapse of the P2 segment (blue arrow) of the posterior mitral leaflet. Aortic valve (AV) in 12th hour (red arrow).

jet is larger and best evaluated in the bicommissural view. LV dyssynchrony is usually present and contributes significantly to FMR.

Patients with hypertrophic cardiomyopathy may have FMR due to papillary muscle hypertrophy and anterior displacement, systolic anterior motion, or even leaflet elongation. The presence of severe diastolic dysfunction and increased LV end-diastolic pressure or the occurrence of AF can result in FMR. Patients with restrictive cardiomyopathy typically have secondary atrioventricular valve regurgitation due to atrial dilation and increased LV end-diastolic pressure. This results in annulus and leaflet enlargement with preserved posterior annular contractility and absence of leaflet tethering.

Diagnostic Evaluation and Severity Classification

Echocardiography can provide information about the underlying etiology as well as the severity. The American Heart Association uses the same severity cutoffs for primary and secondary MR,[20] whereas the European Society of Cardiology recommends lower EROA >20 mm^2 and RV >30 mL as limits for severe FMR with worse prognosis.[21] In patients with reduced LVEF, absolute regurgitant volume may be low due to reduced stroke volume and increased LV and LA pressure. However, regurgitant fraction is increased, indicating severe valvular disease. A recent ESC joint position paper for the management of FMR reconciles the findings of the COAPT and MITRA-FR trials and suggests the use of the COAPT criteria for severe FMR, based on EROA ≥30 mm^2, or Rvol ≥45 mL and/or RF ≥40% when EROA is smaller.[33]

Stress echocardiography with exercise is useful for the evaluation of patients with FMR. Increase in EROA of>13 mm^2 or increase in SPAP to>60 mmHg constitute negative prognostic parameters. The decrease in MR indicates the presence of viable myocardium, and the presence of contractile reserve is a positive prognostic parameter.

Treatment

Optimal medical treatment for HF, revascularization of hibernating myocardium, and cardiac resynchronization therapy are the cornerstones of FMR management.

Surgical intervention usually includes the implantation of an undersized annular ring. Mitral valve replacement and combined surgical repair techniques are under investigation. However, most of the time these patients are at high surgical risk and surgical mitral valve repair has not shown survival benefit.[34] Therefore, transcatheter edge-to-edge mitral valve repair with MitraClip has been used for patients with HF and reduced LVEF, albeit with conflicting results. The COAPT trial has shown significant survival benefit,[35] whereas the Mitra-FR trials showed no mortality benefit with MitraClip.[36] However, these two studies included patients with different characteristics and these results indicate that a subgroup of patients with disproportionate FMR, characterized by low LV end-diastolic

TABLE 14.6: Differences between Atrial Functional and Secondary Ischemic Mitral Regurgitation

	Secondary MR	Atrial Functional MR
Pathophysiology	*Reduced closing force*: Reduced LV contractility Increased LA pressure Reduced annular contraction *Increased tethering force*: LV dilation and dysfunction Papillary muscle displacement Annular dilation	*Reduced closing force*: Preserved LV contractility Increased LA pressure Reduced annular contraction *Leaflet malcoaptation*: Annular dilation and flattening Insufficient leaflet growth Fibrotic leaflet thickening Altered atrial/annular dynamics
Etiology	Ischemic heart disease—myocardial infarction Dilated cardiomyopathy	AF HFpEF Restrictive cardiomyopathy Hypertrophic cardiomyopathy
Diagnosis	Systolic LV dysfunction Restricted leaflet motion and tethering Eccentric or central regurgitant jet Left ventricular dilation	Normal or preserved LV systolic function Normal leaflet motion Central regurgitant jet Severe LA dilation
Management	Optimal medical HF therapy Cardiac resynchronization therapy Revascularization MitraClip	Optimal medical HFpEF therapy, mostly diuretics Sinus rhythm restoration—AF ablation Treatment of HFpEF risk factors (arterial hypertension, diabetes mellitus etc.) Interventional therapy (annuloplasty, MitraClip) under investigation

Abbreviations: AF: atrial fibrillation, HF: heart failure, HFpEF: heart failure with preserved left ventricular ejection fraction, LA: left atrial, LV: left ventricular.

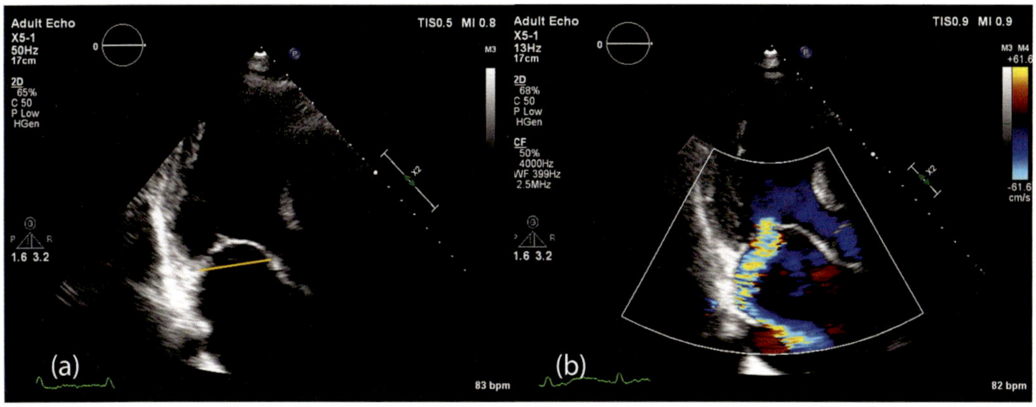

FIGURE 14.10 Two-dimensional and color Doppler of transthoracic echocardiography. Seen in apical 3-chamber view in a patient with ischemic heart disease and secondary mitral regurgitation. Mitral leaflets are tethered and the regurgitant jet is large and eccentric, oriented posteriorly.

and end-systolic volume and large EROA, may benefit from transcatheter interventions.

Treatment of "atrial" FMR in patients with HF and preserved LVEF or AF is not well established. Rhythm control and ablation of AF have been proven to reduce atrial remodeling and FMR.[37] Trials investigating the effect of rhythm restoration on atrial FMR are ongoing.[38]

Indications for surgery in patients with severe FMR include planned coronary artery bypass grafting with LVEF >30% or symptomatic patients with LVEF <30% and viable myocardial segments. For patients who are not candidates for surgical revascularization, interventional therapy might be considered if the patient remains symptomatic despite optimal medical therapy, cardiac resynchronization therapy, and LVEF is >30%.[21] Intermediate to high surgical-risk patients with suitable anatomical and morphological valve characteristics could undergo transcatheter edge-to-edge mitral valve repair (MitraClip). Currently, transcatheter edge-to-edge repair should be considered for patients who remain symptomatic despite optimal medical therapy and cardiac resynchronization therapy with severe secondary MR, suitable valve morphology, LV end-systolic dimension <70 mm and absence of significant RV dysfunction, tricuspid regurgitation, or pulmonary hypertension.[33]

Mitral Stenosis

Epidemiology and Etiology

Although the prevalence of mitral stenosis (MS) has declined over recent decades due to a decline in the incidence of rheumatic fever, it is still a common cause of MS in young people, especially in developing countries, typically affecting the tips of both mitral valve leaflets and sparing the basal segments. In older patients, MS is usually degenerative and characterized by calcification that affects the basal segments while sparing the tips. Other rare causes include congenital MS, carcinoid, lupus, amyloidosis, drugs, chest radiotherapy, functional MS (LA myxoma, thrombus, vegetation, cor triatriatum), and iatrogenic MS after mitral valve repair.[39]

Pathophysiology and Presentation

MS is characterized by HF with normal LV size and contractility. LV preload and cardiac output is reduced. There is an increase in LA pressure and dimensions and an increase in systematic vascular resistance. LA pressure overload results in reduced LA compliance, pulmonary vascular sclerosis, pulmonary hypertension, and RV failure. LA dilation results in AF and embolic episodes due to thrombus formation. If LA pressure exceeds 25 mmHg, acute pulmonary edema can ensue, typically with high cardiac output conditions, e.g., pregnancy, hyperthyroidism, fever, exercise, or AF with high ventricular response. Conditions that raise the end-diastolic LV pressure, e.g., AS, restrictive cardiomyopathy, or HF with reduced LVEF, may lead to underestimation of MS severity, as transmitral peak gradient is reduced.

Severe MS manifests as dyspnea, orthopnea, paroxysmal postural dyspnea, cough and hemoptysis, palpitations, and fatigue. Hoarseness as a result of laryngeal nerve pressure by the enlarged LA can ensue. Typically, symptoms worsen under high-output conditions. MS can also manifest as angina, thromboembolism, respiratory infections, or infective endocarditis. On auscultation, there is loud S1, wide-split S2, and an opening snap. Unless the patient is in AF, a mid-to-late diastolic rumble with presystolic accentuation is best heard at the apex. As severity increases, the murmur becomes longer. ECG may reveal "mitrale" P waves, signs of RV hypertrophy, and AF. Chest radiograph may reveal straightening of left cardiac border, double density sign of right cardiac, upper zone venous enlargement, or pulmonary edema.[39]

Diagnostic Evaluation and Severity Classification

On echocardiography, diastolic doming of anterior mitral leaflet, systolic, anterior movement of posterior mitral leaflet and mitral valve area (MVA) like a "fish mouth" are typical findings of rheumatic MS. In degenerative MS, there is severe calcification of the posterior mitral annulus. LA is enlarged and may content thrombus. Severity classification is summarized in Table 14.7. Clinically significant MS is considered when MVA is <1.5 cm^2 or 1 cm^2/m^2 for patients with large body surface area and is estimated with pressure half-time, continuity equation, or planimetry (Figure 14.11). The Wilkins criteria should be evaluated in candidates for percutaneous mitral commissurotomy and include mobility, calculation, and thickening of leaflets and subvalvular apparatus.[40] 3 D echocardiography is the best method for MVA planimetry and estimation of anatomic abnormalities and Wilkins score. Transesophageal echocardiography is essential during percutaneous commissurotomy.[41]

TABLE 14.7: Stages of Mitral, Tricuspid, and Pulmonary Valve Stenosis

	Mild	Moderate	Severe
Stages of Mitral Stenosis			
Mean PG	<5 mmHg	5–10 mmHg	>10 mmHg
MVA	>1.5 cm^2	1–1.5 cm^2	<1 cm^2
SPAP	<30 mmHg	30–50 mmHg	>50 mmHg
Stages of Tricuspid Stenosis			
Mean PG		<5 mmHg	>5 mmHg
TVA		>2 cm^2	<2 cm^2
Stages of Pulmonic Stenosis			
Vmax	<3 m/s	3–4 m/s	>4 m/s with early- or mid-systolic notch
Peak PG	<36 mmHg	36–64 mmHg	>64 mmHg
Acceleration time			<105 msec

Abbreviations: Mean PG: mean pressure gradient, MVA: mitral valve area, SPAP: systolic pulmonary artery pressure, TVA: tricuspid valve area, Vmax: maximum transpulmonary valve velocity.

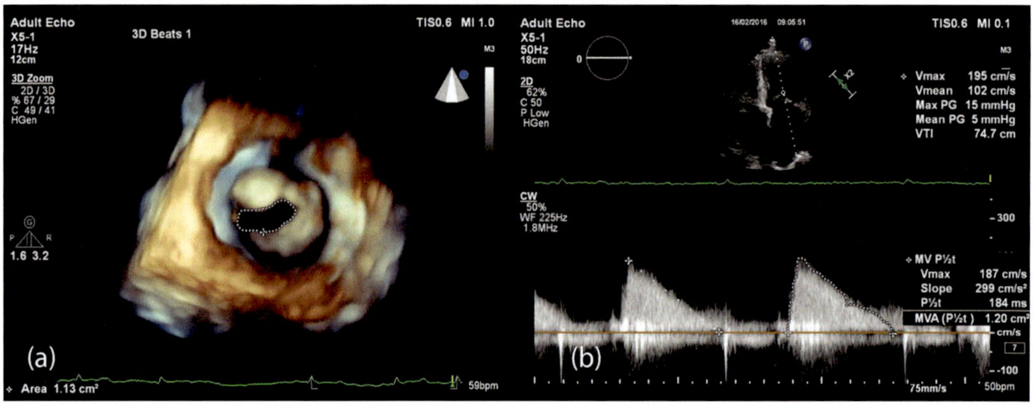

FIGURE 14.11 Echocardiographic imaging of severe mitral stenosis. (a) Three-dimensional transesophageal and (b) 2D-echocardiography with continuous wave Doppler in a patient with severe mitral stenosis. Mitral valve area is estimated about 1.2 cm^2 both with planimetry and with pressure half-time method. Mean pressure gradient is calculated at 5 mmHg.

Stress echocardiography is useful in asymptomatic severe MS or in symptomatic moderate MS. Exercise is the preferred method, although dobutamine can be used instead. The occurrence of symptoms, the increase in mean transmitral gradient>15 mmHg with exercise or>18 mmHg with dobutamine and the increase in SPAP>60 mmHg indicate severe MS.[42]

Treatment

Medical therapy includes rate control, loop diuretics for symptoms, and anticoagulation with vitamin K antagonists for patients who have suffered an embolic event, are in AF, or have severely enlarged LA (>50 mm or >60 mL/m^2) and dense contrast despite sinus rhythm. Exercise is not recommended for patients with severe MS or SPAP >50 mmHg.

Interventional treatment includes percutaneous or surgical mitral commissurotomy and mitral valve replacement. Young patients with rheumatic mitral disease, without severe calcification, Wilkins score <8, and absence of LA thrombus are appropriate candidates for percutaneous commissurotomy. Transcatheter valve implantation is a promising method for older adults with degenerative MS.[21]

Interventional treatment is recommended for symptomatic patients with clinically significant MS (defined as MVA <1.5 cm^2). Asymptomatic patients with severe MS should be considered for interventional treatment if the risk for thromboembolism or hemodynamic decompensation is high. History of systemic embolism, dense LA contrast, or paroxysmal AF are conditions with high thromboembolic risk. Resting SPAP >50 mmHg, trying for pregnancy, or need for non-cardiac surgery are cases at high risk of hemodynamic decompensation.

Tricuspid Regurgitation

Etiology and Epidemiology

The tricuspid valve has three leaflets: the anterior, which is the longest, the posterior, and the septal, which is the shortest. Two papillary muscles, the anterior and the medial, support the leaflets. Chordae tendineae from the anterior papillary muscle support the anterior and posterior leaflets and those from the median support the posterior and the septal leaflets. The septal wall segment provides chordae tendineae to the anterior and the septal leaflet. Typically, the tricuspid is located slightly more apically than the mitral valve but less than 8 mm/m^2.

Trivial tricuspid regurgitation (TR) is common even in normal subjects. TR can be primary or secondary. Secondary TR, as a consequence of RV dilation or dysfunction, is more common, accounting for 90% of cases.[43] Primary TR can result from rheumatic disease, Ebstein's anomaly, atrioventricular septal defect, carcinoid disease, connective tissue disease, leaflet prolapse, trauma, device implantation (iatrogenic), tumors (e.g., myxoma), infective endocarditis, or drugs (ergotamine, methysergide, "ecstasy," fenfluramine).[44] Importantly, primary TR can be aggravated by secondary TR due to RV dilation.

Pathophysiology and Presentation

TR results in RV volume overload. However, RV and RA intracardiac pressures are low and the RV myocardial wall is thin. Subsequently, TR results in RV dilation without hypertrophy. As TR increases in severity, RV end-diastolic pressure equals RA pressure and causes systematic venous congestion. Right ventricular dilation can result in RV dysfunction and increased RV end-diastolic pressure. The shift of the interventricular septum toward LV and the reduced LV preload result in prevention of LV filling and reduction in cardiac output.

TR can be tolerated well for a long time. Symptoms occur when low cardiac output and systemic venous congestion ensue. Symptoms of RV failure include fatigue, anorexia, hepatalgia, weight loss, dyspnea, and palpitations. Signs of RV failure are peripheral edema, ascites, cachexia, jaundice, and positive hepatojugular sign. There is holosystolic murmur, best heard left parasternal in the 3rd to 4th intercostal space, which typically increases with inspiration (Carvallo sign). In very severe TR, the murmur is not heard. RV S3 and S4 may be heard and increase with inspiration. The ECG may demonstrate right bundle branch block or AF.[11] Chest radiogram may show cardiomegaly due to enlarged right heart chambers.

Diagnostic Evaluation and Severity Classification

On echocardiography, leaflet morphology may reveal the etiology of TR. Right-sided volume overload causes dilation of the RV and RA and diastolic flattening ("D-shape") of the interventricular septum. Table 14.8 summarizes the classification of TR severity. In severe TR, there is a large regurgitant jet, large coaptation defect or flail valve, and marked tethering of the leaflets (Figure 14.12). In patients with very severe tricuspid annulus dilation and massive TR, equalization of RV and RA pressures renders estimation of SPAP using the TR regurgitant jet inaccurate. With 3-D echo, the tricuspid valve appears to be circular due to dilation of the annulus. RV end-diastolic and end-systolic volume and TR regurgitant volume can be estimated with accuracy comparable to that of cardiac MRI (Table 14.8). Stress echocardiography may have a role for secondary TR, as exercise-induced increase in SPAP >60 mmHg is associated with adverse prognosis. (In contrast, increase in SPAP >30 mmHg for patients with pulmonary arterial hypertension is associated with improved outcome, indicating presence of RV contractile reserve). On cardiac catheterization, increased RV end-diastolic pressure and high C-V waves with blunt X and deep Y waves in RV pressure waveform are typical for severe TR.

Treatment

Treatment includes diuretics for symptomatic relief. No medication has been shown to reduce mortality for patients with severe TR and right HF. Surgical treatment includes annuloplasty ring, tricuspid valve repair (bicuspidation or double-orifice repair), and valve replacement.[45] Due to increased risk of thrombosis, bioprosthetic valves are preferred over mechanical.

Transcatheter interventions are increasingly performed for TR. Edge-to-edge valve repair has been successfully performed in severe, secondary TR. MitraClip is the most used technique, although other leaflet coaptation devices are under development. Transcatheter annuloplasty devices aim at reducing annular dilation (Table 14.9).[46]

Patients undergoing cardiac surgery with severe or moderate primary TR without RV dysfunction are candidates for tricuspid valve intervention.[47] Asymptomatic patients with severe primary TR and progressive RV dilation or early signs of RV dysfunction should be referred for tricuspid valve intervention. Patients with secondary TR and right annular dilation (>40 mm in echocardiography study or >70 mm during surgery) are candidates for surgical intervention if they have other indications for cardiac surgery. Secondary TR after successful treatment of left heart valve disease, in the absence of LV dysfunction, and with symptoms of progressive RV dysfunction or dilation, may be an indication for intervention.[21]

Pulmonary Regurgitation

Trivial pulmonary regurgitation (PR) is common in healthy individuals. "Congenital" PR is encountered after tetralogy of Fallot repair or balloon valvulotomy for pulmonary stenosis (PS).[48] Pulmonary hypertension, infective endocarditis, carcinoid, and iatrogenic causes can lead to PR, which can be asymptomatic for years.[49] Chronic RV volume overload results in signs and symptoms of right HF (peripheral edema, ascites,

TABLE 14.8: Echocardiographic Severity Stratification of Tricuspid Regurgitation

Stages of TR	Mild	Moderate	Severe	Massive	Torrential
Central jet area (cm^2)	<5	5–10	>10	>10	>10
Vena contracta (cm)	-	<0.7	7–13.9	14–20	>20
Continuous wave signal of regurgitant jet	Soft and parabolic	Dense and variable contour	Dense/triangular with early peaking	Dense/triangular with early peaking. Peak TR vel <2/ms	-
Hepatic vein systolic flow	Dominance	Blunting	Reversal	Reversal	Reversal
PISA radius (mm)			>9	>9	>9
Tricuspid E-wave dominant (cm/s)	<1	<1	>1	>1	>1
EROA (mm)		<40	40–59	60–79	≥80
EROA estimated with 3-D echocardiogram		<75	75–94	95–114	≥115
Rvol (mL/beat)			45–59	60–74	≥75

Note: Vena contracta is estimated at Nyquist limit 50–60 cm/s.

Abbreviations: EROA: effective regurgitant orifice area (estimated as $2\pi r^2$ × aliasing velocity / maximum velocity of regurgitant jet, where r is PISA radius), PISA: proximal isovelocity surface area, estimated at Nyquist limit of 28 cm/s, Rvol: regurgitant volume (equals EROA × VTI of the regurgitant jet, where VTI is time-velocity interval).

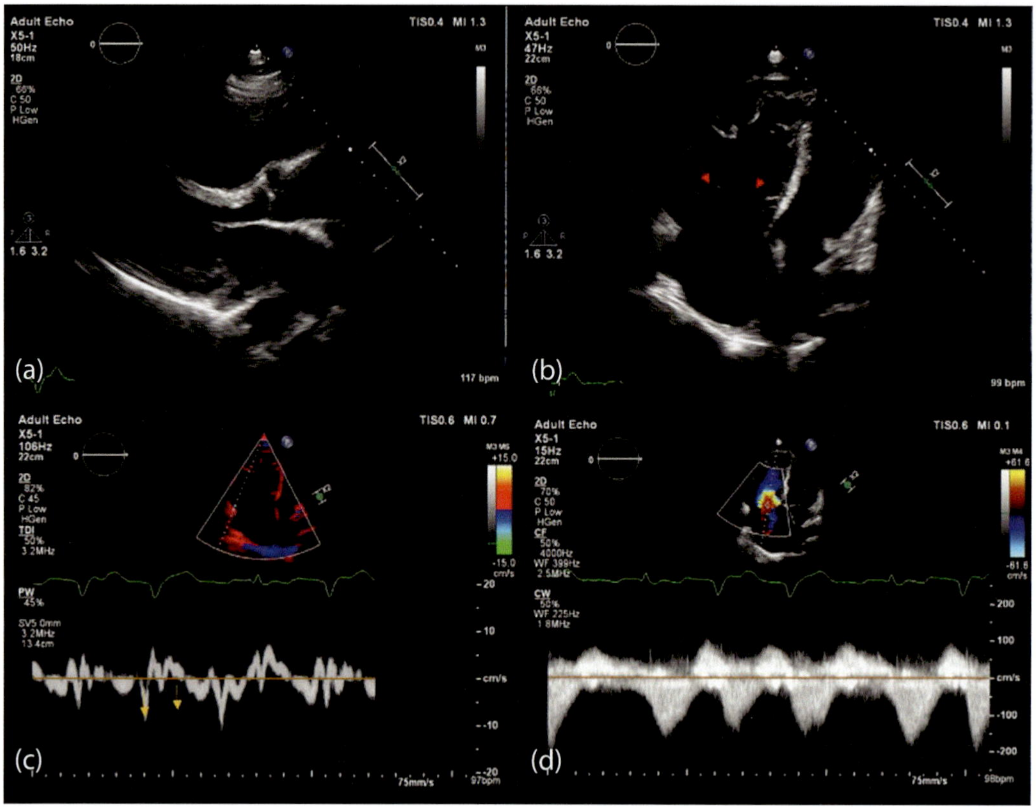

FIGURE 14.12 Severe tricuspid regurgitation of a patient with ischemic cardiac disease and an old infarction of the RV. (a) Right ventricular dilation and diastolic flattering of interventricular septum. (b) Large coaptation defect due to annulus dilation. (c) Reduced systolic annular tissue Doppler indicative of reduced right ventricular systolic function. (d) Continuous wave Doppler is dense and triangular with maximum velocity 2 cm/s, indicative of massive tricuspid regurgitation.

TABLE 14.9: Transcatheter Tricuspid Valve Therapies Currently in Use or Under Development

Tricuspid Valve Repair	
Leaflet	MitraClip
	PASCAL
	FORMA
Annuloplasty	Trialign
	TriCinch
	Cardioband
	Iris
	Minimally invasive annuloplasty (MIA) device
	Transatrial intrapericardial tricuspid annuloplasty (TRAIPTA)
	Pledget-assisted suture tricuspid annuloplasty (PASTA)
Tricuspid Valve Replacement	
Orthotopic	SAPIEN XT/SAPIEN 3 valves
	GATE tricuspid valve stent
	Trisol valve
	LUXValve
	TriCares valve
Heterotopic	SAPIEN XT/SAPIEN 3 valves
	TricValve (superior and inferior cava valves)

fatigue), and palpitations. The diastolic murmur increases with inspiration and Graham-Steel diastolic decrescendo murmur is heard when SPAP is >70 mmHg. There is usually wide QRS complex on ECG, which may also reveal atrial tachycardia or non-sustained ventricular tachycardia. There is RV and RA dilation on echocardiography, with PR jet and concomitant TR jet. Continuous wave Doppler is dense with early equalization of RA and RV end-diastolic pressure and short pressure half-time (Figure 14.13).

Treatment with percutaneous implantation of the bioprosthetic Melody (Medtronic Inc., Minneapolis, MN, USA) valve is recommended for symptomatic patients with severe PR, atrial or ventricular arrhythmias, RV dysfunction (fractional area change <40%) or severe dilation (end-diastolic volume >160

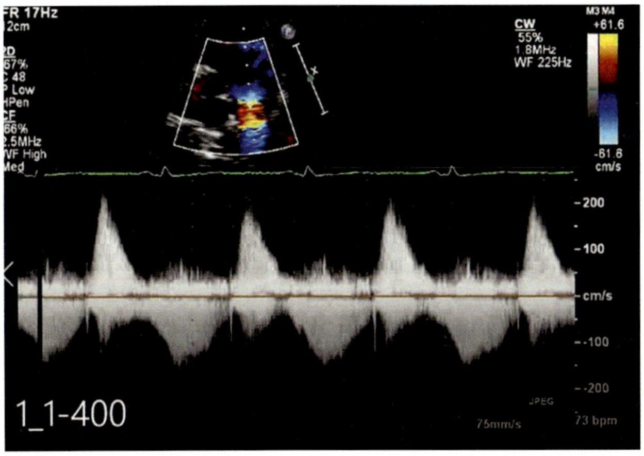

FIGURE 14.13 Severe pulmonary regurgitation. Continuous wave Doppler of a patient with severe pulmonary regurgitation with dense signal and very short pressure half-time.

mL/m^2 or end-systolic volume >82 mL/m^2), progressive TR, QRS prolongation >180 msec or annual increase of ≥3.5 ms, and patients undergoing interventional therapy for left heart valve disease.[50,51]

Mulivalvular Disease

The evaluation of patients with HF symptoms and multivalvular disease, a common scenario, is challenging. First, a primary valvular abnormality can result in another, secondary valvular abnormality. AS can result in MR due to increased LV end-diastolic pressure. MS can cause TR due to pulmonary hypertension. In the absence of anatomical abnormalities of the valve, MR or TR decrease in severity after AS or MS treatment.

On the other hand, systemic diseases, e.g., rheumatic fever, degenerative, autoimmune diseases, Marfan's syndrome, or infective endocarditis can affect multiple valves. In these cases, individual valvular disease severity may be under- or overestimated. For example, AR might underestimate MS severity and AS may overestimate MR severity.[21] In a patient with combined valve stenosis and regurgitation, it is very important to characterize which is the more severe, based on valve morphology and the consequences on the atrium and ventricle.

Finally, HF with reduced and preserved LVEF can cause both secondary MR and TR. Grading valvular disease severity is difficult, since symptoms may be due to underlying HF. Three-dimensional echocardiography is a valuable imaging modality and may give important information about anatomical abnormalities. For asymptomatic patients with severe multiple valvular abnormalities, or for patients with symptoms disproportionate to the severity of the valvular disease, exercise echocardiography might give useful information, while keeping in mind that, during exercise, interaction between valves increases. The management of these patients is difficult, as greater age and multiple comorbidities render concomitant replacement of two or more valves a major undertaking, with substantial periprocedural and late mortality. Therefore, careful individualization of treatment plan is needed in these cases.

References

1. Podlesnikar T, Delgado V, Bax JJ. Imaging of valvular heart disease in heart failure. *Card Fail Rev.* 2018;4:78–86.
2. Ennezat PV, Marechaux S, Pibarot P, Le Jemtel TH. Secondary mitral regurgitation in heart failure with reduced or preserved left ventricular ejection fraction. *Cardiology.* 2013;125:110–7.
3. Unger P, Clavel MA, Lindman BR, Mathieu P, Pibarot P. Pathophysiology and management of multivalvular disease. *Nat Rev Cardiol.* 2016;13:429–40.
4. Bhatia N, Basra SS, Skolnick AH, Wenger NK. Aortic valve disease in the older adult. *J Geriatr Cardiol.* 2016;13:941–4.
5. Martinsson A, Li X, Andersson C, et al. Temporal trends in the incidence and prognosis of aortic stenosis: A nationwide study of the Swedish population. *Circulation.* 2015;131:988–94.
6. Carita P, Coppola G, Novo G, et al. Aortic stenosis: Insights on pathogenesis and clinical implications. *J Geriatr Cardiol.* 2016;13:489–98.
7. Joseph J, Naqvi SY, Giri J, Goldberg S. Aortic stenosis: Pathophysiology, diagnosis, and therapy. *Am J Med.* 2017;130:253–63.
8. Carabello BA. Evaluation and management of patients with aortic stenosis. *Circulation.* 2002;105:1746–50.
9. Ramaraj R, Sorrell VL. Degenerative aortic stenosis. *BMJ.* 2008;336:550–5.
10. Maganti K, Rigolin VH, Sarano ME, Bonow RO. Valvular heart disease: Diagnosis and management. *Mayo Clin Proc.* 2010;85:483–500.
11. Edhouse J, Thakur RK, Khalil JM. ABC of clinical electrocardiography. Conditions affecting the left side of the heart. *BMJ.* 2002;324:1264–7.
12. Clavel MA, Magne J, Pibarot P. Low-gradient aortic stenosis. *Eur Heart J.* 2016;37:2645–57.
13. Hachicha Z, Dumesnil JG, Bogaty P, Pibarot P. Paradoxical low-flow, low-gradient severe aortic stenosis despite preserved ejection fraction is associated with higher afterload and reduced survival. *Circulation.* 2007;115:2856–64.
14. Sannino A, Grayburn PA. Mitral regurgitation in patients with severe aortic stenosis: Diagnosis and management. *Heart.* 2018;104:16–22.
15. Rafique AM, Biner S, Ray I, et al. Meta-analysis of prognostic value of stress testing in patients with asymptomatic severe aortic stenosis. *Am J Cardiol.* 2009;104:972–7.
16. Marechaux S, Hachicha Z, Bellouin A, et al. Usefulness of exercise-stress echocardiography for risk stratification of true asymptomatic patients with aortic valve stenosis. *Eur Heart J.* 2010;31:1390–7.
17. Nishimura RA, Carabello BA. Hemodynamics in the cardiac catheterization laboratory of the 21st century. *Circulation.* 2012;125:2138–50.
18. Boon NA, Bloomfield P. The medical management of valvar heart disease. *Heart.* 2002;87:395–400.
19. Czarny MJ, Resar JR. Diagnosis and management of valvular aortic stenosis. *Clin Med Insights Cardiol.* 2014;8:15–24.
20. Nishimura RA, Otto CM, Bonow RO, et al. 2017 AHA/ACC focused update of the 2014 AHA/ACC guideline for the management of patients with valvular heart disease: A report of the American College of Cardiology/American Heart Association Task Force on Clinical Practice Guidelines. *Circulation.* 2017;135:e1159–e1195.
21. Falk V, Baumgartner H, Bax JJ, et al. 2017 ESC/EACTS guidelines for the management of valvular heart disease. *Eur J Cardiothorac Surg.* 2017;52:616–64.
22. Duchnowski P, Hryniewiecki T, Kusmierczyk M, Szymanski P. Performance of the EuroSCORE II and the Society of Thoracic Surgeons score in patients undergoing aortic valve replacement for aortic stenosis. *J Thorac Dis.* 2019;11:2076–81.
23. Dewaswala N, Chait R. *Aortic regurgitation.* StatPearls, Treasure Island, FL; 2020.
24. Lancellotti P, Tribouilloy C, Hagendorff A, et al. European Association of Echocardiography recommendations for the assessment of valvular regurgitation. Part 1: Aortic and pulmonary regurgitation (native valve disease). *Eur J Echocardiogr.* 2010;11:223–44.
25. Lancellotti P, Magne J. Stress echocardiography in regurgitant valve disease. *Circ Cardiovasc Imaging.* 2013;6:840–9.
26. Carpentier A, Chauvaud S, Fabiani JN, et al. Reconstructive surgery of mitral valve incompetence: Ten-year appraisal. *J Thorac Cardiovasc Surg.* 1980;79:338–48.
27. Douedi S, Douedi H. *Mitral regurgitation.* StatPearls, Treasure Island, FL; 2020.
28. Shiota T. Role of modern 3D echocardiography in valvular heart disease. *Korean J Intern Med.* 2014;29:685–702.
29. Koprivanac M, Kelava M, Alansari S, et al. Degenerative mitral valve disease-contemporary surgical approaches and repair techniques. *Ann Cardiothorac Surg.* 2017;6:38–46.
30. Colli A, Adams D, Fiocco A, et al. Transapical NeoChord mitral valve repair. *Ann Cardiothorac Surg.* 2018;7:812–20.
31. Katz WE, Conrad Smith AJ, Crock FW, Cavalcante JL. Echocardiographic evaluation and guidance for MitraClip procedure. *Cardiovasc Diagn Ther.* 2017;7:616–32.
32. Flynn CD, Wilson-Smith AR, Yan TD. Novel mitral valve technologies-transcatheter mitral valve implantation: A systematic review. *Ann Cardiothorac Surg.* 2018;7:716–23.

33. Coats AJS, Anker SD, Baumbach A, et al. The management of secondary mitral regurgitation in patients with heart failure: A joint position statement from the Heart Failure Association (HFA), European Association of Cardiovascular Imaging (EACVI), European Heart Rhythm Association (EHRA), and European Association of Percutaneous Cardiovascular Interventions (EAPCI) of the ESC. *Eur Heart J.* 2021;42:1254–69.
34. Nappi F, Avatar Singh SS, Santana O, Mihos CG. Functional mitral regurgitation: An overview for surgical management framework. *J Thorac Dis.* 2018;10:4540–55.
35. Stone GW, Lindenfeld J, Abraham WT, et al. Transcatheter mitral-valve repair in patients with heart failure. *N Engl J Med.* 2018;379:2307–18.
36. Iung B, Armoiry X, Vahanian A, et al. Percutaneous repair or medical treatment for secondary mitral regurgitation: Outcomes at 2 years. *Eur J Heart Fail.* 2019;21:1619–27.
37. Gertz ZM, Raina A, Saghy L, et al. Evidence of atrial functional mitral regurgitation due to atrial fibrillation: Reversal with arrhythmia control. *J Am Coll Cardiol.* 2011;58:1474–81.
38. Mauri L, Garg P, Massaro JM, et al. The EVEREST II Trial: Design and rationale for a randomized study of the evalve mitraclip system compared with mitral valve surgery for mitral regurgitation. *Am Heart J.* 2010;160:23–9.
39. Shah SN, Sharma S. *Mitral stenosis.* StatPearls, Treasure Island, FL; 2020.
40. Omran AS, Arifi AA, Mohamed AA. Echocardiography in mitral stenosis. *J Saudi Heart Assoc.* 2011;23:51–8.
41. Sarath Babu D, Ranganayakulu KP, Rajasekhar D, Vanajakshamma V, Pramod Kumar T. Assessment of mitral valve commissural morphology by transoesophageal echocardiography predicts outcome after balloon mitral valvotomy. *Indian Heart J.* 2013;65:269–75.
42. Yavagal ST, Deshpande N, Admane P. Stress echo for evaluation of valvular heart disease. *Indian Heart J.* 2014;66:131–8.
43. Mangieri A, Montalto C, Pagnesi M, et al. Mechanism and implications of the tricuspid regurgitation: From the pathophysiology to the current and future therapeutic options. *Circ Cardiovasc Interv.* 2017;10:e005043.
44. Mulla S, Asuka E, Siddiqui WJ. *Tricuspid regurgitation (tricuspid insufficiency).* StatPearls, Treasure Island, FL; 2020.
45. De Bonis M, Taramasso M, Lapenna E, Alfieri O. Management of tricuspid regurgitation. *F1000Prime Rep.* 2014;6:58.
46. Kolte D, Elmariah S. Current state of transcatheter tricuspid valve repair. *Cardiovasc Diagn Ther.* 2020;10:89–97.
47. Demir OM, Regazzoli D, Mangieri A, et al. Transcatheter tricuspid valve replacement: Principles and design. *Front Cardiovasc Med.* 2018;5:129.
48. Stout KK, Daniels CJ, Aboulhosn JA, et al. 2018 AHA/ACC guideline for the management of adults with congenital heart disease: Executive summary: A report of the American College of Cardiology/American Heart Association Task Force on Clinical Practice Guidelines. *J Am Coll Cardiol.* 2019;73:1494–563.
49. Saji AM, Sharma S. *Pulmonary regurgitation.* StatPearls, Treasure Island, FL; 2020.
50. Ferraz Cavalcanti PE, Sa MP, Santos CA, et al. Pulmonary valve replacement after operative repair of tetralogy of Fallot: Meta-analysis and meta-regression of 3,118 patients from 48 studies. *J Am Coll Cardiol.* 2013;62:2227–43.
51. Geva T. Indications and timing of pulmonary valve replacement after tetralogy of Fallot repair. *Semin Thorac Cardiovasc Surg Pediatr Card Surg Annu.* 2006:11–22.

Chapter 15
THE MANAGEMENT OF PATIENTS WITH HEART FAILURE WITH PRESERVED EJECTION FRACTION (HFpEF)

Jodie L. Kenes, Richard B. Stacey, and Bharathi Upadhya

Introduction

In contrast to heart failure (HF) with reduced ejection fraction (HFrEF), the incidence of HF with preserved ejection fraction (HFpEF) is increasing,[1] potentially due to the combination of aging of the population and increasing prevalence of cardiometabolic disorders (see also Chapter 2). By 2020, the relative prevalence of HFpEF and HFrEF are predicted to be 69% and 31%, respectively, turning HFpEF into the most common HF phenotype.[2] The health and economic impact of HFpEF is at least as great as that of HFrEF, with similar HF hospitalization rates and substantial mortality.[3,4] After HF hospitalization, 5-year survival of HFpEF is a dismal 35%, worse than most cancers.[3] Despite the importance of HFpEF, our understanding of its pathophysiology remains incomplete. Recently, the concept of HFpEF has evolved from a "cardio-centric" model to a syndrome that involves multiple cardiovascular (CV) and non-CV mechanisms. The impact of multiple comorbidities typical of older HFpEF patients further promotes phenotypic heterogeneity and multi-factorial pathophysiology. As a result, there are currently few therapies for HFpEF, as most approved therapies for HFrEF have been demonstrated to be ineffective for HFpEF. In this chapter, we summarize the current guidelines regarding management of HFpEF and provide an overview of emerging treatments that are being tested in clinical trials and novel therapeutic targets that may arise from advances in understanding the pathophysiology of HFpEF.

General Approach to Treating HFpEF

Management goals in patients with HFpEF include relief of symptoms, improvement in functional capacity, prevention of acute exacerbations, and increased survival. A systematic approach should comprise several elements: diagnosis and staging of disease, a search for reversible etiology, judicious use of medications, patient education, enhancement of self-management skills, coordination of care across disciplines, and effective follow-up. A multidisciplinary approach to management reduces acute exacerbations leading to hospitalization, improves quality of life, reduces total costs, and increases survival. Older adults with HF often have severe deconditioning with severe exercise intolerance and should be encouraged to undertake regular moderate physical activity. In Figure 15.1, we summarize a practical approach for the management of HFpEF based on the evidence that is available to date.

Published Guidelines for Treatment of HFpEF

Due to paucity of large trials demonstrating morbidity and mortality benefit for the treatment of HFpEF, the American College of Cardiology and American Heart Association (ACC/AHA) consensus guideline recommendations are relatively sparse regarding management of HFpEF. In patients with symptomatic HFpEF, diuretics are recommended to relieve symptoms due to volume overload (class I).[5] Control of hypertension is suggested as an important treatment strategy for HFpEF (class I).[5] The blood pressure (BP) goals in the ACC/AHA HF guideline are similar to those in the general population. However, a lower systolic BP target of 130 mmHg is recommended in the 2017 ACC/AHA HF guideline update, based on the results of the Systolic Blood Pressure Intervention (SPRINT) trial.[5–7] The ACC/AHA HF guidelines support the use of beta-blockers, angiotensin-converting enzyme inhibitors (ACEIs), and angiotensin receptor blockers (ARBs) for hypertension (class IIa), and consider ARBs and aldosterone antagonists as reasonable options for decreasing hospitalizations in HFpEF (class IIb). The HF Society of America guidelines recommend that ACEIs or ARBs be considered in all patients with HFpEF and symptomatic atherosclerotic disease or diabetes and one additional risk factor.[8] Beta-blockers are recommended for patients with HFpEF and a history of myocardial infarction, hypertension. or atrial fibrillation. The 2017 update states that treatment of anemia with erythropoietin analogs provides no benefit (class III), while iron replacement can be considered in selected patients (class IIb), although patients with HFpEF were not specifically included in the cited trials.[5] Other ACC/AHA recommendations include treatment of common comorbidities, including overt myocardial ischemia, restoration and maintenance of sinus rhythm, control of heart rate in patients with permanent atrial fibrillation, and formal sleep assessment in patients with suspicion of sleep-disordered breathing or excessive daytime sleepiness. European Society of Cardiology (ESC) guidelines have similar recommendations.[9]

Therapeutic Targets in HFpEF

Management of Comorbidities and Prevention of HFpEF

An important component of treating a patient with HFpEF is treating the contributing factors and comorbidities that are frequently present and which significantly impact the clinical course, such as obesity, hypertension, coronary artery disease, diabetes, chronic obstructive lung disease, anemia, chronic kidney disease, and sleep-disordered breathing.[10]

Hypertension

Hypertension is the most prevalent risk factor for HF and precedes the diagnosis of HF in 75–85% of cases.[3] In the Antihypertensive and Lipid-Lowering Treatment to Prevent Heart Attack (ALLHAT) Trial, which compared four initial antihypertensive medication strategies, patients randomized to chlorthalidone had the lowest incidence of overall HF and of HFpEF specifically.[11] Several other hypertension trials, including SPRINT, have shown reduction in incident HF with treatment of hypertension, although these trials did not differentiate between incident HFpEF and HFrEF.[7] Considering the age distribution in these trials and the age-dependent relative

DOI: 10.1201/9780429244544-18

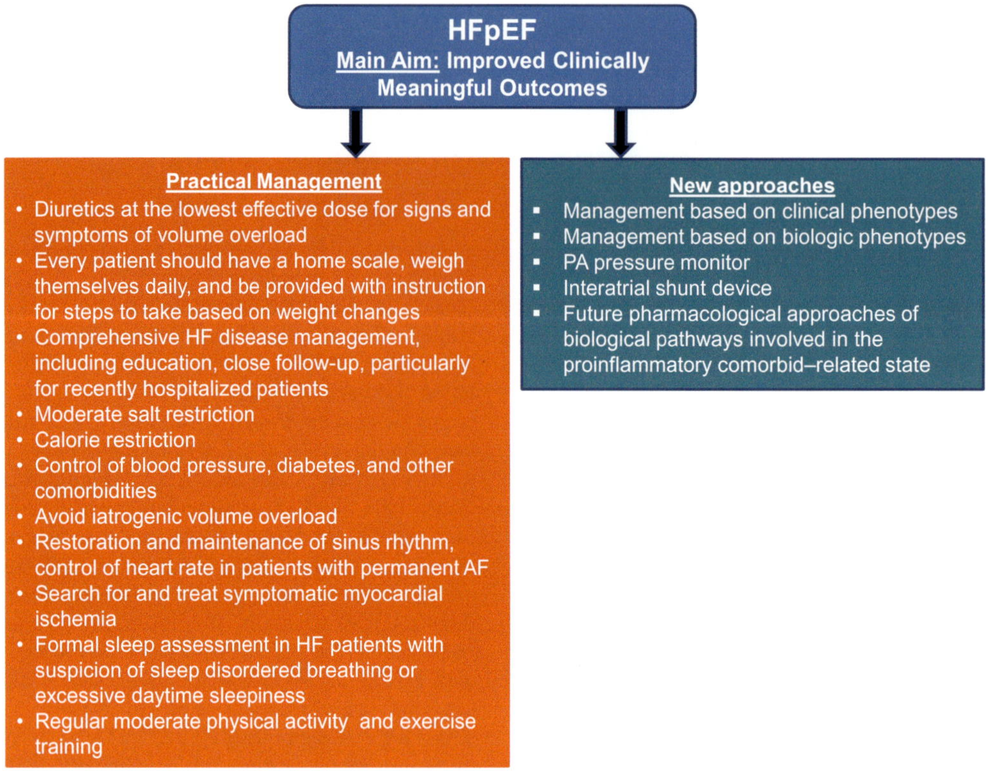

FIGURE 15.1 A practical approach to the management of HFpEF.

incidence of HFpEF, control of hypertension may be the single most important prevention strategy for HFpEF.

Metabolic Risk Factors

Patients with HFpEF have a high prevalence of obesity and diabetes. Approximately 85% of older HFpEF patients are overweight or obese, a rate twice that of the general population, and the HFpEF epidemic has largely paralleled the obesity epidemic.[12] Increased adiposity promotes inflammation, hypertension, insulin resistance, and dyslipidemia, and impairs cardiac, arterial, skeletal muscle, and physical function,[13–15] all of which are common in HFpEF and contribute to its pathophysiology.[16] Recently, studies in patients with type 2 diabetes showed reduced risk of HF hospitalization in patients receiving either empagliflozin or dapagliflozin, which are novel sodium-glucose cotransporter 2 inhibitors.[17,18] In a pooled analysis of 51,000 participants from the Women's Health Initiative, Multiethnic Study of Atherosclerosis, and Cardiovascular Health Study cohorts, the risk of incident HFpEF increased in a dose-dependent manner as body mass index increased and leisure-time physical activity declined.[19]

Non-Pharmacological Targets in HFpEF

Exercise Training in HFpEF

Aerobic exercise training increases both peak oxygen consumption (VO_2) by 2.1–3.0 mL/kg/min and health-related quality of life (HRQoL) in patients with HFpEF,[20–25] and it has become an accepted adjunct therapy for these patients.[26] To date, several trials have examined the efficacy of exercise training to improve peak VO_2, 6-min walk distance, and HRQoL in HFpEF (Table 15.1).[23–25,27–32] A critical question in these studies is the mechanism underlying the training-related improvement in exercise capacity. This needs careful measurements, not only of peak exercise VO_2, but also of its determinants, cardiac output (CO) and arterial–venous oxygen content difference (A-VO_2diff.) before and after an intervention.[33] These factors should be measured simultaneously during exercise along with peak Vo_2, and this is feasible with a number of techniques that have been developed.[33–36] The central effects of exercise training in HFpEF have been minimal in the few studies to date.[10,30] In addition, Fujimoto et al. showed no evidence of a beneficial effect of exercise training on the diastolic properties (LV compliance—assessed by invasive measurements) of LV in HFpEF elderly patients.[37] Additionally, a meta-analysis showed that exercise training in patients with HFpEF is associated with an improvement in VO_2 and HRQoL without significant changes in LV systolic (assessed by EF) or diastolic function (assessed by E/A ratio and early deceleration time).[20,38] Glaringly, Haykowsky et al. showed that 84% of the improvement in VO_2 after 16 weeks of exercise training was attributed to increases in peak A-VO_2diff.[29] This result was confirmed by Fu et al. who found that an exercise-training-mediated increase in peak VO_2 was secondary to the increased A-VO_2diff as peak heart rate, stroke volume index, and cardiac index were unchanged after training.[24] In fact, Bhella et al. recently reported that elderly HFpEF patients have baseline-impaired skeletal muscle oxidative metabolism, which can be favorably shifted by exercise training to more efficient muscle O_2 utilization.[28] Taken together, these data suggest that the majority of exercise training-related improvements in exercise capacity in HFpEF may be related to microvascular and/or skeletal muscle adaptations that increase diffusive oxygen transport and/or utilization by the active muscles.[39,40]

Exercise intervention trials for clinically stable patients with HF have primarily focused on continuous moderate-intensity

TABLE 15.1: **Clinical Trials of Exercise Therapy in HFpEF**

First Author or Trial Acronym	Intervention	HFpEF Patient Type	LVEF	Primary Endpoint	Trial Result
PARIS/Kitzman et al.[27]	Exercise training (n=53)	Aged 70±6 years, 87% female, ambulatory HF patients with NYHA class II–III symptoms, LVEF ≥50%	61±5% (Mean±SD)	Peak VO_2	*Improved peak and submaximal exercise capacity This benefit was not associated with any measurable change in resting LV structure or function
PARIS II/Haykowsky[29]	Exercise training (n=40)	Aged 69±6 years, 82% female, ambulatory HF patients with NYHA class II–III symptoms, LVEF ≥50%	61±5% (Mean±SD)	Peak VO_2	*Improved peak VO_2. Arterial-venous oxygen difference was primary contributor to improved peak VO_2
Kitzman et al.[28]	Exercise training (n=63)	Age 70±7 years, 76% female, ambulatory HF patients, NYHA class II–III, LVEF ≥50%	58±6% (Mean±SD)	Peak VO_2, 6MWD	*Improved peak VO_2 without altering endothelial function
SECRET-1 / Kitzman et al.[23]	Caloric restriction and exercise training (n=100)	Aged 67±5 years, 41% female, ambulatory HF patients with NYHA class II-III symptoms LVEF ≥50%	61±6 % (Mean±SD)	Peak VO_2 and Quality of Life	*Increased peak $\dot{V}O_2$ and the effects may be additive *Quality of life by KCCQ was improved, and benefit was greatest for caloric restriction
Ex-DHF trial[30]	Exercise training (n=64)	Aged 65±7 years, 56% female symptomatic, ambulatory NYHA II/III symptoms, echo-DD, LVEF ≥50%	68±7% (Mean±SD)	Peak VO_2	*Improved exercise capacity and quality of life (KCCQ) Benefits associated with atrial reverse remodeling and improved LV diastolic function
Smart et al.[31]	Exercise training (n=25)	Aged 64±8 years, 48% female, well compensated HF, LVEF >45%	57±10% (Mean±SD)	Peak VO_2	Improved Peak VO_2 No significant changes in diastolic, systolic function, Quality-of-life life by KCCQ and depression scores
Fu et al.[24]	Exercise training (n=30)	Aged 61±3 years, 33% female, NYHA class II/III HF, LVEF ≥50% with episodes of acute pulmonary edema.	58±2% (Mean±SD)	Peak VO_2	Improved Peak VO_2 Improved diastolic function with reduction of the E/e' ratio Improved quality of life scores
Angadi et al.[25]	Exercise training (n=9)	Aged 69±6 years, 11% female, NYHA class II/III HF, ECHO-DD, LVEF ≥50%	65±5% (Mean±SD)	Peak VO_2	Improved Peak VO_2 Improved diastolic dysfunction
Alves et al.[10]	Exercise training (n=31)	Aged 63±11 years, 29% female, admission with clinical signs of HF	56±3% (Mean±SD)	Exercise tolerance (METS), LVEF and E/e'	*Improved exercise tolerance, cardiac systolic and diastolic function

* Significant improvement ($P<0.05$).
Abbreviations: HFpEF = heart failure with preserved ejection fraction; LVEF = left ventricular ejection fraction; n = number of participants; NYHA = New York Heart Association; HF = heart failure; ECHO = echocardiographically assessed; DD = diastolic dysfunction; SD = standard deviation; MWD = minute walk distance; VO_2 = oxygen consumption; KCCQ = Kansas City Cardiomyopathy Questionnaire; E = mitral early diastolic velocity; e' = mitral annular velocity.

aerobic training (MICT).[41] In five HFpEF studies, this was performed 3–5 days per week for between one and five months. This exercise prescription is in line with the AHA exercise guidelines for overall CV health. Resistant training was included as an adjunctive modality to standard aerobic exercise training in one trial of HFpEF.[30] High-intensity interval training, a potent short-term training method characterized by brief, intermittent bursts of vigorous, aerobic exercise interspersed with periods of low-intensity active recovery, has been examined in two small trials of HFpEF patients.[24,25] However, the magnitude of improvement (mean change: +2.2 mL/kg/min peak VO_2) is similar to that observed following MICT (mean change: +1.9 mL/kg/min peak VO_2). To date, the safety and efficacy of high-intensity interval training in patients with HFpEF has not been studied. A large, multicenter trial (OptimEx-CLIN study) is currently ongoing to establish whether 12 months of high-intensity interval training is superior to moderate-intensity training for improving peak VO_2 in patients with HFpEF.[42]

Dietary Modifications

Because increased body adiposity promotes inflammation and impairs cardiac, arterial, renal, and skeletal muscle function, weight loss could be beneficial in the large proportion of patients with the obese HFpEF phenotype. Among obese, older patients with clinically stable HFpEF, weight loss via caloric restriction diet was feasible, appeared safe, and significantly improved exercise capacity and HRQoL, and the effect was additive to exercise training (Figure 15.2).[23] Caloric restriction improved HRQoL much more than did exercise training. The improvements from caloric restriction were associated with reduced total body and skeletal muscle adipose and reduced inflammation. Table 15.2 summarizes trials evaluating dietary modifications and other non-pharmacological approaches to HFpEF.

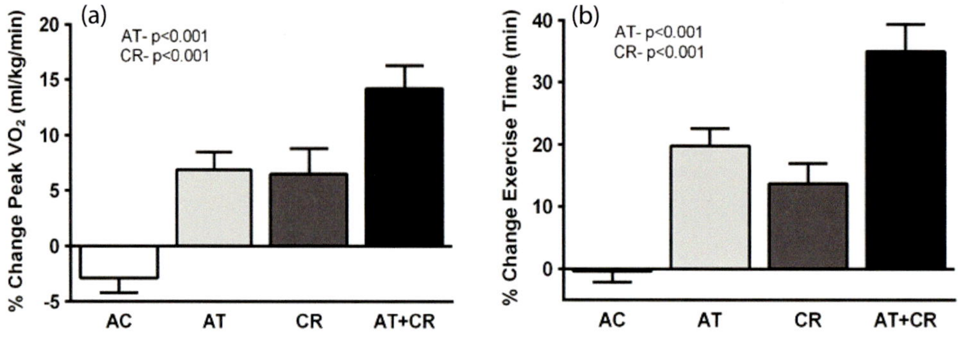

FIGURE 15.2 Effects of a 20-week caloric restriction (CR) diet vs aerobic exercise training (AT) on exercise capacity and quality of life in HFpEF. The graph displays % changes ± standard errors at 20 weeks relative to baseline by a randomized group for (a) peak VO_2 ($mL{\cdot}kg^{-1}{\cdot}min^{-1}$) and (b) Kansas City Cardiomyopathy Questionnaire Score. (Reproduced with permission from Upadhya et al., *J Am Geriatr Soc* 2017;65:2431–40.)

Device Therapy

The CardioMEMS device is a wireless, implanted pulmonary artery pressure monitor implanted in the distal pulmonary artery through right heart catheterization. Patients transmit hemodynamic data using a wireless radiofrequency transmitter. The CardioMEMS Heart Sensor Allows Monitoring of Pressures to Improve Outcomes in New York Heart Association (NYHA) Functional Class III HF (CHAMPION) trial showed a significant reduction in HF hospitalizations (Table 15.2).[43] In HFpEF specifically, the CardioMEMS device reduced decompensation leading to hospitalization compared with standard HF management strategies.[44]

Given that increases in left atrial (LA) pressure and pulmonary venous congestion are shown to herald HF events in patients with HFpEF, creating a controlled left-to-right interatrial shunt to allow LA decompression could be a rational nonpharmacological strategy for alleviating symptoms (Figure 15.3). The Reduce Elevated LA Pressure in Patients with HF (REDUCE LAP-HF) study, a phase 1 study designed to assess the safety and performance of the device in patients with HFpEF and NYHA II-IV symptoms, despite optimal medical or device therapy, demonstrated reductions in LA pressure during exercise with improvements in functional capacity and HRQoL six and 12 months after implantation.[45] Recently, the phase 2 randomized, sham-controlled REDUCE LAP-HF I trial published short-term results and showed decreases in pulmonary capillary wedge pressure (Table 15.2).[46]

A case report and modeling analysis suggest that cardiac resynchronization therapy in patients with HFpEF could potentially lead to improvement in functional class and exercise capacity.[47] Chronotropic incompetence, i.e., blunted heart rate response during exercise, is a significant, independent contributor to exercise intolerance in HFpEF.[48–50] The Restoration of Chronotropic CompEtence in HF PatientS with Normal Ejection FracTion (RESET), designed to evaluate rate-adaptive pacing in symptomatic mild-to-moderate HFpEF with chronotropic incompetence, was not completed due to slow enrollment.[50] The concept is being examined in an ongoing trial, Rate-Adaptive Atrial Pacing in Diastolic HF (RAPID; NCT02145351). Another pilot study has evaluated the implantation of a coronary sinus lead for active vs inactive LA pacing in six patients with HFpEF NYHA III/IV under optimal medical treatment. After three months, there was significant improvement in functional capacity and diastolic function.[51]

Cardiac contractility modulation devices deliver a strong electrical current during the refractory period into the septum, thus triggering molecular remodeling. A recent case series in HFpEF found that soon after initiating cardiac contractility modulation, patients experienced improvements in NYHA class, functional capacity, and HRQOL and showed significant reductions in the diastolic filling index.[52] Baroreflex activation therapy, which is produced by stimulating the carotid sinuses using an implanted device (Rheos, CVRx, Maple Grove, MN, USA), is being studied for the treatment of hypertension. The safety and efficacy of baroreflex activation therapy in HFpEF is being examined in the HOPE4HF (Hope for Heart Failure: NCT00957073) trial.[53] Renal denervation, which improved LV hypertrophy (LVH) and diastolic LV function in a small series with refractory hypertension,[54] was investigated in the Renal Denervation in HF with Preserved EF (RDT-PEF) trial; however, the study appeared statistically underpowered (Table 15.2).[52]

Sleep-disordered breathing is believed to cause LVH, biventricular systolic and diastolic function, endothelial dysfunction, proinflammatory state, and increased arterial stiffness;[55–59] all factors linked to the development of HFpEF. Non-invasive positive airway pressure therapy with adaptive servo-ventilation (ASV) is designed to normalize ventilation in patients with central and obstructive sleep apnea, and is typically better tolerated than continuous positive airway pressure.[60] Although ASV was associated with increased CV mortality in patients with HFrEF treated for predominantly central apnea, there was a sign of possible benefit in patients with LVEF 36%–45% in the ASV for Central Sleep Apnea in Systolic HF (SERVE-HF) trial.[61] This finding was further supported by the CV Improvements With Minute Ventilation-targeted ASV Therapy in HF(CAT-HF) trial and Yoshihisa et al. (Table 15.2).[62,63] As a result, this concept will be further evaluated in a registry and/or a randomized clinical trial of ASV in HFpEF.

Pharmacological Targets

For HFpEF, trials have been based on initial assumptions regarding features that were thought to be both specific to and universally present in HFpEF, such as LVH, diastolic dysfunction, and cardiac fibrosis. However, the results from a large number of studies have questioned these assumptions.[64,65] In a recent trial of well-characterized HFpEF patients, only 8% of patients had LVH at baseline and only 50% had severe diastolic function at rest.[66] This indicates that LVH may not be a fundamental requirement for development of HFpEF. Other studies

TABLE 15.2: **Clinical Trials of Non-Pharmacological Therapies in HFpEF**

First Author or Trial Acronym	Intervention	HFpEF Patient Type	LVEF	Primary Endpoint	Trial Result
Hummel et al.[80]	Sodium-restricted DASH diet (n=13)	Age 72±10 years, 98% female. Stable compensated HF with treated hypertension. LVEF ≥50%	66±18% (Mean±SD)	LV diastolic function, arterial function and ventricular vascular coupling	*Favorable changes in ventricular diastolic function, arterial elastance, and ventricular-arterial coupling.
Eggebeen et al.[81]	Beet root juice, 6.1 mmol inorganic nitrate (n=20)	Aged 69±7 years of age, ambulatory HF patients with NYHA class II–III symptoms, LVEF ≥50%	Mean LVEF not available	Submaximal aerobic endurance	*Improved submaximal endurance
Zamani et al.[82]	Nitrate-rich beetroot juice, 12.9 mmol (n=17)	Aged 66±9, 12% female, symptomatic HF, echo: L VEF >50%, DD, elevated NT-pro-BNP or PCWP >12 mmHg on prior cardiac catheterization	64±9% (Mean±SD)	Exercise efficiency/ Peak VO_2	*Improves peak VO_2 in subjects with HFpEF by significant reduction in systemic vascular resistance
CHAMPION[43]	CardioMEMs sensor (n=550)	Aged 62±13 years, 29% female, NYHA class III, hospitalization for HF in past 12 months. LVEF ≥40%	62±23% (Mean±SD)	HF hospitalization	*Significant and large reduction in hospitalization for patients with NYHA class III HF
REDUCE LAP-HF[45]	Transcatheter interatrial shunt device (n=68)	Aged 69±8 years, 61% female, NYHA class II–IV symptoms, PCWP at rest >15 mmHg and during exercise >25 mmHg measured invasively, LVEF >40%	47±7% (Mean±SD)	PCWP	*Reduced PCWP during exercise *Improved NYHA class, 6-min walk distance, health related quality of life
REDUCE LAP –HF[83]	Transcatheter interatrial shunt device (n=44)	Aged 70±9 years, 50% female, NYHA class II–IV, PCWP at rest >15 mmHg and during exercise >25 mmHg measured invasively, LVEF >40%	59±8% (Mean±SD)	PCWP	*Reduced PCWP during exercise
Yoshihisa et al.[63]	Adaptive servo-ventilation (n=36)	64±16 years, 11% female, NYHA class II–IV HF, stable clinical status, with moderate to severe sleep disorder breathing LVEF >50%	56±7% (Mean±SD)	Improvement in symptoms, cardiac function, and arterial function	*Improved NYHA class, left atrial volume, BNP, diastolic function. Fewer patients had CV events or HF admission with intervention
CAT HF[62]	Minute ventilation adaptive servo-ventilation (n=126)	Aged 61±14 years, 26% female, hospitalized HF, BNP ≥300 pg/mL, with moderate to severe sleep apnea	24 (19%) HFpEF 55±6% (Mean±SD)	Composite global rank score (hierarchy of death, CV hospitalizations, and % changes in 6MWD	No overall difference in outcome between the two groups. *In HFpEF: risk of primary composite endpoint was reduced by 62%
RDT-PEF[52]	Renal denervation (n=25)	Aged 74±6 years, 40% female, NYHA class II–III HF, ECHO-DD, BNP ≥35 ng/mL, LVEF ≥50%	Not available	NYHA class, Peak VO_2, quality of life score, BNP, E/e', LV remodeling	Terminated early because of difficulties in recruitment—underpowered

* Significant improvement (P<0.05).

Abbreviations: DASH = dietary approaches to stop hypertension; HFpEF = heart failure with preserved ejection fraction; LVEF = left ventricular ejection fraction; n = number of participants; NYHA = New York Heart Association; HF = heart failure; ECHO = echocardiographically assessed; DD = diastolic dysfunction; SD = standard deviation; VO_2 = oxygen consumption; KCCQ = Kansas City Cardiomyopathy Questionnaire; NT pro-BNP = N terminal, B-type natriuretic peptide; PCWP = pulmonary capillary wedge pressure; BNP = B-type natriuretic peptide; CV = cardiovascular; LA = left atrium; RDT = renal denervation therapy; E = mitral early diastolic velocity; e' = mitral annular velocity.

of patients with documented HF and LVEF >50% showed that many patients appear to have modest diastolic dysfunction under resting conditions.[13,66] In addition, fibrosis in HFpEF appears to be relatively modest.[67] Finally, pharmacologic interventions that were beneficial in HFrEF on the basis of severe underlying, neurohormonal abnormalities met with limited success in HFpEF, as neurohormonal derangements appeared more limited in breadth and severity in HFpEF.[68–70]

Emerging concepts in HFpEF suggest that the disorder is far more complex, and likely a highly integrated multisystem disorder. In this new paradigm, aging, along with multiple comorbidities, may initiate and/or aggravate chronic systemic inflammation. This may affect myocardial remodeling and dysfunction through a signaling cascade, beginning with microvascular endothelial inflammation and capillary rarefaction (Figure 15.4).[71,72] This new paradigm led to the design of the Optimizing The Management of HFpEF in the Elderly by Optimizing Comorbidities(OPTIMIZE-HFpEF) study, which aimed to determine whether the combination of systematic screening and optimal management of prespecified comorbidities associated with HFpEF improved outcomes.[73]

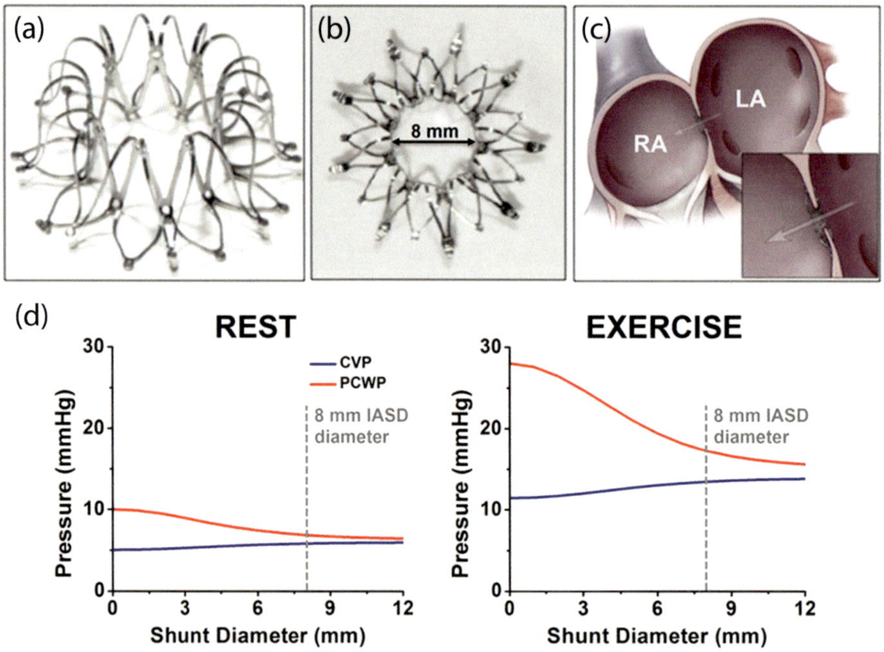

FIGURE 15.3 (a) Corvia Interatrial Shunt Device (IASD) System II. (b) "En face" view of the IASD System II (single size, internal diameter = 8 mm). (c) The IASD creates an interatrial shunt that unloads the left atrium by shunting blood from the higher-pressure left atrium to the lower-pressure right atrium. (d) Simulation studies have shown that an 8-mm internal diameter for the shunt device is optimal in maximally reducing left atrial pressure without overloading the right heart (i.e., keeping pulmonary-to-systemic flow relatively low at a 1.2–1.3 range). CVP indicates central venous pressure (right atrial pressure). (Reproduced with permission from Feldman et al., *Circulation* 2018;137:364–75.)

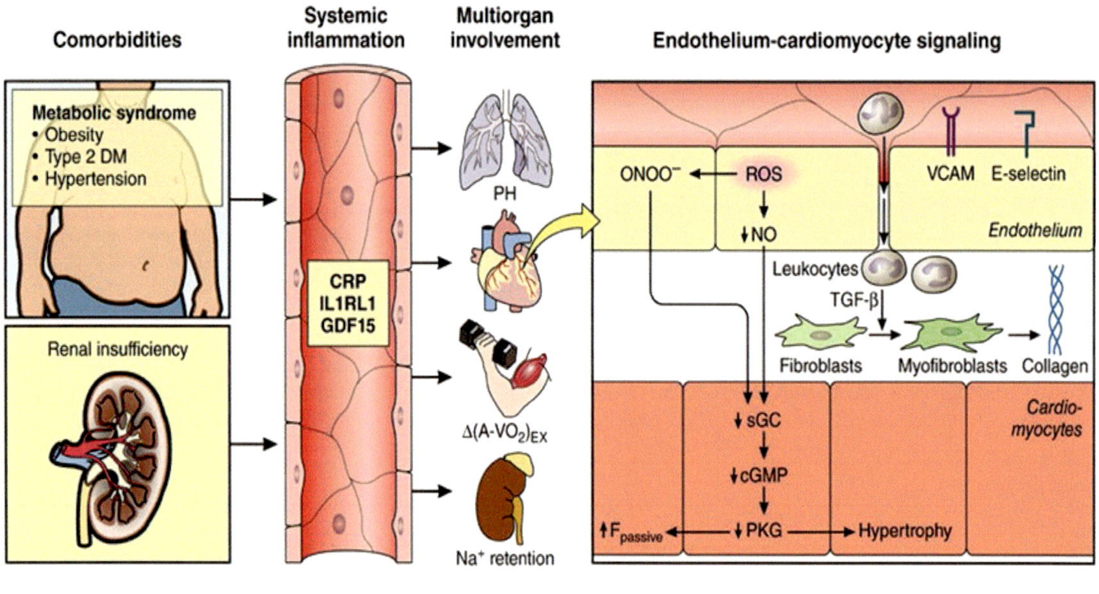

FIGURE 15.4 Systemic and myocardial signaling in HFpEF. Comorbidities induce systemic inflammation, evident from elevated plasma levels of inflammatory biomarkers, such as soluble interleukin-1 receptor-like 1 (IL-1RL1), C-reactive protein (CRP), and growth differentiation factor 15 (GDF15). Chronic inflammation affects the lungs, myocardium, skeletal muscle, and kidneys, leading to diverse HFpEF phenotypes with variable involvement of pulmonary hypertension (PH), myocardial remodeling, deficient skeletal muscle oxygen extraction (ΔA-VO$_2$) during exercise (Ex), and renal Na+ retention. Myocardial remodeling and dysfunction begin with coronary endothelial microvascular inflammation manifest from endothelial expression of adhesion molecules, such as vascular cell adhesion molecule (VCAM) and E-selectin. Expression of adhesion molecules attracts infiltrating leukocytes secreting transforming growth factor β (TGF-β), which converts fibroblasts to myofibroblasts with enhanced interstitial collagen deposition. Endothelial inflammation also results in the presence of reactive oxygen species (ROS), reduced nitric oxide (NO) bioavailability, and production of peroxynitrite (ONOO$^-$). This reduces soluble guanylate cyclase (sGC) activity, cyclic guanosine monophosphate (cGMP) concentration, and the favorable effects of protein kinase G (PKG) on cardiomyocyte stiffness and hypertrophy. HFpEF indicates heart failure with preserved ejection fraction. (Reproduced with permission from Shah et al., *Circulation* 2016;134:73–90.)

TABLE 15.3: Clinical Trials of Pharmacological Therapies in HFpEF

First Author or Trial Acronym	Intervention	HFpEF Patient Type	LVEF	Primary Endpoint	Trial Result
CHARM-Preserved[84]	Candesartan (n=3023)	Aged 67±11 years, 40% female, NYHA class II–IV HF and LVEF >40%. Prior cardiac hospitalization	54±9% (Mean±SD)	CV death or HF admission	No benefit with respect to CV death *Fewer HF admissions
The PEP-CHF[85]	Perindopril (n=850)	Aged 76±5 years, 55% female, diagnosis of HF and treated with diuretics and an Echo-DD. Prior cardiac hospitalization LVEF >40%	65 (56–66)% Median with Interquartile range	All-cause mortality and HF admission	No benefit with respect to mortality orHF admission *Fewer HF admissions, improved symptoms and exercise capacity
I-PRESERVE[86]	Irbesartan (n=4128)	Aged 72±7 years, 60% female, hospitalized for HF during the previous six months and have current NYHA class II-IV symptoms. LVEF >45%	60±9 % (Mean±SD)	Death from any cause or hospitalization for a CV cause	No benefit to risk of death or hospitalization from CV causes No improvement in quality of life
PIE-I / Kitzman et al.[87]	Enalapril (n=71)	Elderly (70±1 years), predominant female (80%) with compensated HF. LVEF ≥50%	66±6% (Mean±SD)	Peak VO_2 and 6MWD	No benefit toward peak exercise capacity or in submaximal exercise performance, aortic distensibility
TOPCAT[88]	Spironolactone (n=3445)	Aged 69 years (Median), 52% female, symptomatic HF. Patients had a HF hospitalization within previous 12 months and elevated BNP within 60 days before randomization. LVEF >45%	56 (51–61)% Median with Interquartile range	CV death or aborted cardiac arrest, HF hospitalization	No benefit with primary outcome *Modest decline HF hospitalization
Aldo-DHF[89]	Spironolactone (n=422)	Aged 67±8 years, 52% female, ambulatory patients/ NYHA class II–III symptoms, grade 1 DD and normal or near-normal BNP levels. LVEF >50%	67±8% (Mean±SD)	Peak VO_2, change in E/e’	Exercise capacity and quality-of-life measures remained unchanged. *LV remodeling, neurohumoral activation were improved
RAAM-PEF[90]	Eplerenone (n=44)	Aged 71±10 years, 7% female, symptomatic NYHA class II–III, increased BNP within 60 days. LVEF ≥50%	62±5% (Mean±SD)	6MWD	No improvement in exercise capacity *Reduction in serum markers of collagen turnover
Kosmala et al.[91]	Spironolactone (n=150)	Age 67±9 years; 85% female, NYHA class II–III, DD, and baseline increased exercise E/e′ ratio, LVEF >50%	73 (7075)% Median with interquartile range	Peak VO_2 and exertional E/e′ ratio	*Improved exercise capacity *Reduced exercise-induced echocardiographically increased LV filling pressure
Upadhya et al.[92]	Spironolactone (n=80)	Elderly (71±1 years), predominant female (80%) with compensated HF	63±1% (Mean±SD)	Peak VO_2, 6MWD and arterial function	Did not improve exercise capacity, quality of life, LV mass, or arterial stiffness
J-DHF[93]	Carvedilol (low-dose) (n=245)	72±10 years, 42% female, ambulatory, NYHA class II–III symptoms, grade I DD, and normal or near-normal BNP levels, LVEF >40%	62±10% (Mean±SD)	Death or HF hospitalization	No benefit with death or HF hospitalization
ELANDD[94]	Nebivolol (n=116)	Aged 67±10 years, 65% female, ambulatory, NYHA class II-III, grade I DD, and normal or near-normal BNP levels. LVEF >45%	62±8% (Mean±SD)	6MWD	Did not improve 6MWD Did not improve peak VO_2, quality of life
NEAT-HFPEF trial[95]	Isosorbide mononitrate (n=110)	Age 69±9 years, 57% female, ambulatory, prior admission for HF within 12 months or increased invasive LV filling pressure or elevated BNP or echo-DD, LVEF ≥50%	62±8% (Mean±SD)	Daily activity level, 6MWD	Those who received isosorbide mononitrate were less active and did not have better quality of life than did patients who received placebo
Borlaug et al.[96]	Inhaled sodium nitrite (n=26)	Age 70±9 years, 54% female, elevated PCWP at rest (>15 mmHg) and with exercise (≥25 mmHg). LVEF ≥50%	62±4% (Mean±SD)	PCWP during exercise	*Acute administration reduces biventricular filling pressures and PAP at rest and during exercise

(Continued)

TABLE 15.3 (Continued): Clinical Trials of Pharmacological Therapies in HFpEF

First Author or Trial Acronym	Intervention	HFpEF Patient Type	LVEF	Primary Endpoint	Trial Result
INDIE-HFpEF[97]	Inhaled inorganic nitrite (n=105)	Age 68±9 years, 56% female, elevated PCWP at rest (≥15 mmHg) and with exercise (≥25 mmHg), elevated, prior admission for HF within 12 months or elevated BNP or echo-DD, LVEF ≥50%	LVEF ≥50%	Peak VO_2	No significant difference in primary endpoint No significant effect on daily activities
RELAX[98]	Sildenafil (n=216)	Aged 69 years (median), 48% female, elevated BNP or elevated, invasive LV filling pressure. LVEF >50%	60 (55–65)% Median with interquartile range	Peak VO_2	No significant improvement in exercise capacity or clinical status
Guazzi et al.[99,100]	Sildenafil (n=44)	Aged 72 years (median), 20% female, HF signs and symptoms, DD, invasively measured PASP >40 mmHg, LVEF ≥50%	60±4% (Mean±SD)	Mean PAP, RV function	*Improvement in PAP, RV function and dimension, LV ventricular relaxation and distensibility
Hoendermis et al.[101]	Sildenafil (n=52)	Aged 74±10 years, 71% was female, NYHA class II–IV HF, mean PAP >25 mmHg PCWP >15 mmHg. LVEF ≥45%	58±4% (Mean±SD)	Change in mean PAP	Did not improve any invasive parameters
RELAX-AHF trial[42]	Serelaxin (IV infusion) Recombinant human relaxin-2 (n=161)	Aged 75±10 years, 58% female, hospitalized with acute decompensated HF	281 (26%) had HFpEF 59±7 (Mean±SD)	Dyspnea, mortality at 180 days	Failed to improve post-discharge readmission rate *Significant 37% reduction in 180-day cardiovascular and all-cause mortality and was well tolerated
DILATE -1[102]	Riociguat (soluble guanylate cyclase stimulator) (n=36)	Mean age 71 years, 61% female, stable symptomatic HF, mean PASP ≥25 mmHg and PCWP >15 mmHg. LVEF >50%	62±7% (Mean±SD)	Change in mean PAP	No significant effect on mean PAP
SOCRATES-PRESERVED[103]	Vericiguat (soluble guanylate cyclase stimulator) (n=477)	73±10, 48% female, NYHA class II–IV, LVEF ≥45%, increased BNP ≥100 pg/mL or NT-proBNP levels ≥300 pg/mL ECHO evidence of DD, LVEF ≥45%	57 (53–61)% Median with interquartile range	Change in NT-proBNP Change in LA volume	No change in NT-proBNP and LA volume *Improvements in quality of life
DIAMOND / Little et al.[104]	Alagebrium chloride (n=23)	Mean age 71 years, 57% female, stable ambulatory NYHA class II–III. LVEF >50%	65±4% (Mean±SD)	Peak VO_2	No change in peak VO_2 *Decreased LV mass and improved LV diastolic filling and quality of life
RALI-DHF[105]	Ranolazine (n=20)	Age 71±2 years, 80% female, NYHA class II–III HF, Echo-DD, NT-pro BNP >220 pg/mL, resting LVEDP ≥18 mmHg, LVEF ≥45%	66±2% (Mean±SD)	LVEDP, PCWP	*Some improvement in hemodynamics: PAP No improvement in relaxation parameters
Zile et al.[106]	Sitaxsentan (selective endothelin type A antagonist) (n=192)	Age 65±11 years, female 63%, NYHA class II–III HF, Echo-DD, LVEF ≥50%	62±12% (Mean±SD)	Change in treadmill exercise time	*Increased exercise tolerance. No improvement in LV mass or diastolic function
PARAMOUNT[66]	LCZ696(ARNI) (n=301)	Age 71±9 years, 57% female, NYHA class II–III HF, NT-pro BNP >400 pg/nL and be on a diuretic therapy. LVEF >45%	58±7% (Mean±SD)	Change in NT-proBNP	*Significant reduction in NT-proBNP
Kosmala et al.[107]	Ivabradine (n=61)	Aged 67±9 years, 82% female, ambulatory patients, NYHA class II–III, grade I DD, normal or near-normal BNP levels. LVEF >50%	67±7% (Mean±SD)	Peak VO_2, Peak E/e'	*Increased exercise capacity, with a contribution from improved LV filling pressure response to exercise

* Significant improvement ($P<0.05$).

Abbreviations: HFpEF = heart failure with preserved ejection fraction; n = number of participants; NYHA = New York Heart Association; HF = heart failure; LVEF = left ventricular ejection fraction; SD = standard deviation; CV = cardiovascular; DD = diastolic dysfunction; VO_2 = oxygen consumption; MWD = minute walk distance; BNP = B-type natriuretic peptide; E = mitral early diastolic velocity; e' = mitral annular velocity; LV = left ventricle; PCWP = pulmonary capillary wedge pressure; PASP = pulmonary artery systolic pressure; RV = right ventricle; MAP = mean pulmonary artery pressure; NT pro BNP = N terminal, B-type natriuretic peptide; LA = left atrium LVEDP = left ventricular end diastolic pressure; ARNI = angiotensin receptor-neprilysin.

As noted above, one potentially unifying mechanistic theory for cardiac dysfunction in HFpEF is comorbidity-driven systemic and microvascular inflammation leading to a number of sequela including oxidative stress, which reduces NO bioavailability, that impairs soluble guanylate cyclase (sGC) activity, which produces less cGMP, and thus, reduces PKG signaling.[71] Several trials have assessed the role of this pathway in HFpEF with limited success (Table 15.3). Another method to augment cGMP/PKG signaling is by stimulating the natriuretic-peptide receptor sGC pathway. One method in clinical use is to block the peptidase neprilysin, which reduces natriuretic-peptide proteolytic cleavage as one of its effects, thereby increasing cGMP/PKG signaling.[74] LCZ696, a new combination drug of the angiotensin II type-1 receptor blocker valsartan and the neprilysin inhibitor pro-drug AHU377, exerts a powerful vasodilatory and natriuresis effect by blocking angiotensin II activity, while also augmenting plasma levels of natriuretic peptides. LCZ696 has been shown to improve mortality in HFrEF. In the Prospective Comparison of ARNI with ARB on Management of HF trial (PARAMOUNT), with LCZ696 significantly lowering NT-pro-B-type natriuretic peptide. At 36 weeks, LA size decreased and there was a trend toward improved functional class.[66] Currently, LCZ696 is being tested in the large-scale Efficacy and Safety of LCZ696 Compared to Valsartan on Morbidity and Mortality in HFpEF (PARAGON) trial (NCT01920711). Table 15.3 summarizes the pharmacological therapies tested to date in HFpEF. Table 15.4 summarizes ongoing or planned trials with respect to HFpEF.

Phenotype-Specific Treatment

One likely explanation for the lack of success in HFpEF trials is the incompatibility of the one-size-fits-all trial design approach with the highly heterogeneous HFpEF population.[75] Indeed, manifestations can vary markedly from patient to patient[76] even within a specific HFpEF patient population.[77] Recently, Shah et al. have proposed the existence of specific phenotypes of HFpEF, which provides a framework to tailor future trials.[78] By utilizing a matrix combining predisposition phenotypes with clinical presentation phenotypes, clinicians may better provide individual care for patients with HFpEF (Figure 15.5).[75] This concept was recently expanded upon by Lewis et al.[46] These authors suggest that determining the underlying pathobiologic disease mechanisms ultimately leads to specific clinical phenotypes. This can drive discernment of the "biological phenotype" from the "clinical phenotypes" and further enhance the potential gains from individualized approaches on the basis of enhanced phenotypic categorization.

TABLE 15.4: Ongoing or Planned Trials in HFpEF

ClinicalTrials.gov Identifier	Intervention	HFpEF Patient Type	Primary Endpoint	Estimated Completion Date
NCT02713126	Inhaled sodium nitrite	≥50 years, NYHA class II–1V, prior hospitalization for HF or Echo-DD or NT-pro BNP >400 pg/mL or resting LVEDP ≥18 mmHg with LVEF ≥50%	Change in exercise capacity, measured by peak VO_2	4/2020
NCT01542502 D-HART2	Anakinra recombinant human IL-1 receptor antagonist	Age >21 years, NYHA class II–III HF, increased LVEDP >16 measured invasively, Echo- DD, BNP >200 pg/mL, LVEF >50%, CRP >2.0 mg/L	Peak VO_2	7/2017
NCT01920711 PARAGON	LCZ696	Aged ≥50 years, HF, NYHA class II–III HF, Echo-DD, NT-pro BNP >400 pg/nL and be on a diuretic therapy. LVEF ≥45%	CV death and HF hospitalization	3/2019
PARALLAX NCT03066804	LCZ696	Aged ≥45 years, NYHA class II–III HF, NT-pro BNP >220 pg/μL and h/o HF on a diuretic therapy. LVEF ≥45%	Change in NT pro-BNP	1/2018
NCT02145351 RAPID	Rate adaptive atrial pacing using a dual-chamber pacemaker	>18 years, NYHA class III 1V, prior hospitalization for HF, NT-pro BNP ≥400 pg/mL or resting LVEDP >20 mmHg, peak VO_2 ≤60% age-/sex-adjusted normal value with LVEF ≥50%	Peak VO_2	5/2018
NCT03098979 PANACHE	Neladenoson bialanate (Partial Adenosine A1 Receptor Agonist)	≥45 years, h/o of HF with NYHA class II–IV, LVEF ≥45%, elevated NT-proBNP	6MWD	6/2018
NCT03030235 PRESERVED-HF	Dapagliflozin SGLT-2 inhibitors	≥19 years, Type II DM, NYHA class II–IV, LVEF ≥45% NT-proBNP ≥300 pg/mL or BNP ≥100 pg/mL.	Change in NT-proBNP	3/2019
FAIR-HFpEF NCT03074591	Intravenous iron (ferric carboxymaltose)	≥18 years, ambulatory HF NYHA class II or III treated with a diuretic, raised plasma levels of natriuretic peptides, hemoglobin >9.0 g/dL and ≤14.0 g/dL, Echo-DD, LVEF ≥45%	6MWD	7/2019
SERENADE NCT03153111	Macitentan (endothelin receptor antagonist)	≥18 years, h/o HF on oral diuretic, LVEF ≥40%, Echo-DD, HF hospitalization within 12 months, PCWP or LVEDP >15 mmHg, elevated NT-proBNP, pulmonary vascular disease or RV dysfunction	Change in NT-proBNP	5/2020
SOUTHPAW NCT03037580	Oral treprostinil (prostacyclin analogue)	≥18 years, LVEF ≥50%, PH documented in RHC within 90 days of screening	Change in 6MWD	7/2020

Abbreviations: HFpEF = heart failure with preserved ejection fraction; n = number of participants; NYHA = New York Heart Association; HF = heart failure; Echo-DD = echocardiographic evidence of diastolic dysfunction; NT-pro BNP = N terminal B-type natriuretic peptide; LVEDP = left ventricular end diastolic pressure; LVEF = left ventricular ejection fraction; VO_2 = oxygen consumption; IL= interleukin; BNP = B-type natriuretic peptide; CRP = C-reactive protein; CV = cardiovascular; PCWP = pulmonary capillary wedge pressure; MWD = minute walk distance; DM = diabetes; RV = right ventricle; PH = pulmonary hypertension.

HFpEF Clinical Presentation Phenotypes

HFpEF Predisposition Phenotypes	Lung Congestion	+Chronotropic Incompetence	+Pulmonary Hypertension (CpcPH)	+Skeletal muscle weakness	+Atrial Fibrillation
Overweight/obesity/ metabolic syndrome/ type 2 DM	• **Diuretics (loop diuretic in DM)** • **Caloric restriction** • Statins • Inorganic nitrite/nitrate • Sacubitril • Spironolactone	+Rate adaptive atrial pacing	+Pulmonary vasodilators (e.g. PDE5I)	**+Exercise training program**	+Cardioversion + Rate Control **+Anticoagulation**
+Arterial hypertension	+ACEI/ARB	+ACEI/ARB +Rate adaptive atrial pacing	+ACEI/ARB +Pulmonary vasodilators (e.g. PDE5I)	+ACEI/ARB **+Exercise training program**	+ACEI/ARB +Cardioversion + Rate Control **+Anticoagulation**
+Renal dysfunction	+Ultrafiltration if needed	+Ultrafiltration if needed +Rate adaptive atrial pacing	+Ultrafiltration if needed +Pulmonary vasodilators (e.g. PDE5I)	+Ultrafiltration if needed **+Exercise training program**	+Ultrafiltration if needed +Cardioversion + Rate Control **+Anticoagulation**
+CAD	+ACEI +Revascularization	+ACEI +Revascularization +Rate adaptive atrial pacing	+ACEI +Revascularization +Pulmonary vasodilators (e.g. PDE5I)	+ACEI +Revascularization **+Exercise training program**	+ACEI +Revascularization +Cardioversion + Rate Control **+Anticoagulation**

FIGURE 15.5 Phenotype-specific HFpEF treatment strategy using a matrix of predisposition phenotypes and clinical presentation phenotypes. (Reproduced with permission from Upadhya et al., *Heart Fail Rev* 2018;23:609–29.)

Future Directions

The development of novel pharmacological agents for treating HFpEF can be centered on our understanding of the two strategies that have been shown to improve clinically meaningful outcomes in HFpEF, namely exercise training and cardiac rehabilitation.[79] Both of these interventions have broad, pleotropic, systemic, and anti-inflammatory effects, as well as favorable effects on multiple organ systems, including effects on arterial, cardiac, and skeletal muscle.[79] Future clinical trials may need to stratify HFpEF into distinct clinical groups. As suggested by Shah et al., phenomapping could be helpful for improved classification of HFpEF patients in terms of effective targeted therapies and may lead to the development of future clinical trials with more tailored design.[78] Approaches that can identify HFpEF sub-phenotypes, determine the underlying mechanism(s), and then create targeted interventions for these specific subtypes may be clinically fruitful. In addition, successful development of a robust HFpEF animal model could further aid in treatment discoveries and help to address the growing HFpEF epidemic.

Conclusion

HFpEF is the most common form of HF in the community. Its prevalence is increasing, and its prognosis has not improved. The effective pharmacological treatment of HFpEF remains challenging. Based on emerging evidence, HFpEF is likely a complex, multi-factorial, systemic syndrome driven by age-related processes, inflammation, chronic comorbidities, and multi-organ involvement with substantial clinical heterogeneity. Clearly, HFpEF patients may benefit from being further classified based on disease mechanism, phenotype, and etiology. Efforts are underway to utilize these concepts to identify novel therapeutic targets, improve the design of future clinical trials, and develop effective clinical management algorithms.

Potential Financial Conflicts of Interest

Dr. Upadhya has received research funding from Novartis and Corvia.

References

1. Tsao CW, Lyass A, Enserro D, et al. Temporal trends in the incidence of and mortality associated with heart failure with preserved and reduced ejection fraction. *JACC Heart Fail.* 2018;6:678–85.
2. Steinberg BA, Zhao X, Heidenreich PA, et al. Trends in patients hospitalized with heart failure and preserved left ventricular ejection fraction: Prevalence, therapies, and outcomes. *Circulation.* 2012;126:65–75.
3. Owan TE, Hodge DO, Herges RM, et al. Trends in prevalence and outcome of heart failure with preserved ejection fraction. *N Engl J Med.* 2006;355:251–9.
4. Nichols GA, Reynolds K, Kimes TM, Rosales AG, Chan WW. Comparison of risk of re-hospitalization, allcCause mortality, and medical care resource utilization in patients with heart failure and preserved versus reduced ejection fraction. *Am J Cardiol.* 2015;116:1088–92.
5. Yancy CW, Jessup M, Bozkurt B, et al. 2017 ACC/AHA/HFSA focused update of the 2013 ACCF/AHA guideline for the management of heart failure: A report of the American College of Cardiology/American Heart Association Task Force on Clinical Practice Guidelines and the Heart Failure Society of America. *J Am Coll Cardiol.* 2017;70:776–803.
6. Wright JT, Jr., Williamson JD, Whelton PK, et al. A randomized trial of intensive versus standard blood-pressure control. *N Engl J Med.* 2015;373:2103–16.
7. Upadhya B, Rocco M, Lewis CE, et al. Effect of intensive blood pressure treatment on heart failure events in the systolic blood pressure reduction intervention trial. *Circ Heart Fail.* 2017;10:e003613.
8. Lindenfeld J, Albert NM, Boehmer JP, et al. Executive summary: HFSA 2010 comprehensive heart failure practice guideline. *J Card Fail.* 2010;16:475–539.
9. Ponikowski P, Voors AA, Anker SD, et al. 2016 ESC guidelines for the diagnosis and treatment of acute and chronic heart failure: The Task Force for the diagnosis and treatment of acute and chronic heart failure of the European Society of Cardiology (ESC). Developed with the special contribution of the Heart Failure Association (HFA) of the ESC. *Eur J Heart Fail.* 2016;18:891–975.
10. Alves AJ, Ribeiro F, Goldhammer E, et al. Exercise training improves diastolic function in heart failure patients. *Med Sci Sports Exerc.* 2012;44:776–85.

11. Davis BR, Kostis JB, Simpson LM, et al. Heart failure with preserved and reduced left ventricular ejection fraction in the antihypertensive and lipid-lowering treatment to prevent heart attack trial. *Circulation.* 2008;118:2259–67.
12. Ndumele CE, Coresh J, Lazo M, et al. Obesity, subclinical myocardial injury, and incident heart failure. *JACC Heart Fail.* 2014;2:600–7.
13. Haykowsky MJ, Kouba EJ, Brubaker PH, et al. Skeletal muscle composition and its relation to exercise intolerance in older patients with heart failure and preserved ejection fraction. *Am J Cardiol.* 2014;113:1211–6.
14. Beavers KM, Beavers DP, Houston DK, et al. Associations between body composition and gait-speed decline: Results from the health, aging, and body composition study. *Am J Clin Nutr.* 2013;97:552–60.
15. Normandin E, Houston DK, Nicklas BJ. Caloric restriction for treatment of geriatric obesity: Do the benefits outweigh the risks? *Curr Opin Cardiol.* 2015;4:143–55.
16. Sharma K, Kass DA. Heart failure with preserved ejection fraction: Mechanisms, clinical features, and therapies. *Circ Res.* 2014;115:79–96.
17. Fitchett D, Inzucchi SE, Cannon CP, et al. Empagliflozin reduced mortality and hospitalization for heart failure across the spectrum of cardiovascular risk in the EMPA-REG OUTCOME trial. *Circulation.* 2019;139:1384–95.
18. Furtado RHM, Bonaca MP, Raz I, et al. Dapagliflozin and cardiovascular outcomes in patients with type 2 diabetes mellitus and previous myocardial infarction. *Circulation.* 2019;139:2516–27.
19. Pandey A, LaMonte M, Klein L, et al. Relationship between physical activity, body mass index, and risk of heart failure. *J Am Coll Cardiol.* 2017;69:1129–42.
20. Pandey A, Parashar A, Kumbhani D, et al. Exercise training in patients with heart failure and preserved ejection fraction: Meta-analysis of randomized control trials. *Circ Heart Fail.* 2015;8:33–40.
21. Tucker WJ, Nelson MD, Beaudry RI, et al. Impact of exercise training on peak oxygen uptake and its determinants in heart failure with preserved ejection fraction. *Card Fail* Rev. 2016;2:95–101.
22. Tucker WJ, Lijauco CC, Hearon CM, Jr., et al. Mechanisms of the improvement in peak VO_2 with exercise training in heart failure with reduced or preserved ejection fraction. *Heart Lung Circ.* 2018;27:9–21.
23. Kitzman DW, Brubaker P, Morgan T, et al. Effect of caloric restriction or aerobic exercise training on peak oxygen consumption and quality of life in obese older patients with heart failure with preserved ejection fraction: a randomized clinical trial. *JAMA.* 2016;315:36–46.
24. Fu TC, Yang NI, Wang CH, et al. Aerobic interval training elicits different hemodynamic adaptations between heart failure patients with preserved and reduced ejection fraction. *Am J Phys Med Rehabil.* 2016;95:15–27.
25. Angadi SS, Mookadam F, Lee CD, et al. High-intensity interval training vs. moderate-intensity continuous exercise training in heart failure with preserved ejection fraction: A pilot study. *J Appl Physiol (1985).* 2015;119:753–8.
26. Heart Failure Society of A, Lindenfeld J, Albert NM, et al. HFSA 2010 comprehensive heart failure practice guideline. *J Card Fail.* 2010;16:e1–194.
27. Kitzman DW, Brubaker PH, Morgan TM, Stewart KP, Little WC. Exercise training in older patients with heart failure and preserved ejection fraction: A randomized, controlled, single-blind trial. *Circ Heart Fail.* 2010;3:659–67.
28. Kitzman DW, Brubaker PH, Herrington DM, et al. Effect of endurance exercise training on endothelial function and arterial stiffness in older patients with heart failure and preserved ejection fraction: A randomized, controlled, single-blind trial. *J Am Coll Cardiol.* 2013;62:584–92.
29. Haykowsky MJ, Brubaker PH, Stewart KP, et al. Effect of endurance training on the determinants of peak exercise oxygen consumption in elderly patients with stable compensated heart failure and preserved ejection fraction. *J Am Coll Cardiol.* 2012;60:120–8.
30. Edelmann F, Gelbrich G, Dungen HD, et al. Exercise training improves exercise capacity and diastolic function in patients with heart failure with preserved ejection fraction: Results of the Ex-DHF (Exercise training in Diastolic Heart Failure) pilot study. *J Am Coll Cardiol.* 2011;58:1780–91.
31. Smart NA, Haluska B, Jeffriess L, Leung D. Exercise training in heart failure with preserved systolic function: A randomized controlled trial of the effects on cardiac function and functional capacity. *Congest Heart Fail.* 2012;18:295–301.
32. Gary RA, Sueta CA, Dougherty M, et al. Home-based exercise improves functional performance and quality of life in women with diastolic heart failure. *Heart Lung.* 2004;33:210–8.
33. Kitzman DW. Understanding results of trials in heart failure with preserved ejection fraction: Remembering forgotten lessons and enduring principles. *J Am Coll Cardiol.* 2011;57:1687–9.
34. Sullivan MJ, Higginbotham MB, Cobb FR. Exercise training in patients with severe left ventricular dysfunction. Hemodynamic and metabolic effects. *Circulation.* 1988;78:506–15.
35. Haykowsky MJ, Brubaker PH, John JM, et al. Determinants of exercise intolerance in elderly heart failure patients with preserved ejection fraction. *J Am Coll Cardiol.* 2011;58:265–74.
36. Borlaug BA, Olson TP, Lam CS, et al. Global cardiovascular reserve dysfunction in heart failure with preserved ejection fraction. *J Am Coll Cardiol.* 2010;56:845–54.
37. Fujimoto N, Prasad A, Hastings JL, et al. Cardiovascular effects of 1 year of progressive endurance exercise training in patients with heart failure with preserved ejection fraction. *Am Heart J.* 2012;164:869–77.
38. Taylor RS, Davies EJ, Dalal HM, et al. Effects of exercise training for heart failure with preserved ejection fraction: A systematic review and meta-analysis of comparative studies. *Int J Cardiol.* 2012;162:6–13.
39. Erbs S, Hollriegel R, Linke A, et al. Exercise training in patients with advanced chronic heart failure (NYHA IIIb) promotes restoration of peripheral vasomotor function, induction of endogenous regeneration, and improvement of left ventricular function. *Circ Heart Fail.* 2010;3:486–94.
40. Esposito F, Reese V, Shabetai R, Wagner PD, Richardson RS. Isolated quadriceps training increases maximal exercise capacity in chronic heart failure: The role of skeletal muscle convective and diffusive oxygen transport. *J Am Coll Cardiol.* 2011;58:1353–62.
41. O'Connor CM, Whellan DJ, Lee KL, et al. Efficacy and safety of exercise training in patients with chronic heart failure: HF-ACTION randomized controlled trial. *JAMA.* 2009;301:1439–50.
42. Filippatos G, Teerlink JR, Farmakis D, et al. Serelaxin in acute heart failure patients with preserved left ventricular ejection fraction: Results from the RELAX-AHF trial. *Eur Heart J.* 2014;35:1041–50.
43. Abraham WT, Adamson PB, Bourge RC, et al. Wireless pulmonary artery haemodynamic monitoring in chronic heart failure: A randomised controlled trial. *Lancet.* 2011;377:658–66.
44. Adamson PB, Abraham WT, Bourge RC, et al. Wireless pulmonary artery pressure monitoring guides management to reduce decompensation in heart failure with preserved ejection fraction. *Circ Heart Fail.* 2014;7:935–44.
45. Hasenfuss G, Hayward C, Burkhoff D, et al. A transcatheter intracardiac shunt device for heart failure with preserved ejection fraction (REDUCE LAP-HF): A multicentre, open-label, single-arm, phase 1 trial. *Lancet.* 2016;387:1298–304.
46. Lewis GA, Schelbert EB, Williams SG, et al. biological phenotypes of heart failure with preserved ejection fraction. *J Am Coll Cardiol.* 2017;70:2186–200.
47. Penicka M, Kocka V, Herman D, Trakalova H, Herold M. Cardiac resynchronization therapy for the causal treatment of heart failure with preserved ejection fraction: Insight from a pressure-volume loop analysis. *Eur J Heart Fail.* 2010;12:634–6.
48. Brubaker PH, Joo KC, Stewart KP, et al. Chronotropic incompetence and its contribution to exercise intolerance in older heart failure patients. *J Cardiopulm Rehabil.* 2006;26:86–9.
49. Borlaug BA, Melenovsky V, Russell SD, et al. Impaired chronotropic and vasodilator reserves limit exercise capacity in patients with heart failure and a preserved ejection fraction. *Circulation.* 2006;114:2138–47.
50. Kass DA, Kitzman DW, Alvarez GE. The restoration of chronotropic competence in heart failure patients with normal ejection fraction (RESET) study: Rationale and design. *J Card Fail.* 2010;16:17–24.
51. Laurent G, Eicher JC, Mathe A, et al. Permanent left atrial pacing therapy may improve symptoms in heart failure patients with preserved ejection fraction and atrial dyssynchrony: A pilot study prior to a national clinical research programme. *Eur J Heart Fail.* 2013;15:85–93.
52. Patel HC, Rosen SD, Hayward C, et al. Renal denervation in heart failure with preserved ejection fraction (RDT-PEF): A randomized controlled trial. *Eur J Heart Fail.* 2016;18:703–12.
53. Georgakopoulos D, Little WC, Abraham WT, Weaver FA, Zile MR. Chronic baroreflex activation: A potential therapeutic approach to heart failure with preserved ejection fraction. *J Card Fail.* 2011;17:167–78.
54. Brandt MC, Mahfoud F, Reda S, et al. Renal sympathetic denervation reduces left ventricular hypertrophy and improves cardiac function in patients with resistant hypertension. *J Am Coll Cardiol.* 2012;59:901–9.
55. Dursunoglu D, Dursunoglu N, Evrengul H, et al. Impact of obstructive sleep apnoea on left ventricular mass and global function. *Eur Respir J.* 2005;26:283–8.
56. Usui Y, Takata Y, Inoue Y, et al. Severe obstructive sleep apnea impairs left ventricular diastolic function in non-obese men. *Sleep Med.* 2013;14:155–9.
57. Lattimore JL, Wilcox I, Skilton M, Langenfeld M, Celermajer DS. Treatment of obstructive sleep apnoea leads to improved microvascular endothelial function in the systemic circulation. *Thorax.* 2006;61:491–5.
58. Golbin JM, Somers VK, Caples SM. Obstructive sleep apnea, cardiovascular disease, and pulmonary hypertension. *Proc Am Thorac Soc.* 2008;5:200–6.
59. Romero-Corral A, Somers VK, Pellikka PA, et al. Decreased right and left ventricular myocardial performance in obstructive sleep apnea. *Chest.* 2007;132:1863–70.

60. Oldenburg O, Schmidt A, Lamp B, et al. Adaptive servoventilation improves cardiac function in patients with chronic heart failure and Cheyne-Stokes respiration. *Eur J Heart Fail.* 2008;10:581–6.
61. Eulenburg C, Wegscheider K, Woehrle H, et al. Mechanisms underlying increased mortality risk in patients with heart failure and reduced ejection fraction randomly assigned to adaptive servoventilation in the SERVE-HF study: Results of a secondary multistate modelling analysis. *Lancet Respir Med.* 2016;4:873–81.
62. O'Connor CM, Whellan DJ, Fiuzat M, et al. Cardiovascular outcomes with minute ventilation-targeted adaptive servo-ventilation therapy in heart failure: The CAT-HF trial. *J Am Coll Cardiol.* 2017;69:1577–87.
63. Yoshihisa A, Suzuki S, Yamaki T, et al. Impact of adaptive servo-ventilation on cardiovascular function and prognosis in heart failure patients with preserved left ventricular ejection fraction and sleep-disordered breathing. *Eur J Heart Fail.* 2013;15:543–50.
64. Zile MR, Gottdiener JS, Hetzel SJ, et al. Prevalence and significance of alterations in cardiac structure and function in patients with heart failure and a preserved ejection fraction. *Circulation.* 2011;124:2491–501.
65. Katz DH, Beussink L, Sauer AJ, et al. Prevalence, clinical characteristics, and outcomes associated with eccentric versus concentric left ventricular hypertrophy in heart failure with preserved ejection fraction. *Am J Cardiol.* 2013;112:1158–64.
66. Solomon SD, Zile M, Pieske B, et al. The angiotensin receptor neprilysin inhibitor LCZ696 in heart failure with preserved ejection fraction: A phase 2 double-blind randomised controlled trial. *Lancet.* 2012;380:1387–95.
67. Su MY, Lin LY, Tseng YH, et al. CMR-verified diffuse myocardial fibrosis is associated with diastolic dysfunction in HFpEF. *JACC Cardiovasc Imaging.* 2014;7:991–7.
68. Kitzman DW, Little WC, Brubaker PH, et al. Pathophysiological characterization of isolated diastolic heart failure in comparison to systolic heart failure. *JAMA.* 2002;288:2144–50.
69. Maisel A. B-type natriuretic peptide levels: Diagnostic and prognostic in congestive heart failure: What's next? *Circulation.* 2002;105:2328–31.
70. Anjan VY, Loftus TM, Burke MA, et al. Prevalence, clinical phenotype, and outcomes associated with normal B-type natriuretic peptide levels in heart failure with preserved ejection fraction. *Am J Cardiol.* 2012;110:870–6.
71. Paulus WJ, Tschope C. A novel paradigm for heart failure with preserved ejection fraction: Comorbidities drive myocardial dysfunction and remodeling through coronary microvascular endothelial inflammation. *J Am Coll Cardiol.* 2013;62:263–71.
72. Normandin E, Houston DK, Nicklas BJ. Caloric restriction for treatment of geriatric obesity: Do the benefits outweigh the risks? *Curr Opin Cardiol.* 2015;4:143–55.
73. Fu M, Zhou J, Thunstrom E, et al. Optimizing the management of heart failure with preserved ejection fraction in the elderly by targeting comorbidities (OPTIMIZE-HFPEF). *J Card Fail.* 2016;22:539–44.
74. McMurray JJ, Packer M, Desai AS, et al. Angiotensin-neprilysin inhibition versus enalapril in heart failure. *N Engl J Med.* 2014;371:993–1004.
75. Shah SJ, Kitzman DW, Borlaug BA, et al. Phenotype-specific treatment of heart failure with preserved ejection fraction. *Circulation.* 2016;134:73–90.
76. Packer M. Can bain natriuretic peptide be used to guide the management of patients with heart failure and a preserved ejection fraction? *Circ Heart Fail.* 2011;4:538–40.
77. Shah AM, Solomon SD. Phenotypic and pathophysiological heterogeneity in heart failure with preserved ejection fraction. *Eur Heart J.* 2012;33:1716–7.
78. Shah SJ, Katz DH, Selvaraj S, et al. Phenomapping for novel classification of heart failure with preserved ejection fraction. *Circulation.* 2015;131:269–79.
79. De Keulenaer GW, Segers VFM, Zannad F, Brutsaert DL. The future of pleiotropic therapy in heart failure. Lessons from the benefits of exercise training on endothelial function. *Eur J Heart Fail.* 2017;19:603–14.
80. Hummel SL, Seymour EM, Brook RD, et al. Low-sodium DASH diet improves diastolic function and ventricular-arterial coupling in hypertensive heart failure with preserved ejection fraction. *Circ Heart Fail.* 2013;6:1165–71.
81. Eggebeen J, Kim-Shapiro DB, Haykowsky M, et al. One week of daily dosing with beetroot juice improves submaximal endurance and blood pressure in older patients with heart failure and preserved ejection fraction. *JACC Heart Fail.* 2016;4:428–37.
82. Redfield MM, Anstrom KJ, Levine JA, et al. Isosorbide mononitrate in heart failure with preserved ejection fraction. *N Engl J Med.* 2015;373:2314–24.
83. Feldman T, Mauri L, Kahwash R, et al. Transcatheter interatrial shunt device for the treatment of heart failure with preserved ejection fraction (REDUCE LAP-HF I [Reduce Elevated Left Atrial Pressure in Patients With Heart Failure]): A phase 2, randomized, Sham-controlled trial. *Circulation.* 2018;137:364–75.
84. Yusuf S, Pfeffer MA, Swedberg K, et al. Effects of candesartan in patients with chronic heart failure and preserved left-ventricular ejection fraction: The CHARM-preserved trial. *Lancet.* 2003;362:777–81.
85. Cleland JG, Tendera M, Adamus J, et al. The perindopril in elderly people with chronic heart failure (PEP-CHF) study. *Eur Heart J.* 2006;27:2338–45.
86. Massie BM, Carson PE, McMurray JJ, et al. Irbesartan in patients with heart failure and preserved ejection fraction. *N Engl J Med.* 2008;359:2456–67.
87. Kitzman DW, Hundley WG, Brubaker PH, et al. A randomized double-blind trial of enalapril in older patients with heart failure and preserved ejection fraction: Effects on exercise tolerance and arterial distensibility. *Circ Heart Fail.* 2010;3:477–85.
88. Pitt B, Pfeffer MA, Assmann SF, et al. Spironolactone for heart failure with preserved ejection fraction. *N Engl J Med.* 2014;370:1383–92.
89. Edelmann F, Wachter R, Schmidt AG, et al. Effect of spironolactone on diastolic function and exercise capacity in patients with heart failure with preserved ejection fraction: The Aldo-DHF randomized controlled trial. *JAMA.* 2013;309:781–91.
90. Deswal A, Richardson P, Bozkurt B, Mann DL. Results of the randomized aldosterone antagonism in heart failure with preserved ejection fraction trial (RAAM-PEF). *J Card Fail.* 2011;17:634–42.
91. Kosmala W, Rojek A, Przewlocka-Kosmala M, et al. Effect of aldosterone antagonism on exercise tolerance in heart failure with preserved ejection fraction. *J Am Coll Cardiol.* 2016;68:1823–34.
92. Upadhya B, Hundley WG, Brubaker PH, et al. Effect of spironolactone on exercise tolerance and arterial function in older adults with heart failure with preserved ejection fraction. *J Am Geriatr Soc.* 2017;65:2374–82.
93. Yamamoto K, Origasa H, Hori M, Investigators JD. Effects of carvedilol on heart failure with preserved ejection fraction: The Japanese Diastolic Heart Failure Study (J-DHF). *Eur J Heart Fail.* 2013;15:110–8.
94. Conraads VM, Metra M, Kamp O, et al. Effects of the long-term administration of nebivolol on the clinical symptoms, exercise capacity, and left ventricular function of patients with diastolic dysfunction: Results of the ELANDD study. *Eur J Heart Fail.* 2012;14:219–25.
95. Redfield MM, Anstrom KJ, Levine JA, et al. Isosorbide mononitrate in heart failure with preserved ejection fraction. *N Engl J Med.* 2015;373:2314–24.
96. Borlaug BA, Melenovsky V, Koepp KE. Inhaled sodium nitrite improves rest and exercise hemodynamics in heart failure with preserved ejection fraction. *Circ Res.* 2016;119:880–6.
97. Borlaug BA, Anstrom KJ, Lewis GD, et al. Effect of inorganic nitrite vs placebo on exercise capacity among patients with heart failure with preserved ejection fraction: The INDIE-HFpEF randomized clinical trial. *JAMA.* 2018;320:1764–73.
98. Redfield MM, Chen HH, Borlaug BA, et al. Effect of phosphodiesterase-5 inhibition on exercise capacity and clinical status in heart failure with preserved ejection fraction: A randomized clinical trial. *JAMA.* 2013;309:1268–77.
99. Guazzi M, Vicenzi M, Arena R, Md G. Pulmonary hypertension in heart failure with preserved ejection fraction: A target of phosphodiesterase-5 inhibition in a 1-year study. *Circulation.* 2011;124:164–74.
100. Guazzi M, Bandera F, Forfia P. Sildenafil and exercise capacity in heart failure. *JAMA.* 2013;310:432.
101. Hoendermis ES, Liu LC, Hummel YM, et al. Effects of sildenafil on invasive haemodynamics and exercise capacity in heart failure patients with preserved ejection fraction and pulmonary hypertension: A randomized controlled trial. *Eur Heart J.* 2015;36:2565–73.
102. Bonderman D, Pretsch I, Steringer-Mascherbauer R, et al. Acute hemodynamic effects of riociguat in patients with pulmonary hypertension associated with diastolic heart failure (DILATE-1): A randomized, double-blind, placebo-controlled, single-dose study. *Chest.* 2014;146:1274–85.
103. Pieske B, Maggioni AP, Lam CSP, et al. Vericiguat in patients with worsening chronic heart failure and preserved ejection fraction: Results of the SOluble guanylate Cyclase stimulatoR in heArT failurE patientS with PRESERVED EF (SOCRATES-PRESERVED) study. *Eur Heart J.* 2017;38:1119–27.
104. Little WC, Zile MR, Kitzman DW, et al. The effect of alagebrium chloride (ALT-711), a novel glucose cross-link breaker, in the treatment of elderly patients with diastolic heart failure. *J Card Fail.* 2005;11:191–5.
105. Maier LS, Layug B, Karwatowska-Prokopczuk E, et al. RAnoLazIne for the treatment of diastolic heart failure in patients with preserved ejection fraction: The RALI-DHF proof-of-concept study. *JACC Heart Fail.* 2013;1:115–22.
106. Zile MR, Bourge RC, Redfield MM, et al. Randomized, double-blind, placebo-controlled study of sitaxsentan to improve impaired exercise tolerance in patients with heart failure and a preserved ejection fraction. *JACC Heart Fail.* 2014;2:123–30.
107. Kosmala W, Dj H, Rojek A, et al. Effect of if-channel inhibition on hemodynamic status and exercise tolerance in heart failure with preserved ejection fraction: A randomized trial. *J Am Coll Cardiol.* 2013;62:1330–8.

Chapter 16
HEART FAILURE WITH RECOVERED EJECTION FRACTION (HFrecEF) AND HEART FAILURE WITH MIDRANGE EJECTION FRACTION (HFmrEF)

Amil M. Shah and Jenine E. John

Introduction

The clinical syndrome of heart failure (HF) occurs at any left ventricular (LV) ejection fraction (LVEF). Whereas early HF clinical trials included patients with this syndrome across the LVEF spectrum,[1,2] subsequent large-scale therapeutic trials restricted enrollment based on LVEF, initially enrolling those with marked systolic dysfunction (typically LVEF <30–40%)[3,4] as a way to enrich risk for high-risk patients.[5] This led to a robust evidence base for therapies in these patients, who were subsequently labeled HF with reduced ejection fraction (HFrEF). The increasing recognition of prevalence, morbidity, and mortality of HF among patients with an LVEF above the range included in these trials motivated therapeutic trials focused on these patients. Although this group of patients has broadly been labeled HF with preserved ejection fraction (HFpEF), large trials have enrolled patients with LVEF >40–45%.[6–10] Subsequent guidelines have formalized HFrEF as HF with an LVEF <40% and HFpEF as HF with an LVEF >50%. Although this categorization was initially pragmatic, it has proven clinically useful also, as drugs that are effective in HFrEF have not been shown to be clearly beneficial in HFpEF.

This chapter will address two groups of HF patients that are not clearly addressed based on the existing evidence base for HFpEF and HFrEF (Table 16.1). LVEF is a dynamic, rather than a static, value (Figure 16.1). In the first part of this chapter, we will discuss the subset of patients with a low LVEF that subsequently improves to normal, termed HF with recovered ejection fraction (HFrecEF). We will then discuss the subgroup of HF patients with an LVEF in the border zone between HFpEF and HFrEF, i.e., LVEF 40–50%, who have recently been labeled HF with midrange ejection fraction (HFmrEF; Figure 16.2). We will explore the recent data that provides some guidance on how to manage these two important groups of HF patients.

LVEF: Ascertainment and Definition of "Normal"

One inherent difficulty in studying patients with HFrecEF and HFmrEF is the physiologic and measurement-associated variability in LVEF itself. LVEF is most assessed by two-dimensional echocardiography both clinically and for clinical trial inclusion, because it is widely available, relatively inexpensive, and carries minimal risk. Even in a highly controlled laboratory setting, the intra-observer variability in LVEF, assessed as one standard deviation (SD) of the mean difference in repeat measurements, was 5–6% and the coefficient of variation was 8–10%.[11] LVEF variability, when assessed clinically and when accounting for interobserver differences, may well be higher. In one study, the interobserver variability, defined as the 2-SD limit of the between-assessment difference for LVEF, was 14%.[12] Contrast and 3-dimensional echocardiography may improve the reliability of LVEF measurement, but are infrequently used in clinical practice.[12,13] Similarly, among imagers with appropriate expertise, alternative imaging modalities, such as radionuclide ventriculography or cardiac magnetic resonance imaging (CMR), can provide greater precision in assessing LVEF, but are not routinely used clinically.[12,14] In a clinical setting, it is unlikely that any cine imaging modality will reliably reduce LVEF variability greatly. This inherent measurement variability will contribute to changes in LVEF assessed on serial imaging studies. It also makes the diagnosis of HFmrEF particularly challenging given the narrow LVEF range defining this syndrome (ten percentage points) relative to the precision of the measure. These caveats must be kept in mind when considering the data regarding HFrecEF and HFmrEF discussed below.

The interpretation of these categories is also made challenging by the unclear definition of normal LVEF. Whereas HFpEF is defined by clinical guidelines based on LVEF >50%, the American Society of Echocardiography and the European Association of Cardiovascular Imaging define the lower limit of normal LVEF as 52% for men and 54% for women.[15] The Normal Reference Range for Echocardiography (NORRE) study found a lower reference value for LVEF of 56% in men and 57% in women, with a modest age-associated increase in the lower reference value in both genders.[16] Data from the Multi-Ethnic Study of Atherosclerosis (MESA) and the Framingham Heart Study indicate increased risk of incident HF with LVEF 50–55% compared to >55%.[17,18] Furthermore, there may be regional differences. In the EchoNoRMAL study, the lower reference for LVEF among European men was 49% to 50%, whereas the lower limit among East Asian women was 57%.[19] This variability further questions the meaning of "preserved" and "midrange" LVEF relative to LV systolic performance, which it is intended to reflect.

HF with Recovered LVEF

Definition

A subset of HF patients demonstrates an improvement in LVEF over time, possibly due to the natural history of the underlying disease process, guideline-directed medical therapies (GDMT) for HF, or both (Figure 16.3). The term "recovery" has been used to refer to improvement in or normalization of LV function, defined using varying LVEF cutoffs. The 2013 American College of Cardiology Foundation/American Heart Association (ACCF/AHA) guidelines for HF management define "HFpEF, improved" as a subset of patients who had prior HFrEF and who experienced an improvement in their LVEF to above 40%.[20] Some studies define improvement using a higher LVEF cutoff, or using a relative improvement in the LVEF. More recently, it has been increasingly appreciated that true recovery of the myocardium is rare, and that "remission" is a more appropriate term to describe gross normalization of LVEF.[21] Based on available evidence, a recent expert panel proposed the following working definition of HFrecEF: 1) documentation of LVEF <40% at baseline; 2) ≥10% absolute improvement in LVEF; and 3) a 2nd measurement of LVEF >40%.[22]

DOI: 10.1201/9780429244544-19

TABLE 16.1: Definitions of HFrEF, HFpEF, HFmrEF

HF with Reduced Ejection Fraction (HFrEF)	HF with LVEF <40%
HF with Midrange Ejection Fraction (HFmrEF)	HF with LVEF between 40% and 50%
HF with Preserved Ejection Fraction (HFpEF)	HF with LVEF ≥50%
HF with Recovered Ejection Fraction (HFrecEF)	HF that has improved, for example, to an LVEF >40% (if the patient continues to have HF, they may also be referred to as having HFmrEF or HFpEF)

Note: Some studies use different LVEF cutoffs than those listed in the table.
Abbreviations: HF: heart failure; LVEF: left ventricular ejection fraction.

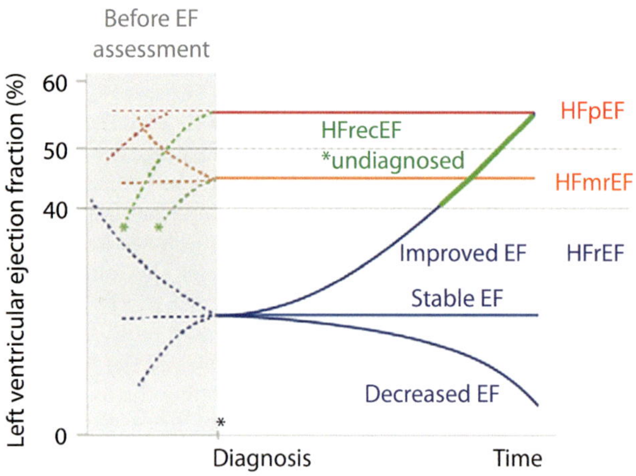

FIGURE 16.1 Illustration of LVEF trajectories in HF. Patients often transition between HFpEF, HFmrEF, and HFrEF, and a patient's LVEF trajectory has implications for their prognosis. (Reproduced with permission from Nijst et al. *Prog Cardiovasc Dis*. 2017;60:226–36.)

Impact on LVEF of Guideline-Directed Therapies for HFrEF

In the Survival and Ventricular Enlargement (SAVE) trial, captopril attenuated the increase in LV size one year after a myocardial infarction, with an associated 35% relative risk reduction in major cardiovascular events.[23] Beta-blockers are associated with improvement in LVEF beyond that accomplished with ACE-inhibitors alone. In a meta-analysis of β-blocker trials for HFrEF, which largely included patients already on ACE-inhibitors, metoprolol increased LVEF by 3.8±0.5 percentage points and carvedilol increased LVEF by 6.5±0.5 percentage points vs placebo.[24] Spironolactone and sacubitril-valsartan also contribute to reverse remodeling.[25,26] Among appropriately selected patients with HFrEF and wide QRS, cardiac resynchronization therapy (CRT) is associated with marked LV reverse remodeling and improvements in LVEF in some patients. CRT is associated with a mean improvement in LVEF of 6 to 11% across studies, and predictors of greater improvement include non-ischemic etiology, left bundle branch morphology, and longer QRS duration (i.e., >150 ms).[27,28] Finally, as will be discussed in greater detail later in this chapter, patients with Stage D HF undergoing mechanical unloading with left ventricular assist devices (LVADs) may experience LV reverse remodeling, even when LV dysfunction is severe.[29]

Predictors of Recovery

There have been numerous attempts to characterize HFrecEF patients and to identify predictors of LVEF recovery in HFrEF patients. A Canadian study examined 10,641 patients diagnosed with HF in a community setting and with two echocardiograms at least six months apart.[30] Less than one-third of the patients (3,124) had HFrEF, defined as an LVEF ≤40%, and these patients demonstrated high rates of GDMT use. Over a median follow-up of 17 months, 38% of the participants showed a ≥10% improvement in LVEF to a mean of 46.4±10.6%. Predictors of improvement included female sex, younger age, atrial fibrillation, and hypertension. Concordant with these findings, an observational study of 674 incident HFrEF patients diagnosed with HF between 1984 and 2009 in Olmsted County found that 39% of the patients had at least one subsequent LVEF of at least 50%.[31] Factors associated with an increase in LVEF included female gender, younger age, absence of coronary artery disease, and use of evidence-based medications.

Cardiovascular imaging can help assess the potential for myocardial recovery. Late gadolinium enhancement (LGE) on CMR identifies areas of myocardial scarring, and areas with LGE are less likely to improve with beta-blockers, particularly with increasing transmurality of the LGE.[32] Areas with LGE through >75% of the myocardial wall are generally considered to be non-viable. Myocardial viability can also be assessed with dobutamine echocardiography, single-photon emission computed tomography (SPECT), and positron emission tomography (PET). In a sub-study of the Surgical Treatment for Ischemic Heart Failure (STICH) trial, only the patients that showed viability based on dobutamine echocardiography or SPECT were found to have an increase in LVEF with either medical therapy or coronary artery bypass grafting (CABG).[33] Despite this, the role of viability testing in predicting clinical outcomes of CABG is unclear.[33,34]

Recovery by Etiology of Heart Failure

The etiology of myocardial dysfunction influences the potential for recovery. Patients with non-ischemic cardiomyopathy are more likely to have myocardial recovery than those with ischemic cardiomyopathy. There are variations in the rates of recovery among the different types of non-ischemic cardiomyopathy.

Myocarditis

Patients with fulminant myocarditis have markedly higher rates of cardiac death and heart transplantation compared with acute myocarditis, both short-term and at 7-year follow-up.[35] Patients with fulminant myocarditis also appear less likely to achieve an LVEF of at least 55% following recovery: 71% compared with 91% for patients with acute myocarditis at a median follow-up of 22 months.[36] Acute myocarditis patients are often studied with patients with idiopathic dilated cardiomyopathy, given the finding that the two groups have similar long-term outcomes.[37] The Intervention in Myocarditis and Acute Cardiomyopathy (IMAC2) study enrolled patients with either idiopathic dilated (including peripartum) cardiomyopathy

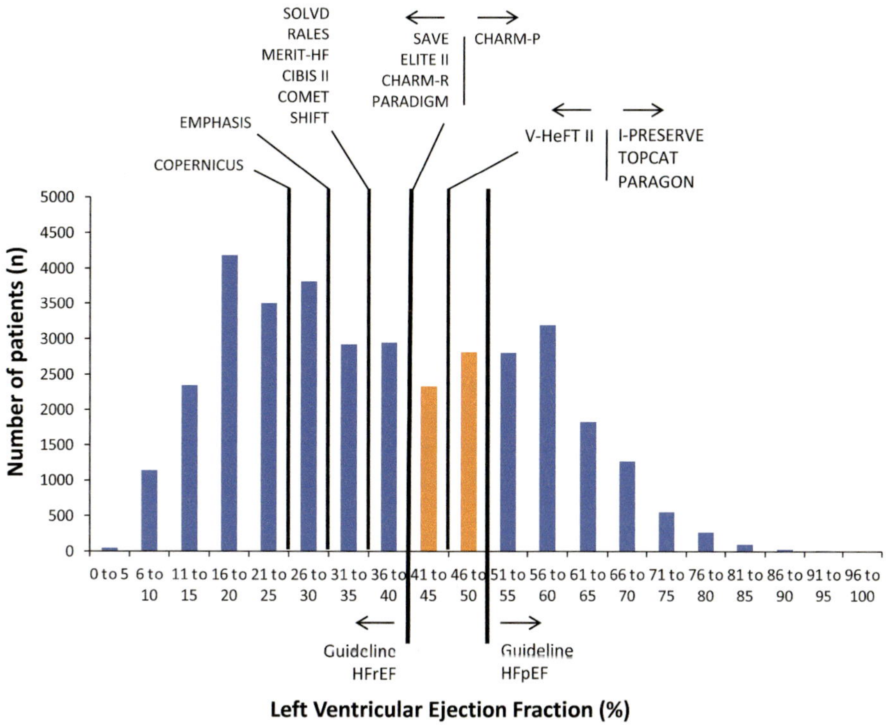

FIGURE 16.2 Distribution of LVEF in hospitalized HF patients in the OPTIMIZE-HF Registry. Guidelines generally specify an LVEF of 40% as the upper cutoff of HFrEF, and 50% as the lower cutoff of HFpEF, leaving the range of LVEF between 40% and 50% as HFmrEF. The LVEF cutoffs used for the inclusion criteria of landmark HF clinical trials are shown. (Reproduced with permission from Fonarow et al. *J Am Coll Cardiol.* 2007;50:768–77.)

or myocarditis who had an LVEF ≤40% and <six months of symptoms.[38] The mean age was 45±14 years and the baseline mean LVEF was 24+8%. At six months, mean LVEF was 40+12%. Among the small number of patients with biopsy-confirmed lymphocytic myocarditis, mean LVEF at six months was 49+8%. Seventy percent of the patients had an increase in LVEF of ≥10 percentage points, and 25% reached a LVEF of ≥50%. Smaller baseline LV end-diastolic dimension (LVEDD) was the strongest predictor of higher LVEF at six months, independent of baseline LVEF or sex. Non-Black race was also a predictor of higher LVEF at six months, despite similarly high rates of HF medication use among Black and non-Black patients. Studies of idiopathic dilated cardiomyopathy suggest that increases in LV volume, abnormalities in diastolic function, and decreased exercise tolerance persist despite normalization of LVEF, and many exhibit deterioration years later.[39,40]

Peripartum Cardiomyopathy

Patients with peripartum cardiomyopathy are frequently found to have recovery of systolic dysfunction. Compared to non-Black patients, Black patients appear less likely to experience normalization of LVEF (57% vs 76%, respectively),[41] and when LVEF normalization does occur, it appears to take longer (median of 265 days vs 126 days, respectively). Notably, some patients take greater than one year to demonstrate recovery.[42,43] Additional factors that predict the lack of LVEF recovery include lower LVEF at presentation, higher LVEDD, presence of right ventricular dysfunction, and increased extracellular volume on CMR.[41,44] Despite normalization of LVEF, HF recurs with subsequent pregnancy in one-fifth of patients.[45] Though patients often maintain a normal LVEF after recovery from peripartum cardiomyopathy in the absence of a subsequent pregnancy, there are rare reports of late recurrent deterioration.[43]

Alcoholic Cardiomyopathy

Alcoholic cardiomyopathy appears to be another cause of cardiomyopathy with frequent normalization of LVEF, and patients with this condition may often be miscategorized as having idiopathic dilated cardiomyopathy. Although studies show that those who continue to drink heavily do not have improvements in their ejection fraction, nearly half of those who abstain from alcohol or reduce their intake to moderate amounts have an LVEF improvement of at least 10 percentage points to at least 40%, and this improvement is associated with good outcomes.[46] The median time to this LVEF improvement after abstaining from alcohol is 28 months (9.6 to 30.9), and the improvement appears largely sustained over a three-year follow-up period in the absence of relapse of alcoholism.[46,47] Predictors of LVEF improvement include use of beta-blocker therapy, suggesting that, beyond reduction of alcohol intake, HF medications may be beneficial for these patients.

Tachycardia-Induced Cardiomyopathy

The recovery of systolic function with treatment of tachycardia occurs over weeks to months.[48] Outcomes of patients with tachycardia-induced cardiomyopathy are generally quite good.[49] However, although it often takes years for tachycardia-induced cardiomyopathy to first develop, decline in LVEF can recur within months with recurrence of arrhythmia, suggesting that the initial myocardial recovery is not complete.[50] Imaging studies have shown that patients with normalization of systolic function continue to have subtle abnormalities in cardiac structure and function, including diffuse fibrosis.[51,52]

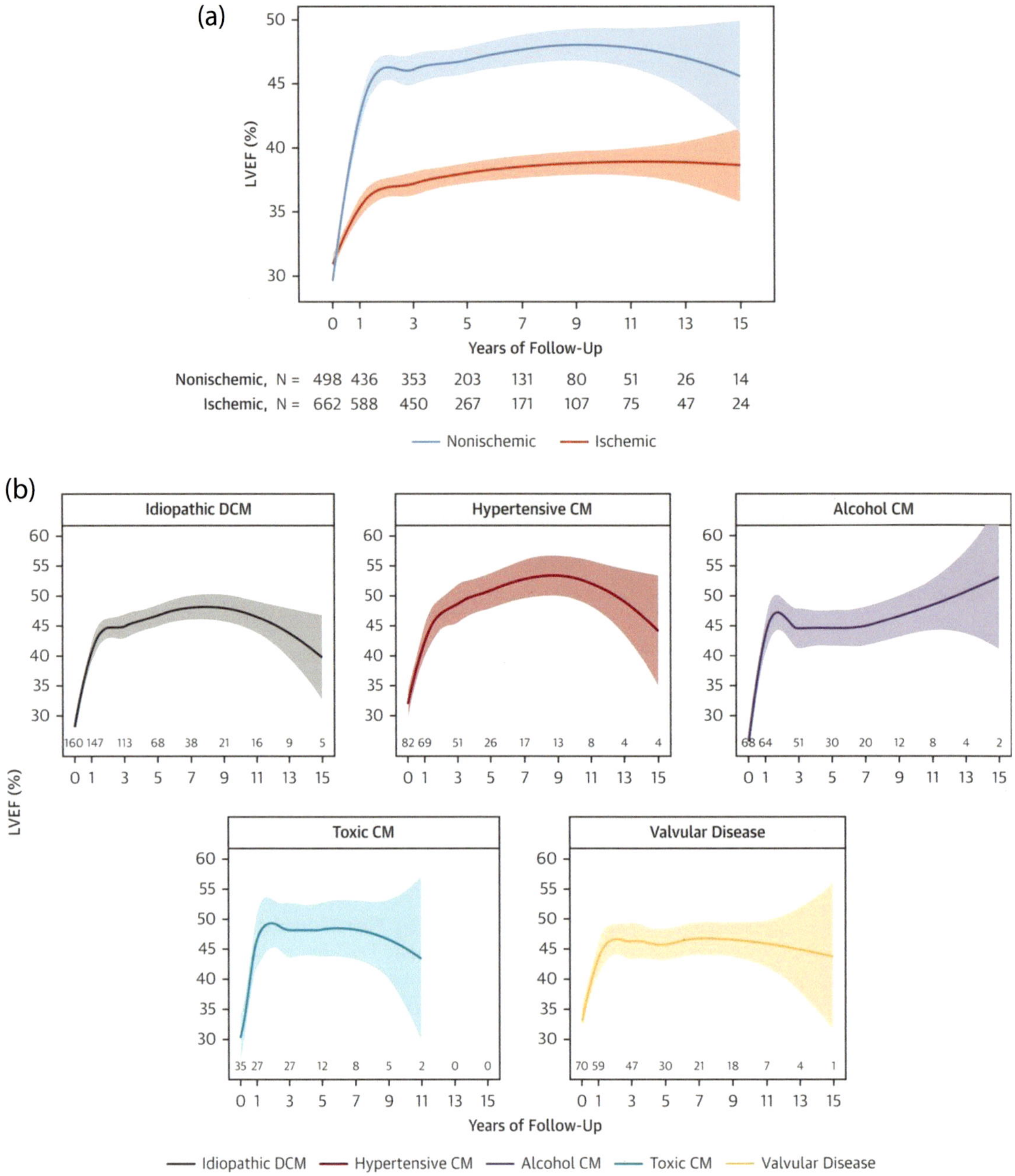

FIGURE 16.3 Loess curves of the LVEF trajectory in HFrEF patients over long-term follow-up, separated by etiology of HF. Patients with non-ischemic cardiomyopathy often have a more pronounced increase in LVEF in the first year after diagnosis compared with patients with ischemic cardiomyopathy. (Reproduced with permission from Lupon et al. *J Am Coll Cardiol.* 2018; 72:591–601.)

There have been rare reports of sudden death among relatively young patients with recovery of LVEF after tachycardia-induced cardiomyopathy.[50] The patients at risk appear to be those with severely reduced systolic function at presentation, and where the patient's tachyarrhythmia was atrial fibrillation. Given these cases, some consider it warranted to continue neurohormonal antagonists after normalization of LVEF.[53]

Hyperthyroidism

Systolic dysfunction from hyperthyroidism is generally reversible.[54] However, in one study of 15 patients with HFrEF from hyperthyroidism, five continued to have persistent systolic dysfunction at one-year follow-up despite treatment for hyperthyroidism and control of tachycardia.[55]

Management of HFrecEF

Much of the effect of HF management on increasing LVEF appears to occur within the first year.[56] Whether patients should be continued on HF medications once recovery is achieved, and for how long, is unclear. The most robust data come from the pilot, randomized TRED-HF trial.[57] In this study, medications were gradually withdrawn in 51 patients with dilated cardiomyopathy with HFrecEF at a median of five years after initial diagnosis and two years after recovery of LVEF. HFrecEF was defined as recovery from LVEF <40% to LVEF ≥50% with no symptoms, N-terminal pro-B-type natriuretic peptide (NT-proBNP) <250 ng/mL, and normalization of LV end-diastolic volume (LVEDV). Only 12% were taking a loop diuretic at enrollment. Within six months of drug withdrawal, 40% of patients had a relapse defined as a reduction in LVEF of more than 10% to less than 50%, an increase in LVEDV by more than 10% to above the normal range, a 2-fold rise in NT-proBNP to >400 ng/mL, or clinical evidence of HF. Most relapses occurred within eight weeks of discontinuing their last medication. Predictors of relapse were older age, prescription of >two HF medications, prescription of a mineralocorticoid receptor antagonist, higher NT-proBNP, and decreased peak global radial strain. The mean decrease in LVEF was −12.0% (95% confidence interval (CI) −16.6 to −7.4) among the patients who relapsed, and it also decreased among patients who did not experience relapse, with a mean decrease of −3.5% (95% CI −5.8 to −1.1). Among the eight patients with a potentially reversible cause of their HF, three (38%) experienced relapses. Of note, a deterioration in LVEF often predated a rise in NT-proBNP, so the authors note that reproducible LVEF measurements, such as with CMR, may be important if withdrawal is considered under certain circumstances.

Future studies may fine-tune the risk stratification of HFrecEF patients to guide whether some patients can safely have their medications discontinued. Among HFrecEF patients, worse global longitudinal strain (GLS) on echocardiography,[58] presence of left bundle branch block, and persistently elevated LVEDD have all been associated with subsequent LVEF deterioration after improvement of LVEF to at least 45%.[59] However, currently, no predictor demonstrates adequate predictive utility for clinical use. Furthermore, some HFrecEF patients have been found to develop relapse throughout a decade of follow-up despite high rates of continued medication use, suggesting that these patients should have prolonged close monitoring.

Recovery in LVAD Patients

While LVADs have traditionally been thought of as a destination therapy or as a bridge to transplantation, their role as a bridge to recovery is increasingly appreciated. Patients with advanced HF are often poorly tolerant of neurohormonal antagonist medications and are often better able to tolerate these medications following LVAD implantation. There is accumulating evidence that aggressive medical management may allow some LVAD patients to recover LV function to the point of being able to have the device explanted.[60,61] Approximately 1% of the LVAD patients in the North American Interagency Registry for Mechanically Assisted Circulatory Support (INTERMACS) database have undergone explantation of their device for myocardial recovery.[62] Predictors of myocardial recovery included female sex, lower body mass index, lower body surface area, non-ischemic etiology of HF, and shorter duration of disease (Figure 16.2).[63] Rates of LVAD explantation were highest among patients with myocarditis (7.7%), followed by peripartum cardiomyopathy (4.4%), and adriamycin-induced dilated cardiomyopathy (4.1%). Interestingly, whereas the patients who exhibited complete recovery (defined by LVAD explantation) had lower pre-implantation use of neurohormonal medications compared with patients without recovery, they had greater use of these drugs during LVAD support, raising the possibility of neurohormonal antagonist medications being an important mechanism of myocardial recovery (Figure 16.3). Small-scale studies using protocols for medication up-titration and active surveillance for recovery have yielded promising LVAD explantation results.[64,65] A striking 50–60% of patients in these studies recovered and were able to undergo LVAD explantation. However, in a recent German study that evaluated a protocol for LVAD explantation among 424 patients with an LVAD greater than six months, LVEF ≥45% and LVEDD <55 mm (or <3.2 mm/m² body surface area), only 14 patients (3.3%) underwent explantation.[66] Notably, no patient with ischemic cardiomyopathy met explantation criteria, consistent with findings from another, similar study.[67]

Research on the extent of myocardial improvement required for successful LVAD explantation without recurrence of HF is ongoing, using data from turn-down echocardiography, and analysis of serum and apical cores obtained during LVAD implantation to determine molecular, cellular, and histological predictors of sustained recovery.

HF with Midrange LVEF

Definition and Epidemiology

In 2016, the European Society of Cardiology (ESC) guidelines established the use of the term HF with midrange LVEF to refer to HF patients with LVEF of 40% to 49%.[68] This group of patients had previously been called "HF with borderline LVEF" or "HF with mildly reduced LVEF." The stated purpose was to stimulate research to better understand this group of patients with HF, who had frequently been excluded from studies of HFrEF or HFpEF. Some argue that HFmrEF is a distinct entity between HFrEF and HFpEF, comprised mostly of patients with improvement of prior HFrEF.[69] Regardless, given that existing trials have found that treatments that are effective for HFrEF are not clearly effective for HFpEF, better understanding of this group of patients may provide greater insights into optimal treatment approaches.

Data from community-based studies and HF registries suggest that HFmrEF accounts for 10% of incident HF cases and 14–21% of prevalent HF. In pooled data from community cohorts, among 28,820 HF-free participants followed for a median of 12 years, 10% of incident HF cases fell into the HFmrEF category.[70] Data from the Get with the Guidelines-Heart Failure registry (GWTG-HF) demonstrated that 14% of the patients hospitalized for HF between 2005 and 2011 were HFmrEF,[71] whereas 21% of HF cases in the Swedish Heart Failure Registry were HFmrEF.[72] Similarly, in a Japanese registry of inpatients and outpatients with HF, 17% had HFmrEF.[73]

Characteristics

Data from several large-scale HF studies demonstrate that patients with HFmrEF have a clinical profile that is intermediate between HFrEF and HFpEF patients, with the notable exception of coronary artery disease (CAD) prevalence, which appears to closely approximate HFrEF (Figure 16.4).[72,74–76] In the ESC Heart Failure Long-Term Registry, the HFmrEF group resembled the HFrEF group in terms of prevalence of CAD but also in features such as age (younger than HFpEF) and gender (higher proportion of men than HFpEF).[77] Notably, the risk of ischemic events also appears higher in HFmrEF and HFrEF patients than in HFpEF patients, independent of a history of CAD.[75] The prevalence of atrial fibrillation and chronic kidney disease (CKD) also appears to be intermediate between HFpEF and HFrEF.[78–80] In a study of patients with HF referred for cardiopulmonary exercise testing (CPET), performance metrics on CPET were closer to those seen in HFpEF.[81] Similarly, a biomarker analysis of the TIME-CHF trial found that HFmrEF

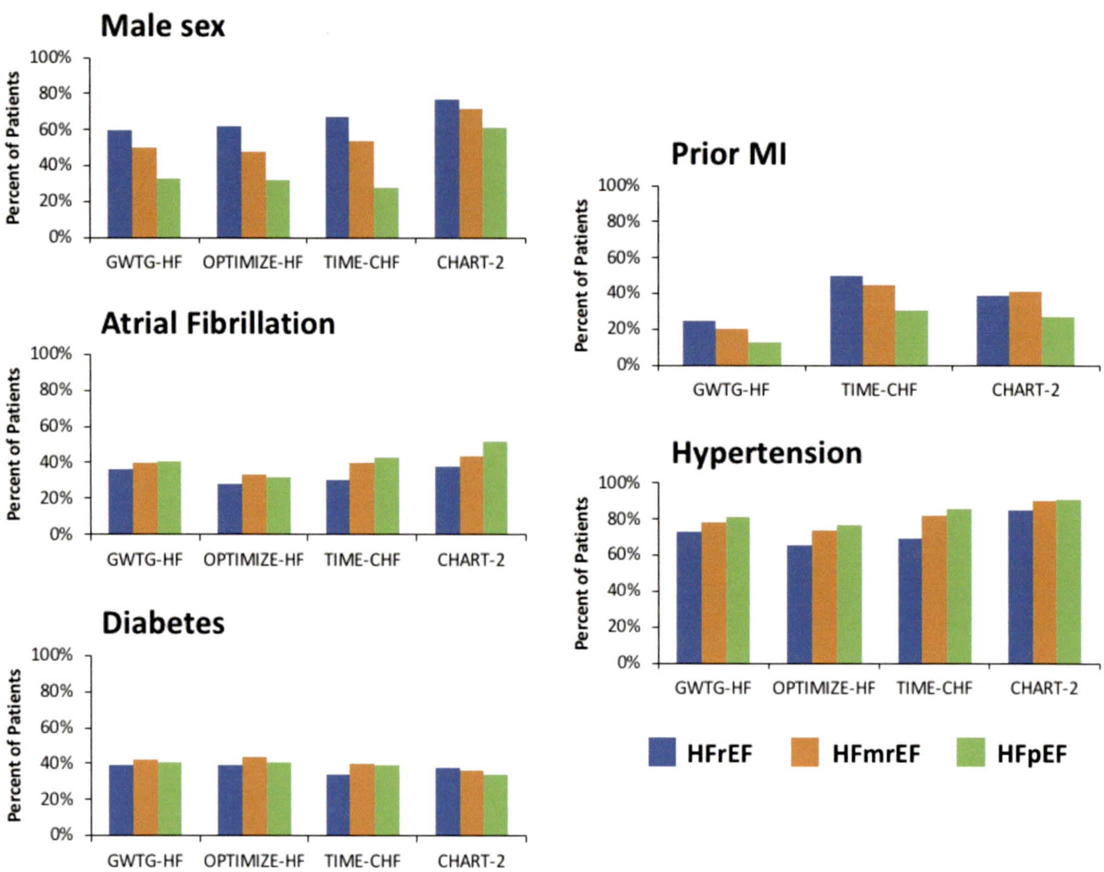

FIGURE 16.4 Prevalence of comorbidities in HFrEF, HFmrEF, and HFpEF. The prevalence of comorbid conditions in HFmrEF is generally intermediate between those of HFrEF and HFpEF. (Based on data from Cheng et al. *Am Heart J.* 2014;168:721–30; Fonarow et al. *J Am Coll Cardiol.* 2007;50:768–77; Rickenbacher et al. *Eur J Heart Fail.* 2017;19:1586–96; Tsuji et al. *Eur J Heart Fail.* 2017;19:1258–69.)

(defined as an LVEF of 41% to 49%) had a profile that was more similar to HFpEF than HFrEF.[82] However, another analysis of patients with acute HF found similarities in the biomarker profile of HFmrEF to both HFrEF and HFpEF,[83] but only 13% of patients included in the analysis had HFpEF.

Prognosis

Data from large-scale registry studies and meta-analyses suggest that the mortality associated with HFmrEF is likely similar to HFpEF and lower than HFrEF (Figure 16.5). In the GWTG-HF registry, the one-year mortality was slightly lower for HFmrEF and HFpEF than for HFrEF.[71] In the Swedish Heart Failure Registry, after multivariable adjustment, prognosis was similar in HFmrEF and HFpEF, and better than for HFrEF at 30 days, one year, and three years.[72] This is similar to the findings of the Meta-analysis Global Group in Chronic Heart Failure (MAGGIC) group.[84] Similar findings were also observed with respect to all-cause and CV mortality in a large-scale meta-analysis of 12 observational studies and prospective trials.[76] This study also noted that the risk of HF hospitalization in HFmrEF was intermediate between HFrEF and HFpEF. Notably, however, five-year follow-up data from GWTG-HF demonstrate that five-year mortality was similar across all three HF categories at approximately 75%, and the median survival was 2.1 years.[85] Furthermore, HFrEF and HFmrEF patients had slightly higher five-year HF readmission rates than did HFpEF patients (48%, 45%, and 40%, respectively) as well as higher five-year CV readmission rates (64%, 63%, and 59%, respectively).[85]

Transitions in LVEF Categories

As LVEF is dynamic, patients often transition from other HF categories to HFmrEF, or transition from HFmrEF to other categories (Figure 16.6). This is an important source of heterogeneity among HFmrEF patients, as trajectory of the LVEF is prognostically relevant (Figure 16.7). Existing data from single-center studies suggest that 35–70% of patients with prevalent HFmrEF had a prior reduced LVEF, and 10–50% of patients experienced deterioration of LVEF from >50%.[86,87] In a study of 944 patients undergoing clinically indicated cardiopulmonary exercise testing at a tertiary medical center, 61% of HFmrEF patients had recovered from a prior LVEF <40%.[88] These patients had similar clinical characteristics and cardiopulmonary exercise-testing parameters to HFmrEF patients without prior low LVEF, but demonstrated a lower incidence of the composite of death, LVAD implantation, and heart transplantation over a median follow-up period of 4.4 years. Furthermore, among 448 HFmrEF patients at a single referral center, patients whose LVEF improved from <40% to mid-range were at lower risk of subsequent all-cause mortality and hospitalization and of cardiovascular mortality and HF hospitalization compared with those whose LVEF had deteriorated from >50%.[87] Studies following changes in LVEF among patients with HFmrEF suggest that only a minority

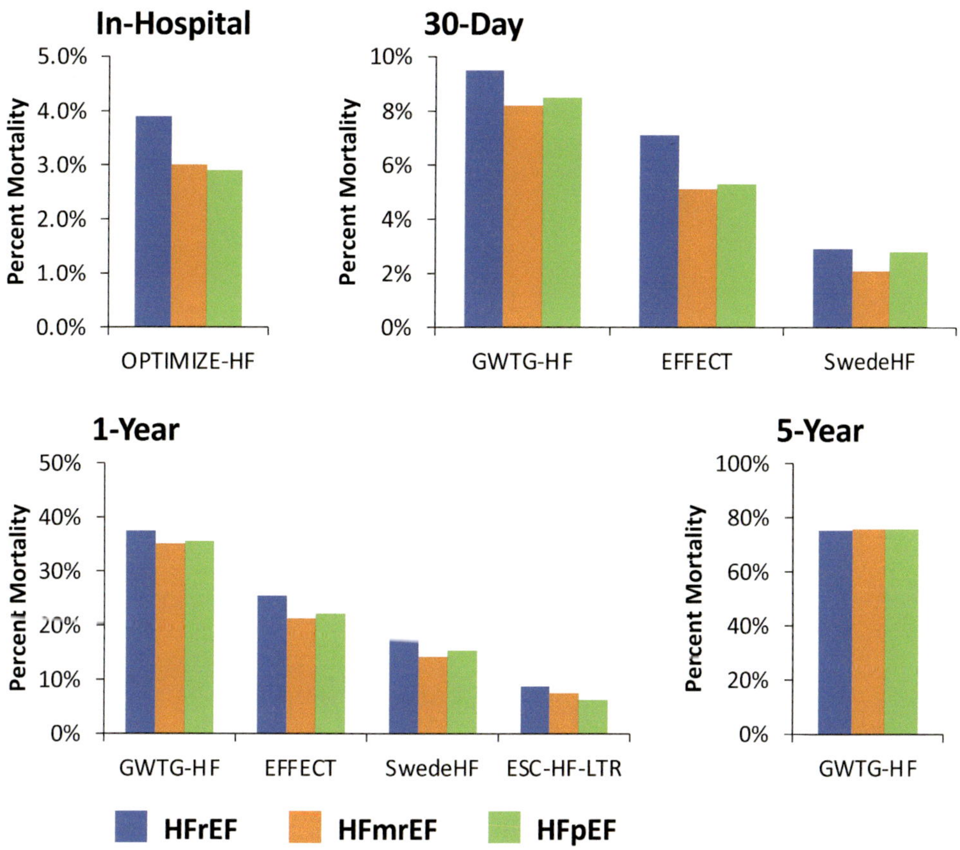

FIGURE 16.5 Prevalence of mortality in HFrEF, HFmrEF, and HFpEF. The prognosis of HFmrEF is similar to that of HFpEF, and mortality at five years is similar across all three categories of HF. (Based on data from Fonarow et al. *J Am Coll Cardiol.* 2007;50:768–77; Cheng et al. *Am Heart J.* 2014;168:721–30; Bhatia et al. *N Engl J Med.* 2006;355:260–9; Koh et al. *Eur J Heart Fail.* 2017;19:1624–34; Chioncel et al. *Eur J Heart Fail.* 2017;19:1574–85; Shah K et al. *J Am Coll Cardiol.* 2017;70:2476–86.)

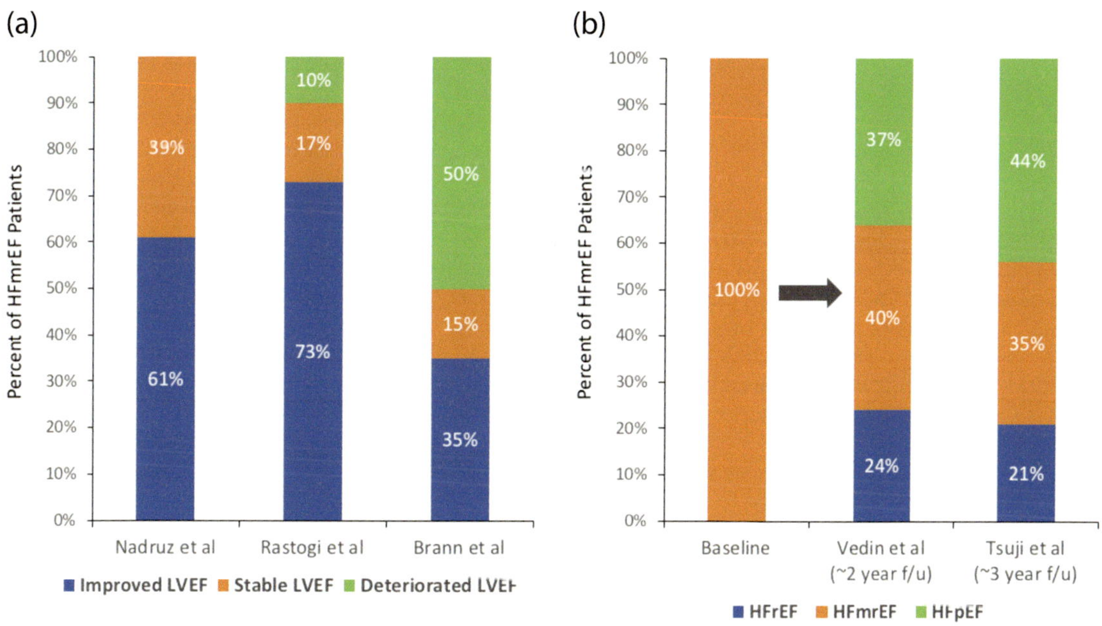

FIGURE 16.6 Transitions in LVEF to and from HFmrEF. (a) Proportion of prevalent HFmrEF patients who have had HFmrEF as a result of improvement from HFrEF, stable HFmrEF, and deterioration of HFpEF. (b) Proportion of HFmrEF patients who subsequently have HFrEF, HFmrEF, and HFpEF on follow-up. (Based on data from Nadruz et al. *Circ Heart Fail.* 2016;9:e002826; Rastogi et al. *Eur J Heart Fail.* 2017;19:1597–605; Brann et al. *JAMA Cardiol.* 2020;e202081; Vedin et al. *Circ Heart Fail.* 2017;10:e003875; Tsuji et al. *Eur J Heart Fail.* 2017;19:12581269.)

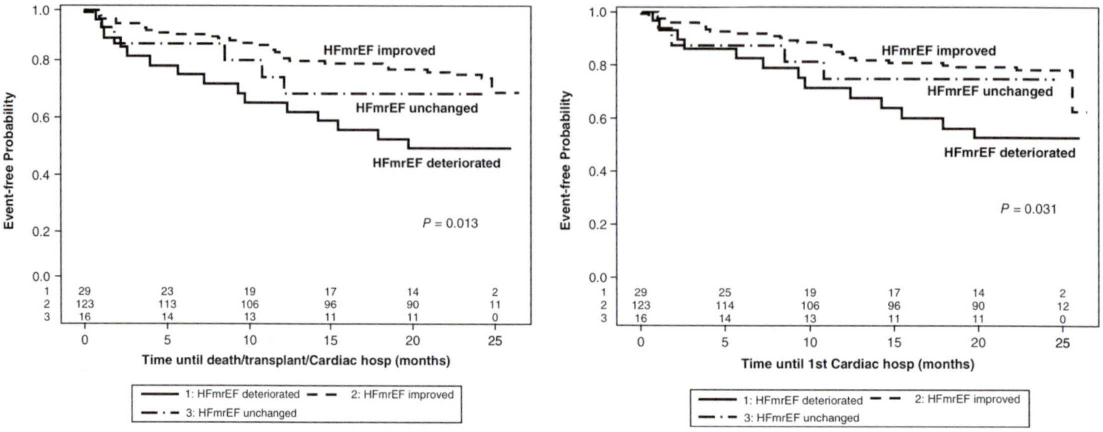

FIGURE 16.7 Impact of prior LVEF on prognosis in HFmrEF. (a) Kaplan-Meier curves of time to death, transplantation, or cardiac hospitalization. HFmrEF patients are divided into three groups based on whether their HFmrEF is the result of improvement in LVEF, unchanged LVEF, or deterioration of LVEF. There was a significant difference between HFmrEF improved and HFmrEF deteriorated. (b) Kaplan-Meier curves of time to first cardiac hospitalization for the three groups of HFmrEF patients. There was a significant difference between HFmrEF improved and HFmrEF deteriorated. (Reproduced with permission from Rastogi et al. *Eur J Heart Fail.* 2017;19:1597–605.)

remain in the HFmrEF range. At two- to three-year follow-ups, approximately 20–25% of HFmrEF patients have a subsequent deterioration to HFrEF, 35–45% increase in LVEF to the normal range, and LVEF remains midrange in only 35–40%.[56,73,75] Patients with HFmrEF who subsequently deteriorate to HFrEF demonstrate higher subsequent mortality compared with HFmrEF patients without deterioration or with improvement.[73]

Treatment

As with HFrEF and HFpEF patients, treating comorbid conditions and managing volume overload with diuretics are important in the management of HFmrEF. There are limited data available regarding whether medications that are effective in HFrEF treatment are also beneficial with respect to HFmrEF. However, post-hoc analyses of clinical trial data and meta-analyses suggest likely efficacy of several of these drug classes in HFmrEF (Figure 16.8).

Beta-Blockers

One meta-analysis assessed the individual patient data from 11 beta-blocker randomized, clinical trials.[89] In an unadjusted analysis, randomization to beta-blocker was associated with lower all-cause and CV mortality in HFmrEF patients in sinus rhythm. When the analysis was adjusted for patient characteristics, such as prior myocardial infarction, beta-blockers significantly reduced the risk of cardiovascular death over a median of 1.3 years of follow-up (hazard ratio 0.48, 95% confidence interval 0.24–0.97) but not all-cause mortality. Beta-blockers also improved the LVEF in these patients. In this meta-analysis, among patients in atrial fibrillation, beta-blockers improved the LVEF in HFmrEF patients but did not improve prognosis for any of the HF categories. Of note, 44% of the HFmrEF patients were drawn from SENIORS trial, which did not have an LVEF inclusion criterion. In SENIORS, the beta-1-selective blocker nebivolol reduced the composite outcome of death or cardiovascular hospitalization among elderly HF patients,[90] with no heterogeneity of effect between patients with LVEF ≤35% (median LVEF 30%) vs >35% (median LVEF 46%). Although nebivolol is used for HF treatment in several countries, it has not been approved for this indication by the US Food and Drug Administration.

Renin-Angiotensin-Aldosterone System Antagonists

A *post-hoc* analysis of the CHARM Programme found that candesartan reduced the composite of cardiovascular death and HF hospitalization as well as first and recurrent HF hospitalizations in HFrEF and HFmrEF patients, but not in HFpEF patients.[91] Similarly, an analysis of the Swedish Heart Failure Registry reported that the use of renin-angiotensin-aldosterone system (RAAS) antagonists was associated with a lower mortality in HF patients with an LVEF of at least 40%. Seventy-four percent of the patients in the analysis were on an ACE-inhibitor, and 38% had HFmrEF. There was no interaction with ejection fraction, but the hazard ratio was significant in the subgroup of patients with LVEF 40% to 49% but not in the subgroup with LVEF ≥50%.[92]

The TOPCAT trial tested the efficacy of spironolactone vs placebo in patients with HF and an LVEF ≥45%. Although the primary composite of CV mortality, HF hospitalization, or aborted cardiac arrest was not met, spironolactone did reduce a pre-specified secondary endpoint of HF hospitalization. Based on this, the 2017 American HF guidelines provided a class IIb recommendation (may be reasonable to consider) for the use of aldosterone receptor antagonists in patients with HF with an LVEF ≥45%, elevated BNP levels or HF admission within one year, and no contraindication to aldosterone receptor antagonists.[93] In a *post-hoc* analysis of TOPCAT, LVEF significantly modified the treatment effect of spironolactone such that spironolactone efficacy appeared greatest among patients at the lower end of the LVEF spectrum. Therefore, it may be reasonable to consider spironolactone in treating HFmrEF patients.[94]

Most recently, the PARAGON-HF trial evaluated the angiotensin receptor-neprilysin inhibitor sacubitril/valsartan for patients with HF and LVEF ≥45%. Although the study narrowly missed its primary endpoint of CV death and total HF hospitalizations, a prespecified analysis suggested benefit among participants with an LVEF between 45% and 57%.[10] If this finding is confirmed in further studies, it would support treating HFmrEF patients with sacubitril/valsartan.

Digoxin

An analysis of the Digitalis Investigation Group (DIG) trial, which investigated the use of digoxin in HF patients with sinus rhythm, assessed 1195 patients with HFmrEF (LVEF 40% to

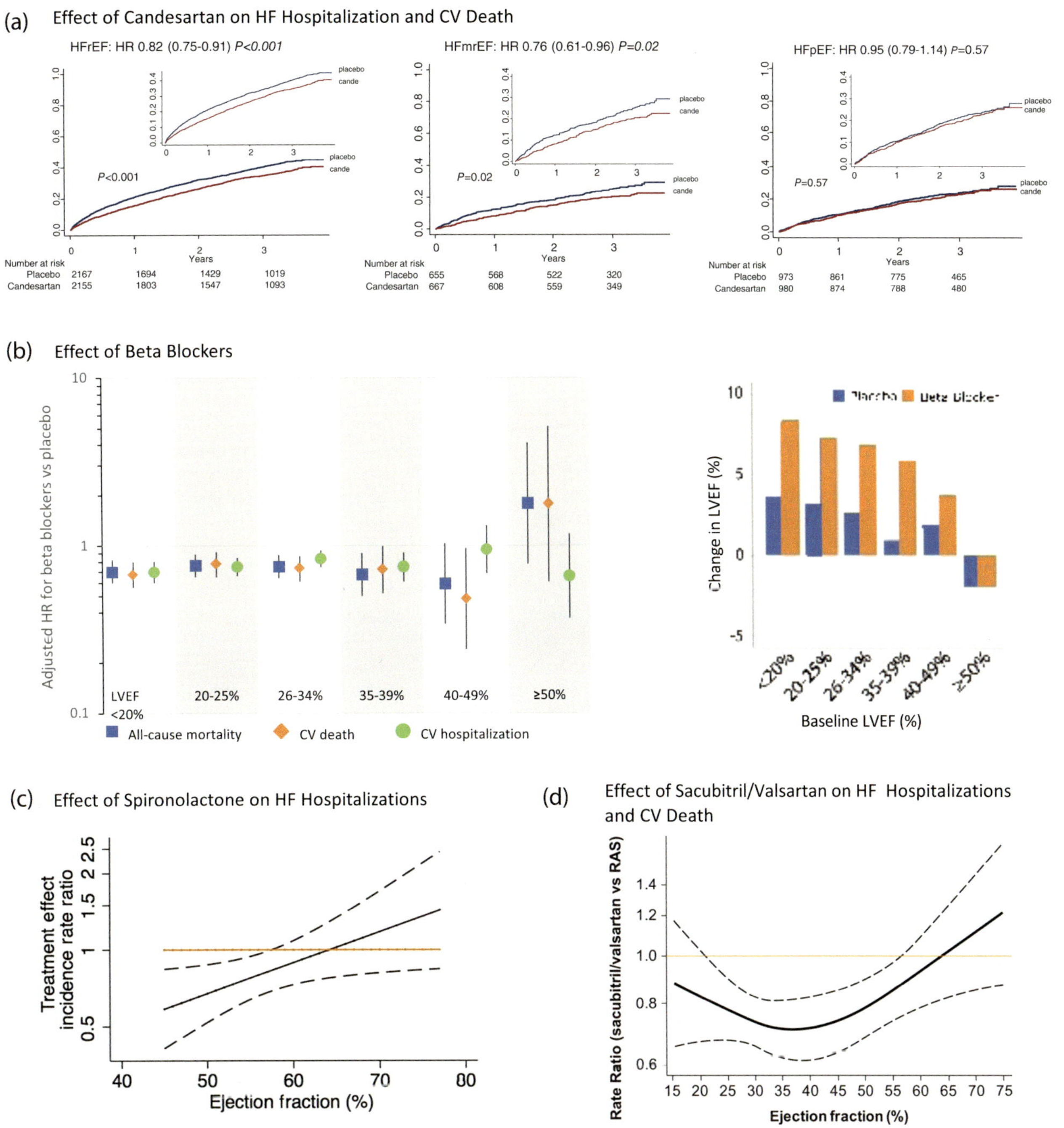

FIGURE 16.8 Effect of HF medications in HFmrEF. (a) Kaplan-Meier curves from the CHARM Programme on the effect of the angiotensin II receptor blocker (ARB) candesartan for the outcome of time to cardiovascular death or first HF hospitalization. (b) Data from a meta-analysis of 11 beta-blocker trials, assessing efficacy of beta-blockers vs placebo in patients in sinus rhythm. Left panel shows hazard ratios with 95% confidence intervals for beta-blockers vs placebo, separated by baseline LVEF. Hazard ratios are adjusted for age, gender, previous MI, systolic blood pressure, heart rate, use of ACE-inhibitors/ARBs, and use of diuretics. Right panel shows change in LVEF with beta-blocker use over median follow-up of one year, according to baseline LVEF. (c) Treatment effect of spironolactone for the outcome of HF hospitalization in the TOPCAT trial, according to baseline LVEF. (d) Treatment effect of sacubitril/valsartan for the outcome of HF hospitalization and CV death, according to baseline LVEF. (Reproduced with permission from Lund et al. *Eur J Heart Fail.* 2018;20:1230–9; Cleland et al. *Eur Heart J.* 2018;39:1230–9; Solomon et al. *Eur Heart J.* 2016;37:455–62; Solomon et al. *Circulation.* 2020;141:352–361.)

49%).[95] Digoxin did not appear to be as beneficial in treating HFmrEF patients as in HFrEF patients.

Biomarker-Guided Treatment Strategies

The TIME-CHF trial randomly assigned HF patients age 60 years or more with at least New York Heart Association (NYHA) class II symptoms, a history of HF hospitalization in the preceding year, and an N-terminal-prohormone BNP (NT-proBNP) level greater than twice the upper normal limit to either a symptom-guided strategy or an NT-proBNP-guided strategy for 18 months.[74] Participants with HFrEF and HFmrEF (LVEF 40% to 49%) had higher NT-proBNP levels than the

HFpEF participants. In the symptom-guided group, HF treatment was titrated to reduce symptoms to NYHA class II or less, and in the NT-proBNP-guided group, the treatment was titrated to additionally reduce N-terminal-pro hormone BNP (NT-proBNP) to less than twice the upper limit of normal. The NT-proBNP-guided strategy was more beneficial than the symptom-guided strategy in reducing HF hospitalizations among HFrEF and HFmrEF patients, but not among HFpEF patients.

Device Therapy

Guidelines recommend implantable cardioverter defibrillator (ICD) implantation for primary prevention of sudden cardiac death in selected patients with an LVEF of ≤35% or among patients with non-sustained ventricular tachycardia due to prior MI, LVEF of ≤40%, and inducible sustained ventricular tachycardia on an electrophysiological study.[20] No current guidelines or compelling randomized clinical data support the use of ICDs for primary prevention among patients with HFmrEF. Intriguing observational data suggest that CMR LGE may help risk stratification of dilated cardiomyopathy patients with an LVEF ≥40%, and that electrophysiology studies may be helpful for post-myocardial infarction patients with an LVEF ≥40%,[96–98] but these strategies have yet to be evaluated in larger trials.

CRT is recommended for select HF patients with an LVEF ≤35%, but its utility in treating patients with HFmrEF is unclear. The BLOCK HF trial compared CRT to right ventricular pacing in patients with atrioventricular (AV) block (I–III), NYHA class I to III HF, and an LVEF ≤50%.[99,100] Nearly 70% of the CRT group had an LVEF >35%, with a mean LVEF of 40%. CRT was found to reduce the risk of adverse clinical events and improve left ventricular end-systolic volume index. A subsequent systematic review assessed four studies to evaluate the utility of CRT compared to right ventricular pacing for heart block or after AV node ablation for atrial fibrillation specifically in HF patients with an LVEF >35%.[101] Results from BLOCK-HF were not included in this analysis. Compared with patients who underwent right ventricular pacing, patients with CRT had smaller LV volumes and a higher LVEF after a mean of 1.9 years, but no differences were detected in quality of life or mortality. Similar effects were seen with His bundle pacing, another form of physiological pacing that is emerging as a potential alternative to CRT for treating HF. Based on these data, the ACC/AHA/HRS Guidelines on the Evaluation and Management of Patients With Bradycardia and Cardiac Conduction Delay provide a class IIa recommendation to choose CRT or His bundle pacing over right ventricular pacing for patients with an LVEF between 36% and 50% who are expected to require ventricular pacing more than 40% of the time.[102]

The guidelines also provide a class IIb recommendation for CRT in patients with HF, an LVEF of 36% to 50%, and a left bundle branch block with QRS duration of ≥150 ms. This is based on limited data including *post-hoc* findings from the Predictors of Response to CRT (PROSPECT) study. In this observational study of the utility of echocardiographic dyssynchrony to predict response to CRT in patients with NYHA class III–IV HF symptoms, QRS duration of ≥130 ms, and an LVEF of ≤35%, 20% of the participants were found to have an LVEF >35% on core laboratory measurement.[103] The mean LVEF of this group was 43%. The improvements in the clinical composite score and left ventricular end-systolic volume index with CRT were found to be similar between patients with an LVEF ≤35% compared with those with an LVEF >35%.[104] Two trials designed to examine the utility of CRT in HF patients with left bundle branch block and LVEF between 36% and 50% failed to recruit a sufficient number of participants, which underscores the difficulty of performing trials on HFmrEF patients.[105]

Conclusion

The definitions of HFrecEF and HFmrEF are evolving. HFrecEF is a phenomenon that is fortunately more common as the therapeutic approaches to heart failure evolve. As we study more of these patients, we gain greater understanding of how to manage them in the long term. The HFmrEF category was created because divisions based on ejection fraction left a border zone for which the optimal management was unclear. In the future, we may be able to decide more definitively that HFmrEF should be treated like HFrEF, or we may be able to better refine how to treat individual patients based on LVEF trajectory or biomarkers. For both HFrecEF and HFmrEF, there are many questions that remain unexplored. Ongoing research on the characteristics of patients with these disease states on a clinical, cellular, and molecular scale holds the promise of greater insight into their effective management.

References

1. Cohn JN, Archibald DG, Ziesche S, et al. Effect of vasodilator therapy on mortality in chronic congestive heart failure. Results of a Veterans Administration Cooperative Study. *N Engl J Med.* 1986;314(24):1547–52. doi:10.1056/NEJM198606123142404
2. CONSENSUS Trial Study Group. Effects of enalapril on mortality in severe congestive heart failure. Results of the Cooperative North Scandinavian Enalapril Survival Study (CONSENSUS). *N Engl J Med.* 1987;316(23):1429–35. doi:10.1056/NEJM198706043162301
3. SOLVD Investigators, Yusuf S, Pitt B, Davis CE, Hood WB, Cohn JN. Effect of enalapril on survival in patients with reduced left ventricular ejection fractions and congestive heart failure. *N Engl J Med.* 1991;325(5):293–302. doi:10.1056/NEJM199108013250501
4. Pitt B, Zannad F, Remme WJ, et al. The effect of spironolactone on morbidity and mortality in patients with severe heart failure. Randomized Aldactone Evaluation Study Investigators. *N Engl J Med.* 1999;341(10):709–17. doi:10.1056/NEJM199909023411001
5. Pfeffer MA, Shah AM, Borlaug BA. Heart failure with preserved ejection fraction in perspective. *Circ Res.* 2019;124(11):1598–617. doi:10.1161/CIRCRESAHA.119.313572
6. Yusuf S, Pfeffer MA, Swedberg K, et al. Effects of candesartan in patients with chronic heart failure and preserved left-ventricular ejection fraction: the CHARM-preserved trial. *Lancet Lond Engl.* 2003;362(9386):777–81. doi:10.1016/S0140-6736(03)14285-7
7. Cleland JGF, Tendera M, Adamus J, et al. The perindopril in elderly people with chronic heart failure (PEP-CHF) study. *Eur Heart J.* 2006;27(19):2338–45. doi:10.1093/eurheartj/ehl250
8. Massie BM, Carson PE, McMurray JJ, et al. Irbesartan in patients with heart failure and preserved ejection fraction. *N Engl J Med.* 2008;359(23):2456–67. doi:10.1056/NEJMoa0805450
9. Pitt B, Pfeffer MA, Assmann SF, et al. Spironolactone for heart failure with preserved ejection fraction. *N Engl J Med.* 2014;370(15):1383–92. doi:10.1056/NEJMoa1313731
10. Solomon SD, McMurray JJV, Anand IS, et al. Angiotensin-neprilysin inhibition in heart failure with preserved ejection fraction. *N Engl J Med.* 2019;381(17):1609–20. doi:10.1056/NEJMoa1908655
11. Shah AM, Cheng S, Skali H, et al. Rationale and design of a multicenter echocardiographic study to assess the relationship between cardiac structure and function and heart failure risk in a biracial cohort of community-dwelling elderly persons: the Atherosclerosis Risk in Communities study. *Circ Cardiovasc Imaging.* 2014;7(1):173–81. doi:10.1161/CIRCIMAGING.113.000736
12. Malm S, Frigstad S, Sagberg E, Larsson H, Skjaerpe T. Accurate and reproducible measurement of left ventricular volume and ejection fraction by contrast echocardiography: a comparison with magnetic resonance imaging. *J Am Coll Cardiol.* 2004;44(5):1030–5. doi:10.1016/j.jacc.2004.05.068
13. Jenkins C, Bricknell K, Chan J, Hanekom L, Marwick TH. Comparison of two- and three-dimensional echocardiography with sequential magnetic resonance imaging for evaluating left ventricular volume and ejection fraction over time in patients with healed myocardial infarction. *Am J Cardiol.* 2007;99(3):300–6. doi:10.1016/j.amjcard.2006.08.026

14. Bellenger NG, Burgess MI, Ray SG, et al. Comparison of left ventricular ejection fraction and volumes in heart failure by echocardiography, radionuclide ventriculography and cardiovascular magnetic resonance; are they interchangeable? *Eur Heart J.* 2000;21(16):1387–96. doi:10.1053/euhj.2000.2011
15. Lang RM, Badano LP, Mor-Avi V, et al. Recommendations for cardiac chamber quantification by echocardiography in adults: an update from the American Society of Echocardiography and the European Association of Cardiovascular Imaging. *Eur Heart J Cardiovasc Imaging.* 2015;16(3):233–70. doi:10.1093/ehjci/jev014
16. Kou S, Caballero L, Dulgheru R, et al. Echocardiographic reference ranges for normal cardiac chamber size: results from the NORRE study. *Eur Heart J Cardiovasc Imaging.* 2014;15(6):680–90. doi:10.1093/ehjci/jet284
17. Yeboah J, Rodriguez CJ, Qureshi W, et al. Prognosis of low normal left ventricular ejection fraction in an asymptomatic population-based adult cohort: the multiethnic study of atherosclerosis. *J Card Fail.* 2016;22(10):763–8. doi:10.1016/j.cardfail.2016.03.013
18. Tsao CW, Lyass A, Larson MG, et al. Prognosis of adults with borderline left ventricular ejection fraction. *JACC Heart Fail.* 2016;4(6):502–10. doi:10.1016/j.jchf.2016.03.003
19. Echocardiographic Normal Ranges Meta-Analysis of the Left Heart Collaboration. Ethnic-specific normative reference values for echocardiographic LA and LV size, LV mass, and systolic function: the EchoNoRMAL study. *JACC Cardiovasc Imaging.* 2015;8(6):656–65. doi:10.1016/j.jcmg.2015.02.014
20. Yancy CW, Jessup M, Bozkurt B, et al. 2013 ACCF/AHA guideline for the management of heart failure: a report of the American College of Cardiology Foundation/American Heart Association Task Force on Practice Guidelines. *J Am Coll Cardiol.* 2013;62(16):e147–239. doi:10.1016/j.jacc.2013.05.019
21. Mann DL, Barger PM, Burkhoff D. Myocardial recovery and the failing heart: myth, magic, or molecular target? *J Am Coll Cardiol.* 2012;60(24):2465–72. doi:10.1016/j.jacc.2012.06.062
22. Wilcox JE, Fang JC, Margulies KB, Mann DL. Heart failure with recovered left ventricular ejection fraction: JACC scientific expert panel. *J Am Coll Cardiol.* 2020;76(6):719–34. doi:10.1016/j.jacc.2020.05.075
23. St John Sutton M, Pfeffer MA, Plappert T, et al. Quantitative two-dimensional echocardiographic measurements are major predictors of adverse cardiovascular events after acute myocardial infarction. The protective effects of captopril. *Circulation.* 1994;89(1):68–75. doi:10.1161/01.cir.89.1.68
24. Packer M, Antonopoulos GV, Berlin JA, Chittams J, Konstam MA, Udelson JE. Comparative effects of carvedilol and metoprolol on left ventricular ejection fraction in heart failure: results of a meta-analysis. *Am Heart J.* 2001;141(6):899–907. doi:10.1067/mhj.2001.115584
25. Januzzi JL, Prescott MF, Butler J, et al. Association of change in N-terminal pro-B-type natriuretic peptide following initiation of sacubitril-valsartan treatment with cardiac structure and function in patients with heart failure with reduced ejection fraction. *JAMA.* Published online September 2, 2019:1–11. doi:10.1001/jama.2019.12821
26. Tsutamoto T, Wada A, Maeda K, et al. Effect of spironolactone on plasma brain natriuretic peptide and left ventricular remodeling in patients with congestive heart failure. *J Am Coll Cardiol.* 2001;37(5):1228–33. doi:10.1016/s0735-1097(01)01116-0
27. Sutton MGSJ, Plappert T, Hilpisch KE, Abraham WT, Hayes DL, Chinchoy E. Sustained reverse left ventricular structural remodeling with cardiac resynchronization at one year is a function of etiology: quantitative Doppler echocardiographic evidence from the Multicenter InSync Randomized Clinical Evaluation (MIRACLE). *Circulation.* 2006;113(2):266–72. doi:10.1161/CIRCULATIONAHA.104.520817
28. Solomon SD, Foster E, Bourgoun M, et al. Effect of cardiac resynchronization therapy on reverse remodeling and relation to outcome: multicenter automatic defibrillator implantation trial: cardiac resynchronization therapy. *Circulation.* 2010;122(10):985–92. doi:10.1161/CIRCULATIONAHA.110.955039
29. Levin HR, Oz MC, Chen JM, Packer M, Rose EA, Burkhoff D. Reversal of chronic ventricular dilation in patients with end-stage cardiomyopathy by prolonged mechanical unloading. *Circulation.* 1995;91(11):2717–20. doi:10.1161/01.cir.91.11.2717
30. Ghimire A, Fine N, Ezekowitz JA, Howlett J, Youngson E, McAlister FA. Frequency, predictors, and prognosis of ejection fraction improvement in heart failure: an echocardiogram-based registry study. *Eur Heart J.* 2019;40(26):2110–7. doi:10.1093/eurheartj/ehz233
31. Dunlay SM, Roger VL, Weston SA, Jiang R, Redfield MM. Longitudinal changes in ejection fraction in heart failure patients with preserved and reduced ejection fraction. *Circ Heart Fail.* 2012;5(6):720–6. doi:10.1161/CIRCHEARTFAILURE.111.966366
32. Bello D, Shah DJ, Farah GM, et al. Gadolinium cardiovascular magnetic resonance predicts reversible myocardial dysfunction and remodeling in patients with heart failure undergoing beta-blocker therapy. *Circulation.* 2003;108(16):1945–53. doi:10.1161/01.CIR.0000095029.57483.60
33. Panza JA, Ellis AM, Al-Khalidi HR, et al. Myocardial viability and long-term outcomes in ischemic cardiomyopathy. *N Engl J Med.* 2019;381(8):739–48. doi:10.1056/NEJMoa1807365
34. Redfors B, Stone GW. Myocardial viability and CABG surgery: a Bayesian appraisal of STICH. *Nat Rev Cardiol.* 2019;16(12):702–3. doi:10.1038/s41569-019-0292-0
35. Ammirati E, Veronese G, Brambatti M, et al. Fulminant versus acute nonfulminant myocarditis in patients with left ventricular systolic dysfunction. *J Am Coll Cardiol.* 2019;74(3):299–311. doi:10.1016/j.jacc.2019.04.063
36. Ammirati E, Cipriani M, Lilliu M, et al. Survival and left ventricular function changes in fulminant versus nonfulminant acute myocarditis. *Circulation.* 2017;136(6):529–45. doi:10.1161/CIRCULATIONAHA.117.026386
37. Grogan M, Redfield MM, Bailey KR, et al. Long-term outcome of patients with biopsy-proved myocarditis: comparison with idiopathic dilated cardiomyopathy. *J Am Coll Cardiol.* 1995;26(1):80–4. doi:10.1016/0735-1097(95)00148-s
38. McNamara DM, Starling RC, Cooper LT, et al. Clinical and demographic predictors of outcomes in recent onset dilated cardiomyopathy: results of the IMAC (Intervention in Myocarditis and Acute Cardiomyopathy)-2 study. *J Am Coll Cardiol.* 2011;58(11):1112–8. doi:10.1016/j.jacc.2011.05.033
39. Semigran MJ, Thaik CM, Fifer MA, Boucher CA, Palacios IF, Dec GW. Exercise capacity and systolic and diastolic ventricular function after recovery from acute dilated cardiomyopathy. *J Am Coll Cardiol.* 1994;24(2):462–70. doi:10.1016/0735-1097(94)90304-2
40. Merlo M, Pyxaras SA, Pinamonti B, Barbati G, Di Lenarda A, Sinagra G. Prevalence and prognostic significance of left ventricular reverse remodeling in dilated cardiomyopathy receiving tailored medical treatment. *J Am Coll Cardiol.* 2011;57(13):1468–76. doi:10.1016/j.jacc.2010.11.030
41. McNamara DM, Elkayam U, Alharethi R, et al. Clinical outcomes for peripartum cardiomyopathy in North America: results of the IPAC study (Investigations of Pregnancy-Associated Cardiomyopathy). *J Am Coll Cardiol.* 2015;66(8):905–14. doi:10.1016/j.jacc.2015.06.1309
42. Irizarry OC, Levine LD, Lewey J, et al. Comparison of clinical characteristics and outcomes of peripartum cardiomyopathy between African American and Non-African American women. *JAMA Cardiol.* 2017;2(11):1256–60. doi:10.1001/jamacardio.2017.3574
43. Sliwa K, Petrie MC, Hilfiker-Kleiner D, et al. Long-term prognosis, subsequent pregnancy, contraception and overall management of peripartum cardiomyopathy: practical guidance paper from the Heart Failure Association of the European Society of Cardiology Study Group on Peripartum Cardiomyopathy. *Eur J Heart Fail.* 2018;20(6):951–62. doi:10.1002/ejhf.1178
44. Blauwet LA, Delgado-Montero A, Ryo K, et al. Right ventricular function in peripartum cardiomyopathy at presentation is associated with subsequent left ventricular recovery and clinical outcomes. *Circ Heart Fail.* 2016;9(5). doi:10.1161/CIRCHEARTFAILURE.115.002756
45. Elkayam U, Tummala PP, Rao K, et al. Maternal and fetal outcomes of subsequent pregnancies in women with peripartum cardiomyopathy. *N Engl J Med.* 2001;344(21):1567–71. doi:10.1056/NEJM200105243442101
46. Amor-Salamanca A, Guzzo-Merello G, González-López E, et al. Prognostic impact and predictors of ejection fraction recovery in patients with alcoholic cardiomyopathy. *Rev Espanola Cardiol Engl Ed.* 2018;71(8):612–9. doi:10.1016/j.rec.2017.11.032
47. Nicolás JM, Fernández-Solà J, Estruch R, et al. The effect of controlled drinking in alcoholic cardiomyopathy. *Ann Intern Med.* 2002;136(3):192–200. doi:10.7326/0003-4819-136-3-200202050-00007
48. Cruz FE, Cheriex EC, Smeets JL, et al. Reversibility of tachycardia-induced cardiomyopathy after cure of incessant supraventricular tachycardia. *J Am Coll Cardiol.* 1990;16(3):739–44. doi:10.1016/0735-1097(90)90368-y
49. Brembilla-Perrot B, Ferreira JP, Manenti V, et al. Predictors and prognostic significance of tachycardiomyopathy: insights from a cohort of 1269 patients undergoing atrial flutter ablation. *Eur J Heart Fail.* 2016;18(4):394–401. doi:10.1002/ejhf.482
50. Nerheim P, Birger-Botkin S, Piracha L, Olshansky B. Heart failure and sudden death in patients with tachycardia-induced cardiomyopathy and recurrent tachycardia. *Circulation.* 2004;110(3):247–52. doi:10.1161/01.CIR.0000135472.28234.CC
51. Dandamudi G, Rampurwala AY, Mahenthiran J, Miller JM, Das MK. Persistent left ventricular dilatation in tachycardia-induced cardiomyopathy patients after appropriate treatment and normalization of ejection fraction. *Heart Rhythm.* 2008;5(8):1111–4. doi:10.1016/j.hrthm.2008.04.023
52. Ling L, Kalman JM, Ellims AH, et al. Diffuse ventricular fibrosis is a late outcome of tachycardia-mediated cardiomyopathy after successful ablation. *Circ Arrhythm Electrophysiol.* 2013;6(4):697–704. doi:10.1161/CIRCEP.113.000681
53. Gopinathannair R, Etheridge SP, Marchlinski FE, Spinale FG, Lakkireddy D, Olshansky B. Arrhythmia-induced cardiomyopathies: mechanisms, recognition, and management. *J Am Coll Cardiol.* 2015;66(15):1714–28. doi:10.1016/j.jacc.2015.08.038

54. Boccalandro C, Boccalandro F, Orlander P, Wei CF. Severe reversible dilated cardiomyopathy and hyperthyroidism: case report and review of the literature. *Endocr Pract Off J Am Coll Endocrinol Am Assoc Clin Endocrinol.* 2003;9(2):140–6. doi:10.4158/EP.9.2.140
55. Siu C-W, Yeung C-Y, Lau C-P, Kung AWC, Tse H-F. Incidence, clinical characteristics and outcome of congestive heart failure as the initial presentation in patients with primary hyperthyroidism. *Heart Br Card Soc.* 2007;93(4):483–7. doi:10.1136/hrt.2006.100628
56. Lupón J, Gavidia-Bovadilla G, Ferrer E, et al. Dynamic trajectories of left ventricular ejection fraction in heart failure. *J Am Coll Cardiol.* 2018;72(6):591–601. doi:10.1016/j.jacc.2018.05.042
57. Halliday BP, Wassall R, Lota AS, et al. Withdrawal of pharmacological treatment for heart failure in patients with recovered dilated cardiomyopathy (TRED-HF): an open-label, pilot, randomised trial. *Lancet Lond Engl.* 2019;393(10166):61–73. doi:10.1016/S0140-6736(18)32484-X
58. Adamo L, Perry A, Novak E, Makan M, Lindman BR, Mann DL. Abnormal global longitudinal strain predicts future deterioration of left ventricular function in heart failure patients with a recovered left ventricular ejection fraction. *Circ Heart Fail.* 2017;10(6). doi:10.1161/CIRCHEARTFAILURE.116.003788
59. de Groote P, Delour P, Mouquet F, et al. The effects of beta-blockers in patients with stable chronic heart failure. Predictors of left ventricular ejection fraction improvement and impact on prognosis. *Am Heart J.* 2007;154(3):589–95. doi:10.1016/j.ahj.2007.05.013
60. Marinescu KK, Uriel N, Mann DL, Burkhoff D. Left ventricular assist device-induced reverse remodeling: it's not just about myocardial recovery. *Expert Rev Med Devices.* 2017;14(1):15–26. doi:10.1080/17434440.2017.1262762
61. Klotz S, Danser AHJ, Foronjy RF, et al. The impact of angiotensin-converting enzyme inhibitor therapy on the extracellular collagen matrix during left ventricular assist device support in patients with end-stage heart failure. *J Am Coll Cardiol.* 2007;49(11):1166–74. doi:10.1016/j.jacc.2006.10.071
62. Kormos RL, Cowger J, Pagani FD, et al. The Society of Thoracic Surgeons Intermacs database annual report: evolving indications, outcomes, and scientific partnerships. *J Heart Lung Transplant Off Publ Int Soc Heart Transplant.* 2019;38(2):114–26. doi:10.1016/j.healun.2018.11.013
63. Topkara VK, Garan AR, Fine B, et al. Myocardial recovery in patients receiving contemporary left ventricular assist devices: results from the Interagency Registry for Mechanically Assisted Circulatory Support (INTERMACS). *Circ Heart Fail.* 2016;9(7). doi:10.1161/CIRCHEARTFAILURE.116.003157
64. Birks EJ, George RS, Hedger M, et al. Reversal of severe heart failure with a continuous-flow left ventricular assist device and pharmacological therapy: a prospective study. *Circulation.* 2011;123(4):381–90. doi:10.1161/CIRCULATIONAHA.109.933960
65. Birks EJ, Drakos SG, Lowes BD, et al. Outcome and primary endpoint results from a prospective multi-center study of myocardial recovery using LVADs: remission from stage D heart failure (RESTAGE-HF). *J Heart Lung Transplant.* 2018;37(4):S142. doi:10.1016/j.healun.2018.01.342
66. Knierim J, Heck R, Pieri M, et al. Outcomes from a recovery protocol for patients with continuous-flow left ventricular assist devices. *J Heart Lung Transplant Off Publ Int Soc Heart Transplant.* 2019;38(4):440–8. doi:10.1016/j.healun.2018.11.001
67. Maybaum S, Mancini D, Xydas S, et al. Cardiac improvement during mechanical circulatory support: a prospective multicenter study of the LVAD Working Group. *Circulation.* 2007;115(19):2497–505. doi:10.1161/CIRCULATIONAHA.106.633180
68. Ponikowski P, Voors AA, Anker SD, et al. 2016 ESC guidelines for the diagnosis and treatment of acute and chronic heart failure: the Task Force for the diagnosis and treatment of acute and chronic heart failure of the European Society of Cardiology (ESC)Developed with the special contribution of the Heart Failure Association (HFA) of the ESC. *Eur Heart J.* 2016;37(27):2129–200. doi:10.1093/eurheartj/ehw128
69. Wilcox JE, Fonarow GC, Yancy CW, et al. Factors associated with improvement in ejection fraction in clinical practice among patients with heart failure: findings from IMPROVE HF. *Am Heart J.* 2012;163(1):49–56.e2. doi:10.1016/j.ahj.2011.10.001
70. Bhambhani V, Kizer JR, Lima JAC, et al. Predictors and outcomes of heart failure with mid-range ejection fraction. *Eur J Heart Fail.* 2018;20(4):651–9. doi:10.1002/ejhf.1091
71. Cheng RK, Cox M, Neely ML, et al. Outcomes in patients with heart failure with preserved, borderline, and reduced ejection fraction in the Medicare population. *Am Heart J.* 2014;168(5):721–730.e3. doi:10.1016/j.ahj.2014.07.008
72. Koh AS, Tay WT, Teng THK, et al. A comprehensive population-based characterization of heart failure with mid-range ejection fraction. *Eur J Heart Fail.* 2017;19(12):1624–34. doi:10.1002/ejhf.945
73. Tsuji K, Sakata Y, Nochioka K, et al. Characterization of heart failure patients with mid-range left ventricular ejection fraction-a report from the CHART-2 study. *Eur J Heart Fail.* 2017;19(10):1258–69. doi:10.1002/ejhf.807
74. Rickenbacher P, Kaufmann BA, Maeder MT, et al. Heart failure with mid-range ejection fraction: a distinct clinical entity? Insights from the trial of intensified versus standard medical therapy in elderly patients with congestive heart failure (TIME-CHF). *Eur J Heart Fail.* 2017;19(12):1586–96. doi:10.1002/ejhf.798
75. Vedin O, Lam CSP, Koh AS, et al. Significance of ischemic heart disease in patients with heart failure and preserved, midrange, and reduced ejection fraction: a nationwide cohort study. *Circ Heart Fail.* 2017;10(6). doi:10.1161/CIRCHEARTFAILURE.117.003875
76. Lauritsen J, Gustafsson F, Abdulla J. Characteristics and long-term prognosis of patients with heart failure and mid-range ejection fraction compared with reduced and preserved ejection fraction: a systematic review and meta-analysis. *ESC Heart Fail.* 2018;5(4):685–94. doi:10.1002/ehf2.12283
77. Chioncel O, Lainscak M, Seferovic PM, et al. Epidemiology and one-year outcomes in patients with chronic heart failure and preserved, mid-range and reduced ejection fraction: an analysis of the ESC Heart Failure Long-Term Registry. *Eur J Heart Fail.* 2017;19(12):1574–1585. doi:10.1002/ejhf.813
78. Zafrir B, Lund LH, Laroche C, et al. Prognostic implications of atrial fibrillation in heart failure with reduced, mid-range, and preserved ejection fraction: a report from 14964 patients in the European Society of Cardiology Heart Failure Long-Term Registry. *Eur Heart J.* 2018;39(48):4277–84. doi:10.1093/eurheartj/ehy626
79. Sartipy U, Dahlström U, Fu M, Lund LH. Atrial fibrillation in heart failure with preserved, mid-range, and reduced ejection fraction. *JACC Heart Fail.* 2017;5(8):565–74. doi:10.1016/j.jchf.2017.05.001
80. Löfman I, Szummer K, Dahlström U, Jernberg T, Lund LH. Associations with and prognostic impact of chronic kidney disease in heart failure with preserved, mid-range, and reduced ejection fraction. *Eur J Heart Fail.* 2017;19(12):1606–14. doi:10.1002/ejhf.821
81. Nadruz W, West E, Sengeløv M, et al. Prognostic value of cardiopulmonary exercise testing in heart failure with reduced, midrange, and preserved ejection fraction. *J Am Heart Assoc.* 2017;6(11). doi:10.1161/JAHA.117.006000
82. Sanders-van Wijk S, van Empel V, Davarzani N, et al. Circulating biomarkers of distinct pathophysiological pathways in heart failure with preserved vs. reduced left ventricular ejection fraction. *Eur J Heart Fail.* 2015;17(10):1006–14. doi:10.1002/ejhf.414
83. Tromp J, Khan MAF, Mentz RJ, et al. Biomarker profiles of acute heart failure patients with a mid-range ejection fraction. *JACC Heart Fail.* 2017;5(7):507–17. doi:10.1016/j.jchf.2017.04.007
84. Meta-analysis Global Group in Chronic Heart Failure (MAGGIC). The survival of patients with heart failure with preserved or reduced left ventricular ejection fraction: an individual patient data meta-analysis. *Eur Heart J.* 2012;33(14):1750–7. doi:10.1093/eurheartj/ehr254
85. Shah KS, Xu H, Matsouaka RA, et al. Heart failure with preserved, borderline, and reduced ejection fraction: 5-year outcomes. *J Am Coll Cardiol.* 2017;70(20):2476–86. doi:10.1016/j.jacc.2017.08.074
86. Rastogi A, Novak E, Platts AE, Mann DL. Epidemiology, pathophysiology and clinical outcomes for heart failure patients with a mid-range ejection fraction. *Eur J Heart Fail.* 2017;19(12):1597–605. doi:10.1002/ejhf.879
87. Brann A, Janvanishstaporn S, Greenberg B. Association of prior left ventricular ejection fraction with clinical outcomes in patients with heart failure with midrange ejection fraction. *JAMA Cardiol.* Published online June 17, 2020. doi:10.1001/jamacardio.2020.2081
88. Nadruz W, West E, Santos M, et al. Heart failure and midrange ejection fraction: implications of recovered ejection fraction for exercise tolerance and outcomes. *Circ Heart Fail.* 2016;9(4):e002826. doi:10.1161/CIRCHEARTFAILURE.115.002826
89. Cleland JGF, Bunting KV, Flather MD, et al. Beta-blockers for heart failure with reduced, mid-range, and preserved ejection fraction: an individual patient-level analysis of double-blind randomized trials. *Eur Heart J.* 2018;39(1):26–35. doi:10.1093/eurheartj/ehx564
90. Flather MD, Shibata MC, Coats AJS, et al. Randomized trial to determine the effect of nebivolol on mortality and cardiovascular hospital admission in elderly patients with heart failure (SENIORS). *Eur Heart J.* 2005;26(3):215–25. doi:10.1093/eurheartj/ehi115
91. Lund LH, Claggett B, Liu J, et al. Heart failure with mid-range ejection fraction in CHARM: characteristics, outcomes and effect of candesartan across the entire ejection fraction spectrum. *Eur J Heart Fail.* 2018;20(8):1230–9. doi:10.1002/ejhf.1149
92. Lund LH, Benson L, Dahlström U, Edner M. Association between use of renin-angiotensin system antagonists and mortality in patients with heart failure and preserved ejection fraction. *JAMA.* 2012;308(20):2108–17. doi:10.1001/jama.2012.14785
93. Yancy CW, Jessup M, Bozkurt B, et al. 2017 ACC/AHA/HFSA focused update of the 2013 ACCF/AHA guideline for the management of heart failure: a report of the American College of Cardiology/American Heart Association Task Force on Clinical Practice Guidelines and the Heart Failure Society of America. *Circulation.* 2017;136(6):e137–61. doi:10.1161/CIR.0000000000000509

94. Solomon SD, Claggett B, Lewis EF, et al. Influence of ejection fraction on outcomes and efficacy of spironolactone in patients with heart failure with preserved ejection fraction. *Eur Heart J.* 2016;37(5):455–62. doi:10.1093/eurheartj/ehv464
95. Abdul-Rahim AH, Shen L, Rush CJ, et al. Effect of digoxin in patients with heart failure and mid-range (borderline) left ventricular ejection fraction. *Eur J Heart Fail.* 2018;20(7):1139–45. doi:10.1002/ejhf.1160
96. Halliday BP, Gulati A, Ali A, et al. Association between midwall late gadolinium enhancement and sudden cardiac death in patients with dilated cardiomyopathy and mild and moderate left ventricular systolic dysfunction. *Circulation.* 2017;135(22):2106–15. doi:10.1161/CIRCULATIONAHA.116.026910
97. Gatzoulis KA, Tsiachris D, Arsenos P, et al. Arrhythmic risk stratification in post-myocardial infarction patients with preserved ejection fraction: the PRESERVE EF study. *Eur Heart J.* 2019;40(35):2940–9. doi:10.1093/eurheartj/ehz260
98. Arsenos P, Gatzoulis KA, Doundoulakis I, et al. Arrhythmic risk stratification in heart failure mid-range ejection fraction patients with a non-invasive guiding to programmed ventricular stimulation two-step approach. *J Arrhythmia.* 2020. doi:10.1002/joa3.12416
99. Curtis AB, Worley SJ, Adamson PB, et al. Biventricular pacing for atrioventricular block and systolic dysfunction. *N Engl J Med.* 2013;368(17):1585–93. doi:10.1056/NEJMoa1210356
100. Curtis AB, Worley SJ, Chung ES, Li P, Christman SA, St John Sutton M. Improvement in clinical outcomes with biventricular versus right ventricular pacing: the BLOCK HF study. *J Am Coll Cardiol.* 2016;67(18):2148–57. doi:10.1016/j.jacc.2016.02.051
101. Slotwiner DJ, Raitt MH, Del-Carpio Munoz F, Mulpuru SK, Nasser N, Peterson PN. Impact of physiologic pacing versus right ventricular pacing among patients with left ventricular ejection fraction greater than 35%: a systematic review for the 2018 ACC/AHA/HRS guideline on the evaluation and management of patients with bradycardia and cardiac conduction delay: a report of the American College of Cardiology/American Heart Association Task Force on Clinical Practice Guidelines and the Heart Rhythm Society. *Circulation.* 2019;140(8):e483–503. doi:10.1161/CIR.0000000000000629
102. Kusumoto FM, Schoenfeld MH, Barrett C, et al. 2018 ACC/AHA/HRS guideline on the evaluation and management of patients with bradycardia and cardiac conduction delay: a report of the American College of Cardiology/American Heart Association Task Force on Clinical Practice Guidelines and the Heart Rhythm Society. *Circulation.* 2019;140(8):e382–482. doi:10.1161/CIR.0000000000000628
103. Chung ES, Leon AR, Tavazzi L, et al. Results of the predictors of response to CRT (PROSPECT) trial. *Circulation.* 2008;117(20):2608–16. doi:10.1161/CIRCULATIONAHA.107.743120
104. Chung ES, Katra RP, Ghio S, et al. Cardiac resynchronization therapy may benefit patients with left ventricular ejection fraction >35%: a PROSPECT trial substudy. *Eur J Heart Fail.* 2010;12(6):581–7. doi:10.1093/eurjhf/hfq009
105. Hai OY, Mentz RJ, Zannad F, et al. Cardiac resynchronization therapy in heart failure patients with less severe left ventricular dysfunction. *Eur J Heart Fail.* 2015;17(2):135–43. doi:10.1002/ejhf.208

Chapter 17
THE ADVANCED HEART FAILURE PATIENT

Eran Kalmanovich, Philippe Gaudard, and François Roubille

Epidemiology

Despite recent progress and implementation of evidence-based medical and device therapies, the prevalence of heart failure (HF) continues to increase (see Chapter 2), and, as HF survival improves, more patients deteriorate into the advanced stages of the disease.

Although it is currently estimated that advanced HF constitutes about 1–10% of the overall HF population,[1] the actual numbers could be much higher. The true prevalence of advanced HF is difficult to determine, mainly due to varying and changing definitions and difficulties in identifying these patients. Many patients with advanced HF are not listed in registries for advanced treatments, often due to age or disqualifying factors.[2,3] Additionally, most evidence on advanced HF is derived from HF with reduced ejection fraction (HFrEF), whereas information on HF with preserved ejection fraction (HFpEF) is lacking.[4] In all, the proportion of patients with advanced HF may be as high as 25% of the HF population.[2,3,5]

The prognosis of advanced HF is unfavorable. In the Olmsted County registry, the five-year survival for patients with stage D HF was 20%, compared to 78% for stage C1 and 60% for the more advanced stage C2 patients (see Chapter 2 for definition of HF stages).[6] The Randomized Evaluation of Mechanical Assistance for the Treatment of Congestive Heart Failure (REMATCH) trial reported mortality rates nearing 75% at one year and virtually no survival at two years in medically treated stage D patients. In a recent cohort study, one out of eight outpatients with stage C HFrEF progressed to stage D after three years, whereas another one of eight died before progressing to stage D despite receiving care in a center with a dedicated HF program[7] In another recent study, three-year mortality among patients identified as stage D vs non-Stage D was 43.7% vs 17.0% (age-adjusted HR 3.17; 95% confidence interval (CI) 1.94–5.18; $P<0.001$).[8]

Definitions of Advanced Heart Failure

Distinguishing patients with advanced HF from those who are sub-optimally or inadequately treated remains a major clinical challenge. Progression of chronic HF is often subtle and underappreciated. Patients with advanced HF are a heterogeneous group, ranging from ambulatory patients with mild symptoms responsible for limited functional exertion to hospitalized patients with cardiogenic shock requiring vasoactive therapy and/or mechanical circulatory support. Most persistent symptoms and recurrent hospitalizations are related to congestion. Although this is often the result of underutilized medical therapy or patient intolerance to recommended doses, progression of the disease should be considered in these cases also.

Over the years, various classification systems to define advanced HF have emerged. Each one addressed the problem from a different perspective, with limited consensus.[3] A recent position statement of the European HFA from 2018 proposed revised criteria for advance HF (Table 17.1).[1] The revised criteria identify patients with advanced HF independent of LVEF. Although most of these patients do have HFrEF, the new criteria recognize that patients with HFpEF or HF and midrange LVEF (HFmrEF) can also progress to advanced disease. Other etiologies, e.g., malignant ventricular arrhythmias, isolated right ventricular dysfunction, or uncorrectable valvular and congenital heart lesions are also considered.[1] In addition, the role of comorbidities in aggravating or masking HF status and ultimately limiting or modifying therapeutic options is recognized.[1]

Medical Therapy

Increased understanding of the neurohormonal process underlying HF progression and the introduction of corresponding pharmacological therapies (including β-blockers and renin-angiotensin-aldosterone inhibitors), in conjunction with device therapy, has led to a dramatic reduction in HF progression and mortality. Nonetheless, as the number of HF patients increases, so does the need for additional treatments, with an increased proportion of patients requiring advanced therapies. The 2013 American College of Cardiology (ACC)/American Heart Association (AHA) and the 2016 European Society of Cardiology (ESC) guidelines for the management of chronic HF recommend initiating therapy for all symptomatic patients, regardless of the severity of the HF, despite the limited numbers of patients with advanced HF enrolled in the major randomized control trials (RCTs). Most trials included patients based on left ventricular ejection fraction (LVEF) and New York Heart Association (NYHA) class and excluded patients at the most severe end of the spectrum. In HF registries, most patients with advanced HF previously followed a long course consisting of guideline-recommended and individually optimized medical therapy with diuretics, β-blockers, angiotensin-converting enzyme inhibitor (ACEi) or angiotensin receptor blockers (ARB), and, in some cases, digoxin.[5,9] Most of these patients cannot tolerate target doses of neurohormonal medications, leading to dose reduction or even discontinuation, which itself has been recognized as an indicator of advanced disease status and poor prognosis.[1,10]

The management of patients with advanced HF includes complex medication regimens, frequent clinical and laboratory follow-ups, together with lifestyle modification and exercise-based rehabilitation, and should be individually adjusted. The long-term objective is to prolong life but (1) improvement of functional capacity and quality of life and (2) prevention of readmissions and acute decompensations are important intermediate goals. As mortality is high, timely patient selection for advanced therapies (heart transplant or mechanical support) or palliative measures is crucial.

Beta-Blockers

Beta-blockers (or β-blockers) are a cornerstone of HF treatment, and their efficacy for chronic compensated HFrEF has been well established in pivotal trials, demonstrating an overall reduction in mortality (14–35%) in symptomatic patients with HFrEF (see also Chapters 5 and 10). Therefore, β-blockers are

DOI: 10.1201/9780429244544-20

TABLE 17.1: Updated HFA-ESC Criteria for Defining Advanced Heart Failure

All the following criteria must be present despite optimal guideline-directed treatment:

1. Severe and persistent symptoms of heart failure [NYHA class III (advanced) or IV].
2. Severe cardiac dysfunction is defined by a reduced LVEF ≤30%, isolated RV failure (e.g., ARVC), non-operable severe valve abnormalities, congenital abnormalities, persistently high (or increasing) BNP or NT-proBNP values, or data of severe diastolic dysfunction or LV structural abnormalities according to the ESC definition of HFpEF and HFmrEF.9.
3. Episodes of pulmonary or systemic congestion requiring high-dose intravenous diuretics (or diuretic combinations) or episodes of low-output-requiring inotropes or vasoactive drugs or malignant arrhythmias causing more than one unplanned visit or hospitalization in the past 12 months.
4. Severe impairment of exercise capacity with inability to exercise or low 6MWTD (<300 m) or pVO_2 (<12–14 mL/kg/min) estimated to be of cardiac origin.

Note: In addition to the above, extra-cardiac organ dysfunction due to heart failure (e.g., cardiac cachexia, liver, or kidney dysfunction) or type 2 pulmonary hypertension may be present but are not necessary. Criteria 1 and 4 can be met in patients who have cardiac dysfunction (as described in criterion #2), but who also have substantial limitation due to other conditions (e.g., severe pulmonary disease, non-cardiac cirrhosis, or, most commonly, renal disease with mixed etiology). These patients still have limited quality of life and survival due to advanced disease and warrant the same intensity of evaluation as someone in whom the only disease is cardiac, but the therapeutic options for the former patients are usually more limited.

Abbreviations: ARVC, arrhythmogenic right ventricular cardiomyopathy; BNP, B-type natriuretic peptide; ESC, European Society of Cardiology; HFA, Heart Failure Association; HFmrEF, heart failure with midrange ejection fraction; HFpEF, heart failure with preserved ejection fraction; LV, left ventricular; LVEF, left ventricular ejection fraction; NT-proBNP, N-terminal pro-B-type natriuretic peptide; NYHA, New York Heart Association; pVO_2, peak exercise oxygen consumption; RV, right ventricular; 6MWTD, 6-minute walk test distance.

Source: Adapted from Crespo-Leiro et al., *European Journal of Heart Failure* 2018;20(11):1505–35.

recommended for all patients with stable or symptomatic HFrEF (Table 17.2). No large-scale RCTs have evaluated long-term β-blocker therapy in patients with advanced HF, and the evidence for benefit comes from post-hoc analyses of major trials. In these analyses, patients with NYHA IV symptoms from the CIBIS-II trial and patients with NYHA III–IV symptoms and LVEF <25% from the MERIT-HF trial derived mortality benefit from β-blockers like other NYHA class groups.[11,12] Metoprolol reduced HF hospitalizations by 45% and improved NYHA class compared to placebo. The COPERNICUS trial tested efficacy of carvedilol against placebo specifically in severe HF (2,289 patients with LVEF <25% and NYHA class III–IV symptoms), but excluded those requiring intravenous inotropic or vasodilatory therapy, advanced renal failure, and blood pressure <85 mmHg). The treatment group experienced a 35% reduction in all-cause mortality compared with placebo.[13]

Patients with advanced HF are often unable to tolerate β-blockers at large doses or at all. In the REMATCH trial, 129 patients who were ineligible for heart transplant were randomized to receive a left ventricular assist device (LVAD) (n=68) or optimal medical management (n=61), of which only 22% tolerated β-blockers. In COPERNICUS, although low blood pressure was a risk marker and a frequent reason to withhold β-blockers, the benefit of carvedilol was similar in patients with low and preserved systolic blood pressure prior to treatment.[14] The negative chronotropic effect appears to be a key to the positive effects of β-blockers. In the placebo group of the Systolic Heart Failure Treatment with the If Inhibitor Ivabradine Trial (SHIFT), which enrolled patients with HFrEF in NYHA classes II–IV, a heart rate of >86 beats per minute was associated with a two-fold higher incidence of the primary endpoint of cardiovascular death and hospitalization for HF compared to <72 beats per minute; the risk was calculated to be 3% higher for every beat per minute higher baseline heart rate.[15] Another analysis suggests that the benefit of β-blockers is directly related not to the dosage, but rather to the degree of heart rate reduction.[16] Therefore, it is imperative to initiate β-blockers usage to treat advanced HF as the benefits outweigh the risks.

When initiating β-blockers, it is important to start with a low dose and gradually up-titrate during subsequent visits every two to four weeks (Table 17.2). Self-evaluation and remote monitoring can help with titration. Initiation of β-blockers can lead to worsening of HF, due mostly to congestion. In this case, the first step would be to increase the dose of either the diuretic or the ACEi, although the main limitation in practice remains low blood pressure. If that does not help, it may be necessary to reduce the dose of β-blocker. In the case of symptomatic hypotonia related to β-blocker usage, the dose of vasodilating agents and/or diuretics should be reduced first and β-blockers should only be reduced or discontinued if there is still no improvement. Importantly, β-blockers should not be discontinued during hospitalization for HF unless the patient is hemodynamically unstable, has evidence of end-organ hypoperfusion, and/or requires intravenous inotropic support with β-adrenergic agonists, although, if necessary, the dose may be temporarily reduced. Discontinuation should be avoided as reintroduction is always challenging in practice. Another option when inotropic support is required is to use drugs with a different mechanism of action, for example, levosimendan or milrinone.[16,17] The evidence suggests that continuation of β-blockers in patients hospitalized with decompensated HF is associated with lower post-discharge mortality and improved treatment rates; in contrast, β blocker withdrawal is associated with higher mortality (adjusted HR 2.3; 95% CI 1.2–4.6, P=0.013).[18] In a meta-analysis of five observational studies and one RCT, β-blocker discontinuation in patients admitted with acute decompensation was associated with higher in-hospital mortality, short-term mortality, and the combined endpoint of short-term readmission or mortality.[19] It is important to reintroduce β-blockers once the patient is stable and appropriately decongested, even at low doses, as evidence suggests that reintroduction leads to improved clinical outcomes and better patient compliance.[20,21]

Angiotensin-Converting Enzyme Inhibitors and Angiotensin Receptor Blockers

Accumulated data on ACEis have shown that these agents improve long-term prognosis in all patients with HF, including those with advanced HF, acting by inducing both vasodilation and neurohormonal antagonism. All HF guidelines recommend ACEIs as a first-line treatment for all patients with LVEF ≤40% to reduce mortality (Table 17.2). In case of ACEi intolerance, ARBs present as a suitable alternative (Table 17.2).

Intolerance to ACEi and/or ARB due to deteriorating renal function or hypotension is reported in up to one-third of

TABLE 17.2: Common Medications in the Management of Chronic Heart Failure

Drug	Start Dose	Target Dose
ACEi		
Enalapril	1.25–2.5 mg BID	10 mg BID/20 mg BID
Lisinopril	2.5–5 mg daily	20–35 mg daily
Perindopril	2–4 mg daily	4–8 mg daily
Ramipril	1.25–2.5 mg BID	5 mg BID
ARB		
Candesartan	4–8 mg daily	32 mg daily
Valsartan	40 mg BID	160 mg BID
Beta-Blockers		
Carvedilol	3.125 mg BID	25 mg BID 50 mg BID (>85kg)
Bisoprolol	1.25 mg daily	10 mg daily
Metoprolol CR/XL	12.5–25 mg daily	200 mg daily
MRA		
Spironolactone	12.5 mg daily	50 mg daily
Eplerenone	25 mg daily	50 mg daily
ARNI		
Sacubutril/Valsartan	50–100 mg BID	200 mg BID
I_f Inhibitor		
Ivabradine	2.5–5 mg BID	7.5 mg BID
Vasodilators		
Isosorbide dinitrate	20 mg TID	40 mg TID
Hydralazine	37.5 mg TID	75–100 mg TID-QID
Diuretics		
Furosemide	20–500 mg BID or TID	Lowest dose possible in stable compensated HF
Torsemide	5–200 mg QD or BID	
Bumetanide	0.5–5 mg BID or TID	
Hydrochlorothiazide	12.5–50 mg QD	
Metolazone	2.5–10 mg QD or BID	

Abbreviations: ACEi, angiotensinogen-converting enzyme inhibitor; ARB, angiotensin receptor blocker; MRA, mineralocorticoid receptor antagonist; ARNI, angiotensin receptor-neprilysin inhibitors; HF, heart failure; BID, bis in die (twice daily); TID, ter in die (three times daily); QD, quaque die (once daily).

patients with advanced HF and portends increased mortality risk.[22] In practice, every effort should be taken to start β-blockers and ACEis simultaneously and titrate doses together. Adding β-blockers to ACEis or ARBs has been shown to reduce mortality by 30–40% and mortality and rehospitalization combined by 20–40%.[23]

Mineralocorticoid Receptor Antagonists

Mineralocorticoid receptor antagonists (MRAs) are indicated in patients with NYHA class III–IV HF caused by LV systolic dysfunction (Table 17.2). In the Randomized Aldactone Evaluation Study (RALES), the first large-scale mortality trial of MRAs, 1,663 patients with NYHA IV symptoms within six months prior to randomization or NYHA III or IV symptoms at time of enrolment received either placebo or spironolactone. A 30% reduction in all-cause mortality and a 35% reduction in HF hospitalization was observed in the spironolactone arm compared with the placebo. The effective dose range of spironolactone was 12.5 mg to 25 mg.[24] However, this trial was conducted before β-blocker trials; therefore, only 11% of patients were treated with β-blockers at enrollment. Soon after RALES, there was a steep increase in hospitalization rates and deaths due to hyperkalemia reported by HF registries, thus undermining the effectiveness of MRAs.[25] Patients >75-year-old, male, those with diabetes or renal dysfunction (creatinine >2.0 mg/dL), and those treated with multiple renin-angiotensin-aldosterone system inhibitors are at higher risk of adverse outcomes.[26] Nevertheless, those at high risk of adverse outcomes are those in the advanced HF group and might benefit the most. This is a common observation in the field of HF (and probably medicine in general). The sickest patients are the most difficult to treat but also benefit the most from interventions; these patients require careful consideration of therapies and close clinical and laboratory monitoring.

Angiotensin Receptor and Neprilysin Inhibitors

The landmark Prospective Comparison of ARNI with ACEi to Determine Impact on Global Mortality and Morbidity in Heart Failure (PARADIGM-HF) trial included 8,442 patients with mild-to-moderate HFrEF, 2,018 (24%) of whom were in NYHA class III and only 60 (0.7%) in NYHA class IV. The trial compared the long-term effects of the single-molecule angiotensin receptor and neprilysin inhibitor (ARNI) sacubitril-valsartan with enalapril (Table 17.2). ARNI therapy reduced HF admission and death by 20% compared to the ACEi alone. A subgroup analysis showed that NYHA classification did not affect the primary outcome.[27] However, the small number of patients in NYHA class IV precludes the generalization of the

PARADIGM findings to the advanced HF population. While ARNI appears to be a promising treatment, data on patients with advanced HF are still lacking. The ongoing LCZ696 In Advanced Heart Failure (LIFE) trial will determine whether sacubitril-valsartan will improve levels of N-terminal pro-B-type natriuretic peptide (NT-proBNP), compared with valsartan, in patients with advanced HFrEF after 24 weeks of therapy (NCT02816736).

Digoxin

The use of cardiac glycosides in treating patients with chronic HF, especially those in sinus rhythm, remains controversial. The Digitalis Investigation Group (DIG) trial showed a neutral effect on mortality with a trend toward reduced hospital admissions compared with placebo.[28] A DIG post-hoc analysis showed a decrease in mortality among those with low digoxin serum concentrations.[29] Several meta-analyses showed a neutral or even adverse effect of digoxin on mortality in patients with HFrEF and sinus rhythm or atrial fibrillation.[30] However, a meta-analysis indicated that digoxin withdrawal was associated with increased HF hospitalization and decompensation in patients with stable HFrEF (RR 1.30; 95% CI 1.16–1.46), but had no impact on all-cause mortality (RR 1.00; 95% CI 0.90–1.12).[31–33] A new trial, DIGIT-HF, is currently in progress to compare digoxin vs placebo in treating HFrEF (NYHA III–IV and LVEF ≤40%, or NYHA II and LVEF ≤30%) in patients both with and without AF. One theory regarding the lack of consensus regarding digoxin is that patients treated with digoxin tend to have more comorbidities and/or more advanced HF, thereby introducing confounding factors, which likely impact mortality. Therefore, despite the controversy, both European and American guidelines recommend digoxin as a last-line therapy in patients with HFrEF and persistent symptoms due to its beneficial effects on symptoms and hospital admissions.

Nitrates and Hydralazine

The concept behind using nitrates together with hydralazine was to achieve a nitroprusside-like effect with a combined preload and afterload reduction, caused by the predominant venodilatory effect of organic nitrates and the arterial dilatory effect of hydralazine (Table 17.2). The Vasodilator-Heart Failure Trial (V-HeFT I) compared isosorbide dinitrate and hydralazine (ID+H) vs placebo and demonstrated a trend toward reduced mortality in the ID+H group (44% vs 38.7%; P=0.09). The V-HeFT II trial compared ID+H to enalapril (804 patients) and revealed a trend toward improved mortality with enalapril (38.2% vs 32.8%; P=0.08).[34] However, the ID+H arm had greater improvement in LVEF and exercise tolerance.[34] These studies showed that ACEi use in patients with NYHA II–III HF provides greater survival benefit than direct vasodilation.[35] In a retrospective analysis of the V-HeFT trials, African Americans derived significantly greater mortality benefit from ID+H vs placebo or enalapril, compared with European-Americans. This led to the African American Heart Failure (A-HeFT) Trial, which randomized 1,040 African Americans with class III–IV HFrEF on diuretics, ACEi, and β-blockers, to ID+H or placebo. At 10 months, ID+H had reduced mortality by 43% and first HF hospitalization by 33%.[36] However, in a meta-analysis, when used alone, ID+H was associated with higher all-cause mortality compared to ACEi (OR 1.35; 95% CI 1.03–1.76; P=0.03), and cardiovascular mortality (OR 1.37; 95% CI 1.04–1.81; P=0.03).[37] Therefore, the current recommendation is to use ID+H only in symptomatic HFrEF patients who cannot tolerate either ACEi or ARB (or they are contraindicated) or in African American men.[38, 39]

Ivabradine

Ivabradine is a selective inhibitor of the hyperpolarization-activated cyclic nucleotide-gated or I_f channels.[40] It reduces sinoatrial nodal discharge, thus reducing heart rate and prolonging diastolic depolarization without any negative inotropic effects.[41] Due to the findings of SHIFT and additional subgroup analyses, ivabradine has been approved for patients with LVEF <5%, sinus rhythm with a heart rate of ≥75, and symptomatic HF (NYHA II–IV) to reduce HF hospitalization risk.[41–43] However, few patients with advanced HF were included in SHIFT, and therefore data on the efficacy of ivabradine in this population are limited. Nevertheless, considering the relatively minor effect of ivabradine on blood pressure, which might limit use of β-blockers in advanced HF, this agent could have a role for patients whose tachycardia persists despite use of maximally tolerated β-blockers.[44]

Sodium-Glucose Co-Transporter 2 Inhibitors

Sodium-glucose co-transporter 2 inhibitors (SGLT2i) have emerged as a novel therapy in patients with HFrEF. The DAPA-HF (Dapagliflozin and Prevention of Adverse-Outcomes in Heart Failure) trial and the EMPEROR-Reduced (EMPagliflozin outcomE tRial in Patients With chrOnic heaRt Failure With Reduced Ejection Fraction) trial evaluated the effects of dapagliflozin and empagliflozin, respectively, in patients with HFrEF regardless of the presence of diabetes.[45,46] Both trials demonstrated a significant reduction in the composite of first HF hospitalization or cardiovascular death. Subsequent meta-analyses including these trials demonstrated that these agents also reduce the risk of all-cause mortality and cardiovascular mortality in HFrEF (see also Chapters 10 and 22 for more information on SGLT2i).[47]

As with previous pharmacological trials, the mean LVEF was around 27 % and 30% in the EMPEROR-Reduced and DAPA-HF trials, respectively. Fewer than 30% of the study population were NYHA class IIII and less than 1% were NYHA class IV in each trial. Nonetheless, Zannad et al. showed that SGLT2i had a positive effect even in patients with NYHA class III–IV.[47] SGLT2i has a safe profile, with low risks of hypotension and favorable renal effects, making these agents a good treatment option for advanced HF patients who are intolerant to, e.g., ACEi, ARBs, or ARNI due to their blood pressure-lowering effects. In post hoc analyses of DAPA-HF and EMPEROR-Reduced, the SGLT2i effects were independent of ARNI use.[47]

In other post-hoc analyses of the SGLT2i trials, a consistently positive effect has been demonstrated, even in patients with an eGFR <60 mL/min per 1·73 m². Together with the data from the Dapagliflozin in Patients with Chronic Kidney Disease (DAPA-CKD) trial, in which patients with eGFR as low as 25 mL/min per 1·73 m² had favorable renal and cardiovascular outcomes,[48] there is significant evidence for benefit from SGLT2i use in the high-risk group of advanced HF patients who are often intolerant to side-effects of RAAS inhibitors or have a concomitant renal functional deterioration which limits the treatment options.

Device Therapy for Advanced HF

Therapeutic Implantable Devices

Therapeutic implantable devices for patients with HF include implantable cardioverter-defibrillators (ICDs) and cardiac resynchronization therapy (CRT)—see also Chapter 10. Both devices have established indications in HF management, improved long-term mortality and morbidity, and have been investigated extensively. Currently, "primary" ICD implantation, i.e., with the goal of primary prevention of sudden cardiac death, is indicated for NYHA class II–III patients with HF and LVEF≤35% who have a projected survival of over one year. "Secondary" implantation is indicated for all patients with HF who have experienced hemodynamically unstable ventricular arrhythmias.[49] ICD implantation in advanced HF should be individualized, as this therapy might not alter the outlook and, in fact, frequent shocks might worsen both hemodynamic status and quality of life.[50,51] In all, patients with advanced HF can benefit from ICD and CRT devices but more evidence is needed, particularly for ICDs; as most CRT pivotal trials did include subjects with advanced HF (NYHA class III–IV), the current recommendations support the use of CRT in this population.

Monitoring Implantable Devices

Early detection of impending decompensation, even before clinical symptoms appear, and timely intervention to avert clinical decompensation and hospital admission, has been the holy grail of HF management. The low sensitivity of clinical and circulating markers, together with the disappointing results of telemonitoring, have led to the implementation of more advanced technologies for this purpose.[52–54] CardioMEMS (St. Jude Medical, Inc., Saint Paul, MN, USA) is an implantable wireless sensor, placed through right heart catheterization in the pulmonary artery, that continuously monitors pulmonary artery pressure and transmits data to the caring physician. CardioMEMS can identify changes in intracardiac pressure promptly and allows timely pharmacological management. The multi-center CardioMEMS Heart Sensor Allows Monitoring of Pressure to Improve Outcomes in NYHA Class III Heart Failure Patients (CHAMPION) trial randomized 550 patients with NYHA class III symptoms to receive either the device or usual care. Medications were adjusted based on data generated by the sensor. A 28% reduction of HF hospitalization in six months and a 37% reduction in 15 months was observed without increasing other causes of hospitalization.[54, 55] The recent ESC guidelines recommend this technology for patients with NYHA III symptoms and HF hospitalization in the past year, regardless of LVEF.[38] There are no reports utilizing CardioMEMS specifically in the advanced HF population, although it is an appealing option and it is reasonable to assume that these patients would derive benefit from this technology. Additional information for monitoring devices which have been approved or are under investigation is provided in Chapter 6.

Revascularization and Valvular Disease Approaches

Surgical and transcatheter procedures in patients with advanced HF are challenging. On one hand, HFrEF itself confers high procedural risk because of delicate hemodynamics, whereas patients with HFpEF are prone to peri-procedural complications due to age and comorbidities. On the other hand, interventions are required in certain cases to mitigate myocardial damage due to coronary artery disease (CAD) or valvular abnormalities. Breakthroughs in interventional and structural cardiology offer new approaches for percutaneous or hybrid procedures for treating this high-risk population.

Strategies for Revascularization

Together with high blood pressure, CAD is the most common etiology leading to HF,[56] and ischemic HF patients have worse outcomes[57,58] than other etiologies. The Surgical Treatment for Ischemic Heart Failure (STICH) trial compared the efficacy of revascularization by coronary artery bypass grafting (CABG) with standard medical therapy in patients with CAD and LVEF ≤35%. The ten-year results showed lower all-cause mortality with the addition of CABG (HR 0.70; 95% CI 0.58–0.84; P<0.001).[59] Although CABG benefits this HF population, a comparison between CABG and percutaneous coronary intervention (PCI) in these patients is lacking.[60] Early observational studies comparing PCI vs CABG in patients with HF reported that mortality was similar or slightly better with CABG.[61,62] However, in most of these reports, few patients had LVEF below 30–35% and advanced HF was not specifically defined, with the exception of a retrospective analysis of everolimus-eluting stents vs CABG in patients with multivessel disease and LVEF <35%; in that study, mortality was similar in the PCI and CABG arms (HR 1.01, 95% CI 0.81–1.28, P=0.91).[63] A meta-analysis of eight observational studies involving 10,268 patients with CAD and reduced LVEF treated either with CABG or PCI with drug-eluting stents demonstrated higher risk of all-cause mortality (HR 1.36, 95% CI 1.16–1.60), cardiac mortality (HR 2.20, 95% CI 1.63–2.95), myocardial infarction (HR 1.69, 95% CI 1.28–2.24), and repeat revascularization (HR 4.95, 95% CI 3.28–7.46) in patients undergoing PCI. A subgroup analysis of patients with LVEF <35% or left main and/or multivessel disease yielded results similar to the main analysis.[64] The small number of patients in these studies, the lack of large RCTs, and the continuously evolving percutaneous and surgical technologies (leading to results on outdated practices by the time a study is published) make it difficult to reliably assess the optimal revascularization strategy for patients with advanced ischemic HF. The 2014 ESC/EACTS guidelines on myocardial revascularization support coronary reperfusion, mainly CABG, for all patients with LVEF ≤35% and left main artery disease or left main equivalent disease,[65] a finding which is consistent with the 2018 ESC-HFA expert opinion statement for advanced HF.[1] Therefore, a heart team approach is required to individualize the revascularization strategy, after careful evaluation of the patient's clinical status and coronary anatomy, anticipated completeness of revascularization, coexisting valvular disease, and co-morbidities. In advanced HF with unacceptably high surgical risk, PCI under short-term mechanical circulatory support (e.g., with an Impella device) is a reasonable alternative.[1] Observational studies reported improved survival with early revascularization when compared with medical therapy in the presence of hibernating myocardium, and therefore evaluation for a viable myocardium is recommended.[65] Also, it is important to note that the indication for revascularization in this population is not driven by angina refractory to medical therapy or ischemia, but also by symptomatic ventricular arrythmias or aborted sudden cardiac death.

Valvular Surgery and Percutaneous Solutions

Valvular etiologies of HF or valvular dysfunction due to ventricular dysfunction, e.g., functional mitral regurgitation (FMR), are discussed in detail in Chapter 15. Both AHA and ESC recommend intervention early in the process for patients with aortic or mitral disease and signs of myocardial dysfunction.[66] The presence of FMR is common in patients with advanced HF of both ischemic and non-ischemic etiology and heralds a poor prognosis.[67] Until recently, mitral valve repair remained a last-resort option for FMR non-responsive to optimal medical therapy, CRT, and revascularization. However, transcatheter mitral valve repair using the MitraClip device has transformed this field. Two RCTs, Percutaneous Repair with the MitraClip Device for Severe Functional/Secondary Mitral Regurgitation (MITRA-FR) and Cardiovascular Outcomes Assessment of the MitraClip Percutaneous Therapy for HF Patients with Functional Mitral Regurgitation (COAPT), assessed the efficacy and safety of MitraClip in patients with HFrEF and severe FMR. The two trials reported different efficacy findings, sparking intense debate. Critics of the two studies argued that, although they both targeted the same disease entity, the difference in the population of patients recruited for the trials yielded different results.[68] Therefore, the proposed criteria for patient selection include (1) ≥ moderate-to-severe (3+) FMR defined as effective regurgitant orifice area ≥30 mm^2 and/or regurgitant volume >45 mL; (2) LVEF 20–50% and LVEDD <70 mm; (3) persistent HF symptoms (NYHA ≥ II) despite optimal medical treatment with CRT and coronary revascularization, where appropriate.[68] The role of surgical or transcatheter interventions for valvular dysfunction in advanced HF continues to evolve.

Rehabilitation

In clinical trials, exercise training in patients with HFrEF demonstrated a wide range of clinical and physiological benefits, including improved quality of life and exercise capacity, favorable effects on neurohumoral, inflammatory, metabolic, and autonomic function, and improvement in endothelial, skeletal muscle, and cardiac remodeling.[69–71] Most of these trials have focused on patients with advanced HF by definition, with LVEF ≤25%, demonstrating also a modest improvement in survival and hospitalization rates.[72] A recent Cochrane review reported that exercise-based rehabilitation has no short-term (up to 12 months) effect on mortality but reduces risk of hospitalization and yields improvements in quality of life. It was suggested that exercise training might reduce mortality in the longer term and that the benefits of exercise may depend on age, gender, and HF severity.[73] Due to these findings, we recommend that patients take part in a rehabilitation program as part of a comprehensive treatment program. Exercise training is further discussed in Chapter 11.

Management of Acute Decompensation in Advanced Heart Failure

Patients with advanced HF present a terminal pathophysiological process. Therefore, these patients are prone to frequent clinical deterioration, due to congestion or low cardiac output, with or without end-organ compromise. On one hand, vasoconstrictors and inotropes may improve hemodynamics in the short term and help reverse end-organ dysfunction; on the other hand, these agents exert adverse pathophysiological effects and are associated with worse prognosis. Their use, however, is justified in refractory decompensation, as a bridge to temporary or long-term mechanical circulatory support (MCS), heart transplant, or palliative therapy. Co-morbidities, e.g., worsening renal function or resistance to diuresis, can further complicate treatment of congestion in these patients.

Nitrates

Nitrates (as vasodilators) are considered the second most often used agent after diuretics in acute decompensated HF for symptomatic relief, although the evidence for their effectiveness is limited. These agents are most useful in patients with acute decompensated HF and normal or high blood pressure, owing to their hemodynamic effect on the venous and arterial systems, leading to quick pre-load and afterload reduction. The recent ESC HF guidelines recommend the use of nitrates as a continuous infusion in patients with acute HF and systolic blood pressure >110 mmHg and to use with caution in patients with systolic blood pressure between 90 and 110 mmHg.[38] Nitrates in cardiogenic shock cases should be avoided and used only at the discretion of the treating physician in select cases.[74,75]

Diuretics

Diuretics are recommended for all symptomatic patients with HF, despite the lack of RCT evidence.[38] In a meta-analysis of 14 trials (525 participants total), seven of which were placebo-controlled and seven of which compared diuretics to other treatment options such as ACEi or digoxin, diuretic use was associated with lower mortality (OR 0.24, 95% CI 0.07–0.83; P=0.02).[76] On the other hand, data from the Prospective Randomized Amlodipine Survival Evaluation (PRAISE),[77] SOLVD,[78] and DIG studies, and the ADHERE Registry,[4] suggest that large doses of diuretics are associated with higher mortality in HF populations.

Most patients with advanced HF who are treated with diuretics eventually develop diuretic resistance, defined as impaired sensitivity to diuretics, resulting in reduced natriuresis and diuresis, therefore limiting the possibility to achieve euvolemia. Diuretic resistance associated with worsening renal function is an indicator of advanced HF and the need for more advanced therapies.[79] Diuretic resistance may be, in part, the result of an adaptive response to the volume depletion, leading to increased activity of the RAAS and the sympathetic nervous system, nephron remodeling, pre-existing renal dysfunction, and changing pharmacokinetics.[80] Although net fluid output and body weight are practical markers of diuretic response, the correlation between body weight and volume redistribution is poor.[81,82] A recent consensus statement supports assessment of natriuresis alongside diuresis to judge diuretic response.[80] Sequential nephron blockade, i.e., a combination of different types of diuretics, can have a strong synergistic effect on diuresis and natriuresis. Thiazide and thiazide-like diuretics, acetazolamide, mineralocorticoid receptor antagonists (MRAs), and other agents, e.g., sodium-glucose cotransporter 2 inhibitors, can be combined with loop diuretics.

Thiazide and thiazide-like diuretics act by blocking the sodium-chloride co-transporter in the distal convoluted tubule, thus increasing sodium secretion by the distal nephron. The addition of metolazone was an integral part of the stepped pharmacologic algorithm in the CARRESS-HF-trial, which resulted in the recommendation of thiazides as a second-line agent in both American and European guidelines.[38] Observational studies support the effectiveness of thiazides in patients with reduced glomerular filtration rate (<30 mL/min/1.73 m^2), which can be an advantage in patients with advanced HF.

In the Aldosterone Targeted Neurohormonal Combined with Natriuresis Therapy in Heart Failure (ATHENA-HF) trial, spironolactone 100 mg daily was not superior to 25 mg (or placebo) in reducing NT-proBNP or increasing urine output after 96 h in patients with acute HF. On the other hand, spironolactone was safe and useful in offsetting the hypokalemic effect of potassium-wasting loop and thiazide diuretics. This may result in more patients with HFrEF being discharged on optimized therapy.[83] Acetazolamide is a carbonic anhydrase inhibitor that inhibits sodium reabsorption in the proximal tubule. Observational studies demonstrated its ability to boost the diuretic response in combination with loop diuretics.[84]

In summary, achieving euvolemia is a major challenge in advanced HF. Various strategies have been proposed based on circulating, imaging, or sensor-derived markers, e.g., BNP or NT-proBNP,[85] echocardiographic parameters[86,87] or bio-impedance.[88,89] However, all have had a neutral effect at best on rehospitalization or cardiovascular outcomes, except for CardioMEMS which proved to decrease HF hospitalizations through better diuretic management.[90] Furthermore, recent trials tried to discontinue loop diuretics without worsening of dyspnea or reintroduction of higher diuretic doses in stable, less sick patients, in an attempt to reduce the potential detrimental effects of loop diuretics on chronic HF.[91] In advanced HF, our approach upon decongestion is to reduce the diuretics to the lowest dose possible; this might help the use of other neurohormonal blocker therapy in doses closer to the current guideline recommendations and avoid side effects of diuretics.

Inotropic Support

Current inotropic drugs include β-adrenergic receptor agonists, phosphodiesterase inhibitors (PDEi), and calcium sensitizers. These agents are frequently used in acute decompensated HF with signs of hypoperfusion with or without evidence of pulmonary congestion.[42] The most used inotropic drugs are dobutamine, milrinone, and levosimendan (which is available only in Europe). The hemodynamic effects of these agents are well studied and summarized in Table 17.3. Inotropes improve both symptoms and hemodynamics, although continuous use of these agents in refractory HF has been associated with adverse effects on mortality.

Dobutamine, a β-adrenergic receptor agonist, increases intracellular cAMP, which activates protein kinase A, leading to calcium-channel opening and sarcoplasmic reticulum calcium release. Dobutamine increases cardiac output (CO) and decreases pulmonary capillary wedge pressure (PCWP) in patients with HF, and therefore is recommended for patients with low CO and reduced organ perfusion. Concomitant use of β-blockers is not recommended as it may attenuate the benefits of both agents.[92] However, as first demonstrated in a post-hoc analysis of the Flolan International Randomized Survival Trial (FIRST), dobutamine infusion was associated with higher mortality (70.5% vs 37.1%; $P<0.001$) compared with other treatments.[93] Subsequent studies confirmed this association between dobutamine and increased mortality, especially with prolonged administration and/or the administration of relatively high doses (i.e., >5 μg/kg/min).

Milrinone, a PDEi, inhibits cAMP breakdown within the cell, thereby increasing cAMP levels, and produces similar effects on myocytes as β1-adrenergic agonists. However, PDEis have a more direct effect on cAMP levels than dobutamine, and thus PDEis have a significant vasodilatory effect on vascular smooth muscle cells. This may cause hypotension and further peripheral and/or coronary hypoperfusion. However, milrinone may be preferred in patients with systemic hypertension, pulmonary hypertension, low CO, or hypoperfusion symptoms.[94] In OPTIME-CHF, an RCT that evaluated milrinone vs placebo, demonstrated that milrinone (relative to placebo) did not significantly alter in-hospital or two-month mortality rates (3.8% vs 2.3% and 10.3% vs 8.9%, respectively). Milrinone was associated with more hypotension and arrhythmias.[94] A subsequent OPTIME-CHF trial analysis reported higher mortality with milrinone in patients with ischemic cardiomyopathy.[95]

Levosimendan, a calcium sensitizer, improves cardiomyocyte responsiveness to intracellular calcium. However, unlike digoxin or PDEi, it has no impact on intracellular calcium concentrations. Levosimendan acts on K^+-dependent ATP channels in cardiac mitochondria and vascular smooth muscle cells, thereby producing cardioprotective and vasodilatory effects, respectively. The net effect of levosimendan is increased CO (through enhanced systolic and diastolic left ventricular function), vasodilatation leading to increased peripheral perfusion, and reduced natriuretic peptide levels.[96] Levosimendan has an active metabolite, OR-1896, with similar effects but different pharmacokinetics; levosimendan has a half-life of about 1 h, whereas its metabolite reaches peak plasma concentrations two to three days after infusion, thus prolonging the therapeutic effects beyond the infusion period.[97] This effect allows for the use of levosimendan as a bridge to other therapies or in dobutamine weaning. Levosimendan in acute HF leads to marked symptom relief. A meta-analysis of ~5500 patients in 45 RCTs demonstrated a reduction in mortality with levosimendan.[98]

In conclusion, whereas inotropes improve hemodynamics and symptoms in acute HF, reports of increased mortality rates and adverse outcomes following inotrope treatment have raised concerns regarding the long-term use of these agents in advanced HF.[99]

TABLE 17.3: Comparison of Inotropic and Vasoactive Agents Used in Decompensated Heart Failure

Medication	Activity				Dose Range	Hemodynamic Effects						
	α1	β1	β2	DA		CO/CI	SVR	PVR	PCWP	MAP	HR	VO_2
Dopamine		+	–	++	1–5 μg/kg/min	⇔	⇔	⇔	⇔	⇔	⇔	⇔
	+	++	–	++	5–15 μg/kg/min	⇧	⇧	⇔⇧	⇔⇧	⇔⇩	⇧	⇧
	+	++	–	++	>15 μg/kg/min	⇧	⇧	⇔⇧	⇧	⇔⇧	⇧⇧	⇧
Dobutamine	–/+	+++	+	–	2–20 μg/kg/min	⇧⇧	⇔⇩	⇩	⇔⇩	⇩⇔	⇧	⇧
Epinephrine	++	+++	++	–	0.01–0.1 μg/kg/min	⇧⇧	⇧	⇔⇧	⇧	⇧⇧	⇧⇧	⇧
Norepinephrine	+++	++	–	–	0.5–30 μg /min	⇧⇩	⇧⇧	⇔⇧	⇧	⇧⇧	⇧	⇧
Milrinone	PDE inhibitor				50 μg/kg bolus, 0.375–0.75 μg/kg/min	⇧⇧	⇩⇩	⇩	⇩⇩	⇩⇔	⇧	⇔
Levosimendan	calcium sensitizer				6–24 μg/kg/min bolus, 0.25–0.75 μg/kg/min	⇧⇧⇧	⇩⇩	⇩	⇩⇩	⇩	⇧	⇔
Phenylephrine	+++	–	–	–	0.5–5 μg/kg/min	⇩	⇧	⇔	⇧	⇧	⇩	⇧
Vasopressin	ADH antagonist				0.04 U/min	⇔⇩	⇧	⇔	⇧	⇧	⇔	⇔

Abbreviations: ⇧, increase; ⇩, decrease; ⇔, no change; DA, Dopamine agonist; CO, cardiac output; CI, cardiac index; SVR, systemic vascular resistance; PVR, pulmonary vascular resistance; PCWP, pulmonary capillary wedge pressure; MAP, mean arterial pressure; HR, heart rate; VO_2, myocardial oxygen demand.

Non-Pharmacological Therapies for Congestion

Driven by a machine-generated transmembrane pressure gradient, ultrafiltration removes plasma water across a semipermeable membrane. This technique lowers right atrial pressure and PCWP and can therefore result in sustained symptomatic improvement. However, the available evidence does not support the use of ultrafiltration as a first-line therapy. In the CARRESS-HF trial, ultrafiltration was inferior to stepped pharmacotherapy.[100] A meta-analysis of eight RCTs comparing ultrafiltration to diuretics did not show any significant difference in survival or renal function; only a trend toward a lower readmission rate in patients treated with ultrafiltration was reported. Therefore, the current recommendation is to use ultrafiltration should pharmacotherapy fail to resolve congestion.[1,38,80]

The evidence to support ultrafiltration in advanced HF is scarce. In a highly selected group of 63 patients with advanced HF (LVEF 26±15%), worsening renal function (creatinine 1.9±0.8 mg/dL), elevated mean central venous pressure and PCWP, and low cardiac index (1.8 L/min/m^2; 18% were treated with inotropes at baseline), ultrafiltration led to reduction in filling pressures and increase in cardiac index in the first 48 h. After initiation of ultrafiltration, 59% of patients required conversion to continuous dialysis during the hospital stay, and 14% were dependent on dialysis at discharge. In-hospital mortality was high, with 19 (30%) of 63 patients dying before discharge and six additional patients discharged to palliative care.[101] In a small RCT, 30 NYHA class III–IV patients with acute HF and congestion were randomized to receive either continuous diuretic infusion or ultrafiltration; greater weight loss, greater clinical improvement at 36 h, and more favorable biomarkers (NT-proBNP and aldosterone) and hemodynamics (increased stroke volume index and cardiac index and decreased systemic vascular resistance) were observed with ultrafiltration, but mortality was not affected.[102] Another option is peritoneal ultrafiltration, which, unlike intravenous ultrafiltration, can be used daily. Several small cohorts have demonstrated moderate improvement in functional and clinical parameters with peritoneal ultrafiltration.[103,104]

Temporary Mechanical Circulatory Support (MCS)

Temporary, short-term MCS is recommended for patients with cardiogenic shock, chronic HF with acute decompensation refractory to maximal medical therapy, multi-organ failure, sepsis, or ventilator dependence to optimize hemodynamics and evaluate neurologic status, as per the 2013 Lung and Heart Transplantation guidelines and AHA and ESC consensus statement.[1,105,106] The ideal MCS device allows for rapid percutaneous access, enables both hemodynamic support and myocardial protection, and has a low rate of procedural complications (limb ischemia, embolization, infection, and hemolysis). MCS can support the LV alone, RV alone, or both ventricles, and can also support oxygenation depending on the modality (Table 17.4).[107] From intra-aortic balloon counter-pulsation pump, to Impella and TandemHeart, to extracorporeal membrane oxygenation and Centrimag, devices offer increasing support, but also require more invasive vascular access, leading to more complications. Temporary MCS requires expertise in acute care and should be used as a bridge to recovery or bridge to decisions for other solutions (i.e., long-term MCS, heart transplant, or palliative care). Despite increasing use of MCS, randomized evidence is limited. Furthermore, most of these trials focused on patients with cardiogenic shock due to myocardial infarction.[108–110] Recent registries have shown that temporary MCS may be used to bridge critically ill candidates directly to heart transplantation in a setting of short waitlist times.[111,112] The options for temporary MCS are further discussed in detail in Chapter 9.

Advanced Therapies for Advanced HF

Long-Term Mechanical Circulatory Support

Long-term MCS devices, mainly LVADs, have emerged as alternatives to heart transplantation and have been shown to enhance quality of life and reduce mortality compared to medical therapy in inotrope-dependent patients or in patients who have contraindications for heart transplant (Figure 17.1).[38,113,114] The growing number of patients with HF, combined with improved medical therapy, has led to an increase in the number of patients surviving and progressing to advanced HF.

TABLE 17.4: Comparison of Temporary Mechanical Circulatory Support Devices

	IABP	ECMO	TandemHeart	Impella 2.5	Impella CP	Impella 5.0
Pump mechanism	Pneumatic	Centrifugal	Centrifugal	Axial	Axial	Axial
Cannula size	7–9 Fr	18–21 Fr inflow; 15-22 Fr outflow	21 Fr inflow; 15–17 Fr outflow	13 Fr	14 Fr	22 Fr
Insertion technique	Descending aorta via the temporal artery	Peripheral approach—Inflow cannula into the right atrium via the femoral/jugular vein. Outflow cannula into the descending aorta via the femoral artery Central approach	Inflow cannula into the left atrium via femoral vein and transseptal puncture and 15–17 Fr outflow cannula into the femoral artery	Cather placed retrogradely across the aortic valve via the femoral artery		Catheter placed retrogradely across the aortic valve via surgical cutdown of the femoral/ subclavian artery
Hemodynamic support	0.5–1.0 L min	Up to 10 L/min	4 L min	2.5 L/min	4 L/min	5 L/min
Implantation time	+	++	+++	++	++	+++
Risk of limb ischemia	+	+++	++	++	++	++
Anticoagulation	+	+++	+++	+	+	+
Hemolysis	+	++	++	++	++	++
Post-implantation management complexity	+	+++	++++	++	++	++

Source: Adapted from Werdan et al., *European Heart Journal* 2014;35:156–67, by permission from Oxford University Press and European Society of Cardiology.

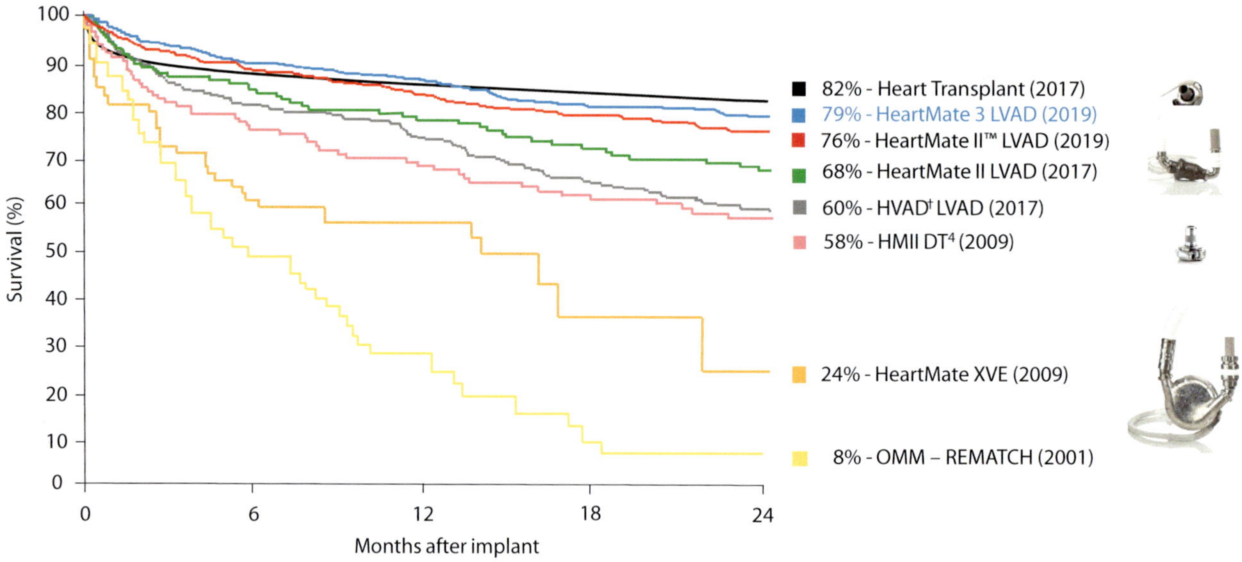

FIGURE 17.1 A historical perspective of survival for patients with end-stage heart failure who partook in randomized clinical trials. The yellow lines depict the survival associated with optimal medical therapy and pulsatile technology. Eight years after the completion of the REMATCH trial, the pulsatile technology has been completely abandoned in favor of smaller continuous-flow pumps, which has translated into not only a dramatic improvement in survival, as seen in the purple, green, and red curves, but also a drastic improvement in quality of life. Current devices are associated with a two-year survival of 83%, which is comparable to that of heart transplantation.

TABLE 17.5: Comparison of Common LVADs

Device Type	HeartMate II	Heartmate III	HeartWare HVAD System
Rotation per minute	6,000–15,000	3,000–9,000	2,400–3,200
Rotor design	Axial	Centrifugal	Centrifugal
Pump position	Pump pocket	Intrapericardial	Intrapericardial
Weight (g)	292	220	145
Bearing system	Ball in a cup	Magnetic levitation	Magnetic levitation
Artificial pulsatility		+	
FDA approved indication	BTT (2008) DT (2010)	BTT (2017) DT (2017)	BTT (2012) DT (2017)

Abbreviations: BTT, bridge to transplant; DT, destination therapy.

Despite the transplant waitlist continuing to grow, survival has improved, mainly due to increased use of MCS.[115,116] The older, pneumatically driven and pulsatile-flow pumps were large and required extensive surgical dissection. These devices suffered from high failure rates and poor survival of the patients. In contrast, the newer generation, continuous-flow LVADs have smaller pumps, incorporating axial and centrifugal pump technology. Due to their small size, there is a significantly lower risk of pocket infections. Currently, >98% of LVAD implants are non-pulsatile devices, which are the current standard of care.[115,116]

The most commonly implanted devices are the axial-flow HeartMate II device (Thoratec, Abbott Laboratories), the centrifugal-flow HeartWare HVAD device (Medtronic), and the newer-generation centrifugal-flow HeartMate 3 (Thoratec, Abbott Laboratories), which has a fully magnetically levitated rotor (Table 17.5).[117–119] In the pivotal HeartMate II trial, the continuous-flow HeartMate II LVAD significantly improved stroke- and reoperation-free survival at two years in patients with advanced HF who were ineligible for transplantation as compared with a pulsatile device (46% vs 11%; P<0.001), leading to the approval of HeartMate II as destination therapy.[117] The ENDURANCE trial compared HVAD to HeartMate II as destination therapy in patients with advanced HF not eligible for a heart transplant. The trial demonstrated the non-inferiority of HVAD for stroke- and reoperation-free survival at two years, although the rate of stroke in HVAD was higher.[120] In a post-hoc analysis, better blood pressure management was associated with reduced stroke rates in patients with HVAD.[121] In the Multicenter Study of MagLev Technology in Patients Undergoing Mechanical Circulatory Support Therapy With HeartMate 3 (MOMENTUM) trial, the fully magnetically levitated, centrifugal-flow HeartMate III (Figure 17.2) was superior to HeartMate II for stroke- and reoperation-free survival at two years (76.9% vs 64.8%; P<0.001).[122] All three devices (HeartMate II and III and HVAD) are approved by FDA both for bridge-to-transplant and destination therapy use (Figure 17.3).

Although there are currently no consensus guidelines for LVAD implantation, criteria have been developed to help optimize patient selection and outcomes. Patients should be considered for LVAD therapy if they have experienced severe symptoms for more than two months despite optimal medical and device therapy, along with one of the following: LVEF <25% and peak oxygen consumption less than 12 mL/kg/min; two or more hospitalizations due to HF during the previous 12 months, without an obvious precipitating cause; dependence

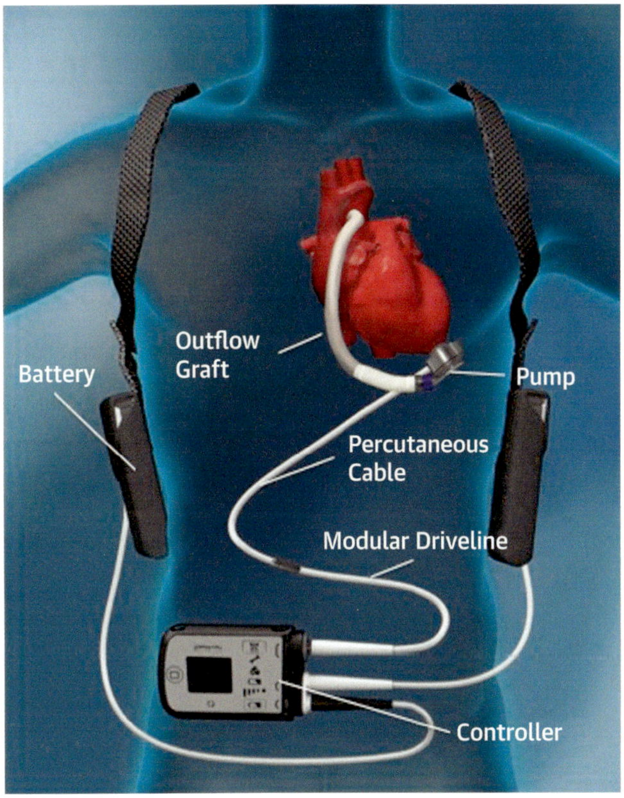

FIGURE 17.2 The fully magnetically levitated left ventricular assist system (LVAS). The blood pump is positioned within the pericardial space, with its integral inflow conduit in the left ventricle and outflow graft attached to the ascending aorta. The percutaneous power cable is tunneled through the abdominal wall and is attached to the system controller that receives power from two lithium-ion batteries. (Reproduced with permission from Netuka et al., *J Am Coll Cardiol* 2015;66(23):2579–89.)

or frequent need for intravenous inotropic therapy.[38] Because of limited head-to-head data, it is difficult to compare LVADs. Device selection should be made according to patient anatomy and local surgical expertise. Besides the ischemic and hemorrhagic strokes mentioned, there are other major, non-surgical adverse events and complications that can occur after LVAD transplantation. These include bleeding complications, device thrombosis, renal impairment, multi-organ failure, and infections, which have been the primary causes of death in some series.[123–128] Therefore, long-term MCS management necessitates a multidisciplinary team approach with experience in MCS, in centers that may improve patient survival.

Heart Transplant

Heart transplant remains the standard for surgical intervention in refractory advanced HF, despite the absence of RCTs due to limited donor heart availability.[129] With proper patient selection, heart transplant significantly increases survival, exercise capacity, and quality of life compared to medical therapy.[42,130] In a recent report from the United States, one-year survival after heart transplant was 90.8% for males and 90.6% for females, and five-year survival was 77.5% for males and 75.6% for females.[115] Other registries worldwide have reported similar results on short- and long-term outcomes.[131–134] Acute and chronic rejection and autoimmune vasculopathy pose major post-transplantation challenges, followed by the consequences of the complications of immunosuppressive therapy in the long term (i.e., infection, hypertension, renal failure, diabetes, and malignancy).[130]

Palliative Treatment (see also Chapter 18)

Palliative care should be an integral part of any HF management program and should be discussed early in the process with patients suffering from advanced HF, especially when life expectancy is limited, or whenever the patients and family choose.[1,135] Palliative care as part of a multidisciplinary team including primary care, specialist services, advanced HF service, and social and psychological support, should be involved in the shared care of these patients[136] Discontinuation of

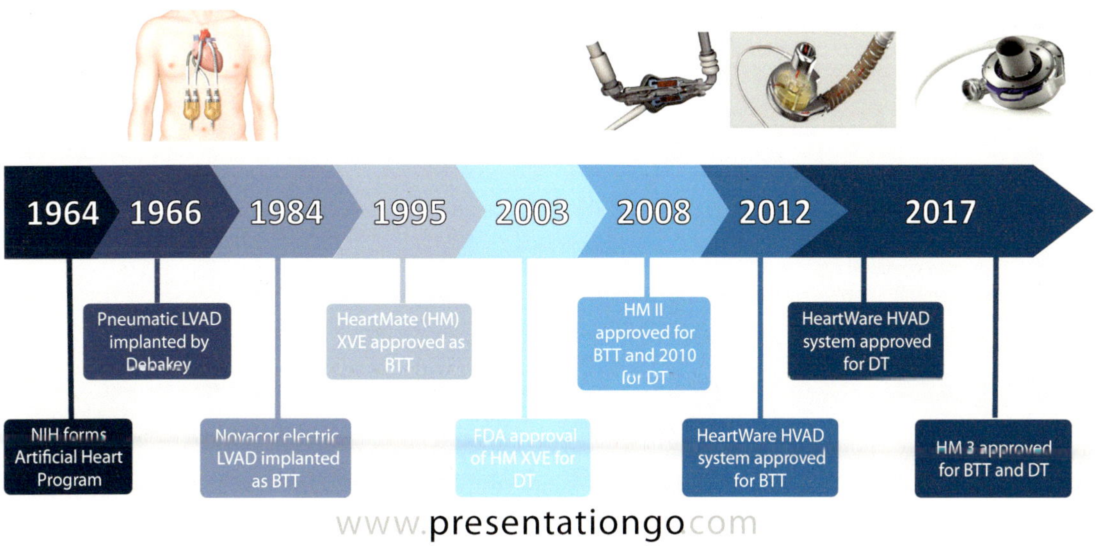

FIGURE 17.3 The evolution of long-term mechanical circulatory support.

devices and advanced therapies, e.g., ICD, MCS, immunosuppressive therapy, can be considered based on the wishes of the patients and their families. Palliative care can take place either in primary care or in hospice, depending on patient and family preferences and healthcare system resources.[135,137,138]

Conclusion

Advanced HF is a final common pathway for a syndrome affecting increasing numbers of patients in recent decades. In previous years, the definition and prevalence of advanced HF have changed, together with the development of new treatment options. Still, the management of advanced HF is based more on expert consensus rather than RCTs. Most RCTs concerning medical management have a low representation of stage D/NYHA IV patients. Therefore, the evidence for optimal dosing and effectiveness of medical therapies is still limited. Titration of standard medication in advanced HF should be done with care and close surveillance facilitated by imaging, intravascular pressure monitoring devices (e.g., CardioMEMS), and biomarkers (e.g., NT-proBNP).

Many patients with advanced HF have co-morbidities that may lead to inadequate response to medical therapy as outpatients or during hospitalization. At some point, most patients will need parenteral treatment, ultrafiltration, or even MCS to achieve euvolemia and stable hemodynamics. More and more patients will need advanced therapies, as the access to heart transplant is limited by the number of donors. The use of MCS in the short or long term has become a turning point in the treatment of patients with advanced HF, as advances in these technologies have reduced mortality and morbidity. Further research is needed to understand better the natural history and the biological base of transition to advanced HF. Better understanding of the interaction between the failing heart, neurohormonal processes, and end-organ dysfunction will allow us to evaluate patients for medical and surgical management or palliative care in a timely manner according to the patient's beliefs and preferences.

References

1. Crespo-Leiro MG, Metra M, Lund LH, et al. Advanced heart failure: a position statement of the Heart Failure Association of the European Society of Cardiology. *Eur J Heart Fail.* 2018;20:1505–35.
2. Fang JC, Ewald GA, Allen LA, et al. Advanced (stage D) heart failure: a statement from the Heart Failure Society of America Guidelines Committee. *J Card Fail.* 2015;21:519–34.
3. Bjork JB, Alton KK, Georgiopoulou VV, Butler J, Kalogeropoulos AP. Defining advanced heart failure: a systematic review of criteria used in clinical trials. *J Card Fail.* 2016;22:569–77.
4. Costanzo MR, Mills RM, Wynne J. Characteristics of "Stage D" heart failure: insights from the Acute Decompensated Heart Failure National Registry Longitudinal Module (ADHERE LM). *Am Heart J.* 2008;155:339–47.
5. Chaudhry SP, Stewart GC. Advanced heart failure: prevalence, natural history, and prognosis. *Heart Fail Clin.* 2016;12:323–33.
6. Ammar KA, Jacobsen SJ, Mahoney DW, et al. Prevalence and prognostic significance of heart failure stages: application of the American College of Cardiology/American Heart Association heart failure staging criteria in the community. *Circulation.* 2007;115:1563–70.
7. Kalogeropoulos AP, Samman-Tahhan A, Hedley JS, et al. Progression to Stage D heart failure among outpatients with Stage C heart failure and reduced ejection fraction. *JACC Heart Fail.* 2017;5:528–37.
8. Hedley JS, Samman-Tahhan A, McCue AA, et al. Definitions of Stage D heart failure and outcomes among outpatients with heart failure and reduced ejection fraction. *Int J Cardiol.* 2018;272:250–4.
9. Norton C, Georgiopoulou VV, Kalogeropoulos AP, Butler J. Epidemiology and cost of advanced heart failure. *Prog Cardiovasc Dis.* 2011;54:78–85.
10. Metra M, Ponikowski P, Dickstein K, et al. Advanced chronic heart failure: a position statement from the Study Group on Advanced Heart Failure of the Heart Failure Association of the European Society of Cardiology. *Eur J Heart Fail.* 2007;9:684–94.
11. Erdmann E, Lechat P, Verkenne P, Wiemann H. Results from post-hoc analyses of the CIBIS II trial: effect of bisoprolol in high-risk patient groups with chronic heart failure. *Eur J Heart Fail.* 2001;3:469–79.
12. Hjalmarson A, Goldstein S, Fagerberg B, et al. Effects of controlled-release metoprolol on total mortality, hospitalizations, and well-being in patients with heart failure: the Metoprolol CR/XL Randomized Intervention Trial in congestive heart failure (MERIT-HF). MERIT-HF Study Group. *JAMA.* 2000;283:1295–302.
13. Packer M, Fowler MB, Roecker EB, et al. Effect of carvedilol on the morbidity of patients with severe chronic heart failure: results of the carvedilol prospective randomized cumulative survival (COPERNICUS) study. *Circulation.* 2002;106:2194–9.
14. Rouleau JL, Roecker EB, Tendera M, et al. Influence of pretreatment systolic blood pressure on the effect of carvedilol in patients with severe chronic heart failure: the Carvedilol Prospective Randomized Cumulative Survival (COPERNICUS) study. *J Am Coll Cardiol.* 2004;43: 1423–9.
15. Bohm M, Swedberg K, Komajda M, et al. Heart rate as a risk factor in chronic heart failure (SHIFT): the association between heart rate and outcomes in a randomised placebo-controlled trial. *Lancet.* 2010;376:886–94.
16. Mebazaa A, Nieminen MS, Packer M, et al. Levosimendan vs dobutamine for patients with acute decompensated heart failure: the SURVIVE randomized trial. *JAMA.* 2007;297:1883–91.
17. Metra M, Nodari S, D'Aloia A, et al. Beta-blocker therapy influences the hemodynamic response to inotropic agents in patients with heart failure: a randomized comparison of dobutamine and enoximone before and after chronic treatment with metoprolol or carvedilol. *J Am Coll Cardiol.* 2002;40:1248–58.
18. Fonarow GC, Abraham WT, Albert NM, et al. Influence of beta-blocker continuation or withdrawal on outcomes in patients hospitalized with heart failure: findings from the OPTIMIZE-HF program. *J Am Coll Cardiol.* 2008;52:190–9.
19. Prins KW, Neill JM, Tyler JO, Eckman PM, Duval S. Effects of beta-blocker withdrawal in acute decompensated heart failure: a systematic review and meta-analysis. *JACC Heart Fail.* 2015;3:647–53.
20. Bristow MR, Gilbert EM, Abraham WT, et al. Carvedilol produces dose-related improvements in left ventricular function and survival in subjects with chronic heart failure. MOCHA Investigators. *Circulation.* 1996;94:2807–16.
21. Jondeau G, Neuder Y, Eicher JC, et al. B-CONVINCED: Beta-blocker CONtinuation Vs. INterruption in patients with Congestive heart failure hospitalizED for a decompensation episode. *Eur Heart J.* 2009;30:2186–92.
22. Kittleson M, Hurwitz S, Shah MR, et al. Development of circulatory-renal limitations to angiotensin-converting enzyme inhibitors identifies patients with severe heart failure and early mortality. *J Am Coll Cardiol.* 2003;41:2029–35.
23. Packer M. Current role of beta-adrenergic blockers in the management of chronic heart failure. *Am J Med.* 2001;110 Suppl 7A:81S–94S.
24. Pitt B, Zannad F, Remme WJ, et al. The effect of spironolactone on morbidity and mortality in patients with severe heart failure. Randomized Aldactone Evaluation Study Investigators. *N Engl J Med.* 1999;341:709–17.
25. McMurray JJ, O'Meara E. Treatment of heart failure with spironolactone--trial and tribulations. *N Engl J Med.* 2004;351:526–8.
26. Desai A. Hyperkalemia associated with inhibitors of the renin-angiotensin-aldosterone system: balancing risk and benefit. *Circulation.* 2008;118:1609–11.
27. McMurray JJ, Packer M, Desai AS, et al. Angiotensin-neprilysin inhibition versus enalapril in heart failure. *N Engl J Med.* 2014;371: 993–1004.
28. Digitalis Investigation Group. The effect of digoxin on mortality and morbidity in patients with heart failure. *N Engl J Med.* 1997;336:525–33.
29. Rathore SS, Curtis JP, Wang Y, Bristow MR, Krumholz HM. Association of serum digoxin concentration and outcomes in patients with heart failure. *JAMA.* 2003;289:871–8.
30. Vamos M, Erath JW, Hohnloser SH. Digoxin-associated mortality: a systematic review and meta-analysis of the literature. *Eur Heart J.* 2015;36:1831–8.
31. Uretsky BF, Young JB, Shahidi FE, et al. Randomized study assessing the effect of digoxin withdrawal in patients with mild to moderate chronic congestive heart failure: results of the PROVED trial. PROVED investigative group. *J Am Coll Cardiol.* 1993;22:955–62.
32. Packer M, Gheorghiade M, Young JB, et al. Withdrawal of digoxin from patients with chronic heart failure treated with angiotensin-converting-enzyme inhibitors. RADIANCE study. *N Engl J Med.* 1993;329:1–7.
33. Hopper I, Samuel R, Hayward C, Tonkin A, Krum H. Can medications be safely withdrawn in patients with stable chronic heart failure? Systematic review and meta-analysis. *J Card Fail.* 2014;20:522–32.
34. Cohn JN, Johnson G, Ziesche S, et al. A comparison of enalapril with hydralazine-isosorbide dinitrate in the treatment of chronic congestive heart failure. *N Engl J Med.* 1991;325:303–10.

35. Elkayam U, Bitar F. Effects of nitrates and hydralazine in heart failure: clinical evidence before the African American heart failure trial. *Am J Cardiol.* 2005;96:37i–43i.
36. Taylor AL, Ziesche S, Yancy C, et al. Combination of isosorbide dinitrate and hydralazine in blacks with heart failure. *N Engl J Med.* 2004;351:2049–57.
37. Farag M, Mabote T, Shoaib A, et al. Hydralazine and nitrates alone or combined for the management of chronic heart failure: a systematic review. *Int J Cardiol.* 2015;196:61–9.
38. Ponikowski P, Voors AA, Anker SD, et al. 2016 ESC guidelines for the diagnosis and treatment of acute and chronic heart failure: the Task Force for the diagnosis and treatment of acute and chronic heart failure of the European Society of Cardiology (ESC)Developed with the special contribution of the Heart Failure Association (HFA) of the ESC. *Eur Heart J.* 2016;37:2129–200.
39. Yancy CW, Jessup M, Bozkurt B, et al. 2013 ACCF/AHA guideline for the management of heart failure: a report of the American College of Cardiology Foundation/American Heart Association Task Force on Practice Guidelines. *J Am Coll Cardiol.* 2013;62:e147–239.
40. Roubille F, Tardif JC. New therapeutic targets in cardiology: heart failure and arrhythmia: HCN channels. *Circulation.* 2013;127:1986–96.
41. Chaudhary R, Garg J, Krishnamoorthy P, et al. Ivabradine: heart failure and beyond. *J Cardiovasc Pharmacol Ther.* 2016;21:335–43.
42. Ponikowski P, Voors AA, Anker SD, et al. 2016 ESC guidelines for the diagnosis and treatment of acute and chronic heart failure: the Task Force for the diagnosis and treatment of acute and chronic heart failure of the European Society of Cardiology (ESC). Developed with the special contribution of the Heart Failure Association (HFA) of the ESC. *Eur J Heart Fail.* 2016;18:891–975.
43. Swedberg K, Komajda M, Bohm M, et al. Ivabradine and outcomes in chronic heart failure (SHIFT): a randomised placebo-controlled study. *Lancet.* 2010;376:875–85.
44. Gallet R, Ternacle J, Damy T, et al. Hemodynamic effects of Ivabradine in addition to dobutamine in patients with severe systolic dysfunction. *Int J Cardiol.* 2014;176:450–5.
45. McMurray JJV, Solomon SD, Inzucchi SE, et al. Dapagliflozin in patients with heart failure and reduced ejection fraction. *N Engl J Med.* 2019;381:1995–2008.
46. Packer M, Anker SD, Butler J, et al. Cardiovascular and renal outcomes with empagliflozin in heart failure. *N Engl J Med.* 2020;383:1413–24.
47. Zannad F, Ferreira JP, Pocock SJ, et al. SGLT2 inhibitors in patients with heart failure with reduced ejection fraction: a meta-analysis of the EMPEROR-reduced and DAPA-HF trials. *Lancet.* 2020;396:819–29.
48. Heerspink HJL, Stefansson BV, Correa-Rotter R, et al. Dapagliflozin in patients with chronic kidney disease. *N Engl J Med.* 2020;383:1436–46.
49. Brignole M, Auricchio A, Baron-Esquivias G, et al. 2013 ESC guidelines on cardiac pacing and cardiac resynchronization therapy: the task force on cardiac pacing and resynchronization therapy of the European Society of Cardiology (ESC). Developed in collaboration with the European Heart Rhythm Association (EHRA). *Europace.* 2013;15:1070–118.
50. Moss AJ, Zareba W, Hall WJ, et al. Prophylactic implantation of a defibrillator in patients with myocardial infarction and reduced ejection fraction. *N Engl J Med.* 2002;346:877–83.
51. Bardy GH, Lee KL, Mark DB, et al. Amiodarone or an implantable cardioverter-defibrillator for congestive heart failure. *N Engl J Med.* 2005;352:225–37.
52. Cavusoglu Y, Alper AT, Altay H, et al. Natriuretic peptides in clinical practice. *Anatol J Cardiol.* 2019;21:1–40.
53. Chow SL, Maisel AS, Anand I, et al. Role of biomarkers for the prevention, assessment, and management of heart failure: a scientific statement from the American Heart Association. *Circulation.* 2017;135:e1054–e1091.
54. Ong MK, Romano PS, Edgington S, et al. Effectiveness of remote patient monitoring after discharge of hospitalized patients with heart failure: the better effectiveness after transition—heart failure (BEAT-HF) randomized clinical trial. *JAMA Intern Med.* 2016;176:310–8.
55. Abraham WT, Stevenson LW, Bourge RC, et al. Sustained efficacy of pulmonary artery pressure to guide adjustment of chronic heart failure therapy: complete follow-up results from the CHAMPION randomised trial. *Lancet.* 2016;387:453–61.
56. Crespo-Leiro MG, Anker SD, Maggioni AP, et al. Heart Failure Association (HFA) of the European Society of Cardiology (ESC). European Society of Cardiology Heart Failure Long-Term Registry (ESC-HF-LT): 1-year follow-up outcomes and differences across regions. *Eur J Heart Fail.* 2016;18:613–25.
57. Purek L, Laule-Kilian K, Christ A, et al. Coronary artery disease and outcome in acute congestive heart failure. *Heart.* 2006;92:598–602.
58. Badar AA, Perez-Moreno AC, Hawkins NM, et al. Clinical characteristics and outcomes of patients with angina and heart failure in the CHARM (Candesartan in Heart Failure Assessment of Reduction in Mortality and Morbidity) Programme. *Eur J Heart Fail.* 2015;17:196–204.
59. Velazquez EJ, Lee KL, Deja MA, et al. Coronary-artery bypass surgery in patients with left ventricular dysfunction. *N Engl J Med.* 2011;364:1607–16.
60. Aksut B, Starling R, Kapadia S. Stable coronary artery disease and left ventricular dysfunction: the role of revascularization. *Catheter Cardiovasc Interv.* 2017;90:777–83.
61. Investigators B. The final 10-year follow-up results from the BARI randomized trial. *J Am Coll Cardiol.* 2007;49:1600–6.
62. Gioia G, Matthai W, Gillin K, et al. Revascularization in severe left ventricular dysfunction: outcome comparison of drug-eluting stent implantation versus coronary artery by-pass grafting. *Catheter Cardiovasc Interv.* 2007;70:26–33.
63. Bangalore S, Guo Y, Samadashvili Z, Blecker S, Hannan EL. Revascularization in patients with multivessel coronary artery disease and severe left ventricular systolic dysfunction: everolimus-eluting stents versus coronary artery bypass graft surgery. *Circulation.* 2016;133:2132–40.
64. Cui K, Zhang D, Lyu S, et al. Meta-analysis comparing percutaneous coronary revascularization using drug-eluting stent versus coronary artery bypass grafting in patients with left ventricular systolic dysfunction. *Am J Cardiol.* 2018;122:1670–6.
65. StephanWindecker, Kolh P, Alfonso F, et al. 2014 ESC/EACTS guidelines on myocardial revascularization. *Rev Esp Cardiol (Engl Ed).* 2015; 68:144.
66. Singh M, Sporn ZA, Schaff HV, Pellikka PA. ACC/AHA versus ESC guidelines on prosthetic heart valve management: JACC guideline comparison. *J Am Coll Cardiol.* 2019;73:1707–18.
67. Kaneko H, Suzuki S, Uejima T, et al. Functional mitral regurgitation and left ventricular systolic dysfunction in the recent era of cardiovascular clinical practice, an observational cohort study. *Hypertens Res.* 2014;37:1082–7.
68. Pibarot P, Delgado V, Bax JJ. MITRA-FR vs. COAPT: lessons from two trials with diametrically opposed results. *Eur Heart J Cardiovasc Imaging.* 2019;20:620–4.
69. Keteyian SJ, Pina IL, Hibner BA, Fleg JL. Clinical role of exercise training in the management of patients with chronic heart failure. *J Cardiopulm Rehabil Prev.* 2010;30:67–76.
70. Crimi E, Ignarro LJ, Cacciatore F, Napoli C. Mechanisms by which exercise training benefits patients with heart failure. *Nat Rev Cardiol.* 2009;6:292–300.
71. Erbs S, Hollriegel R, Linke A, et al. Exercise training in patients with advanced chronic heart failure (NYHA IIIb) promotes restoration of peripheral vasomotor function, induction of endogenous regeneration, and improvement of left ventricular function. *Circ Heart Fail.* 2010;3:486–94.
72. O'Connor CM, Whellan DJ, Lee KL, et al. Efficacy and safety of exercise training in patients with chronic heart failure: HF-ACTION randomized controlled trial. *JAMA.* 2009;301:1439–50.
73. Taylor RS, Sagar VA, Davies EJ, et al. Exercise-based rehabilitation for heart failure. *Cochrane Database Syst Rev.* 2014:Cd003331.
74. Kimura M, Kohno T, Murata M, et al. Oral nitrate administration ameliorates cardiogenic shock due to eclipsed mitral regurgitation. *Cardiology.* 2016;134:327–30.
75. Lenders GD, Jorens PG, De Meyer T, et al. Coronary spasm after the topical use of cocaine in nasal surgery. *Am J Case Rep.* 2013;14:76–9.
76. Faris RF, Flather M, Purcell H, Poole-Wilson PA, Coats AJ. Diuretics for heart failure. *Cochrane Database Syst Rev.* 2012:Cd003838.
77. Neuberg GW, Miller AB, O'Connor CM, et al. Diuretic resistance predicts mortality in patients with advanced heart failure. *Am Heart J.* 2002;144:31–8.
78. Domanski M, Norman J, Pitt B, et al. Diuretic use, progressive heart failure, and death in patients in the Studies Of Left Ventricular Dysfunction (SOLVD). *J Am Coll Cardiol.* 2003;42:705–8.
79. Mielniczuk LM, Tsang SW, Desai AS, et al. The association between high-dose diuretics and clinical stability in ambulatory chronic heart failure patients. *J Card Fail.* 2008;14:388–93.
80. Mullens W, Damman K, Harjola VP, et al. The use of diuretics in heart failure with congestion - a position statement from the Heart Failure Association of the European Society of Cardiology. *Eur J Heart Fail.* 2019;21:137–55.
81. Testani JM, Hanberg JS, Cheng S, et al. Rapid and highly accurate prediction of poor loop diuretic natriuretic response in patients with heart failure. *Circ Heart Fail.* 2016;9:e002370.
82. Testani JM, Brisco MA, Kociol RD, et al. Substantial discrepancy between fluid and weight loss during acute decompensated heart failure treatment. *Am J Med.* 2015;128:776–83 e4.
83. Butler J, Hernandez AF, Anstrom KJ, et al. Rationale and design of the ATHENA-HF trial: aldosterone targeted neurohormonal combined with natriuresis therapy in heart failure. *JACC Heart Fail.* 2016;4: 726–35.
84. Imiela T, Budaj A. Acetazolamide as add-on diuretic therapy in exacerbations of chronic heart failure: a pilot study. *Clin Drug Investig.* 2017;37:1175–81.
85. Pruett AE, Lee AK, Patterson JH, et al. Evolution of biomarker guided therapy for heart failure: current concepts and trial evidence. *Curr Cardiol Rev.* 2015;11:80–9.

86. Ricci JE, Kalmanovich E, Robert C, et al. Management of acute heart failure: contribution of daily bedside echocardiographic assessment on therapy adjustment with impact measure on the 30-day readmission rate (JECICA). *Contemp Clin Trials Commun.* 2018;12:103–8.
87. Thavendiranathan P, Yingchoncharoen T, Grant A, et al. Prediction of 30-day heart failure-specific readmission risk by echocardiographic parameters. *Am J Cardiol.* 2014;113:335–41.
88. Maier SKG, Paule S, Jung W, et al. Evaluation of thoracic impedance trends for implant-based remote monitoring in heart failure patients - results from the (J-)HomeCARE-II study. *J Electrocardiol.* 2019;53:100–8.
89. Conraads VM, Tavazzi L, Santini M, et al. Sensitivity and positive predictive value of implantable intrathoracic impedance monitoring as a predictor of heart failure hospitalizations: the SENSE-HF trial. *Eur Heart J.* 2011;32:2266–73.
90. Abraham WT, Adamson PB, Bourge RC, et al. Wireless pulmonary artery haemodynamic monitoring in chronic heart failure: a randomised controlled trial. *Lancet.* 2011;377:658–66.
91. da Rosa PR, Rohde LE, Doebber M, et al. Rational and design of a randomized, double-blind, multicenter trial to evaluate the safety and tolerability of furosemide withdrawal in stable chronic outpatients with heart failure: the ReBIC-1 trial. *Am Heart J.* 2017;194:125–31.
92. Hasenfuss G, Teerlink JR. Cardiac inotropes: current agents and future directions. *Eur Heart J.* 2011;32:1838–45.
93. O'Connor CM, Gattis WA, Uretsky BF, et al. Continuous intravenous dobutamine is associated with an increased risk of death in patients with advanced heart failure: insights from the Flolan International Randomized Survival Trial (FIRST). *Am Heart J.* 1999;138:78–86.
94. Cuffe MS, Califf RM, Adams KF, Jr., et al. Short-term intravenous milrinone for acute exacerbation of chronic heart failure: a randomized controlled trial. *JAMA.* 2002;287:1541–7.
95. Felker GM, Benza RL, Chandler AB, et al. Heart failure etiology and response to milrinone in decompensated heart failure: results from the OPTIME-CHF study. *J Am Coll Cardiol.* 2003;41:997–1003.
96. Nieminen MS, Akkila J, Hasenfuss G, et al. Hemodynamic and neurohumoral effects of continuous infusion of levosimendan in patients with congestive heart failure. *J Am Coll Cardiol.* 2000;36:1903–12.
97. Kivikko M, Antila S, Eha J, Lehtonen L, Pentikainen PJ. Pharmacokinetics of levosimendan and its metabolites during and after a 24-hour continuous infusion in patients with severe heart failure. *Int J Clin Pharmacol Ther.* 2002;40:465–71.
98. Landoni G, Biondi-Zoccai G, Greco M, et al. Effects of levosimendan on mortality and hospitalization. A meta-analysis of randomized controlled studies. *Crit Care Med.* 2012;40:634–46.
99. Thackray S, Easthaugh J, Freemantle N, Cleland JG. The effectiveness and relative effectiveness of intravenous inotropic drugs acting through the adrenergic pathway in patients with heart failure-a meta-regression analysis. *Eur J Heart Fail.* 2002;4:515–29.
100. Bart BA, Goldsmith SR, Lee KL, et al. Ultrafiltration in decompensated heart failure with cardiorenal syndrome. *N Engl J Med.* 2012;367:2296–304.
101. Patarroyo M, Wehbe E, Hanna M, et al. Cardiorenal outcomes after slow continuous ultrafiltration therapy in refractory patients with advanced decompensated heart failure. *J Am Coll Cardiol.* 2012;60:1906–12.
102. Giglioli C, Landi D, Cecchi E, et al. Effects of ULTRAfiltration vs. DIureticS on clinical, biohumoral and haemodynamic variables in patients with deCOmpensated heart failure: the ULTRADISCO study. *Eur J Heart Fail.* 2011;13:337–46.
103. Viglino G, Neri L, Feola M. Peritoneal ultrafiltration in congestive heart failure-findings reported from its application in clinical practice: a systematic review. *J Nephrol.* 2015;28:29–38.
104. Courivaud C, Kazory A, Crepin T, et al. Peritoneal dialysis reduces the number of hospitalization days in heart failure patients refractory to diuretics. *Perit Dial Int.* 2014;34:100–8.
105. Feldman D, Pamboukian SV, Teuteberg JJ, et al. The 2013 International Society for Heart and Lung Transplantation Guidelines for mechanical circulatory support: executive summary. *J Heart Lung Transplant.* 2013;32:157–87.
106. Peura JL, Colvin-Adams M, Francis GS, et al. Recommendations for the use of mechanical circulatory support: device strategies and patient selection: a scientific statement from the American Heart Association. *Circulation.* 2012;126:2648–67.
107. Ouweneel DM, Henriques JP. Percutaneous cardiac support devices for cardiogenic shock: current indications and recommendations. *Heart.* 2012;98:1246–54.
108. van Diepen S, Katz JN, Albert NM, et al. Contemporary management of cardiogenic shock: a scientific statement from the American Heart Association. *Circulation.* 2017;136:e232–68.
109. Brown JL, Estep JD. Temporary percutaneous mechanical circulatory support in advanced heart failure. *Heart Fail Clin.* 2016;12:385–98.
110. Mandawat A, Rao SV. Percutaneous mechanical circulatory support devices in cardiogenic shock. *Circ Cardiovasc Interv.* 2017;10.
111. Barge-Caballero E, Almenar-Bonet L, Gonzalez-Vilchez F, et al. Clinical outcomes of temporary mechanical circulatory support as a direct bridge to heart transplantation: a nationwide Spanish registry. *Eur J Heart Fail.* 2018;20:178–86.
112. Yin MY, Wever-Pinzon O, Mehra MR, et al. Post-transplant outcome in patients bridged to transplant with temporary mechanical circulatory support devices. *J Heart Lung Transplant.* 2019;38:858–69.
113. Pieri M, Pappalardo F. Impella RP in the treatment of right ventricular failure: what we know and where we go. *J Cardiothorac Vasc Anesth.* 2018;32:2339–43.
114. Gosev I, Kiernan MS, Eckman P, et al. Long-term survival in patients receiving a continuous-flow left ventricular assist device. *Ann Thorac Surg.* 2018;105:696–701.
115. Benjamin EJ, Blaha MJ, Chiuve SE, et al. Heart disease and stroke statistics-2017 update: a report from the American Heart Association. *Circulation.* 2017;135:e146–603.
116. McCarthy PM, Sabik JF. Implantable circulatory support devices as a bridge to heart transplantation. *Semin Thorac Cardiovasc Surg.* 1994;6:174–80.
117. Slaughter MS, Rogers JG, Milano CA, et al. Advanced heart failure treated with continuous-flow left ventricular assist device. *N Engl J Med.* 2009;361:2241–51.
118. Sheikh FH, Russell SD. HeartMate(R) II continuous-flow left ventricular assist system. *Expert Rev Med Devices.* 2011;8:11–21.
119. Han JJ, Acker MA, Atluri P. Left ventricular assist devices. *Circulation.* 2018;138:2841–51.
120. Rogers JG, Pagani FD, Tatooles AJ, et al. Intrapericardial left ventricular assist device for advanced heart failure. *N Engl J Med.* 2017;376:451–60.
121. Milano CA, Rogers JG, Tatooles AJ, et al. HVAD: the ENDURANCE supplemental trial. *JACC Heart Fail.* 2018;6:792–802.
122. Mehra MR, Uriel N, Naka Y, et al. A fully magnetically levitated left ventricular assist device - final report. *N Engl J Med.* 2019;380:1618–27.
123. Stulak JM, Davis ME, Haglund N, et al. Adverse events in contemporary continuous-flow left ventricular assist devices: a multi-institutional comparison shows significant differences. *J Thorac Cardiovasc Surg.* 2016;151:177–89.
124. Topkara VK, Kondareddy S, Malik F, et al. Infectious complications in patients with left ventricular assist device: etiology and outcomes in the continuous-flow era. *Ann Thorac Surg.* 2010;90:1270–7.
125. Tuncer ON, Kemaloglu C, Erbasan O, et al. Outcomes and readmissions after continuous flow left ventricular assist device: heartmate II versus heartware ventricular assist device. *Transplant Proc.* 2016;48:2157–61.
126. Akhter SA, Badami A, Murray M, et al. Hospital readmissions after continuous-flow left ventricular assist device implantation: incidence, causes, and cost analysis. *Ann Thorac Surg.* 2015;100:884–9.
127. Haglund NA, Davis ME, Tricarico NM, Keebler ME, Maltais S. Readmissions after continuous flow left ventricular assist device implantation: differences observed between two contemporary device types. *ASAIO J.* 2015;61:410–6.
128. Forest SJ, Bello R, Friedmann P, et al. Readmissions after ventricular assist device: etiologies, patterns, and days out of hospital. *Ann Thorac Surg.* 2013;95:1276–81.
129. Kittleson MM, Kobashigawa JA. Cardiac transplantation: current outcomes and contemporary controversies. *JACC Heart Fail.* 2017;5:857–68.
130. Mehra MR, Canter CE, Hannan MM, et al. The 2016 International Society for Heart Lung Transplantation listing criteria for heart transplantation: a 10-year update. *J Heart Lung Transplant.* 2016;35:1–23.
131. Lee HY, Jeon ES, Kang SM, Kim JJ. Initial report of the Korean Organ Transplant Registry (KOTRY): heart transplantation. *Korean Circ J.* 2017;47:868–76.
132. Lund LH, Khush KK, Cherikh WS, et al. The Registry of the International Society for Heart and Lung Transplantation: thirty-fourth adult heart transplantation report-2017; focus theme: allograft ischemic time. *J Heart Lung Transplant.* 2017;36:1037–46.
133. Lee HY, Oh BH. Heart transplantation in Asia. *Circ J.* 2017;81:617–21.
134. Peled Y, Freimark D, Har-Zahav Y, et al. Trends and outcomes in heart transplantation over the past three decades: a single tertiary center experience in Israel. *Isr Med Assoc J.* 2018;20:567–72.
135. Klinedinst R, Kornfield ZN, Hadler RA. Palliative care for patients with advanced heart disease. *J Cardiothorac Vasc Anesth.* 2019;33:833–43.
136. Teuteberg JJ, Teuteberg WG. *Palliative Care for Patients with Heart Failure.* American College of Cardiology; 2016 https://www.acc.org/latest-in-cardiology/articles/2016/02/11/08/02/palliative-care-for-patients-with-heart-failure.
137. Cross SH, Kamal AH, Taylor DH, Jr., Warraich HJ. Hospice use among patients with heart failure. *Card Fail Rev.* 2019;5:93–98.
138. Wordingham SE, McIlvennan CK. Palliative care for patients on mechanical circulatory support. *AMA J Ethics.* 2019;21:E435–42.

Chapter 18
PALLIATIVE CARE AND ADVANCED DIRECTIVES IN HEART FAILURE

Melissa I. Owen and Debbie A. Gunter

Introduction

Palliative care is defined as a holistic approach to care that improves quality of life through the prevention and relief of suffering in patients with chronic and potentially life-limiting illnesses. The early focus of palliative care was on patients with oncological diagnoses, specifically on the terminal phases of the disease.[1] Advanced heart failure (HF) patients present with multiple symptoms, including dyspnea, pain, anxiety, depression, and fatigue, all of which impact quality of life.[2] HF patients also have an uncertain illness trajectory. These factors make patients with advanced HF ideal candidates for palliative care. The objectives of this chapter are to:

1. Describe benefits of palliative care in heart failure patients
2. Apply principles of primary palliative care and referral for specialty care
3. Utilize evidence-based practice approaches for symptom management in patients
4. Explore advanced-care planning in heart failure patients

History and Benefits of Palliative Care

Providing supportive care for patients with chronic diseases is not a new concept, and research has demonstrated concerning findings. In the 1990s, the Institute of Medicine released the report "Approaching Death: Improving Care at the End of Life," which focused on themes associated with the care of patients with life-threatening illnesses. Themes included unrelieved symptoms, knowledge gaps in end-of-life care, and inadequate training and preparation for clinicians to manage these patients appropriately. Recommendations to address these issues were also made, such as clinicians committing to improving care for dying patients and addressing systematic problems to improve quality of life and remove barriers to care provision.[3]

The Study to Understand Prognoses and Preferences for Outcomes and Risks of Treatment (SUPPORT) was a controlled trial that sought to improve decision making in end-of-life care. This study found that less than 50% of physicians knew when their patients wanted to avoid CPR, and there was no significant improvement despite targeted interventions to improve communication after six months.[4] To combat some of these issues, the Robert Wood Johnson Foundation ran the "Last Acts" campaign from 1995–2005. "Last Acts" sought to improve communication and decision making for patients at end-of-life, and to change culture and attitudes around death in America.[5] Finally, in 2006, hospice and palliative medicine was recognized as a medical specialty.[6]

The focus of palliative care has shifted from end-of-life care to providing holistic care across the spectrum of illness. However, a barrier to the incorporation of palliative care, specifically in non-oncologic patients, has been the persistent association by both clinicians and patients that palliative care is synonymous with hospice. Hospice is just one possible intervention, and palliative care is intended to be implemented for any acute or chronic illness that impacts a patient's quality of life, regardless of the life expectancy. A landmark study found that patients with non-small cell lung cancer who received palliative care lived longer than those who did not.[7] A randomized, control trial for patients with HF also identified a clinically significant improvement in quality of life, depression, anxiety, and spiritual well-being in the group randomized to receive palliative care.[8]

Clinical Application of Palliative Care Principles

All clinicians have a responsibility to provide palliative care to patients, and interventions may vary based upon the clinician's level of specialization and knowledge of palliative care. Palliative care is often described as primary or specialty. Primary or generalist palliative care is the responsibility of all clinicians who do not specialize in palliative care, including cardiology practitioners. Specialty palliative care includes care provided by a clinician who is certified in Palliative Medicine or Nursing, with the addition of an interdisciplinary team to support patient needs.[9] Table 18.1 summarizes the varying functions primary palliative care and specialty palliative care physicians aim to deliver within several domains of HF management.[10]

The National Consensus Project (NCP) for Quality Palliative Care: Clinical Practice Guidelines for Quality Palliative Care are a set of guidelines developed to establish a standard for excellence in palliative care provision. The NCP guidelines identify eight domains of care. These include: 1) structures and processes of care, 2) physical aspects of care, 3) psychological and psychiatric aspects of care, 4) social aspects of care, 5) spiritual, religious, and existential aspects of care, 6) cultural aspects of care, 7) care for the patient nearing the end of life, and 8) ethical and legal aspects of care.[11]

All clinicians, regardless of specialty, need to be able to assess physical and psychological symptoms burden, functional status, social concerns such as access to food and transportation, spiritual distress, quality of life, and conversations related to advance care planning, as well as to initiate a timely referral to hospice if indicated. Clinicians should also develop a patient-centered treatment plan with which to address concerns related to these areas. In addition to providing palliative care interventions, clinicians need to know when to refer patients for specialty palliative services. Common indications for referral to specialty palliative care include: 1) complex or unresolved physical or psychological symptom burden, 2) management of complex family dynamics, and 3) unique or complicated advance care planning needs.

Current cardiology clinical practice guidelines recommend palliative care for advanced HF patients.[12,13] In 2013, the Center for Medicare Services instituted a requirement for a palliative care specialist to be part of the interdisciplinary team for patients undergoing evaluation for Ventricular Assist Device (VAD) placement.[14] Early in the disease trajectory for all patients, discussions about health status, expectations surrounding disease progression, and prognosis should occur with patients and families.

DOI: 10.1201/9780429244544-21

TABLE 18.1: Primary Palliative Care versus Specialist Palliative Care for Patients with HF

Domains		Primary Palliative Care (PPC)	When to Refer to Specialist Palliative Care (SPC)
Symptom Management	**Shortness of breath**	Maximize HF therapies to relieve congestion	Debilitating refractory dyspnea despite PPC interventions
	Pain	Maximize antianginal medications and recommend activity modification for anginal pain Acetaminophen or single- agent opioid therapy for somatic pain Referral to physical therapy for musculoskeletal pain, if possible	Pain refractory to PPC interventions Neuropathic pain
	Depressed mood	Treat low mood from an adjustment reaction by referral for psychotherapy or initiation of anti-depressant medication if appropriate	Symptoms of major depressive disorder such as incapacitating hopelessness and anhedonia requiring medical management
	Anxiety	Treat mild anxiety with referral to psychologist for help with relaxation techniques and psychotherapy or initiation of anxiolytic medication if appropriate	Debilitating anxiety or panic symptoms that prevent the patient from participating in regular activities
	Nausea	Adjust HF therapies Consider adding single-agent anti- emetic	Ongoing symptoms despite PPC interventions
	Fatigue	Maximize HF therapies Referral to cardiac rehabilitation Evaluate and treat for insomnia Evaluate for sleep-disordered breathing, if indicated	Ongoing symptoms despite PPC Patients unable to participate in cardiac rehabilitation SPC can provide pharmacotherapy for fatigue
	Insomnia	Education on sleep hygiene Treat mild associated anxiety with psychotherapy and relaxation techniques	Refractory to PPC interventions SPC can provide pharmacotherapy for insomnia and/or associated anxiety and advanced education on sleep hygiene
Communication	**Discussing code status**	Patients with clear wishes and an understanding of prognosis after CPR	Patients unable to verbalize understanding of their illness and prognosis after CPR
	Advanced care planning	Patients with clear wishes has already identified a surrogate and family/surrogates who support those wishes	Patients unable to verbalize understanding of their illness and prognosis Patients and families who are in disagreement about the patient's end-of- life choices Disagreement about the chosen surrogate or the patient is ambivalent about choice
	Discussions to withdraw life-sustaining therapies	Patients and/or surrogates who verbalize a clear understanding of the patient's prognosis with and without therapy and can base decisions made on patient's goals and values	Patients and/or surrogates unable to verbalize clear understanding of prognosis Patients and/or surrogates who are in disagreement (conflict) about the treatment that best matches patient's goals and values Surrogates with lack of insight into patient's goals and values
	Request for assisted suicide	Referral to specialist level palliative care	SPC to navigate complex request and explore other options
Psychosocial support	**Patient support**	Supportive listening Referral to HF team social worker	Refer to SPC when needs exceed the expertise of HF social worker, especially around issues of end-of-life care such as counseling parents on how to talk to their children
	Caregiver support	Supportive listening Referral to HF team social worker	Refer to SPC when needs exceed the expertise of the HF social worker, especially when caregiver has significant needs or the patient and caregiver are in conflict
Care coordination		Communication with other providers caring for the patient Straightforward referral for home hospice for patients with good support at home and without complex medical or social needs	Complex hospice or home care referral for patients who require placement in facilities with need for complex medical management (e.g., palliative home inotropes)

Abbreviations: CPR: cardiopulmonary resuscitation; HF: heart failure; PPC: primary palliative care; SPC: specialty palliative care.
Source: Adapted from Gelfman et al. Primary palliative care for heart failure: What is it? How do we implement it? *Heart Fail Rev.* 2017;22(5):611–20.

Symptom Management

Patients with advanced HF experience a high symptom burden that is similar to those with advanced cancer.[15] Palliative care is often underutilized in patients with HF and symptoms may go untreated as the disease progresses, leading to physical, emotional, and spiritual distress.[15,16] In order to help reduce symptom burden and maintain quality of life, a combination of pharmacologic and non-pharmacologic interventions needs to be utilized by the clinician. There are several standardized symptom assessment tools that have been used with HF patients, including the Edmonton Symptom Assessment Scale, the Heart Failure Symptom Survey, the Memorial Symptom Assessment Scale-HF, and the Kansas City Cardiomyopathy Questionnaire.[17–21] Symptoms commonly reported in advanced HF include dyspnea, pain, depression, anxiety, anorexia, cachexia, fatigue, and others.

Patients with advanced HF suffer from extensive symptoms beyond the typical manifestations of HF. Patients often normalize their suffering as a normal part of everyday existence, and clinicians may fail to ask the right questions to allow patients to accurately quantify symptoms and distress.[22] As a result, symptoms are under-recognized and under-treated despite a predictable pattern of progression that parallels a worsening of the HF syndrome. Heightened awareness, formal assessment, and empiric treatment of symptoms can markedly improve quality of life for patients with advanced HF. Palliative care specialists can be helpful in managing symptoms that are unrelieved through primary clinician management.[15]

Common Heart Failure Symptom Evaluation and Interventions

Dyspnea

Dyspnea is defined as the subjective experience of breathing discomfort and is often described as an uncomfortable awareness of breathing or breathlessness (American Thoracic Society). It is one of the hallmark symptoms in advanced HF. The etiology and experience of dyspnea arises from multiple physiological, psychological, social, and environmental factors. The frequency and severity increase as HF progresses. The pathology of dyspnea is multifactorial and may include the reduction of lung or gas exchange capacity, muscle weakness, airway obstruction, degeneration of neurons, reduced blood diffusing capacity, and anxiety and/or depression.[23] Dyspnea can only be perceived by the person experiencing it. Patients may describe it as air hunger, shortness of breath, and/or having to work harder to breathe. Clinicians may objectively observe an increased respiratory rate, use of accessory muscles, and a distressed facial expression. In addition, many patients with advanced disease experience episodic dyspnea, which is poorly understood and often develops without any identifiable trigger. In advanced HF patients, the estimates of dyspnea vary between 18 and 88% with a recent average of 60% of patients being affected.[24]

Dyspnea is a multidimensional symptom resulting from multiple mechanisms and it may not respond equally to pharmacologic and non-pharmacologic treatments. Therefore, a comprehensive multidisciplinary approach, composed of physical, emotional, social, and spiritual aspects of refractory breathlessness, is recommended. Dyspnea can be managed in multiple ways. To choose the most appropriate approach or combination of interventions, clinicians should consider several aspects, including the underlying disease, the onset of symptoms, the stage and the trajectory of disease, and the emotional response of the patient.

Management of dyspnea in advanced HF should first focus on hemodynamic optimization through current guideline-directed therapies to maintain euvolemia. This involves the use of diuretics, sodium, and fluid restriction as appropriate, afterload reduction, and positive inotropic agents as indicated. Dyspnea is considered to be refractory when it persists despite optimal treatment of the underlying disease. When refractory dyspnea occurs, palliative treatment options including pharmacologic and non-pharmacologic measures should be maximized.[16]

Pharmacological measures include opioids and benzodiazepines or other anti-anxiolytics. It is important to note that the use of bronchodilators in patients with advanced HF is not recommended if there is no co-existing chronic obstructive pulmonary disease.[25] In adult patients with compensated HF receiving optimum treatment, the use of opioids as adjuvant therapy is shown to be of some benefit in terms of dyspnea perception.[22] Dyspnea relief occurs through altering the perception of dyspnea by the nervous system, improving exercise tolerance, and reducing anxiety. Several recent literature reviews regarding the use of opioids in advanced or terminal illness concluded that some low-quality evidence shows benefit from the use of oral or parenteral opioids to palliate dyspnea, but no evidence to support the use of nebulized opioids. There is a need, however, for randomized, controlled clinical trials with a larger number of patients and medium- to long-term follow-up is necessary to determine not only the effectiveness of pharmacological treatment on dyspnea, but also the impact of these interventions on the quality of life of patients with advanced HF.[16]

Opioids should be selected based on patient-specific variables including renal and hepatic function. At lower doses of opioids, there is no alteration in respiratory drive, but, with higher doses, respiratory depression and decreased level of consciousness can occur. Patients with severe dyspnea are more likely to respond to opioid therapy. Consistent use of opioids decreases gastrointestinal motility and requires close attention to be paid to bowel function and usually the initiation of an aggressive bowel regimen.[16]

Benzodiazepines can be utilized when symptoms of anxiety and panic have accompanied dyspnea. Anxiety can be either the consequence or a contributing cause of dyspnea. Like opioids, data are conflicting about the role of these medications. A recent Cochrane review concluded that there is no evidence for or against benzodiazepines for the relief of dyspnea in patients with advanced cancer and chronic obstructive pulmonary disease (COPD); however, HF was not mentioned.[26] Reduction in anxiety symptoms has been achieved with benzodiazepines. Benzodiazepines and other anxiolytics may be considered second- or third-line treatments when opioids and other non-pharmacologic treatments fail to provide adequate control of dyspnea. Caution is advised when initiating benzodiazepines to control anxiety secondary to dyspnea along with opioid therapy. The Food and Drug Administration announced changes to the labeling of all benzodiazepines and opioids, warning that concurrent therapy poses a heightened risk of central nervous system depression including respiratory depression, coma, and death.[27]

Non-pharmacologic interventions in advanced HF patients include improved air flow, supplemental oxygen, reduction of physical demand, meditation, guided imagery, breathing techniques, positioning, environmental modifications, and medical devices. However, most research in this area has produced little scientifically positive data and more research is needed.[28] A fan near the face increases airflow across the nose and mouth and has demonstrated a significant reduction in breathlessness. Supplemental oxygen may be helpful for patients with documented hypoxemia but has not been shown to be beneficial in patients with normal oxygenation.[29]

Pain

More than half of all patients with HF acknowledge that pain consistently contributes to their suffering. Pain reports increase with NYHA class, affecting 89% of those with class IV symptoms, and worsens over time, afflicting up to 75% of patients with HF in the final six months of life. Over time, pain that persists becomes even more closely tied to psychosocial and emotional factors. Pain may be caused by multiple etiologies, including cardiac and non-cardiac causes.[30] Distressing sequelae from unrelieved pain include poor medication compliance, poor self-care, depression, anxiety, sleeplessness, fear, reduced cognitive functioning, hopelessness, and increased suicidal ideation. Unrelieved pain can lead to poor outcomes including increased hospital readmissions, reduced functional status, and decreased quality of life. Pain frequently clusters with other symptoms in HF patients, and adequate treatment of pain can lead to improvement in those pain symptoms.[16]

Physical pain can be nociceptive, resulting from damage to non-neuronal tissue, or neuropathic, resulting from damage to the body's peripheral sensors. Nociceptive pain can be further divided into somatic pain and visceral pain. Somatic pain is usually musculoskeletal or superficial in nature, causing throbbing, aching, or stabbing. Visceral pain on the other hand, is described as an internal pain brought on by stretch, ischemia, or inflammation, and manifests as deep, diffuse, and dull discomfort. Assessment of pain in the advanced HF patient should be the same as in any other patient complaining of pain. Pharmacological and non-pharmacological measures should be used.[31]

When treating pain, cardiac ischemia should be ruled out. Other etiologies of pain can prove more challenging to manage if the underlying cause is unclear. Some common analgesics are also relatively contraindicated in the treatment of advanced HF. Opioids are recommended for moderate to severe pain, either alone or with concomitant use of other drugs. Although limited data suggest that chronic opioid administration slightly increases adverse cardiovascular events in healthy patients, expert consensus argues that the benefits of using opioids to effectively manage symptoms in the HF population outweigh the risks of under-treated pain. Although oral and intravenous non-steroidal anti-inflammatories (NSAIDs) are generally contraindicated in HF patients, topically applied NSAIDs are effective; compared with systemic administration, the topical absorption has minimal effects on the cardiovascular system. NSAIDs are generally recommended for mild somatic or visceral pain.[16,32]

For neuropathic pain, there are several different classes of medications available, though they all must be considered carefully in the HF population due to their potential for significant side effects. Topical lidocaine is effective for localized peripheral neuropathic pain and causes very few side effects. Medications such as gabapentin and pregabalin are often effective for neuropathic pain, but they must be dose-adjusted for patients with renal insufficiency, may increase fluid retention, and often have significant potential for drug–drug interaction. Tricyclic antidepressants can also be quite effective for neuropathic pain but are usually not a safe choice in patients with HF because they can cause negative effects, including prolongation of the QT interval and myocardial contractility depression. Serotonin-norepinephrine reuptake inhibitors are another class of medications that could be helpful for treating neuropathic pain.[33]

Depression

Depression is extremely common in the general population but occurs even more frequently among patients with HF. Studies document that 21–36% of patients with HF have a mood disorder, but this number rises as high as 70% when limited to HF in-patients. Depression in patients with HF can be particularly challenging to diagnose. Symptoms of depression are often unmasked only when pursued by heightened suspicion, as the fatigue, poor appetite, and sleep disturbances of depression may all be attributed to the comorbid HF.

HF patients with depression have been shown to have higher readmission rates, decreased functional status, and increased mortality rates. Less than 25% of cardiac patients with major depression are diagnosed with depression despite its high prevalence and clinical significance. Of those diagnosed, only 50% are treated. Treatment of depression may not improve morbidity and mortality but may improve quality of life. A combination of pharmacologic and cognitive therapy is recommended for all patients. Choosing an antidepressant in this population should be guided by efficacy as well as side effect profiles.[34]

Recommended pharmacologic therapies may include serotonin reuptake inhibitors (SSRIs), serotonin-norepinephrine reuptake inhibitors (SNRIs), and tetracyclic and tricyclic antidepressants. Multiple clinical trials have evaluated the efficacy of SSRIs in HF, and these drugs are commonly prescribed. Of the SSRIs studied in HF patients, citalopram, escitalopram, and sertraline have lower risk of drug–drug interactions than paroxetine or fluoxetine. All SSRIs have the potential to slow heart rate slightly and can infrequently increase bleeding risk. Neither of these risks is clinically significant alone but they may be concerning if other medications that increase these risks are concurrently prescribed. When starting an SSRI, it is important to monitor patients with renal dysfunction for worsening hyponatremia and fluid retention.[34]

The class of SNRIs includes venlafaxine, desvenlafaxine, and duloxetine. These have not been studied for treating depression in patients with HF and are generally not used as a first-line therapy. Because of norepinephrine stimulation, increases in blood pressure and cardiac arrhythmias are possible. Mirtazapine, a tetracyclic, can be useful in some patients who are also experiencing concomitant poor appetite or sleeping difficulties with their depression. However, mirtazapine is considered a second-line treatment as doses of 15 mg per day or greater are indicated for depression and increased noradrenergic activity at these doses could theoretically lead to worsening of HF. Mirtazapine has also been associated with mild increases in the QT interval. Tricyclic antidepressants are only recommended with expert consultation due to the possibility of negative inotropy, QT-prolongation, and significant antimuscarinic side effects.[34]

Fatigue

Fatigue is common in advanced HF patients, with a prevalence ranging from 50% to 96%. Fatigue is strongly associated with depression and reduced quality of life. The underlying cause is likely related to many contributing factors, including low cardiac output, decreased systemic tissue perfusion, depression, deconditioning, insomnia, and cachexia. Treatments for fatigue often focus on behavioral changes to directly target an underlying cause and may include exercise, scooter use, dietary modification, adjusted diuretic scheduling, upright sleep positioning with a wedge or hospital bed, if necessary, use of a continuous positive airway pressure machine, or nocturnal supplemental oxygen. Treatments should be targeted to these, but often, despite these, fatigue continues as the disease progresses. Corticosteroids may provide temporary relief of fatigue in doses of 2 to 20 mg daily, but these benefits typically only last for four to six weeks. Long-term use is not a viable option due to side effects. Stimulants have also been studied for improving fatigue and depression in patients with cancer, HIV, and other advanced diseases, but they have not been studied in patients with advanced HF. Side effects of increased heart rate, blood pressure, afterload, and risk of ventricular arrhythmias need to be monitored closely in this population.[35]

Gastrointestinal Distress

Patients with HF frequently experience a wide variety of gastrointestinal symptoms, including nausea, vomiting, anorexia, and constipation.

Nausea and vomiting can be attributed to low forward cardiac output and poor intestinal blood flow, as well as right-sided volume overload, hepatic congestion, and gut wall edema. Nausea can also be exacerbated by cardiac medications, such as aspirin, spironolactone, amiodarone, digoxin, and opioids. Consideration should be given as to whether any of these medications can be discontinued as a first-line approach. Commonly used anti-emetic medications, including prochlorperazine, promethazine, ondansetron, and metoclopramide, can be effective at reducing nausea, but they can prolong the QT interval and require close monitoring; they may be contraindicated if a patient has a prolonged QT interval. If this occurs, possible use of dronabinol or benzodiazepines may be trialed.[36]

Constipation is also a common complaint and likely due to fluid restriction, diuretic use, comorbid diabetic gastroparesis, or opioids. Interventions may include dietary changes, osmotic agents, stool softeners, stimulant laxatives, and motility agents. Anorexia or diminished oral intake results from early satiety, ascites, fatigue, and depression. Metoclopramide and mirtazapine, which could help stimulate appetite, both have the potential to cause QT prolongation, so their use is often limited in the advanced HF patient. Megestrol should be avoided because it increases thromboembolism risk in this already sedentary population. Educating the patient and family regarding the need for very small meals or snacks at more frequent intervals is suggested.[36]

Advance Care Planning

Advance care planning (ACP) is an ongoing process. It involves conversations designed to facilitate communication between individuals and clinicians to identify and document medical and personal care preferences which are consistent with personal values if a person becomes too ill in the future to express their wishes. In this dynamic process, patients can identify a person(s) they trust to help ensure that their health care wishes are respected if they lose the ability to speak for themselves.[37] The ACP process helps answer two key questions:

1. If you are unable to or do not wish to participate in the decision-making process related to your health, what would you want us to think about when making decisions about your care?
2. If you are unable to or do not wish to participate in the decision-making process related to your health, who would you want us to speak with?

These conversations are imperative for advanced HF patient care, where medical technology has given clinicians the ability to prolong life by artificial means. Advances in HF treatments have created their own ethical dilemmas that need careful consideration and communication with patients, especially when treatments might be of limited benefit.[37] Complex shared decision making becomes increasingly significant as HF progresses, particularly when patients are faced with options such as transplant and mechanical circulatory support, which may not align well with their overall goals or preferences.[38]

HF clinicians can integrate palliative care strategies by incorporating several important components of planning and decision making for HF patients.[37] These components include understanding the patient's perspective and care preferences, explaining what is medically feasible, and integrating these considerations into the overall care plan. Use of defined triggers for ACP can help prompt important patient–caregiver conversations. Guidelines advocate an annual review of HF status and future care preferences.[39]

For patients to effectively participate in ACP, they need knowledge about their life-limiting illness and possible outcomes, including information about their illness trajectory and the benefits and risks of different treatment interventions such as home inotrope therapy, VADs, transplantation, internal cardiac defibrillators, and cardiopulmonary resuscitation. This information will help them to identify their preferences. A key element of the ACP process is discussing when to start and stop treatments. Patient decision making relies heavily on the thoroughness of each discussion about current and future benefits and burdens of proposed treatments.[37]

Shared decision making occurs when the clinician and the patient work together to make health care decisions that are best for the patient. The ideal decision considers evidence-based information about available options, presented in a way that patients can understand, the clinician's knowledge and experience, and the patient's values and preferences. Shared decision making in health care has now been actualized into a model/approach that any clinician can utilize.[40] The SHARE approach incorporates these five steps:

1. **S**eek your patient's participation
2. **H**elp your patient explore and compare treatment options
3. **A**ssess your patient's values and preferences
4. **R**each a decision with your patient
5. **E**valuate your patient's decision(s)

Many clinicians are reluctant to have these discussions and believe the patient should initiate the conversation.[41] A consequence of clinicians not having these discussions is that people with life-limiting illnesses, who have been receiving care throughout the course of their illness, will reach the end-stage of the disease without ever having had an honest conversation about what is happening.[37] For HF patients, opinions differ as to whose responsibility it is to discuss with patients, with 66% of cardiology clinicians citing that the responsibility is that of the primary care physician, while 57% of primary care physicians believe the converse.[37,42] Patients are often hesitant to start these conversations, but usually express relief when they do come up. Patients need time to think about and reflect on what has been discussed and talk with family members. Decisions can change along the disease course and clinicians need to be prepared to discuss implications.[43]

Important factors for the patient that play a role in the ACP process include religion, spirituality, and culture. Each religion has its own values, beliefs, and practices, which will influence the patient's concept of their illness and possible treatment decisions. Spirituality is part of how a person thinks about the world and themselves and is inherent in the decision-making process. Cultural norms can influence many aspects of the ACP process including who participates in the discussion, who makes decisions, what type of decisions are made, and what

TABLE 18.2: Primary Palliative Care Training Opportunities

Program	Target Population	Modules	Costs	Time Commitment	Format
CAPC Online	Health care professionals who care for patients with serious illness	Pain management Communication skills Symptom management	Part of CAPC membership for all staff (~$3,500 per organization)	40+ modules	Online
EPEC	Health care professionals and caregivers	Communication skills Ethical decision making Psychosocial considerations Symptom management	Conference: ~ $750 Each online module: $30	1.5 days (in-person) 16 modules with 30 screens per module (online)	In-person workshops and conferences Online
ELNEC	Undergraduate and graduate nursing faculty CE providers and staff development educators Hospice nurses Homecare nurses APRN/staff nurses working in acute care settings	Nursing care at the end of life Pain management Symptom management Ethical/legal issues; cultural considerations in end-of-life care Communication loss, grief, bereavement Preparation for and care at the time of death	$625 plus travel and lodging	Two days with optional additional half-day	In-person trainings ELNEC online for undergraduate nursing students
CardioTalk	Physicians and advance practice RNs	Giving bad news. Conducting family conferences Defining goals of care Responding to emotion Discussing code status Respecting and supporting religious and spiritual beliefs Withdrawing life- sustaining therapies	$600 plus travel and lodging	Two days	In-person

Abbreviations: APRN: Advanced Practice Registered Nurse; CAPC: Center to Advance Palliative Care; CE: continuing education; ELNEC: End of Life Nursing Education Consortium; EPEC: Education in Palliative and End of Life Care; RN: Registered Nurse.
Source: Adapted from Gelfman et al. Primary palliative care for heart failure: What is it? How do we implement it? *Heart Fail Rev.* 2017;22(5):611–20.

rituals might be important at end of life.[37] ACP is based on Western medical culture that values patient autonomy, which can be contrary to a patient or family's cultural beliefs.[44]

Family members and significant others are an important part of the ACP process. Patients should decide who should participate in the discussions, if able. How the ACP process proceeds can be variable, depending on the patient circumstances. There is no set way, and clinicians need to be prepared for variations in the process. However, certain topics should be covered during the ACP process, including surrogate decision makers, cardiopulmonary resuscitation, and device deactivation, as applicable.[45]

The appointment of a health care decision maker is the patient's decision, assuming the patient has decision-making capacity. If the patient does not have decision-making capacity, and there is no written designation of a decision maker, most countries have a legal process which outlines who can assist the health care team in making health care decisions.[46]

In advanced HF patients, the use of device-based therapies, such as implantable cardioverter defibrillators and cardiac resynchronization therapy, and advanced therapies, such as home inotrope infusions, VADs, and transplantation, increases significantly. Discussions around these therapies require thorough explanations, including risks and benefits. Challenges encountered by clinicians initiating conversations regarding discontinuing devices or therapies can be due to clinician discomfort, lack of counseling prior to implantation, and patient misconceptions. Planning for device deactivation or therapy discontinuation should start before implantation.[47–49]

Several national organizations and associations recognize the importance of resources and tools to facilitate discussion for both patients and clinicians, and these are usually free and available on the internet.[37] There are also several sample conversations available to clinicians in having discussions with patients regarding general ACP, changes in condition, delivering difficult news, prognosis, do-not-rescuscitate status, quality of life, discontinuation of therapies.[50,51] Additionally, there are several national programs designed as palliative care training opportunities for health care providers; Table 18.2 summarizes these resources.[10]

ACP conversations can help provide patients and families with opportunities to make choices, discuss personal values and goals, provide direction to the health care team, and identify a proxy decision maker(s).[52] The ACP process may change over the illness trajectory, but, at the core, the need for open, honest, and ongoing communication between all involved in caring for the person remains the highest priority.[39]

Conclusion

Palliative care is essential for patients with HF.[53] Clinicians need to be knowledgeable in symptom assessment and management, able to facilitate difficult discussions, and open to patient and family input.[37] Clinicians also need to recognize when a patient's condition has become too complex for primary palliative care and when to initiate a referral to the specialty clinician in a timely manner.

References

1. Clark D. From margins to centre: a review of the history of palliative care in cancer. *Lancet Oncol.* 2007 May;8(5):430–8.
2. Shah A, et al. An evaluation of the prevalence and severity of pain and other symptoms in acute decompensated heart failure. *J Palliat Med.* 2013 Jan;16(1):87–90.
3. Institute of Medicine (US) Committee on Care at the End of Life. Approaching death: improving care at the end of life--a report of the Institute of Medicine. *Health Serv Res.* 1998 Apr;33(1):1–3.
4. Connors A, et al. A controlled trial to improve care for seriously ill hospitalized patients: the study to understand prognoses and preferences for outcomes and risks of treatments (SUPPORT). *JAMA.* 1995;274(20):1591–8.

5. DeMilto L. Assessment of last acts program provides recommendations for future direction. *RWJF: Program Results Report.* 2002 Oct.
6. Ruder D. From specialty to shortage. *Harvard Magazine.* 2015 Mar-Apr.
7. Temel J, et al. Early palliative care for patients with metastatic non-small-cell lung cancer. *N Engl J Med.* 2010 Aug;363(8):733–42.
8. Rogers J, et al. Palliative care in heart failure: the PAL-HF randomized, controlled clinical trial. *J Am Coll Cardiol.* 2017 Jul;70(3):331–41.
9. Quill T, Abernethy A. Generalist plus specialist palliative care — creating a more sustainable model. *N Engl J Med.* 2013 Mar;368(13):1173–5.
10. Gelfman L, et al. Primary palliative care for heart failure: what is it? How do we implement it? *Heart Fail Rev.* 2017;22(5):611–20.
11. National Consensus Project for Quality Palliative Care. 2018 Oct.
12. Yancy C, et al. 2013 ACCF/AHA guideline for the management of heart failure: a report of the American College of Cardiology Foundation/American Heart Association task force on practice guidelines. *Circulation.* 2013 Oct 15;128(16):e240–327.
13. Braun L, et al. Palliative care and cardiovascular disease and stroke: a policy statement from the American Heart Association/American Stroke Association. *Circulation.* 2016 Sep 13;134(11):e198–225.
14. Jacques L, et al. 2013. Centers for Medicare and Medicaid Services, National Coverage Analysis and Decision Memo. Decision memo for ventricular assist devices for bridge-to-transplant and destination therapy. 2013 Oct. 1–64.
15. Alpert C, et al. Symptom burden in heart failure: assessment, impact on outcomes, and management. *Heart Fail Rev.* 2017 Jan;22(1):25–39.
16. Stewart D, McPherson M. Symptom management challenges in heart failure: pharmacotherapy considerations. *Heart Fail Rev.* 2017 Sep;22(5):525–34.
17. Zambroski C, et al. Impact of symptom prevalence and symptom burden on quality of life in patients with heart failure. *Eur J Cardiovasc Nurs.* 2005 Sep;4(3):198–206.
18. Nekolaichuk C, et al. The Edmonton symptom assessment system: a 15-year retrospective review of validation studies (1991–2006). *Palliat Med.* 2008 Mar;22(2):111–22.
19. Pozehl B, et al. Heart failure symptom survey: validity and reliability. *J Card Fail.* 2006 Aug;12(6):S100.
20. Green C, et al. Development and evaluation of the Kansas City cardiomyopathy questionnaire: a new health status measure for heart failure. *J Am Coll Cardiol.* 2000 Apr;35(5):1245–55.
21. Kelkar A, et al. Utility of patient-reported outcome instruments in heart failure. *JACC Heart Fail.* 2016 Mar;4(3):165–75.
22. Wilson J, McMillan S. Symptoms experienced by heart failure patients in hospice care. *J Hosp Palliat Nurs.* 2013 Feb;15(1):13–21.
23. Parshall M, et al. An official American Thoracic Society statement: update on the mechanisms, assessment, and management of dyspnea. *Am J Respir Crit Care Med.* 2012 Feb 15;185(4):435–52.
24. Kupper N, et al. Determinants of dyspnea in chronic heart failure. *J Card Fail.* 2016 Mar;22(3):201–9.
25. Barnes H, et al. Opioids for the palliation of refractory breathlessness in adults with advanced disease and terminal illness. *Cochrane Database Syst Rev.* 2016 Mar;3:CD011008.
26. Simon S, et al. Benzodiazepines for the relief of breathlessness in advanced malignant and non-malignant diseases in adults. *Cochrane Database Syst Rev.* 2016 Oct;10.CD007354.
27. U.S. Food and Drug Administration. FDA requires strong warning of opioid analgesics, prescription opioid cough products, and benzodiazepine labeling related to serious risks and death from combined use. August 31, 2016.
28. Kwekkeboom K, Bratzke L. A systematic review of relaxation, meditation, and guided imagery strategies for symptom management in heart failure. *J Cardiovasc Nurs.* 2016 Sep-Oct;31(5):457–68.
29. Qian Y, et al. Fan therapy for the treatment of dyspnea in adults: a systematic review. *J Pain Symptom Manage.* 2019 Sep;58(3):481–6.
30. Goodlin S, et al. Investigating pain in heart failure patients: the pain assessment, incidence, and nature in heart failure (PAIN-HF) study. *J Card Fail.* 2012 Oct;18(10):776–83.
31. Skelly A, et al. Noninvasive nonpharmacological treatment for chronic pain: a systematic review. Agency for Healthcare Research and Quality (US), Rockville (MD); 2018. PMID: 30179389.
32. Lin T-C, et al. Comparative risk of cardiovascular outcomes between topical and oral nonselective NSAIDs in Taiwanese patients with rheumatoid arthritis. *J Am Heart Assoc.* 2017;6(11):e006874.
33. Alemzadeh-Ansari M, et al. Chronic pain in chronic heart failure: a review article. *J The Univ Heart Ctr.* 2017 Apr;12(2):49–56.
34. Sokoreli I, et al. Depression and anxiety as predictors of mortality among heart failure patients: systematic review and meta-analysis. *Heart Fail Rev.* 2016 Jan;21(1):49–63.
35. Perez-Moreno A, et al. Fatigue as a predictor of outcome in patients with heart failure: analysis of CORONA (Controlled Rosuvastatin Multinational Trial in Heart Failure). *JACC Heart Fail.* 2014 Apr;2(2):187–97.
36. Lowey S. Palliative care in the management of patients with advanced heart failure. In: M. Islam, ed. *Heart failure: from research to clinical practice.* New York City: Springer; 2017: 295–311.
37. Wittenberg E, et al. *Textbook of palliative care communication.* New York: Oxford University Press; 2016.
38. Teuteberg J, Teuteberg W. *Palliative care for patients with heart failure.* Washington DC: American College of Cardiology; 2016.
39. Meyers D, Goodlin S. End-of-life decisions and palliative care in advanced heart failure. *Can J Cardiol.* 2016 Sep;32(9):1148–56.
40. The SHARE Approach: A Model for Shared Decisionmaking - Fact Sheet. Content last reviewed September 2020. Agency for Healthcare Research and Quality, Rockville, MD. https://www.ahrq.gov/health-literacy/professional-training/shared-decision/tools/factsheet.html.
41. Malhotra C, et al. Impact of advance care planning on the care of patients with heart failure: study protocol for a randomized controlled trial. *Trials.* 2016 Jun;17(1):285.
42. Dunlay S, et al. A survey of clinician attitudes and self-reported practices regarding end-of-life care in heart failure. *Palliat Med.* 2015 Mar;29(3):260–7.
43. Bodtke S, Ligon K. *Hospice and palliative medicine handbook: a clinical guide.* Scotts Valley: CreateSpace Independent Publishing Platform; 2016.
44. Lee M, et al. A systematic review of advance directives and advance care planning in Chinese people from eastern and western cultures. *J Hosp Palliat Nurs.* 2014 Apr;16(2):75–85.
45. Liao M, et al. Knowledge of and attitudes toward advance directives in patients with advanced heart failure. *J Hosp Palliat Nurs.* 2019 Feb;21(1):80–9.
46. American Heart Association. *Planning for advanced heart failure.* 2017 May.
47. LeMond L, Goodlin S. Management of heart failure in patients nearing the end of life – there is so much more to do. *Card Fail Rev.* 2015 Apr;1(1):547–55.
48. Karches K, Sulmasy D. Ethical considerations for turning off pacemakers and defibrillators. *Card Electrophysiol Clin.* 2015 Sep;7(3):547–55.
49. Fang J, et al. Advanced (Stage D) heart failure: a statement from the Heart Failure Society of America Guidelines Committee. *J Card Fail.* 2015 Jun;21(6):519–34.
50. Cardiosmart. Planning your care. *Palliative Care.* 2018 Mar.
51. Heart Failure Society of America Patient Education. *Module 9: Advance care planning.* 2017.
52. Kates J. Advance care planning conversations. *J Am Acad Nurse Pract.* 2017;13(7):e321–3.
53. Kavalieratos D, et al. Palliative care in heart failure: rationale, evidence, and future priorities. *J Am Coll Cardiol.* 2017 Oct;70(15):1919–30.

Section IV
Managing Cardiovascular Comorbidities in Heart Failure

DOI: 10.1201/9780429244544-22

Chapter 19
MANAGEMENT OF HYPERTENSION IN HEART FAILURE

Jesse Kane, Clive Goulbourne, and Hal A. Skopicki

Introduction

Systemic arterial hypertension (hypertension) is the most prevalent and modifiable factor for both the development of heart failure (HF) and the amelioration of HF-related morbidity and mortality.[1] Globally, about one in four adults have hypertension resulting in a nearly 50% increase in the total number of healthy life-years lost.[2] The Framingham Heart Study noted a two- to three-fold increase in the incidence of HF in hypertensive vs normotensive patients,[3] while patients with hypertension who develop acutely decompensated HF are at dramatically higher risk of subsequent cardiovascular events and death.[4]

A prominent long-term driver of left ventricular hypertrophy and HF with preserved ejection fraction (HFpEF), hypertension is a deleterious comorbidity of both HFpEF and HF with reduced ejection fraction (HFrEF), and acts as a driver for both progression and exacerbations of these diseases. More often, hypertension occurs as a comorbidity of HF,[5–7] and, in most instances, complicates attempts to optimize overall cardiovascular function, end-organ preservation, and quality of life.

Definitions of Hypertension

Hypertension is the most common cardiovascular disease worldwide and, when poorly controlled, markedly increases the risk of multiple cardiovascular events, including HF. Contributing to the complexity of diagnosis is the challenge of disease detection, which is dependent on the method, time, number, and duration of measurements. Whereas hypertension is most commonly diagnosed based on repeated blood pressure (BP) measurements in a clinical office setting, the future undoubtedly will center around device-based home and ambulatory monitoring, which limit the effect of bias from a single BP measurement.[8]

Another challenge lies in defining the disease. Hypertension should be contextualized by predicted atherosclerotic cardiovascular risk, as people with higher cardiovascular risk derive the most benefit from BP-lowering treatments.[9,10] The association between BP and cardiovascular risk is continuous, starting well within the normotensive range, reportedly as low as 115/75 mmHg.[11,12] In practice, the European Society of Hypertension (ESH),[13] the International Society of Hypertension (ISH)[14] and the Asian guideline committees[15,16] have recently reaffirmed a threshold of ≥140/90 mmHg for the diagnosis of hypertension. The American College of Cardiology (ACC) and American Heart Association (AHA) utilize a different cut-off and definition system, with stage 1 hypertension as systolic BP (SBP) 130–139 mmHg or diastolic BP (DBP) 80–89 mmHg, and stage 2 as SBP >140 mmHg or DBP ≥90 mmHg.[17] Supporting evidence is based on work demonstrating that these cutoffs identify adults at higher risk for HF events.[18] Figure 19.1 summarizes the differences in the European vs American guidelines for the diagnosis and management of hypertension.

Heart Failure Risk Assessment in Hypertension

Patients with hypertension are at increased risk of HF and appropriate treatment of hypertension drastically reduces this risk. For this reason, the ACC/AHA guidelines for HF designate hypertension as Stage A HF, i.e., patients are at risk of HF, with the goal of emphasizing prevention Figure 19.2). Patients with target organ damage from hypertension, for example, left ventricular hypertrophy (LVH), have preclinical (Stage B) HF and are at heightened risk of HF, Figure 19.2. In these patients, close attention to management of hypertension is warranted, with the goal of reversing structural damage to the heart.[19]

Beyond the accurate diagnosis and definition of hypertension, the use of advanced cardiac imaging and biomarkers may provide insight into the risk of progression into hypertensive heart disease and HFpEF.[20] Progression may be associated with wall strain-inducing cardiac fibroblast production of collagen[21–23] and myocardial scarring, suggesting that cardiac magnetic resonance (CMR) may be useful in identifying the progressive nature of fibrosis, separating those into hypertension with and without progression to HF. Of note, LVH may not be an adequate marker of hypertensive heart disease. Studies of BP treatment that resulted in lower cardiovascular event rates were not significantly associated with changes in left ventricular (LV) mass, function, or fibrosis.[24] In the SPRINT-HEART study, only 9% of men and 13% of women had abnormal LV mass by CMR myocardial native T1 values when compared with healthy controls[25] and studies in patients with hypertensive heart disease have found that patients with concentric LV remodeling had normal native T1.[26] This suggests that the development of myocardial fibrosis in hypertensive heart disease may not be linearly related to BP.

Thus, mechanisms beyond ventricular remodeling and LVH may hold further insight into mechanisms of HFpEF development. An analysis of SPRINT-HEART has shown that treatment resulted in a significantly attenuated increase in carotid-femoral pulse wave velocity, a measure of aortic stiffness,[27] suggesting increased afterload and vascular distensibility. Possible mechanisms include increased arterial stiffness,[28] oxidative stress,[29] systemic inflammation[30] and microvasculature/endothelial changes[31] providing targets for future therapies and means of monitoring progression of disease.

Treatment of Hypertension to Prevent Heart Failure

The vast majority (90–95%) of patients with hypertension are considered to have primary or essential hypertension with a complex multifactorial etiology related to genetic predisposition, environment, and diet. However, it remains important to recognize secondary causes of hypertension that are amenable to direct intervention, such as renal artery stenosis, sleep apnea, coarctation of the aorta, pheochromocytoma, mineralocorticoid excess, and primary hyperaldosteronism.

DOI: 10.1201/9780429244544-23

Guideline Differences	American College of Cardiology/American Heart Association (ACC/AHA)		European Society of Cardiology/European Society of Hypertension (ESC/ESH)	
Level of blood pressure (BP) defining hypertension	Systolic (mm Hg) and/or	Diastolic (mm Hg)	Systolic (mm Hg) and/or	Diastolic (mm Hg)
Office/Clinic BP	≥ 130	≥ 80	≥ 140	≥ 90
Daytime mean	≥ 130	≥ 80	≥ 135	≥ 85
Nighttime mean	≥ 110	≥ 65	≥ 120	≥ 70
24-hour mean	≥ 125	≥ 75	≥ 130	≥ 80
Home BP mean	≥ 130	≥ 80	≥ 135	≥ 85
BP targets for treatment	< 130/80 mm Hg		Systolic targets < 140 mm Hg and close to 130 mm Hg	
Initial Combination Therapy	Initial single-pill combination therapy in patients > 20/10 mm Hg above BP goal		Initial single-pill combination therapy in patients ≥ 140/90 mm Hg	
Hypertensive requiring intervention	> 130/80 mm Hg		≥ 140/90 mm Hg	

Guideline Similarities	ACC/AHA	ESC/ESH
Importance of home BP monitoring	• Take BP at home, twice in the morning and twice in the evening, in the week before clinic • Bring the BP machine in annually for validation	
Therapy	• Restrict beta blockers to patients with comorbidities or other indications • Initial single pill combination as initial therapy	
Follow-up	• Detect poor adherence and focus on improvement • BP telemonitoring and digital health solutions recommended	

FIGURE 19.1 Comparison of American and European society definitions and management of hypertension. *Abbreviations*: ACC = American College of Cardiology; AHA = American Heart Association; BP = blood pressure; ESC = European Society of Cardiology; ESH = European Society of Hypertension. (Reproduced with permission from Bakris et al. *J Am Coll Cardiol.* 2019;73(23):3018–26.)

Therapeutic interventions should begin with identifying potential lifestyle modifications before progressing to pharmacologic therapies. Lifestyle modifications that effectively lower BP are increased physical activity,[32] lowered dietary sodium[33, 34] and higher potassium consumption,[35] limiting alcohol intake,[36] weight loss[37] and enhanced dietary intake of whole grains, vegetables, nuts, seeds, and fruits[38] with a reduction in foods high in sugar and saturated fats,[39,40] as well as relaxation/mindfulness-based techniques.[41] Improving sleep disturbances for BP control is an area of ongoing investigation.[42,43]

Management of hypertension is complex due to underlying pathophysiology. On a background of genetic and environmental influences, clinicians must manage an admixture of neurohumoral mediators and vascular modulation through natriuretic peptides and the renin-angiotensin-aldosterone, sympathetic nervous, inflammatory, and immune systems.[44] Even the gut microbiome may be involved.[45]

At least three classes of agents are considered first-line agents by most societies: thiazide diuretics, angiotensin-converting enzyme inhibitors (ACEis) or angiotensin II receptor blockers (ARBs) and dihydropyridine calcium channel blockers (CCBs). Thiazide-like (e.g., chlorthalidone) and thiazide diuretics promote a natriuresis with intravascular volume reduction through inhibition of distal tubular Na^+ and Cl^- co-transporters. Care must be taken to monitor for side effects including hypokalemia, hyponatremia, and worsening glucose metabolism. ACEi and ARBs are preferred initial therapies for hypertension in HF with comparable abilities to reduce cardiovascular risk.[46] Renal dysfunction, hyperkalemia, cough, and potentially life-threatening angioedema (the latter two being primarily associated with ACEi) are potential side effects.

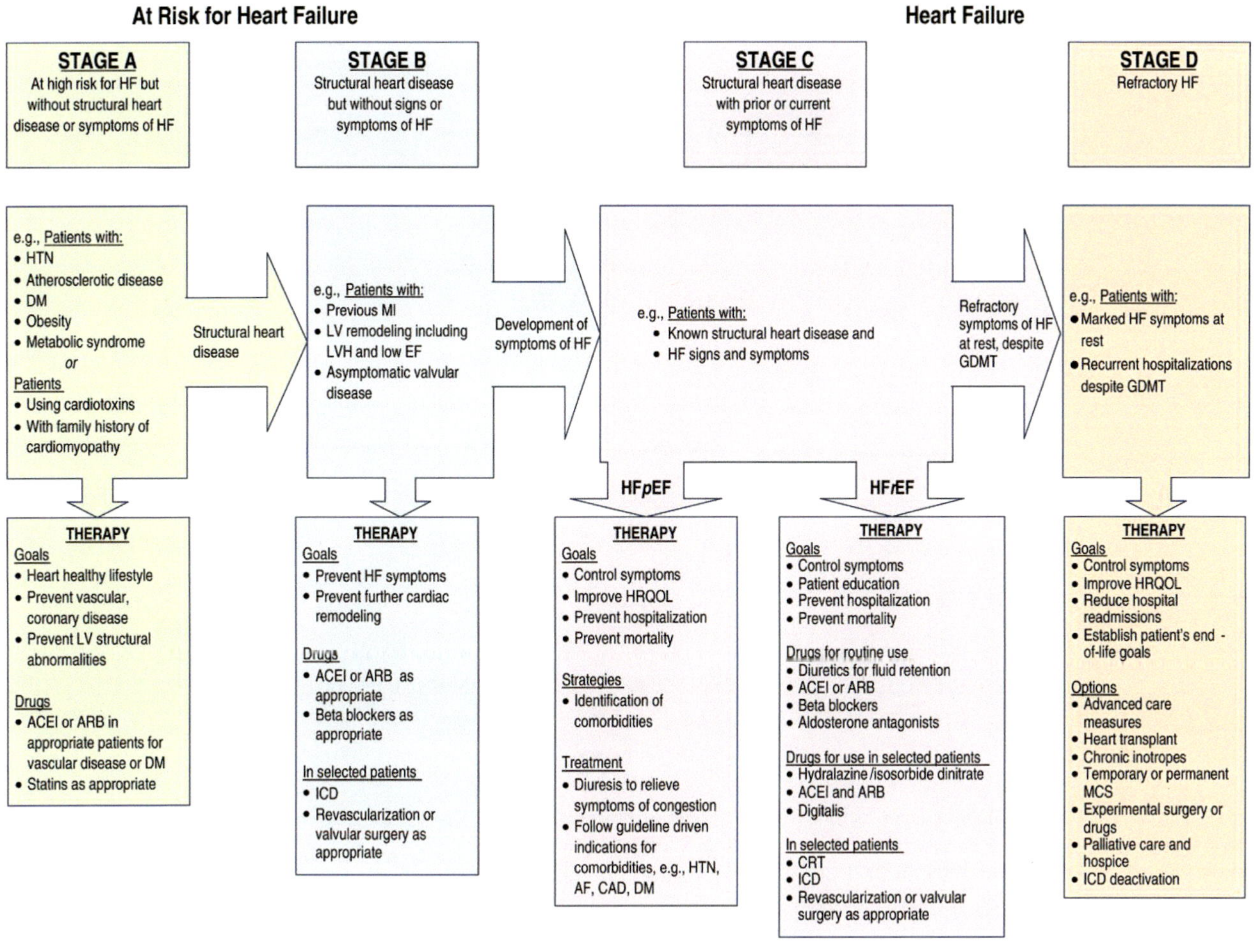

FIGURE 19.2 Steps in the development of HF and recommended therapy by stage. *Abbreviations*: ACEI, angiotensin-converting enzyme inhibitor; AF, atrial fibrillation; ARB, angiotensin-receptor blocker; CAD, coronary artery disease; CRT, cardiac resynchronization therapy; DM, diabetes mellitus; EF, ejection fraction; GDMT, guideline-directed medical therapy; HF, heart failure; HFpEF, heart failure with preserved ejection fraction; HFrEF, heart failure with reduced ejection fraction; HRQoL, health-related quality of life; HTN, hypertension; ICD, implantable cardioverter-defibrillator; LV, left ventricular; LVH, left ventricular hypertrophy; MCS, mechanical circulatory support; and MI, myocardial infarction. (Adapted with permission from Hunt et al. *J Am Coll Cardiol.* 2009;53:e9.)

CCBs cause vasodilation by blocking vascular smooth muscle L-type calcium channels and can cause peripheral edema due to peripheral arterial vasodilation, especially amlodipine.

The SPRINT trial demonstrated that an aggressive treatment approach, targeting an SBP less than 120 mmHg (compared with less than 140 mmHg) in patients without diabetes or prior stroke, significantly lowered the occurrence of the primary composite endpoint of myocardial infarction (MI), stroke, incident HF, or cardiovascular death, driven by a 36% reduction in acute decompensated HF events (Figure 19.3).[4] Recent studies have suggested that the use of certain antihypertensives (ACEi) and their combination with thiazides[47] in patients at increased cardiovascular risk may protect against the appearance of HF.[48] Yet, this advantage was not reproduced with the ARB valsartan in the VALUE trial.[49] Whether the choice of first-line agents makes a difference in those at lower risk requires further prospective investigation based on the results of the HOPE-3 trial[50] and the LEGEND study.[51]

Interestingly, the 2020 International Society of Hypertension removed thiazide or thiazide-type diuretic directs from its first line agents, opting instead for just ACEi, ARB, and/or a calcium channel blockade.[14] The elimination of the thiazide-like diuretics was met with much consternation[52,53] since the data used to make the changes were regionally based, without significant Black, Latino, or Asian population representation. Therefore, many clinicians, including the current authors, suggest their continued use based on the demonstrated benefits of thiazide or thiazide-type diuretics in preventing LVH, HF, myocardial infarction, and aortic aneurysm.

Refractory hypertension should signal the need for agents that may target additional pathways. The PATHWAY2 study suggested a beneficial role of the mineralocorticoid antagonist spironolactone (compared with placebo, bisoprolol, and doxazosin) in improving cardiovascular outcomes in drug-resistant hypertension.[54] More patients achieved controlled (<130/80 mmHg) BP with spironolactone, whereas eplerenone also effectively improved BP[55] and was as effective as amlodipine in lowering systolic BP and pulse pressure in older patients with hypertension and widened pulse pressure.[56]

Recent work has noted similar central BP and arterial stiffness in refractory hypertension,[57] and thus adding more vasodilators may not yield optimal control. ESH guidelines

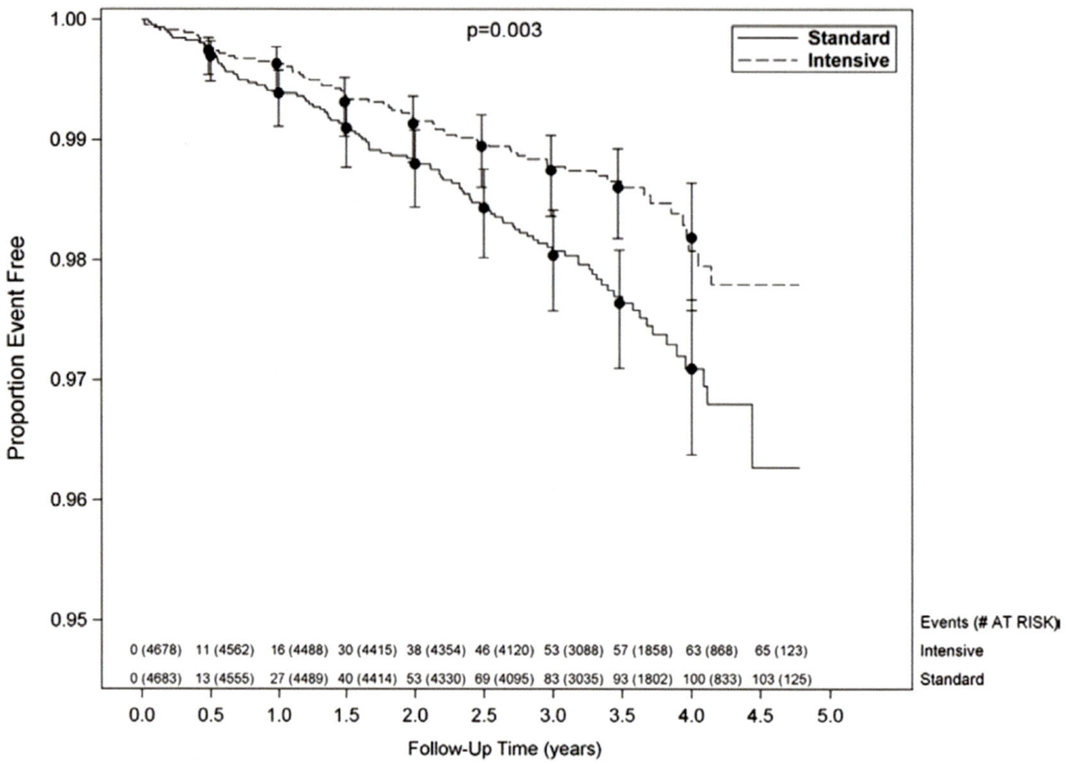

FIGURE 19.3 Kaplan–Meier curves for the SPRINT (Systolic Blood Pressure Reduction Intervention Trial) acute decompensated heart failure outcome by treatment group. Vertical bars indicate 95% confidence intervals. P value is from a Cox proportional hazards model stratified by clinical site. Number at risk and number of events are shown every six months. (Reproduced with permission from Upadhya et al. *Circ Heart Fail.* 2017;10:e003613.)

recommend torsemide in hypertensive patients.[58] However, apart from mineralocorticoid receptor antagonists and thiazides, it is our experience that other diuretics are of limited benefit and studies suggest that volume retention persists despite these therapies.[59] Therefore, sympathetic blockers (non-selective β-blockers, centrally acting α_2 antagonists, e.g., clonidine) may benefit select populations with refractory hypertension.[60,61]

Finally, it is critical to note the need to not overtreat hypertension. The risks of overaggressive treatment of hypertension include hypotension, falls, syncope, acute kidney injury, electrolyte abnormalities, bradycardia, and potential sudden death due to arrhythmias.

Hypertension as a Comorbidity/Target in Heart Failure: HFpEF vs HFrEF

The link between treatment of hypertension and HF necessitates an understanding of the contributions of BP to left ventricular hypertrophy, diastolic dysfunction, atrial dysfunction, coronary microvascular disease, endothelial dysfunction, myocardial injury, and fibrosis. No randomized studies have been performed to assess the effect of targeted BP control based on the diagnoses of either HFpEF or HFrEF.

Treatment of Heart Failure in the Setting of Acute Hypertension

In acute HF, the presence of severe hypertension is often associated with underlying HFpEF but HFrEF may also be present. Treatment of severe, hypertensive HF has not been systematically studied and remains challenging as underlying ischemia, infarct, renal insufficiency, and electrolyte and metabolic abnormalities are usually also present. Moreover, neither specific medication classes nor strategies have been endorsed by major societies or their guideline writing committees.

In HFpEF, the acute redistribution of intravascular volume into the extravascular space accounts for the abrupt presentation of pulmonary edema. Nitrates, vasodilators, and beta-blockers with alpha blocking activity, along with respiratory support, are suggested in the acute phase. Diuresis, in patients with acute HF and reduced LVEF, should be used after the above therapies in this scenario.

Both nitroglycerin and nitroprusside induce vasodilation through activation of calcium-sensitive potassium channels, mediated by nitric oxide through cyclic GMP.[62] Nitroprusside is a potent, first-line agent in hypertension with HF, with a rapid onset (within 1 min) and a duration of action of 10 min. However, targeted BP control may require a continuous infusion that should not be continued for more than 2–3 days. Potentially fatal cyanide toxicity can result from nitroprusside metabolism and should be assessed by monitoring for lactic acidosis and mental status changes.[63] Nitroglycerin has a rapid onset (within 5 min) with effects resolving within 10–20 min after cessation. At lower doses, it is a selective venodilator but can also decrease cardiac output. Low-dose administration may be used as an adjunct to IV antihypertensive therapy in hypertensive emergencies associated with acute coronary syndromes or acute pulmonary edema. Common adverse effects of IV nitroglycerin include hypotension, hypoxemia from ventilation perfusion mismatching, methemoglobinemia, reflex tachycardia, and tachyphylaxis.

Nicardipine is a highly vascular selective CCB with an onset of action in 5–15 min, a duration of action of 4–6 h and a half-life of approximately 8 h.[64] Of note, nicardipine has been shown to reduce both cardiac and cerebral ischemia.[65] The CCB clevidipine appears to be safe and efficacious in lowering acute BP to control hypertensive HF. In a randomized, open-label, active-controlled trial of patients presenting with presumed acute HF and an SBP ≥160 mmHg, IV clevidipine, when compared with nicardipine and additional nitroglycerin, achieved target BP more often and was less likely to require additional therapy for treating BP.[66] Common side effects are headache, abdominal pain, flushing, myalgia, and nausea.

Intravenous enalaprilat has also shown efficacy in reducing BP in the emergency room but should be used carefully in patients with underlying renal disease. In a retrospective study of hypertensive patients presenting to the emergency department with hypertensive HF, IV enalaprilat, with or without IV furosemide and nitroglycerin, resulted in a decrease in mean SBP of ~31 mmHg with an approximate 2% incidence of hypotension despite enalaprilat's prolonged half-life (about 35 hours).[67]

Labetalol is a competitive α_1- and β_1/β_2-adrenergic antagonist.[68] It can modulate BP within 2–5 min, with action lasting ~4 hours. Because of non-selective β blockade, labetalol should be avoided with patients with asthma, high-degree heart block, or severe bradycardia, and high doses should be avoided in HF treatment.

Hydralazine is a direct arteriolar vasodilator that has the potential to induce reflex tachycardia and coronary artery steal syndrome and can have deleterious outcomes in patients with significant underlying coronary artery disease or aortic dissection. When utilized in these scenarios, concomitant beta-blocker use should be considered. Hydralazine has an intermediated onset of action within 10–30 min and its effects last up to 12–24 hours.[69,70]

Treatment of Chronic Hypertension in HFpEF

In chronic HFpEF, hypertension increases the risk of disease progression and clinical deterioration. Although multiple classes of agents have been utilized to manage hypertension in HFpEF, no therapy has been able to demonstrate long-term morbidity and mortality benefits. However, based on mechanisms and multiple anecdotal or retrospective assessments, a variety of medications are routinely employed.

The 2017 ACC/AHA/Heart Failure Society of America (HFSA) guideline update recommends that patients with HFpEF and persistent hypertension after management of volume overload should be treated to SBP <130 mmHg.[71] Notably, the use of nitrates in the HFpEF has been associated with a signal of harm and therefore is discouraged. As high-quality evidence for optimal antihypertensive therapy of HFpEF is limited, with inhibition of the renin-angiotensin-aldosterone system with ACEi, ARB, mineralocorticoid receptor antagonist (MRA), and possibly angiotensin receptor neprilysin inhibitor (ARNI) being suggested as the preferred initial choice.

MRAs inhibit aldosterone's activation of the epithelial sodium channel. Through this mechanism, MRAs inhibit sodium retention, endothelial dysfunction, vasoconstriction, vascular remodeling, and fibrosis.[72] For patients with HFpEF in the TOPCAT study,[73] spironolactone did not significantly reduce the incidence of the primary composite outcome of death from cardiovascular causes or hospitalization. There was, however, a significant reduction in hospitalization for HF in the Americas, where the protocol was followed more rigorously.[74] Based on these results, the 2017 ACC/AHA/HFSA guideline update added new recommendations for the use of MRAs in the management of HFpEF.[71] Third-generation MRAs, including finerenone and canrenone, are non-steroidal compounds with both high selectivity and high potency to inhibit the mineralocorticoid receptor, enhanced concentration in both the kidney and heart (spironolactone and eplerenone remain primarily in the kidney) with beneficial effects on progressive myocardial fibrosis and potentially lower incidence of hyperkalemia.[75] The FINEARTS-HF study will assess the role of finerenone on reduction of cardiovascular death and HF events, including HF hospitalizations and urgent visits with HF issues in patients with HFpEF.[76]

Two large trials of angiotensin receptor blockers, CHARM-preserved (candesartan) and I-PRESERVE (irbesartan), one for angiotensin-converting enzyme inhibition, PEP-CHF (perindopril), and one trial (PARAGON-HF) for angiotensin receptor-neprilysin inhibition (sacubitril-valsartan) have shown no significant benefit for the combined endpoint of mortality and HF hospitalization.[77–80] However, the rates of hospitalization for both perindopril and candesartan were lower than for the control groups.

The PARAMOUNT study demonstrated that sacubitril/valsartan reduced NT-proBNP compared with valsartan in patients with HF and LVEF >45%.[81] Given this finding, the PARAGON-HF study was conducted, but showed no significant benefit for the combined endpoint of mortality and HF hospitalization[80]. However, in a pre-specified subgroup analysis, sacubitril-valsartan reduced the risk of HF hospitalization more in women than in men.

Finally, despite the significant role of intravenous nitrates in acute hypertension with HF,[78,82] oral nitrates have shown a disappointing lack of efficacy in chronic HFpEF with hypertension.[83]

Chronic Hypertension and HFrEF

Although HFrEF may result from chronic hypertension and, less frequently, acute hypertension, hypertension most commonly exists as a comorbidity of both acute and chronic HFrEF. The 2017 ACC/AHA/HFSA guidelines for the management of HF give a class I recommendation for the titration of medical therapy to attain an SBP of <130 mmHg in patients with HFrEF and hypertension.[71] However, this is based on expert opinion extrapolated from data involving studies of patients with significant cardiovascular disease or who were deemed high risk for cardiovascular complications.[84–86]

It is therefore something of a paradox that studies have suggested that a higher BP prior to pharmacotherapy is a predictor of better survival in patients with HF.[87] A subgroup analysis of the PARADIGM-HF trial[88] showed a U-shaped relationship between SBP and the rate of HF hospitalization. Patients with SBP <120 mmHg or SBP >140 mmHg were more likely to be hospitalized for HF exacerbations.[85] Other studies have noted an increased risk for poor clinical outcomes (all-cause mortality, cardiovascular mortality, HF hospitalizations) with both elevated and reduced BP.[89–91]

Therefore, BP reduction, in and of itself, should not be thought of as a target for HFrEF management, rather that goals of therapy should be directed towards maximally tolerated HFrEF medication dosages. Table 19.1 summarizes the pivotal clinical trials that have shown benefit with agents that also lower BP in patients with HFrEF.[92–102]

TABLE 19.1: HFrEF Clinical Trials Depicting Effect of Medical Therapy on Blood Pressure, Mortality, and Hospitalizations

Trial	Intervention	Control	BP Effect	Intervention Target Dose	CV Mortality	HF Hospitalization	All-Cause Mortality
COPERNICUS[92]	Carvedilol	Placebo	↓	25 mg twice daily	NA	↓	↓
COMET[93]	Carvedilol	Metoprolol Tartrate	↓	25 mg twice daily	↓	NA	↓
MERIT-HF[94]	Metoprolol Succinate	Placebo	↑	200mg once daily	↓	NA	↓
CIBIS-II[95]	Bisoprolol	Placebo	↔	10 mg once daily	↓	↓	↓
SOLVD[96]	Enalapril	Placebo	↓	10 mg twice daily	↓	↓	↓
Val-HeFT[97]	Valsartan	Placebo	↓	160 mg twice daily	NA	↓	↔
CHARM-Added[98]	Candesartan	Placebo	↓	32 mg once daily	↓	↓	↔
EMPHASIS-HF[99]	Eplerenone	Placebo	↓	50 mg once daily	↓	↓	↓
RALES[100]	Spironolactone	Placebo	↔	25–50 mg twice daily	↓	↓	↓
PARADIGM-HF[101]	Sacubitril/Valsartan	Enalapril	↓	97/103 mg twice daily	↓	↓	↓
A-HeFT[102]	ISDN/Hydralazine	Placebo	↓	40/75 mg twice daily	NA	↓	↓

Abbreviations: BP: blood pressure; CV: cardiovascular; NA: information not available; HF: heart failure; ISDN: isosorbide dinitrate.

Outpatient Management of Hypertension in HFrEF

Generally, treatment of HFrEF includes several classes of antihypertensive agents, such as ARNIs, ACEis, ARBs, beta-blockers, and MRAs. Sodium-glucose co-transport protein 2 (SGLT2) inhibitors, which were initially approved as anti-diabetic agents, and the soluble guanylate cyclase stimulator vericiguat have also recently been added to the armamentarium. When optimized or in the presence of persistent hypertension, most HF physicians advocate additional medications to reach normotensive ranges.

There are several specific beta-blockers which have proven mortality benefits for HFrEF patients, including bisoprolol, carvedilol, metoprolol succinate, and nebivolol.[103] However, questions remain regarding whether there are differential benefits to each medication. Potential areas of exploration include the impact of vasodilatory effects of certain beta-blockers (i.e., α-adrenergic receptor inhibition by carvedilol vs NO-mediated vasodilation by nebivolol) or the β_1 specificity of bisoprolol.

The additional role of hydralazine-nitrate is supported by the A-HeFT (African-American Heart Failure Trial) which reported improvement in quality of life, LVEF, LV remodeling, and survival with the addition of combination hydralazine-isosorbide dinitrate in self-described Black patients with HfrEF.[104,105] Mechanistically, the nitrate is believed to induce vasodilation by phosphorylating proteins involved in intracellular calcium mobilization. Yet tolerance to that effect rapidly develops (within several hours). The tolerance is prevented or reversed by hydralazine, resulting in a synergistic effect with the nitrate. For those who are intolerant to or who meet the criteria for the use of either ARNIs, ACE inhibitors, or ARBs, the combination of hydralazine-nitrates may be more effective than withholding vasodilatory therapy. Compared to placebo, the combination was shown to reduce the risk of dying[106] and hospitalization was equal to that with ACEI.[107,108]

Amlodipine, a CCB, has few negative inotropic effects and studies have shown neither benefit nor harm when used in patients with NYHA class II or III HF.[106,109,110] Therefore, when background HFrEF therapy proves inadequate to simultaneously control BP, amlodipine may be a reasonable choice.

Physicians in general are reluctant to give additional antihypertensive treatment to HF patients who have the potential to become hypotensive, especially elderly patients.[111] Questions remain as to what degree of concern is warranted. In PARADIGM-HF, a trial of sacubitril-valsartan vs optimal medical therapy, hypotension occurred in 14% vs 9.2% of patients, with number needed to harm of 21, and higher rates of symptomatic hypotension with SBP<90 mmHg (2.7% vs 1.4%). Yet this did not necessitate discontinuation of therapy. Moreover, an analysis in the Seniors trial showed that, whereas patients who began the study with an SBP≤130 mmHg fared worse than those with a higher initial SBP, both higher- and lower-BP groups derived similar benefits from beta-blocker treatment on the composite outcome of death or cardiovascular hospital admission.[112] Thus, choice of medication and dosing should be carefully considered based on individual patient needs.

Treatment of Hypertension in Acute Decompensated HFrEF

For HFrEF patients admitted with acutely decompensated HF, decongestion, with the maintenance of end-organ perfusion, and not BP control, is the goal of therapy. Although higher BP on admission in acute decompensated HF patients is associated with improved survival,[113] there is a potential J-shaped relationship between discharge SBP and long-term mortality.[114] The mortality rate increased significantly only at lower BP, with only a trend for an increased mortality at higher SBP, while readmission risk increased with both SBP and DBP.

As outlined in other chapters, optimization of standard therapy has been shown to result in the best clinical outcomes for all patients in the long term. Clinically, this means optimization of afterload, preload, and wedge pressure, while maintaining end-organ perfusion. To offer the greatest probability of survival, the goal should be an adequate BP with a minimal need for vasoconstriction to maintain end organ perfusion.

Newer mineralocorticoid antagonists have enhanced theoretical benefits, given a greater ability to reduce BP and afterload. In HFrEF patients with worsening chronic HF, concomitant type 2 diabetes mellitus, and/or CKD, finerenone was associated with a significant reduction in death from any cause, cardiovascular hospitalizations, and emergency presentation for worsening HF until day 90 when compared with eplerenone in the ARTs-HF (MinerAlocorticoid Receptor antagonist Tolerability Study-Heart Failure) trial.[115] A systemic review also reported that finerenone had fewer treatment-related adverse events, including lower serum potassium levels and higher eGFR vs steroidal MRAs.[116]

The use of additional agents to treat residual hypertension and afterload remains speculative. In the setting of elevated natriuretic peptides, the current authors routinely use hydralazine and amlodipine followed by clonidine[117] for BP control, although data are lacking. Supportive data, for instance in A-HeFT, showed that, in preselected patients, hydralazine-nitrates could decrease the number of hospitalizations and reduce hospital length of stay compared with standard therapy alone.[118] Similar to patients without HF, care is required not to overtreat hypertension.[119]

Conclusion

Our understanding of the interplay between hypertension and HF is still evolving. Whereas the past decades have brought breakthroughs in HF management, there is still much to be explored when concomitant hypertension is involved. Novel insights into the modulation of immune and inflammatory processes, the gut microbiome, renal and cervical ganglion, and endothelial plasticity against known contributors to intracellular volume and vascular reactivity will undoubtedly guide further interventions to optimize clinical outcomes.

References

1. Virani SS, Alonso A, Benjamin EJ, et al. Heart disease and stroke statistics–2020 update: a report from the American Heart Association. *Circulation*. 2020;141:e139–596.
2. Forouzanfar MH, Liu P, Roth GA, et al. Global burden of hypertension and systolic blood pressure of at least 110 to 115 mm Hg, 1990–2015. *Jama*. 2017;317:165–82.
3. Levy D, Larson MG, Vasan RS, Kannel WB, Ho KK. The progression from hypertension to congestive heart failure. *Jama*. 1996;275:1557–62.
4. Upadhya B, Lovato LC, Rocco M, et al. Heart failure prevention in older patients using intensive blood pressure reduction: potential role of diuretics. *JACC Heart Fail*. 2019;7:1032–41.
5. RuDusky BM. Heart failure and comorbidities. *JACC Heart Fail*. 2015;3:1003.
6. Murad K, Goff DC, Jr., Morgan TM, et al. Burden of comorbidities and functional and cognitive impairments in elderly patients at the initial diagnosis of heart failure and their impact on total mortality: the cardiovascular health study. *JACC Heart Fail*. 2015;3:542–50.
7. Stanaway JD, Afshin A, Gakidou E, et al. Global, regional, and national comparative risk assessment of 84 behavioural, environmental and occupational, and metabolic risks or clusters of risks for 195 countries and territories, 1990–2017: a systematic analysis for the global burden of disease study 2017. *The Lancet*. 2018;392:1923–94.
8. Bello NA, Schwartz JE, Kronish IM, et al. Number of measurements needed to obtain a reliable estimate of home blood pressure: results from the improving the detection of hypertension study. *Journal of the American Heart Association*. 2018;7:e008658.
9. Blood Pressure Lowering Treatment Trialists' Collaboration. Blood pressure-lowering treatment based on cardiovascular risk: a meta-analysis of individual patient data. *Lancet*. 2014;384:591–8.
10. Bress AP, Greene T, Derington CG, et al. Patient selection for intensive blood pressure management based on benefit and adverse events. *J Am Coll Cardiol*. 2021;77:1977–90.
11. Lewington S, Clarke R, Qizilbash N, Peto R, Collins R. Age-specific relevance of usual blood pressure to vascular mortality: a meta-analysis of individual data for one million adults in 61 prospective studies. *Lancet*. 2002;360:1903–13.
12. Neaton JD, Wentworth D. Serum cholesterol, blood pressure, cigarette smoking, and death from coronary heart disease. Overall findings and differences by age for 316,099 white men. Multiple Risk Factor Intervention Trial Research Group. *Arch Intern Med*. 1992;152:56–64.
13. Williams B, Mancia G, Spiering W, et al. 2018 ESC/ESH guidelines for the management of arterial hypertension: the task force for the management of arterial hypertension of the European Society of Cardiology (ESC) and the European Society of Hypertension (ESH). *European Heart Journal*. 2018;39:3021–104.
14. Unger T, Borghi C, Charchar F, et al. International society of hypertension global hypertension practice guidelines. *Hypertension*. 2020;75:1334–57.
15. Joint Committee for Guideline Revision. 2018 Chinese guidelines for prevention and treatment of hypertension-a report of the revision committee of chinese guidelines for prevention and treatment of hypertension. *J Geriatr Cardiol*. 2019;16:182–241.
16. Umemura S, Arima H, Arima S, et al. The Japanese Society of Hypertension guidelines for the management of hypertension (JSH 2019). *Hypertens Res*. 2019;42:1235–481.
17. Whelton PK, Carey RM, Aronow WS, et al. 2017 ACC/AHA/AAPA/ABC/ACPM/AGS/APhA/ASH/ASPC/NMA/PCNA guideline for the prevention, detection, evaluation, and management of high blood pressure in adults: executive summary: a report of the American College of Cardiology/American Heart Association Task Force on clinical practice guidelines. *Hypertension*. 2018;71:1269–324.
18. Kaneko H, Yano Y, Itoh H, et al. Association of blood pressure classification using the 2017 American College of Cardiology/American Heart Association blood pressure guideline with risk of heart failure and atrial fibrillation. *Circulation*. 2021;143:2244–53.
19. Kalogeropoulos AP, Goulbourne C, Butler J. Diagnosis and prevention of hypertensive heart failure. *Heart Fail Clin*. 2019;15:435–45.
20. Stacey RB, Hundley WG. Integrating measures of myocardial fibrosis in the transition from hypertensive heart disease to heart failure. *Curr Hypertens Rep*. 2021;23:22.
21. López B, Ravassa S, González A, et al. Myocardial collagen cross-linking is associated with heart failure hospitalization in patients with hypertensive heart failure. *J Am Coll Cardiol*. 2016;67:251–60.
22. Heymans S, González A, Pizard A, et al. Searching for new mechanisms of myocardial fibrosis with diagnostic and/or therapeutic potential. *Eur J Heart Fail*. 2015;17:764–71.
23. Ferreira JP, Rossignol P, Pizard A, et al. Potential spironolactone effects on collagen metabolism biomarkers in patients with uncontrolled blood pressure. *Heart*. 2019;105:307.
24. Upadhya B, Rocco MV, Pajewski NM, et al. Effect of intensive blood pressure reduction on left ventricular mass, structure, function, and fibrosis in the SPRINT-HEART. *Hypertension*. 2019;74:276–84.
25. Haykowsky MJ, Nicklas BJ, Brubaker PH, et al. Regional adipose distribution and its relationship to exercise intolerance in older obese patients who have heart failure with preserved ejection fraction. *JACC Heart Fail* 2018;6:640–9.
26. Rodrigues JC, Amadu AM, Dastidar AG, et al. Comprehensive characterisation of hypertensive heart disease left ventricular phenotypes. *Heart*. 2016;102:1671–9.
27. Upadhya B, Pajewski NM, Rocco MV, et al. Effect of intensive blood pressure control on aortic stiffness in the SPRINT-HEART. *Hypertension*. 2021;77:1571–80.
28. Seravalle G, Lonati L, Buzzi S, et al. Sympathetic nerve traffic and baroreflex function in optimal, normal, and high-normal blood pressure states. *J Hypertens*. 2015;33:1411–7.
29. Baradaran A, Nasri H, Rafieian-Kopaei M. Oxidative stress and hypertension: possibility of hypertension therapy with antioxidants. *J Res Med Sci*. 2014;19:358–67.
30. Ikdahl E, Rollefstad S, Hisdal J, et al. Sustained improvement of arterial stiffness and blood pressure after long-term rosuvastatin treatment in patients with inflammatory joint diseases: results from the RORA-AS study. *PLoS One*. 2016;11:e0153440.
31. Feihl F, Liaudet L, Waeber B, Levy BI. Hypertension: a disease of the microcirculation? *Hypertension*. 2006;48:1012–7.
32. Cornelissen VA, Smart NA. Exercise training for blood pressure: a systematic review and meta-analysis. *J Am Heart Assoc*. 2013;2:e004473.
33. He FJ, Li J, Macgregor GA. Effect of longer term modest salt reduction on blood pressure: cochrane systematic review and meta-analysis of randomised trials. *BMJ*. 2013;346:f1325.
34. Sacks FM, Svetkey LP, Vollmer WM, et al. Effects on blood pressure of reduced dietary sodium and the dietary approaches to stop hypertension (DASH) diet. *N Engl J Med*. 2001;344:3–10.
35. Aburto NJ, Hanson S, Gutierrez H, et al. Effect of increased potassium intake on cardiovascular risk factors and disease: systematic review and meta-analyses. *BMJ*. 2013;346:f1378.
36. Roerecke M, Kaczorowski J, Tobe SW, et al. The effect of a reduction in alcohol consumption on blood pressure: a systematic review and meta-analysis. *Lancet Public Health*. 2017;2:e108–20.
37. Semlitsch T, Krenn C, Jeitler K, et al. Long-term effects of weight-reducing diets in people with hypertension. *Cochrane Database Syst Rev*. 2021;2:Cd008274.
38. Appel LJ, Moore TJ, Obarzanek E, et al. A clinical trial of the effects of dietary patterns on blood pressure. *N Engl J Med*. 1997;336:1117–24.
39. Gay HC, Rao SG, Vaccarino V, Ali MK. Effects of different dietary interventions on blood pressure: systematic review and meta-analysis of randomized controlled trials. *Hypertension*. 2016;67:733–9.
40. Cicero AFG, Grassi D, Tocci G, et al. Nutrients and nutraceuticals for the management of high normal blood pressure: an evidence-based consensus document. *High Blood Press Cardiovasc Prev*. 2019;26:9–25.
41. Matthews KA, Katholi CR, McCreath H, et al. Blood pressure reactivity to psychological stress predicts hypertension in the CARDIA study. *Circulation*. 2004;110:74–8.
42. Iftikhar IH, Valentine CW, Bittencourt LR, et al. Effects of continuous positive airway pressure on blood pressure in patients with resistant hypertension and obstructive sleep apnea: a meta-analysis. *J Hypertens*. 2014;32:2341–50; discussion 2350.
43. McEvoy RD, Antic NA, Heeley E, et al. CPAP for prevention of cardiovascular events in obstructive sleep apnea. *N Engl J Med*. 2016;375:919–931.

44. Oparil S, Acelajado MC, Bakris GL, et al. Hypertension. *Nat Rev Dis Primers*. 2018;4:18014.
45. Wilck N, Matus MG, Kearney SM, et al. Salt-responsive gut commensal modulates T(H)17 axis and disease. *Nature*. 2017;551:585–9.
46. Turnbull F. Effects of different blood-pressure-lowering regimens on major cardiovascular events: results of prospectively-designed overviews of randomised trials. *Lancet*. 2003;362:1527–35.
47. ALLHAT Officers and Coordinators for the ALLHAT Collaborative Research Group. Major outcomes in high-risk hypertensive patients randomized to angiotensin-converting enzyme inhibitor or calcium channel blocker vs diuretic: the antihypertensive and lipid-lowering treatment to prevent heart attack trial (ALLHAT). *Jama*. 2002;288:2981–97.
48. Ferreira JP, Gregson J, Böhm M, et al. Blood pressure reduction and antihypertensive treatment choice: a post-hoc analysis of the SPRINT trial. *Clinical Cardiology*. 2021;44:665–674.
49. Julius S, Kjeldsen SE, Weber M, et al. Outcomes in hypertensive patients at high cardiovascular risk treated with regimens based on valsartan or amlodipine: the VALUE randomised trial. *Lancet*. 2004;363:2022–31.
50. Lonn EM, Bosch J, López-Jaramillo P, et al. Blood-pressure lowering in intermediate-risk persons without cardiovascular disease. *N Engl J Med*. 2016;374:2009–20.
51. Suchard MA, Schuemie MJ, Krumholz HM, et al. Comprehensive comparative effectiveness and safety of first-line antihypertensive drug classes: a systematic, multinational, large-scale analysis. *Lancet*. 2019;394:1816–26.
52. Kjeldsen SE, Narkiewicz K, Burnier M, Oparil S. The International Society of Hypertension Guidelines 2020 - a new drug treatment recommendation in the wrong direction? *Blood Press*. 2020;29:264–6.
53. Kjeldsen SE, Narkiewicz K, Burnier M, Oparil S. Was it optimal to drop a diuretic as a first-line choice of drug treatment in the 2020 International Society of Hypertension Guidelines? *Blood Press*. 2020;29:341–3.
54. Williams B, MacDonald TM, Morant S, et al. Spironolactone versus placebo, bisoprolol, and doxazosin to determine the optimal treatment for drug-resistant hypertension (PATHWAY-2): a randomised, double-blind, crossover trial. *Lancet*. 2015;386:2059–68.
55. Tam TS, Wu MH, Masson SC, et al. Eplerenone for hypertension. *Cochrane Database Syst Rev*. 2017;2:Cd008996.
56. White WB, Duprez D, St Hillaire R, et al. Effects of the selective aldosterone blocker eplerenone versus the calcium antagonist amlodipine in systolic hypertension. *Hypertension*. 2003;41:1021–6.
57. Cai A, Siddiqui M, Judd EK, Oparil S, Calhoun DA. Aortic blood pressure and arterial stiffness in patients with controlled resistant and non-resistant hypertension. *J Clin Hypertens (Greenwich)*. 2020;22:167–73.
58. Kjeldsen SE, Narkiewicz K, Burnier M, Oparil S. Practice guidelines for the management of arterial hypertension of the European Society of Hypertension. *Blood Press*. 2018;27:313.
59. Velasco A, Siddiqui M, Kreps E, et al. Refractory hypertension is not attributable to intravascular fluid retention as determined by intracardiac volumes. *Hypertension*. 2018;72:343–9.
60. Augustyniak RA, Tuncel M, Zhang W, Toto RD, Victor RG. Sympathetic overactivity as a cause of hypertension in chronic renal failure. *J Hypertens*. 2002;20:3–9.
61. Grassi G, Mark A, Esler M. The sympathetic nervous system alterations in human hypertension. *Circ Res*. 2015;116:976–90.
62. Archer SL, Huang JM, Hampl V, et al. Nitric oxide and cGMP cause vasorelaxation by activation of a charybdotoxin-sensitive K channel by cGMP-dependent protein kinase. *Proc Natl Acad Sci U S A*. 1994;91:7583–7.
63. Schulz V. Clinical pharmacokinetics of nitroprusside, cyanide, thiosulphate and thiocyanate. *Clin Pharmacokinet*. 1984;9:239–51.
64. Finger JR, Kurczewski LM, Brophy GM. Clevidipine versus nicardipine for acute blood pressure reduction in a neuroscience intensive care population. *Neurocrit Care*. 2017;26:167–73.
65. Lambert CR, Hill JA, Nichols WW, Feldman RL, Pepine CJ. Coronary and systemic hemodynamic effects of nicardipine. *Am J Cardiol*. 1985;55:652–6.
66. Peacock WF, Chandra A, Char D, et al. Clevidipine in acute heart failure: results of the a study of blood pressure control in acute heart failure-a pilot study (PRONTO). *Am Heart J*. 2014;167:529–36.
67. Ayaz SI, Sharkey CM, Kwiatkowski GM, et al. Intravenous enalaprilat for treatment of acute hypertensive heart failure in the emergency department. *International Journal of Emergency Medicine*. 2016;9:28.
68. Baum T, Sybertz EJ. Pharmacology of labetalol in experimental animals. *Am J Med*. 1983;75:15–23.
69. O'Malley K, Segal JL, Israili ZH, et al. Duration of hydralazine action in hypertension. *Clin Pharmacol Ther*. 1975;18:581–6.
70. Ludden TM, Shepherd AM, McNay JL, Lin MS. Hydralazine kinetics in hypertensive patients after intravenous administration. *Clin Pharmacol Ther*. 1980;28:736–42.
71. Yancy CW, Jessup M, Bozkurt B, et al. 2017 ACC/AHA/HFSA focused update of the 2013 ACCF/AHA guideline for the management of heart failure: a report of the American College of Cardiology/American Heart Association Task Force on Clinical Practice Guidelines and the Heart Failure Society of America. *Circulation*. 2017;136:e137–61.
72. McCurley A, Jaffe IZ. Mineralocorticoid receptors in vascular function and disease. *Molecular and Cellular Endocrinology*. 2012;350: 256–65.
73. Pitt B, Pfeffer MA, Assmann SF, et al. Spironolactone for heart failure with preserved ejection fraction. *New Engl J Med*. 2014;370:1383–92.
74. Pfeffer MA, Claggett B, Assmann SF, et al. Regional variation in patients and outcomes in the treatment of preserved cardiac function heart failure with an aldosterone antagonist (TOPCAT) trial. *Circulation*. 2015;131:34–42.
75. Pitt B, Kober L, Ponikowski P, et al. Safety and tolerability of the novel non-steroidal mineralocorticoid receptor antagonist BAY 94–8862 in patients with chronic heart failure and mild or moderate chronic kidney disease: a randomized, double-blind trial. *Eur Heart J*. 2013;34: 2453–63.
76. A multicenter, randomized, double-blind, parallel-group, placebo-controlled study to evaluate the efficacy and safety of finerenone on morbidity and mortality in participants with heart failure (NYHA II-IV) and left ventricular ejection fraction ≥ 40% (LVEF ≥ 40%).
77. Yusuf S, Pfeffer MA, Swedberg K, et al. Effects of candesartan in patients with chronic heart failure and preserved left-ventricular ejection fraction: the CHARM-preserved trial. *Lancet*. 2003;362:777–81.
78. Massie BM, Carson PE, McMurray JJ, et al. Irbesartan in patients with heart failure and preserved ejection fraction. *N Engl J Med*. 2008;359:2456–67.
79. Cleland JG, Tendera M, Adamus J, et al. The perindopril in elderly people with chronic heart failure (PEP-CHF) study. *Eur Heart J*. 2006;27:2338–45.
80. Solomon SD, McMurray JJV, Anand IS, et al. Angiotensin–Neprilysin inhibition in heart failure with preserved ejection fraction. *New Engl J Med*. 2019;381:1609–20.
81. Solomon SD, Zile M, Pieske B, et al. The angiotensin receptor neprilysin inhibitor LCZ696 in heart failure with preserved ejection fraction: a phase 2 double-blind randomised controlled trial. *Lancet*. 2012;380:1387–95.
82. Adamson PB, Abraham WT, Bourge RC, et al. Wireless pulmonary artery pressure monitoring guides management to reduce decompensation in heart failure with preserved ejection fraction. *Circ Heart Fail*. 2014;7:935–44.
83. Redfield MM, Anstrom KJ, Levine JA, et al. Isosorbide mononitrate in heart failure with preserved ejection fraction. *New Engl J Med*. 2015;373:2314–24.
84. Chi G, Jamil A, Jamil U, et al. Effect of intensive versus standard blood pressure control on major adverse cardiac events and serious adverse events: a bivariate analysis of randomized controlled trials. *Clin Exp Hypertens*. 2018;10:1–8.
85. Böhm M, Schumacher H, Teo KK, et al. Achieved blood pressure and cardiovascular outcomes in high-risk patients: results from ONTARGET and TRANSCEND trials. *Lancet*. 2017;389:2226–37.
86. SPRINT Research Group, Wright JT Jr, Williamson JD, Whelton PK, et al. A randomized trial of intensive versus standard blood-pressure control. *New Engl J Med*. 2015;373:2103–2116.
87. Kalantar-Zadeh K, Block G, Horwich T, Fonarow GC. Reverse epidemiology of conventional cardiovascular risk factors in patients with chronic heart failure. *J Am Coll Cardiol*. 2004;43:1439–44.
88. McMurray JJV, Packer M, Desai AS, et al. Angiotensin–Neprilysin inhibition versus enalapril in heart failure. *New Engl J Med*. 2014;371:993–1004.
89. Lip GY, Skjøth F, Overvad K, Rasmussen LH, Larsen TB. Blood pressure and prognosis in patients with incident heart failure: the Diet, Cancer and Health (DCH) cohort study. *Clin Res Cardiol*. 2015;104:1088–96.
90. Schmid FA, Schlager O, Keller P, et al. Prognostic value of long-term blood pressure changes in patients with chronic heart failure. *Eur J Heart Fail*. 2017;19:837–842.
91. Arundel C, Lam PH, Gill GS, et al. Systolic blood pressure and outcomes in patients with heart failure with reduced ejection fraction. *J Am Coll Cardiol*. 2019;73:3054–63.
92. Eichhorn EJ, Bristow MR. The carvedilol prospective randomized cumulative survival (COPERNICUS) trial. *Curr Contr Trials Cardiovasc Med*. 2001;2:20–23.
93. Poole-Wilson PA, Swedberg K, Cleland JG, et al. Comparison of carvedilol and metoprolol on clinical outcomes in patients with chronic heart failure in the Carvedilol Or Metoprolol European Trial (COMET): randomised controlled trial. *Lancet*. 2003;362:7–13.
94. MERIT-HF Study Group. Effect of metoprolol CR/XL in chronic heart failure: metoprolol CR/XL Randomised Intervention Trial in Congestive Heart Failure (MERIT-HF). *Lancet*. 1999;353:2001–7.
95. CIBIS-II Investigators and Committees. The Cardiac Insufficiency Bisoprolol Study II (CIBIS-II): a randomised trial. *Lancet*. 1999;353:9–13.
96. SOLVD Investigators, Yusuf S, Pitt B, et al. Effect of enalapril on survival in patients with reduced left ventricular ejection fractions and congestive heart failure. *N Engl J Med*. 1991;325:293–302.
97. Cohn JN, Tognoni G, Valsartan heart failure trial I. A randomized trial of the angiotensin-receptor blocker valsartan in chronic heart failure. *N Engl J Med*. 2001;345:1667–75.

98. McMurray JJ, Ostergren J, Swedberg K, et al. Effects of candesartan in patients with chronic heart failure and reduced left-ventricular systolic function taking angiotensin-converting-enzyme inhibitors: the CHARM-Added trial. *Lancet*. 2003;362:767–71.
99. Zannad F, McMurray JJ, Krum H, et al. Eplerenone in patients with systolic heart failure and mild symptoms. *N Engl J Med*. 2011;364:11–21.
100. Pitt B, Zannad F, Remme WJ, et al. The effect of spironolactone on morbidity and mortality in patients with severe heart failure. Randomized Aldactone Evaluation Study Investigators. *N Engl J Med*. 1999;341:709–17.
101. McMurray JJ, Packer M, Desai AS, et al. Angiotensin-neprilysin inhibition versus enalapril in heart failure. *N Engl J Med*. 2014;371: 993–1004.
102. Taylor AL, Ziesche S, Yancy C, et al. Combination of isosorbide dinitrate and hydralazine in blacks with heart failure. *N Engl J Med*. 2004;351:2049–57.
103. Flather MD, Shibata MC, Coats AJ, et al. Randomized trial to determine the effect of nebivolol on mortality and cardiovascular hospital admission in elderly patients with heart failure (SENIORS). *Eur Heart J*. 2005;26:215–25.
104. Taylor AL, Ziesche S, Yancy C, et al. Combination of isosorbide dinitrate and hydralazine in blacks with heart failure. *New Engl J Med*. 2004;351:2049–57.
105. Cohn JN, Tam SW, Anand IS, et al. Isosorbide dinitrate and hydralazine in a fixed-dose combination produces further regression of left ventricular remodeling in a well-treated black population with heart failure: results from A-HeFT. *J Card Fail*. 2007;13:331–9.
106. Cohn JN, Archibald DG, Ziesche S, et al. Effect of vasodilator therapy on mortality in chronic congestive heart failure. Results of a Veterans Administration Cooperative Study. *N Engl J Med*. 1986;314:1547–52.
107. Cohn JN, Johnson G, Ziesche S, et al. A comparison of enalapril with hydralazine–isosorbide dinitrate in the treatment of chronic congestive heart failure. *N Engl J Med*. 1991;325:303–10.
108. Carson P, Ziesche S, Johnson G, Cohn JN. Racial differences in response to therapy for heart failure: analysis of the vasodilator-heart failure trials. Vasodilator-Heart Failure Trial Study Group. *J Card Fail*. 1999;5:178–87.
109. de Vries RJ, van Veldhuisen DJ, Dunselman PH. Efficacy and safety of calcium channel blockers in heart failure: focus on recent trials with second-generation dihydropyridines. *Am Heart J*. 2000;139:185–94.
110. Packer M, O'Connor CM, Ghali JK, et al. Effect of amlodipine on morbidity and mortality in severe chronic heart failure. Prospective Randomized Amlodipine Survival Evaluation Study Group. *N Engl J Med*. 1996;335:1107–14.
111. Remme WJ, McMurray JJV, Hobbs FDR, et al. Awareness and perception of heart failure among European cardiologists, internists, geriatricians, and primary care physicians. *Eur Heart J*. 2008;29:1739–52.
112. Montero-Perez-Barquero M, Flather M, Roughton M, et al. Influence of systolic blood pressure on clinical outcomes in elderly heart failure patients treated with nebivolol: data from the SENIORS trial. *Eur J Heart Fail*. 2014;16:1009–1015.
113. Gheorghiade M, Abraham WT, Albert NM, et al. Systolic blood pressure at admission, clinical characteristics, and outcomes in patients hospitalized with acute heart failure. *JAMA*. 2006;296:2217–26.
114. Lee SE, Lee HY, Cho HJ, et al. Reverse J-curve relationship between on-treatment blood pressure and mortality in patients with heart failure. *JACC Heart Fail*. 2017;5:810–9.
115. Filippatos G, Anker SD, Böhm M, et al. A randomized controlled study of finerenone vs. eplerenone in patients with worsening chronic heart failure and diabetes mellitus and/or chronic kidney disease. *Eur Heart J*. 2016;37:2105–14.
116. Pei H, Wang W, Zhao D, et al. The use of a novel non-steroidal mineralocorticoid receptor antagonist finerenone for the treatment of chronic heart failure: a systematic review and meta-analysis. *Medicine (Baltimore)*. 2018;97:e0254.
117. Azevedo ER, Newton GE, Parker JD. Cardiac and systemic sympathetic activity in response to clonidine in human heart failure. *J Am Coll Cardiol*. 1999;33:186–91.
118. Angus DC, Linde-Zwirble WT, Tam SW, et al. Cost-effectiveness of fixed-dose combination of isosorbide dinitrate and hydralazine therapy for blacks with heart failure. *Circulation*. 2005;112:3745–53.
119. Böhm M, Ferreira JP, Mahfoud F, et al. Myocardial reperfusion reverses the J-curve association of cardiovascular risk and diastolic blood pressure in patients with left ventricular dysfunction and heart failure after myocardial infarction: insights from the EPHESUS trial. *Eur Heart J*. 2020;41:1673–83.

Chapter 20
MANAGEMENT OF ATRIAL FIBRILLATION IN PATIENTS WITH HEART FAILURE

Panagiotis Korantzopoulos and Aris Bechlioulis

Epidemiology of Atrial Fibrillation in Heart Failure

Atrial fibrillation (AF) is the most common arrhythmia, affecting one in four middle-aged adults in the Western world (Figure 20.1),[1] with a greater prevalence in the elderly, especially in the presence of conditions such as hypertension, obesity, diabetes, coronary artery disease, valvular heart disease, and heart failure (HF).[1,2] AF has been associated with a one-and-a-half- to two-fold greater mortality, mainly attributed to death due to stroke, but also to HF and sudden death.[1,3,4] AF is also associated with increased morbidity, including HF-related events.[5] Left ventricular (LV) dysfunction is found in nearly 20–30% of patients with AF, with the majority of patients with HF and AF having preserved LV function.[1,6,7]

In many patients, HF and AF coexist, implying the presence of common risk factors and common pathophysiological pathways.[1,8,9] HF has been shown to occur in 33%, 44%, and 54% of patients with paroxysmal, persistent, and permanent AF, respectively,[10] indicating a high risk of HF in patients with AF.[11] The increased HF risk associated with AF tends to be higher for HF with preserved (HFpEF) vs reduced (HFrEF) ejection fraction.[12] On the other hand, the prevalence of AF is high in HF patients and further increases with HF progression and functional status impairment. For example, AF occurs in 5% of patients with New York Heart Association (NYHA) class I symptoms but reaches>50% in NYHA class IV patients.[13] Indeed, AF is the most common arrhythmia in patients with HF and is related to an increased thromboembolic risk, impaired cardiac function, and worse symptoms.[14]

Even though the development of HF as a result of persistent, usually rapid AF may be associated with a benign prognosis (tachycardia-induced cardiomyopathy),[15,16] the diagnosis of new-onset AF in chronic HF patients is associated with a worse prognosis. AF may be a marker of more advanced HF but may also cause direct impairment of cardiac function.[1,14,17,18] In fact, the coexistence of AF and HF is associated with increased mortality compared to either entity alone.[19] In asymptomatic HF (stage B) with LV systolic dysfunction, newly diagnosed AF or prevalent AF (especially paroxysmal AF) has also been associated with increased morbidity and mortality.[20] Moreover, implantable cardioverter defibrillator (ICD) recipients with HFrEF and prevalent AF exhibit increased mortality and higher rates of appropriate and inappropriate ICD therapies compared with their non-AF counterparts.[21] In patients with HFpEF, AF is associated with worse exercise capacity, impaired contractile reserve, and increased mortality.[22, 23] Whether this association is causal or AF is a bystander to abnormal diastolic function requires further investigation.[22] In a recent meta-analysis, AF was associated with a higher mortality in HFrEF compared with HFpEF patients, with similar risk of thromboembolic stroke and hospitalizations for HF.[18] On the other hand, in a large registry, AF was independently associated with increased risk of adverse outcomes only in HF with preserved and mid-range ejection fraction but not in HFrEF patients.[24] It has been suggested that AF may affect prognosis differently according to HF phenotype; AF may be an independent predictor of mortality in HFpEF and not in HFrEF, where it is considered a marker of more advanced disease.[25–27] The striking similarity of risk factors between HFpEF and AF, e.g., age and other age-related comorbidities (i.e., hypertension, obesity, and sleep apnea) suggests an important role for AF in the pathophysiology of HFpEF.[28]

Brief Pathophysiology

The pathophysiology of AF in the setting of HF is complex, as HF has several different etiologies and substrates and various associated abnormalities and comorbidities. In addition, HF and AF share many risk factors. In addition to local triggers, atrial electrophysiological and structural abnormalities that constitute atrial remodeling seem to play an important role in AF development and persistence.[29,30] The molecular pathways implicated in the initiation and perpetuation of AF show a high diversity and variability across different substrates.[29,30] In the setting of HF, increased intracardiac filling pressures, the activation of the renin-angiotensin-aldosterone system, the activation of the sympathetic nervous system, and the associated inflammation and oxidative stress observed in HF promote arrhythmogenesis as well as atrial structural and electrical remodeling (Figure 20.2).[29–34] Structural atrial remodeling mainly consists of atrial fibrosis and myocyte apoptosis that affect cardiac conduction and create the substrate for micro-reentry. Electrical remodeling consists of shortening of the effective refractory period (ERP), loss of rate adaptation, and prolongation of atrial conduction.[29,30] Collectively, these changes shorten the wavelength (ERP × conduction velocity) and promote the development of multiple atrial wavelets (reentrant circuits).

Heart rate irregularity has been associated with abnormalities in calcium handling,[30,35] whereas atrial tachycardia per se promotes calcium overload. On the other hand, HF is associated with diastolic calcium leak that provokes delayed afterdepolarizations and electrical remodeling.[35] These abnormalities favor both the development of AF by calcium-mediated triggered activity (ectopic firing mostly from pulmonary veins) as well as the maintenance and perpetuation of AF, mainly by downregulation of the L-type calcium channel and other ionic channel alterations that provoke shortening of the atrial ERP.[35]

Furthermore, the development of AF adversely affects cardiac hemodynamics due to loss of atrial mechanical systole, which contributes 15–20% of cardiac output as well as that due to irregular ventricular contraction and atrioventricular (AV) dyssynchrony. Because of these abnormalities, along with sympathetic system activation, AF may cause arrhythmia-induced cardiomyopathy even with adequate rate control.[36,37] Rapid rates reduce diastolic LV filling time and impair coronary perfusion, leading to a further impairment of LV function.[36,37] AF per se aggravates electrophysiological and structural remodeling ("AF begets AF") leading to a vicious circle.[29, 30] Interestingly, in some instances, the cause-effect relationship

DOI: 10.1201/9780429244544-24

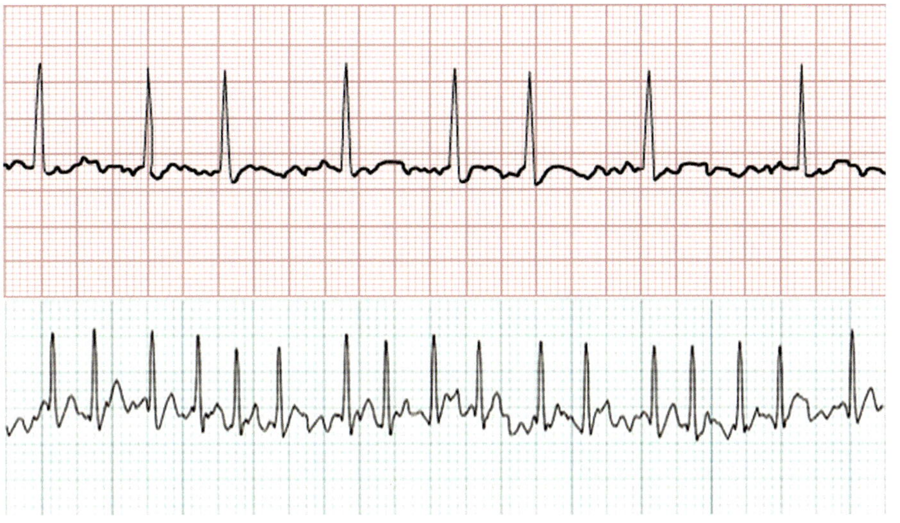

FIGURE 20.1 Atrial fibrillation on electrocardiogram.

between HF and AF is not clear.[38] The absence of an obvious cause of HF along with a poorly controlled AF points to arrhythmia-induced cardiomyopathy. However, this working diagnosis can be confirmed only by the marked improvement of LV function after aggressive rate and rhythm control of AF.

As discussed, HFpEF and AF share several risk factors, e.g., hypertension, diabetes, obesity, metabolic syndrome, obstructive sleep apnea, and coronary artery disease.[32,39] The ventricular stiffness and diastolic dysfunction observed in HFpEF result in increased atrial stretch and remodeling that is similar to HFrEF.[32] Most aforementioned pathophysiological processes, including neurohormonal activation, atrial fibrosis, inflammation, oxidative stress, abnormal calcium handling, electrophysiological remodeling, and autonomic imbalance, are also implicated in HFpEF.

Management of HF in Patients with Atrial Fibrillation

In patients who have both AF and HF, the main goals of treatment are to prevent adverse outcomes, improve symptoms, and maintain a good quality of life. In those presenting acutely with AF and HF, the guidelines recommend focusing on euvolemia, acute rate control aiming for an initial heart rate target of <110 bpm, use of anticoagulants, inhibition of the renin–angiotensin–aldosterone system, and early consideration of rhythm control.[14]

Heart Failure Medications

The current HF guidelines do not suggest major deviations from pharmacological therapy standards for the treatment of HFrEF in the presence of concomitant AF. However, in pivotal HF trials, patients with AF were typically older with more comorbidities and longer duration of HF symptoms, all of which may reduce the beneficial effects of HF medications. Analyses of large-scale, randomized trials demonstrated that beta-blockers, angiotensin-converting enzyme inhibitors, angiotensin II receptor blockers, and eplerenone all reduce AF incidence in patients with HFrEF, whereas ivabradine may increase AF incidence.[40–45]

Current recommendations support the use of beta-blockers in all patients with HFrEF, regardless of AF. Beta-blockers have been associated with significantly lower mortality but have no effect on hospitalizations in patients with HFrEF and AF, irrespective of the pattern or burden of AF.[14,46] In a recent meta-analysis of observational and randomized trials, beta-blockers were associated with a 22% decrease in mortality in patients with AF and HFrEF without a benefit in HF hospitalizations.[47] Interestingly, other meta-analyses of randomized trials revealed no mortality benefit with beta-blockers in patients with HFrEF and AF (regardless of baseline heart rate and treatment-achieved heart rate), in contrast to those in sinus rhythm.[48,49] Differences among studies in terms of methodology and patient characteristics may account for these discrepant findings. Additionally, it is not known whether the dose and titration schemes used in patients with HFrEF and sinus rhythm are equally effective in their counterparts with HFrEF and AF. The AF target heart rate for HFrEF patients with AF may be different; in a previous study, strict heart rate control (<80 bpm at rest) was not associated with a worse outcome compared with lenient heart rate control (<110 bpm at rest).[50] Current HF guidelines recommend a target resting heart rate of 60–100 bpm in HFrEF patients and AF using beta-blockers as a first-line treatment followed by digoxin for a better rate control.[14]

Digoxin is indicated in patients with HF and AF when heart rate is inadequately controlled with beta-blockers, and in symptomatic HFrEF unresponsive to first- and second-line treatments to reduce HF rehospitalizations, irrespective of AF.[14] In a single, randomized trial (DIG) and other observational studies in HFrEF, the use of digoxin was related to fewer HF rehospitalizations without any effect on mortality,[51,52] whereas a beneficial effect on mortality was suggested in patients with low plasma levels of digoxin.[51,53] However, several retrospective analyses on the use of digoxin in patients with AF and/or HF (including mostly observational studies), have shown that digoxin use is associated with increased mortality.[54–56] However, digoxin is more likely to be prescribed in patients with AF and HF who have more advanced disease; have greater difficulty in controlling ventricular rate in persistent/permanent states rather than in paroxysmal AF; and are intolerant to beta-blockers or unsuitable for other modalities, e.g., cardiac resynchronization therapy (CRT). In these patients, mortality risk is likely to be higher, independent of digoxin use.[57]

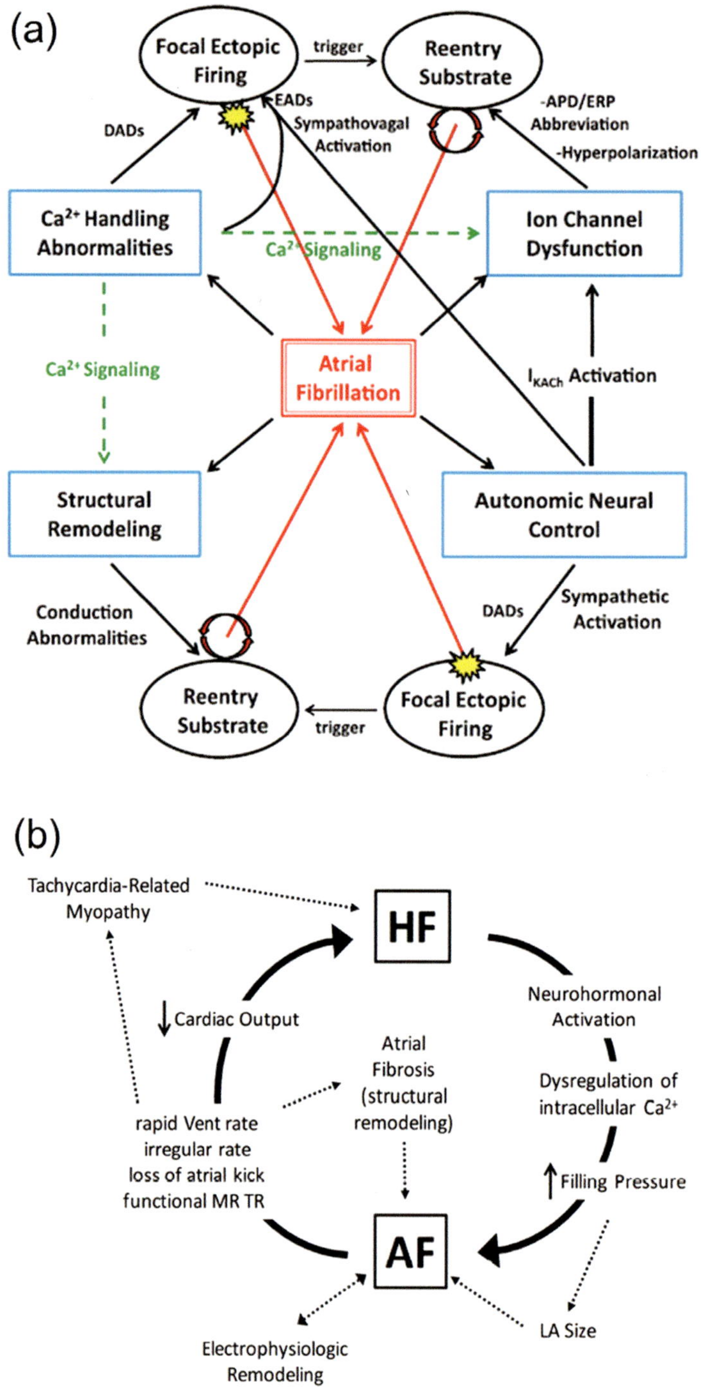

FIGURE 20.2 Various mechanisms underlying the pathophysiology of atrial fibrillation (a) (adapted from Andrade J, et al. The clinical profile and pathophysiology of atrial fibrillation: relationships among clinical features, epidemiology, and mechanisms. *Circ Res.* 2014 Apr 25;114(9):1453–68) and the interrelation between atrial fibrillation and heart failure syndrome (b) (adapted from Skanes AC, Tang ASL. Atrial fibrillation and heart failure: Untangling a modern Gordian knot. *Can J Cardiol.* 2018 Nov;34(11):1437–48). *Abbreviations*: APD, action potential duration; DAD, delayed afterdepolarization; EAD, early afterdepolarization; ERP, effective refractory period; HF, heart failure; AF, atrial fibrillation; LA, left atrium.

Cardioversion of Atrial Fibrillation in Heart Failure Patients

Cardioversion is indicated in patients with HF and AF, either urgently in the case of the presence of hemodynamic instability, or electively in the case of the presence of persistent symptoms attributed to AF.[1,14] Over half of inpatients undergoing cardioversion for AF have HF.[58] Unfortunately, recurrence of AF after successful cardioversion is a frequent problem (~50% at six months), particularly in patients with HF.[59,60]

Synchronized direct-current electrical cardioversion can be used to convert AF to sinus rhythm and can be performed safely in sedated patients usually with intravenous midazolam and/or propofol with continuous monitoring of blood pressure and oximetry during the procedure. The use of biphasic defibrillators and anterior–posterior electrode positions (especially in patients with implantable rhythm devices) is associated with a greater efficacy in sinus rhythm restoration.[1] When anti-arrhythmic drug therapy is planned to maintain sinus rhythm following cardioversion, it seems prudent to start pharmacological therapy (usually amiodarone) a few weeks before cardioversion in order to increase the efficacy of the cardioversion.[1]

Antiarrhythmic drugs can achieve restoration of sinus rhythm in patients with AF (pharmacological cardioversion) without the need for sedation or fasting state, but are usually associated with longer hospitalization times. In patients with AF and HF, the use of class I antiarrhythmic agents and dronedarone is contraindicated. Vernakalant can be used in patients with mild HF (NYHA class I or II, moderate HFrEF or HFmrEF/HFpEF, or abnormal left ventricular hypertrophy), including those with ischemic heart disease, provided they do not present with hypotension or severe aortic stenosis. Dofetilide is a class III medication that may be used for AF cardioversion in HF patients but requires prolonged in-hospital stay and is currently not approved in Europe.[61] Amiodarone is currently the drug of choice for pharmacological cardioversion in patients with AF and HF.[1]

Cardioversion has been associated with an increased risk of embolic stroke in patients not on anticoagulation therapy. All patients planned for immediate cardioversion should receive immediate anticoagulation. Patients who have been in AF for longer than 48 h should start anticoagulation therapy for at least three weeks before cardioversion, whereas, in the case of an urgent cardioversion in a patient with AF lasting >48 hours, a transesophageal echocardiogram is recommended to reduce the possibility of left atrial thrombi before cardioversion.[1]

Cardiac Resynchronization Therapy (CRT)

CRT has been consistently demonstrated to improve prognosis in selected patients with HF and sinus rhythm,[14] but its benefit seems to be attenuated in patients with AF.[14,62,63] Frequent AF episodes may lead to HF progression in CRT recipients and responders due to loss of biventricular pacing.[64] AV nodal ablation may be the most effective adjunctive treatment in these cases. On the other hand, modern CRT algorithms in patients in sinus rhythm may reduce AF burden, especially in CRT responders.[65,66]

Thromboprophylaxis

The thromboembolic risk in patients with AF and HF is higher than in patients without HF, irrespective of reduced or preserved ejection fraction.[67,68] Anticoagulation in patients with HF and AF is mandatory, with the goal to reduce strokes and other thromboembolic events. The relative efficacy and safety of direct oral anticoagulants (DOACs) compared with warfarin in the setting of AF and HF has been clearly demonstrated in subgroups of large, randomized trials of dabigatran, rivaroxaban, and apixaban in AF (30–60% of participants had HF) (Table 20.1).[69,70] No significant difference in the effect of DOACs vs warfarin on strokes and hemorrhagic complications was observed for patients with HF vs without HF.[71] The type of HF (HFrEF or HFpEF) does not affect choice of anticoagulant. However, anticoagulation for AF in patients with HF should be individualized and choice of oral anticoagulant

TABLE 20.1: Characteristics of the Direct Oral Anticoagulants

	Dabigatran Exetilate	Rivaroxaban	Apixaban	Edoxaban
Mode of action	Oral direct thrombin inhibitor	Oral direct factor Xa inhibitor	Oral direct factor Xa inhibitor	Oral direct factor Xa inhibitor
Clinical study (year)	RE-LY (2009)	ROCKET-AF (2011)	ARISTOTLE (2011)	ENGAGE AF-TIMI 48 (2013)
Follow-up, years	2	1.9	1.8	2.8
$CHADS_2$	2.1	3.5	2.1	2.8
Age, years	71.5	73	70	72
Males, %	63.6	61.3	64.5	62.7
Heart failure, %	32	62.5	44	57.5
Bioavailability	3–7%	60–80%	50%	60%
Time to peak, h	1.5–3	2–4	3	1–2
Half-life, h	12–17	7–13	12	10–14
Prodrug	Yes	No	No	No
Renal clearance, %	80	35	25	50
Requires CYP450	No	Yes	Yes	Minimal
Plasma protein binding, %	35	95	87	55
Dose	150 mg bid 110 mg bid if >75–80 years, verapamil, or increased bleeding risk	20 mg od 15 mg od if CrCl <50 mL/min	5 mg bid 2.5 mg bid if ≥2 of the following: age ≥80 years, body weight ≤60 kg or serum creatinine ≥1.5 mg/dL	60 mg od 30 mg od if CrCl <50 mL/min or body weight ≤60 kg or verapamil or quinidine
Special considerations	Avoid if CrCl <30 mL/min; pH-dependent intestinal absorption which is reduced by proton pump inhibitors	Avoid if CrCl <15 mL/min; should be taken after food for optimum effect	Avoid if CrCl <15 mL/min	Avoid if CrCl <15 mL/min or >95 mL/min
Coagulation assay	TT, ECT	Anti-Xa activity*	Anti-Xa activity*	Anti-Xa activity*
Reversal agent	Idarucizumab	4F-PCC	4F-PCC	4F-PCC

* Anti-factor Xa activity assay calibrated to specific anticoagulant agent.

Abbreviations: CHADS, Congestive heart failure-Hypertension-Age-Diabetes-Stroke; CYP, cytochrome P; CrCl, creatinine clearance; TT, thrombin time; ECT, ecarin clotting time; 4F-PCC, 4 factor prothrombin complex concentrate.

should consider multiple comorbidities and polypharmacy, both prevalent in HF populations. For example, chronic renal failure is quite common in patients with HF and must be considered when choosing anticoagulation therapy (warfarin or DOACs) and for appropriate dosing.[72] Warfarin may be suboptimal in cases of advanced HF with frequent hospitalizations, and therefore novel anticoagulants would seem more suitable in these situations.[73]

Management of Atrial Fibrillation: Rhythm or Rate Control

Pharmacological Therapy

Pharmacological therapy of AF aims at rate and/or rhythm control, with the goal of hemodynamic and clinical improvement. Rate control is particularly important in cases of fast ventricular response. Adequate ventricular rate control increases diastolic LV filling and reduces risk of further deterioration due to arrhythmia-induced cardiomyopathy. However, the latter risk is not completely abolished, as the irregularity of the underlying rhythm may still have a significant impact on LV function. On the other hand, effective long-term rhythm control is not feasible in most cases. Pharmacologic therapies, such as antiarrhythmic drugs, have limited efficacy in the maintenance of sinus rhythm in HF. Moreover, the safety profile and the side effects of antiarrhythmic agents, especially in frail HF patients who have several comorbidities, limit their widespread use. Apart from ion channel blocking drugs, agents with favorable hemodynamic, antifibrotic, or other pleiotropic effects may have a role in a rhythm control strategy. Optimal medical therapy of HF per se may be quite effective in reducing AF burden, especially agents that inhibit the renin-angiotensin-aldosterone system, which have been shown to reduce the incidence of AF in HFrEF when administered in optimal doses,[74] although no such benefit was shown in HFpEF patients.[74] Furthermore, aldosterone receptor antagonists may be effective in AF prevention, especially in the HFrEF setting.[75]

The choice between rhythm and rate control strategies in AF has been the subject of several trials. Early consideration of rhythm control in the setting of HF may have significant impact on long-term outcomes, and on AF perpetuation and persistence, as suggested by the current guidelines.[1] In the AFFIRM trial, in patients with persistent AF, rate control was not inferior to rhythm control (with anti-arrhythmic drugs) in terms of reducing morbidity and mortality.[76] HF progression as assessed by deterioration in NYHA functional class is more pronounced with a rate control strategy in AF patients with HFrEF, but is comparable to rhythm control in AF patients with HFpEF. Hence, rhythm control, with the goal of reducing HF progression, may be desirable in patients with HFrEF and AF.[77] In two large-scale trials in patients with AF and HFrEF (AF-CHF and DIAMOND, respectively), rhythm control using amiodarone or dofetilide did not result in reductions in mortality or morbidity compared with rate control.[61, 78] However, the percentage of patients that achieved rhythm control with drugs in these trials was extremely low, whereas, in the subgroup of patients that actually achieved and maintained optimal rhythm control, an improvement in survival was shown.[61] Moreover, antiarrhythmic drugs carry a high risk of adverse effects, including pro-arrhythmia and negative inotropic effects, that potentially worsen HF status. In fact, only amiodarone is recommended in this setting but its frequent extra-cardiac adverse effects limit its use.[1,14] Amiodarone reduces the incidence of AF, facilitates cardioversion, reduces AF recurrence, and helps control symptoms in patients with paroxysmal AF if beta-blockers fail (Figure 20.3).[14] On the other hand, dronedarone (a drug with electrophysiological properties that are similar to those of amiodarone) is contraindicated in patients with AF and HF[14] since clinical studies in patients with HF and AF have shown that dronedarone was associated with increased mortality and worsening of heart failure.[79–81]

The Role of Catheter Ablation

Catheter ablation for AF seems to have greater efficacy than antiarrhythmic drugs for rhythm control.[1] Recent trials have shown catheter ablation to be superior to pharmacological therapy as a rhythm control strategy in patients with HFrEF, in terms of sinus rhythm maintenance, as well as in left ventricular ejection fraction (LVEF) and functional status improvements. These findings reinforce the hypothesis that AF may aggravate the underlying cardiomyopathy despite adequate rate control. The recently published landmark CASTLE-AF study randomized symptomatic patients with HFrEF and paroxysmal or persistent AF with LVEF $\leq$35% to either catheter ablation or medical therapy (rate or rhythm control) in addition to guideline-based therapy for HF.[82] All patients had been implanted with an ICD or CRT-D device, with automatic remote-monitoring capabilities. The study demonstrated that AF ablation significantly reduced all-cause mortality (relative reduction of 47%) and HF hospitalizations (relative reduction of 44%) after a median follow-up of 37 months. There were also improvements in LVEF (median absolute increase of 8% in the ablation group vs 0.2% in the medical therapy group; P=0.005).[82] Of note, 63.1% of patients in the ablation group and 21.7% in the medical therapy group (P<0.001) were in sinus rhythm at 60 months.[82] In a similar population, the AATAC randomized trial showed that catheter ablation is superior to amiodarone in patients with cardiomyopathy and persistent AF in terms of freedom from AF, quality of life, HF admissions, and mortality after a two-year follow-up period.[83] Furthermore, the CAMERA-MRI trial randomized patients with ischemic cardiomyopathy (mean LVEF 33%) and persistent AF to ablation (pulmonary vein isolation and posterior wall isolation) or medical rate control therapy.[84] The absolute LVEF improvement was 18±13% in the ablation group compared to 4.4±13% in the medical therapy group (P<0.0001); catheter ablation also resulted in improved NYHA class and brain natriuretic peptide levels.[84] The absence of fibrosis on cardiac magnetic resonance imaging was predictive of greater LVEF improvement. Recent meta-analyses support the superiority of ablation over medical therapy for AF in patients with HF in terms of LVEF and functional status improvement as well as for mortality reduction (Table 20.2).[82–90] The relative value of AF ablation in ischemic vs non-ischemic cardiomyopathy is not known.

The effect of catheter ablation in patients with AF and HFpEF has been less studied, although small studies suggest similar effectiveness in terms of procedural characteristics, arrhythmia recurrence, and functional improvement.[91] Reduction of AF burden and clinical improvement seems to be comparable in patients with HFrEF vs HFpEF.[92] In a small study, patients with HFpEF and AF who underwent catheter ablation for rhythm control had fewer HF hospitalizations and left atrial and ventricular remodeling without any effect on mortality, compared with a rate control strategy.[93]

Improved risk stratification is needed to identify patients with AF and HF who might benefit the most from catheter ablation. For this purpose, several clinical and imaging risk factors

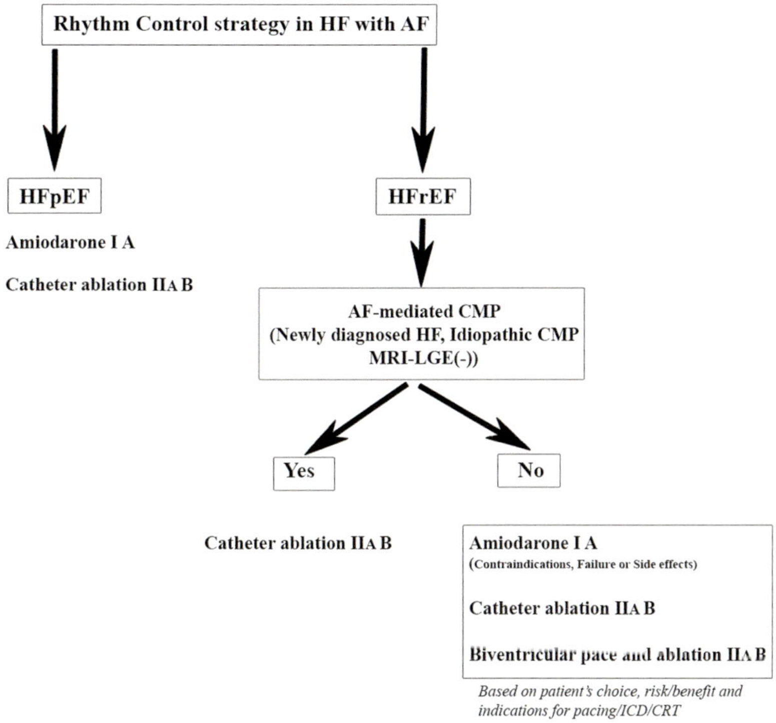

FIGURE 20.3 Rhythm control strategy in patients with concomitant heart failure and atrial fibrillation based on guideline recommendations. *Abbreviations*: HF, heart failure; AF, atrial fibrillation; HFpEF, heart failure with preserved ejection fraction; HFrEF, heart failure with reduced ejection fraction; CMP, cardiomyopathy; MRI-LGE, magnetic resonance imaging late gadolinium enhancement; ICD, implantable cardioverter defibrillator; CRT, cardiac resynchronization therapy. (Adapted from Kirchhof P, et al. Eur Heart J. 2016 Oct 7;37(38):2893–962 and Ponikowski P, et al. *Eur Heart J.* 2016 Jul 14;37(27):2129–200.)

have been proposed (Table 20.3).[94] Importantly, ablation procedures in recent clinical trials were performed in high-volume centers, whereas different strategies and modalities were used across the studies. Moreover, the studied populations included relatively young males with moderate LV dysfunction and relatively short duration of AF, while the follow-up period was not long. Catheter ablation appears to be more beneficial in patients with HFrEF earlier in the course of disease (NYHA class II, LVEF >25%), who do not have advanced, irreversible myocardial damage (i.e., extensive fibrosis).[82,84] The presence of AF by itself is associated with structural and functional abnormalities of the left atrium, which are not entirely resolved by restoration of sinus rhythm, whereas catheter ablation can cause further injury to the atrium as a result of replacement of the normal myocardium with scar. Catheter ablation may be associated with up to 30–35% replacement of left atrium by fibrotic tissue. These changes may be well tolerated in relatively healthy patients with paroxysmal AF, but, in patients with HF and severe structural atrial changes, ablation-related injury may further impair atrial function with subsequent worsening of HF. Although the fibrotic atrium in HF is an ideal substrate for the development of AF, it may be a suboptimal substrate for catheter ablation, as these patients are unlikely to derive long-term benefits from the procedure.[95]

In general, a single ablation procedure is safe and effective in AF patients with HF and decreased EF <50%; >70% of patients remain on sinus rhythm after three years of follow-up.[96] AF recurrences in the post-ablation period are commonly treated by electrical cardioversion with or without amiodarone administration. Amiodarone is often continued for at least 8–12 weeks after ablation to reduce early AF recurrences (hybrid rhythm control strategy) and has been hypothesized to act synergistically with ablation therapy, increasing the maintenance of sinus rhythm. The management of patients with HFrEF and recurrent AF (>3 months) after an initial ablation procedure should be individualized. A repeat procedure may be reasonable in patients with previous clinical improvement after ablation, in whom amiodarone was proven ineffective or contraindicated. A biventricular ablate-and-pace strategy should also be considered in these patients.[94]

Ablate-and-Pace Strategy

AV junction ablation and pacemaker implantation are indicated for refractory patients who have failed rhythm control and medical rate control for AF.[97] Besides a more robust control of ventricular rate, this strategy also provides regularization of the R-R intervals. It seems to be a safe and effective approach for reducing symptoms and improving quality of life in this population.[97] AV junction ablation should not be performed in cases with a reversible cause of rapid AF, e.g., hyperthyroidism, acute myocardial infarction, and electrolyte abnormalities. An increase in LVEF in patients with systolic dysfunction has been observed following the "ablate-and-pace" approach,[97] and survival benefit has been reported for patients with HF who undergo AV ablation and receive CRT.[98] In patients with HF and AF who receive CRT, AV junction ablation leads to maximal biventricular pacing and therefore, optimal benefits.[98] Another option for patients with insufficient rate control or failed AF catheter ablation is AV junction ablation combined with His bundle pacing,[99] a strategy that can provide long-term clinical benefits in selected patients with HF and AF.[99]

TABLE 20.2: Synopsis of Landmark, Randomized Clinical Trials for Catheter Ablation of Atrial Fibrillation in Patients with Heart Failure and Reduced Ejection Fraction

Study	Khan et al. 2008, PABA-CHF	MacDonald et al. 2011	Jones et al. 2013, ARC-HF	Hunter et al. 2014, CAMTAF	Di Biase et al. 2016, AATAC	Prabhu et al. 2017, CAMERA-MRI	Marrouche et al. 2018, CASTLE-AF
Sample size, N (ablation/medical)	41/40	22/19	26/26	26/24	102/101	33/33	179/184
Mean age, years (ablation/medical)	60/61	62/64	64/62	55/60	62/60	59/62	64/64 (median)
Setting	Multicenter	Single-center	Multicenter	Single-center	Multicenter	Multicenter	Multicenter
Ablation technique	PVI ± linear lesions & CFAE	PVI ± linear lesions & CFAE ± CVTI	PVI ± linear lesions ± CFAE ± CVTI	PVI with CFAE ± linear lesions ± CVTI	PVI ± LAPWI ± SVCI ± CFAE	PVI ± LAPWI	PVI ± LAPWI ± SVCI ± CFAE (operator discretion)
Freedom from AF at follow-up, % (ablation/medical)	88/0	50/0	84/0	73/0	71/36	100/0	63/22
Medical strategy	AV nodal ablation & CRT	Rate control with BB and digoxin	Rate control with BB and digoxin	Rate control	Amiodarone	Rate control	Rate or Rhythm control
Primary outcome	Composite of LVEF, distance on 6MWT and QoL assessment	Change in LVEF	Change in peak V_{O2} or functional capacity	Change in LVEF	AF recurrence	Change in LVEF	Death from any cause or hospitalization due to worsening of heart failure
Inclusion criteria	Symptomatic drug resistant AF, NYHA II–III HF, LVEF <40%	Persistent AF, NYHA II–IV HF despite optimal therapy for at least 3 months, LVEF <35%	Persistent AF, NYHA II–IV HF on optimal tx, LVEF <35%	Persistent AF, NYHA II–IV HF, LVEF <50%	Persistent AF, dual chamber ICD/CRT-D, NYHA II–III HF, LVEF <40% within the past 6 months	Persistent AF, 18–85 years old, NYHA ≥II, LVEF ≤45%, on baseline CMR, no significant CAD or other cause of LV dysfunction	Persistent or paroxysmal AF, no response to, unacceptable side effects from or unwillingness to take anti-arrhythmic drugs, NYHA II–IV HF, LVEF <35%
Paroxysmal AF, %	49	0	0	0	0	0	32.5
LVEF, %	28	18	23	33	29	35	32
Follow-up	6 months	6 months	12 months	6 months	24 months	6 months	38 months
Ischemic HF, %	71	49	33	26	62	NA	47
NYHA II-III, %	100	100	100	100	NA	NA	87
Time since AF diagnosis	47 months	54 months	51 months	NA	8.2 months	NA	NA
Amiodarone, %	NA	NA	34	54	0	24	28
ACE-I/ARB, % (ablation/medical)	NA	95	98	NA	92	94	94
BB, % (ablation/medical)	NA	88	92	NA	76	97	92
MRA, % (ablation/medical tx)	NA	32	37	NA	45	33	NA
ICD/CRT, % (ablation/medical tx)	49	NA	27	NA	100	NA	100
Result	Superior QoL, functional status, and LVEF improvement	No difference in LVEF change, functional status, QoL, natriuretic peptides	No difference in LVEF change; improved exercise performance, QoL, natriuretic peptides	Superior QoL, functional capacity and LVEF improvement	72% free from arrhythmia, improved LVEF, distance in 6MWT and QoL	Improvement in LVEF	Improvement in composite endpoint of death and heart failure hospitalization

Abbreviations: 6MWT: 6-minute walk test; AF: atrial fibrillation; AV: atrioventricular; BB: beta-blocker; CAD: coronary artery disease; CFAE: complex fractionated atrial electrograms; CMR: cardiac magnetic resonance; CRT: cardiac resynchronization therapy; CRT-D cardiac resynchronization therapy-defibrillation; CVTI: cavotricuspid isthmus; HF: heart failure; ICD: implantable cardioverter-defibrillator; LAPWI: left atrial posterior wall isolation; LVEF: left ventricular ejection fraction; NYHA: New York Heart Association; PVI: pulmonary vein isolation; SVCI superior vena cava isolation; QoL: quality of life.

TABLE 20.3: Factors Favoring Ablation vs Medical Therapy or Ablate-and-Pace Strategy in Patients with Heart Failure and Atrial Fibrillation

Factors Favoring AF Catheter Ablation *High Benefit*	Factors Favoring Medical Therapy or Ablate-and-Pace Therapy *Low Benefit*
Low peri-procedural risk	High peri-procedural risk
High-volume, experienced centers	Low-volume, less-experienced centers
Young age (<65 years)	Elderly patients (>80 years)
No or few comorbidities	Many comorbidities
Recent onset AF	Long history of HF >> AF history
Recent onset AF with fast heart rate	Long-standing persistent AF with controlled heart rate
	Failed repeat ablation for persistent AF
Idiopathic cardiomyopathy	Ischemic or valvular cardiomyopathy
LV ejection fraction >25%	LV ejection fraction <25%
LA diameter <55 mm	LA diameter >55 mm
Negative LV MRI-LGE	Positive LV MRI-LGE
LA fibrosis ≤10%	LA fibrosis >10%

Abbreviations: AF, atrial fibrillation; HF, heart failure; LV, left ventricular; LA, left atrium; MRI-LGE, magnetic resonance imaging–late gadolinium enhancement.

Conclusions, Controversies, and Research Opportunities

HF and AF represent two epidemics in cardiovascular medicine that are highly prevalent and which feed each other. The coexistence of HF and AF adversely affects morbidity and mortality and has a significant impact on healthcare resource utilization and costs. The true burden of AF in HF is not known, as many episodes, especially in older patients, may be asymptomatic. The ideal diagnostic pathway for estimation of AF burden in the setting of HF is unclear, but close surveillance is warranted. The role of external or internal loop recorders in high-risk HF patients not implanted with a cardiac rhythm device needs further clarification.

An increasing body of evidence supports the value of AF ablation in the HF setting, with reduced morbidity and mortality. However, the available evidence indicates that this modality may have limited value for older patients with severely depressed LVEF and/or longer duration of AF (>2 years). Interestingly, contemporary imaging modalities that can estimate the extent of atrial and ventricular fibrosis, such as MRI, may guide our therapeutic decisions regarding rate vs rhythm control strategies as well as interventional management.

In addition to standard antiarrhythmic drugs, signaling pathways involved in atrial fibrosis, oxidative stress, and inflammation are potential pharmacological targets. Also, microRNAs, which have been implicated in both AF and HF pathogenesis, represent potential therapeutic targets. Several issues need to be addressed in future studies regarding the diagnosis (imaging and natriuretic peptides) and management of HFpEF in the presence of AF.

Given that several comorbidities such as obesity, sleep apnea, diabetes, and chronic kidney disease are associated with atrial remodeling and AF, it is reasonable to assume that tailored therapies targeting these conditions may have a favorable effect on both HF and AF. Multitarget pharmacological interventions and catheter ablation, as well as risk factors and lifestyle modifications at an early stage where atrial remodeling is not extensive, seem to be the most effective therapeutic approaches in patients with HF and AF.

References

1. Kirchhof P, Benussi S, Kotecha D, et al. 2016 ESC guidelines for the management of atrial fibrillation developed in collaboration with EACTS. *Eur Heart J.* 2016;37:2893–962.
2. McManus DD, Rienstra M, Benjamin EJ. An update on the prognosis of patients with atrial fibrillation. *Circulation.* 2012;126:e143–6.
3. Benjamin EJ, Wolf PA, D'Agostino RB, et al. Impact of atrial fibrillation on the risk of death: the Framingham Heart Study. *Circulation.* 1998;98:946–52.
4. Kotecha D, Holmes J, Krum H, et al. Efficacy of beta blockers in patients with heart failure plus atrial fibrillation: an individual-patient data meta-analysis. *Lancet.* 2014;384:2235–43.
5. Ruddox V, Sandven I, Munkhaugen J, et al. Atrial fibrillation and the risk for myocardial infarction, all-cause mortality and heart failure: a systematic review and meta-analysis. *Eur J Prev Cardiol.* 2017;24:1555–66.
6. Chamberlain AM, Gersh BJ, Alonso A, et al. No decline in the risk of heart failure after incident atrial fibrillation: a community study assessing trends overall and by ejection fraction. *Heart Rhythm.* 2017;14:791–8.
7. Pandey A, Kim S, Moore C, et al. Predictors and prognostic implications of incident heart failure in patients with prevalent atrial fibrillation. *JACC Heart Fail.* 2017;5:44–52.
8. Guha K, McDonagh T. Heart failure epidemiology: European perspective. *Curr Cardiol Rev.* 2013;9:123–7.
9. Kotecha D, Piccini JP. Atrial fibrillation in heart failure: what should we do? *Eur Heart J.* 2015;36:3250–7.
10. Chiang CE, Naditch-Brule L, Murin J, et al. Distribution and risk profile of paroxysmal, persistent, and permanent atrial fibrillation in routine clinical practice: insight from the real-life global survey evaluating patients with atrial fibrillation international registry. *Circ Arrhythm Electrophysiol.* 2012;5:632–9.
11. Vermond RA, Geelhoed B, Verweij N, et al. Incidence of atrial fibrillation and relationship with cardiovascular events, heart failure, and mortality: a community-based study from the Netherlands. *J Am Coll Cardiol.* 2015;66:1000–7.
12. Santhanakrishnan R, Wang N, Larson MG, et al. Atrial fibrillation begets heart failure and vice versa: temporal associations and differences in preserved versus reduced ejection fraction. *Circulation.* 2016;133:484–92.
13. Maisel WH, Stevenson LW. Atrial fibrillation in heart failure: epidemiology, pathophysiology, and rationale for therapy. *Am J Cardiol.* 2003;91:2D–8D.
14. Ponikowski P, Voors AA, Anker SD, et al. 2016 ESC guidelines for the diagnosis and treatment of acute and chronic heart failure: the Task Force for the diagnosis and treatment of acute and chronic heart failure of the European Society of Cardiology (ESC)Developed with the special contribution of the Heart Failure Association (HFA) of the ESC. *Eur Heart J.* 2016;37:2129–200.
15. Smit MD, Moes ML, Maass AH, et al. The importance of whether atrial fibrillation or heart failure develops first. *Eur J Heart Fail.* 2012;14:1030–40.
16. Calvo N, Bisbal F, Guiu E, et al. Impact of atrial fibrillation-induced tachycardiomyopathy in patients undergoing pulmonary vein isolation. *Int J Cardiol.* 2013;168:4093–7.

17. Mamas MA, Caldwell JC, Chacko S, et al. A meta-analysis of the prognostic significance of atrial fibrillation in chronic heart failure. *Eur J Heart Fail.* 2009;11:676–83.
18. Kotecha D, Chudasama R, Lane DA, Kirchhof P, Lip GY. Atrial fibrillation and heart failure due to reduced versus preserved ejection fraction: a systematic review and meta-analysis of death and adverse outcomes. *Int J Cardiol.* 2016;203:660–6.
19. Ziff OJ, Carter PR, McGowan J, et al. The interplay between atrial fibrillation and heart failure on long-term mortality and length of stay: insights from the United Kingdom ACALM registry. *Int J Cardiol.* 2018;252:117–121.
20. Mogensen UM, Jhund PS, Abraham WT, et al. Type of atrial fibrillation and outcomes in patients with heart failure and reduced ejection fraction. *J Am Coll Cardiol.* 2017;70:2490–500.
21. Naka KK, Bazoukis G, Bechlioulis A, et al. Association between atrial fibrillation and patient-important outcomes in heart failure patients with implantable cardioverter-defibrillators: a systematic review and meta-analysis. *Eur Heart J Qual Care Clin Outcomes.* 2019;5:96–104.
22. Elshazly MB, Senn T, Wu Y, et al. Impact of atrial fibrillation on exercise capacity and mortality in heart failure with preserved ejection fraction: insights from cardiopulmonary stress testing. *J Am Heart Assoc.* 2017;6(11):e006662.
23. Sartipy U, Savarese G, Dahlstrom U, Fu M, Lund LH. Association of heart rate with mortality in sinus rhythm and atrial fibrillation in heart failure with preserved ejection fraction. *Eur J Heart Fail.* 2019;21:471–9.
24. Zafrir B, Lund LH, Laroche C, et al. Prognostic implications of atrial fibrillation in heart failure with reduced, mid-range, and preserved ejection fraction: a report from 14 964 patients in the European Society of Cardiology Heart Failure Long-Term Registry. *Eur Heart J.* 2018;39:4277–84.
25. Linssen GC, Rienstra M, Jaarsma T, et al. Clinical and prognostic effects of atrial fibrillation in heart failure patients with reduced and preserved left ventricular ejection fraction. *Eur J Heart Fail.* 2011;13:1111–20.
26. Cheng M, Lu X, Huang J, et al. The prognostic significance of atrial fibrillation in heart failure with a preserved and reduced left ventricular function: insights from a meta-analysis. *Eur J Heart Fail.* 2014;16:1317–22.
27. Paolillo S, Agostoni P, Masarone D, et al. Prognostic role of atrial fibrillation in patients affected by chronic heart failure. Data from the MECKI score research group. *Eur J Intern Med.* 2015;26:515–20.
28. Kotecha D, Lam CS, Van Veldhuisen DJ, et al. Heart failure with preserved ejection fraction and atrial fibrillation: vicious twins. *J Am Coll Cardiol.* 2016;68:2217–28.
29. Andrade J, Khairy P, Dobrev D, Nattel S. The clinical profile and pathophysiology of atrial fibrillation: relationships among clinical features, epidemiology, and mechanisms. *Circ Res.* 2014;114:1453–68.
30. Heijman J, Algalarrondo V, Voigt N, et al. The value of basic research insights into atrial fibrillation mechanisms as a guide to therapeutic innovation: a critical analysis. *Cardiovasc Res.* 2016;109:467–79.
31. Korantzopoulos P, Goudevenos JA. Aldosterone signaling in atrial fibrillation another piece in the puzzle of atrial remodeling. *J Am Coll Cardiol.* 2010;55:771–3.
32. Skanes AC, Tang ASL. Atrial fibrillation and heart failure: untangling a modern gordian knot. *Can J Cardiol.* 2018;34:1437–48.
33. Korantzopoulos P, Letsas K, Fragakis N, Tse G, Liu T. Oxidative stress and atrial fibrillation: an update. *Free Radic Res.* 2018;52:1199–209.
34. Sugumar H, Nanayakkara S, Prabhu S, et al. Pathophysiology of atrial fibrillation and heart failure: dangerous interactions. *Cardiol Clin.* 2019;37:131–8.
35. Denham NC, Pearman CM, Caldwell JL, et al. Calcium in the pathophysiology of atrial fibrillation and heart failure. *Front Physiol.* 2018;9:1380.
36. Sugumar H, Prabhu S, Voskoboinik A, Kistler PM. Arrhythmia induced cardiomyopathy. *J Arrhythm.* 2018;34:376–83.
37. Huizar JF, Ellenbogen KA, Tan AY, Kaszala K. Arrhythmia-induced cardiomyopathy: JACC state-of-the-art review. *J Am Coll Cardiol.* 2019;73:2328–44.
38. Batul SA, Gopinathannair R. Atrial fibrillation in heart failure: a therapeutic challenge of our times. *Korean Circ J.* 2017;47:644–62.
39. Patel RB, Vaduganathan M, Shah SJ, Butler J. Atrial fibrillation in heart failure with preserved ejection fraction: insights into mechanisms and therapeutics. *Pharmacol Ther.* 2017;176:32–39.
40. Vermes E, Tardif JC, Bourassa MG, et al. Enalapril decreases the incidence of atrial fibrillation in patients with left ventricular dysfunction: insight from the Studies Of Left Ventricular Dysfunction (SOLVD) trials. *Circulation.* 2003;107:2926–31.
41. Maggioni AP, Latini R, Carson PE, et al. Valsartan reduces the incidence of atrial fibrillation in patients with heart failure: results from the Valsartan Heart Failure Trial (Val-HeFT). *Am Heart J.* 2005;149:548–57.
42. McMurray J, Kober L, Robertson M, et al. Antiarrhythmic effect of carvedilol after acute myocardial infarction: results of the Carvedilol Post-Infarct Survival Control in Left Ventricular Dysfunction (CAPRICORN) trial. *J Am Coll Cardiol.* 2005;45:525–30.
43. Ducharme A, Swedberg K, Pfeffer MA, et al. Prevention of atrial fibrillation in patients with symptomatic chronic heart failure by candesartan in the Candesartan in heart failure: assessment of reduction in mortality and morbidity (CHARM) program. *Am Heart J.* 2006;151:985–91.
44. Swedberg K, Zannad F, McMurray JJ, et al. Eplerenone and atrial fibrillation in mild systolic heart failure: results from the EMPHASIS-HF (Eplerenone in Mild Patients Hospitalization And SurvIval Study in Heart Failure) study. *J Am Coll Cardiol.* 2012;59:1598–603.
45. Martin RI, Pogoryelova O, Koref MS, et al. Atrial fibrillation associated with ivabradine treatment: meta-analysis of randomised controlled trials. *Heart.* 2014;100:1506–10.
46. Cadrin-Tourigny J, Shohoudi A, Roy D, et al. Decreased mortality with beta-blockers in patients with heart failure and coexisting atrial fibrillation: an AF-CHF substudy. *JACC Heart Fail.* 2017;5:99–106.
47. Ma G, Fang Q, Wang F. The effect of beta-blockers on mortality in patients with heart failure and atrial fibrillation: a meta-analysis of observational cohort and randomized controlled studies. *Cardiol J.* 2018;26:744–52.
48. Kotecha D, Flather MD, Altman DG, et al. Heart rate and rhythm and the benefit of beta-blockers in patients with heart failure. *J Am Coll Cardiol.* 2017;69:2885–96.
49. Rienstra M, Damman K, Mulder BA, et al. Beta-blockers and outcome in heart failure and atrial fibrillation: a meta-analysis. *JACC Heart Fail.* 2013;1:21–8.
50. Mulder BA, Van Veldhuisen DJ, Crijns HJ, et al. Lenient vs. strict rate control in patients with atrial fibrillation and heart failure: a post-hoc analysis of the RACE II study. *Eur J Heart Fail.* 2013;15:1311–8.
51. Rathore SS, Curtis JP, Wang Y, Bristow MR, Krumholz HM. Association of serum digoxin concentration and outcomes in patients with heart failure. *JAMA.* 2003;289:871–8.
52. Lam PH, Bhyan P, Arundel C, et al. Digoxin use and lower risk of 30-day all-cause readmission in older patients with heart failure and reduced ejection fraction receiving beta-blockers. *Clin Cardiol.* 2018;41:406–412.
53. Ahmed A, Rich MW, Love TE, et al. Digoxin and reduction in mortality and hospitalization in heart failure: a comprehensive post hoc analysis of the DIG trial. *Eur Heart J.* 2006;27:178–86.
54. Shah M, Avgil Tsadok M, Jackevicius CA, et al. Relation of digoxin use in atrial fibrillation and the risk of all-cause mortality in patients >/=65 years of age with versus without heart failure. *Am J Cardiol.* 2014;114:401–6.
55. Lopes RD, Rordorf R, De Ferrari GM, et al. Digoxin and mortality in patients with atrial fibrillation. *J Am Coll Cardiol.* 2018;71:1063–74.
56. Vamos M, Erath JW, Benz AP, Lopes RD, Hohnloser SH. Meta-analysis of effects of digoxin on survival in patients with atrial fibrillation or heart failure: an update. *Am J Cardiol.* 2019;123:69–74.
57. Bavendiek U, Aguirre Davila L, Koch A, Bauersachs J. Assumption versus evidence: the case of digoxin in atrial fibrillation and heart failure. *Eur Heart J.* 2017;38:2095–9.
58. Steinberg BA, Schulte PJ, Hofmann P, et al. Outcomes after nonemergent electrical cardioversion for atrial arrhythmias. *Am J Cardiol.* 2015;115:1407–14.
59. Nergardh AK, Rosenqvist M, Nordlander R, Frick M. Maintenance of sinus rhythm with metoprolol CR initiated before cardioversion and repeated cardioversion of atrial fibrillation: a randomized double-blind placebo-controlled study. *Eur Heart J.* 2007;28:1351–7.
60. Lip GY, Lane DA. Assessing bleeding risk in atrial fibrillation with the HAS-BLED and ORBIT scores: clinical application requires focus on the reversible bleeding risk factors. *Eur Heart J.* 2015;36:3265–7.
61. Pedersen OD, Bagger H, Keller N, et al. Efficacy of dofetilide in the treatment of atrial fibrillation-flutter in patients with reduced left ventricular function: a Danish investigations of arrhythmia and mortality on dofetilide (diamond) substudy. *Circulation.* 2001;104:292–6.
62. Gasparini M, Steinberg JS, Arshad A, et al. Resumption of sinus rhythm in patients with heart failure and permanent atrial fibrillation undergoing cardiac resynchronization therapy: a longitudinal observational study. *Eur Heart J.* 2010;31:976–83.
63. Wilton SB, Leung AA, Ghali WA, Faris P, Exner DV. Outcomes of cardiac resynchronization therapy in patients with versus those without atrial fibrillation: a systematic review and meta-analysis. *Heart Rhythm.* 2011;8:1088–94.
64. Nakajima I, Noda T, Kanzaski H, et al. Development of heart failure from transient atrial fibrillation attacks in responders to cardiac resynchronization therapy. *JACC Clin Electrophysiol.* 2018;4:1227–34.
65. Birnie D, Hudnall H, Lemke B, et al. Continuous optimization of cardiac resynchronization therapy reduces atrial fibrillation in heart failure patients: results of the adaptive cardiac resynchronization therapy trial. *Heart Rhythm.* 2017;14:1820–5.
66. Hsu JC, Birnie D, Stadler RW, et al. Adaptive cardiac resynchronization therapy is associated with decreased risk of incident atrial fibrillation compared to standard biventricular pacing: a real-world analysis of 37,450 patients followed by remote monitoring. *Heart Rhythm.* 2019;16:983–9.

67. Sobue Y, Watanabe E, Lip GYH, et al. Thromboembolisms in atrial fibrillation and heart failure patients with a preserved ejection fraction (HFpEF) compared to those with a reduced ejection fraction (HFrEF). *Heart Vessels.* 2018;33:403–12.
68. Mentias A, Briasoulis A, Shantha G, Alvarez P, Vaughan-Sarrazin M. Impact of heart failure type on thromboembolic and bleeding risk in patients with atrial fibrillation on oral anticoagulation. *Am J Cardiol.* 2019;123:1649–53.
69. Boos CJ, Nam M, Camm AJ. Novel oral anticoagulants and stroke prevention in atrial fibrillation and chronic heart failure. *Heart Fail Rev.* 2014;19:391–401.
70. Xiong Q, Lau YC, Senoo K, et al. Non-vitamin K antagonist oral anticoagulants (NOACs) in patients with concomitant atrial fibrillation and heart failure: a systemic review and meta-analysis of randomized trials. *Eur J Heart Fail.* 2015;17:1192–200.
71. Savarese G, Giugliano RP, Rosano GM, et al. Efficacy and safety of novel oral anticoagulants in patients with atrial fibrillation and heart failure: a meta-analysis. *JACC Heart Fail.* 2016;4:870–80.
72. Brown LAE, Boos CJ. Atrial fibrillation and heart failure: factors influencing the choice of oral anticoagulant. *Int J Cardiol.* 2017;227:863–8.
73. Lee TC, Qian M, Lip GYH, et al. Heart failure severity and quality of warfarin anticoagulation control (from the WARCEF trial). *Am J Cardiol.* 2018;122:821–7.
74. Chaugai S, Meng WY, Ali Sepehry A. Effects of RAAS blockers on atrial fibrillation prophylaxis: an updated systematic review and meta-analysis of randomized controlled trials. *J Cardiovasc Pharmacol Ther.* 2016;21:388–404.
75. Liu T, Korantzopoulos P, Shao Q, et al. Mineralocorticoid receptor antagonists and atrial fibrillation: a meta-analysis. *Europace.* 2016;18:672–8.
76. Van Gelder IC, Hagens VE, Bosker HA, et al. A comparison of rate control and rhythm control in patients with recurrent persistent atrial fibrillation. *N Engl J Med.* 2002;347:1834–40.
77. Slee A, Saad M, Saksena S. Heart failure progression and mortality in atrial fibrillation patients with preserved or reduced left ventricular ejection fraction. *J Interv Card Electrophysiol.* 2019;55:325–31.
78. Roy D, Talajic M, Nattel S, et al. Rhythm control versus rate control for atrial fibrillation and heart failure. *N Engl J Med.* 2008;358:2667–77.
79. Kober L, Torp-Pedersen C, McMurray JJ, et al. Increased mortality after dronedarone therapy for severe heart failure. *N Engl J Med.* 2008;358:2678–87.
80. Connolly SJ, Camm AJ, Halperin JL, et al. Dronedarone in high-risk permanent atrial fibrillation. *N Engl J Med.* 2011;365:2268–76.
81. Chatterjee S, Ghosh J, Lichstein E, Aikat S, Mukherjee D. Meta-analysis of cardiovascular outcomes with dronedarone in patients with atrial fibrillation or heart failure. *Am J Cardiol.* 2012;110:607–13.
82. Marrouche NF, Brachmann J, Andresen D, et al. Catheter ablation for atrial fibrillation with heart failure. *N Engl J Med.* 2018;378:417–27.
83. Di Biase L, Mohanty P, Mohanty S, et al. Ablation versus amiodarone for treatment of persistent atrial fibrillation in patients with congestive heart failure and an implanted device: results from the AATAC multicenter randomized trial. *Circulation.* 2016;133:1637–44.
84. Prabhu S, Taylor AJ, Costello BT, et al. Catheter ablation versus medical rate control in atrial fibrillation and systolic dysfunction: the CAMERA-MRI study. *J Am Coll Cardiol.* 2017;70:1949–61.
85. Smer A, Salih M, Darrat YH, et al. Meta-analysis of randomized controlled trials on atrial fibrillation ablation in patients with heart failure with reduced ejection fraction. *Clin Cardiol.* 2018;41:1430–8.
86. Virk SA, Bennett RG, Chow C, et al. Catheter ablation versus medical therapy for atrial fibrillation in patients with heart failure: a meta-analysis of randomised controlled trials. *Heart Lung Circ.* 2019;28:707–18.
87. Khan MN, Jais P, Cummings J, et al. Pulmonary-vein isolation for atrial fibrillation in patients with heart failure. *N Engl J Med.* 2008;359:1778–85.
88. MacDonald MR, Connelly DT, Hawkins NM, et al. Radiofrequency ablation for persistent atrial fibrillation in patients with advanced heart failure and severe left ventricular systolic dysfunction: a randomised controlled trial. *Heart.* 2011;97:740–7.
89. Jones DG, Haldar SK, Hussain W, et al. A randomized trial to assess catheter ablation versus rate control in the management of persistent atrial fibrillation in heart failure. *J Am Coll Cardiol.* 2013;61:1894–903.
90. Hunter RJ, Berriman TJ, Diab I, et al. A randomized controlled trial of catheter ablation versus medical treatment of atrial fibrillation in heart failure (the CAMTAF trial). *Circ Arrhythm Electrophysiol.* 2014;7:31–8.
91. Black-Maier E, Ren X, Steinberg BA, et al. Catheter ablation of atrial fibrillation in patients with heart failure and preserved ejection fraction. *Heart Rhythm.* 2018;15:651–7.
92. Ichijo S, Miyazaki S, Kusa S, et al. Impact of catheter ablation of atrial fibrillation on long-term clinical outcomes in patients with heart failure. *J Cardiol.* 2018;72:240–6.
93. Machino-Ohtsuka T, Seo Y, Ishizu T, et al. Relationships between maintenance of sinus rhythm and clinical outcomes in patients with heart failure with preserved ejection fraction and atrial fibrillation. *J Cardiol.* 2019;74:235–44.
94. Richter S, Di Biase L, Hindricks G. Atrial fibrillation ablation in heart failure. *Eur Heart J.* 2019;40:663–71.
95. Packer M. Electrophysiological interventions in the treatment of chronic heart failure: a comparison of the strength of evidence supporting cardiac resynchronization for electrical conduction delay and catheter ablation for atrial fibrillation. *Eur J Heart Fail.* 2019;21:398–401.
96. Bazoukis G, Letsas KP, Tse G, et al. Predictors of arrhythmia recurrence in patients with heart failure undergoing left atrial ablation for atrial fibrillation. *Clin Cardiol.* 2018;41:63–7.
97. Vlachos K, Letsas KP, Korantzopoulos P, et al. A review on atrioventricular junction ablation and pacing for heart rate control of atrial fibrillation. *J Geriatr Cardiol.* 2015;12:547–54.
98. Steinberg JS. Role of atrioventricular junctional ablation and cardiac resynchronization therapy in patients with chronic atrial fibrillation. *Card Electrophysiol Clin.* 2019;11:147–54.
99. Huang W, Su L, Wu S. Pacing treatment of atrial fibrillation patients with heart failure: his bundle pacing combined with atrioventricular node ablation. *Card Electrophysiol Clin.* 2018;10:519–35.

Chapter 21
VENTRICULAR ARRHYTHMIAS IN HEART FAILURE

Antonis S. Manolis, Antonis A. Manolis, and Theodora A. Manolis

Introduction

Ventricular arrhythmias culminating in cardiac arrest make a considerable contribution to mortality in patients with heart failure (HF). Ventricular arrhythmias include complex ventricular ectopic activity, such as frequent or multifocal premature ventricular complexes (PVCs) and runs of non-sustained (either monomorphic or polymorphic) ventricular tachycardia (NSVT), which are potentially malignant, and malignant or life-threatening ventricular arrhythmias, such as sustained (monomorphic or polymorphic) ventricular tachycardia (VT) and ventricular fibrillation (VF), responsible for sudden cardiac death (SCD).

Pathogenetic Mechanisms

Ventricular arrhythmias in HF are a consequence of altered cardiomyocyte properties. Myocardial tissue composition in HF facilitates sustained ventricular arrhythmias.[1] Ventricular ectopic activity in HF is multifactorial,[2] and is related to the type of underlying structural heart disease (ischemic or non-ischemic cardiomyopathy), myocardial ischemia, presence of scar or fibrosis, neurohumoral activation (autonomic nervous system, renin-angiotensin-aldosterone system), worsening congestion, electrolyte abnormalities, proarrhythmic drugs, calcium overload, and genetic susceptibility. Areas of scar or fibrosis affect regional conduction patterns and serve as islands of reentry circuits, the commonest mechanism of sustained ventricular tachyarrhythmias. Ischemia and sympathetic activation can lead to abnormal automaticity, the second most common mechanism. A focal non-reentry mechanism may also contribute to ventricular tachyarrhythmias in patients with ischemic or non-ischemic cardiomyopathy (NICM), probably from triggered activity arising from either early afterdepolarizations or delayed afterdepolarizations, giving rise to polymorphic ventricular tachyarrhythmias or VF. Under certain conditions, monomorphic VT can also degenerate into VF in a sick myocardium. Thus, the leading immediate causes of SCD are VT and VF. Although these two ventricular tachyarrhythmias (VT and VF) have been traditionally ascribed to two different mechanisms (reentry for VT and multiple wandering wavelet hypothesis for VF), some investigators believe that both may emanate from a single mechanism, i.e., self-organized electrical waves forming "rotors," with the rotor of VT being stationary and having a frequency of rotation that allows 1:1 excitation of both ventricles, and the rotor of VF, either drifting or stationary, having a very high frequency, resulting in multiple areas of intermittent block and giving rise to complex patterns of propagation.[3]

Premature Ventricular Complexes (PVCs)

Based on prior reviews, 60–90% of patients with HF have ventricular arrhythmias in the form of PVCs.[4] Factors that may point to worse prognosis in patients with PVCs may comprise the type of underlying structural heart disease, a high PVC burden (>2000 PVCs/24 h), complex PVCs (couplets, triplets, and NSVT), increased number of morphologies, increasing number of PVCs with exercise, non-outflow tract PVC, short coupling interval of PVCs ("R-on-T"), and PVCs with broader QRS complexes.[5,6]

Non-Sustained Ventricular Tachycardia (NSVT)

A high proportion of HF patients (40–80%) will manifest runs of NSVT.[7] Although some studies suggested that patients who died suddenly had significantly more episodes of NSVT compared with survivors and those who died from HF,[8] many studies have indicated that asymptomatic runs of NSVT on a Holter monitor may not predict SCD in moderate-to-severe HF,[9,10] and are not an independent predictor of mortality,[7] implying that suppression of these arrhythmias may not improve survival. Rather, patients with NSVT have worse left ventricular (LV) function.[10] When in doubt about the clinical significance of NSVT, an electrophysiology study with programmed ventricular stimulation may help in risk stratification;[11] in patients with inducible sustained VT, an implantable cardioverter defibrillator (ICD) should be offered.

This lack of association between ventricular arrhythmias and sudden death has been ascribed to two possible reasons.[12] First, complex ventricular arrhythmias may be a nonspecific manifestation of a decompensating myocardium rather than an indication of a specific arrhythmogenic substrate. This is in keeping with the observation that patients with mild HF who have NSVT are more likely to develop progression of HF rather than sudden death. Second, sudden death may be related to events other than a malignant arrhythmia, such as myocardial ischemia or electromechanical dissociation. Neither outcome can be predicted by a prior history of ventricular arrhythmias on a Holter monitor.

An exception to the above may relate to runs of rapid NSVT (Figure 21.1). A sub-analysis of the SCD-HeFT trial showed that rapid NSVT (mean number of beats: 26; mean cycle length: 259 ms) in HF patients was independently associated with appropriate ICD shocks and all-cause mortality.[13] Compared with patients without rapid NSVT, those with rapid NSVT were less likely to be taking beta-blockers. The authors suggested that clinical evaluation of patients with rapid NSVT should include intensification of medical therapy, particularly beta-blockers.

Sustained Monomorphic Ventricular Tachycardia

The most common anatomic substrate for sustained monomorphic VT is chronic coronary artery disease (CAD), usually associated with prior myocardial infarction (MI), which is the common arrhythmogenic substrate for reentry responsible for sustained monomorphic VT (Figure 21.2).[14] Sustained monomorphic VT may also occur in NICM; in these cases, the

DOI: 10.1201/9780429244544-25

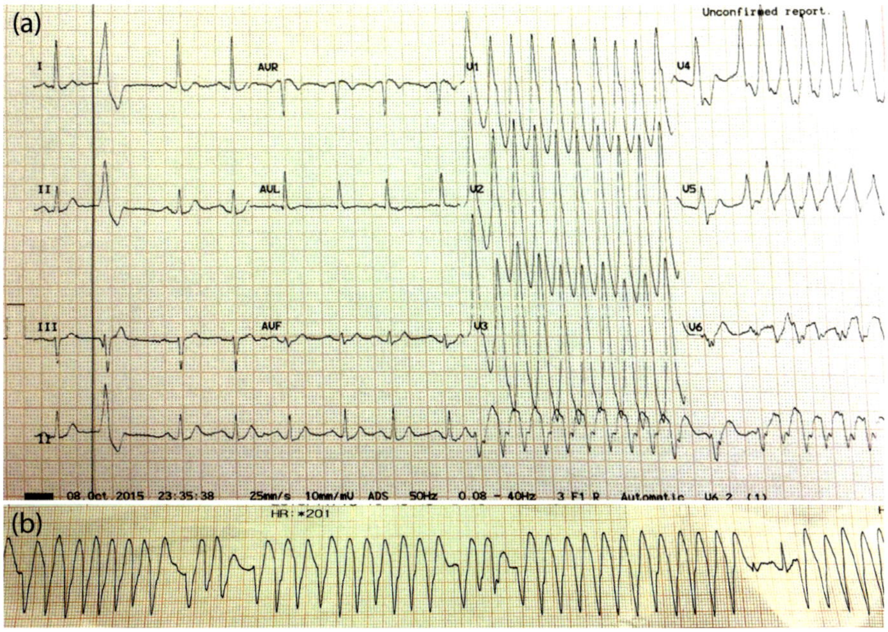

FIGURE 21.1 A 53-year-old man with a history of hypertension presented with symptomatic runs of very rapid (220–250 bpm) non-sustained ventricular tachycardia lasting for <15 s (panels a and b). Coronary angiography revealed normal coronary arteries and the left ventricular ejection fraction was measured at ~45%, attributed to non-ischemic cardiomyopathy. The patient had failed treatment with beta-blockers and sotalol and was placed on amiodarone with adequate response; he finally received an implantable cardioverter defibrillator for back-up. He fared well over the ensuing two years on medical therapy.

pathophysiologic basis is considered to be patchy or segmental fibrosis.[15] Cardiac arrest as a result of polymorphic VT and/or VF is much more common than hemodynamically tolerated sustained monomorphic VT in patients with either dilated or hypertrophic cardiomyopathies. Sustained monomorphic VT is not a feature of hypertrophic cardiomyopathy (HCM), except for the apical variety of HCM.[16]

Sustained monomorphic VT is reproducible with programmed ventricular stimulation during an electrophysiology study (Figure 21.3). This is considered the most specific arrhythmic response indicating the presence of a functional reentry circuit and is probably clinically significant, regardless of the type of underlying structural heart disease.[17] The sensitivity and specificity of an electrophysiology study is much higher in ischemic cardiomyopathy (ICM). In the presence of wall motion abnormalities, LV aneurysm, or a lower LV ejection fraction (LVEF), the development of a sustained monomorphic VT is more likely.

The overall prevalence of reentrant monomorphic VT is not known, because VT can precede SCD and therefore cannot be ascertained. It is more prevalent in diseases more likely to have scar, including prior MI, NICM, infiltrative diseases, and myocarditis. In an ICD cohort with underlying structural heart disease, including both primary and secondary prevention patients, over a mean of 11±3 months, 81% of occurring ventricular tachyarrhythmias were attributable to VT amenable to antitachycardia pacing, implying reentrant monomorphic VT.[18]

Patients with CAD and prior MI may present with sustained monomorphic VT or full-blown cardiac arrest due to a sustained monomorphic VT, that has degenerated into VF, or due to initial polymorphic VT/VF.[19,20] This latter group usually has severe CAD, normal LVEF, and ischemia responsible for the VF; in these cases, an electrophysiology study is less useful. Sustained VT may appear in the first year after an MI (~25%), but in most patients appears many years later (Figure 21.2). The patient's clinical status does not appear to determine the initial occurrence of VT but is an important factor in recurrent episodes of VT. Recurrences seem to be more frequent in the setting of overt HF, possibly related to electrolyte imbalance, high catecholamine state, or drug toxicity acting as VT triggers.

Polymorphic Ventricular Tachycardia and Ventricular Fibrillation

Torsades de Pointes

Polymorphic VT in the form of torsade de pointes (TdP) may occur in HF patients as a result of a proarrhythmic drug effect or an electrolyte abnormality and may be self-terminating or may occasionally degenerate into VF.[21] There is a long list of cardiac drugs (antiarrhythmic agents, e.g., amiodarone and sotalol) and non-cardiac (antibiotics, antidepressants) that prolong the corrected QT interval (QTc) interval (www.qtdrugs.org) (Figure 21.4). QTc prolongation is common in HF and can be profound. QTc prolongation is reported to occur mainly at low heart rates, explaining the finding that many cases of SCD occur at lower rather than higher heart rates, and suggesting that QTc prolongation may be an important mechanism in ventricular tachyarrhythmias leading to SCD in subjects with impaired LV function.[22] Furthermore, electrolyte abnormalities (e.g., hypokalemia and hypomagnesemia), which are common in HF patients receiving diuretics, may also enhance the risk of or lead to TdP. Therefore, it is important to closely monitor and maintain potassium levels at 4.0–5.2 mEq/L, or even higher, at 4.5–5.5 mEq/L.[23]

Amiodarone has been considered safer than other antiarrhythmic agents and the least proarrhythmic, and is often used in HF patients e.g., for rate/rhythm control in atrial fibrillation

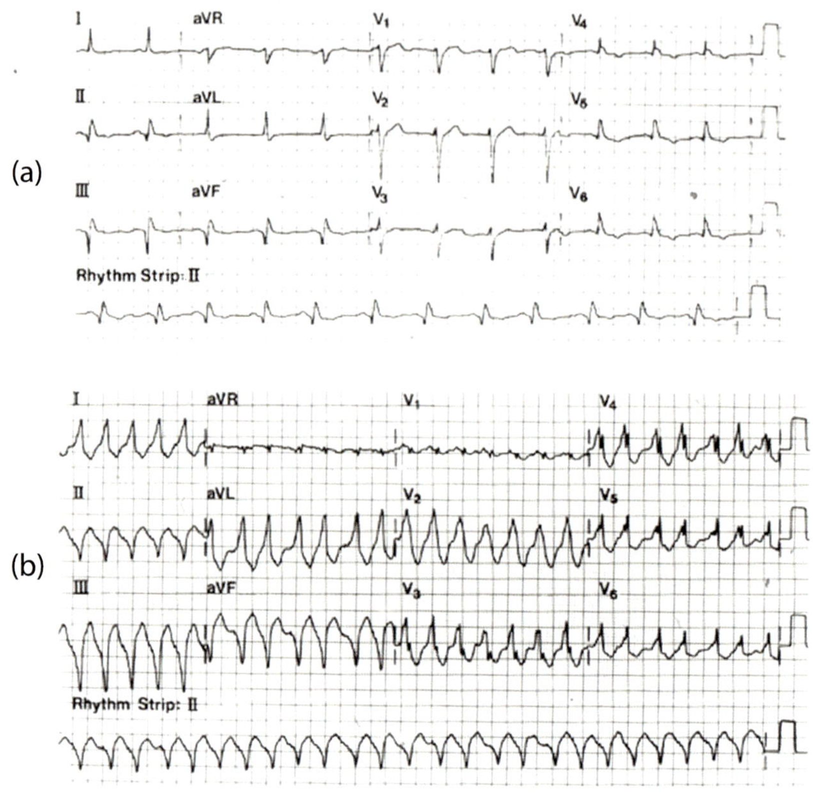

FIGURE 21.2 A 52-year-old man had sustained a large inferior myocardial infarction (note the Q-waves in the inferior leads on ECG in panel a) for which he had received no reperfusion or revascularization therapy. Ten years later, he presented with sustained monomorphic ventricular tachycardia (panel b). A chronic total occlusion of the proximal right coronary artery was found on coronary angiography. He received an ICD which has delivered successful electrical therapies several times over the subsequent 20 years. Left ventricular ejection fraction was 40% with NYHA class II symptoms of heart failure successfully managed medically. At one point, he sustained an electrical storm for which he underwent successful radiofrequency ablation of the clinical and two other forms of inducible ventricular tachycardia. His arrhythmias remained quiescent on amiodarone for a while but recurred at 18 months and periodically thereafter were treated successfully by the ICD, either with antitachycardia pacing or occasionally via ICD shocks. *Abbreviations*: ICD = implantable cardioverter defibrillator; NYHA = New York Heart Association.

(AF) and to treat VT. However, it has been reported that the risk of SCD is markedly increased in amiodarone recipients with in those without prior history of TdP (55% vs 15%).[24] It is thus prudent to strictly avoid using amiodarone in patients with prior history of TdP. With regard to sotalol, this drug is blatantly proarrhythmic, with proarrhythmia reported in ~4% of patients, and TdP in ~2.5%, while ~1% of patients are forced to discontinue the drug as a result of worsened HF due to its negative inotropic effect.[25]

Importantly, the trials that have shown these dismal results had excluded patients with poor LV systolic function and/or overt HF. Thus, a much higher risk is expected in HF patients, which should dictate total avoidance of sotalol in HF patients.

Acute management of TdP includes immediate withdrawal of the offending agent and correction of the electrolyte abnormality, if present. However, TdP will stop recurring only after administration of intravenous (IV) magnesium sulfate, but mainly after temporary pacing at 90–110 ppm.[26] IV isoproterenol may also be a temporizing measure, but one needs to swiftly establish overdrive cardiac pacing at these higher rates, either by inserting a temporary pacing wire or, in patients fitted with a pacemaker or ICD, by increasing their pacing rate. Of course, in cases of TdP degenerating into VF, immediate defibrillation and full resuscitative measures will be needed (Figure 21.4).

Polymorphic VT without Long QT

In patients with ischemia or acute MI, polymorphic VT may occur in the absence of a prolonged QTc and can degenerate into VF.[27] In such cases, β-adrenergic blockers, correction of electrolyte abnormalities, and prompt myocardial reperfusion are required. Polymorphic VT/VF may also occur in patients with NICM or HCM. If such arrhythmias are observed in the absence of ischemia or other reversible or correctable causes, an ICD will be needed to protect the patient from SCD.

Ventricular Fibrillation (VF)

Sustained polymorphic or monomorphic VT that degenerates into VF is a common cause of out-of-hospital cardiac arrest in HF patients; in other cases, VF may be the initial ventricular tachyarrhythmia (VTA).[28] Management of such cases follows advanced cardiac life support (ACLS) guidelines, with defibrillation to restore sinus rhythm.[29] For patients successfully resuscitated, further evaluation is required to identify and treat underlying structural heart disease (e.g., reperfusion, revascularization, etc.) and potential causes of the VTA. If a transient reversible or correctable cause, such as acute MI, is not identified, patients should receive an ICD for SCD prevention. For those who are not ICD candidates, chronic amiodarone therapy may be employed.

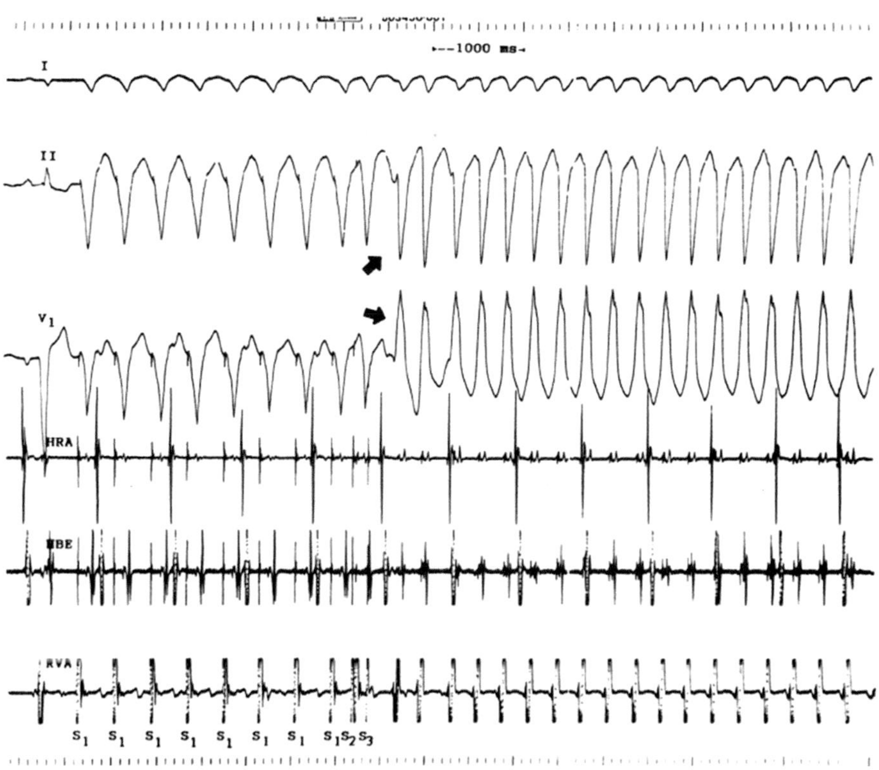

FIGURE 21.3 Electrophysiology study: programmed electrical stimulation with delivery of ventricular extrasystoles (S2/S3) after a train of eight paced beats (S1) reproducibly induces sustained monomorphic VT (arrows) most predictably in patients with underlying coronary artery disease in the setting of a prior myocardial infarction, who present with sustained monomorphic VT as their clinical arrhythmia. *Abbreviation*: VT = ventricular tachycardia.

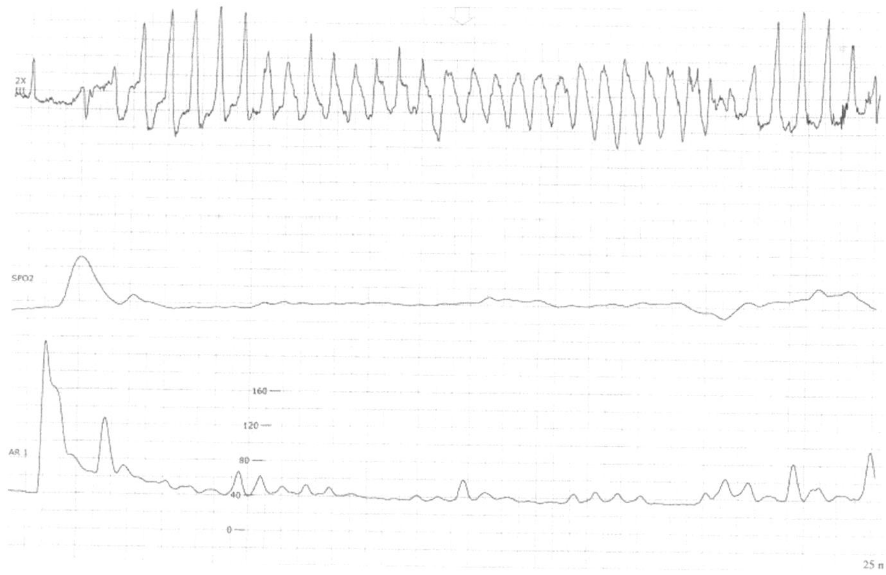

FIGURE 21.4 An 87-year-old patient with HFpEF who had been on amiodarone for AF and had a baseline prolonged QT (600 ms) but without prior history of VAs, while in hospital for HF exacerbation, received a quinolone antibiotic (ciprofloxacin) for a urinary tract infection. A day later, he developed cardiac arrest as a result of polymorphic VT in the form of TdP (upper panel) degenerating into VF. Note the immediate collapse of oximetry (mid panel) and blood pressure (lower panel) with the onset of TdP. No electrolyte abnormality or ischemia was documented. The patient had no further arrhythmic episodes after discontinuation of the antibiotic. *Abbreviations*: AF = atrial fibrillation; HF = heart failure; HFpEF = heart failure with preserved ejection fraction; TdP = torsade de pointes; VAs = ventricular arrhythmias; VT = ventricular tachycardia. (Reproduced with permission from Manolis et al., *Hospital Chronicles* 2011;6(1):50–1.)

Heart Failure with Reduced Ejection Fraction (HFrEF)

Data analyzing mortality and mode of death in patients with HFrEF in relation to New York Heart Association (NYHA) functional class indicate that the proportion of sudden deaths generally decreases with increasing severity of HF according to NYHA functional class (64% in NYHA class II, 59% in NYHA class III, and 33% in NYHA class IV). Conversely, the proportion of patients who die from worsening pump failure increases with increasing severity of HF (12% in NYHA class II, 26% in NYHA class III, and 56% in NYHA class IV).[30] On the other hand, the risk of SCD increases with the severity of HF according to LVEF; a percentual increase in SCD victims is noted at lower LVEF (0.41% in LVEF >50%, 1.2% in LVEF 40–50%, 2.2% in LVEF 30–40 and 5.1% in LVEF <30%), indicating a higher risk with poorer pump function.[31] CAD is by far the most common cause of SCD.

Heart Failure with Preserved Ejection Fraction (HFpEF)

Patients with heart failure with preserved ejection fraction (HFpEF) are a heterogeneous group associated with a plethora of comorbidities that leads to variable, but substantial, sudden death risk.[32,33] The mortality burden of HFpEF (10–30% annually), mainly ascribed to cardiovascular (CV) causes (50–70%), is lower than with HFrEF, but clearly increased compared with age- and comorbidity-matched controls without HF. Among CV deaths, sudden death and HF death are the leading cardiac modes of death in HFpEF clinical trials, although non-CV deaths constitute a higher proportion of deaths in patients with HFpEF than in those with HFrEF. Importantly, and in contrast to HFrEF, the contribution of ventricular tachyarrhythmias to sudden death has not been clearly demonstrated in patients with HFpEF, and thus the underlying mechanism of sudden death may be different in these patients. Thus, sudden death could be sudden cardiac death (SCD), either arrhythmic SCD (most commonly attributable to VT/VF and less commonly to bradyarrhythmias or pulseless electrical activity), or non-arrhythmic SCD, whereas sudden death could also be due to non-cardiac causes, such as pulmonary disease, acute hemorrhage, etc.

Ischemic Heart Disease

As mentioned, chronic ischemic heart disease, usually associated with prior MI and LV aneurysm formation, is the most common cardiac disorder associated with VT, particularly sustained monomorphic VT. Of those presenting with sustained monomorphic VT, ≈25% have their first episode within the first year following MI with a subsequent 3–5% per year incidence of VT occurrence over the following 15 years. Some investigators report that late-occurring sustained monomorphic VT most often occurs following inferior wall MI (Figure 21.2). One cannot predict which patients may develop VT early or late post-MI; importantly, in either case, the occurrence of VT is usually associated with a large infarction, severe LV dysfunction, the presence of an aneurysm, or significant CAD.[34,35] This type of clinical VT is reproducibly inducible via programmed ventricular stimulation in a high percentage (75–90%) in patients with CAD[34,36] compared to the percentage of inducible VT in patients with NICM.[37]

Polymorphic VT may self-terminate or become sustained; it is generally poorly tolerated. Sustained polymorphic VT is consistently associated with hemodynamic compromise and may degenerate into VF, most commonly observed in ischemic heart disease, followed by other forms of structural heart disease. As mentioned, when associated with prolonged QTc, it is referred to as TdP. The most common setting for polymorphic VT is acute ischemia and acute MI.[38,39] Electrolyte abnormalities and drug toxicity may exacerbate polymorphic ventricular tachyarrhythmias.

Non-Ischemic Cardiomyopathy

Sudden cardiac death (SCD) in patients with non-ischemic dilated cardiomyopathy (NICM) is mainly due to sustained ventricular tachyarrhythmias.[40] Guidelines rely on a LVEF cut-off of 35% to propose management schemes for this group of patients, practically focused on ICD implantation in patients with an LVEF ≤35%; however, LVEF is plagued by a low specificity to discern pump failure death from SCD. Furthermore, SCD can also occur in patients with HFpEF or patients with normal or mildly depressed LVEF.[32] Thus, it is indispensable to employ other markers to improve the prognostic stratification of SCD.

Myocardial fibrosis has emerged as a potent new marker for ventricular arrhythmias and SCD in patients with NICM. Areas of myocardial fibrosis may produce electrical heterogeneity and slow conduction zones in the myocardial tissue and constitute a substrate for reentry, favoring ventricular arrhythmias. Myocardial fibrosis is best evaluated with cardiac magnetic resonance (CMR) imaging wherein late gadolinium enhancement (LGE) identifies the areas and the distribution of fibrosis.[41] LGE in patients with NICM has been linked to increased mortality, HF hospitalization, and SCD and can assist in guiding risk stratification and management.[41]

PVC-Induced Cardiomyopathy

PVC-induced CM (PVC-CM) is defined as the development of LV dysfunction caused by frequent PVCs. However, PVC-CM can be superimposed on a known CM and lead to worsening of LVEF by at least 10% conferred by frequent PVCs. A PVC burden of >10% is often considered significant enough to trigger PVC-CM.[42] Others have considered a >10,000 PVC burden over 24 h as the risk factor for PVC-CM.[1] Radiofrequency ablation plays an important role in treating PVC-CM.[43]

Comorbidities and Uncorrected Structural Heart Disease

Patients with HF have an increased prevalence of cardiovascular and non-cardiovascular comorbidities.[33,44] The risk of ventricular arrhythmias is increased by coexisting comorbidities, such as ischemia, electrolyte disturbances, obstructive sleep apnea,[45] hypoxemia, chronic obstructive pulmonary disease,[46] catecholamine excess, chronic kidney disease,[47] diabetes,[48] or hepatic dysfunction.[49,50] Furthermore, the pro-arrhythmic effects of several cardiac and non-cardiac medications need also to be considered. The risk of ventricular arrhythmias and SCD is also very high in patients with underlying significant non-revascularized CAD, non-corrected valvular or congenital heart disease, or other mechanical problems (LV aneurysm or pseudoaneurysm).[51,52]

Diagnosis and Risk Stratification

Patients with HF have an increased risk of death. Ventricular arrhythmias are predominant in these patients and the question arises whether they are predictive of SCD. HF symptoms, as categorized by NYHA class and the low LVEF (≤35%), remain the most important risk factors of death in HF patients. Limited evidence indicates that runs of NSVT may also be an independent predictor of increased mortality due to SCD in patients with severe HF[53] particularly if they have a rapid rate.[13]

Other tests, such as microvolt T-wave alternans, heart rate variability, baroreflex sensitivity, and/or late potentials, may contain some prognostic information, although their positive prognostic value remains low.[1] Invasive EP studies with programmed ventricular stimulation (Figure 21.3) have an indication in ischemic CM, where demonstration of inducible monomorphic VT is associated with a high risk for SCD, but with a very limited clinical predictive value in NICM.[15,54]

The presence of myocardial scarring on CMR using gadolinium, as well as semi-quantitative measurement of adrenergic innervation by I-123 metaiodobenzylguanidine (MIBG) scans, may predict ventricular arrhythmias and identify high-risk patients,with emerging data about the utility of such non-invasive testing being encouraging.[55,56] This appears to relate to mechanisms of heterogenous myocardial conduction and local reentry promoted by myocardial scar or fibrosis that may ultimately lead to SCD. Importantly, this non-invasive risk stratifier may be also useful in patients with LVEF >35%, where there is greater and direr need for SCD risk stratification.

In keeping with the evidence provided by studies and meta-analyses on the usefulness of CMR for risk stratification,[57] the new ACC/AHA guidelines on SCD recommend that in patients with NICM, CMR with LGE can be useful for assessing the risk of SCD (class IIa, level of evidence B).[26] Whether such patients should be submitted to ICD implantation with or without the performance of an EP study awaits further investigation.

Role of Electrophysiology Study

Although a low LVEF (≤35%) and NYHA class are employed as the prime risk stratifiers in patients with HF, they remain problematic in identifying patients at truly high risk of SCD as they mainly identify patients at overall high cardiac mortality risk and not patients specifically at risk of SCD, who could maximally benefit from ICD implantation.[58] Also, all other tools and scores proposed at times for risk stratification are not specific for SCD, as all of them suffer from low positive predictive values. Combining these tests (e.g., late potentials, NSVT on Holter monitor, heart rate variability, T-wave alternans, etc.) may increase the predictive value but the number of patients having some or all of them positive sharply diminishes.

Among all of these imperfect tools, an EP study appears to be the only well-established risk stratification tool specifically for SCD, but this test also suffers from relatively low predictive values, while its major drawback is its invasive nature. Current indications for an EP study for SCD risk stratification include patients with underlying structural heart disease (ischemic CM or NICM) and an LVEF >35% or who do not meet indications for a primary prevention ICD, when they present with symptoms suggestive of ventricular tachyarrhythmias, including palpitations, presyncope, or syncope.[26,58–61] An EP study can also be used before catheter ablation of the arrhythmia substrate to guide and determine the results of the procedure. Finally, an EP study may be used to determine the mechanism of a wide complex tachycardia.[26,58,61,62] Current guidelines employ low LVEF (≤35%) as the principal risk stratifier for ICD implantation without the performance of an EP study.

Of the EP study results, only the induction of sustained monomorphic VT is considered to be a specific finding, whereas the induction of polymorphic VT or VF are considered to be non-specific findings.[63,64] Some investigators may consider that the reproducible induction of polymorphic VT/VF with one or two ventricular extrastimuli may have some clinical significance.[63] In general, induction of polymorphic VA with programmed ventricular stimulation applied at the RV outflow tract, particularly with the use of three ventricular extrastimuli, is considered to be a non-specific finding. The sensitivity and specificity of EP study is always higher in patients with CAD compared with patients with NICM. Although a positive EP study with inducible monomorphic VT may predict the occurrence of clinical monomorphic VT, its ability to predict polymorphic VT or VF is limited.

In patients with normal QTc and CAD, who have clinical polymorphic VT and/or VF, this VTA can be induced ~60–85% of the time by programmed stimulation.[65–67] Although this type of induced VA may be a nonspecific response to aggressive stimulation (e.g., with use of three ventricular extrastimuli at the RV outflow tract or very short coupling intervals, e.g., <180 ms), when induced by one to two ventricular extrastimuli and especially if reproducibly inducible, it may suggest structural basis of the VTA (functional or anatomic), indicating that the induced VA is likely to be clinically meaningful.[65]

Management

Management of ventricular arrhythmias in HF is multifaceted as one has to provide optimal medical therapy for HF, maintain electrolyte balance, avoid proarrhythmic drugs, correct underlying ischemia and other structural problems (e.g., revascularization, valve surgery, etc., as needed), implant an ICD or a CRT-D device per guideline recommendations and, in certain cases, consider catheter ablation when PVC-induced CM is suspected or when an electrical storm occurs, and finally consider mechanical support and/or heart transplant in refractory and advanced HF cases.

Medical Therapy

Standard HF Therapy

All HF patients presenting with ventricular ectopic activity should have the standard HF therapy with an ACEi or ARB, beta-blocker, and MRA optimized (class I, Level of Evidence-LOE A indication). According to the European HF guidelines,[33] treatment with beta-blocker, MRA, and sacubitril/valsartan reduces the risk of sudden death and is recommended for patients with HFrEF and ventricular arrhythmias (class I, LOE A).[30,68–73] Beta-blockers have been shown to reduce total mortality by ~35%, and SCD by ~40–45% in HF patients.[30,69] According to the American guidelines on management of ventricular arrhythmias and prevention of SCD, patients with HFrEF (LVEF ≤40%) should receive treatment with a beta-blocker, an MRA, and either an ACEi, an ARB, or an angiotensin receptor-neprilysin inhibitor to reduce SCD and all-cause mortality (class I, LOE A).[26]

The angiotensin receptor neprilysin inhibitor (ARNI), sacubitril/valsartan, was superior to enalapril in reducing both SCDs (hazard ratio-HR 0.80; p=0.008) and deaths from worsening HF (HR 0.79; p=0.034) in the PARADIGM-HF trial.[74,75] This beneficial effect might be related to cardiac reverse remodeling.[76] In a small study of 120 HF patients with ICD (NYHA class≥II; LVEF <40%), sacubitril-valsartan significantly decreased NSVT episodes (5.4±0.5 vs 15±1.7 in angiotensin inhibition; p<0.002), sustained VT, and appropriate ICD shocks (0.8% vs 6.7%; p<0.02).[77]

Antiarrhythmic Drugs

Routine use of antiarrhythmic agents is not recommended in patients with HF and ventricular arrhythmias because of safety concerns (worsening HF, proarrhythmia, and death) (class III, LOE A). Amiodarone (often in combination with a beta-blocker) may be used to suppress symptomatic ventricular arrhythmias (class IIa, LOE C), but it may adversely affect prognosis, especially in patients with more severe HF.[78,79] Practically, only amiodarone has been proven to be acceptable in the HFrEF population.[80]

Among the other antiarrhythmic agents, class I and III agents are all contraindicated in HF patients, including sotalol, which is a beta-blocker but also possesses class III antiarrhythmic effects, thus having significant potential for proarrhythmia.[81] Of the newer agents, ranolazine, which is an inhibitor of the late sodium current and additionally has effects on the sodium-dependent calcium channels during ischemia, has, in smaller studies, shown promising antiarrhythmic effects,[82,83] but larger-scale studies are needed, especially in HF patients.

Statins

Statins have not been shown to consistently ameliorate the incidence of ventricular arrhythmias in patients with HF; studies have provided conflicting results. In the CORONA trial,[84] ischemic HF patients and in the GISSI-HF trial,[85] any-cause HF patients had no reduction in SCD incidence with use of a statin (rosuvastatin 10 mg daily). However, in MADIT-CRT, in non-ischemic HF patients, the incidence of life-threatening VA was significantly lower in statin-users than in non-users.[86] Similarly, in the SCD-HeFT trial, mortality risk was significantly lower in those taking a statin (hazard ratio-HR, 0.70) in all prespecified subgroups, namely ischemic cardiomyopathy (HR 0.69), NICM (HR 0.67), ICD (HR 0.66), non-ICD (HR 0.71), NYHA II (HR 0.62), and NYHA III (HR 0.79).[87] On the other hand, a large real-world practice cohort study reported a 43% risk reduction of VT/VF/SCD and a 28% risk reduction of total mortality with statin use, with equal benefit in both ischemic and non-ischemic HF patients.[88] The authors concluded that the pleiotropic effects of statins might contribute to its antiarrhythmic properties.

Surgical/Interventional Therapies

Correction of underlying structural heart disease is of paramount importance in achieving optimal overall and antiarrhythmic management of the HF patient. It has been amply shown that revascularization has a durable antiarrhythmic and SCD-protective effect.[51,89,90] Similarly, surgical or transcatheter correction of underlying valvular disease has great overall and antiarrhythmic benefits.[91,92] For the patient with acute coronary syndrome, who develops HF and ventricular arrhythmias, timely reperfusion and urgent revascularization are crucial and lifesaving. [93] Furthermore, patients with acute MI, who undergo successful primary PCI, benefit not only acutely but also long-term by the reduced possibility incurred by successful reperfusion of developing an LV scar or aneurysm which is the substrate for future malignant VA events and SCD. [94]

Implantable Cardioverter Defibrillator

In patients with HFrEF/HFpEF and malignant ventricular tachyarrhythmias (clinical VT/VF or recurrent syncope with inducible SuVT), ICDs reduce mortality by 20–24% over the long term (two to five years) follow-up (secondary prevention) and constitute the current treatment of choice (Table 21.1). A meta-analysis of the three major secondary prevention trials showed a significant reduction in total mortality with ICD therapy compared with the best antiarrhythmic drug therapy (amiodarone) with a net HR of 0.72 (p=0.0006). [95] For the outcome of SCD, the HR was 0.50 (p<0.0001). Thus, patients with HF who develop sustained VTA (either sustained monomorphic or polymorphic VT, VF, or recurrent syncope with inducible sustained VT in the EP study) are candidates for ICD (Figure 21.5), as long as they have a reasonable life expectancy (more than one year), irrespective of their LVEF status.

For primary prevention of SCD in high-risk patients with HFrEF, ICDs also play a major role in specific patient groups who have not yet developed a malignant VTA. These groups comprise patients with a low LVEF of≤35% and prior MI where all-cause mortality was reduced by 54% over 27 months (MADIT

TABLE 21.1: Indications for Implantable Cardioverter Defibrillator Implantation in Patients with Heart Failure

Primary Prevention

- Patients with asymptomatic LV systolic dysfunction (LVEF <30%) of ischemic origin, who are at least 40 days after an acute MI (class I/LOE B)
- Patients with asymptomatic NICM (LVEF <30%), who receive optimal medical therapy, in order to prevent SCD and prolong life (class I/LOE B)
- An ICD is recommended to reduce the risk of SCD and all-cause mortality in patients with symptomatic HF (NYHA Class II–III), and an LVEF ≤35% despite three months or more of optimal medical therapy, provided they are expected to survive substantially longer than one year with good functional status, and they have: (a) IHD (unless they have had an MI in the prior 40 days) (class I/LOE A); (b) DCM (class I/LOE B)

Secondary Prevention

- An ICD is recommended to reduce the risk of SCD and all-cause mortality in patients who have recovered from a VA (VT/VF) causing hemodynamic instability, and who are expected to survive for more than one year with good functional status (class I/LOE A)

Notes: ICD implantation is not recommended within 40 days of an MI as implantation at this time does not improve prognosis (class III). ICD therapy is not recommended in patients in NYHA class IV with severe symptoms refractory to pharmacological therapy unless they are candidates for CRT, a ventricular assist device, or cardiac transplantation.

Abbreviations: HF = heart failure; ICD = implantable cardioverter defibrillator; IHD = ischemic heart disease; LOE = level of evidence; LV = left ventricular; LVEF = left ventricular ejection fraction; MI = myocardial infarction; NICM = non-ischemic cardiomyopathy; NYHA = New York Heart Association; SCD = sudden cardiac death; VA = ventricular arrhythmia; VF = ventricular fibrillation; VT = ventricular tachycardia.

Source: Adapted from Yancy et al., *J Am Coll Cardiol* 2013:e147–239.

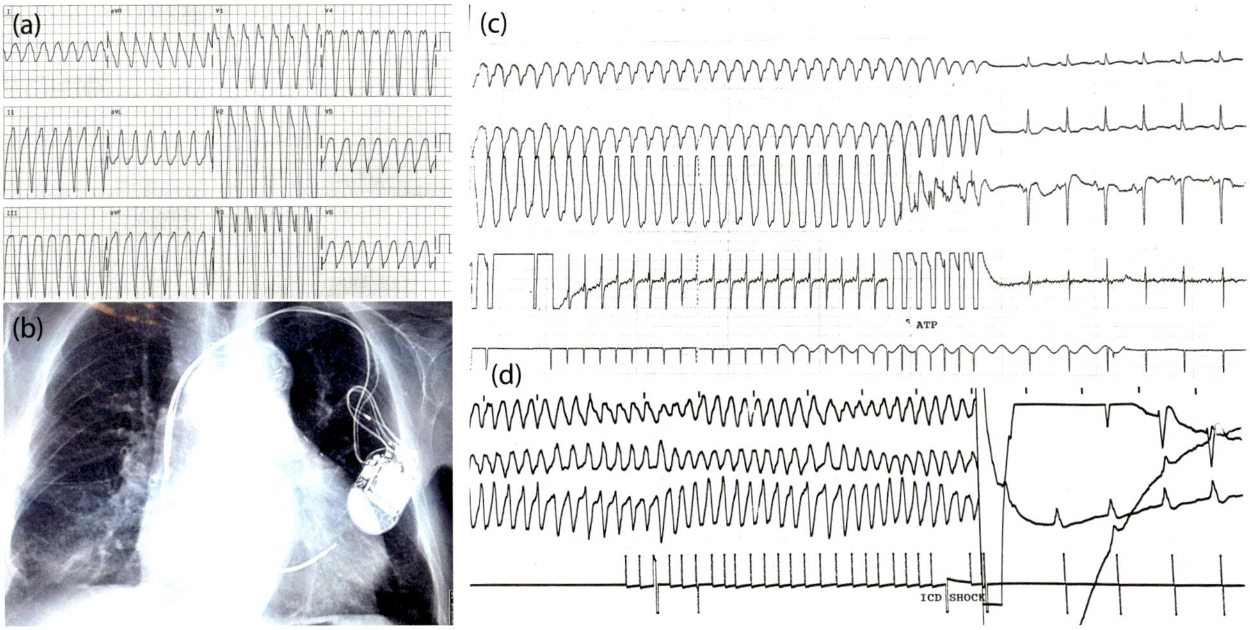

FIGURE 21.5 For patients with sustained VT (panel a), ICD implantation (panel b) is the standard prophylaxis for SCD (secondary prevention). The device can either painlessly convert VT with ATP (panel c) or, when needed (failed ATP or very fast VT or VF), it can deliver a shock and restore the rhythm (panel d). *Abbreviations*: ATP = antitachycardia pacing; ICD = implantable cardioverter defibrillator; VF = ventricular fibrillation; VT = ventricular tachycardia; SCD = sudden cardiac death.

trial);[96] patients with an LVEF <30% and prior MI where total mortality was reduced by 29% over two years (MADIT II study) (NYHA class was I–III in both studies);[97] and patients with a low LVEF (≤35%) and either ischemic CM or NICM, where total mortality was reduced by 24% over five years with the ICD (p=0.007) (SCD-HeFT study; NYHA class II or III).[78] In SCD-HeFT, the greatest benefit was observed in patients with NYHA class II HF, while NYHA class III patients had a high mortality rate due to pump failure, which may have offset the benefit of the ICD. It should be noted that ICD offers protection but no cure as it may avert SCD, but not prevent VTA. Therefore, ICD therapy needs to be accompanied by optimal medical therapy and, in ~50% of patients, there may be a need for amiodarone in addition to beta-blockers to reduce symptomatic VTA.

Particularly for patients with NICM, optimal HF therapy should precede the decision for ICD implantation by ≥3 months. The SCD-HeFT trial (n=792) provided clear evidence that favored ICD over amiodarone in prevention of SCD in NICM (hazard ratio 0.77, p=0.007).[78] Recently, the DANISH trial (n=1,116, LVEF <35%) raised concerns about the role of ICDs in primary prevention of SCD in patients with NICM. ICDs reduced SCD from 8.4% to 4.3% over a mean of 5.6 years, but with no difference in all-cause mortality.[98] However, this trial differed from previous trials as over 50% (58%) of patients in both (ICD and medical) arms received CRT (CRT-D or CRT-P). Subsequent meta-analyses that included the DANISH trial did confirm survival benefit from ICD implantation in NICM patients (22–25% relative risk reduction in mortality).[99,100] The majority of data involved patients with NYHA class II–ambulatory IV patients; hence, there is uncertainty about the utility of ICD in NICM patients with class I or class IV HF symptoms. Finally, a special group of familial NICM patients includes patients with laminopathies caused by mutations mainly in the lamin A/C gene, who appear to have a high risk of SCD, especially when they are men and have NSVT on Holter monitor, LVEF <45%, and non-missense mutations.[101] However, even lamin A/C patients with preserved (>45%) LVEF are at high risk of malignant ventricular arrhythmias in the presence of significant conduction disorders (hazard ratio 5.20; p=0.03).[102]

Cardiac Resynchronization Therapy

For patients having indication for an ICD, a CRT-D device is recommended in those also having symptoms of HF of NYHA class II, III, or ambulatory IV, an LVEF of ≤35%, and a QRS duration of ≥120 ms.[33,103] This mode of therapy is particularly effective for HF patients with left bundle branch block (LBBB) and a QRS duration >150 ms (Figure 21.6). To ensure effective CRT, biventricular pacing needs to constitute >95–98% of ventricular pacing. CRT has been associated with a reduction of VTA and consequent ICD therapies as it improves LV function.[104]

For patients in whom an LV lead cannot be placed for various reasons and thus biventricular pacing cannot be achieved, one may resort to bifocal RV pacing or His or parahisian pacing.[105] His bundle pacing, currently an elaborate procedure, may represent the preferred approach in the future.

Catheter Ablation

In patients with LV dysfunction suspected to be caused by PVCs or NSVTs ("PVC- or tachycardia-induced CM") catheter ablation should be considered (Table 21.2).[61,106,107] A high PVC burden (>24% or >10,000/24 h) in patients with LV dysfunction and a rather short coupling interval of the PVCs (<300 ms) suggest PVC-induced cardiomyopathy.[1,108] In such patients, catheter ablation can suppress PVCs and restore LV function.[43]

Occasionally, an electrical storm from polymorphic VT/VF may develop either in the subacute phase of MI or much later after the index event, and PVCs may be identified as the triggers; catheter ablation of such PVCs triggering these arrhythmias can successfully abolish electrical storm and become a life-saving procedure.[109]

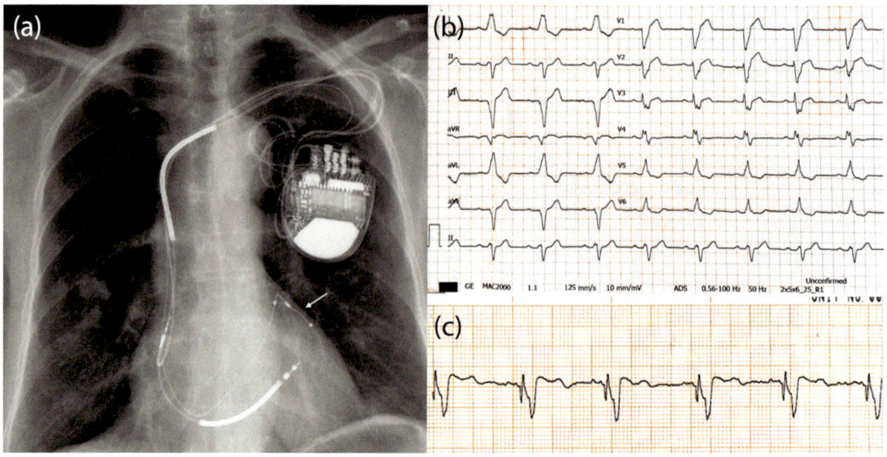

FIGURE 21.6 Cardiac resynchronization therapy (CRT) is effected via biventricular pacing and is best combined with a defibrillator device (CRT-D) rather than just a pacemaker (CRT-P); current technology allows for the use of a quadripolar left ventricular lead placed at a posterolateral coronary venous branch (white arrow, panel a) for optimization of pacing and avoidance of phrenic nerve stimulation. The best results (responder patient) are obtained when a patient with left bundle branch block and QRS duration >150 ms (panel b) is selected who has New York Heart Association class II to ambulatory IV symptoms of heart failure and when biventricular pacing results in shortening of the paced QRS duration (panel c).

In patients with recurrent VT, despite complete revascularization and optimal medical treatment, radiofrequency catheter ablation should be considered. Recurrent VT can be treated effectively with catheter ablation, which may reduce VT recurrence in both ischemic and non-ischemic cardiomyopathy.[40,110] However, all these patients need to have a backup ICD.[111] Urgent catheter ablation will be needed in patients presenting with incessant VT or an electrical storm resulting in ICD shocks (Figure 21.7). Catheter ablation is recommended in rare patients with NICM and bundle branch re-entry VT which is refractory to medical therapy.[112]

Ventricular Arrhythmias Early Post-Myocardial Infarction

In the case of a patient with a large MI who was not fortunate enough to have timely successful reperfusion and remained with compromised LV function (LVEF <35–40%), and who, according to RCTs, [113, 114] is not a candidate for a prophylactic ICD before the first 40 days have elapsed, management plans to bridge these first 40 days should include optimal medical therapy comprising beta-blockers, ACEi or ARBs, and eplerenone.[115] Utilization of the wearable cardioverter defibrillator during this period did not lead to significantly lower rate of the primary endpoint of arrhythmic death than the control.[116]

However, for those with large anterior MI and LV dysfunction, runs of NSVT, symptoms of palpitations, presyncope, or syncope, a targeted approach to SCD protection, with performance of a pre-discharge EP study, could be adopted with early implantation of an ICD for those with inducible VT.[115,117,118] For patients with recent MI who develop malignant ventricular tachyarrhythmias >48 hours after the index MI in the absence of reversible or correctable causes, an ICD should be implanted for secondary prevention.[119]

Advanced Heart Failure / LV Assist Devices / Heart Transplant

Among antiarrhythmic drugs, only amiodarone may be used to reduce ventricular arrhythmias in HF patients, although concern has been raised that its use may be associated with increased mortality.[120] Catheter ablation may also be effective in achieving VA suppression in this group of patients. Advanced therapies required for intractable progressive pump failure or refractory ventricular arrhythmias include heart transplantation and durable mechanical circulatory support with LV assist devices (LVADs), as long as these high-risk patients are reasonable candidates for these surgical therapies.[120]

Recently, a consensus statement from the American Heart Association was issued that reviews the available evidence and provides guidance on the management of arrhythmias in LVAD recipients, as well as on procedural interventions and cardiovascular implantable electronic devices (CIED) and CRT programming strategies.[121] Among other considerations and suggestions, they indicate that available evidence shows no survival benefit for ICD therapy or CRT in patients with a continuous flow (CF)-LVAD. Because sustained ventricular arrhythmias in patients with an LVAD are often well tolerated and given the adverse consequences of recurrent and painful ICD shocks, a conservative programming strategy should be used with the aim of minimizing ICD shocks. Recurrent ventricular arrhythmias in a patient with a CF-LVAD should prompt evaluation to rule out a suction event or other reversible causes such as electrolyte disturbances and drug proarrhythmia. VT ablation should be considered in patients with an LVAD with recurrent, drug-resistant ventricular arrhythmias resulting in hemodynamic compromise or recurrent ICD shocks.

Electrical Storm

Electrical storm (ES), defined as three or more sustained episodes of VT, VF, or appropriate ICD discharges over a period of 24 h, is a life-threatening condition in patients with various forms of ischemic CM or NICM and is associated with increased mortality.[122] It requires hospitalization to control ventricular tachyarrhythmias and manage hemodynamically unstable patients via medical or interventional therapy. Triggers, such as electrolyte abnormalities, proarrhythmic

TABLE 21.2: Indications for Catheter Ablation of VAs in Patients with Heart Failure

Ablation of PVCs

- In patients with CM suspected to be caused by frequent and predominantly monomorphic PVCs and for whom AADs are ineffective, not tolerated, or not preferred for long-term therapy (class I, LOE B-NR)
- In patients with SHD in whom frequent PVCs are suspected to be contributing to a CM and for whom AADs are ineffective, not tolerated, or not preferred for long-term therapy (class IIa/LOE B-NR 2)
- In non-responders to CRT with very frequent unifocal PVCs limiting optimal biventricular pacing despite pharmacological therapy (class IIa/LOE CL-D)
- Ablation of PVCs triggering an electrical storm (ES) with polymorphic VT/VF may successfully abolish ES

Ablation of VT

- In patients with IHD who experience recurrent MMVT despite chronic amiodarone therapy (class I/LOE B-R)
- In patients with IHD and recurrent symptomatic MMVT despite AAD therapy, or when AAD therapy is contraindicated or not tolerated, catheter ablation is recommended to reduce recurrent VT (class I/LOE B-NR)
- In patients with IHD and VT storm refractory to AAD therapy (class I/LOE B-NR)
- In selected patients with AHF and incessant VAs, immediate angiography (with resultant revascularization, if needed) and EP testing with radiofrequency ablation may be considered (class I/LOE B)
- In patients with IHD and recurrent MMVT, in whom AADs are not desired, catheter ablation can be useful (class IIa/LOE C-EO)
- In patients with IHD and an ICD who experience a first episode of MMVT, catheter ablation may be considered to reduce the risk of recurrent VT or ICD therapies (class IIb/LOE A).
- In patients with prior MI and recurrent episodes of symptomatic suVT for whom prior endocardial catheter ablation has not been successful and who have ECG, endocardial mapping, or imaging evidence of a subepicardial VT substrate, epicardial ablation may be considered (class IIb/LOE C-LD)
- In patients with NICM and recurrent SuMMVT for whom antiarrhythmic medications are ineffective, contraindicated, or not tolerated, catheter ablation is useful for reducing recurrent VT and ICD shocks (class I/LOE B-NR)
- In patients with NICM and electrical storm refractory to AAD therapy (class I/LOE B-NR)
- In patients with NICM, epicardial catheter ablation of VT can be useful after failure of endocardial ablation or as the initial ablation approach when there is a suspicion of an epicardial substrate or circuit (class IIa/LOE B-NR)
- In patients with cardiac sarcoidosis and recurrent VT despite medical therapy, catheter ablation can be useful to reduce the risk of VT recurrence and ICD shocks (class IIa/LOE B-NR)
- In patients with NICM and recurrent SuMMVT for whom antiarrhythmic medications are not desired, catheter ablation can be useful for reducing recurrent VT and ICD shocks (class IIa/LOE C-EO)
- In patients with NICM related to lamin A/C (LMNA) mutations and recurrent VT, catheter ablation may be considered as a palliative strategy for short-term arrhythmia control (class IIb/LOE B-NR)
- In patients with BBR VT (class I/LOE B-NR)
- In select patients at risk of requiring HS, a decision to proceed with catheter ablation of VA should be made in collaboration with specialists in advanced heart failure management (class I/LOE C-EO)
- In select patients, HS with a percutaneous VAD and ECMO during VT ablation can be useful to avoid acute hemodynamic deterioration (class IIa/LOE B-NR)
- Mechanical HS may be considered in selected cases to allow mapping and ablation of unstable VTs (class IIb/LOE B-NR)

Abbreviations: AAD = antiarrhythmic drug(s); AHF = acute heart failure; BBR = bundle branch reentry; CM = cardiomyopathy; CRT = cardiac resynchronization therapy; ECMO = extracorporeal membrane oxygenation; EP = electrophysiology; ES = electrical storm; HS = hemodynamic support; ICD = implantable cardioverter defibrillator; IHD = ischemic heart disease; LOE = level of evidence; MMVT = monomorphic ventricular tachycardia; NICM = non-ischemic cardiomyopathy; PVCs = premature ventricular complexes; SHD = structural heart disease; SuVT = sustained ventricular tachycardia; SuMMVT = sustained monomorphic ventricular tachycardia; VA = ventricular arrhythmia; VAD = ventricular assist device; VT = ventricular tachycardia.
Source: Adapted from Cronin et al., *Heart Rhythm* 2020;17:e155-e205.

drugs, ischemia, or worsening HF, or risk factors, such as suboptimal HF therapy or chronic kidney disease (CKD), need to be identified and managed. A key component in managing ES is the reduction of elevated sympathetic tone by maximizing the dose of beta-blockers, usually in combination with amiodarone and other antiarrhythmic drugs or invasive adrenergic blockade[123] and implantation of an intra-aortic balloon pump, when needed for treating hemodynamic instability. The role of catheter ablation therapy of VT-producing ES is important and potentially life-saving (Figure 21.7).[107,124] Occasionally, ES may be due to PVCs which focally trigger polymorphic VT/VF, and catheter ablation can abolish ES.[109] In some cases, CRT, with acceptable efficacy and safety, has been applied when decompensation of HF has been identified as a trigger of ES.[125] The long-term benefit of CRT seems to be due to the improved hemodynamics, as CRT-responders perform markedly better over long-term follow-up.

Ventricular Arrhythmias in Acute Heart Failure

Ventricular arrhythmias, particularly VT, are common in acute HF. In the ADHERE trial, among 105,388 patients with acute HF, 8% presented with VT and 1% developed VF.[126] Ventricular arrhythmias requiring defibrillation or resuscitation was higher (6%) in those admitted to the intensive care unit. In the VMAC trial, among 489 patients with acute HF, 13% had sustained VT and 6% developed VF.[127] In the OPTIME-CHF trial, among 949 patients, 6% developed arrhythmias of which half were ventricular arrhythmias.[128] Mortality during index hospitalization was 26% in the arrhythmia group and 1.8% in the no-arrhythmia group (p=0.001). The authors concluded

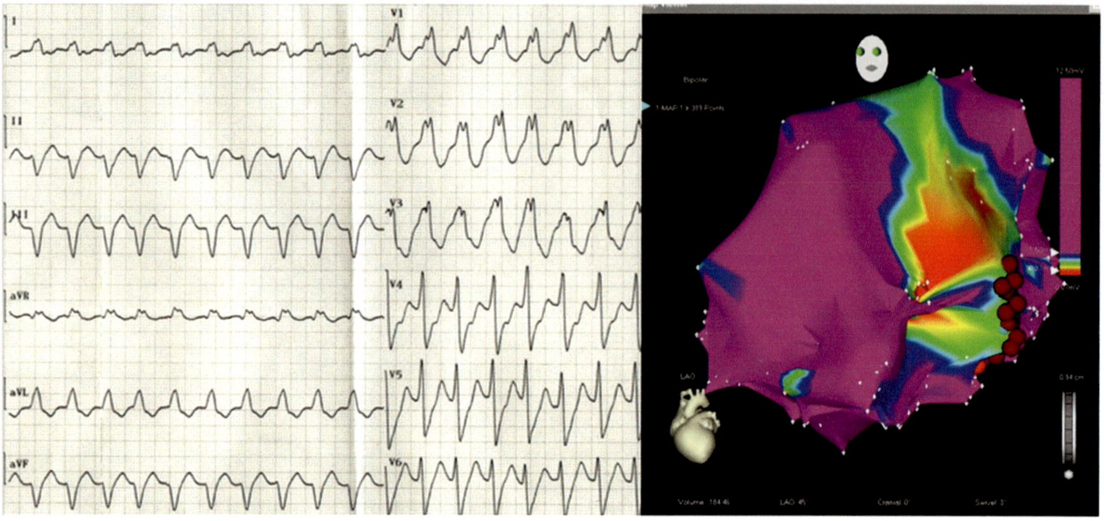

FIGURE 21.7 When a patient has frequent recurrences of ventricular arrhythmias leading to more than three ICD electrical therapies clustered over 24 hours or when the arrhythmia is incessant and usually of slow rate (left panel: sustained monomorphic VT of RBBB morphology, cycle length 480 ms or rate 125 bpm in a 65-year-old patient with ischemic cardiomyopathy and LVEF ~23%), the condition is defined as an electrical or ventricular arrhythmia storm, usually not responding to antiarrhythmic drugs and optimized medical care, where RF ablation is an effective rescue therapy, guided by EP entrainment techniques and facilitated with use of electroanatomical mapping that identifies areas of slow conduction and low-voltage electrical activity where the application of RF energy (vertical cluster of dots, right panel) can terminate and successfully ablate the arrhythmia. *Abbreviations*: EP = electrophysiology; LVEF = left ventricular ejection fraction; RBBB = right bundle branch block; RF = radiofrequency; VT = ventricular tachycardia.

that new arrhythmia during an exacerbation of HF identifies a high-risk group with higher intrahospital and 60-day morbidity and mortality.

The use of inotropic agents has been considered proarrhythmic in acute HF as a result of the beta-adrenergic effects of catecholamines (dopamine, dobutamine) or of the enhanced calcium influx into the cell as a result of an increase in cyclic AMP by phosphodiesterase inhibitors (milrinone).[129,130] On the other hand, patients receiving beta-blockers have been reported to have a lower burden of ventricular arrhythmias during acute HF exacerbation.[131] Generally, chronic maintenance therapy in HF patients presenting with acute decompensation should be continued during hospitalization unless contraindications exist.[33]

Conclusion

With the possible exception of rapid-rate NSVT, asymptomatic complex ventricular arrhythmias (frequent/multifocal PVCs and/or runs of NSVT) may not independently predict SCD in HF patients, as they may just be a nonspecific manifestation of a decompensating myocardium. On the other hand, sustained VTA portend a poor prognosis and need to be managed aggressively.

Among the standard HF therapies, beta-blockers, angiotensin system blockers (ACEi/ARBs), ARNIs, and MRAS play a protective role against VTA and SCD. Conventional antiarrhythmic drugs and other potentially proarrhythmic extracardiac drugs (e.g., QTc-prolonging agents) should be avoided. In HF patients, only amiodarone, as the antiarrhythmic drug which is devoid of a negative inotropic effect and has the least proarrhythmic risk, may be used to reduce VTA, albeit with some concern about its long-term impact on survival. For symptomatic sustained VTA and/or aborted SCD, ICDs have the greatest benefit for secondary prevention, while primary prevention is currently based on an LVEF ≤30–35% justifying prophylactic ICD implantation in both ischemic CM and NICM. When indicated, CRT has been associated with a reduction in ventricular tachyarrhythmias and consequent ICD therapies as it improves LV function. For patients with LVEF >35% and/or HFpEF, the target remains to treat comorbidities and selectively implant an ICD as based on the results of an EP study (inducible sustained VTA) and/or genetics (e.g., lamin A/C CM); CMR-detected myocardial fibrosis is emerging as a new and potent SCD risk marker and stratifier. The role of catheter ablation is important in cases of VA-induced CM and is lifesaving in cases of an electrical storm. Finally, in cases of intractable and progressive pump failure and/or refractory VTA, heart transplantation and durable mechanical circulatory support with LVADs play an important role, as long as these high-risk patients are reasonable candidates for these surgical therapies.

References

1. Lip GY, Heinzel FR, Gaita F, et al. European Heart Rhythm Association/Heart Failure Association joint consensus document on arrhythmias in heart failure, endorsed by the Heart Rhythm Society and the Asia Pacific Heart Rhythm Society. *Eur J Heart Fail.* 2015;17:848–74.
2. Tomaselli GF, Zipes DP. What causes sudden death in heart failure? *Circ Res.* 2004;95:754–63.
3. Samie FH, Jalife J. Mechanisms underlying ventricular tachycardia and its transition to ventricular fibrillation in the structurally normal heart. *Cardiovasc Res.* 2001;50:242–50.
4. Cleland JG, Chattopadhyay S, Khand A, Houghton T, Kaye GC. Prevalence and incidence of arrhythmias and sudden death in heart failure. *Heart Fail Rev.* 2002;7:229–42.
5. Arnar DO, Mairesse GH, Boriani G, et al. Management of asymptomatic arrhythmias: a European Heart Rhythm Association (EHRA) consensus document, endorsed by the Heart Failure Association (HFA), Heart

Rhythm Society (HRS), Asia Pacific Heart Rhythm Society (APHRS), Cardiac Arrhythmia Society of Southern Africa (CASSA), and Latin America Heart Rhythm Society (LAHRS). *Europace*. 2019;21:844–5.
6. Manolis AS. *Ventricular premature beats*. UpToDate; 2019.
7. Singh SN, Fisher SG, Carson PE, Fletcher RD. Prevalence and significance of nonsustained ventricular tachycardia in patients with premature ventricular contractions and heart failure treated with vasodilator therapy. Department of Veterans Affairs CHF STAT Investigators. *J Am Coll Cardiol*. 1998;32:942–7.
8. Meinertz T, Hofmann T, Kasper W, et al. Significance of ventricular arrhythmias in idiopathic dilated cardiomyopathy. *Am J Cardiol*. 1984;53:902–7.
9. Teerlink JR, Jalaluddin M, Anderson S, et al. Ambulatory ventricular arrhythmias in patients with heart failure do not specifically predict an increased risk of sudden death. PROMISE (Prospective Randomized Milrinone Survival Evaluation) Investigators. *Circulation*. 2000;101:40–6.
10. von Olshausen K, Schafer A, Mehmel HC, et al. Ventricular arrhythmias in idiopathic dilated cardiomyopathy. *Br Heart J*. 1984;51:195–201.
11. Manolis AS, Estes NA, 3rd. Value of programmed ventricular stimulation in the evaluation and management of patients with nonsustained ventricular tachycardia associated with coronary artery disease. *Am J Cardiol*. 1990;65:201–5.
12. Packer M. Lack of relation between ventricular arrhythmias and sudden death in patients with chronic heart failure. *Circulation*. 1992;85 Supplement:I50–6.
13. Chen J, Johnson G, Hellkamp AS, et al. Rapid-rate nonsustained ventricular tachycardia found on implantable cardioverter-defibrillator interrogation: relationship to outcomes in the SCD-HeFT (Sudden Cardiac Death in Heart Failure Trial). *J Am Coll Cardiol*. 2013;61:2161–8.
14. Josephson ME, Almendral JM, Buxton AE, Marchlinski FE. Mechanisms of ventricular tachycardia. *Circulation*. 1987;75:Iii41–7.
15. Hsia HH, Marchlinski FE. Electrophysiology studies in patients with dilated cardiomyopathies. *Card Electrophysiol Rev*. 2002;6:472–81.
16. Wilson P, Marks A, Rastegar H, Manolis AS, Estes NA, 3rd. Apical hypertrophic cardiomyopathy presenting with sustained monomorphic ventricular tachycardia and electrocardiographic changes simulating coronary artery disease and left ventricular aneurysm. *Clin Cardiol*. 1990;13:885–7.
17. De Ferrari GM, Rordorf R, Frattini F, et al. Predictive value of programmed ventricular stimulation in patients with ischaemic cardiomyopathy: implications for the selection of candidates for an implantable defibrillator. *Europace*. 2007;9:1151–7.
18. Wathen MS, DeGroot PJ, Sweeney MO, et al. Prospective randomized multicenter trial of empirical antitachycardia pacing versus shocks for spontaneous rapid ventricular tachycardia in patients with implantable cardioverter-defibrillators: pacing fast ventricular tachycardia reduces shock therapies (PainFREE Rx II) trial results. *Circulation*. 2004;110:2591–6.
19. Adhar GC, Larson LW, Bardy GH, Greene HL. Sustained ventricular arrhythmias: differences between survivors of cardiac arrest and patients with recurrent sustained ventricular tachycardia. *J Am Coll Cardiol*. 1988;12:159–65.
20. Stevenson WG, Brugada P, Waldecker B, Zehender M, Wellens HJ. Clinical, angiographic, and electrophysiologic findings in patients with aborted sudden death as compared with patients with sustained ventricular tachycardia after myocardial infarction. *Circulation*. 1985;71:1146–52.
21. Jebberi Z, Marazzato J, De Ponti R, et al. Polymorphic wide QRS complex tachycardia: differential diagnosis. *Card Electrophysiol Clin*. 2019;11:333–44.
22. Davey PP, Barlow C, Hart G. Prolongation of the QT interval in heart failure occurs at low but not at high heart rates. *Clin Sci (Lond)*. 2000;98:603–10.
23. Macdonald JE, Struthers AD. What is the optimal serum potassium level in cardiovascular patients? *J Am Coll Cardiol*. 2004;43:155–61.
24. Middlekauff HR, Stevenson WG, Saxon LA, Stevenson LW. Amiodarone and torsades de pointes in patients with advanced heart failure. *Am J Cardiol*. 1995;76:499–502.
25. O'Callaghan PA, McGovern BA. Evolving role of sotalol in the management of ventricular tachyarrhythmias. *Am J Cardiol*. 1996;78:54–60.
26. Al-Khatib SM, Stevenson WG, Ackerman MJ, et al. 2017 AHA/ACC/HRS guideline for management of patients with ventricular arrhythmias and the prevention of sudden cardiac death: a report of the American College of Cardiology/American Heart Association Task Force on Clinical Practice Guidelines and the Heart Rhythm Society. *J Am Coll Cardiol*. 2018;72:e91–220.
27. Passman R, Kadish A. Polymorphic ventricular tachycardia, long Q-T syndrome, and torsades de pointes. *Med Clin North Am*. 2001;85:321–41.
28. Link MS, Berkow LC, Kudenchuk PJ, et al. Part 7: adult advanced cardiovascular life support: 2015 American Heart Association Guidelines Update for Cardiopulmonary Resuscitation and Emergency Cardiovascular Care. *Circulation*. 2015;132 Supplement 2:S444–64.
29. Narayan SM, Wang PJ, Daubert JP. New concepts in sudden cardiac arrest to address an intractable epidemic: JACC state-of-the-art review. *J Am Coll Cardiol*. 2019;73:70–88.
30. MERIT-HF Study Group. Effect of metoprolol CR/XL in chronic heart failure: Metoprolol CR/XL Randomised Intervention Trial in Congestive Heart Failure (MERIT-HF). *Lancet*. 1999;353:2001–7.
31. Gorgels AP, Gijsbers C, de Vreede-Swagemakers J, Lousberg A, Wellens HJ. Out-of-hospital cardiac arrest--the relevance of heart failure. The Maastricht Circulatory Arrest Registry. *Eur Heart J*. 2003;24:1204–9.
32. Manolis AS, Manolis AA, Manolis TA, Melita H. Sudden death in heart failure with preserved ejection fraction and beyond: an elusive target. *Heart Fail Rev*. 2019;24:847–66.
33. Ponikowski P, Voors AA, Anker SD, et al. 2016 ESC guidelines for the diagnosis and treatment of acute and chronic heart failure: the Task Force for the diagnosis and treatment of acute and chronic heart failure of the European Society of Cardiology (ESC)Developed with the special contribution of the Heart Failure Association (HFA) of the ESC. *Eur Heart J*. 2016;37:2129–200.
34. Marchlinski FE, Waxman HL, Buxton AE, Josephson ME. Sustained ventricular tachyarrhythmias during the early postinfarction period: electrophysiologic findings and prognosis for survival. *J Am Coll Cardiol*. 1983;2:240–50.
35. Buxton AE, Hafley GE, Lehmann MH, et al. Prediction of sustained ventricular tachycardia inducible by programmed stimulation in patients with coronary artery disease. Utility of clinical variables. *Circulation*. 1999;99:1843–50.
36. Roy D, Marchand E, Theroux P, et al. Long-term reproducibility and significance of provokable ventricular arrhythmias after myocardial infarction. *J Am Coll Cardiol*. 1986;8:32–9.
37. Gonska BD, Bethge KP, Kreuzer H. Programmed ventricular stimulation in coronary artery disease and dilated cardiomyopathy: influence of the underlying heart disease on the results of electrophysiologic testing. *Clin Cardiol*. 1987;10:294–304.
38. Choudhuri I, Pinninti M, Marwali MR, Sra J, Akhtar M. Polymorphic ventricular tachycardia-part I: structural heart disease and acquired causes. *Curr Probl Cardiol*. 2013;38:463–96.
39. Wolfe CL, Nibley C, Bhandari A, Chatterjee K, Scheinman M. Polymorphous ventricular tachycardia associated with acute myocardial infarction. *Circulation*. 1991;84:1543–51.
40. Ebert M, Richter S, Dinov B, Zeppenfeld K, Hindricks G. Evaluation and management of ventricular tachycardia in patients with dilated cardiomyopathy. *Heart Rhythm*. 2019;16:624–31.
41. Ganesan AN, Gunton J, Nucifora G, McGavigan AD, Selvanayagam JB. Impact of late gadolinium enhancement on mortality, sudden death and major adverse cardiovascular events in ischemic and nonischemic cardiomyopathy: a systematic review and meta-analysis. *Int J Cardiol*. 2018;254:230–7.
42. Huizar JF, Ellenbogen KA, Tan AY, Kaszala K. Arrhythmia-induced cardiomyopathy: JACC state-of-the-art review. *J Am Coll Cardiol*. 2019;73:2328–44.
43. Latchamsetty R, Bogun F. Premature ventricular complex-induced cardiomyopathy. *JACC Clin Electrophysiol*. 2019;5:537–50.
44. Lawson CA, Solis-Trapala I, Dahlstrom U, et al. Comorbidity health pathways in heart failure patients: a sequences-of-regressions analysis using cross-sectional data from 10,575 patients in the Swedish Heart Failure Registry. *PLoS Med*. 2018;15:e1002540.
45. Marinheiro R, Parreira L, Amador P, et al. Ventricular arrhythmias in patients with obstructive sleep apnea. *Curr Cardiol Rev*. 2019;15:64–74.
46. van den Berg ME, Stricker BH, Brusselle GG, Lahousse L. Chronic obstructive pulmonary disease and sudden cardiac death: a systematic review. *Trends Cardiovasc Med*. 2016;26:606–13.
47. Whitman IR, Feldman HI, Deo R. CKD and sudden cardiac death: epidemiology, mechanisms, and therapeutic approaches. *J Am Soc Nephrol*. 2012;23:1929–39.
48. Movahed MR, Hashemzadeh M, Jamal M. Increased prevalence of ventricular fibrillation in patients with type 2 diabetes mellitus. *Heart Vessels*. 2007;22:251–3.
49. Ayesta A, Martinez-Selles H, Bayes de Luna A, Martinez-Selles M. Prediction of sudden death in elderly patients with heart failure. *J Geriatr Cardiol*. 2018;15:185–92.
50. Mozos I. Arrhythmia risk in liver cirrhosis. *World J Hepatol*. 2015;7:662–72.
51. Holmes DR, Jr., Davis KB, Mock MB, et al. The effect of medical and surgical treatment on subsequent sudden cardiac death in patients with coronary artery disease: a report from the Coronary Artery Surgery Study. *Circulation*. 1986;73:1254–63.
52. Taniguchi T, Morimoto T, Shiomi H, et al. Sudden death in patients with severe aortic stenosis: observations from the CURRENT AS Registry. *J Am Heart Assoc*. 2018;7:e008397.
53. Doval HC, Nul DR, Grancelli HO, et al. Nonsustained ventricular tachycardia in severe heart failure. Independent marker of increased mortality due to sudden death. GESICA-GEMA Investigators. *Circulation*. 1996;94:3198–203.

54. Chung FP, Lin CY, Lin YJ, et al. Ventricular arrhythmias in nonischemic cardiomyopathy. *J Arrhythm.* 2018;34:336–46.
55. Zeidan-Shwiri T, Yang Y, Lashevsky I, et al. Magnetic resonance estimates of the extent and heterogeneity of scar tissue in ICD patients with ischemic cardiomyopathy predict ventricular arrhythmia. *Heart Rhythm.* 2015;12:802–8.
56. Christensen TE, Kjaer A, Hasbak P. The clinical value of cardiac sympathetic imaging in heart failure. *Clin Physiol Funct Imaging.* 2014;34:178–82.
57. Manolis AS. Sudden death risk stratification in non-ischemic dilated cardiomyopathy using old and new tools: a clinical challenge. *Expert Rev Cardiovasc Ther.* 2017;15:315–25.
58. Manolis AS. The diminished role of an electrophysiology study in the current guidelines for sudden cardiac death. *Rhythmos.* 2018;13:1–5.
59. Hilfiker G, Schoenenberger AW, Erne P, Kobza R. Utility of electrophysiological studies to predict arrhythmic events. *World J Cardiol.* 2015;7:344–50.
60. Muresan L, Cismaru G, Martins RP, et al. Recommendations for the use of electrophysiological study: update 2018. *Hellenic J Cardiol.* 2019;60:82–100.
61. Priori SG, Blomstrom-Lundqvist C, Mazzanti A, et al. 2015 ESC guidelines for the management of patients with ventricular arrhythmias and the prevention of sudden cardiac death: the task force for the management of patients with ventricular arrhythmias and the prevention of sudden cardiac death of the European Society of Cardiology (ESC). Endorsed by: Association for European Paediatric and Congenital Cardiology (AEPC). *Eur Heart J.* 2015;36:2793–867.
62. Kusumoto FM, Bailey KR, Chaouki AS, et al. Systematic review for the 2017 AHA/ACC/HRS guideline for management of patients with ventricular arrhythmias and the prevention of sudden cardiac death: a report of the American College of Cardiology/American Heart Association Task Force on Clinical Practice Guidelines and the Heart Rhythm Society. *J Am Coll Cardiol.* 2018;72:1653–1676.
63. Daubert JP, Zareba W, Hall WJ, et al. Predictive value of ventricular arrhythmia inducibility for subsequent ventricular tachycardia or ventricular fibrillation in Multicenter Automatic Defibrillator Implantation Trial (MADIT) II patients. *J Am Coll Cardiol.* 2006;47:98–107.
64. Brembilla-Perrot B, Suty-Selton C, Claudon O, et al. Significance of inducible ventricular flutter-fibrillation after myocardial infarction. *Pacing Clin Electrophysiol.* 2005;28:938–43.
65. Spielman SR, Farshidi A, Horowitz LN, Josephson ME. Ventricular fibrillation during programmed ventricular stimulation: incidence and clinical implications. *Am J Cardiol.* 1978;42:913–8.
66. Schoenfeld MH, McGovern B, Garan H, et al. Determinants of the outcome of electrophysiologic study in patients with ventricular tachyarrhythmias. *J Am Coll Cardiol.* 1985;6:298–306.
67. Swerdlow CD, Bardy GH, McAnulty J, et al. Determinants of induced sustained arrhythmias in survivors of out-of-hospital ventricular fibrillation. *Circulation.* 1987;76:1053–60.
68. Pitt B, Zannad F, Remme WJ, et al. The effect of spironolactone on morbidity and mortality in patients with severe heart failure. Randomized Aldactone Evaluation Study Investigators. *N Engl J Med.* 1999;341:709–17.
69. The Cardiac Insufficiency Bisoprolol Study II (CIBIS-II): a randomised trial. *Lancet.* 1999;353:9–13.
70. Packer M, Fowler MB, Roecker EB, et al. Effect of carvedilol on the morbidity of patients with severe chronic heart failure: results of the carvedilol prospective randomized cumulative survival (COPERNICUS) study. *Circulation.* 2002;106:2194–9.
71. Flather MD, Shibata MC, Coats AJ, et al. Randomized trial to determine the effect of nebivolol on mortality and cardiovascular hospital admission in elderly patients with heart failure (SENIORS). *Eur Heart J.* 2005;26:215–25.
72. Zannad F, McMurray JJ, Krum H, et al. Eplerenone in patients with systolic heart failure and mild symptoms. *N Engl J Med.* 2011;364:11–21.
73. McMurray JJ, Packer M, Desai AS, et al. Angiotensin-neprilysin inhibition versus enalapril in heart failure. *N Engl J Med.* 2014;371:993–1004.
74. Desai AS, McMurray JJ, Packer M, et al. Effect of the angiotensin-receptor-neprilysin inhibitor LCZ696 compared with enalapril on mode of death in heart failure patients. *Eur Heart J.* 2015;36:1990–7.
75. Manolis AS, Manolis TA, Manolis AA, Melita H. Neprilysin inhibitors: filling a gap in heart failure management, albeit amidst controversy and at a significant cost. *Am J Cardiovasc Drugs.* 2019;19:21–36.
76. Martens P, Nuyens D, Rivero-Ayerza M, et al. Sacubitril/valsartan reduces ventricular arrhythmias in parallel with left ventricular reverse remodeling in heart failure with reduced ejection fraction. *Clin Res Cardiol.* 2019;108:1074–82.
77. de Diego C, Gonzalez-Torres L, Nunez JM, et al. Effects of angiotensin-neprilysin inhibition compared to angiotensin inhibition on ventricular arrhythmias in reduced ejection fraction patients under continuous remote monitoring of implantable defibrillator devices. *Heart Rhythm.* 2018;15:395–402.
78. Bardy GH, Lee KL, Mark DB, et al. Amiodarone or an implantable cardioverter-defibrillator for congestive heart failure. *N Engl J Med.* 2005;352:225–37.
79. Torp-Pedersen C, Metra M, Spark P, et al. The safety of amiodarone in patients with heart failure. *J Card Fail.* 2007;13:340–5.
80. Ezekowitz JA, O'Meara E, McDonald MA, et al. Comprehensive update of the Canadian Cardiovascular Society Guidelines for the management of heart failure. *Can J Cardiol.* 2017;33:1342–433.
81. Waldo AL, Camm AJ, deRuyter H, et al. Effect of d-sotalol on mortality in patients with left ventricular dysfunction after recent and remote myocardial infarction. The SWORD Investigators. Survival With Oral d-Sotalol. *Lancet.* 1996;348:7–12.
82. Verrier RL, Kumar K, Nieminen T, Belardinelli L. Mechanisms of ranolazine's dual protection against atrial and ventricular fibrillation. *Europace.* 2013;15:317–24.
83. Polytarchou K, Manolis AS. Ranolazine and its antiarrhythmic actions. *Cardiovasc Hematol Agents Med Chem.* 2015;13:31–9.
84. Kjekshus J, Apetrei E, Barrios V, et al. Rosuvastatin in older patients with systolic heart failure. *N Engl J Med.* 2007;357:2248–61.
85. Tavazzi L, Maggioni AP, Marchioli R, et al. Effect of rosuvastatin in patients with chronic heart failure (the GISSI-HF trial): a randomised, double-blind, placebo-controlled trial. *Lancet.* 2008;372:1231–9.
86. Buber J, Goldenberg I, Moss AJ, et al. Reduction in life-threatening ventricular tachyarrhythmias in statin-treated patients with nonischemic cardiomyopathy enrolled in the MADIT-CRT (Multicenter Automatic Defibrillator Implantation Trial with Cardiac Resynchronization Therapy). *J Am Coll Cardiol.* 2012;60:749–55.
87. Dickinson MG, Ip JH, Olshansky B, et al. Statin use was associated with reduced mortality in both ischemic and nonischemic cardiomyopathy and in patients with implantable defibrillators: mortality data and mechanistic insights from the Sudden Cardiac Death in Heart Failure Trial (SCD-HeFT). *Am Heart J.* 2007;153:573–8.
88. Liao YC, Hsieh YC, Hung CY, et al. Statin therapy reduces the risk of ventricular arrhythmias, sudden cardiac death, and mortality in heart failure patients: a nationwide population-based cohort study. *Int J Cardiol.* 2013;168:4805–7.
89. Hugenholtz PG, Serruys PW, Laird-Meeter K, Roelandt JR. Revascularization as a means of reducing sudden death. *Eur Heart J.* 1986; 7 Suppl A:181–6.
90. Ngaage DL, Cale AR, Cowen ME, Griffin S, Guvendik L. Early and late survival after surgical revascularization for ischemic ventricular fibrillation/tachycardia. *Ann Thorac Surg.* 2008;85:1278–81.
91. Gohlke-Barwolf C, Peters K, Petersen J, et al. Influence of aortic valve replacement on sudden death in patients with pure aortic stenosis. *Eur Heart J.* 1988;9 Suppl E:139–41.
92. Leon MB, Smith CR, Mack M, et al. Transcatheter aortic-valve implantation for aortic stenosis in patients who cannot undergo surgery. *N Engl J Med.* 2010;363:1597–607.
93. Mehta RH, Starr AZ, Lopes RD, et al. Incidence of and outcomes associated with ventricular tachycardia or fibrillation in patients undergoing primary percutaneous coronary intervention. *JAMA.* 2009;301:1779–89.
94. Shiga T, Hagiwara N, Ogawa H, et al. Sudden cardiac death and left ventricular ejection fraction during long-term follow-up after acute myocardial infarction in the primary percutaneous coronary intervention era: results from the HIJAMI-II registry. *Heart.* 2009;95:216–20.
95. Connolly SJ, Hallstrom AP, Cappato R, et al. Meta-analysis of the implantable cardioverter defibrillator secondary prevention trials. AVID, CASH and CIDS studies. Antiarrhythmics vs Implantable Defibrillator study. Cardiac Arrest Study Hamburg. Canadian Implantable Defibrillator Study. *Eur Heart J.* 2000;21:2071–8.
96. Moss AJ, Hall WJ, Cannom DS, et al. Improved survival with an implanted defibrillator in patients with coronary disease at high risk for ventricular arrhythmia. Multicenter Automatic Defibrillator Implantation Trial Investigators. *N Engl J Med.* 1996;335:1933–40.
97. Moss AJ, Zareba W, Hall WJ, et al. Prophylactic implantation of a defibrillator in patients with myocardial infarction and reduced ejection fraction. *N Engl J Med.* 2002;346:877–83.
98. Kober L, Thune JJ, Nielsen JC, et al. Defibrillator implantation in patients with nonischemic systolic heart failure. *N Engl J Med.* 2016;375: 1221–30.
99. Beggs SAS, Jhund PS, Jackson CE, McMurray JJV, Gardner RS. Non-ischaemic cardiomyopathy, sudden death and implantable defibrillators: a review and meta-analysis. *Heart.* 2018;104:144–50.
100. El Moheb M, Nicolas J, Khamis AM, et al. Implantable cardiac defibrillators for people with non-ischaemic cardiomyopathy. *Cochrane Database Syst Rev.* 2018;12:Cd012738.
101. van Rijsingen IA, Arbustini E, Elliott PM, et al. Risk factors for malignant ventricular arrhythmias in lamin a/c mutation carriers a European cohort study. *J Am Coll Cardiol.* 2012;59:493–500.

102. Anselme F, Moubarak G, Savoure A, et al. Implantable cardioverter-defibrillators in lamin A/C mutation carriers with cardiac conduction disorders. *Heart Rhythm.* 2013;10:1492–8.
103. Yancy CW, Jessup M, Bozkurt B, et al. 2017 ACC/AHA/HFSA focused update of the 2013 ACCF/AHA guideline for the management of heart failure: a report of the American College of Cardiology/American Heart Association Task Force on Clinical Practice Guidelines and the Heart Failure Society of America. *J Am Coll Cardiol.* 2017;70:776–803.
104. Galve E, Oristrell G, Acosta G, et al. Cardiac resynchronization therapy is associated with a reduction in ICD therapies as it improves ventricular function. *Clin Cardiol.* 2018;41:803–8.
105. Manolis AS, Koulouris S, Tsiachris D. Electrophysiology catheter-facilitated coronary sinus cannulation and implantation of cardiac resynchronization therapy systems. *Hellenic J Cardiol.* 2018;59:26–33.
106. Deyell MW, Park KM, Han Y, et al. Predictors of recovery of left ventricular dysfunction after ablation of frequent ventricular premature depolarizations. *Heart Rhythm.* 2012;9:1465–72.
107. Cronin EM, Bogun FM, Maury P, et al. HRS/EHRA/APHRS/LAHRS expert consensus statement on catheter ablation of ventricular arrhythmias: executive summary. *Heart Rhythm.* 2020;17:e155–e205.
108. Baman TS, Lange DC, Ilg KJ, et al. Relationship between burden of premature ventricular complexes and left ventricular function. *Heart Rhythm.* 2010;7:865–9.
109. Peichl P, Cihak R, Kozeluhova M, et al. Catheter ablation of arrhythmic storm triggered by monomorphic ectopic beats in patients with coronary artery disease. *J Interv Card Electrophysiol.* 2010;27:51–9.
110. Betensky BP, Marchlinski FE. Outcomes of catheter ablation of ventricular tachycardia in the setting of structural heart disease. *Curr Cardiol Rep.* 2016;18:68.
111. Frankel DS, Mountantonakis SE, Robinson MR, et al. Ventricular tachycardia ablation remains treatment of last resort in structural heart disease: argument for earlier intervention. *J Cardiovasc Electrophysiol.* 2011;22:1123–8.
112. Tchou P, Jazayeri M, Denker S, et al. Transcatheter electrical ablation of right bundle branch. A method of treating macroreentrant ventricular tachycardia attributed to bundle branch reentry. *Circulation.* 1988;78:246–57.
113. Hohnloser SH, Kuck KH, Dorian P, et al. Prophylactic use of an implantable cardioverter-defibrillator after acute myocardial infarction. *N Engl J Med.* 2004;351:2481–8.
114. Steinbeck G, Andresen D, Seidl K, et al. Defibrillator implantation early after myocardial infarction. *N Engl J Med.* 2009;361:1427–36.
115. Manolis AS. The clinical challenge of preventing sudden cardiac death immediately after acute ST-elevation myocardial infarction. *Expert Rev Cardiovasc Ther.* 2014;12:1427–37.
116. Olgin JE, Pletcher MJ, Vittinghoff E, et al. Wearable cardioverter-defibrillator after myocardial infarction. *N Engl J Med.* 2018;379:1205–15.
117. Zaman S, Sivagangabalan G, Narayan A, et al. Outcomes of early risk stratification and targeted implantable cardioverter-defibrillator implantation after ST-elevation myocardial infarction treated with primary percutaneous coronary intervention. *Circulation.* 2009;120:194–200.
118. Russo AM, Stainback RF, Bailey SR, et al. ACCF/HRS/AHA/ASE/HFSA/SCAI/SCCT/SCMR 2013 appropriate use criteria for implantable cardioverter-defibrillators and cardiac resynchronization therapy: a report of the American College of Cardiology Foundation appropriate use criteria task force, Heart Rhythm Society, American Heart Association, American Society of Echocardiography, Heart Failure Society of America, Society for Cardiovascular Angiography and Interventions, Society of Cardiovascular Computed Tomography, and Society for Cardiovascular Magnetic Resonance. *Heart Rhythm.* 2013;10:e11–58.
119. Ibanez B, James S, Agewall S, et al. 2017 ESC guidelines for the management of acute myocardial infarction in patients presenting with ST-segment elevation: the Task Force for the management of acute myocardial infarction in patients presenting with ST-segment elevation of the European Society of Cardiology (ESC). *Eur Heart J.* 2018;39:119–77.
120. Santangeli P, Rame JE, Birati EY, Marchlinski FE. Management of ventricular arrhythmias in patients with advanced heart failure. *J Am Coll Cardiol.* 2017;69:1842–60.
121. Gopinathannair R, Cornwell WK, Dukes JW, et al. Device therapy and arrhythmia management in left ventricular assist device recipients: a scientific statement from the American Heart Association. *Circulation.* 2019;139:e967–89.
122. Metaxa S, Koulouris S, Manolis AS. Electrical storm: clinical management. In: A. S. K. et al., ed. *Cardiac arrhythmias.* London: Springer-Verlag; 2014: 293–304.
123. Manolis AA, Manolis TA, Apostolopoulos EJ, Apostolaki NE, Melita H, Manolis AS. The role of the autonomic nervous system in cardiac arrhythmias: the neuro-cardiac axis, more foe than friend? *Trends Cardiovasc Med.* 2021;31:290–302.
124. Leal RT, Monteiro GC, da Silva Menezes Junior A. Catheter ablation in the treatment of electrical storm: integrative review. *Indian Pacing Electrophysiol J.* 2017;17:140–5.
125. Guerra F, Palmisano P, Dell'Era G, et al. Cardiac resynchronization therapy and electrical storm: results of the OBSERVational registry on long-term outcome of ICD patients (OBSERVO-ICD). *Europace.* 2018;20:979–85.
126. Adams KF, Jr., Fonarow GC, Emerman CL, et al. Characteristics and outcomes of patients hospitalized for heart failure in the United States: rationale, design, and preliminary observations from the first 100,000 cases in the Acute Decompensated Heart Failure National Registry (ADHERE). *Am Heart J.* 2005;149:209–16.
127. Publication Committee for the VMAC Investigators (Vasodilatation in the Management of Acute CHF). Intravenous nesiritide vs nitroglycerin for treatment of decompensated congestive heart failure: a randomized controlled trial. *JAMA.* 2002;287:1531–40.
128. Benza RL, Tallaj JA, Felker GM, et al. The impact of arrhythmias in acute heart failure. *J Card Fail.* 2004;10:279–84.
129. Burger AJ, Horton DP, LeJemtel T, et al. Effect of nesiritide (B-type natriuretic peptide) and dobutamine on ventricular arrhythmias in the treatment of patients with acutely decompensated congestive heart failure: the PRECEDENT study. *Am Heart J.* 2002;144:1102–8.
130. Amsallem E, Kasparian C, Haddour G, Boissel JP, Nony P. Phosphodiesterase III inhibitors for heart failure. *Cochrane Database Syst Rev.* 2005:Cd002230.
131. Aronson D, Burger AJ. Concomitant beta-blocker therapy is associated with a lower occurrence of ventricular arrhythmias in patients with decompensated heart failure. *J Card Fail.* 2002;8:79–85.

Section V
Non-Cardiac Comorbidities and Heart Failure

DOI: 10.1201/9780429244544-26

Chapter 22
THE MANAGEMENT OF PATIENTS WITH HEART FAILURE AND DIABETES

Tiffany Dong and Salim S. Hayek

Epidemiology of Heart Failure in Patients with Diabetes Mellitus

Prevalence and Incidence of Heart Failure in Patients with Diabetes

In the, Rubler and colleagues coined the term "diabetic cardiomyopathy," defining it as myocardial dysfunction in patients with diabetes mellitus (DM) independent of coronary, valvular, or hypertrophic causes.[1] Diabetics are at 2–5 times higher risk of developing heart failure (HF) than the general population.[2] In the United States, the prevalence of HF among Medicare beneficiaries (≥65 years old) with type 2 diabetes (T2DM) was 22.3% in 1994, and the annual incidence was 12.6% in subsequent years, with similar rates by sex and race but accelerating with age.[3] The incidence of HF in type 1 diabetics (T1DM) was 3.0% over a median of nine years and an annualized incidence of 0.34%.[4] Poor glycemic control in T1DM is strongly associated with the risk of incident HF, rising 30% for every 1% increase in HbA1c.[4] Although intensive glucose control has led to a decrease in the rate of cardiovascular complications of T1DM, the burden of HF remains significant.[5]

Diabetes, Glycemic Control, and Prognosis in Heart Failure

While DM is associated with atherosclerotic disease, HF can occur in diabetics in the absence of coronary artery disease.[6] Ischemic cardiomyopathy, however, confers a poorer prognosis in patients with DM, compared with non-ischemic cardiomyopathy.[7] Diabetes increases the rate of HF hospitalizations,[8] and is associated with a more than two-fold higher risk of all-cause and cardiovascular death in patients with HF and either reduced or preserved left ventricular (LV) ejection fraction.[9]

Glycemic control has not been consistently shown to improve indices of cardiac function. In one study of patients with DM and underlying impaired LV systolic and diastolic function, who underwent optimization of their blood glucose for one year with a median reduction in HbA1c of 2.4%, LV systolic and diastolic functions, as measured by global longitudinal strain and septal e' velocities, were improved.[10] However, other studies contradict these findings,[11,12] as intensive glycemic control does not appear to reduce the progression of HF.[13,14] For example, intensive glycemic control to an HbA1c of 6% in the ACCORD trial was associated with an increase in mortality of 22%.[15] These findings suggest that the increase in risks attributed to DM is not due solely to poor glycemic control.

Pathogenesis of Heart Failure in Patients with Diabetes

Although comorbidities associated with DM, such as hypertension, dyslipidemia, and vascular disease, increase the risk of developing HF, the diabetic milieu itself directly alters both the structure and function of the myocardium (Figure 22.1).[16] Insulin resistance promotes free fatty acid release and decreased myocardial glucose uptake. The accumulation of free fatty acids and associated metabolites induces cardiac myocyte apoptosis and inflammation in both the myocardium and the vasculature.[17] Furthermore, DM is associated with impaired contractility attributed to alterations in cardiomyocyte calcium handling through increased oxidative stress and changes in enzyme isoforms.[18]

In addition to these direct effects on the myocardium, DM worsens HF indirectly through amplification of neurohormonal responses.[19] Diabetes exacerbates the sympathetic drive and neurohormonal imbalance that are key to the development of HF. Autonomic neuropathy is a common complication of DM and causes parasympathetic denervation, leaving a heightened sympathetic response.[19] Diabetes has also been associated with higher levels of angiotensin II, inducing apoptosis, inflammation, and oxidative stress, and lastly myocardial fibrosis, often seen in autopsy studies of diabetics.[18,20]

Effectiveness of Conventional Heart Failure Therapies in Patients with Diabetes

Evidence-based therapy is effective in patients with HF, regardless of the presence of DM. A meta-analysis showed survival benefit and decreased hospitalization rates with carvedilol in patients with or without DM, without a significant difference in benefit between groups.[21] Analyses from the MERIT-HF and CIBIS II trials showed that metoprolol succinate decreased hospitalization rates while bisoprolol was associated with lower mortality rates in both diabetics and non-diabetics.[22,23]

Similarly, angiotensin-converting enzyme inhibitors (ACEis) and angiotensin receptor blockers (ARB) improve both hospitalizations and mortality to a similar extent in patients with or without diabetes. Diabetes-based subgroup analyses from the pivotal SAVE, SOLVD, and TRACE trials demonstrated a mortality reduction with captopril, enalapril, and trandolapril, respectively, for patients with diabetes, and SOLVD demonstrated decreased rate of HF hospitalizations.[24–26] Mineralocorticoid receptor antagonists also showed mortality benefit, with both spironolactone and eplerenone reducing mortality in patients with diabetes.[27,28] Thus far, no clinical trials have compared the effectiveness of hydralazine and isosorbide dinitrate between patients with or without DM.

Therapies for Diabetes Mellitus and Their Impact on the Prevention and Treatment of Heart Failure

Better glycemic control improves myocardial contractility in non-insulin-dependent diabetes for both ischemic and non-ischemic heart disease.[12] Although the exact mechanism remains unknown, possible explanations include improved microvascular perfusion, less endothelial dysfunction, and more effective myocardial energy substrate use.[12] The impact on outcomes is, however, mixed. The ORIGIN trial, which

DOI: 10.1201/9780429244544-27

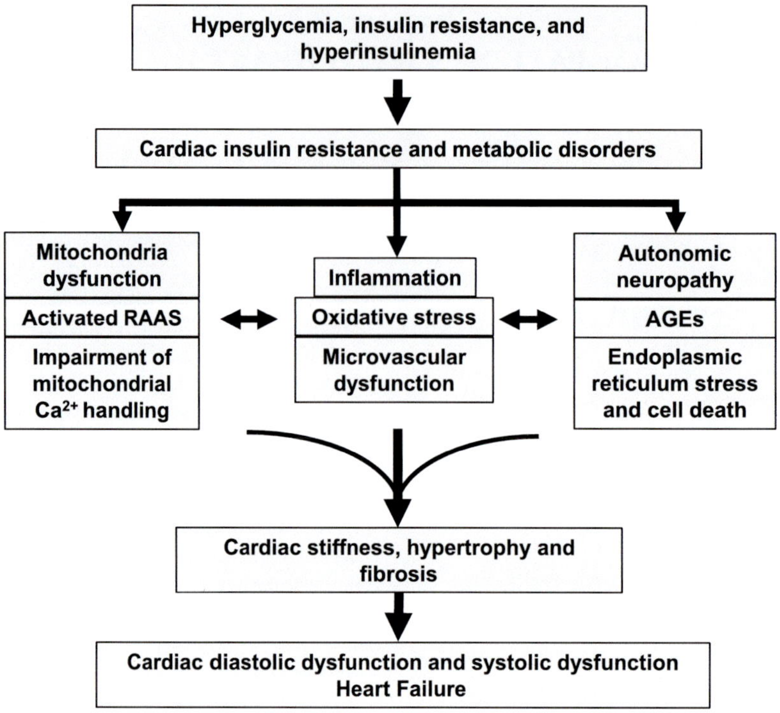

FIGURE 22.1 Pathophysiological mechanisms of diabetic cardiomyopathy. *Abbreviations*: AGEs = advanced glycation end-products; RAAS = renin-angiotensin-aldosterone system. (Modified with permission from Jia et al. *Circ Res* 2018;122:624–38.)

randomized 12,537 patients with impaired insulin sensitivity or diabetes to receive either insulin glargine or standard care, showed a non-significant trend in terms of decreasing HF hospitalizations in insulin-treated patients.[15] However, trials prior to ORIGIN failed to show improved HF outcomes with intensive insulin control.[14,29] Although certain medications for diabetes lower cardiovascular events (Table 22.1), evidence of improvement in HF outcomes was lacking, until the advent of sodium-glucose cotransporter 2 (SGLT-2) inhibitors.[30–32]

Sodium-Glucose Cotransporter 2 Inhibitors

SGLT-2 Inhibitors as a Novel Therapy for Heart Failure and Diabetes

The EMPA-REG OUTCOME trial was the first study to provide evidence of improved HF outcomes with a drug (empagliflozin), the target population of which was diabetics. Empagliflozin belongs to the SGLT-2 inhibitor family. In the kidneys, SGLT-2 serves as a sodium-glucose cotransporter and reabsorbs about 90% of the glucose, while promoting natriuresis. SGLT-2 inhibitors block this channel, enhancing glucosuria. Worsening hyperglycemia augments their function, whereas lower glucose level diminishes their efficacy, decreasing the risk of hypoglycemia with SGLT-2 inhibitors alone. However, the risk of hypoglycemia increases when SGLT-2 inhibitors are combined with insulin or insulin secretagogues, such as sulfonylureas.[33]

The EMPA-REG trial ultimately demonstrated both a reduction in major adverse cardiac events (MACE) and a decrease in HF hospitalizations in response to empagliflozin. The study randomized approximately 7,000 patients to three groups: empagliflozin 10 mg, empagliflozin 25 mg, or placebo, with a median treatment period of 2.6 years. The prevalence of HF was 11% and most patients were on established HF therapies such as beta-blockers, ACE inhibitors, and ARBs prior to enrolling. After a follow-up period of three years, combined figures from patients in the two empagliflozin groups had lower rates of three-point MACE (nonfatal myocardial infarction, cerebrovascular accident, or cardiovascular death) with a number needed to treat (NNT) of 62. Furthermore, the secondary outcome of decreased HF hospitalizations was also significant in the combined empagliflozin groups with a hazard ratio (HR) of 0.65 (95% confidence interval [CI]: 0.50–0.85) and an NNT of 71. This finding held true regardless of age, race, kidney function, and use of cardiovascular or other antidiabetic medications. In addition, the empagliflozin arms had fewer subjects initiated on loop diuretics during the course of the study, suggestive of a lower incidence of new HF with this SGLT-2 inhibitor.[34] Based on these findings, the American College of Cardiology recommended initiating empagliflozin in patients with diabetes and comorbid HF or at high risk of developing HF.[34]

The DECLARE TIMI 58 trial showed that dapagliflozin significantly reduced HF hospitalization (HR 0.83; NNT 125). The study randomized 17,160 patients with T2DM to either dapagliflozin 10 mg daily or placebo. Median follow-up was 4.2 years and approximately 10% of patients had HF. The primary endpoints were MACE, HF hospitalizations, or cardiovascular death. Unlike the EMPA-REG study, this study failed to achieve the reduction in MACE. However, along with a reduction in HF hospitalizations, they did find a lower incidence of cardiovascular death. DECLARE TIMI failed to achieve the secondary endpoints of improving renal function or all-cause mortality; however, patients with estimated glomerular filtration rate (eGFR) <60 mL/min/1.73 m^2 were excluded.[35] These two trials strengthen the argument for SGLT-2 inhibitors to reduce HF hospitalizations for patients with diabetes and HF. In a meta-analysis of DECLARE TIMI 58 and EMPA-REG, SGLT-2 inhibitors decreased the risk of cardiovascular death, myocardial

TABLE 22.1: Diabetes Drugs: Mechanism of Action and Effects on Heart Failure

Drug Class	Mechanism of Action	Effects in HF
Metformin	• Decreases hepatic gluconeogenesis • Promotes glucose uptake by skeletal muscle • Decreases TGs and VLDL; increases HDL	• Lower mortality in HF • Reduces cardiac hypertrophy • Increases cardiac glucose uptake
Sulfonylureas	• Binds to SU receptor and closes K channels on pancreatic beta cells • Increases intracellular calcium that causes release of insulin	• No increased cardiovascular risk compared to metformin • Role in HF is not established
Thiazolidinediones	• Activates PPAR-γ in adipose tissue • Decreases hepatic glucose uptake, production, and gluconeogenesis • Promotes glucose uptake by skeletal muscle • Promotes adipogenesis	• Increases fluid retention and weight gain in HF
GLP-I	• Binds GLP-I receptors • Leads to glucose-dependent insulin secretion • Possibly leads to increase B cell proliferation and survival • Prolongs gastric emptying leading to increase satiety and weight loss	• Reduced cardiovascular events but no change in HF hospitalizations • Conflicting results in HF • Mild improvement in EF • Higher rates of hospitalizations in advanced HF
DPP-4 Inhibitors	• Inhibits DPP-4, which leads to increased GLP-I levels and thus causes insulin secretion • Decreases hepatic gluconeogenesis	• Saxagliptin and alogliptin associated with higher HF hospitalization rates
SGLT2 Inhibitors	• Block SGLT2 reabsorption of glucose and thus cause glucosuria	• Canagliflozin reduced HF hospitalizations with increased risk of limb amputations among patients with diabetes and high cardiovascular risk. • Dapagliflozin reduced HF hospitalizations but no reduction in MACE with diabetes and high cardiovascular risk. • Empagliflozin with reduced HF hospitalizations and MACE in patients with diabetes and high cardiovascular risk • Both dapagliflozin and empagliflozin reduce risk of cardiovascular death and HF hospitalizations among patients with HF and reduced ejection fraction
Insulin	• Binds to insulin receptors lowering glucose levels • Reduces hepatic gluconeogenesis	• Long-acting insulin does not increase the risk of cardiovascular events • Insulin use is associated with increased risk of death in heart failure

Abbreviations: DPP-4 = dipeptidyl peptidase-4; EF = ejection fraction; GLP-I = glucagon-like peptide-1; HF = heart failure; MACE = major adverse cardiac events; PPAR-γ = peroxisome proliferator-activated receptor-γ; SGLT-2 = sodium-glucose cotransporter 2.
Source: Adapted from Kenny and Abel. *Circ Res* 2019;24(1):121–41.

infarction, and cerebrovascular accident (CVA), with a relative risk reduction (RRR) of 14% compared to placebo. This meta-analysis also confirmed the reduction in HF hospitalization (RRR 30%). Only empagliflozin was associated with significant reductions in all-cause and cardiovascular mortality (RRR 32%).[36]

Canagliflozin was examined in the CANVAS trial and was shown to reduce HF hospitalizations and combined cardiovascular events (cardiovascular mortality, non-fatal myocardial infarction, and non-fatal CVA), as well as to slow the progression of kidney disease. Canagliflozin was, however, associated with an increased incidence of lower limb amputations.[30]

SGLT-2 Inhibitors as a Novel Therapy for Heart Failure with Reduced Ejection Fraction

Building upon the previous trials, results from the DAPA-HF trial suggest that SGLT2 inhibitors may benefit non-diabetic HF patients.[37] DAPA-HF randomized 4,744 patients with HF with reduced ejection fraction, of whom 42% were diabetic, to dapagliflozin 10 mg daily or placebo. The primary endpoint was a composite of hospitalization for heart failure or need for intravenous diuretics and cardiovascular death. The primary outcome occurred in 16.3% of the dapagliflozin group and 21.2% of the placebo group with an HR 0.74 (95% CI 0.65–0.85; P<0.001). Findings were similar in patients with and without diabetes. Dapagliflozin was also associated with reduction in the secondary endpoints of worsening heart failure, death from cardiovascular death, and all-cause death.

In the EMPEROR-Reduced trial, 3,730 patients with HFrEF with or without diabetes were randomized to receive either 10 mg of empagliflozin or placebo.[38] Empagliflozin achieved a 25% reduction in the primary composite endpoint of CV death or hospitalization for worsening HF (HR 0.75, 0.65–0.86, P<0.001).[38] The total number of hospitalizations for HF was 30% lower in the empagliflozin arm (HR 0.70, 95% CI 0.58–0.85; P<0.001). Importantly, the annual rate of decline in the estimated glomerular filtration rate (a prespecified endpoint in the study) was slower in the empagliflozin arm (−0.55 vs −2.28 mL per minute per 1.73 m^2 per year, P<0.001), and empagliflozin-treated patients had a lower risk of serious renal outcomes.[38]

For more information on the use of SGLT2 inhibitors in patients with HF and reduced ejection fraction, regardless of diabetes, please refer to Chapter 10.

Mechanisms of SGLT-2 Inhibitors as Therapies for Heart Failure

There are multiple theories as to why SGLT-2 inhibition is efficacious in improving HF outcomes, including increase in

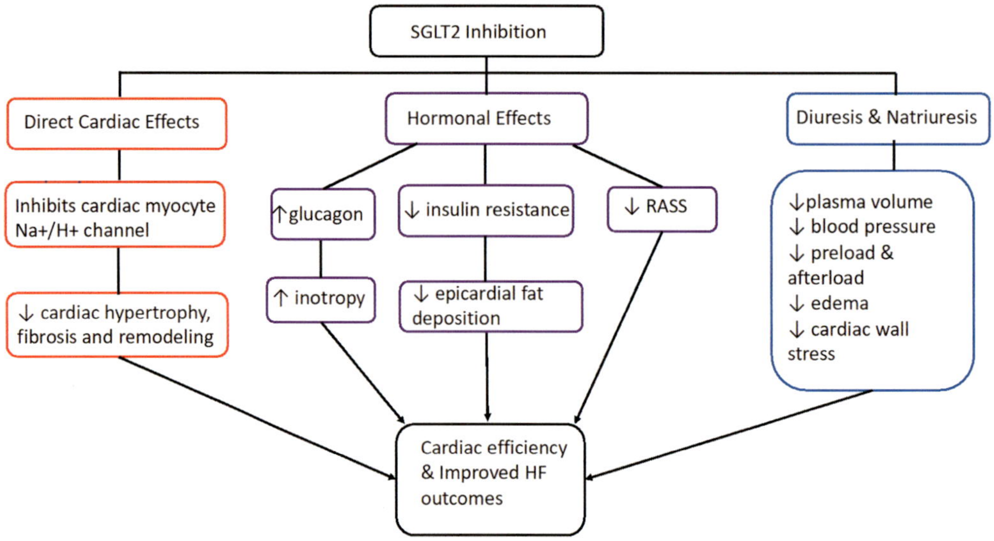

FIGURE 22.2 Mechanisms of action of SGLT-2 inhibitors. *Abbreviations*: RAAS = renin-angiotensin-aldosterone system; SGLT-2 = sodium-glucose cotransporter 2. (Adapted from Wojcik and Warden. *Curr Cardiol Rep* 2019;21:130.)

diuresis as well as natriuresis, improvement in blood pressure, decrease in neurohumoral response, and inhibition of the renin-angiotensin-aldosterone system (RAAS) (Figure 22.2). Although better glycemic control has been associated with improvement in cardiovascular health, SGLT-2 inhibitors may influence pathophysiology through other mechanisms, as the reduction in HbA1c in the EMPA-REG trial was only approximately 0.5% in both the 10 mg and the 25 mg empagliflozin groups. In addition, SGLT-2 inhibitors stimulate secretion of glucagon, increasing production of ketone bodies, which serve as a fuel for the myocardium, ultimately increasing inotropy.[39]

SGLT-2 inhibitors cause both diuresis and natriuresis through increasing both volumes of urine and concentrations of urinary sodium.[40,41] The osmotic diuresis is driven by glycosuria, as SGLT-2 inhibitors block the sodium-glucose cotransporter, whereas the natriuresis occurs because sodium is co-transported with glucose.

Although increased urine output alone could lead to a decrease in blood pressure, SGLT-2 inhibitors also appear to lower blood pressure through vasodilation. Empagliflozin reduces pulse pressure as well as arterial stiffness, through an unknown mechanism.[42,43] However, the decrease in arterial stiffness is consistent with improvement in blood pressure with this drug, and empagliflozin decreased systolic and diastolic blood pressures in the EMPA-REG BP trial.[44] The resulting reduction in afterload may also contribute to the positive impact of empagliflozin on HF outcomes.

The EMPA-REG OUTCOME trial suggests that empagliflozin may have a synergistic effect when combined with ACE inhibitors or ARBs in suppressing the RAAS system.[45] About 80% of the subjects in the EMPA-REG OUTCOME trial were already on ACE inhibitors or ARBs, and had a mean estimated glomerular filtration rate (eGFR) of ≥30 mL/min/1.73 m^2. Those in the empagliflozin groups did have slower progression to macroalbuminuria and to doubling of their serum creatinine. Moreover, empagliflozin was associated with a decrease in eGFR during the initial four weeks, with subsequent recovery, consistent with RAAS inhibition.[46] A possible mechanism by which SGLT-2 inhibitors moderate the RAAS system revolves around decreasing hyperfiltration, one of the first signs of diabetic nephropathy. The RAAS system contributes to glomerular hyperfiltration, which then progresses to glomerular hypertrophy and eventual renal injury.[47] SGLT-2 inhibitors may influence RAAS indirectly by increasing sodium delivery to the juxtaglomerular apparatus with subsequent relief of RAAS activation.[48] Empagliflozin could theoretically improve the cardio-renal axis in HF patients. SGLT2 inhibition is thought to have direct effects on the myocardium through inhibition of the myocardial sodium/hydrogen exchanger, known to be associated with inflammation and thrombosis.[39]

Contraindications and Adverse Events with SGLT-2 Inhibitors

Contraindications for SGLT-2 inhibitors include a history of hypersensitivity reactions, eGFR <30 mL/minute/1.73 m^2, or end-stage renal disease. In terms of adverse reactions, SGLT-2 inhibitors are associated with a higher incidence of genital mycotic infections, and with a higher incidence in females (10%) than males (5%) in the EMPA-REG trial.[32] A meta-analysis of multiple SGLT-2 inhibitors found that empagliflozin increases the risk of urinary tract infections in women more than men.[49] The incidence of hypovolemia was especially high in the elderly.[50] Although diuresis is beneficial for symptomatic relief of HF, adding SGLT-2 inhibitors to an existing diuretic regimen could potentially lead to overdiuresis. However, rates of volume depletion in the empagliflozin and control groups were comparable in the EMPA-REG trial.[32] Patients receiving empagliflozin exhibited an initial increase in creatinine, with subsequent recovery and stabilization of eGFR within four weeks of starting the medication.[51] Empagliflozin, however, slows the progression of chronic kidney disease.[52] Thus, it may be reasonable to initiate this medication while monitoring for renal dysfunction. Ketoacidosis is the other major concern about SGLT-2 inhibitors, as they are associated with euglycemic diabetic ketoacidosis (DKA), and should be avoided in T1DM.[53] Higher rates of DKA were noted with dapagliflozin in the DECLARE trial, but not with empagliflozin in the EMPA-REG trial.[32,35] The American Association of Clinical Endocrinologists and the American College of Endocrinology recommend holding back SGLT-2 inhibitors for at least one

TABLE 22.2: Summary of Practical Recommendations

- Metformin remains the first-line medication for diabetes mellitus type 2.
- For patients with diabetes and high cardiovascular risk, an SGLT2 inhibitor should be started to lower risk of cardiovascular events and HF hospitalizations.
- For patients with HF and reduced ejection fraction, regardless of diabetes, dapagliflozin can be started to reduce cardiovascular mortality and HF hospitalizations; empagliflozin is currently (Q2 2021) under review for the same indication.
- Contraindications to SGLT2 inhibitors include orthostatic hypotension and reduced eGFR: <30 mL/min/1.73 m^2 for dapagliflozin and empagliflozin; end-stage renal disease and dialysis for all SGLT2 inhibitors. Dapagliflozin and empagliflozin not recommended for glycemic control if eGFR <45; canagliflozin if eGFR <30. Follow latest recommendations as data on SGLT2 inhibitors are updated constantly.
- Relative contraindications to SGLT2 inhibitors include history of genital or recurrent urinary tract infections, high risk of DKA, or hypovolemia.
- Liraglutide may be added to reduce cardiovascular adverse outcomes.

Abbreviations: DKA: diabetic ketoacidosis; SGLT2: sodium-glucose cotransporter 2.

day prior to potential precipitants of DKA.[54] Although other SGLT-2 inhibitors have been associated with higher rates of bone fractures and limb amputation, empagliflozin itself has not.[55,56] In summary, SGLT-2 inhibitors should be either avoided or used cautiously in patients with history of mycotic infections, recurrent urinary tract infections, at risk for hypovolemia, or those at high risk of DKA.

Metformin

Metformin is the first-line therapy in patients with T2DM due to its efficacy and safety profile as both monotherapy and in combination.[57] Although metformin should be discontinued for use in patients with acutely decompensated HF, it appears safe to use in chronic HF.[58] Despite being the most widely used diabetes drug, its mechanism of action remains unclear. It lowers glucose by suppressing gluconeogenesis in the liver.[59] Metformin has an all-cause mortality benefit and may be more effective at decreasing the risk of cardiac events than insulin or sulfonylureas.[60] These positive findings carry over into HF treatment, as patients taking metformin have a lower incidence of HF.[61,62] Furthermore, metformin has a possible survival benefit in patients with diabetes and HF compared with other diabetic medications.[63,64] Metformin may improve cardiac health through several mechanisms, including inhibiting cardiac hypertrophy by decreasing protein synthesis,[65] and reducing cardiac fibrosis through lowering collagen synthesis.[66] Considering the availability, safety profile, and low cost of metformin, patients with HF and diabetes should be on metformin as the initial drug of choice.

Other Antidiabetic Medications and Cardiovascular Effects

Studies have shown that the glucagon-like peptide-1 (GLP-1) agonist, liraglutide, is associated with lower rates of all-cause mortality, cardiovascular mortality, non-fatal myocardial infarction, and non-fatal CVA. Liraglutide, however, failed to reduce HF hospitalizations.[31] GLP-1 agonists stimulate the distal ileum to release GLP-1, which raises insulin levels while lowering glucagon, and promotes satiety by delaying gastric emptying.[67] Contraindications to GLP-1 agonist use include hypersensitivity, end-stage renal disease, family or personal history of medullary thyroid cancer, or multiple endocrine neoplasia syndrome type 2 (MEN-2). Adverse events include resting tachycardia, increase in pancreatitis, mood disorders, and renal injury.[68]

Medications to Avoid in Patients with Diabetes and Heart Failure

Whereas empagliflozin, canagliflozin, and liraglutide are beneficial for cardiovascular health, certain medications for DM should be avoided in patients with HF, including thiazolidinediones and saxagliptin. Thiazolidinediones have been associated with worsening edema and carry a boxed warning for symptomatic HF and New York Heart Association class III or IV.[69,70] Both rosiglitazone and troglitazone are associated with pulmonary edema.[71] The PROACTIVE trial found that patients on pioglitazone had higher rates of HF hospitalizations than placebo, despite achieving their primary endpoint of reducing all-cause mortality, non-fatal myocardial infarction, and CVA.[72] The edema associated with this drug class is attributed to activation of peroxisome proliferator-activated receptor γ leading to sodium reabsorption by epithelial sodium channels in renal collecting tubules.[73]

The dipeptidyl peptidase-4 (DPP-4) inhibitors, saxagliptin and alogliptin, have been associated with an increased risk of HF hospitalizations, prompting a statement from the Food and Drug Administration.[74–77] The American Heart Association issued a scientific statement stating that saxagliptin may worsen myocardial dysfunction.[78] Although DPP-4 inhibitors increase GLP-1, they also increase the expression of stromal cell-derived factor-1, leading to cardiac fibrosis.[79]

Conclusion

Patients with DM are at an increased risk of HF. However, these patients respond similarly to HF therapies as do patients without diabetes. Metformin remains the first-line agent for patients with diabetes, including those with HF, given its cardioprotective effects. The advent of novel therapies for diabetes that have a positive impact on HF, such as SGLT-2 inhibitors and GLP-1 agonists, are set to change the landscape of HF treatment in patients with DM. Based on the EMPA-REG, CANVAS, and LEADER trials, the American College of Cardiology recommends the use of SGLT-2 inhibitors in patients with T2DM and established atherosclerotic cardiovascular disease. Based on DAPA-HF, dapagliflozin is recommended for patients with HF and reduced ejection fraction, regardless of diabetes status, and empagliflozin is currently reviewed for the same indication, based on the results of the EMPEROR-Reduced trial (see Chapter 10 for more on SGLT2 inhibitors and HF with reduced ejection fraction). Empagliflozin 10 mg and 25 mg, as well as liraglutide up to 1.8 mg, are currently preferred in patients who are not on dialysis, pregnant, or breastfeeding.[34] Table 22.2 provides a summary of the current recommendations.

References

1. Rubler S, Dlugash J, Yuceoglu YZ, et al. New type of cardiomyopathy associated with diabetic glomerulosclerosis. *Am J Cardiol*. 1972;30:595–602.

2. Nichols GA, Gullion CM, Koro CE, Ephross SA, Brown JB. The incidence of congestive heart failure in type 2 diabetes: an update. *Diabetes Care.* 2004;27:1879–84.
3. Cowie CC, Rust KF, Byrd-Holt DD, et al. Prevalence of diabetes and high risk for diabetes using A1C criteria in the U.S. population in 1988–2006. *Diabetes Care.* 2010;33:562–8.
4. Lind M, Bounias I, Olsson M, et al. Glycaemic control and incidence of heart failure in 20,985 patients with type 1 diabetes: an observational study. *Lancet.* 2011;378:140–6.
5. Konduracka E, Gackowski A, Rostoff P, et al. Diabetes-specific cardiomyopathy in type 1 diabetes mellitus: no evidence for its occurrence in the era of intensive insulin therapy. *Eur Heart J.* 2007;28:2465–71.
6. Hensel KO. Non-ischemic diabetic cardiomyopathy may initially exhibit a transient subclinical phase of hyperdynamic myocardial performance. *Med Hypotheses.* 2016;94:7–10.
7. Johansson I, Dahlstrom U, Edner M, et al. Prognostic implications of type 2 diabetes mellitus in ischemic and nonischemic heart failure. *J Am Coll Cardiol.* 2016;68:1404–16.
8. Shindler DM, Kostis JB, Yusuf S, et al. Diabetes mellitus, a predictor of morbidity and mortality in the Studies of Left Ventricular Dysfunction (SOLVD) Trials and Registry. *Am J Cardiol.* 1996;77:1017–20.
9. Cubbon RM, Adams B, Rajwani A, et al. Diabetes mellitus is associated with adverse prognosis in chronic heart failure of ischaemic and non-ischaemic aetiology. *Diab Vasc Dis Res.* 2013;10:330–6.
10. Leung M, Wong VW, Hudson M, Leung DY. Impact of improved glycemic control on cardiac function in type 2 diabetes mellitus. *Circ Cardiovasc Imaging.* 2016;9:e003643.
11. Jarnert C, Landstedt-Hallin L, Malmberg K, et al. A randomized trial of the impact of strict glycaemic control on myocardial diastolic function and perfusion reserve: a report from the DADD (Diabetes mellitus And Diastolic Dysfunction) study. *Eur J Heart Fail.* 2009;11:39–47.
12. von Bibra H, Hansen A, Dounis V, et al. Augmented metabolic control improves myocardial diastolic function and perfusion in patients with non-insulin dependent diabetes. *Heart.* 2004;90:1483–4.
13. Duckworth W, Abraira C, Moritz T, et al. Glucose control and vascular complications in veterans with type 2 diabetes. *N Engl J Med.* 2009;360:129–39.
14. Patel A, MacMahon S, Chalmers J, et al. Intensive blood glucose control and vascular outcomes in patients with type 2 diabetes. *N Engl J Med.* 2008;358:2560–72.
15. Gerstein HC, Bosch J, Dagenais GR, et al. Basal insulin and cardiovascular and other outcomes in dysglycemia. *N Engl J Med.* 2012;367: 319–28.
16. Metra M, Zaca V, Parati G, et al. Cardiovascular and noncardiovascular comorbidities in patients with chronic heart failure. *J Cardiovasc Med (Hagerstown).* 2011;12:76–84.
17. Cherian S, Lopaschuk GD, Carvalho E. Cellular cross-talk between epicardial adipose tissue and myocardium in relation to the pathogenesis of cardiovascular disease. *Am J Physiol Endocrinol Metab.* 2012;303:E937–49.
18. Dei Cas A, Khan SS, Butler J, et al. Impact of diabetes on epidemiology, treatment, and outcomes of patients with heart failure. *JACC Heart Fail.* 2015;3:136–45.
19. Givertz MM, Sawyer DB, Colucci WS. Antioxidants and myocardial contractility: illuminating the "Dark Side" of beta-adrenergic receptor activation? *Circulation.* 2001;103:782–3.
20. van Hoeven KH, Factor SM. A comparison of the pathological spectrum of hypertensive, diabetic, and hypertensive-diabetic heart disease. *Circulation.* 1990;82:848–55.
21. Shekelle PG, Rich MW, Morton SC, et al. Efficacy of angiotensin-converting enzyme inhibitors and beta-blockers in the management of left ventricular systolic dysfunction according to race, gender, and diabetic status: a meta-analysis of major clinical trials. *J Am Coll Cardiol.* 2003;41:1529–38.
22. Deedwania PC, Giles TD, Klibaner M, et al. Efficacy, safety and tolerability of metoprolol CR/XL in patients with diabetes and chronic heart failure: experiences from MERIT-HF. *Am Heart J.* 2005;149:159–67.
23. Erdmann E, Lechat P, Verkenne P, Wiemann H. Results from post-hoc analyses of the CIBIS II trial: effect of bisoprolol in high-risk patient groups with chronic heart failure. *Eur J Heart Fail.* 2001;3:469–79.
24. Yusuf S, Pitt B, Davis CE, Hood WB, Cohn JN. Effect of enalapril on survival in patients with reduced left ventricular ejection fractions and congestive heart failure. *N Engl J Med.* 1991;325:293–302.
25. Moye LA, Pfeffer MA, Wun CC, et al. Uniformity of captopril benefit in the SAVE Study: subgroup analysis. Survival and Ventricular Enlargement Study. *Eur Heart J.* 1994;15 Suppl B:2–8; discussion 26–30.
26. Gustafsson I, Torp-Pedersen C, Kober L, Gustafsson F, Hildebrandt P. Effect of the angiotensin-converting enzyme inhibitor trandolapril on mortality and morbidity in diabetic patients with left ventricular dysfunction after acute myocardial infarction. Trace Study Group. *J Am Coll Cardiol.* 1999;34:83–9.
27. Pitt B, Remme W, Zannad F, et al. Eplerenone, a selective aldosterone blocker, in patients with left ventricular dysfunction after myocardial infarction. *N Engl J Med.* 2003;348:1309–21.
28. Pitt B, Zannad F, Remme WJ, et al. The effect of spironolactone on morbidity and mortality in patients with severe heart failure. Randomized Aldactone Evaluation Study Investigators. *N Engl J Med.* 1999;341:709–17.
29. Gerstein HC, Miller ME, Byington RP, et al. Effects of intensive glucose lowering in type 2 diabetes. *N Engl J Med.* 2008;358:2545–59.
30. Neal B, Perkovic V, Mahaffey KW, et al. Canagliflozin and cardiovascular and renal events in type 2 diabetes. *N Engl J Med.* 2017;377:644–57.
31. Marso SP, Daniels GH, Brown-Frandsen K, et al. Liraglutide and cardiovascular outcomes in type 2 diabetes. *N Engl J Med.* 2016;375:311–22.
32. Zinman B, Wanner C, Lachin JM, et al. Empagliflozin, cardiovascular outcomes, and mortality in type 2 diabetes. *N Engl J Med.* 2015;373:2117–28.
33. Pham D, Albuquerque Rocha N, McGuire DK, Neeland IJ. Impact of empagliflozin in patients with diabetes and heart failure. *Trends Cardiovasc Med.* 2017;27:144–51.
34. Das SR, Everett BM, Birtcher KK, et al. 2018 ACC expert consensus decision pathway on novel therapies for cardiovascular risk reduction in patients with type 2 diabetes and atherosclerotic cardiovascular disease: a report of the American College of Cardiology Task Force on Expert Consensus Decision Pathways. *J Am Coll Cardiol.* 2018;72:3200–23.
35. Wiviott SD, Raz I, Bonaca MP, et al. Dapagliflozin and cardiovascular outcomes in type 2 diabetes. *N Engl J Med.* 2019;380:347–57.
36. Zelniker TA, Wiviott SD, Raz I, et al. SGLT2 inhibitors for primary and secondary prevention of cardiovascular and renal outcomes in type 2 diabetes: a systematic review and meta-analysis of cardiovascular outcome trials. *Lancet.* 2019;393:31–9.
37. McMurray JJV, Solomon SD, Inzucchi SE, et al. Dapagliflozin in patients with heart failure and reduced ejection fraction. *N Engl J Med.* 2019.
38. Packer M, Anker SD, Butler J, et al. Cardiovascular and renal outcomes with empagliflozin in heart failure. *N Engl J Med.* 2020;383:1413–24.
39. Wojcik C, Warden BA. Mechanisms and evidence for heart failure benefits from SGLT2 inhibitors. *Curr Cardiol Rep.* 2019;21:130.
40. List JF, Woo V, Morales E, Tang W, Fiedorek FT. Sodium-glucose cotransport inhibition with dapagliflozin in type 2 diabetes. *Diabetes Care.* 2009;32:650–7.
41. Heise T, Jordan J, Wanner C, et al. Pharmacodynamic effects of single and multiple doses of empagliflozin in patients with type 2 diabetes. *Clin Ther.* 2016;38:2265–76.
42. Chilton R, Tikkanen I, Cannon CP, et al. Effects of empagliflozin on blood pressure and markers of arterial stiffness and vascular resistance in patients with type 2 diabetes. *Diabetes Obes Metab.* 2015;17:1180–93.
43. Cherney DZ, Perkins BA, Soleymanlou N, et al. The effect of empagliflozin on arterial stiffness and heart rate variability in subjects with uncomplicated type 1 diabetes mellitus. *Cardiovasc Diabetol.* 2014;13:28.
44. Tikkanen I, Narko K, Zeller C, et al. Empagliflozin reduces blood pressure in patients with type 2 diabetes and hypertension. *Diabetes Care.* 2015;38:420–8.
45. Li L, Konishi Y, Morikawa T, et al. Effect of a SGLT2 inhibitor on the systemic and intrarenal renin-angiotensin system in subtotally nephrectomized rats. *J Pharmacol Sci.* 2018;137:220–3.
46. de Boer IH, Kahn SE. SGLT2 inhibitors-sweet success for diabetic kidney disease? *J Am Soc Nephrol.* 2017;28:7–10.
47. Helal I, Fick-Brosnahan GM, Reed-Gitomer B, Schrier RW. Glomerular hyperfiltration: definitions, mechanisms and clinical implications. *Nat Rev Nephrol.* 2012;8:293–300.
48. Cherney DZ, Perkins BA, Soleymanlou N, et al. Renal hemodynamic effect of sodium-glucose cotransporter 2 inhibition in patients with type 1 diabetes mellitus. *Circulation.* 2014;129:587–97.
49. Li D, Wang T, Shen S, et al. Urinary tract and genital infections in patients with type 2 diabetes treated with sodium-glucose co-transporter 2 inhibitors: a meta-analysis of randomized controlled trials. *Diabetes Obes Metab.* 2017;19:348–55.
50. Wu JH, Foote C, Blomster J, et al. Effects of sodium-glucose cotransporter-2 inhibitors on cardiovascular events, death, and major safety outcomes in adults with type 2 diabetes: a systematic review and meta-analysis. *Lancet Diabetes Endocrinol.* 2016;4:411–9.
51. Wanner C, Inzucchi SE, Lachin JM, et al. Empagliflozin and progression of kidney disease in type 2 diabetes. *N Engl J Med.* 2016;375:323–34.
52. Wanner C, Lachin JM, Inzucchi SE, et al. Empagliflozin and clinical outcomes in patients with type 2 diabetes mellitus, established cardiovascular disease, and chronic kidney disease. *Circulation.* 2018;137:119–29.
53. FDA. *FDA revises labels of SGLT2 inhibitors for diabetes to include warnings about too much acid in the blood and serious urinary tract infections.* 2015;2019.
54. Handelsman Y, Henry RR, Bloomgarden ZT, et al. American Association of Clinical Endocrinologists and American College of Endocrinology Position Statement on the association of Sglt-2 inhibitors and diabetic ketoacidosis. *Endocr Pract.* 2016;22:753–62.

55. Inzucchi SE, Iliev H, Pfarr E, Zinman B. Empagliflozin and assessment of lower-limb amputations in the EMPA-REG OUTCOME trial. *Diabetes Care.* 2018;41:e4–e5.
56. Ruanpeng D, Ungprasert P, Sangtian J, Harindhanavudhi T. Sodium-glucose cotransporter 2 (SGLT2) inhibitors and fracture risk in patients with type 2 diabetes mellitus: a meta-analysis. *Diabetes Metab Res Rev.* 2017;33(6):e2903–2906.
57. Foretz M, Guigas B, Bertrand L, Pollak M, Viollet B. Metformin: from mechanisms of action to therapies. *Cell Metab.* 2014;20:953–66.
58. *Glucophage (metformin hydrochloride) [package insert].* Princeton, NJ: Bristol-Myers Squibb Company; 2017.
59. El Messaoudi S, Rongen GA, de Boer RA, Riksen NP. The cardioprotective effects of metformin. *Curr Opin Lipidol.* 2011;22:445–53.
60. Intensive blood-glucose control with sulphonylureas or insulin compared with conventional treatment and risk of complications in patients with type 2 diabetes (UKPDS 33). UK Prospective Diabetes Study (UKPDS) Group. *Lancet.* 1998;352:837–53.
61. Hippisley-Cox J, Coupland C. Diabetes treatments and risk of heart failure, cardiovascular disease, and all cause mortality: cohort study in primary care. *BMJ.* 2016;354:i3477.
62. Crowley MJ, Diamantidis CJ, McDuffie JR, et al. Clinical outcomes of metformin use in populations with chronic kidney disease, congestive heart failure, or chronic liver disease: a systematic review. *Ann Intern Med.* 2017;166:191–200.
63. Eurich DT, McAlister FA, Blackburn DF, et al. Benefits and harms of antidiabetic agents in patients with diabetes and heart failure: systematic review. *BMJ.* 2007;335:497.
64. Aguilar D, Chan W, Bozkurt B, Ramasubbu K, Deswal A. Metformin use and mortality in ambulatory patients with diabetes and heart failure. *Circ Heart Fail.* 2011;4:53–8.
65. Zhang CX, Pan SN, Meng RS, et al. Metformin attenuates ventricular hypertrophy by activating the AMP-activated protein kinase-endothelial nitric oxide synthase pathway in rats. *Clin Exp Pharmacol Physiol.* 2011;38:55–62.
66. Xiao H, Ma X, Feng W, et al. Metformin attenuates cardiac fibrosis by inhibiting the TGFbeta1-Smad3 signalling pathway. *Cardiovasc Res.* 2010;87:504–13.
67. Trujillo JM, Nuffer W, Ellis SL. GLP-1 receptor agonists: a review of head-to-head clinical studies. *Ther Adv Endocrinol Metab.* 2015;6:19–28.
68. Croom KF, McCormack PL. Liraglutide: a review of its use in type 2 diabetes mellitus. *Drugs.* 2009;69:1985–2004.
69. Yki-Jarvinen H. Thiazolidinediones. *N Engl J Med.* 2004;351:1106–18.
70. Tanne JH. FDA places "black box" warning on antidiabetes drugs. *BMJ.* 2007;334:1237.
71. Thomas ML, Lloyd SJ. Pulmonary edema associated with rosiglitazone and troglitazone. *Ann Pharmacother.* 2001;35:123–4.
72. Dormandy JA, Charbonnel B, Eckland DJ, et al. Secondary prevention of macrovascular events in patients with type 2 diabetes in the PROactive Study (PROspective pioglitAzone Clinical Trial In macroVascular Events): a randomised controlled trial. *Lancet.* 2005;366: 1279–89.
73. Guan Y, Hao C, Cha DR, et al. Thiazolidinediones expand body fluid volume through PPARgamma stimulation of ENaC-mediated renal salt absorption. *Nat Med.* 2005;11:861–6.
74. Scirica BM, Bhatt DL, Braunwald E, et al. Saxagliptin and cardiovascular outcomes in patients with type 2 diabetes mellitus. *N Engl J Med.* 2013;369:1317–26.
75. Scirica BM, Braunwald E, Raz I, et al. Heart failure, saxagliptin, and diabetes mellitus: observations from the SAVOR-TIMI 53 randomized trial. *Circulation.* 2014;130:1579–88.
76. Zannad F, Cannon CP, Cushman WC, et al. Heart failure and mortality outcomes in patients with type 2 diabetes taking alogliptin versus placebo in EXAMINE: a multicentre, randomised, double-blind trial. *Lancet.* 2015;385:2067–76.
77. U.S. Food and Drug Administration. *FDA drug safety communication: FDA adds warnings about heart failure risk to labels of type 2 diabetes medicines containing saxagliptin and alogliptin.* May 4, 2016. https://www.fda.gov/drugs/drug-safety-and-availability/fda-drug-safety-communication-fda-adds-warnings-about-heart-failure-risk-labels-type-2-diabetes. Accessed March 28, 2022.
78. Kaul S, Bolger AF, Herrington D, Giugliano RP, Eckel RH. Thiazolidinedione drugs and cardiovascular risks: a science advisory from the American Heart Association and American College of Cardiology Foundation. *Circulation.* 2010;121:1868–77.
79. Packer M. Activation and inhibition of sodium-hydrogen exchanger is a mechanism that links the pathophysiology and treatment of diabetes mellitus with that of heart failure. *Circulation.* 2017;136:1548–59.

Chapter 23
THE PATIENT WITH RENAL DYSFUNCTION

Alexandros Briasoulis, Ily Kristine T. Yumul-Non, and Paulino Alvarez

Interactions between Heart Failure and Kidney Disease

Heart and kidney disease frequently co-exist and the course of one condition often interferes with the course, prognosis, and management of the other,[1] as illustrated by the following observations[2–5] A large proportion of patients with heart failure (HF) have varying degrees of renal dysfunction, varying from mild chronic kidney disease (CKD) to end-stage renal disease (ESRD) requiring dialysis. Patients with CKD carry a larger burden of comorbid cardiovascular conditions than do those without CKD, and a significantly higher risk of HF, myocardial infarction, and stroke. Cardiovascular disease (CVD) accounts for more than 50% of deaths in patients with CKD. Substantial data indicate that not only ESRD, but also Stages 3–4 CKD are associated with a significant increase in CVD risk; hence, CKD can be viewed as a CVD equivalent. Patients with ESRD are at increased risk of cardiovascular and cerebrovascular events. The incidence of cardiovascular mortality and morbidity in the subgroup with kidney disease is about two to ten times that in the general population with normal renal function.[6] The interactions between cardiac and kidney disease are commonly described by the term "cardiorenal" syndrome (CRS). According to the classification proposed by Ronco *et al.*,[7] there are five subtypes of CRS (Figure 23.1): (1) acute HF results in acute kidney injury (AKI); (2) chronic HF (or other chronic cardiac condition) causes CKD; (3) acute worsening of kidney function leads to acute HF; (4) CKD contributes to cardiac dysfunction, which may be manifested by coronary artery disease (CAD), HF, or arrhythmias; and (5) acute or chronic systemic disorders cause both cardiac and renal dysfunction.

Prevalence

Among HF patients, 30 to 60% have CKD stages 3 to 5 (defined as a glomerular filtration rate [GFR] <60 mL/min/1.73 m^2.[8] In the Acute Decompensated Heart Failure National Registry (ADHERE) of hospitalized patients with HF[9] ~30% had serum creatinine >2.0 mg/dL, mean estimated GFR was 55 mL/min/1.73 m^2, and only 9% had a normal estimated GFR (>90 mL/min/1.73 m^2). Furthermore, among hospitalized and ambulatory HF patients, ~30% have serum creatinine ≥1.5 mg/dL or higher, or a serum cystatin C ≥1.56 mg/dL.[10] Worsening renal function, defined as an increase in serum creatinine of >0.3 mg/dL, occurs in ~20 to 30% of patients treated for acute or chronic HF and particularly in those with pre-existing diabetes, uncontrolled hypertension, and CKD, usually within the first three to five days of hospitalization.[11,12]

Diagnosis

Measurement of GFR can be challenging in clinical practice. Therefore, GFR is usually estimated from serum markers. Equations to estimate GFR include[13–15] (1) the Cockcroft-Gault equation; (2) the Modification of Diet in Renal Disease (MDRD) study equation; and (3) the Chronic Kidney Disease Epidemiology Collaboration (CKD-EPI) equation. The most widely used marker to estimate GFR is serum creatinine. However, older and sicker patients often have sarcopenia and therefore reduced creatinine production. Thus, the GFR may be significantly decreased in patients with normal or only mildly elevated serum creatinine. Moreover, the aforementioned equations require that serum creatinine be stable and should not be used to estimate GFR in individuals with rising serum creatinine. In clinical settings with variable creatinine production, use of a confirmatory test, such as estimated GFR from cystatin C or creatinine-cystatin GFR- estimating equations, a 24-h urine sample for creatinine clearance, or measurement of clearance of an exogenous filtration marker (such as radioactive or non-radioactive iothalamate), will provide a more accurate assessment of GFR.[16] Among patients with HF and abnormal GFR, it is important to distinguish between CRS and underlying CKD as the cause. In those who have an elevated serum creatinine and/or a reduced estimated GFR, it is important to distinguish between CRS 1 and 2. The distinction may be challenging as several patients may have CRS 1 in the setting of pre-existing CKD. Markers of underlying CKD include significant proteinuria (more than 0.5–1 g/day), characteristic urine sediment, and diminished kidney size on sonographic evaluation. The blood urea nitrogen/creatinine ratio (BUN/Cr) is frequently used to aid in the differentiation between prerenal renal failure and intrinsic renal disease. An elevated BUN/Cr ratio is typically suggestive of a prerenal etiology and prerenal azotemia and can be caused by reduced cardiac output or volume overload in HF patients. In these settings, an elevated BUN/Cr should not deter diuresis and/or vasodilation if evidence of clinical congestion is present. Measurement of the urine sodium concentration may also be helpful, especially in patients who are not on diuretics. In HF, urine sodium concentration below 30 mEq/L can be expected, because of decreased renal perfusion and activation of the renin-angiotensin-aldosterone system (RAAS) and sympathetic nervous system (SNS), which promote sodium reabsorption.[17,18]

Pathophysiology

Kidney dysfunction in HF patients is multifactorial (Figure 23.2).[19,20] The most important mechanisms are upregulation of RAAS and SNS,[21,22] reduced renal perfusion,[23,24] increased renal venous pressure,[25,26] and right ventricular (RV) dysfunction.[27,28] Impaired left ventricular function leads to reduced stroke volume and cardiac output, arterial underfilling, elevated atrial pressures, and venous congestion. These hemodynamic derangements activate the RAAS and SNS and stimulate the release of antidiuretic hormone and endothelin-1 which, in turn, promote sodium and water retention and systemic vasoconstriction. These mechanisms also lead to the disproportionate reabsorption of urea compared with that of creatinine[21] hence, in the setting of HF, BUN is a surrogate marker of neurohormonal activation.[22] These hemodynamic and neurohormonal derangements create an imbalance

DOI: 10.1201/9780429244544-28

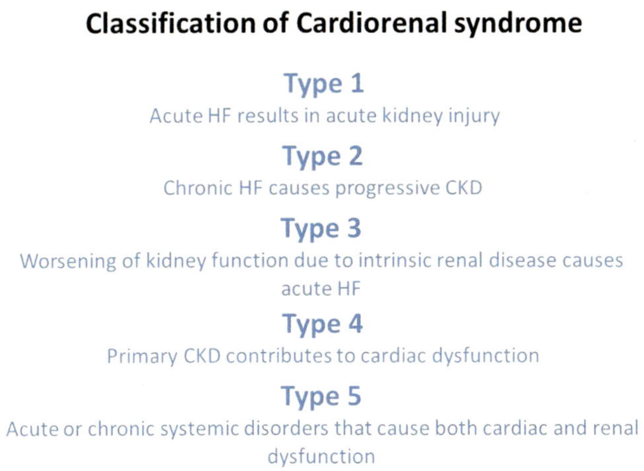

FIGURE 23.1 Classification of cardiorenal syndrome. *Abbreviations*: HF; heart failure, CKD; chronic kidney disease.

between beneficial vasodilatory and natriuretic (natriuretic peptides, nitric oxide, bradykinin) and sodium retentive and vasoconstrictive hormones.[19] Systemic vasoconstriction increases cardiac afterload, reduces cardiac output, and leads to reduced renal perfusion. Although reduced cardiac output was previously considered as the etiology of reduced renal perfusion in CRS 1, evidence from the Evaluation Study of Congestive Heart Failure and Pulmonary Artery Catheterization Effectiveness (ESCAPE) trial suggested no association between cardiac index and either the baseline GFR or worsening renal function (WRF).[23] Moreover, increasing cardiac index did not improve renal function after discharge.[29] Furthermore, CRS 1 patients did not have lower cardiac output or filling pressures.[24] Although reductions in cardiac index lead to reduced renal blood flow, GFR is initially maintained by an increase in the filtration fraction until the cardiac index decreases below 1.5 L/min.[24] On the other hand, increased renal venous pressure due to increasing intra-abdominal or central venous pressure reduces GFR.[30] In patients with HF, an inverse relationship between right atrial pressure (RAP) and GFR is present.[25] The frequency of WRF is lower in patients with a RAP <8 mmHg and the predictive value of RAP is independent of systemic blood pressure, pulmonary capillary wedge pressure, and cardiac index. A similar association has been described between elevated intra-abdominal venous pressure of ≥8 mmHg and decreased GFR that improved after decongestion.[30] Finally, RV dysfunction can adversely affect renal function via (1) elevated RAP leading to increased renal venous pressure and (2) impaired left ventricular filling and preload, due to RV dilatation and interventricular septal bowing, leading to diminished cardiac output.[27,28] Decongestive strategies result in improved RV hemodynamics and GFR by reduction in renal venous pressure and augmented cardiac output. The mechanisms of WRF described above apply not only to patients with HF and reduced ejection fraction (HFrEF) but also to patients with HF with preserved ejection fraction (HFpEF).[31]

Management of Patients with Heart Failure and Acute Kidney Injury

Treatment of acute HF can be complicated by WRF (elevation in BUN and creatinine), which, in turn, affects decisions about diuretic regimens and doses of RAAS antagonists.

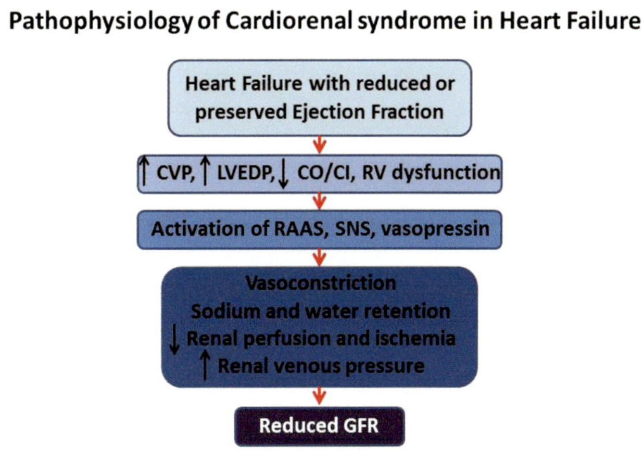

FIGURE 23.2 Pathophysiology of cardiorenal syndrome in heart failure. *Abbreviations*: CVP; central venous pressure, LVEDP; left ventricular end-diastolic pressure, CO; cardiac output, CI; cardiac index, RAAS; renin-angiotensin-aldosterone system, SNS; sympathetic nervous system, GFR; glomerular filtration rate.

Although WRF in acute HF is multifactorial, aggressive diuresis leads to intravascular volume depletion at a rate greater than the refill rate from the extravascular rate, with hemoconcentration being a common cause. However, in the ESCAPE trial,[32] hemoconcentration was related to higher loop diuretic doses, greater volume loss, and improvement in intracardiac filling pressures, and, despite WRF, it was associated with favorable six-month survival. A subsequent analysis of the Efficacy of Vasopressin Antagonism in Heart Failure Outcome Study with Tolvaptan (EVEREST) trial showed that hemoconcentration (≥3% absolute increase in hematocrit) was associated with in-hospital WRF that improved within four weeks of discharge. Hemoconcentration and WRF related to diuresis was associated with improved all-cause mortality and HF hospitalizations.[33] The timing of hemoconcentration and WRF is also important, as early intravascular depletion may not indicate euvolemia, as extravascular fluid has not yet shifted in the intravascular space. Late hemoconcentration (three to six days after initiation of diuretics) may allow greater weight loss, shorter length of stay, and improved survival compared with earlier hemoconcentration.[34] The explanation for these observations is that AKI may not be the underlying mechanism of WRF in the setting of acute HF. An analysis of 599 consecutive hospitalized patients showed that WRF alone, with the use of serum creatinine, was not an independent marker of adverse outcomes, whereas persistent congestion was.[35] Moreover, in a retrospective study of 358 patients with acute HF, WRF was not related to changes in brain-natriuretic peptide (BNP), and the development of WRF did not affect mortality.[36] Although AKI has been associated with an increase in serum creatinine, this association is not always valid. A recent analysis from the Renal Optimization Strategies Evaluation–Acute Heart Failure (ROSE–AHF) trial[37] suggested that worsening of cystatin C or creatinine levels with aggressive diuresis did not correlate with changes in the urine levels of three renal tubular injury biomarkers (N-acetyl-β-D-glucosaminidase [NAG], neutrophil gelatinase-associated lipocalin [NGAL], or kidney injury molecule 1 [KIM-1]), which detect and quantify tubular damage more accurately than serum creatinine.[38–40] The same analysis found no association between these markers and WRF; in fact, increases in tubular injury biomarkers with diuresis were not associated with adverse outcomes.[37] Similar increases in creatinine can be observed with RAAS antagonists. However, an analysis of the Heart failure Endpoint evaluation of Angiotensin II Antagonist Losartan (HEAAL) trial showed that high doses of losartan were associated with improved mortality and HF rehospitalization rates and sustained reduction in GFR compared with a lower losartan dose.[41] Based on the data above, the commonly observed WRF in acute HF should not be automatically considered to be AKI and lead to discontinuation of diuresis and RAAS antagonism. Small-to-moderate changes in creatinine during aggressive diuresis and treatment with RAAS antagonists do not seem to have adverse implications and should not trigger withdrawal of these beneficial interventions. In the setting of asymptomatic reductions in blood pressure and GFR, the goal of diuresis remains to decrease elevated central venous pressures and peripheral edema.

The effect on renal function of other strategies in addition to diuresis (Figure 23.3), used to treat acute HF, is controversial. Intravenous vasodilators, such as nesiritide (a recombinant human BNP) and nitroglycerin combined with intravenous diuresis, were associated with higher rates of WRF in the ADHERE trial.[42] The largest, randomized trial of nesiritide, ASCEND-HF, suggested that this drug results in rates of WRF similar to placebo and did not affect mortality or HF hospitalizations.[43] Finally, an analysis of the ROSE-HF trial confirmed that nesiritide did not improve volume status and hence did not alter renal function in combination with intravenous diuretics.[44] The efficacy of inotropic agents (dobutamine, dopamine, milrinone) in acute HF and WRF has not been established. The hypothesis that short-term administration of these agents may improve cardiac output and decrease renal venous pressure via dilatation of renal blood vessels, leading to increased renal blood flow, was confirmed in small series of patients[45] but failed to improve outcomes compared with intravenous diuretics alone in the Dopamine in Acute Decompensated Heart Failure (DAD-HF) and ROSE-HF trials.[44,46]

Improvement in cardiac function may favorably affect renal function in acute and chronic HF. For example, left ventricular assist devices (LVADs) lead to improved hemodynamic parameters with lower pulmonary arterial and capillary wedge pressures and higher cardiac outputs.[47] Although CRS with eGFR <60 mL/min/1.73 m^2 is found in >50% of patients with acute HF, eGFR improves to >60 mL/min/1.73 m^2 in two-thirds of patients within a month of LVAD implantation.[47,48] However, early improvement of renal function is not maintained at one year after LVAD support.[48]

Based on the above, patients with acute decompensated HF and WRF should be treated with a stepwise approach, including high-dose bolus plus continuous infusion of loop diuretics, or addition of thiazide diuretics if loop diuretics do not result in adequate volume loss, and vasodilator or inotropic therapy with hemodynamic guidance in selected patients. In refractory cases unresponsive to diuretics, ultrafiltration can be used. As demonstrated in the CARESS-HF trial, ultrafiltration was associated with similar weight loss, but increased serum creatinine and higher rate of adverse events compared with stepwise escalation of a loop diuretic-based strategy.[49] Hence, this approach should be reserved for patients not responding to medical therapy rather than being used as first-line therapy for volume control in acute HF.

Management of Patients with Heart Failure and Chronic Kidney Disease

Both HF and CKD have increasing prevalence owing to rising rates of hypertension, diabetes, and other cardiac and CKD risk factors. The Kidney Disease Improving Global Outcomes (KDIGO) guidelines define CKD as either GFR <60 mL/min/1.73 m^2 and/or one or more marker of kidney damage (electrolyte abnormalities due to tubular disorders, urine sediment abnormalities, albuminuria [>30 mg/24 h]), abnormalities detected by histology or imaging, or history of renal transplant. These abnormalities in kidney structure or function must be present for more than three months.[50] CKD may be classified based on GFR, cause, and albuminuria. Data from ADHERE suggested that concurrent CKD was present in >50% of patients admitted with decompensated HF.[51] Similar patterns were described in a meta-analysis of 25 studies of patients with HFrEF and HFpEF that found CKD stages 3 to 5 in 55% of both HF groups[52] with increasing mortality risk with worsening CKD stage or presence of albuminuria. In the Atherosclerosis Risk in Communities study, baseline CKD stage 3 or higher among HF-free participants was associated

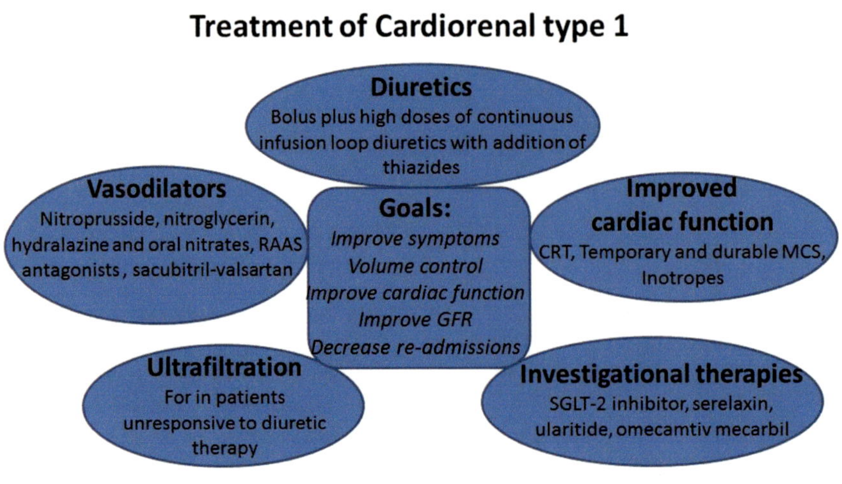

FIGURE 23.3 Treatment approach to cardiorenal type I. *Abbreviations*: CRT, cardiac resynchronization therapy, CKD; chronic kidney disease, MCS; mechanical circulatory support devices, SGLT-2; sodium glucose co-transporter 2.

with a 2-fold increased risk of incident HF compared with individuals with GFR ≥ 90 mL/min/1.73 m^2.[53]

Clinicians may be discouraged from initiating guideline-directed medical therapy (GDMT) for HFrEF in CKD patients, given less clinical data in terms of efficacy of GDMT in this population, multiple comorbid conditions, and increased mortality rates. The main objectives of HF therapy in CKD are to: (1) decrease the preload and afterload and to reduce neurohormonal activation of SNS and RAAS; (2) control risk factors such as hypertension, diabetes, and obstructive sleep apnea, and address myocardial ischemia, if present; (3) improve HF symptoms and disease-related quality of life; and (4) improve cardiac function and decrease HF related-morbidity and mortality. Even though HF management in patients with or without CKD is the same, the risk of hyperkalemia with RAAS antagonists must be strongly considered for patients with serum creatinine level >2.5–3.0 mg/dL and/or eGFR <30 mL/min/1.73 m^2.

Angiotensin Inhibition in Chronic Kidney Disease

Landmark studies in HF management with angiotensin-converting enzyme inhibitors (ACEIs) and angiotensin receptor blockers (ARBs) had represented patients with moderate CKD (eGFRs of 30–59 mL/min/1.73 m^2) but excluded those with advanced CKD. In a post-hoc analysis of the Cooperative North Scandinavian Enalapril Survival Study, which showed improved six-month mortality with enalapril compared with placebo, there was a 10–15% increase in serum creatinine within the first several weeks from a mean baseline of 1.5 mg/dL. These were associated with hypotension or other comorbidities, and in most cases, creatinine returned to within 30% of the baseline with continuation/dose reduction of the ACEI.[54] The Valsartan in Heart Failure Trial (Val-HEFT) excluded patients with serum creatinine >2.5 mg/dL; however, 60% of patients had GFR <60 mL/min/1.73 m^2. A secondary analysis of Val-HEFT in this CKD group showed a lower rate of the first morbid event.[55] A propensity score analysis from the Digitalis Investigation Group trial showed that, among patients with CKD (serum creatinine 1.3–2.5 mg/dL), therapy with ACEI was associated with lower rates of mortality and all-cause hospitalizations.[56] Finally, in patients >75 years of age with HFrEF and CKD (GFR <45 mL/min/1.73 m^2), treatment with ACEI/ARBs is associated with a decreased rate of major adverse cardiac events as long as there is no other formal contraindication to its use.[57]

Studies on HFrEF and more advanced CKD are mostly observational. RAAS inhibition was associated with higher one-year survival in a propensity-matched cohort of patients with HFrEF and CKD stages 4 and 5 with an efficacy similar to those without CKD.[58] A combination of ACEI and ARB significantly increases the risk of adverse effects and should not be used.[59] The KDIGO guidelines recommend a reduced starting dose of ACEI/ARBs and follow-up on potassium levels one week after initiation in patients with CKD stage 3b or higher. Patients with CKD stage 4 or 5 would still benefit from ACEI/ARBs and routine discontinuation is not advised, given the current strategies to manage hyperkalemia.[50] Consultation with a nephrologist would be advisable for those patients with HF and advanced CKD.[60]

Intolerance to Angiotensin Inhibition

The combination of hydralazine and isosorbide dinitrate was associated with improved survival in a post-hoc analysis of Black patients from the Vasodilator Heart Failure Trial (V-HeFT I).[60] In the African-American Heart Failure Trial (A-HeFT), ~17% of patients had CKD and were on background neurohormonal blockade. Among these patients, all-cause mortality, hospitalization for HF, and change in quality-of-life score at six months were significantly better than placebo.[61] Therefore, this combination can be used as an alternative in patients (particularly African Americans) with HFrEF who are unable to tolerate an ACEI or ARB.

Angiotensin Receptor-Neprilysin Inhibitors in Chronic Kidney Disease

The PARADIGM-HF trial suggested a significant benefit of angiotensin receptor-neprilysin inhibitors (ARNIs) on HF symptoms, hospitalizations, cardiovascular and overall mortality.[62] Of note, this trial excluded patients with GFR <30 mL/min/1.73 m^2 and further excluded those with (1) >35% decrease in GFR from the baseline; (2) GFR that decreased to <30 mL/min/1.73 m^2; and (3) potassium >5.5 mEq/L during the run-in period.[62] In a subgroup analysis of this trial (excluding CKD stages 4 and 5), ARNI led to improved cardiovascular outcomes and a slower rate of GFR decrease compared with enalapril.[63] Further studies are warranted to determine whether these findings are applicable to those patients with advanced CKD.

Beta-Blockers in Chronic Kidney Disease

Sympathetic overactivity plays a key role in the development and progression of hypertension and left ventricular hypertrophy in CKD patients. It is thought that adverse cardiovascular events and mortality in these patients can be predicted by high plasma epinephrine levels.[64] The benefits of beta-blockers in patients with CKD had been studied in multiple subgroup analyses. In an analysis of Cardiac Insufficiency Bisoprolol Study II, a decreased risk of HF hospitalization or all-cause mortality was detected in patients with CKD stage 3b or higher.[65] In a secondary analysis of the Metoprolol CR/XL Controlled Randomized Intervention Trial in Chronic Heart Failure trial, treatment with the beta-blocker was associated with a ~60% decrease in total mortality and hospitalizations for HF.[66] In the Study of the Effects of Nebivolol Intervention on Outcomes and Rehospitalization in Seniors with Heart Failure, the primary outcome of all-cause mortality or cardiovascular hospital admission was significantly reduced with nebivolol in the group with CKD.[67] Finally, a meta-analysis of six placebo-controlled trials showed that β-blockers reduced the risk of all-cause and cardiovascular mortality but increased the risk of hypotension and bradycardia.[68]

Beta-blocker use in patients with CKD is supported by the American HF guidelines; the KDIGO guidelines suggest that the dose should be reduced by 50% for those with CKD stages 4 and 5.[50,59]

Aldosterone Antagonists in Chronic Kidney Disease

Several major trials of aldosterone antagonists (AA) in HF had excluded patients with moderate or severe CKD given concerns for hyperkalemia; thus, the effect of AA in this group of patients is not definitive. In contrast, patients on dialysis may be able to tolerate higher potassium levels without clinical manifestations as hyperkalemia will be effectively managed by dialysis.[69]

Both the Randomized Aldactone Evaluation Study (RALES) and the Eplerenone Post-Acute Myocardial Infarction Heart Failure Efficacy and Survival (EPHESUS) trials excluded patients with serum creatinine levels >2.5 mg/dL.[70,71] In a recent, large retrospective study of HF patients with concomitant CKD and/or diabetes mellitus, AA therapy at discharge was associated with a lower long-term risk of all-cause readmission. However, there were greater short-term and long-term risks of readmission secondary to hyperkalemia and WRF.[72]

In CKD stages 3b and 4, doses of spironolactone >25 mg daily should be avoided or used with very close monitoring of potassium levels.[73] In CKD stage 5, AAs should generally be avoided. In consideration of pharmacokinetics, physicians might consider eplerenone over spironolactone, given the former's shorter plasma half-life; one can subsequently deduce that this will allow the kidneys to excrete potassium more efficaciously and thus hyperkalemia will resolve faster.[74]

Diuretics

Loop diuretics are generally the preferred diuretic in patients with renal insufficiency. With a thiazide-type diuretic, the action is attenuated when the GFR is <50 mL/min/1.73 m^2. However, thiazides can be used to augment the effect of loop diuretics in patients with CKD, since the loop diuretic-induced increase in sodium delivery out of the loop of Henle leads to increased distal tubule sodium reabsorption, which is targeted by thiazides. Although furosemide is the most commonly used loop diuretic, bioavailability of the oral formulation is ~50%, with substantial variability[75] Torsemide has a longer half-life than furosemide, whereas both bumetanide and torsemide have more predictable bioavailabilities. Therefore, the response to torsemide or bumetanide may be greater than that to furosemide and this is supported by an open-label, randomized trial of HF patients that showed lower re-admission rates with torsemide than with furosemide.[76] Appropriate dosing of loop diuretics is even more important than the type of diuretic. Patients with HF have a lower response to a given dose of diuretic than normal subjects because of (1) decreased diuretic delivery to the kidney due to reduced renal blood flow; (2) increased sodium reabsorption at other sites due to hypoperfusion and neurohormonal activation; and (3) diminished intestinal absorption of oral loop diuretics in hypervolemic patients.[75] The dose, rather than the frequency of administration, of loop diuretics should be increased gradually to maintain the patient's dry weight.

Fluid loss in response to diuresis leads to decreased intravascular volume and capillary pressure, thus permitting mobilization of edema fluid from the interstitium.[77] Refilling of the vasculature with interstitial fluid occurs in less than one hour. A reduction in GFR with diuresis is not uncommon and suggests a rate of diuresis that exceeds the rate at which interstitial fluid can be mobilized. Furthermore, in some patients, rapid reduction of preload may lead to further neurohormonal activation and a decline in cardiac output. However, many patients have no changes in cardiac output as they are on the flat part of the Frank-Starling curve in which changes in left ventricular end-diastolic pressure have little or no effect on cardiac output. Furthermore, among patients with elevated central venous pressure, diuresis improves renal venous pressure, intra-abdominal pressure, and renal perfusion, and leads to increases in GFR. Monitoring of BUN, serum creatinine, and potassium levels is necessary for patients on loop diuretics. In patients with advanced HF, decreased renal perfusion, upregulation of RAAS, increased renal venous and intra-abdominal pressures, RV dysfunction, and hypoalbuminemia limit the response to conventional diuretic doses. For these patients, oral bumetanide or torsemide can be use in lieu of furosemide, often in combination with thiazide-type diuretics (chlorthalidone, metolazone, or chlorothiazide). In patients whose conditions are refractory to oral diuretics, intravenous administration by either intermittent bolus therapy or continuous intravenous infusion has comparable safety and efficacy in volume control. In patients with HF and CKD which are not responding to these measures, invasive hemodynamic evaluation and optimization of afterload and cardiac output should be attempted before initiation of hemofiltration or hemodialysis.

Novel Potassium Binders

Patiromer and sodium zirconium cyclosilicate are novel potassium binders that may help mitigate hyperkalemia with angiotensin blockade and AA specifically in CKD patients. Patiromer (RLY5016) is a non-absorbed, sodium-free polymer that exchanges calcium for potassium in the gastrointestinal (GI) tract, promoting fecal potassium excretion.[78] In PEARL-HF (Parallel Evaluation of RLY5016 in Heart Failure), patiromer prevented hyperkalemia in HF patients with CKD who had been on an angiotensin blockade regimen and spironolactone (25–50 mg/day).[78] Sodium zirconium cyclosilicate (ZS-9) is a highly selective cation exchanger that entraps potassium in the GI tract, exchanging it for hydrogen and sodium. It can correct hyperkalemia within 48 hours and its effects are noted to be most significant in higher potassium levels at baseline.[79] Prior to administration of either of these agents, careful consideration of potential adverse effects is required, such as constipation, hypomagnesemia and drug interactions (metformin, levothyroxine) with patiromer, or edema with ZS-9. Also, a low-potassium diet and loop diuretics should be attempted first before initiation of these agents.

Implantable Device Therapy

Among patients with advanced CKD, the benefit of a primary prevention implantable cardioverter-defibrillator (ICD) is uncertain. A meta-analysis of three randomized, controlled trials (Multicenter Automatic Defibrillator Implantation Trial [MADIT] I, MADIT-II and Sudden Cardiac Death in Heart Failure Trial [SCD-HeFT]) did not find any survival benefit in patients with CKD stage 4 and 5.[80] In another meta-analysis, including the aforementioned three trials and Defibrillators in Non-Ischemic Cardiomyopathy Treatment Evaluation (DEFINITE), it was also shown that patients with extensive medical comorbidities, including CKD, experience less benefit from primary prevention ICDs.[81] Therefore, implantation should be carefully considered but not withheld if indications are met.

Management of Patients with Heart Failure and End-Stage Renal Disease

HFrEF and ESRD share common risk factors, such as diabetes mellitus, hypertension, coronary artery disease, obesity, and tobacco use. Furthermore, these two highly co-morbid conditions utilize significant amount of health care resources, imposing significant burden on the health care system. Among patients with ESRD, poor volume control, uncontrolled hypertension, progression of coronary artery disease, anemia, electrolytic abnormalities, myocardial fibrosis,[82] and uremic toxins[83,84] lead to development of HF and hospitalization with HF exacerbation. Cardiac dysfunction ranges from left ventricular hypertrophy and left ventricular dilation to asymptomatic systolic dysfunction and eventually symptomatic heart failure in sicker, elderly patients with higher prevalence of comorbidities.

Myocardial fibrosis and hypertrophy, with or without ischemic heart disease, is a frequent pathologic finding and a strong predictor of mortality.[83] Therefore, in these patients, there is a shift from ischemic to non-ischemic etiologies of cardiac death.[84] Approximately one-third of patients with ESRD have HF at initiation of dialysis and 25% of patients with ESRD develop HF while on dialysis.[85] The three-year survival rate of patients on dialysis after diagnosis of HF is lower than 20%.[85,86] Available data on use of optimal medical therapy in patients with coexistent HFrEF and ESRD on dialysis are limited. Most randomized, controlled trials have systematically excluded patients with ESRD with the concern that the investigational drug might lead to potential side effects. Despite the lack of data from randomized, clinical trials supporting the safety and efficacy of HF therapies in patients with ESRD, the National Kidney Foundation Kidney Disease Outcomes Initiative working group guidelines recommend angiotensin-converting enzyme inhibitors (ACEi) or angiotensin receptor blockers (ARB) and β-blockers for all ESRD patients with symptomatic HF who are receiving dialysis and have HF with reduced ejection fraction (HFrEF),[87] based on findings from smaller clinical trials that demonstrated improved outcomes with the use of ACEi/ARB and β-blockers.[88,89] However, a decline in long-term mortality has been noted in previous studies[90] and is related, in part, to greater intensity of dialysis. Most importantly, there is a reported trend toward improved adherence with guideline-directed medical therapies and scheduled follow-ups among ESRD patients with HF.[91]

Studies on the effects of β-blockers on outcomes of patients with ESRD on dialysis, when examined in a randomized, controlled clinical trial of dialysis patients with HF and left ventricular ejection fraction (LVEF) less than 35%, showed that the use of carvedilol was associated with improved LVEF, functional class, cardiovascular death, readmissions, and all-cause mortality. The dialyzability of beta-blockers may be associated with differential effects on outcomes. Beta-blockers that are poorly dialyzed, such as bisoprolol or carvedilol, may provide a survival benefit compared with easily dialyzed beta-blockers such as metoprolol. Overall, beta-blockers appear safe and efficacious in these patients if initiated at low doses and adjusted carefully to avoid hypotensive episodes.[92]

Evidence of benefit from administration of ACEi/ARB in patients with HF and ESRD is scarce. In the randomized Fosinopril in Dialysis (FOSIDIAL) trial, there was a non-significant trend toward fewer cardiovascular events with fosinopril compared with placebo among dialysis patients with LV hypertrophy.[90] Although clinical data from randomized, controlled trials are lacking, the favorable effects of ACE inhibitors on neurohormonal activation and ventricular remodeling may translate into a reduction in cardiovascular events in dialysis patients with LV dysfunction and HF.[93,94] However, careful monitoring of serum potassium concentration is required, as these patients carry a significant risk of hyperkalemia. The use of mineralocorticoid receptor antagonists is controversial in dialysis patients because of the risk of hyperkalemia.[95] Finally, digoxin is not routinely used in dialysis patients because of the higher risk of digoxin toxicity.[96] Newer additions to the therapeutic armamentarium of HF, such as ivabradine and angiotensin receptor-neprilysin inhibitors, have not been tested in patients with ESRD.

Although adherence to guideline-directed medical therapies (ACEi/ARB and β-blockers) among dialysis patients improved significantly over time, the utilization of guideline-recommended implantable cardioverter-defibrillators (ICD) for primary prevention of sudden cardiac death and cardiac resynchronization therapy in these patients remains low. This phenomenon can be explained by the lack of definitive evidence to support the use of device therapy in this group of patients.[91] Most randomized trials that evaluated the benefits of ICD and CRT therapy in HF excluded ESRD patients. As a result, the current American College of Cardiology/AHA/European Society of Cardiology guidelines do not address this issue adequately.[97,98] Furthermore, dialysis patients are at increased risk of device-related infections and vascular complications that may bias the cardiologists against the use of these devices. In these patients with dialysis, the use of subcutaneous ICDs may be associated with lower infection risk[99] and could be the preferred option in cases where pacing or CRT are not necessary.

Patients with ESRD are rarely referred for LVAD implantation with only 1.5% of new patients requiring dialysis before surgery, based on data from the INTERMACS database.[100] A proportion of LVAD recipients who develop AKI and require hemodialysis after implantation will require long-term maintenance hemodialysis. Outpatient hemodialysis (HD) in this setting, albeit safe, can be an important barrier to discharge as many HD are not acquainted with the care of LVAD patients. A previous analysis of outpatient HD sessions in ten LVAD recipients, showed a low interruption rate of HD, low incidence of low-flow alarms and no serious adverse events or deaths.[47,101] Intradialytic hypotension is the main reason to terminate the HD session and some of the hypotensive episodes may be precipitated by catheter-related sepsis. Anecdotal experience suggests that outpatient hemodialysis is safe and feasible in adequately trained hemodialysis centers. Careful assessment of blood pressure with Doppler probes, dosing of antihypertensive medications on non-dialysis days, and use of midodrine in cases of recurrent symptomatic intra-dialytic hypotension are ways to facilitate completion of HD sessions without hypotensive episodes. Although concerns were previously raised, regarding maturation of arterio-venous fistulas in the setting of continuous flow, recent reports suggest normal maturation without hemodynamic or infectious complications.[102]

Conclusion

Both AKI and CKD are common in HFrEF and HFpEF patients and portend poor prognosis. Since there are no available treatments that directly improve renal function, optimization of preload and afterload and neurohormonal activation are the key components of therapy in cases of CRS. The effects of diuretic-induced volume removal on GFR can be variable, hence clinical decision should be based on patients' weight, symptoms, and physical examination as well as on hemodynamic assessment, if indicated. Aggressive decongestion may be associated with lower mortality despite reduction in GFR, and GDMT for HF may improve outcomes in these patients and should not be discontinued or withheld in the absence of serious adverse events. Future randomized, controlled clinical trials should include patients with advanced CKD stages and examine the effects of medical and device therapies on the outcomes of this high-morbidity and high-mortality risk group of patients.

Disclosures

No conflict of interest declared.

References

1. Sarnak MJ, Levey AS, Schoolwerth AC, et al. Kidney disease as a risk factor for development of cardiovascular disease: a statement from the American Heart Association Councils on kidney in cardiovascular disease, high blood pressure research, clinical cardiology, and epidemiology and prevention. *Circulation.* 2003;108(17):2154–69.
2. Ather S, Chan W, Bozkurt B, et al. Impact of noncardiac comorbidities on morbidity and mortality in a predominantly male population with heart failure and preserved versus reduced ejection fraction. *J Am Coll Cardiol.* 2012;59(11):998–1005.
3. Go AS, Chertow GM, Fan D, McCulloch CE, Hsu CY. Chronic kidney disease and the risks of death, cardiovascular events, and hospitalization. *N Engl J Med.* 2004;351(13):1296–305.
4. Chronic Kidney Disease Prognosis C, Matsushita K, van der Velde M, et al. Association of estimated glomerular filtration rate and albuminuria with all-cause and cardiovascular mortality in general population cohorts: a collaborative meta-analysis. *Lancet.* 2010;375(9731):2073–81.
5. Tonelli M, Muntner P, Lloyd A, et al. Risk of coronary events in people with chronic kidney disease compared with those with diabetes: a population-level cohort study. *Lancet.* 2012;380(9844):807–14.
6. Bloembergen WE, Port FK, Mauger EA, Wolfe RA. Causes of death in dialysis patients: racial and gender differences. *J Am Soc Nephrol.* 1994;5(5):1231–42.
7. Ronco C, Haapio M, House AA, Anavekar N, Bellomo R. Cardiorenal syndrome. *J Am Coll Cardiol.* 2008;52(19):1527–39.
8. Ezekowitz J, McAlister FA, Humphries KH, et al. The association among renal insufficiency, pharmacotherapy, and outcomes in 6,427 patients with heart failure and coronary artery disease. *J Am Coll Cardiol.* 2004;44(8):1587–92.
9. Adams KF, Jr., Fonarow GC, Emerman CL, et al. Characteristics and outcomes of patients hospitalized for heart failure in the United States: rationale, design, and preliminary observations from the first 100,000 cases in the Acute Decompensated Heart Failure National Registry (ADHERE). *Am Heart J.* 2005;149(2):209–16.
10. Smith GL, Lichtman JH, Bracken MB, et al. Renal impairment and outcomes in heart failure: systematic review and meta-analysis. *J Am Coll Cardiol.* 2006;47(10):1987–96.
11. Forman DE, Butler J, Wang Y, et al. Incidence, predictors at admission, and impact of worsening renal function among patients hospitalized with heart failure. *J Am Coll Cardiol.* 2004;43(1):61–7.
12. Butler J, Forman DE, Abraham WT, et al. Relationship between heart failure treatment and development of worsening renal function among hospitalized patients. *Am Heart J.* 2004;147(2):331–8.
13. Shoker A, Hossain MA, Koru-Sengul T, Raju DL, Cockcroft D. Performance of creatinine clearance equations on the original Cockcroft-Gault population. *Clin Nephrol.* 2006;66(2):89–97.
14. Levey AS, Bosch JP, Lewis JB, Greene T, Rogers N, Roth D. A more accurate method to estimate glomerular filtration rate from serum creatinine: a new prediction equation. Modification of Diet in Renal Disease Study Group. *Ann Intern Med.* 1999;130(6):461–70.
15. Poggio ED, Wang X, Greene T, Van Lente F, Hall PM. Performance of the modification of diet in renal disease and Cockcroft-Gault equations in the estimation of GFR in health and in chronic kidney disease. *J Am Soc Nephrol.* 2005;16(2):459–66.
16. Knight EL, Verhave JC, Spiegelman D, et al. Factors influencing serum cystatin C levels other than renal function and the impact on renal function measurement. *Kidney Int.* 2004;65(4):1416–21.
17. Groesbeck D, Kottgen A, Parekh R, et al. Age, gender, and race effects on cystatin C levels in US adolescents. *Clin J Am Soc Nephrol.* 2008;3(6):1777–85.
18. Anderson RJ, Linas SL, Berns AS, et al. Nonoliguric acute renal failure. *N Engl J Med.* 1977;296(20):1134–8.
19. Sarraf M, Masoumi A, Schrier RW. Cardiorenal syndrome in acute decompensated heart failure. *Clin J Am Soc Nephrol.* 2009;4(12):2013–26.
20. Liang KV, Williams AW, Greene EL, Redfield MM. Acute decompensated heart failure and the cardiorenal syndrome. *Crit Care Med.* 2008;36(1 Suppl) Suppl:S75–88.
21. Schrier RW, Abraham WT. Hormones and hemodynamics in heart failure. *N Engl J Med.* 1999;341(8):577–85.
22. Kazory A. Emergence of blood urea nitrogen as a biomarker of neurohormonal activation in heart failure. *Am J Cardiol.* 2010;106(5):694–700.
23. Nohria A, Hasselblad V, Stebbins A, et al. Cardiorenal interactions: insights from the ESCAPE trial. *J Am Coll Cardiol.* 2008;51(13):1268–74.
24. Hanberg JS, Sury K, Wilson FP, et al. Reduced cardiac index is not the dominant driver of renal dysfunction in heart failure. *J Am Coll Cardiol.* 2016;67(19):2199–208.
25. Mullens W, Abrahams Z, Francis GS, et al. Importance of venous congestion for worsening of renal function in advanced decompensated heart failure. *J Am Coll Cardiol.* 2009;53(7):589–96.
26. Damman K, van Deursen VM, Navis G, Voors AA, van Veldhuisen DJ, Hillege HL. Increased central venous pressure is associated with impaired renal function and mortality in a broad spectrum of patients with cardiovascular disease. *J Am Coll Cardiol.* 2009;53(7):582–8.
27. Alpert JS. The effect of right ventricular dysfunction on left ventricular form and function. *Chest.* 2001;119(6):1632–3.
28. Testani JM, Khera AV, St John Sutton MG, et al. Effect of right ventricular function and venous congestion on cardiorenal interactions during the treatment of decompensated heart failure. *Am J Cardiol.* 2010;105(4):511–6.
29. Weinfeld MS, Chertow GM, Stevenson LW. Aggravated renal dysfunction during intensive therapy for advanced chronic heart failure. *Am Heart J.* 1999;138(2 Pt 1):285–90.
30. Mullens W, Abrahams Z, Skouri HN, et al. Elevated intra-abdominal pressure in acute decompensated heart failure: a potential contributor to worsening renal function? *J Am Coll Cardiol.* 2008;51(3):300–6.
31. Ter Maaten JM, Damman K, Verhaar MC, et al. Connecting heart failure with preserved ejection fraction and renal dysfunction: the role of endothelial dysfunction and inflammation. *Eur J Heart Fail.* 2016;18(6):588–98.
32. Testani JM, Chen J, McCauley BD, Kimmel SE, Shannon RP. Potential effects of aggressive decongestion during the treatment of decompensated heart failure on renal function and survival. *Circulation.* 2010;122(3):265–72.
33. Greene SJ, Gheorghiade M, Vaduganathan M, et al. Haemoconcentration, renal function, and post-discharge outcomes among patients hospitalized for heart failure with reduced ejection fraction: insights from the EVEREST trial. *Eur J Heart Fail.* 2013;15(12):1401–11.
34. Testani JM, Brisco MA, Chen J, McCauley BD, Parikh CR, Tang WH. Timing of hemoconcentration during treatment of acute decompensated heart failure and subsequent survival: importance of sustained decongestion. *J Am Coll Cardiol.* 2013;62(6):516–24.
35. Metra M, Davison B, Bettari L, et al. Is worsening renal function an ominous prognostic sign in patients with acute heart failure? The role of congestion and its interaction with renal function. *Circ Heart Fail.* 2012;5(1):54–62.
36. Ather S, Bavishi C, McCauley MD, et al. Worsening renal function is not associated with response to treatment in acute heart failure. *Int J Cardiol.* 2013;167(5):1912–17.
37. Ahmad T, Jackson K, Rao VS, et al. Worsening renal function in patients with acute heart failure undergoing aggressive diuresis is not associated with tubular injury. *Circulation.* 2018;137(19):2016–28.
38. Emmens JE, Ter Maaten JM, Matsue Y, et al. Plasma kidney injury molecule-1 in heart failure: renal mechanisms and clinical outcome. *Eur J Heart Fail.* 2016;18(6):641–9.
39. Vaidya VS, Ozer JS, Dieterle F, et al. Kidney injury molecule-1 outperforms traditional biomarkers of kidney injury in preclinical biomarker qualification studies. *Nat Biotechnol.* 2010;28(5):478–85.
40. Park M, Hsu CY, Go AS, et al. Urine kidney injury biomarkers and risks of cardiovascular disease events and all-cause death: the CRIC study. *Clin J Am Soc Nephrol.* 2017;12(5):761–71.
41. Kiernan MS, Gregory D, Sarnak MJ, et al. Early and late effects of high- versus low-dose angiotensin receptor blockade on renal function and outcomes in patients with chronic heart failure. *JACC Heart Fail.* 2015;3(3):214–23.
42. Costanzo MR, Johannes RS, Pine M, et al. The safety of intravenous diuretics alone versus diuretics plus parenteral vasoactive therapies in hospitalized patients with acutely decompensated heart failure: a propensity score and instrumental variable analysis using the Acutely Decompensated Heart Failure National Registry (ADHERE) database. *Am Heart J.* 2007;154(2):267–77.
43. O'Connor CM, Starling RC, Hernandez AF, et al. Effect of nesiritide in patients with acute decompensated heart failure. *N Engl J Med.* 2011;365(1):32–43.
44. Chen HH, Anstrom KJ, Givertz MM, et al. Low-dose dopamine or low-dose nesiritide in acute heart failure with renal dysfunction: the ROSE acute heart failure randomized trial. *JAMA.* 2013;310(23):2533–43.
45. Elkayam U, Ng TM, Hatamizadeh P, Janmohamed M, Mehra A. Renal vasodilatory action of dopamine in patients with heart failure: magnitude of effect and site of action. *Circulation.* 2008;117(2):200–5.
46. Giamouzis G, Butler J, Starling RC, et al. Impact of dopamine infusion on renal function in hospitalized heart failure patients: results of the dopamine in acute decompensated heart failure (DAD-HF) trial. *J Card Fail.* 2010;16(12):922–30.
47. Hasin T, Topilsky Y, Schirger JA, et al. Changes in renal function after implantation of continuous-flow left ventricular assist devices. *J Am Coll Cardiol.* 2012;59(1):26–36.
48. Hasin T, Grupper A, Dillon JJ, et al. Early gains in renal function following implantation of heartmate II left ventricular assist devices may not persist to one year. *ASAIO J.* 2017;63(4):401–7.

49. Bart BA, Goldsmith SR, Lee KL, et al. Ultrafiltration in decompensated heart failure with cardiorenal syndrome. *N Engl J Med.* 2012;367(24):2296–304.
50. Stevens PE, Levin A, Kidney disease: improving global outcomes chronic kidney disease guideline development work Group M. Evaluation and management of chronic kidney disease: synopsis of the kidney disease: improving global outcomes 2012 clinical practice guideline. *Ann Intern Med.* 2013;158(11):825–30.
51. Heywood JT, Fonarow GC, Costanzo MR, et al. High prevalence of renal dysfunction and its impact on outcome in 118,465 patients hospitalized with acute decompensated heart failure: a report from the ADHERE database. *J Card Fail.* 2007;13(6):422–30.
52. McAlister FA, Ezekowitz J, Tarantini L, et al. Renal dysfunction in patients with heart failure with preserved versus reduced ejection fraction: impact of the new Chronic Kidney Disease-Epidemiology Collaboration Group formula. *Circ Heart Fail.* 2012;5(3):309–14.
53. Kottgen A, Russell SD, Loehr LR, et al. Reduced kidney function as a risk factor for incident heart failure: the atherosclerosis risk in communities (ARIC) study. *J Am Soc Nephrol.* 2007;18(4):1307–15.
54. Group CTS. Effects of enalapril on mortality in severe congestive heart failure. Results of the Cooperative North Scandinavian Enalapril Survival Study (CONSENSUS). *N Engl J Med.* 1987;316(23):1429–35.
55. Cohn JN, Tognoni G, Valsartan heart failure trial I. A randomized trial of the angiotensin-receptor blocker valsartan in chronic heart failure. *N Engl J Med.* 2001;345(23):1667–75.
56. Ahmed A, Love TE, Sui X, Rich MW. Effects of angiotensin-converting enzyme inhibitors in systolic heart failure patients with chronic kidney disease: a propensity score analysis. *J Card Fail.* 2006;12(7):499–506.
57. Haas M, Leko-Mohr Z, Erler C, Mayer G. Antiproteinuric versus antihypertensive effects of high-dose ACE inhibitor therapy. *Am J Kidney Dis.* 2002;40(3):458–63.
58. Edner M, Benson L, Dahlstrom U, Lund LH. Association between renin-angiotensin system antagonist use and mortality in heart failure with severe renal insufficiency: a prospective propensity score-matched cohort study. *Eur Heart J.* 2015;36(34):2318–26.
59. Yancy CW, Jessup M, Bozkurt B, et al. 2013 ACCF/AHA guideline for the management of heart failure: a report of the American College of Cardiology Foundation/American Heart Association Task Force on Practice Guidelines. *J Am Coll Cardiol.* 2013;62(16):e147–239.
60. Cohn JN, Archibald DG, Ziesche S, et al. Effect of vasodilator therapy on mortality in chronic congestive heart failure. Results of a Veterans Administration Cooperative Study. *N Engl J Med.* 1986;314(24):1547–52.
61. Taylor AL, Ziesche S, Yancy C, et al. Combination of isosorbide dinitrate and hydralazine in blacks with heart failure. *N Engl J Med.* 2004;351(20):2049–57.
62. McMurray JJ, Packer M, Desai AS, et al. Angiotensin-neprilysin inhibition versus enalapril in heart failure. *N Engl J Med.* 2014;371(11):993–1004.
63. Damman K, Gori M, Claggett B, et al. Renal effects and associated outcomes during angiotensin-neprilysin inhibition in heart failure. *JACC Heart Fail.* 2018;6(6):489–98.
64. Zoccali C, Mallamaci F, Parlongo S, et al. Plasma norepinephrine predicts survival and incident cardiovascular events in patients with end-stage renal disease. *Circulation.* 2002;105(11):1354–9.
65. Castagno D, Jhund PS, McMurray JJ, et al. Improved survival with bisoprolol in patients with heart failure and renal impairment: an analysis of the cardiac insufficiency bisoprolol study II (CIBIS-II) trial. *Eur J Heart Fail.* 2010;12(6):607–16.
66. Ghali JK, Wikstrand J, Van Veldhuisen DJ, et al. The influence of renal function on clinical outcome and response to beta-blockade in systolic heart failure: insights from Metoprolol CR/XL Randomized Intervention Trial in Chronic HF (MERIT-HF). *J Card Fail.* 2009;15(4):310–8.
67. Cohen-Solal A, Kotecha D, van Veldhuisen DJ, et al. Efficacy and safety of nebivolol in elderly heart failure patients with impaired renal function: insights from the SENIORS trial. *Eur J Heart Fail.* 2009;11(9):872–80.
68. Badve SV, Roberts MA, Hawley CM, et al. Effects of beta-adrenergic antagonists in patients with chronic kidney disease: a systematic review and meta-analysis. *J Am Coll Cardiol.* 2011;58(11):1152–61.
69. Chua D, Lo A, Lo C. Spironolactone use in heart failure patients with end-stage renal disease on hemodialysis: is it safe? *Clin Cardiol.* 2010;33(10):604–8.
70. Pitt B, White H, Nicolau J, et al. Eplerenone reduces mortality 30 days after randomization following acute myocardial infarction in patients with left ventricular systolic dysfunction and heart failure. *J Am Coll Cardiol.* 2005;46(3):425–31.
71. Pitt B, Zannad F, Remme WJ, et al. The effect of spironolactone on morbidity and mortality in patients with severe heart failure. Randomized Aldactone Evaluation Study Investigators. *N Engl J Med.* 1999;341(10):709–17.
72. Cooper LB, Lippmann SJ, Greiner MA, et al. Use of mineralocorticoid receptor antagonists in patients with heart failure and comorbid diabetes mellitus or chronic kidney disease. *J Am Heart Assoc.* 2017;6(12):
73. Acquarone N, Castello C, Antonucci G, Lione S, Bellotti P. Pharmacologic therapy in patients with chronic heart failure and chronic kidney disease: a complex issue. *J Cardiovasc Med (Hagerstown).* 2009;10(1):13–21.
74. Pitt B, Pedro Ferreira J, Zannad F. Mineralocorticoid receptor antagonists in patients with heart failure: current experience and future perspectives. *Eur Heart J Cardiovasc Pharmacother.* 2017;3(1):48–57.
75. Choudhury D, Ahmed Z. Drug-associated renal dysfunction and injury. *Nat Clin Pract Nephrol.* 2006;2(2):80–91.
76. Murray MD, Deer MM, Ferguson JA, et al. Open-label randomized trial of torsemide compared with furosemide therapy for patients with heart failure. *Am J Med.* 2001;111(7):513–20.
77. Cotter G, Metra M, Milo-Cotter O, Dittrich HC, Gheorghiade M. Fluid overload in acute heart failure--re-distribution and other mechanisms beyond fluid accumulation. *Eur J Heart Fail.* 2008;10(2):165–9.
78. Pitt B, Anker SD, Bushinsky DA, et al. Evaluation of the efficacy and safety of RLY5016, a polymeric potassium binder, in a double-blind, placebo-controlled study in patients with chronic heart failure (the PEARL-HF) trial. *Eur Heart J.* 2011;32(7):820–8.
79. Packham DK, Rasmussen HS, Lavin PT, et al. Sodium zirconium cyclosilicate in hyperkalemia. *N Engl J Med.* 2015;372(3):222–31.
80. Pun PH, Al-Khatib SM, Han JY, et al. Implantable cardioverter-defibrillators for primary prevention of sudden cardiac death in CKD: a meta-analysis of patient-level data from 3 randomized trials. *Am J Kidney Dis.* 2014;64(1):32–9.
81. Steinberg BA, Al-Khatib SM, Edwards R, et al. Outcomes of implantable cardioverter-defibrillator use in patients with comorbidities: results from a combined analysis of 4 randomized clinical trials. *JACC Heart Fail.* 2014;2(6):623–9.
82. Banerjee D, Ma JZ, Collins AJ, Herzog CA. Long-term survival of incident hemodialysis patients who are hospitalized for congestive heart failure, pulmonary edema, or fluid overload. *Clin J Am Soc Nephrol.* 2007;2(6):1186–90.
83. Mailloux LU, Napolitano B, Bellucci AG, Mossey RT, Vernace MA, Wilkes BM. The impact of co-morbid risk factors at the start of dialysis upon the survival of ESRD patients. *ASAIO J.* 1996;42(3):164–9.
84. Miskulin D, Bragg-Gresham J, Gillespie BW, et al. Key comorbid conditions that are predictive of survival among hemodialysis patients. *Clin J Am Soc Nephrol.* 2009;4(11):1818–26.
85. Harnett JD, Foley RN, Kent GM, Barre PE, Murray D, Parfrey PS. Congestive heart failure in dialysis patients: prevalence, incidence, prognosis and risk factors. *Kidney Int.* 1995;47(3):884–90.
86. Stack AG, Bloembergen WE. A cross-sectional study of the prevalence and clinical correlates of congestive heart failure among incident US dialysis patients. *Am J Kidney Dis.* 2001;38(5):992–1000.
87. K/DOQI Workgroup. K/DOQI clinical practice guidelines for cardiovascular disease in dialysis patients. *Am J Kidney Dis.* 2005;45(4 Suppl 3):S1–153.
88. Cice G, Di Benedetto A, D'Isa S, et al. Effects of telmisartan added to Angiotensin-converting enzyme inhibitors on mortality and morbidity in hemodialysis patients with chronic heart failure a double-blind, placebo-controlled trial. *J Am Coll Cardiol.* 2010;56(21):1701–8.
89. Cice G, Ferrara L, D'Andrea A, et al. Carvedilol increases two-year survivalin dialysis patients with dilated cardiomyopathy: a prospective, placebo-controlled trial. *J Am Coll Cardiol.* 2003;41(9):1438–44.
90. Zannad F, Kessler M, Lehert P, et al. Prevention of cardiovascular events in end-stage renal disease: results of a randomized trial of fosinopril and implications for future studies. *Kidney Int.* 2006;70(7):1318–24.
91. Pandey A, Golwala H, DeVore AD, et al. Trends in the use of guideline-directed therapies among dialysis patients hospitalized with systolic heart failure: findings from the American Heart Association get with the guidelines-heart failure program. *JACC Heart Fail.* 2016;4(8):649–61.
92. Tang CH, Wang CC, Chen TH, Hong CY, Sue YM. Prognostic benefits of carvedilol, bisoprolol, and metoprolol controlled release/extended release in hemodialysis patients with heart failure: a 10-year cohort. *J Am Heart Assoc.* 2016;5(1):e002584.
93. Tokmakova MP, Skali H, Kenchaiah S, et al. Chronic kidney disease, cardiovascular risk, and response to angiotensin-converting enzyme inhibition after myocardial infarction: the Survival And Ventricular Enlargement (SAVE) study. *Circulation.* 2004;110(24):3667–73.
94. Bowling CB, Sanders PW, Allman RM, et al. Effects of enalapril in systolic heart failure patients with and without chronic kidney disease: insights from the SOLVD Treatment trial. *Int J Cardiol.* 2013;167(1):151–6.
95. Zannad F, McMurray JJ, Krum H, et al. Eplerenone in patients with systolic heart failure and mild symptoms. *N Engl J Med.* 2011;364(1):11–21.
96. Chan KE, Lazarus JM, Hakim RM. Digoxin associates with mortality in ESRD. *J Am Soc Nephrol.* 2010;21(9):1550–9.
97. Cannizzaro LA, Piccini JP, Patel UD, Hernandez AF. Device therapy in heart failure patients with chronic kidney disease. *J Am Coll Cardiol.* 2011;58(9):889–96.

98. Friedman DJ, Upadhyay GA, Singal G, et al. Usefulness and consequences of cardiac resynchronization therapy in dialysis-dependent patients with heart failure. *Am J Cardiol.* 2013;112(10):1625–31.
99. El-Chami MF, Levy M, Kelli HM, et al. Outcome of subcutaneous implantable cardioverter defibrillator implantation in patients with end-stage renal disease on dialysis. *J Cardiovasc Electrophysiol.* 2015;26(8):900–4.
100. Kirklin JK, Naftel DC, Pagani FD, et al. Sixth INTERMACS annual report: a 10,000-patient database. *J Heart Lung Transplant.* 2014;33(6):555–64.
101. Demirozu ZT, Etheridge WB, Radovancevic R, Frazier OH. Results of HeartMate II left ventricular assist device implantation on renal function in patients requiring post-implant renal replacement therapy. *J Heart Lung Transplant.* 2011;30(2):182–7.
102. Patel AM, Eduardo Rame J, Rudnick MR. How does the nephrologist manage an LVAD patient on chronic maintenance dialysis? *Semin Dial.* 2014;27(3):284–8.

Chapter 24
THE PATIENT WITH ANEMIA AND IRON DEFICIENCY

Haye H. van der Wal and Peter van der Meer

Introduction

Heart failure (HF) is frequently accompanied by one or more comorbidities, which are associated with poorer quality of life and impaired prognosis. Anemia and iron deficiency are of particular importance, because of their high incidence and severe clinical consequences. Although HF treatment has dramatically improved in recent decades, there is still substantial morbidity and mortality, which is partially attributed to the impact of comorbidities. Thus, comorbidities are an attractive therapeutic target in HF. However, treatment of anemia in HF with erythropoiesis-stimulating agents did not improve outcomes. On the other hand, treating iron deficiency with intravenous iron seems more promising. In this chapter, we describe the etiology and pathophysiology of anemia and iron deficiency in HF, discuss the clinical consequences and diagnostic process, and review established and novel strategies for treatment of anemia and iron deficiency in HF.

Etiology and Pathophysiology

When applying the World Health Organization (WHO) definition of anemia (i.e. hemoglobin <12.0 g/dL in women and <13.0 g/dL in men), the frequency of anemia in patients with HF is around 40%, with a slightly higher prevalence in patients with preserved left ventricular ejection fraction (LVEF).[1–5] The etiology of anemia in HF is multifactorial and includes factors that are common in the general population, including nutritional deficiencies (iron, vitamin B_{12}, and folate), anemia of chronic disease (associated with inflammation), and chronic kidney disease with impaired erythropoietin production (Figure 24.1a). Deficiencies of vitamin B_{12} and folate are relatively rare in an HF population. In a cohort of patients with chronic HF, vitamin B_{12} and folate deficiency were present at frequencies of 5% and 4%, respectively.[6] In contrast, iron deficiency is very common in HF patients and seems to be a major etiological factor for anemia in these patients.[7] Although erythropoietin levels are elevated in HF patients, in most cases they are disproportionately lower than expected with respect to hemoglobin levels, indicating an inadequate erythropoietin response, most likely due to HF-associated renal dysfunction. Furthermore, inflammation is associated with bone marrow resistance to hemopoiesis, leading to increased erythropoietin levels.[8–10] Chronic HF is associated with significant bone marrow dysfunction, beyond erythropoietin resistance.[11] Additionally, the renin-angiotensin system, especially angiotensin II, has been linked to the erythropoietin pathway by stimulating erythropoietin production and erythropoiesis. Consequently, renin-angiotensin system blockers have been linked to development of anemia due to inhibition of erythropoiesis.[12,13] Finally, in patients with HF and volume overload, the consequent hemodilution can cause pseudo-anemia because of a reduction in relative hemoglobin levels despite normal red blood cell volume.

The essential trace element iron is best known for its oxygen-binding capacity in hemoglobin. However, iron also plays a critical role in cellular energetics, as it is an essential component of several mitochondrial respiratory chain complexes and heme-containing enzymes.[14] Thus, tissues with intense metabolism (e.g., skeletal muscle and myocardium) are highly dependent on iron. In both chronic and acute HF, iron deficiency is more prevalent than anemia, being encountered in ~50% of patients with HF, irrespective of LVEF and hemoglobin levels.[2,15] Iron deficiency can be absolute, when total iron stores are depleted, or functional, when iron stores are adequate but not available for systemic use due to entrapment in the reticuloendothelial storage system, leading to defective iron utilization in body tissues.[16] The etiology of iron deficiency is multifactorial and includes malnutrition, drug interactions (e.g., proton-pump inhibitors), impaired duodenal iron uptake due to bowel edema, gastrointestinal blood loss, and chronic low-grade inflammation (Figure 24.1b).[17] The normal distribution of iron within the body is depicted in Figure 24.2.

Clinical Implications

In otherwise healthy individuals, tissue oxygenation is preserved until hemoglobin levels of 5 g/dL are attained by an increase in cardiac output, a compensatory mechanism which is impaired in HF.[18] Thus, anemia in patients with HF can have various consequences related to impaired oxygen delivery, including neurohormonal activation, renal dysfunction, and cardiac remodeling.[19] This leads to aggravation of HF, additional symptoms, and reduced exercise capacity. Irrespective of LVEF, anemia is strongly associated with mortality and HF hospitalization, although the association between hemoglobin levels and outcomes in HF is not linear; both anemia and polycythemia increase the risk of adverse outcomes.[5,20–22]

Iron deficiency is associated with health-related quality of life in HF.[23,24] In a large, international cohort of chronic HF patients, iron deficiency independently predicted mortality (hazard ratio [HR] 1.42; 95% confidence interval (CI) 1.14–1.77; P=0.002), irrespective of hemoglobin levels.[2] In this study, HF severity, N-terminal pro-B-type natriuretic peptide (NT-proBNP) levels, and female sex were correlates of iron deficiency.[2] These findings have been replicated by other observational studies.[25,26] A small direct tissue analysis study on myocardial iron in patients with advanced HF showed decreased myocardial iron content compared with controls, which was not related to hemoglobin content. Moreover, patients with the lowest concentration of myocardial iron showed clearly reduced activity of citric acid cycle enzymes and lower expression of enzymes protecting tissues against reactive oxygen species.[27] Finally, iron deficiency has been associated with peripheral muscle myopathy in HF, which seems to be driven by impaired oxidative mitochondrial capacity.[28]

Diagnosis of Anemia and Iron Deficiency in HF

In routine clinical practice, anemia is diagnosed using hemoglobin or hematocrit levels as surrogate markers for a reduced

DOI: 10.1201/9780429244544-29

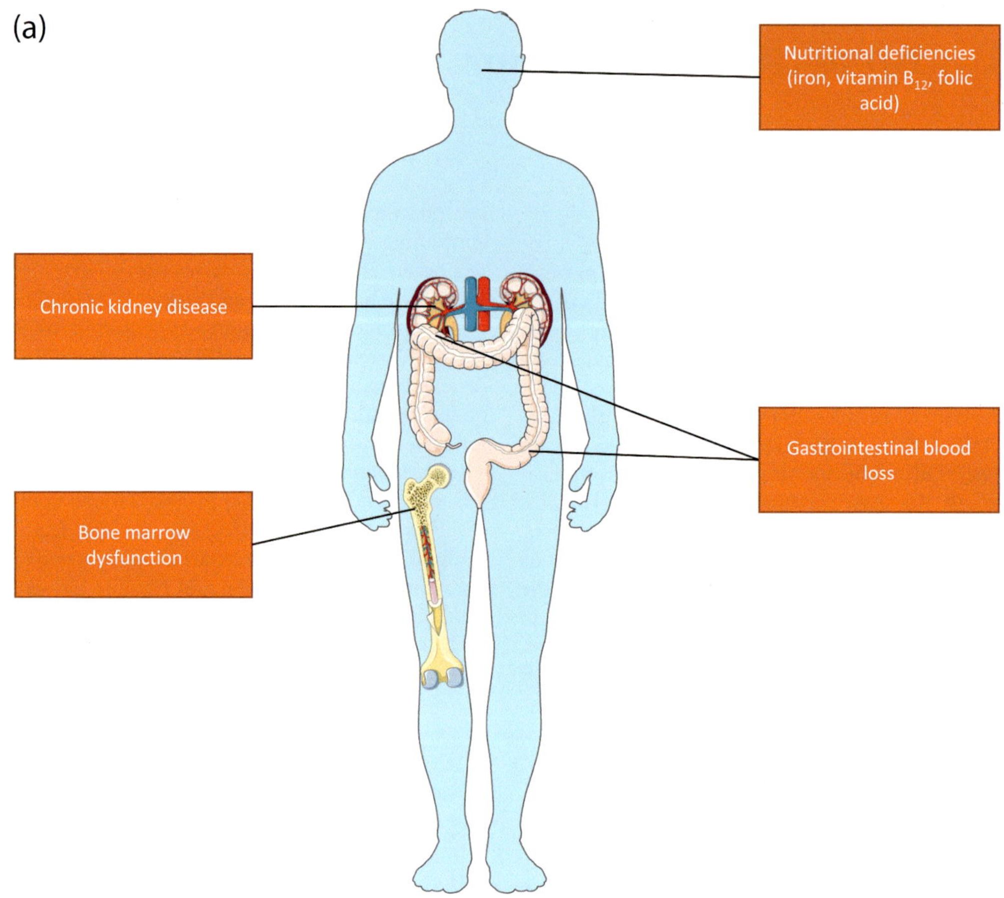

FIGURE 24.1 Etiological factors for anemia and iron deficiency in heart failure. (a) In general, anemia is caused by either a disturbed erythropoiesis, blood loss, hemolysis, or a combination of these factors. Bone marrow dysfunction in heart failure can be due to several underlying causes, including chronic low-grade inflammation, decreased endogenous erythropoietin production associated with chronic kidney disease, or bone marrow resistance to erythropoietin. Furthermore, nutritional deficiencies (iron, vitamin B_{12} and folic acid) may hamper erythropoiesis, leading to anemia. Finally, (chronic) blood loss (e.g., occult gastrointestinal blood loss due to angiodysplasia, gastric ulcers, or malignancy) gradually decreases hemoglobin levels. (b) Iron deficiency and anemia share several etiological factors, including nutritional (iron) deficiency and chronic (gastrointestinal) blood loss. Additionally, iron malabsorption related to intestinal edema or drug interaction (e.g., proton-pump inhibitors) may cause a deterioration in iron status. Finally, chronic, low-grade inflammation may lead to increased production of hepcidin, the key regulator of iron metabolism, which blocks intestinal and reticuloendothelial iron transporters, and further inhibits dietary iron uptake and systemic iron use (see also Figure 24.3).

red cell mass, which is the strict definition of anemia. The most commonly used definition for anemia is a hemoglobin concentration <12 g/dL (7.5 mmol/L) for women and <13 g/dL (8.1 mmol/L) for men.[29] A distinction should be made between "true" anemia (i.e., reduced hemoglobin and erythrocyte count) and pseudo-anemia caused by fluid overload, leading to hemodilution (i.e., reduced hemoglobin with normal erythrocyte count).[10,30,31] Therefore, hemoglobin levels should ideally be measured when the patient is in a euvolemic state. In patients with acute decompensated HF, the absolute change in hemoglobin during intravenous diuretic therapy—indicating hemoconcentration—is an independent predictor of mortality.[1] Other hematological parameters, such as mean corpuscular volume (MCV), red cell distribution width, and reticulocyte count may be normal in anemic patients. In a large, observational cohort of chronic HF patients, MCV was often within the normal range and not significantly associated with either vitamin B_{12} or folate levels. Therefore, MCV should be used cautiously in the differential diagnosis of anemia in chronic HF patients.[6]

The gold standard test for diagnosing iron deficiency is bone marrow aspirate staining (Perls' Prussian blue staining) for iron stores and iron incorporation in erythroblasts (sideroblasts). However, this test is rarely used to diagnose iron deficiency, as it is a rather invasive and painful procedure. Therefore, the diagnosis is generally based on circulating markers. Several markers for iron status can be used in the diagnostic work-up of iron deficiency, including circulating levels of ferritin, iron, transferrin, and transferrin saturation. Ferritin is a protein reflecting body iron stores, and one molecule can bind several thousand iron ions. In the general population, ferritin levels <15–30 µg/L are consistent with iron deficiency.[32] However, ferritin is an acute-phase reactant and its levels can be "falsely" increased in pro-inflammatory conditions. Although higher ferritin cut-off levels are more sensitive for the diagnosis of iron deficiency, the specificity is lower. Iron measured in serum or plasma reflects circulating iron, which is primarily bound to transferrin (an iron transport protein). Circulating iron levels will be low in various

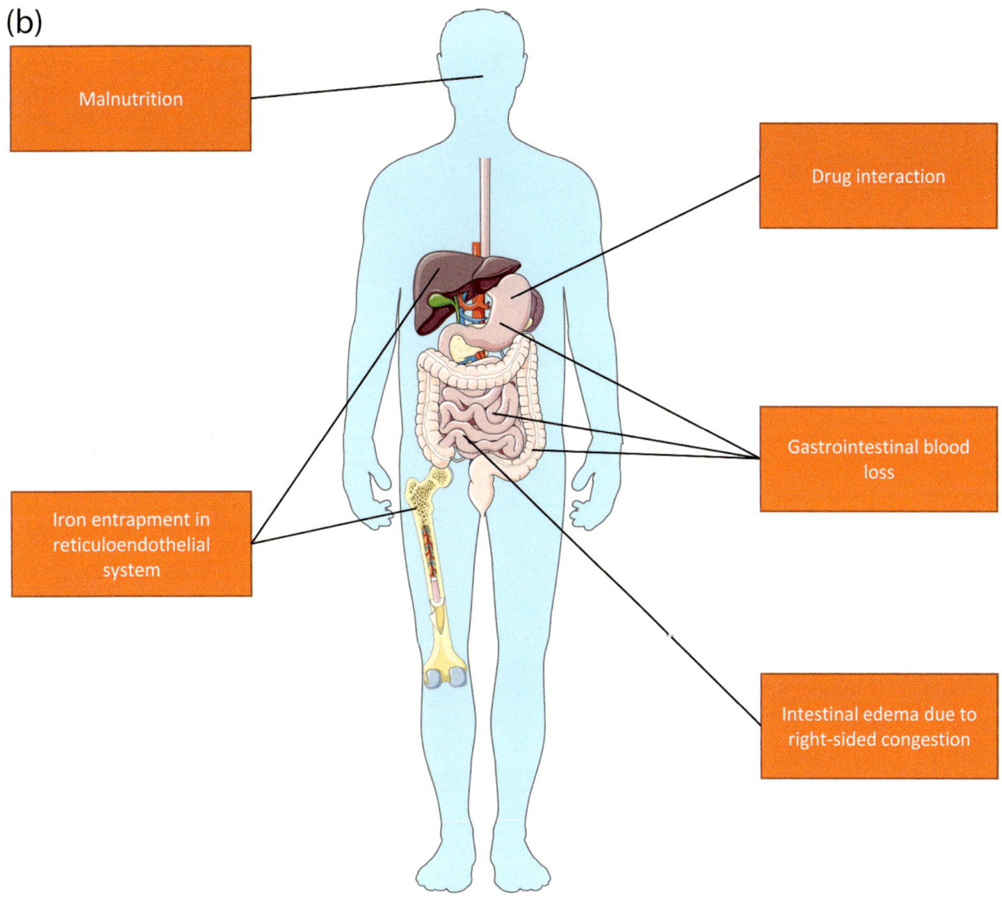

FIGURE 24.1 (Continued)

conditions, including iron deficiency and anemia of chronic disease. Therefore, iron levels must be interpreted in light of other markers reflecting iron status. As circulating iron levels are subject to diurnal variation and are affected by dietary iron intake, serum or plasma iron is ideally measured in the patient in a fasting state. Finally, transferrin saturation is the ratio between circulating iron and transferrin levels. Iron deficiency generally results in a reduced transferrin saturation, although several cut-off levels are used to define iron deficiency.[32]

The diagnosis of iron deficiency in HF can be challenging. Whereas serum ferritin is typically used to diagnose iron deficiency in the general population, the diagnosis of iron deficiency based on ferritin alone can be unreliable in the light of the effects of chronic inflammation seen in patients with HF.[33] Traditionally, iron deficiency in patients with HF is defined as a serum ferritin <100 µg/L or ferritin 100–299 µg/L combined with a transferrin saturation <20%. This "conventional definition" has been used in several clinical trials evaluating intravenous iron therapy in HF. However, this definition has not been validated in patients with HF against the gold standard (bone marrow iron staining) and is rather arbitrary. In a small cohort of patients with HF and reduced (≤45%) ejection fraction (HFrEF), who were scheduled for coronary artery bypass graft surgery, bone marrow iron deficiency was present in ~50%, based on iron staining of sternal bone marrow aspirates.[34] The predictive value of the conventional definition (based on ferritin and transferrin saturation) for iron deficiency was fair, with sensitivity and specificity of 82% and 72%, respectively. A definition based solely on transferrin saturation (<20%) predicted iron deficiency with 94% sensitivity and 84% specificity (area under curve 0.93; 95% CI 0.86–1.00; P<0.05 for the comparison with the conventional definition). In a cohort of outpatients with HF, the transferrin saturation-based definition identified patients with the highest risk of all-cause mortality (multivariable HR, 2.78; 95% CI 1.22–6.34; P=0.015), in contrast to isolated low ferritin <100 µg/L, which was not significantly associated with mortality (multivariable HR, 1.54; 95% CI, 0.45–5.22; P=0.488).[34] Finally, in a meta-analysis of intravenous iron treatment in populations with chronic HF, patients with a transferrin saturation ≥20% did not benefit from intravenous iron supplementation, whereas those with transferrin saturation <20% had improved outcomes when treated with intravenous iron (P for interaction = 0.009).[35]

Novel markers, such as hepcidin and soluble transferrin receptor, are currently used in research and are not yet suitable for clinical practice. The hepatocyte-derived protein hepcidin is considered the main regulator of iron metabolism. By degrading the iron-exporting protein ferroportin 1 in duodenal enterocytes, hepcidin inhibits dietary iron uptake. Hepcidin also traps iron in the iron storage pool (e.g., liver, reticuloendothelial cells) by blocking ferroportin 1, which causes functional iron deficiency.[36] Hepcidin levels are driven by several stimuli, including iron status, inflammation, infection, and renal dysfunction, making interpretation of circulating hepcidin levels in HF difficult (Figure 24.3).[37] Soluble transferrin receptor (sTfR) is the shed fragment of

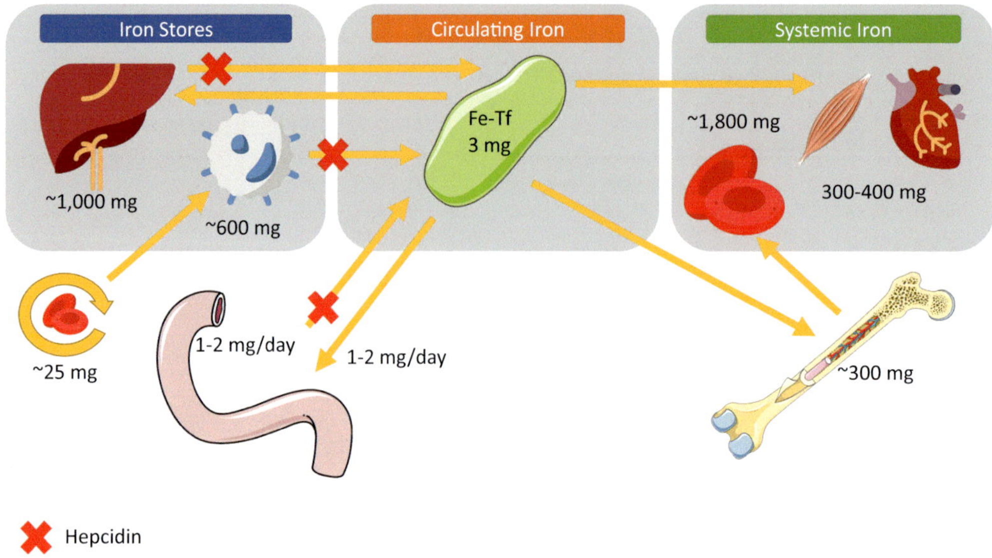

FIGURE 24.2 Distribution and homeostasis of iron. In healthy individuals, total body iron levels are in the range 3–5 g, of which most is incorporated in erythrocytes as heme (~1,800 mg) and stored as ferritin (~1,000 mg). Additionally, significant amounts of iron are present in the reticuloendothelial system (~600 mg), metabolically active tissues (e.g., skeletal muscle, heart muscle, 300–400 mg), and bone marrow (~300 mg). Finally, systemically circulating iron is mainly represented by transferrin-bound iron (~3 mg). The iron system is a relatively closed system as there is no physiological mechanism to excrete iron. In the absence of iron deficiency and iron loss (e.g., gastrointestinal blood loss, menstrual blood loss), dietary iron uptake is therefore only minor (1–2 mg/day). Dietary iron uptake and systemic release of iron is tightly regulated by the liver-derived hormone hepcidin (see Figure 24.3).

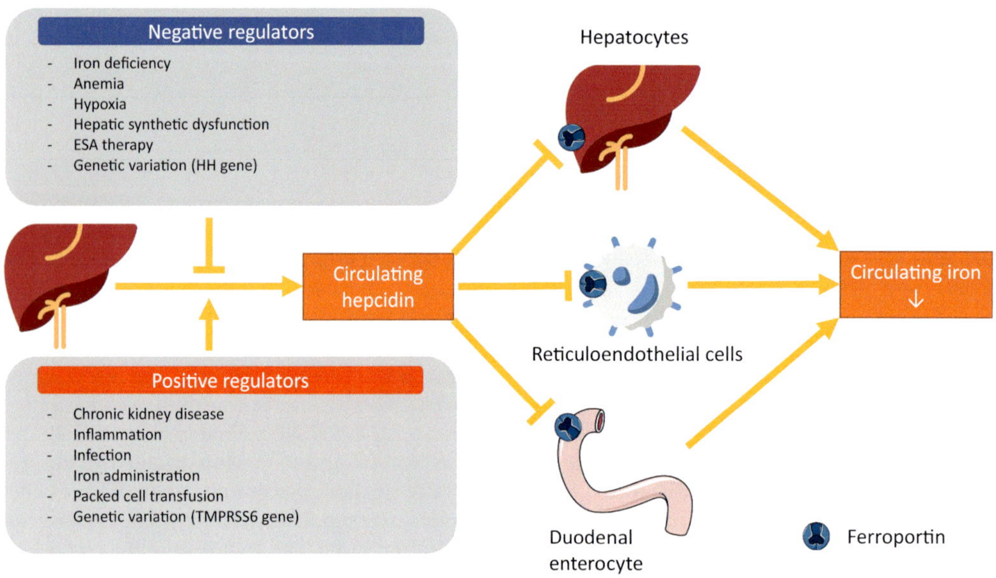

FIGURE 24.3 Regulation and effects of hepcidin. The liver-derived hormone hepcidin is considered the key regulator of iron metabolism. Hepcidin inhibits the iron-exporting protein ferroportin, which is expressed on duodenal enterocytes and cells of the reticuloendothelial system. Elevated hepcidin levels therefore lead to a reduced dietary iron uptake and iron entrapment in the reticuloendothelial system. The expression of circulating hepcidin is controlled by numerous positive and negative regulators, of which iron deficiency and inflammation seem to be the most important in heart failure, as both conditions are very common in patients with heart failure.

transferrin receptor 1. Circulating sTfR levels are inversely related to the degree of cellular iron deficiency. Analysis of sTfR levels is not readily available and reference ranges are highly variable. Nevertheless, the prognostic value of both hepcidin and sTfR has been assessed in a small acute HF cohort. Patients with a combination of low hepcidin (i.e., depleted iron stores) and high sTfR levels (cellular iron deficiency) had the highest mortality after 12 months, with findings being comparable between anemic and non-anemic patients.[38]

Treatment of Anemia in HF

Red Blood Cell Transfusion

No randomized, clinical trials have been conducted on the safety and efficacy of red blood cell (RBC) transfusion in anemic HF patients. Transfusion of RBC may lead to volume overload and ischemic events, which might be caused by platelet and coagulation cascade activation. A recent retrospective study, focusing on risk factors of transfusion-associated circulatory overload in a broad spectrum of intensive care unit patients, showed that HF is a risk factor for adverse events related to transfusion (odds ratio 2.4; 95% CI 1.2–4.6; *P*=0.01).[39] In another study of anemic patients with and without RBC transfusions in an unselected cohort of ~600,000 hospital admissions for HF, transfusion therapy independently predicted mortality (adjusted OR 3.8; 95% CI 3.5–4.1), a finding which might be explained by underlying disease severity of patients receiving RBCs.[40] In patients undergoing cardiac surgery (including ~2,000 patients with LVEF <50%), a restrictive RBC transfusion strategy (i.e., hemoglobin <7.5 g/dL) was non-inferior to a liberal strategy (i.e., hemoglobin <9.5 g/dL) with respect to the composite of mortality, myocardial infarction, stroke, and new-onset renal failure requiring dialysis.[41] In contrast, RBC transfusion seemed safe in a small acute HF cohort who received RBC transfusion compared with matched control patients.[42] Considering the paucity of data on RBC transfusion in patients with HF, a restrictive strategy might be preferred, with the goal of preventing transfusion-related adverse events, especially congestion. Patients with HF receiving RBCs should be closely monitored for signs of fluid overload. Moreover, treatable causes of anemia (e.g., hematinic deficiencies, gastrointestinal blood loss, etc.) should be identified.

Erythropoiesis-Stimulating Agents

Erythropoiesis-stimulating agents (ESA) or exogenous erythropoietin are commonly used to treat anemia in chronic kidney disease. Initially, several smaller trials showed that ESA therapy improved HF-related symptoms, exercise capacity, and quality of life.[43–45] These promising findings prompted the conduct of the large, randomized controlled morbidity and mortality trial "Reduction of Events by Darbepoetin Alfa in Heart Failure" (RED-HF). This trial enrolled 2,278 patients with chronic symptomatic HFrEF and mild-to-moderate anemia (hemoglobin 9.0–12.0 g/dL), who were randomized to either darbepoetin alfa or placebo in a double-blind fashion. The starting dose of darbepoetin alfa was 0.75 µg/kg every two weeks until the target hemoglobin concentration of 13.0 g/dL was reached. In the maintenance phase, darbepoetin alfa was administered monthly to keep hemoglobin levels between 13.0 and 14.5 g/dL. Oral and intravenous iron supplementation were provided in patients with transferrin saturation <20% during follow-up. The primary endpoint was the composite of all-cause mortality and HF-related hospitalization. One month after randomization, hemoglobin level was significantly higher in the ESA group compared with placebo and remained higher throughout the study. However, darbepoetin alfa did not affect the primary endpoint after a median follow-up of 28 months (HR 1.01; 95% CI 0.90–1.13; P=0.87), with no clear benefit toward quality of life (clinical meaningful improvement in Kansas City Cardiomyopathy Questionnaire: 53% in darbepoetin alfa arm vs 48% in placebo; P=0.06). On the contrary, rates of thromboembolic events and ischemic stroke were increased in patients receiving darbepoetin alfa (13.5% vs 10.0% in the placebo arm, P=0.009; 4.5% vs 2.8%, P=0.03, respectively).[46] These findings were similar to a comparable study in patients with anemic chronic kidney disease and diabetes, the "Trial to Reduce Cardiovascular Events With Aranesp Therapy" (TREAT).[47] In a subset of ~1,400 patients with HF from this trial, darbepoetin alfa did not show a significant reduction in mortality (HR 1.10, 95% CI 0.93–1.29) or non-fatal HF-related events (HR 1.02; 95% CI 0.87–1.20).[48] In a post-hoc analysis of RED-HF, non-responders to darbepoetin alfa had a greater risk of mortality and HF hospitalizations compared with responders.[49] Taken together, ESA therapy in HF does not improve outcomes and is associated with an increased risk of thromboembolic events. It is therefore not recommended to use ESAs for the treatment of anemia in HF patients.[50,51]

Novel Treatment Strategies

Given the safety concerns and neutral effects of ESA therapy, other treatment modalities are currently explored to target anemia in HF, besides treating iron deficiency. These strategies mainly focus on enhancing erythropoiesis without using ESAs. Currently, the most promising agents are hypoxia-inducible factor (HIF) stabilizers. HIF is strongly upregulated under hypoxic conditions and directly stimulates endogenous erythropoietin production and expression of several other pathways (e.g., angiogenesis and glucose metabolism). The hypothesis is that stabilizing HIF leads to alleviation of anemia via the endogenous erythropoietin pathway instead of administering ESAs. A few early-phase trials using HIF stabilizers in patients with advanced renal disease showed an improvement in hemoglobin with suppression of hepcidin levels.[52] However, the long-term safety and efficacy of HIF stabilizing are not yet clear and data in patients with HF are currently lacking.

Treatment of Iron Deficiency in HF

Intravenous Iron Therapy

Several moderate-sized trials have studied the effect of intravenous iron in patients with chronic HFrEF (Table 24.1). Initially, small, open-label trials of short duration showed better exercise tolerance and lower NT-proBNP levels in response to intravenous iron administration.[19,53,54] These promising results led to randomized, clinical trials of intravenous iron therapy, mainly in the form of ferric carboxymaltose (FCM) in HFrEF subjects. The "Ferric Carboxymaltose in Patients with Heart Failure and Iron Deficiency" (FAIR-HF) trial enrolled 459 symptomatic patients with chronic HF, at least moderately reduced LVEF, and iron deficiency according to conventional definition. The primary endpoints were patient-reported Patient Global Assessment and New York Heart Association (NYHA) functional class at 24 weeks. Patients randomized to FCM (200 mg intravenous (IV) at baseline, followed by weekly administrations when iron deficiency persisted) showed significant improvement in Patient Global Assessment (odds ratio for better score 2.51; 95% CI 1.75–3.61; P<0.001) and NYHA class (odds ratio for improvement, 2.40; 95% CI 1.55–3.71, P<0.001) compared with placebo, without safety issues. Secondary endpoints, i.e., six-minute walking distance (6MWD) and quality of life, were also improved.[55] These findings were replicated by the "ferric CarboxymaltOse evaluatioN on perFormance in patients with IRon deficiency in coMbination with chronic Heart Failure" (CONFIRM-HF) trial, which enrolled 304 patients with characteristics comparable to those of FAIR-HF. Patients were randomized to either FCM IV (500–2000 mg in the therapy phase, followed by maintenance doses of 500 mg in

TABLE 24.1: Randomized Clinical Trials on Intravenous and Oral Iron Supplementation in Heart Failure

Study	Patients Randomized (n)	Subject Characteristics	Definition of Iron Deficiency	Agent	Primary Endpoint	Follow-Up Duration*	Outcomes
Toblli et al. (2007)	40	NYHA II–IV LVEF ≤35% Hb <12.5 g/dL	TSAT <20% + ferritin <100 μg/L	Iron sucrose (IV)	Δ NT-proBNP Δ CRP	6 months	↓ NT-proBNP ↓ CRP ↑ LVEF ↑ 6MWT distance ↓ Hospitalizations
FERRIC-HF Okonko et al. (2008)	35	NYHA II–III LVEF ≤45% Hb <14.5 g/dL	Ferritin <100 μg/L or ferritin 100–300 μg/L + TSAT <20%	Iron sucrose (IV)	Δ peak VO_2	16 weeks	↑ peak VO_2
FAIR-HF Anker et al. (2009)	459	NYHA II–III LVEF ≤40% Hb 9.5–13.5 g/dL	Ferritin <100 μg/L or ferritin 100–300 μg/L + TSAT <20%	Ferric carboxymaltose (IV)	PGA NYHA functional class	24 weeks	↑ PGA ↓ NYHA functional class
IRON-HF Beck-da Silva et al. (2013)	23	NYHA II–IV LVEF <40% Hb 9–12 g/dL	TSAT <20% + ferritin <500 μg/L	Ferrous sulfate (p.o.)	Δ peak VO_2	3 months	~ peak VO_2 ↑ ferritin, TSAT and Hb
CONFIRM Ponikowski et al. (2015)	301	NYHA II–III LVEF ≤45% Hb <15 g/dL NT-proBNP >400 pg/mL or BNP >100 pg/mL	Ferritin <100 μg/L or ferritin 100–300 μg/L + TSAT <20%	Ferric carboxymaltose (IV)	Δ 6MWT distance	24 weeks†	↑ 6MWT distance ↑ QoL ↓ NYHA functional class ↓ HF hospitalizations
IRONOUT Lewis et al. (2017)	225	NYHA II–IV LVEF ≤40% Hb 9–15 g/dL (males) or 9-13.5 g/dL (females)	Ferritin 15–100 ng/mL or ferritin 101–299 ng/mL + TSAT <20%	Iron polysaccharide (p.o.)	Δ peak VO_2	16 weeks	~ peak VO_2 ~ QoL ~ NT-proBNP
EFFECT-HF Van Veldhuisen et al. (2017)	172	NYHA II-III ↓ peak VO_2 10–20 mL/kg/min	Ferritin <100 μg/L or ferritin 100–300 μg/L + TSAT <20%	Ferric carboxymaltose (IV)	Δ peak VO_2	24 weeks	↑ peak VO_2§
FERRIC-HF II Charles-Edwards et al. (2019)	40	NYHA II–IV LVEF ≤45% 50% anemia	Ferritin <100 μg/L or ferritin 100–300 μg/L + TSAT <20%	Iron isomaltoside (IV)	PCr $t_{1/2}$	2 weeks	↓ PCr $t_{1/2}$

* For primary endpoint.
† Total study follow-up was 52 weeks.
§ No significant difference between study groups when missing data were not imputed.
Abbreviations: 6-MWT = six-minute walk test; BNP = brain natriuretic peptide; CRP = c-reactive protein; Hb = hemoglobin; HF = heart failure; i.v. = intravenous; LVEF = left ventricular ejection fraction; NT-proBNP = N-terminal prohormone brain natriuretic peptide; NYHA = New York Heart Association; p.o. = per os; PCr = phosphocreatine; PGA = patient global assessment; QoL = quality of life; TSAT = transferrin saturation.

patients with persisting iron deficiency) or saline infusion. After 24 weeks, FCM significantly improved 6MWD compared with placebo (primary study endpoint, difference between groups: 33±11; P=0.002), symptoms, and quality of life. Moreover, HF rehospitalization rates were significantly reduced in the FCM group (HR 0.39; 95% CI 0.19–0.82; P=0.009), although this is an exploratory finding since the study was statistically underpowered for this endpoint.[56] Finally, the "Effect of Ferric Carboxymaltose on Exercise Capacity in Patients With Iron Deficiency and Chronic Heart Failure" (EFFECT-HF) specifically focused on the effects of FCM on peak VO_2 in symptomatic HF patients. Patients were randomized to either FCM therapy or standard of care for 24 weeks. After 24 weeks, a favorable effect on peak VO_2 (primary study endpoint) was observed with FCM.[57] All three trials exclusively focused on patients with HF as reduced LVEF; there are currently no data on the effect of intravenous iron therapy in patients with HF and preserved ejection fraction (HFpEF). The safety, efficacy, and effects on exercise capacity of FCM in patients with HFpEF are currently being evaluated in the "Effect of IV Iron in Patients with Heart Failure with Preserved Ejection Fraction" (FAIR-HFpEF) trial (NCT 03074591). This randomized, clinical trial aims to enroll 200 symptomatic HF patients with an LVEF ≥45% and evidence of diastolic dysfunction. This study primarily focuses on 6MWD, assessed 52 weeks after FCM administration.

Several meta-analyses have been published on intravenous iron therapy in patients with chronic HF, of which one used individual patient data of four FCM trials. This meta-analysis included 839 HFrEF patients, of whom 60% were assigned to FCM.[35] Patients receiving FCM had lower rates of cardiovascular events (composite of recurrent cardiovascular hospitalizations and cardiovascular mortality; rate ratio 0.59; 95% CI 0.400–0.88; P=0.009) and less frequent HF hospitalizations (rate ratio 0.41; 95% CI 0.23–0.73; P=0.003), although no safety issues were identified.[35] Currently, four large randomized, clinical trials are evaluating the effects of intravenous iron on mortality and HF hospitalizations, including three trials on FCM and one trial using iron isomaltoside (Table 24.2). Until the results of these studies are available, treatment of iron deficiency in chronic HFrEF patients should be considered to improve exercise capacity, in agreement with HF treatment guidelines.[51,58] Finally, iron supplementation using FCM seems a cost-effective intervention, primarily due to a reduction in hospitalization costs.[59,60]

In brief, current evidence suggests a beneficial effect of intravenous iron on symptoms in patients with chronic HFrEF. Unfortunately, little is known about the mode of action of intravenous iron therapy. Several explanations have been provided. First, hemoglobin levels increased significantly in patients receiving intravenous iron, which—theoretically—implies augmented tissue oxygenation due to improved oxygen-carrying capacity and better exercise tolerance. However, the beneficial effects of intravenous iron therapy on exercise tolerance and other surrogate endpoints were irrespective of anemia at baseline.[35,57] Therefore, it seems reasonable that intravenous iron has direct, non-hematopoietic consequences, on, for example, skeletal and cardiac muscle. Pre-clinical data suggest a link between iron depletion and mitochondrial dysfunction in various cell types, including human cardiomyocytes, which can be reverted by administering iron.[61,62] Furthermore, several in-vivo studies showed that skeletal muscle energetics are impaired in patients with HF and iron deficiency. Again, when treating these patients with intravenous iron, skeletal muscle metabolism improved significantly irrespective of changes in hemoglobin level.[28,63,64]

Oral Iron Therapy

In contrast to intravenous iron therapy, oral iron therapy is easier to administer, inexpensive, and readily available. However, this treatment modality seems less attractive in patients with HF due to several reasons, including gastro-intestinal side-effects, drug–drug interactions, and malabsorption associated with bowel edema and increased hepcidin levels, which hamper dietary iron uptake by blocking the iron-transporting protein ferroportin on enterocytes. Oral iron administration in HF has received limited attention (Table 24.1).[65,66] The "Iron Repletion Effects on Oxygen Uptake in Heart Failure" (IRONOUT) trial was the largest study on oral iron administration in patients with HF. In this placebo-controlled trial, 225 HF patients with an LVEF <40% and iron deficiency (i.e., ferritin 15–100 ng/mL, or ferritin 101–299 ng/mL with a transferrin saturation <20%) received either high-dose oral iron polysaccharide or matching placebo for 16 weeks. The primary endpoint—change in peak oxygen uptake after 16 weeks—was not significantly different between the study arms (between-group difference, 0.30 mL/kg/min; 95% CI −0.27 to 0.87; P=0.30). Patients receiving oral iron did not show improvement in 6MWD, quality of life, or NT-proBNP.[66] Although significant improvements in ferritin levels (+11 ng/mL) and transferrin saturation (+3%) were observed in patients receiving oral iron, the clinical significance is questionable. In comparison, ferritin and transferrin saturation levels increased by ~250 ng/mL and ~10%, respectively, in comparable trials using intravenous iron preparations.[53,55,56,66] This discrepancy between dosage and change in iron indices possibly implies an impaired gastrointestinal iron uptake; indeed, the biochemical response to oral iron therapy was significantly lower in patients with higher hepcidin levels, which may reduce gastrointestinal iron uptake.[66] In short, oral iron supplementation in iron-deficient HFrEF patients does not seem to adequately improve biochemical iron status and has no effect on exercise capacity. Oral treatment of iron deficiency has not been tested in HFpEF patients.

Novel Treatment Strategies

Considering the pivotal role of hepcidin in iron metabolism, antagonizing this peptide might be an alternative therapeutic target for the treatment of iron deficiency. By lowering circulating hepcidin levels or blocking its activity, both dietary iron uptake and systemic iron availability might improve. Indeed, several anti-hepcidin agents have been studied in preclinical and small-scale proof-of-principle studies on iron bioavailability, including synthetic oligonucleotides (lexaptepid), non-anticoagulant heparins, anticalins, spironolactone, and imatinib.[67–71] Prospective trials in humans are needed to assess the clinical value of antihepcidin agents for the treatment of iron deficiency.

Conclusion

Both anemia and iron deficiency are common comorbidities in HF patients and are associated with substantial burdens to patients. The etiology of both comorbidities is related to the systemic consequences of HF (chronic inflammation, renal dysfunction, fluid retention, and malnutrition). Given the neutral effects of ESA therapy on prognosis and its safety concerns (increased risk of thromboembolism and stroke), treatment of anemia in HF patients using ESAs is not recommended. Instead, management of anemia should be focused on identifying the underlying cause, which should be treated, if possible. These include hematinic deficiencies (iron, vitamin

TABLE 24.2: Ongoing Randomized Clinical Trials on Intravenous Iron Supplementation in Acute and Chronic Heart Failure

Study	Estimated Enrollment (n)	Patient Population	Agent	Primary Endpoint	Follow-Up Duration	NCT Identifier
AFFIRM-AHF	1,100	Acute HF LVEF <50%	Ferric carboxymaltose	HF hospitalizations and CV death (composite)	52 weeks	NCT02937454
HEART-FID	3,014	Chronic HF LVEF ≤35%	Ferric carboxymaltose	All-cause mortality HF hospitalizations Δ 6MWT distance	52 weeks*	NCT03037931
IRONMAN	1,300	Chronic HF LVEF <45%	Iron isomaltoside	CV mortality and HF hospitalizations (composite)	≥2.5 years	NCT02642562
FAIR-HF2	1,200	Chronic HF HFrEF	Ferric carboxymaltose	HF hospitalizations and CV death (composite)	≥52 weeks	NCT03036462
FAIR-HFpEF	260	Chronic HF LVEF ≥45% with diastolic dysfunction	Ferric carboxymaltose	Δ 6MWT distance**	52 weeks	–
PREFER-HF	72	Chronic HF LVEF >45%	Ferric carboxymaltose	Δ 6MWT distance	24 weeks	NCT03833336
Myocardial-IRON	50	Chronic HF LVEF <50%	Ferric carboxymaltose	Δ myocardial iron content (CMR)	7 and 30 days	NCT03398681

* Follow-up duration for change in 6-minute walk test is 26 months.
** Assessed after 24 weeks.
Abbreviations: 6MWT= six minute walking test; CMR = cardiac magnetic resonance; CV = cardiovascular; HF = heart failure; LVEF = left ventricular ejection fraction.

B_{12}, and folic acid) and gastrointestinal bleeding. In symptomatic patients with HFrEF and iron deficiency, intravenous iron should be considered to improve symptoms, quality of life, and exercise tolerance, irrespective of anemia. Long-term safety and efficacy characteristics of intravenous iron in HF are currently unknown, although ongoing randomized, clinical trials will evaluate its effects on cardiovascular morbidity and mortality. Currently, little is known about the etiology and clinical consequences of anemia and iron deficiency in HFpEF, a form of HF characterized by the greatest incidence of comorbidities. Whether treatment of anemia and iron deficiency in HFpEF is beneficial still needs to be determined.

References

1. van der Meer P, Postmus D, Ponikowski P, et al. The predictive value of short-term changes in hemoglobin concentration in patients presenting with acute decompensated heart failure. *J Am Coll Cardiol.* 2013;61:1973–81.
2. Klip IT, Comin-Colet J, Voors AA, et al. Iron deficiency in chronic heart failure: an international pooled analysis. *Am Heart J.* 2013;165:575–82.e3.
3. Berry C, Poppe KK, Gamble GD, et al. Prognostic significance of anaemia in patients with heart failure with preserved and reduced ejection fraction: results from the MAGGIC individual patient data meta-analysis. *QJM.* 2016;109:377–82.
4. Streng KW, Nauta JF, Hillege HL, et al. Non-cardiac comorbidities in heart failure with reduced, mid-range and preserved ejection fraction. *Int J Cardiol.* 2018;271:132–9.
5. Groenveld HF, Januzzi JL, Damman K, et al. Anemia and mortality in heart failure patients a systematic review and meta-analysis. *J Am Coll Cardiol.* 2008;52:818–27.
6. van der Wal HH, Comin-Colet J, Klip IT, et al. Vitamin B12 and folate deficiency in chronic heart failure. *Heart.* 2015;101:302–10.
7. Opasich C, Cazzola M, Scelsi L, et al. Blunted erythropoietin production and defective iron supply for erythropoiesis as major causes of anaemia in patients with chronic heart failure. *Eur Heart J.* 2005;26:2232–7.
8. van der Meer P, Lok DJ, Januzzi JL, et al. Adequacy of endogenous erythropoietin levels and mortality in anaemic heart failure patients. *Eur Heart J.* 2008;29:1510–5.
9. Belonje AM, Voors AA, van der Meer P, et al. Endogenous erythropoietin and outcome in heart failure. *Circulation.* 2010;121:245–51.
10. Westenbrink BD, Visser FW, Voors AA, et al. Anaemia in chronic heart failure is not only related to impaired renal perfusion and blunted erythropoietin production, but to fluid retention as well. *Eur Heart J.* 2007;28:166–71.
11. Westenbrink BD, Voors AA, de Boer RA, et al. Bone marrow dysfunction in chronic heart failure patients. *Eur J Heart Fail.* 2010;12:676–84.
12. van der Meer P, Lipsic E, Westenbrink BD, et al. Levels of hematopoiesis inhibitor N-acetyl-seryl-aspartyl-lysyl-proline partially explain the occurrence of anemia in heart failure. *Circulation.* 2005;112:1743–7.
13. Fyhrquist F, Karppinen K, Honkanen T, Saijonmaa O, Rosenlof K. High serum erythropoietin levels are normalized during treatment of congestive heart failure with enalapril. *J Intern Med.* 1989;226:257–60.
14. Usselman RJ, Fielding AJ, Frerman FE, et al. Impact of mutations on the midpoint potential of the [4Fe-4S]+1,+2 cluster and on catalytic activity in electron transfer flavoprotein-ubiquinone oxidoreductase (ETF-QO). *Biochemistry.* 2008;47:92–100.
15. Martens P, Nijst P, Verbrugge FH, et al. Impact of iron deficiency on exercise capacity and outcome in heart failure with reduced, mid-range and preserved ejection fraction. *Acta Cardiol.* 2018;73:115–23.
16. Grote Beverborg N, van der Wal HH, Klip IjT, et al. Differences in clinical profile and outcomes of low iron storage vs defective iron utilization in patients with heart failure: results from the DEFINE-HF and BIOSTAT-CHF studies. *JAMA Cardiol.* 2019;4:696–701.
17. Jankowska EA, von Haehling S, Anker SD, Macdougall IC, Ponikowski P. Iron deficiency and heart failure: diagnostic dilemmas and therapeutic perspectives. *Eur Heart J.* 2013;34:816–29.
18. Weiskopf RB, Viele MK, Feiner J, et al. Human cardiovascular and metabolic response to acute, severe isovolemic anemia. *Jama.* 1998;279:217–21.
19. van Veldhuisen DJ, Anker SD, Ponikowski P, Macdougall IC. Anemia and iron deficiency in heart failure: mechanisms and therapeutic approaches. *Nat Rev.* 2011;8:485–93.
20. Voors AA, Ouwerkerk W, Zannad F, et al. Development and validation of multivariable models to predict mortality and hospitalization in patients with heart failure. *Eur J Heart Fail.* 2017;19:627–34.
21. Sharma R, Francis DP, Pitt B, et al. Haemoglobin predicts survival in patients with chronic heart failure: a substudy of the ELITE II trial. *Eur Heart J.* 2004;25:1021–8.
22. Go AS, Yang J, Ackerson LM, et al. Hemoglobin level, chronic kidney disease, and the risks of death and hospitalization in adults with chronic heart failure: the anemia in chronic heart failure: outcomes and resource utilization (ANCHOR) study. *Circulation.* 2006;113:2713–23.
23. Comin-Colet J, Enjuanes C, Gonzalez G, et al. Iron deficiency is a key determinant of health-related quality of life in patients with chronic heart failure regardless of anaemia status. *Eur J Heart Fail.* 2013;15:1164–72.
24. Enjuanes C, Klip IT, Bruguera J, et al. Iron deficiency and health-related quality of life in chronic heart failure: results from a multicenter European study. *Int J Cardiol.* 2014;174:268–75.
25. Jankowska EA, Rozentryt P, Witkowska A, et al. Iron deficiency: an ominous sign in patients with systolic chronic heart failure. *Eur Heart J.* 2010;31:1872–80.

26. Yeo TJ, Yeo PS, Ching-Chiew Wong R, et al. Iron deficiency in a multi-ethnic Asian population with and without heart failure: prevalence, clinical correlates, functional significance and prognosis. *Eur J Heart Fail.* 2014;16:1125–32.
27. Melenovsky V, Petrak J, Mracek T, et al. Myocardial iron content and mitochondrial function in human heart failure: a direct tissue analysis. *Eur J Heart Fail.* 2017;19:522–30.
28. Melenovsky V, Hlavata K, Sedivy P, et al. Skeletal muscle abnormalities and iron deficiency in chronic heart failure: an exercise (31)P magnetic resonance spectroscopy study of calf muscle. *Circ Fail.* 2018;11:e004800.
29. WHO Scientific Group on Nutritional Anaemias & World Health Organization. Nutritional anaemias. Report of a WHO scientific group. *World Health Organ Tech Rep Ser.* 1968;405:5–37.
30. Adlbrecht C, Kommata S, Hulsmann M, et al. Chronic heart failure leads to an expanded plasma volume and pseudoanaemia, but does not lead to a reduction in the body's red cell volume. *Eur Heart J.* 2008;29:2343–50.
31. Androne AS, Katz SD, Lund L, et al. Hemodilution is common in patients with advanced heart failure. *Circulation.* 2003;107:226–9.
32. Weiss G, Goodnough LT. Anemia of chronic disease. *N Engl J Med.* 2005;352:1011–23.
33. Lok DJ, Klip IT, Lok SI, et al. Incremental prognostic power of novel biomarkers (growth-differentiation factor-15, high-sensitivity C-reactive protein, galectin-3, and high-sensitivity troponin-T) in patients with advanced chronic heart failure. *Am J Cardiol.* 2013;112:831–7.
34. Grote Beverborg N, Klip IjT, Meijers WC, et al. Definition of iron deficiency based on the gold standard of bone marrow iron staining in heart failure patients. *Circ Hear Fail.* 2018;11:e004519. Available from: https://www.ahajournals.org/doi/10.1161/CIRCHEARTFAILURE.117.004519
35. Anker SD, Kirwan BA, van Veldhuisen DJ, et al. Effects of ferric carboxymaltose on hospitalisations and mortality rates in iron-deficient heart failure patients: an individual patient data meta-analysis. *Eur J Heart Fail.* 2018;20:125–33.
36. Anderson GJ, Frazer DM. Current understanding of iron homeostasis. *Am J Clin Nutr.* 2017;106:1559S–1566S.
37. Huang H, Constante M, Layoun A, Santos MM. Contribution of STAT3 and SMAD4 pathways to the regulation of hepcidin by opposing stimuli. *Blood.* 2009;113:3593–9.
38. Jankowska EA, Kasztura M, Sokolski M, et al. Iron deficiency defined as depleted iron stores accompanied by unmet cellular iron requirements identifies patients at the highest risk of death after an episode of acute heart failure. *Eur Heart J.* 2014;35:2468–76.
39. Bosboom JJ, Klanderman RB, Zijp M, et al. Incidence, risk factors, and outcome of transfusion-associated circulatory overload in a mixed intensive care unit population: a nested case-control study. *Transfusion.* 2018;58:498–506.
40. Kao DP, Kreso E, Fonarow GC, Krantz MJ. Characteristics and outcomes among heart failure patients with anemia and renal insufficiency with and without blood transfusions (public discharge data from California 2000–2006). *Am J Cardiol.* 2011;107:69–73.
41. Mazer CD, Whitlock RP, Fergusson DA, et al. Restrictive or liberal red-cell transfusion for cardiac surgery. *N Engl J Med.* 2017;377:2133–44.
42. Garty M, Cohen E, Zuchenko A, et al. Blood transfusion for acute decompensated heart failure--friend or foe? *Am Heart J.* 2009;158:653–8.
43. van Veldhuisen DJ, Dickstein K, Cohen-Solal A, et al. Randomized, double blind, placebo-controlled study to evaluate the effect of two dosing regimens of darbepoetin alfa in patients with heart failure and anaemia. *Eur Heart J.* 2007;28:2208–16.
44. Ghali JK, Anand IS, Abraham WT, et al. Randomized double-blind trial of darbepoetin alfa in patients with symptomatic heart failure and anemia. *Circulation.* 2008;117:526–35.
45. Kotecha D, Ngo K, Walters JA, et al. Erythropoietin as a treatment of anemia in heart failure: systematic review of randomized trials. *Am Heart J.* 2011;161:822–31.e2.
46. Swedberg K, Young JB, Anand IS, et al. Treatment of anemia with darbepoetin alfa in systolic heart failure. *N Engl J Med.* 2013;368:1210–9.
47. Solomon SD, Uno H, Lewis EF, et al. Erythropoietic response and outcomes in kidney disease and type 2 diabetes. *N Engl J Med.* 2010;363:1146–55.
48. Desai A, Lewis E, Solomon S, McMurray JJ, Pfeffer M. Impact of erythropoiesis-stimulating agents on morbidity and mortality in patients with heart failure: an updated, post-TREAT meta-analysis. *Eur J Heart Fail.* 2010;12:936–42.
49. van der Meer P, Grote Beverborg N, Pfeffer MA, et al. Hyporesponsiveness to darbepoetin alfa in patients with heart failure and anemia in the RED-HF study (Reduction of Events by Darbepoetin Alfa in Heart Failure): Clinical and Prognostic Associations. *Circ Fail.* 2018;11:e004431.
50. Members WC, Yancy CW, Jessup M, et al. 2013 ACCF/AHA guideline for the management of heart failure: a report of the American College of Cardiology Foundation/American Heart Association Task Force on practice guidelines. *Circulation.* 2013;128:e240–327.
51. Ponikowski P, Voors AA, Anker SD, et al. 2016 ESC Guidelines for the diagnosis and treatment of acute and chronic heart failure: the Task Force for the diagnosis and treatment of acute and chronic heart failure of the European Society of Cardiology (ESC)Developed with the special contribution of the Heart Failure Association (HFA) of the ESC. *Eur Heart J.* 2016;37:2129–200.
52. Hasegawa S, Tanaka T, Nangaku M. Hypoxia-inducible factor stabilizers for treating anemia of chronic kidney disease. *Curr Opin Nephrol Hypertens.* 2018;27:331–8.
53. Okonko DO, Grzeslo A, Witkowski T, et al. Effect of intravenous iron sucrose on exercise tolerance in anemic and nonanemic patients with symptomatic chronic heart failure and iron deficiency FERRIC-HF: a randomized, controlled, observer-blinded trial. *J Am Coll Cardiol.* 2008;51:103–12.
54. Toblli JE, Lombrana A, Duarte P, Di Gennaro F. Intravenous iron reduces NT-pro-brain natriuretic peptide in anemic patients with chronic heart failure and renal insufficiency. *J Am Coll Cardiol.* 2007;50:1657–65.
55. Anker SD, Comin Colet J, Filippatos G, et al. Ferric carboxymaltose in patients with heart failure and iron deficiency. *N Engl J Med.* 2009;361:2436–48.
56. Ponikowski P, van Veldhuisen DJ, Comin-Colet J, et al. Beneficial effects of long-term intravenous iron therapy with ferric carboxymaltose in patients with symptomatic heart failure and iron deficiencydagger. *Eur Heart J.* 2015;36:657–68.
57. van Veldhuisen DJ, Ponikowski P, van der Meer P, et al. Effect of ferric carboxymaltose on exercise capacity in patients with chronic heart failure and iron deficiency. *Circulation.* 2017;136:1374–83.
58. Yancy CW, Jessup M, Bozkurt B, et al. 2017 ACC/AHA/HFSA focused update of the 2013 ACCF/AHA guideline for the management of heart failure: a report of the American College of Cardiology/American Heart Association Task Force on Clinical Practice Guidelines and the Heart Failure Society of America. *Circulation.* 2017;136:e137–61.
59. Bourguignon S, Faller M, Champs FO, et al. Budget impact of intravenous ferric carboxymaltose in patients with chronic heart failure and iron deficiency in France. *ESC Hear Fail.* 2019;6:559–69.
60. Hofmarcher T, Cabrales Alin D, Linde C. Cost effectiveness of implementing ESC guidelines for treatment of iron deficiency in heart failure in the Nordic countries. *Scand Cardiovasc J.* 2018;52:348–55.
61. Hoes MF, Beverborg NG, Kijlstra JD, et al. Iron deficiency impairs contractility of human cardiomyocytes through decreased mitochondrial function. *Eur J Heart Fail.* 2018;20:910–9.
62. Rensvold JW, Ong SE, Jeevananthan A, et al. Complementary RNA and protein profiling identifies iron as a key regulator of mitochondrial biogenesis. *Cell Rep.* 2013;3:237–45.
63. Charles-Edwards G, Amaral N, Sleigh A, et al. Effect of iron isomaltoside on skeletal muscle energetics in patients with chronic heart failure and iron deficiency. *Circulation.* 2019;139:2386–98.
64. van der Meer P, van der Wal HH, Melenovsky V. Mitochondrial function, skeletal muscle metabolism, and iron deficiency in heart failure. *Circulation.* 2019;139:2399–402.
65. Beck-da-Silva L, Piardi D, Soder S, et al. IRON-HF study: a randomized trial to assess the effects of iron in heart failure patients with anemia. *Int J Cardiol.* 2013;168:3439–42.
66. Lewis GD, Malhotra R, Hernandez AF, et al. Effect of oral iron repletion on exercise capacity in patients with heart failure with reduced ejection fraction and iron deficiency: the IRONOUT HF randomized clinical trial. *Jama.* 2017;317:1958–66.
67. van Eijk LT, John AS, Schwoebel F, et al. Effect of the antihepcidin Spiegelmer lexaptepid on inflammation-induced decrease in serum iron in humans. *Blood.* 2014;124:2643–46.
68. Boyce M, Warrington S, Cortezi B, et al. Safety, pharmacokinetics and pharmacodynamics of the anti-hepcidin Spiegelmer lexaptepid pegol in healthy subjects. *Br J Pharmacol.* 2016;173:1580–8.
69. Poli M, Asperti M, Ruzzenenti P, Naggi A, Arosio P. Non-anticoagulant heparins are hepcidin antagonists for the treatment of anemia. *Molecules.* 2017;22. doi: 10.3390/molecules22040598.
70. Hohlbaum AM, Gille H, Trentmann S, et al. Sustained plasma hepcidin suppression and iron elevation by anticalin-derived hepcidin antagonist in cynomolgus monkey. *Br J Pharmacol.* 2018;175:1054–65.
71. Mleczko-Sanecka K, da Silva AR, Call D, et al. Imatinib and spironolactone suppress hepcidin expression. *Haematologica.* 2017;102: 1173–84.

Chapter 25
MANAGEMENT OF NEUROLOGIC AND PSYCHIATRIC ILLNESS IN THE PATIENT WITH HEART FAILURE

Evangelos Pavlos Myserlis and Grigorios Kalaitzidis

Cognitive Dysfunction in HF Patients

Definitions

Cognition is a term used to describe the ability of an individual to perceive information, learn and remember specific information, and use this knowledge to problem-solve and reason in newly encountered situations. Cognition can be categorized into specific cognitive domains that can be separately defined and evaluated (Table 25.1). Cognitive impairment refers to a global deterioration in cognitive function, which can be assessed using a variety of neuropsychological tests (Table 25.2). Three cognitive impairment syndromes are important in clinical practice: dementia, mild cognitive impairment (MCI), and delirium (Table 25.3). The first two syndromes represent a chronic, gradual decline in cognition and will be discussed as one entity, whereas the latter is an acute change in cognitive function and will be presented separately.

Dementia and MCI in HF Patients

Epidemiological and Clinical Remarks

The prevalence of cognitive impairment in patients with heart failure (HF) has been reported to range from 20% to 80%. Patients with HF have 1.62–2.64 times the odds of developing cognitive dysfunction compared with their healthy counterparts.[1] Coexisting conditions that may be further associated with cognitive dysfunction include atrial fibrillation (AF), hypertension, low left ventricular ejection fraction, high NYHA class, obesity, physical inactivity, chronic obstructive pulmonary disease, depression, sleep apnea, insomnia, poor sleep quality, anemia, renal dysfunction, hyperglycemia, prior stroke, increasing age, and lower education level.[2–11] Cognitive impairment in HF patients is associated with poorer functional status and quality of life, increased mortality, and increased readmission rates.[12]

Diagnostic Evaluation

A wide range of neuropsychological tests has been described for the evaluation of cognition in HF patients.[13] The 2016 European Society of Cardiology (ESC) Guidelines suggest the use of Mini Mental State Examination (MMSE) and the Montreal Cognitive Assessment (MoCA) tool.[14] Although the MMSE is the test most commonly used in HF patients, it is influenced by education level, culture, and language; furthermore, MMSE does not contain a direct evaluation of executive function, which is a key cognitive domain affected in this population and a crucial aspect of self-care. MoCA is more sensitive in detecting MCI in HF patients. An increasing number of studies conclude that MoCA is a better screening tool than MMSE for cognitive impairment in patients with HF, as it explicitly measures executive function and is more sensitive for diagnosing MCI.[15]

It should be highlighted that these tests are simply screening tools that should be administered in the event that the HF management team suspects a cognitive deficit in a patient. If abnormal results are obtained, a comprehensive neuropsychological consultation should be considered.

Therapeutic Management

In general, physicians treating HF patients may be reluctant to prescribe guideline-directed HF medications due to concerns of causing or worsening cognitive dysfunction in a vulnerable population. However, use of appropriate medications for HF is associated with improved cognition, both after discharge and in the short term.[16] Standard in-hospital treatment for HF, leading to restoration of normal glucose, potassium, and hemoglobin levels during hospitalization, is also related to improved cognitive ability at discharge.[17] Of note, upon admission, clinicians should have in mind the reversible causes of cognitive impairment, such as hypothyroidism, vitamin B_{12} deficiency, anticholinergic drugs, depression, infections, and space-occupying lesions.[18]

With regard to specific pharmacologic treatment, angiotensin-converting enzyme inhibitors seem to be associated with improved cognitive function in a dose-dependent manner.[19] Digoxin also seems to be associated with improved cognition.[20] Further data from randomized, controlled trials (RCTs) are necessary to validate these findings.

A considerable amount of research has focused on interventions that increase left ventricular ejection fraction, with the hypothesis that increased cerebral blood flow may improve cognitive function. Cardiac resynchronization therapy has been associated with improved functional and cognitive performance in HF patients, despite previous conflicting results.[21] Left ventricular assist device implantation has been associated with improvements in neurocognitive function in the short, medium, and long term. Specific cognitive domains include memory, processing speed, language, and visuospatial and executive function.[22] However, in a recent study, left ventricular assist devices were associated with cognitive decline after one year, highlighting the importance of careful screening.[23] Enhanced, external counterpulsation has also been found to be associated with improvement in spontaneous naming, attention, and executive function.[24] Percutaneous mitral valve repair with the MitraClip has also been studied as a tool to improve cognitive function in HF, with improvements in memory, executive, and psychosocial functioning.[25] Lastly, improvements in cerebral blood flow and cognitive function have been reported after heart transplantation, especially in the memory component.[26]

The importance of exercise in preserving cognitive function in HF patients has been highlighted by several studies. Good physical activity is associated with enhanced global cognitive function, executive function, attention, and processing speed.[27] Improvements in memory, attention, psychomotor and visual speed, executive function, and global cognitive ability have been reported after participation in cardiac rehabilitation programs, involving sessions of aerobic exercise combined with educational interventions about risk factor management.[28]

DOI: 10.1201/9780429244544-30

TABLE 25.1: A Brief Description of the Cognitive Domains and Common Neuropsychological Tools for Their Evaluation

Cognitive Domain	Neuropsychological Test	Description
Attention	Trail-making test A Attentional matrices	The ability to focus selectively on a stimulus, sustaining that focus, and shifting it at will.
Psychomotor speed	Digit symbol substitution test Trail-making test A Trail-making test B Stroop color word test	The ability to detect and respond to stimuli.
Working memory	Digit span backwards Corsi's block tapping test Short category test	The ability to temporarily store and manage the information required to carry out complex cognitive tasks, such as learning, reasoning, and comprehension.
Learning/memory	Verbal learning test	The process of repetition of stimuli that requires additional mental processing of those stimuli/the ability to recall stimuli.
Speech/language	Boston naming test Benton controlled oral word association test Token test Semantic fluency Controlled oral word association	Symbols used to exchange information.
Visual/spatial/constructional function	Complex figure drawing/copying Benton facial recognition test Judgement of line orientation test Block design test Clock drawing test	The ability to represent, analyze, and mentally manipulate objects and then respond with motor output to visual stimuli.
Executive function	Stroop color word test Trail-making test B Letter fluency Raven's progressive matrices Wisconsin card sorting test Intra-extra dimensional set shift Stockings of Cambridge	A group of complex mental processes and cognitive abilities that control the skills necessary for goal-directed behavior.

TABLE 25.2: Common Neuropsychological Tests Used and Cognitive Domains Assessed

Neuropsychological Test	Cognitive Domain Assessed
Mini Mental State Examination	Orientation Attention/working memory Short-term memory Concentration Language Visuospatial function
Montreal Cognitive Assessment tool	Concentration/attention Visuospatial function Executive function Language Working memory Short-term memory Orientation
Mini-Cog	Memory Executive function Visual/spatial/constructional function
Clock Drawing Task	Executive function Visual/spatial/constructional function

Other non-pharmacological interventions that have been studied include cognitive training, counseling, and educational interventions. Computerized cognitive training programs in HF populations seem to be associated with improvements in processing speed, delayed recall, and working memory.[29] A large RCT evaluating the effects of computerized training on memory is currently being conducted.[30] Lastly, retrieval practice, a form of repeated word recall, was found to be associated with improved memory in HF patients, although not statistically significant.[31]

Regardless of the specific therapeutic option chosen, a multi-level approach to management of cognitive impairment is advised. Coordination at the healthcare system level should ideally aim at: inclusion of more "elderly friendly" approaches, with avoidance of certain medications and urinary catheters; implementation of a formal screening method that identifies and aids patients with cognitive impairment after discharge; and introduction of integrated models that involve both hospital and home care. At the patient level, identification and management of known risk factors, better educational strategies for cognitively impaired HF patients, and close monitoring of this subgroup of patients are equally important.[32] Involvement of family members, caregivers, and other healthcare professionals is crucial in this regard. In conclusion, the management of cognitive impairment in patients with HF should aim to provide effective care both at the hospital and at the community level, by shifting the focus from individual approaches to system-level interventions, with the goal of improving outcomes.[33]

Delirium in HF Patients

Epidemiological and Clinical Remarks

Delirium is a common condition presenting in the in-patient setting, especially in decompensated HF patients. The prevalence of delirium on admission, ranges from 14% to 24%, whereas, during hospitalization, the incidence can rise to 56% among all hospitalized patients.[34] Despite the high

TABLE 25.3: Clinically Relevant Cognitive Impairment Syndromes and Their Clinical Characteristics

Cognitive Impairment Syndromes	Characteristics
Mild cognitive impairment	Intermediate state between normal aging and dementia.
	Performance on neuropsychological tests 1–2 standard deviations (SD) below the education-adjusted cut-offs, in one or more cognitive domains.
Dementia	An acquired, chronic, progressive condition characterized by multiple cognitive deficits that impair social and occupational functioning.
	Performance on neuropsychological tests 2 SD or more below education-adjusted cut-offs in at least one cognitive domain.
Delirium	An acute change in cognitive function; a state of confusion.
	Usually associated with acute illness.

incidence rates, nearly two-thirds of delirium cases remain undiagnosed.[35]

HF is an independent risk factor for the development of delirium.[36] In a patient with HF, simple precipitating factors, such as dehydration, infections, electrolyte abnormalities, or even a dose of sleeping medication can easily lead to this acute state of confusion. Although physicians should not be reluctant to prescribe guideline-based HF medications, they should also be aware that common cardiovascular drugs have been associated with delirium, including beta-blockers, non-dihydropyridine calcium channel blockers, amiodarone, digoxin, and furosemide.[37]

Delirium is associated with increased in-hospital mortality, as well as elevated 30- and 90-day rehospitalization rates, and 90-day mortality after decompensated HF.[38]

Diagnostic Evaluation

The diagnosis of delirium is primarily based on clinical evaluation. When a patient presents with confusion, it is important to determine the onset of this change in cognitive function and whether there is fluctuation in the disease state. The baseline cognitive function of the patient can be evaluated by information from caregivers, if no other recent formal assessment exists. An acute decline in cognition suggests delirium and the patient should be promptly assessed for delirium precipitants, including a potential HF exacerbation. Overview of the medications received and evaluation for potential side effects should not be omitted from the diagnostic process. If no history can be obtained, the patient should be considered delirious until proven otherwise.

In order to aid the diagnosis of delirium, a formal assessment of cognitive function should be conducted. The most widely used delirium screening tool is the Confusion Assessment Method.[39] It is based on four key diagnostic features of delirium, namely (1) acute onset and fluctuating course, (2) inattention, (3) disorganized thinking, and (4) altered level of consciousness.[40]

After delirium has been ruled in, additional testing should be undertaken. This includes complete blood count; measurement of electrolytes; renal, liver, and thyroid function tests; urine and blood cultures; measurement of drug concentrations; arterial blood gas analysis; electrocardiography and chest radiography; lumbar puncture; neuroimaging; and electroencephalography. The approach should be individualized and guided by the patient's history and physical examination findings.

In many cases, it is difficult to differentiate delirium from dementia, due to their common feature of cognitive impairment. In these cases, the main differentiating feature is the acuteness of presentation. Clinicians should also be aware of the two forms of delirium, the hyperactive and the hypoactive form. Notably, the hypoactive form is more common among the elderly and is often unrecognized.

Therapeutic Management

Concerning therapeutic options, most evidence is derived from clinical experience rather than RCTs. The mainstay of treatment for delirium has been the identification and management of precipitating factors, along with non-pharmacologic and pharmacologic measures to eliminate delirium symptoms.

The initial management should be focused around supportive measures: airway protection, prevention of aspiration, maintenance of adequate hydration and nutritional status, early mobilization, avoidance of physical restraints, and addressing the patient's daily care needs.[41] Non-pharmacological measures for symptom management should then be considered: discontinuation or reduction of specific medications; involvement of the family in the care for reorientation and comfort; creation of a comfortable environment with orienting instruments such as familiar objects; allowing uninterrupted periods of sleep with reduced noise and light; correction of sensory deficits with eyeglasses and hearing aids; and minimization of room changes. In cases where the symptoms of delirium are so severe that the safety of the patient is threatened from interruption of lifesaving interventions such as mechanical ventilation, dialysis, or central venous catheters, or when the patient suffers from severe psychotic symptoms, pharmacologic treatment should be considered. The best-studied drug for delirium is the antipsychotic haloperidol.[42] Antipsychotics, benzodiazepines, and antidepressants have also been studied with variable results.[43] Importantly, specifically for HF patients, compensation of uncompensated HF with standard in-hospital treatment has been found to be associated with improved cognition.[44] Once the symptoms of delirium have been controlled, patient care should focus on assessment and management of the underlying risk factors, as previously outlined.

Depression in HF Patients

Epidemiological and Clinical Remarks

The prevalence of depression in patients with HF is ~22%.[45] HF is a strong, independent risk factor for depression.[46] Other factors present in HF patients that can predispose to depression are summarized in Table 25.4. Depression has been shown to be an independent risk factor for increased mortality in HF.[47] Also, it can lead to up to a three-fold increase in the risk of readmission or death in the next three to 12 months after hospitalization for HF.[48] Depression is a strong predictor of short-term health decline, significant deterioration of HF symptoms, and physical and social dysfunction.[49]

TABLE 25.4: Independent Correlates of Suspected Major Depression According to Patient Health Questionnaire 9 (PHQ-9 Score of >11)

Association	Variables	Odds Ratio (OR)	95% CI	P
Independent risk factors for depression	History of depression	3.09	1.98–4.82	<0.001
	NYHA class	2.07 per class	1.52–2.81	<0.001
	Leukocyte count > 8000 mm^{-3}	1.50	1.03–2.17	0.032
	COPD	1.60	1.04–2.50	0.033
Independent protective factors for depression	Hemoglobin	0.87 per g/dL increase	0.79–0.96	0.005
	Statin use	0.66	0.45–0.98	0.039

Abbreviations: CI: confidence interval; COPD: chronic obstructive pulmonary disease; NYHA: New York Heart Association.

TABLE 25.5: Adjunctive Tools for Screening of Depression in CVD Patients

Screening Tool	Study Population	Study	Threshold	Sensitivity (%)	Specificity (%)
BDI	One month post-MI patients	Strik et al.	≥10	81.8	78.7
	Two months post-ACS patients	Frasure-Smith et al.	≥14	91.2	77.5
	Two weeks post-ACS patients	Low et al.	≥10	100.0	75.0
	CAD patients under cardiac rehabilitation	Bunevicius et al.	≥14	89.0	4.0
HADS	One month post-MI patients	Strik et al.	≥13	90.0	84.3
	In-patients with ACS	Tesio et al.	≥13	91.2	76.5
	CAD patients under cardiac rehabilitation	Bunevicius et al.	≥13	82.0	75
HADS-D	One month post-MI patients	Strik et al.	≥4	85.0	74.8
	Recent ACS patients	Bambauer et al.	≥4	96.0	25.0
	CAD patients under cardiac rehabilitation	Bunevicius et al.	≥4	84.0	55.0
SCL-90	One month post-MI patients	Strik et al.	≥25	95.5	74.0
HAMD	One month post-MI patients	Strik et al.	≥15	86.4	93.2

Abbreviations: BDI = Beck Depression Inventory; HADS = Hospital Depression and Anxiety Scale; HADS-D = Depression subscale of HADS; SCL-90 = 90-item Symptom checklist (depression subscale); HAMD = Hamilton Rating scale for depression; MI = myocardial infarction; ACS = acute coronary syndrome; CAD = coronary artery disease.

Diagnostic Evaluation

Diagnosing depression in patients with HF can be challenging. Common symptoms including fatigue, weight changes, loss of appetite, and lack of sleep, can make the diagnosis of depression difficult in patients with HF.[50]

There are many tools used to diagnose depression in HF patients, with the most widely used being the Patient Health Questionnaires (PHQ). The screening for depression in patients with coronary artery disease (CAD) involves a two-step process.[51] The first step is screening with the two-item PHQ (PHQ-2). If the patient is positive on PHQ-2 (mood and anhedonia), the second step is to validate the diagnosis of depression with the PHQ-9. Apart from PHQ, other screening tools also exist (Table 25.5). However, this two-step algorithm is considered to be the best tool available for screening for depression in patients with cardiovascular disease, due to its feasibility, availability in many languages, and wide accessibility.[52]

Specifically for HF, screening is recommended to be carried out regularly during hospitalization.[53] Negative screening results may not exclude the possibility of depression. It is suggested that rescreening is done annually or on a regular basis in cases of stressful life incidents or changes in clinical condition.[54] Moreover, lower thresholds in PHQ for screening have been proposed as more applicable than thresholds in the general population.[55] Finally, taking into account that the diagnosis of depression requires the exclusion of other conditions, patients should be assessed for these conditions (Table 25.6).[56]

Therapeutic Management

Various studies have investigated different treatment options for depression in HF patients, including pharmacotherapy, psychotherapy, and exercise. Nevertheless, there are no specific recommendations available.[14]

Pharmacotherapy with antidepressants is one of the most thoroughly studied interventions.[57] Selective serotonin reuptake inhibitors (SSRIs) are considered to be first-line agents, due to their safety profile and drug interactions in patients with multiple comorbidities.[58] Concerning the efficacy of antidepressants in patients with HF, however, clear conclusions are yet to be made. There are studies reporting improvement in depressive symptoms with antidepressants.[59] However, the two large trials, SADHART-CHF and MOOD-HF, failed to show improvements

TABLE 25.6: Conditions to Exclude for the Diagnosis of Depression

Category	Conditions		Rating Scales/Instruments
Psychiatric conditions	Bipolar disorder		Structured interview and DSM-5 diagnostic checklist
	Psychotic disorder		
	Other psychiatric disorders		
Medical conditions	Hypothyroidism		Laboratory tests
	Obstructive sleep apnea		
	Anemia		
	Folate deficiency		
	B_{12} deficiency		
	Cushing disease		
	Substance use		Michigan Alcohol screening test, drug abuse screening test
Iatrogenic causes	Drugs	Interferon	Medical history
		Glucocorticoids	
		Propranolol	
		Levodopa	
		Oral contraceptives	

with antidepressants compared with placebo.[60,61] In another large study, SSRIs and tricyclic antidepressants (TCAs) were associated with increased cardiovascular mortality.[62] It is worth mentioning that cardiovascular adverse effects are more common with monoamine oxidase inhibitors (MAOIs) (27%), followed by TCAs (15%). SSRIs are associated with a low frequency of cardiovascular side effects (0.08%).[63] Adverse effects include (1) QT prolongation with the potential for life-threatening arrhythmias, most importantly Torsades de pointes (with TCAs); (2) orthostatic hypotension (with TCAs and selective serotonin-norepinephrine reuptake inhibitors [SNRIs]); and (3) hypertension (with SNRIs and MAOIs).[64] Finally, clinicians should be aware of possible drug interactions. The antidepressants fluoxetine and paroxetine are strong CYP2D6 inhibitors, so they can lead to increased activity of beta-blockers.[14] Another possible interaction of SSRIs (fluoxetine and fluvoxamine) is with warfarin, through CYP2C9 inhibition.[65,66]

Treatment approaches other than pharmacotherapy have also been investigated. Cognitive behavioral therapy (CBT) and internet-based CBT have been found to reduce depressive symptoms. However, larger studies are needed to systematically investigate these findings.[67]

Exercise training is another intervention that has been studied in patients with HF.[68] A meta-analysis using inconsistent depression scales as outcome measures found that aerobic exercise in patients with left ventricular ejection fraction <50% could significantly decrease depressive symptoms.[69] Additionally, the HF-ACTION study showed that exercise three times per week over a period of three months could decrease depressive symptoms.[70]

Finally, a multidisciplinary approach focusing on patient education can be important for the treatment of depression. Although cardiologists may already be evaluating and treating depression,[71] the role of primary care providers is important for initial treatment of depression, especially in areas with limited access to mental health care providers.[72] Collaborative care, consisting of a nurse coordinator, a primary care physician, a psychiatrist, and a cardiologist, has been shown to reduce the severity of depression and mortality in depressed HF patients.[73] Lastly, an RCT studying the effect of a structured, collaborative management program, Health Net Care-HF (HNC) for depressed patients with HF, found that HNC decreased mortality in depressed patients with decompensated HF.[74]

Other Neurologic and Psychiatric Comorbidities

Stroke in HF Patients

Approximately 10% to 24% of stroke patients are reported to have HF.[75] The risk of ischemic stroke is two to three times higher in patients with HF than in those without HF.[76] Patients with stroke and HF have increased rates of mortality, severe neurologic deficits, and longer hospital stays, compared with those without HF.[77] Several studies have attempted to develop a strategy to assess stroke risk in HF patients, largely based on the presence or absence of AF. In patients with AF, stroke risk is calculated with the $CHADS_2$ and the CHA_2DS_2-VASc scores.[78] Therapeutic management is similarly based on AF status. In patients with AF, guidelines suggest the use of oral anticoagulants in patients with a CHA_2DS_2-VASc score of at least 2. With a CHA_2DS_2-VASc score of 1, all three options are recommended (use of oral anticoagulants, aspirin, no antithrombotic treatment), with a preference for oral anticoagulants. Since a CHA_2DS_2-VASc score in patients with HF and AF is ≥ 1, oral anticoagulants should be strongly considered. In patients without AF, findings have been inconclusive with regard to anticoagulation use. In the WASH and HELAS trials, no differences were observed between warfarin, aspirin, or placebo with respect to death, stroke, and myocardial infarction.[79,80] In the WATCH study, warfarin was associated with reduced incidence of ischemic stroke, compared with aspirin or clopidogrel, but the primary outcomes of all-cause mortality, nonfatal myocardial infarction, and non-fatal stroke were similar among all groups.[81] In the most recent and largest WARCEF trial, warfarin was associated with lower risk of ischemic stroke, but also associated with increased major hemorrhagic events.[82] In a subsequent meta-analysis, warfarin was associated with decreased ischemic stroke risk but increased risk for hemorrhage, although intracranial hemorrhage was rare.[83] In light of the above findings, the use of oral anticoagulants in patients with HF and sinus rhythm should be individualized.

Anxiety in HF Patients

The association of anxiety with HF has recently been studied.[84] The effects of anxiety on HF outcomes are controversial. Several studies failed to show a significant association between anxiety and mortality in HF.[85] Nevertheless, screening for anxiety in patients with HF may be important. Anxiety has been linked to higher rates of mortality in CAD patients, which is often the underlying etiology of HF, and anxiety disorders may also lead to poor cardiac outcomes in patients with or without cardiac disease.[86] Anxiety is often under-diagnosed in HF patients.[87] Although HF guidelines do not suggest universal screening for anxiety disorders, it may be useful to screen for generalized anxiety disorder (GAD) in patients with HF.[88] An easy-to-use tool is the 7-item Generalized Anxiety Disorder (GAD-7) or its abbreviated version, the two-item GAD-2.[89] It is suggested that screening be performed only in programs that guarantee initiation and monitoring of treatment.[86] Treatment options include antidepressant pharmacotherapy, mainly SSRIs, CBT, and exercise, with no data supporting the superiority of one treatment strategy over the others.[90]

Controversies and Research Opportunities

Regarding cognitive impairment in HF, several limitations should be taken into consideration. Most data are derived from older hospitalized patients, or from large, population-based cohorts. More data are needed from representative populations of varying age, gender, and educational background.[10] Also, limited information exists about the efficacy or safety of specific medications for cognitive impairment in HF. No large-scale HF trial has included cognitive function as an outcome, with the exception of a few recent studies investigating the efficacy of the new angiotensin receptor-neprilysin inhibitor sacubitril-valsartan (LCZ696).[1] In PARADIGM-HF, no adverse events associated with cognitive function were reported.[91] Two ongoing trials of LCZ696 independently use either the MMSE or a detailed neuropsychological battery.[92]

Similarly, for delirium, several research opportunities exist for future investigation. Diagnosis, severity, and subtype classification can be refined with improved measurement and identification tools. Neuroimaging studies, as well as newly developed biomarkers (deliriomics) can be used to facilitate diagnosis, risk stratification, and prognosis.[41]

Concerning the data on depression in patients with HF, there are limitations that must be taken into account, as well as corresponding research opportunities. For example, there are several limitations concerning the diagnosis of depression in HF patients. Although the American Heart Association (AHA) suggests the use of PHQ in patients with CAD for diagnosis of depression, there are no specific AHA guidelines for the diagnosis of depression in HF patients. Of note, the ESC suggests the use of Beck's Depression Inventory or Cardiac Depression Scale as tools for the diagnosis of depression in patients with HF. More data are needed to evaluate the efficacy of antidepressant pharmacotherapy in patients with HF; there are also controversies pertinent to the adverse effects and cardiovascular mortality associated with these agents.[93] Finally, multidisciplinary approaches, with patient-focused education for patients with HF and depression, need further investigation.[94]

References

1. Cannon JA, Moffitt P, Perez-Moreno AC, et al. Cognitive impairment and heart failure: systematic review and meta-analysis. *J Card Fail.* 2017;23(6):464–75.
2. Alosco ML, Spitznagel MB, Cohen R, et al. Obesity and cognitive dysfunction in heart failure: the role of hypertension, type 2 diabetes, and physical fitness. *Eur J Cardiovasc Nurs.* 2015;14(4):334–41.
3. Alosco ML, Spitznagel MB, Josephson R, Hughes J, Gunstad J. COPD is associated with cognitive dysfunction and poor physical fitness in heart failure. *Heart Lung.* 2015;44(1):21–6.
4. Alosco ML, Spitznagel MB, Raz N, et al. The interactive effects of cerebral perfusion and depression on cognitive function in older adults with heart failure. *Psychosom Med.* 2013;75(7):632–9.
5. Hjelm C, Stromberg A, Arestedt K, Brostrom A. Association between sleep-disordered breathing, sleep-wake pattern, and cognitive impairment among patients with chronic heart failure. *Eur J Heart Fail.* 2013;15(5):496–504.
6. Knecht KM, Alosco ML, Spitznagel MB, et al. Sleep apnea and cognitive function in heart failure. *Cardiovasc Psychiatry Neurol.* 2012;2012:402079.
7. Myserlis PG, Malli A, Kalaitzoglou DK, et al. Atrial fibrillation and cognitive function in patients with heart failure: a systematic review and meta-analysis. *Heart Fail Rev.* 2017;22(1):1–11.
8. Alosco ML, Brickman AM, Spitznagel MB, et al. The independent association of hypertension with cognitive function among older adults with heart failure. *J Neurol Sci.* 2012;323(1–2):216–20.
9. Jurgens CY, Faulkner KM, Lee CS. Phenotypic profiling of cognitive impairment risk among patients with heart failure: a literature review of the usefulness of cardiac-related variables. *Eur J Cardiovasc Nurs.* 2013;12(2):109–31.
10. Vogels RL, Scheltens P, Schroeder-Tanka JM, Weinstein HC. Cognitive impairment in heart failure: a systematic review of the literature. *Eur J Heart Fail.* 2007;9(5):440–9.
11. Harkness K, Demers C, Heckman GA, McKelvie RS. Screening for cognitive deficits using the Montreal cognitive assessment tool in outpatients >/=65 years of age with heart failure. *Am J Cardiol.* 2011;107(8): 1203–7.
12. Alosco ML, Spitznagel MB, Cohen R, et al. Reduced cognitive function predicts functional decline in patients with heart failure over 12 months. *Eur J Cardiovasc Nurs.* 2014;13(4):304–10.
13. Cameron J, Kure CE, Pressler SJ, Ski CF, Clark AM, Thompson DR. Diagnostic accuracy of cognitive screening instruments in heart failure: a systematic review. *J Cardiovasc Nurs.* 2016;31(5):412–24.
14. Ponikowski P, Voors AA, Anker SD, et al. 2016 ESC guidelines for the diagnosis and treatment of acute and chronic heart failure: the task force for the diagnosis and treatment of acute and chronic heart failure of the European Society of Cardiology (ESC). Developed with the special contribution of the Heart Failure Association (HFA) of the ESC. *Eur J Heart Fail.* 2016;18(8):891–975.
15. Alagiakrishnan K, Mah D, Dyck JR, Senthilselvan A, Ezekowitz J. Comparison of two commonly used clinical cognitive screening tests to diagnose mild cognitive impairment in heart failure with the golden standard European Consortium Criteria. *Int J Cardiol.* 2017;228: 558–62.
16. Almeida OP, Tamai S. Clinical treatment reverses attentional deficits in congestive heart failure. *BMC Geriatr.* 2001;1(1):2.
17. Sanford A, Morley JE. Are the new guidelines for cholesterol and hypertension age friendly? *J Am Med Dir Assoc.* 2014;15(6):373–5.
18. Morley JE. Mild cognitive impairment-a treatable condition. *J Am Med Dir Assoc.* 2014;15(1):1–5.
19. Zuccala G, Onder G, Marzetti E, et al. Use of angiotensin-converting enzyme inhibitors and variations in cognitive performance among patients with heart failure. *Eur Heart J.* 2004;26(3):226–33.
20. Laudisio A, Marzetti E, Pagano F, Cocchi A, Bernabei R, Zuccala G. Digoxin and cognitive performance in patients with heart failure: a cohort, pharmacoepidemiological survey. *Drugs Aging.* 2009;26(2):103–12.
21. Fumagalli S, Pieragnoli P, Ricciardi G, et al. Cardiac resynchronization therapy improves functional status and cognition. *Int J Cardiol.* 2016;219:212–7.
22. Bhat G, Yost G, Mahoney E. Cognitive function and left ventricular assist device implantation. *J Heart Lung Transplant.* 2015;34(11):1398–405.
23. Fendler TJ, Spertus JA, Gosch KL, et al. Incidence and predictors of cognitive decline in patients with left ventricular assist devices. *Circ Cardiovasc Qual Outcomes.* 2015;8(3):285–91.
24. Kozdag G, Iseri P, Gokce G, et al. Treatment with enhanced external counterpulsation improves cognitive functions in chronic heart failure patients. *Turk Kardiyol Dern Ars.* 2013;41(5):418–28.
25. Terhoeven V, Nikendei C, Cranz A, et al. Effects of MitraClip on cognitive and psychological function in heart failure patients: the sicker the better. *Eur J Med Res.* 2019;24(1):14.
26. Gruhn N, Larsen FS, Boesgaard S, et al. Cerebral blood flow in patients with chronic heart failure before and after heart transplantation. *Stroke.* 2001;32(11):2530–3.
27. Fulcher KK, Alosco ML, Miller L, et al. Greater physical activity is associated with better cognitive function in heart failure. *Health Psychol.* 2014;33(11):1337.
28. Gary RA, Brunn K. Aerobic exercise as an adjunct therapy for improving cognitive function in heart failure. *Cardiol Res Pract.* 2014;2014:157508.

29. Kua ZJ, Valenzuela M, Dong Y. Can computerized cognitive training improve cognition in patients with heart failure?: A review. *J Cardiovasc Nurs.* 2019;34(2):E19–27.
30. Cameron J, Rendell PG, Ski CF, et al. PROspective MEmory Training to improve HEart failUre Self-care (PROMETHEUS): study protocol for a randomised controlled trial. *Trials.* 2015;16(1):196.
31. Viveiros J, Sethares K, Shapiro A. Repeated recall as an intervention to improve memory performance in heart failure patients. *Eur J Cardiovasc Nurs.* 2017;16(8):724–32.
32. Harkness K, Heckman GA, McKelvie RS. The older patient with heart failure: high risk for frailty and cognitive impairment. *Expert Rev Cardiovasc Ther.* 2012;10(6):779–95.
33. Cannon JA, McMurray JJ, Quinn TJ. "Hearts and minds": association, causation and implication of cognitive impairment in heart failure. *Alzheim Res Ther.* 2015;7(1):22.
34. Inouye SK. Delirium in older persons. *N Engl J Med.* 2006;354(11):1157–65.
35. Harkness K, Heckman GA, McKelvie RS. The older patient with heart failure: high risk for frailty and cognitive impairment. *Expert Rev Cardiovasc Ther.* 2012;10(6):779–95.
36. Mathillas J, Olofsson B, Lövheim H, Gustafson Y. Thirty-day prevalence of delirium among very old people: a population-based study of very old people living at home and in institutions. *Arch Gerontol Geriatr.* 2013;57(3):298–304.
37. Keller S, Frishman WH. Neuropsychiatric effects of cardiovascular drug therapy. *Cardiol Rev.* 2003;11(2):73–93.
38. Uthamalingam S, Gurm GS, Daley M, Flynn J, Capodilupo R. Usefulness of acute delirium as a predictor of adverse outcomes in patients> 65 years of age with acute decompensated heart failure. *Am J Cardiol.* 2011;108(3):402–8.
39. O'Mahony R, Murthy L, Akunne A, Young J, Guideline Development Group. Synopsis of the National Institute for Health and Clinical Excellence guideline for prevention of delirium. *Ann Intern Med.* 2011;154(11):746–51.
40. Inouye SK, van Dyck CH, Alessi CA, Balkin S, Siegal AP, Horwitz RI. Clarifying confusion: the confusion assessment method. A new method for detection of delirium. *Ann Intern Med.* 1990;113(12):941–8.
41. Inouye SK, Westendorp RG, Saczynski JS. Delirium in elderly people. *The Lancet.* 2014;383(9920):911–22.
42. Breitbart W, Marotta R, Platt MM, et al. A double-blind trial of haloperidol, chlorpromazine, and lorazepam in the treatment of delirium in hospitalized AIDS patients. *Focus.* 2005;153(2):231–340.
43. Inouye SK. Delirium in older persons. *New Engl J Med.* 2006;354(11): 1157–65.
44. Kindermann I, Fischer D, Karbach J, et al. Cognitive function in patients with decompensated heart failure: the Cognitive Impairment in Heart Failure (CogImpair-HF) study. *Eur J Heart Fail.* 2012;14(4):404–13.
45. Rutledge T, Reis VA, Linke SE, Greenberg BH, Mills PJ. Depression in heart failure a meta-analytic review of prevalence, intervention effects, and associations with clinical outcomes. *J Am Coll Cardiol.* 2006;48(8):1527–37.
46. Angermann CE, Gelbrich G, Stork S, et al. Somatic correlates of comorbid major depression in patients with systolic heart failure. *Int J Cardiol.* 2011;147(1):66–73.
47. Fan H, Yu W, Zhang Q, et al. Depression after heart failure and risk of cardiovascular and all-cause mortality: a meta-analysis. *Prev Med.* 2014;6336–42.
48. Jani BD, Mair FS, Roger VL, Weston SA, Jiang R, Chamberlain AM. Comorbid depression and heart failure: a community cohort study. *PLoS One.* 2016;11(6):e0158570.
49. Rumsfeld JS, Havranek E, Masoudi FA, et al. Depressive symptoms are the strongest predictors of short-term declines in health status in patients with heart failure. *J Am Coll Cardiol.* 2003;42(10):1811–7.
50. Ghosh RK, Ball S, Prasad V, Gupta A. Depression in heart failure: intricate relationship, pathophysiology and most updated evidence of interventions from recent clinical studies. *Int J Cardiol.* 2016;224170–177.
51. Lichtman JH, Bigger JT, Jr., Blumenthal JA, et al. Depression and coronary heart disease: recommendations for screening, referral, and treatment: a science advisory from the American Heart Association Prevention Committee of the Council on Cardiovascular Nursing, Council on Clinical Cardiology, Council on Epidemiology and Prevention, and Interdisciplinary Council on Quality of Care and Outcomes Research: endorsed by the American Psychiatric Association. *Circulation.* 2008;118(17):1768–75.
52. Jha MK, Qamar A, Vaduganathan M, Charney DS, Murrough JW. Screening and management of depression in patients with cardiovascular disease: JACC state-of-the-art review. *J Am Coll Cardiol.* 2019;73(14):1827–45.
53. Panel PMIDCPG. AAFP guideline for the detection and management of post-myocardial infarction depression. *Ann Fam Med.* 2009;7(1):71–9.
54. Jha MK, Qamar A, Vaduganathan M, Charney DS, Murrough JW. Screening and management of depression in patients with cardiovascular disease: JACC state-of-the-art review. *J Am Coll Cardiol.* 2019;73(14):1827–45.
55. Haddad M, Walters P, Phillips R, et al. Detecting depression in patients with coronary heart disease: a diagnostic evaluation of the PHQ-9 and HADS-D in primary care, findings from the UPBEAT-UK study. *PLoS One.* 2013;8(10):e78493.
56. American Psychiatric Association. *Diagnostic and statistical manual of mental disorders (DSM-5).* Washington, DC: American Psychiatric Publishing; 2013.
57. Stahl SM. *Essential psychopharmacology: the prescriber's guide.* Cambridge, UK: Cambridge University Press; 2005.
58. Watson K, Summers KM. Depression in patients with heart failure: clinical implications and management. *Pharmacotherapy.* 2009;29(1):49–63.
59. Angermann CE, Gelbrich G, Stork S, et al. Effect of escitalopram on all-cause mortality and hospitalization in patients with heart failure and depression: the MOOD-HF randomized clinical trial. *JAMA.* 2016;315(24):2683–93.
60. Angermann CE, Gelbrich G, Störk S, et al. Effect of escitalopram on all-cause mortality and hospitalization in patients with heart failure and depression: the MOOD-HF randomized clinical trial. *JAMA.* 2016;315(24):2683–93.
61. O'Connor CM, Jiang W, Kuchibhatla M, et al. Safety and efficacy of sertraline for depression in patients with heart failure: results of the SADHART-CHF (Sertraline Against Depression and Heart Disease in Chronic Heart Failure) trial. *J Am Coll Cardiol.* 2010;56(9):692–9.
62. Fosb l EL, Gislason GH, Poulsen HE, et al. Prognosis in heart failure and the value of β-blockers are altered by the use of antidepressants and depend on the type of antidepressants used. *Circ Heart Fail.* 2009;2(6):582–90.
63. Spindelegger CJ, Papageorgiou K, Grohmann R, et al. Cardiovascular adverse reactions during antidepressant treatment: a drug surveillance report of German-speaking countries between 1993 and 2010. *Int J Neuropsychopharmacol.* 2015;18(4):pyu080.
64. Roose SP, Miyazaki M. Pharmacologic treatment of depression in patients with heart disease. *Psychosom Med.* 2005;67 Suppl 1S54-57.
65. Benfield P, Ward A. Fluvoxamine. A review of its pharmacodynamic and pharmacokinetic properties, and therapeutic efficacy in depressive illness. *Drugs.* 1986;32(4):313–34.
66. Dent LA, Orrock MW. Warfarin-fluoxetine and diazepam-fluoxetine interaction. *Pharmacotherapy.* 1997;17(1):170–2.
67. Lundgren J, Andersson G, Dahlstrom O, Jaarsma T, Kohler AK, Johansson P. Internet-based cognitive behavior therapy for patients with heart failure and depressive symptoms: a proof of concept study. *Patient Educ Couns.* 2015;98(8):935–42.
68. Cooney G, Dwan K, Mead G. Exercise for depression. *JAMA.* 2014;311(23):2432–3.
69. Tu RH, Zeng ZY, Zhong GQ, et al. Effects of exercise training on depression in patients with heart failure: a systematic review and meta-analysis of randomized controlled trials. *Eur J Heart Fail.* 2014;16(7):749–57.
70. Blumenthal JA, Babyak MA, O'Connor C, et al. Effects of exercise training on depressive symptoms in patients with chronic heart failure: the HF-ACTION randomized trial. *JAMA.* 2012;308(5):465–74.
71. Feinstein RE, Blumenfield M, Orlowski B, Frishman WH, Ovanessian S. A national survey of cardiovascular physicians' beliefs and clinical care practices when diagnosing and treating depression in patients with cardiovascular disease. *Card Rev.* 2006;14(4):164–9.
72. U.S. Department of Health and Human Services. *National and regional projections of supply and demand for primary care practitioners: 2013–2025.* Rockville, MD: National Center for Health Workforce Analysis; 2016. https://bhw.hrsa.gov/sites/default/files/bhw/health-workforce-analysis/research/projections/primary-care-national-projections2013-2025.pdf.
73. Bekelman DB, Plomondon ME, Carey EP, et al. Primary results of the patient-centered disease management (PCDM) for heart failure study: a randomized clinical trial. *JAMA Intern Med.* 2015;175(5):725–32.
74. Gelbrich G, Stork S, Kreissl-Kemmer S, et al. Effects of structured heart failure disease management on mortality and morbidity depend on patients' mood: results from the interdisciplinary network for heart failure study. *Eur J Heart Fail.* 2014;16(10):1133–41.
75. Haeusler KG, Laufs U, Endres M. Chronic heart failure and ischemic stroke. *Stroke.* 2011;42(10):2977–82.
76. Pullicino PM, McClure LA, Wadley VG, et al. Blood pressure and stroke in heart failure in the REasons for Geographic And Racial Differences in Stroke (REGARDS) study. *Stroke.* 2009;40(12):3706–10.
77. Haeusler KG, Laufs U, Endres M. Chronic heart failure and ischemic stroke. *Stroke.* 2011;42(10):2977–82.
78. January CT, Wann LS, Alpert JS, et al. 2014 AHA/ACC/HRS guideline for the management of patients with atrial fibrillation: a report of the American College of Cardiology/American Heart Association Task Force on Practice Guidelines and the Heart Rhythm Society. *J Am Coll Cardiol.* 2014;64(21):e1–76.
79. Cleland JG, Findlay I, Jafri S, et al. The Warfarin/Aspirin Study in Heart failure (WASH): a randomized trial comparing antithrombotic strategies for patients with heart failure. *Am Heart J.* 2004;148(1):157–64.

80. Cokkinos DV, Haralabopoulos GC, Kostis JB, Toutouzas PK, HELAS Investigators. Efficacy of antithrombotic therapy in chronic heart failure: the HELAS study. *Eur J Heart Fail.* 2006;8(4):428–32.
81. Massie BM, Collins JF, Ammon SE, et al. Randomized trial of warfarin, aspirin, and clopidogrel in patients with chronic heart failure: the Warfarin and Antiplatelet Therapy in Chronic Heart Failure (WATCH) trial. *Circulation.* 2009;119(12):1616–24.
82. Homma S, Thompson JL, Pullicino PM, et al. Warfarin and aspirin in patients with heart failure and sinus rhythm. *N Engl J Med.* 2012;366(20):1859–69.
83. Hopper I, Skiba M, Krum H. Updated meta-analysis on antithrombotic therapy in patients with heart failure and sinus rhythm. *Eur J Heart Fail.* 2013;15(1):69–78.
84. Easton K, Coventry P, Lovell K, Carter LA, Deaton C. Prevalence and measurement of anxiety in samples of patients with heart failure: meta-analysis. *J Cardiovasc Nurs.* 2016;31(4):367–79.
85. Pelle AJ, Pedersen SS, Schiffer AA, Szabo B, Widdershoven JW, Denollet J. Psychological distress and mortality in systolic heart failure. *Circ Heart Fail.* 2010;3(2):261–7.
86. Roest AM, Zuidersma M, de Jonge P. Myocardial infarction and generalised anxiety disorder: 10-year follow-up. *Br J Psychiatry.* 2012;200(4):324–9.
87. Huffman JC, Smith FA, Blais MA, Beiser ME, Januzzi JL, Fricchione GL. Recognition and treatment of depression and anxiety in patients with acute myocardial infarction. *Am J Cardiol.* 2006;98(3):319–24.
88. Celano CM, Villegas AC, Albanese AM, Gaggin HK, Huffman JC. Depression and anxiety in heart failure: a review. *Harv Rev Psychiatry.* 2018;26(4):175–84.
89. Spitzer RL, Kroenke K, Williams JB, Lowe B. A brief measure for assessing generalized anxiety disorder: the GAD-7. *Arch Intern Med.* 2006;166(10):1092–7.
90. Angermann CE, Ertl G. Depression, anxiety, and cognitive impairment: comorbid mental health disorders in heart failure. *Curr Heart Fail Rep.* 2018;15(6):398–410.
91. McMurray JJ, Packer M, Desai AS, et al. Angiotensin-neprilysin inhibition versus enalapril in heart failure. *N Engl J Med.* 2014;371(11): 993–1004.
92. Solomon SD, Rizkala AR, Gong J, et al. Angiotensin receptor neprilysin inhibition in heart failure with preserved ejection fraction: rationale and design of the PARAGON-HF trial. *JACC Heart Fail.* 2017;5(7): 471–82.
93. Rajeswaran T, Plymen CM, Doherty AM. The effect of antidepressant medications in the management of heart failure on outcomes: mortality, cardiovascular function and depression–a systematic review. *Int J Psychiatry Clin Pract.* 2018;22(3):164–9.
94. Frasure-Smith N, Lespérance F. Depression and anxiety as predictors of 2-year cardiac events in patients with stable coronary artery disease. *Arch Gen Psych.* 2008;65(1):62–71.

Section VI
The Patient with Right Heart Disease

DOI: 10.1201/9780429244544-31

Chapter 26
PULMONARY HYPERTENSION AND RIGHT VENTRICULAR FAILURE FROM LEFT HEART DISEASE

Anjan Tibrewala and Jonathan D. Rich

Definition

Pulmonary hypertension (PH) is categorized into five groups as designated by the World Health Organization (WHO). Pulmonary hypertension due to left heart failure (HF) is categorized into WHO Group 2 PH.[1,2] The etiology of WHO Group 2 PH may occur under any of the following conditions: (i) heart failure with reduced ejection fraction (HFrEF), (ii) heart failure with preserved ejection fraction (HFpEF), (iii) valvular heart disease, and/or (iv) congenital/acquired cardiovascular conditions that result in an elevation in left-sided pressures.[1]

Traditionally, pulmonary hypertension has been defined by a mean pulmonary artery pressure (mPAP) ≥25 mmHg.[2,3] To qualify hemodynamically as having Group 2 PH, the pulmonary capillary wedge pressure (PCWP) or left ventricular end-diastolic pressure (LVEDP) should also be >15 mmHg.[1,4] In 2018, the 6th World Symposium on Pulmonary Hypertension (WSPH) Task Force proposed lowering the threshold for PH to a mPAP >20 mmHg.[1,5] This recent, though debatable, recommendation was made on the basis of studies demonstrating average mPAP in normal subjects is 14.0 ± 3.3 mmHg, which makes mPAP >20 mmHg about 2 standard deviations above the mean, and findings that mPAP >20 mmHg is associated with adverse outcomes.[1,5]

In the assessment of Group 2 PH, there are several relevant hemodynamic calculations: (i) transpulmonary gradient (TPG) = mPAP–PCWP, (ii) pulmonary vascular resistance (PVR) = TPG/cardiac output, and a lesser used calculation (iii) diastolic pulmonary gradient (DPG) = diastolic PAP–PCWP (Box 26.1). Depending on the above measurements, more recent terminology further categorizes Group 2 PH patients as having either isolated postcapillary PH (Ipc-PH) or combined pre- and postcapillary PH (Cpc-PH).[1,6,7]

BOX 26.1 DEFINITIONS OF MEASUREMENTS FOR DIAGNOSIS OF WHO GROUP 2 PULMONARY HYPERTENSION

Abbreviations: mPAP: mean pulmonary artery pressure, PCWP: pulmonary capillary wedge pressure, dPAP: diastolic pulmonary artery pressure, CO: cardiac output.

Transpulmonary Gradient (TPG) = mPAP − PCWP
Diastolic Pulmonary Gradient (DPG) = dPAP − PCWP

$$\text{Pulmonary Vascular Resistance (PVR)} = \frac{\text{TPG}}{\text{CO}} = \frac{(\text{mPAP} - \text{PCWP})}{\text{CO}}$$

Isolated postcapillary PH occurs when an elevated left atrial pressure results in PH but with a PVR <3 Wood units (WU). Conversely, Cpc-PH occurs when changes occur in the pulmonary vasculature that are deemed to be "out of proportion" to the left atrial pressure. In this scenario, a PVR ≥3 WU is the rule, though it is often also associated with a TPG ≥12 mmHg and/or DPG ≥7 mmHg (Table 26.1).[1,2,6,8]

Pathogenesis

Left heart failure is often associated with abnormalities in left atrial structure and function,[9,10] which result in elevations in left atrial pressure. Consistent with basic principles of fluid mechanics, left atrial pressure elevations are "passively" transmitted to the pulmonary veins and in turn the pulmonary arteries, resulting in PA pressure elevation. Thus, the root cause of pulmonary hypertension due to left heart disease is primarily based on elevations in left atrial pressure and the subsequent hemodynamic and pathologic changes that occur to the pulmonary vasculature.[7,9] Indeed, studies with echocardiographic and invasive hemodynamic data demonstrate associations between pulmonary artery pressure elevations and vascular remodeling with decreased left atrial ejection fraction and increased left atrial stiffness.[10]

Though not entirely understood, as elevations in left atrial pressure persist over time, structural and functional abnormalities may develop in the pulmonary vasculature, which may lead to sufficient remodeling to result in Cpc-PH. In this scenario, although the root cause of PA pressure elevation is still elevations in left atrial pressure, sufficient changes within the pulmonary vasculature itself occur leading to further elevated pressure gradients and resistances.[2,7,9,11] These adaptive changes within the pulmonary vasculature consist of "arterialization" of the pulmonary veins with increased vessel wall thickness, predominantly due to hypertrophy of the medial wall layer.[6,7,9] These changes, including the elevations in pulmonary venous pressure, are subsequently transmitted to the pulmonary capillaries, which induce further changes in the alveolar-capillary unit including an increased production of glycosaminoglycans and deposition of collagen in the extracellular matrix (Figure 26.1).[7,9,12] These changes are largely mediated by growth factors including transforming growth factor, angiotensin-II, tumor necrosis factor-α, and endothelin-1.[6,7] Similarly, these growth factors may also induce "muscularization" of the pulmonary arterioles, leading to intimal hyperplasia and smooth muscle hypertrophy.[7] Furthermore, disequilibrium in nitric oxide (NO) and endothelin-1 (ET-1) levels may also contribute to vasoconstriction and endothelial dysfunction of the arterioles, leading to the increases in PA pressures and PVR.[7,9]

In addition, there may be genetic mutations that predispose or contribute to the development of Group 2 PH.[6] For example, mutations in the bone morphogenic protein receptor 2 (*BMPR2*) gene are associated with 70% of cases of heritable pulmonary arterial hypertension (PAH) and 10–40% of cases of idiopathic PAH.[13,14] Though specific genes have not been identified to be behind Group 2 PH, it is plausible that similar or unrelated genetic underpinnings may play a role in the pathogenesis of Group 2 PH.[6,13–15]

Ultimately, it is the right ventricle (RV) that must overcome downstream changes in the pulmonary vasculature and

DOI: 10.1201/9780429244544-32

TABLE 26.1: Diagnostic Criteria for Different Types of WHO Group 2 Pulmonary Hypertension (PH)

	mPAP	PCWP	PVR	TPG	DPG
WHO Group 2 PH	≥25	≥15			
Isolated postcapillary PH	≥25	≥15	≥3	≥12	≥7
Combined pre- and postcapillary PH	≥25	≥15	<3	<12	<7

Abbreviations: mPAP: mean pulmonary artery pressure, PCWP: pulmonary capillary wedge pressure, PVR: pulmonary vascular resistance, TPG: transpulmonary gradient, DPG: diastolic pulmonary gradient.
Source: Adapted from Simonneau et al. (2019); Galie et al. (2015); Berthelot et al. (2018); Franco (2018).

increases in afterload. To do so, the RV hypertrophies in an effort to maintain adequate contractile function[9,16] However, the afterload-sensitive RV will eventually dilate in response to persistent or further increases in PA pressure. As the RV dilates and its contractile performance diminishes due to RV-PA uncoupling (i.e., the inability of the RV to match increases in afterload), stroke volume is reduced, tricuspid regurgitation develops, and clinical pictures of LV underfilling and right-sided congestion ensue.[7,9,16,17]

Epidemiology and Prognosis

The prevalence of Group 2 PH varies depending on the HF population being studied and the modalities used to make the diagnosis. When using invasive hemodynamic criteria, 60–80% of patients with HFrEF and 50–65% of those with HFpEF have PH.[7,8,18] Among these patients, at least 12–24% have Cpc-PH, but the figure may approach 50% of patients, depending on the Cpc-PH definition being used[7,18–20] With respect to advanced HF, studies have shown that patients with worse NYHA functional class, lower cardiac index, and higher right atrial pressure are increasingly likely to have PH.[21,22] By extrapolation, it would be estimated that those with advanced HF would have a prevalence of PH that is at least within the 60–80% range seen in HFrEF, if not higher.

The presence of Group 2 PH confers an increased risk of adverse outcomes compared with HF patients without PH. For example, a 5 mmHg increase in PASP is associated with a 9% increase in risk of mortality when accounting for the presence of HF among other covariates.[22] Similarly, a 10 mmHg increase in estimated PASP is associated with a 37% increased risk of all-cause mortality, left ventricular assist device (LVAD) implantation, or urgent heart transplantation within a median follow-up time of 2.6 years.[23] Moreover, patients with Cpc-PH have been shown to have the lowest survival rate among all patients with Group 2 PH (Figure 26.2).[7,18,19,24] In one study evaluating both HFrEF and HFpEF patients, the median survival of patients with Cpc-PH was 78 and 54 months, respectively, compared with 110 and 102 months, respectively, in those with isolated postcapillary PH.[18,19] In fact, Cpc-PH patients have been shown to have an overall survival rate approaching the poor prognosis seen in those patients with Group 1 PAH.[7,19] In addition, advanced HF patients with Cpc-PH, as defined by an elevated PVR, have an increased risk of early and late mortality following cardiac transplantation.[25,26] Thus, in advanced HF, the presence of PH, particularly Cpc-PH, should be considered an indicator of end-organ damage.

Diagnosis

Transthoracic Echocardiography

Transthoracic echocardiography (TTE) is often used as a screening tool for PH. The estimation of PASP is based on Doppler evaluation of peak tricuspid regurgitation velocity combined with an estimate of right atrial pressure based on size and collapsibility of the inferior vena cava.[2] An estimated PASP ≥40 mmHg in the presence of RV dilation, RV dysfunction, flattening or abnormal motion of the intraventricular septum, right atrial enlargement, tricuspid regurgitation, pulmonic regurgitation, and/or pericardial effusion are findings consistent with possible PH.[2,27]

However, under- or overestimation of PASP occurs frequently when using TTE. In fact two separate studies demonstrated that Doppler echocardiography estimates of PASP are inaccurate in approximately 50% when compared with the reference standard of invasive measurement during right heart catheterization (RHC).[28,29] Much of the inaccuracies that occur with TTE are due to limitations of Doppler estimates of a tricuspid regurgitation jet, use of the modified Bernoulli equation, assumptions regarding lack of pulmonic stenosis, effects of respiration, and difficulties in estimating right atrial pressure.[28–30] Thus, whereas echocardiography may be used as a preliminary tool for identifying patients with an increased likelihood of having PH, its use is insufficient to definitively diagnose PH. In any patient in which a diagnosis of PH is being considered, invasive testing is required to reach a definitive diagnosis.

Right Heart Catheterization

Invasive hemodynamics derived from RHC are essential to confirm the diagnosis and determine the subtype of PH.[2,3,31] In HF patients, and particularly in those at an advanced stage, determining the presence of Group 2 PH, assessing its severity, and response to provocative testing are critical aspects of HF assessment and have important therapeutic implications. As described above, Group 2 PH occurs across a spectrum from passive elevations to those with pulmonary vascular remodeling. However, the degree to which the elevated PA pressures are acutely reversible cannot be definitively determined without provocative vasodilator testing. Intravenous nitroprusside is a logical agent which is often used for vasodilator challenge in patients with advanced HF due largely to its potent systemic vasodilatory properties and the rapid onset and offset of its action. However, caution should be used to avoid significant, inducible systemic hypotension to levels of systolic blood pressure <85 mmHg, as arriving at a reliable determination of PH reversibility in such a context is difficult.[3,26,31–33] In patients with both low blood pressure and low cardiac output, acute testing with intravenous milrinone has been shown to be a reasonable alternative to nitroprusside.[34] Agents such as inhaled nitric oxide (iNO) should always be avoided in cases of advanced left heart failure because of the risk of inducing an acute rise in left atrial pressure and flash pulmonary edema.[3] The role of a fluid challenge during RHC for evaluation of Group 2 PH is typically of little clinical

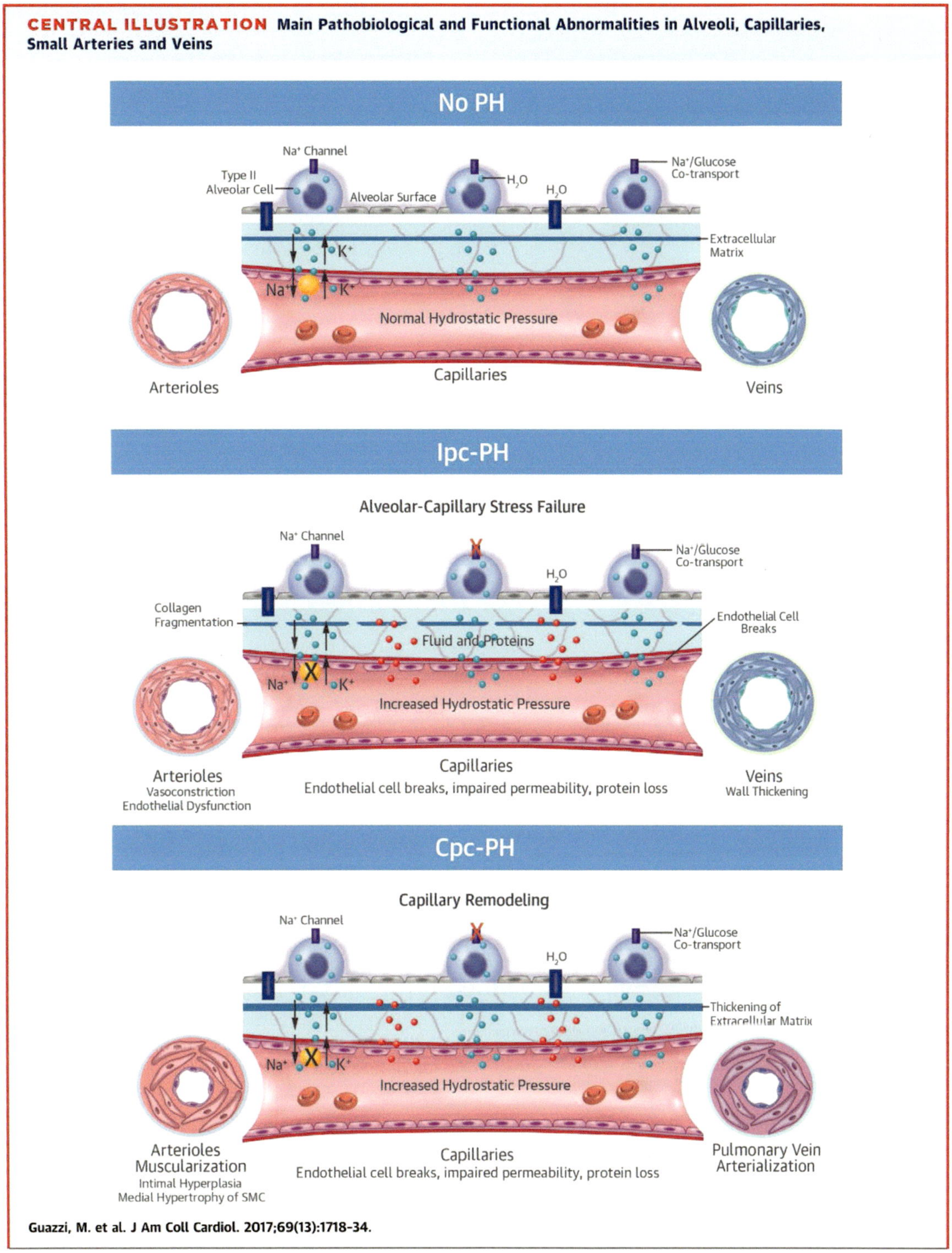

FIGURE 26.1 Pathogenesis of isolated postcapillary pulmonary hypertension (Ipc-PH) and combined pre- and postcapillary pulmonary hypertension (Cpc-PH). In Ipc-PH, there is vasoconstriction and endothelial dysfunction of the arterioles combined with thickening of the pulmonary veins. In Cpc-PH, there is progression to thickening of the extracellular matrix, hyperplasia and hypertrophy of arterioles, and arterialization of pulmonary veins. (Reproduced with permission from Guazzi and Naeije, *J Am Coll Cardiol.* 2017;69(13):1718–34.)

utility and not without safety concerns, analogous to the use of iNO.

As referenced above, determining the presence, severity, and reversibility of PH in patients with advanced HF has significant therapeutic and prognostic implications. For instance, a PASP ≥50 mmHg in conjunction with PVR >3 WU or TPG >15 mmHg is associated with RV failure and increased mortality following cardiac transplantation.[25,26,31,33,35,36] On the other hand, if the PVR can be reduced to <3 WU with a vasodilator challenge during RHC, most patients can safely proceed

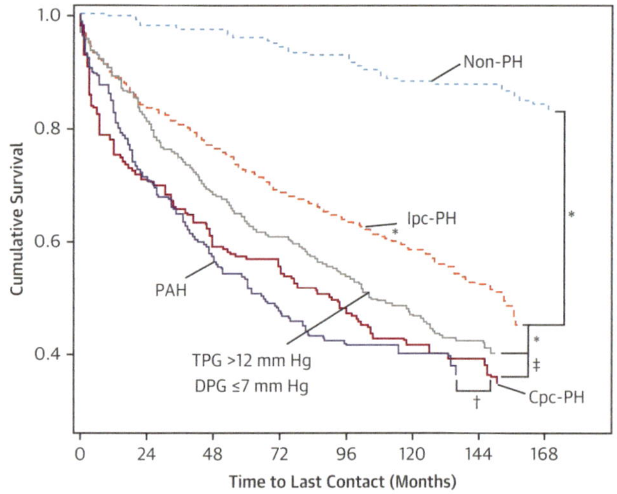

FIGURE 26.2 Prognosis of patients with pulmonary arterial hypertension (PAH), combined pre- and postcapillary pulmonary hypertension (Cpc-PH), isolated pre- and postcapillary hypertension (Ipc-PH), and no pulmonary hypertension (PH). Notably, patients with PAH and Cpc-PH are associated with relatively similar survival, which is worse than for those with Ipc-PH or no PH. (Reproduced with permission from Guazzi and Naeije, *J Am Coll Cardiol.* 2017;69(13):1718–34.)

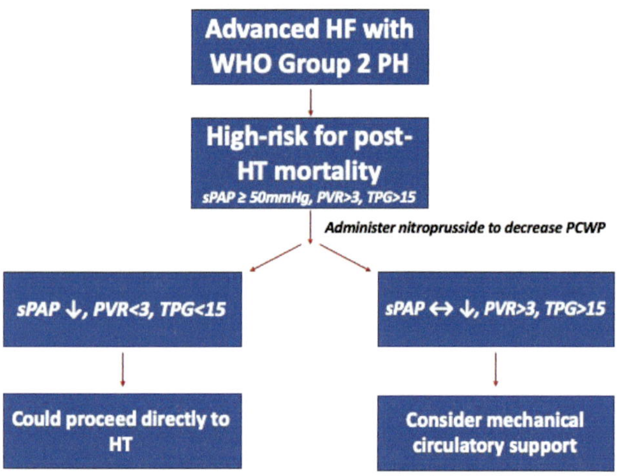

FIGURE 26.3 Algorithm for patients with advanced heart failure (HF) and Group 2 pulmonary hypertension (PH) including the use of vasodilator testing and implications for possible treatment options. *Abbreviations*: HT: heart transplantation, sPAP: systolic pulmonary artery pressure, PVR: pulmonary vascular resistance, TPG: transpulmonary gradient.

directly to cardiac transplantation without suffering a significant risk of post-operative RV failure.[9,26,31] If the PVR and/or TPG remains elevated despite vasodilator testing, a strategy of mechanical support is often considered as a bridge to potential future transplantation.[7,31,33] Although a majority of patients with advanced HF and Group 2 PH demonstrate reversibility with vasodilator challenge, an "unmasking" of a component of pulmonary vascular disease (i.e., precapillary PH) can be observed in those patients thought to have Ipc-PH. This phenomenon occurs as the PCWP is lowered disproportionately to changes in the PA pressure, which results in an actual increase rather than the expected decrease in the PVR or TPG. For these patients as well, proceeding directly to cardiac transplantation must be considered with caution and a bridging strategy should at least be considered (Figure 26.3).[25,31,33,37–39]

Treatment

Pharmacotherapy

The goals of pharmacotherapy of Group 2 PH are to: (a) aggressively treat the underlying left heart disease, (b) reduce congestion, and (c) optimize treatment of non-cardiac comorbidities (e.g., chronic obstructive lung disease, obstructive sleep apnea) with the intended effects of reducing PA pressures and preserving or improving RV function.[3,7] Because Group 2 PH is typically due to elevations in left-sided filling pressures, the mainstay of treatment in most cases must be focused on the aggressive, guideline-directed management of the underlying left heart disease and not the PH itself.[2]

The primary classes of medications used to treat PAH (i.e., Group 1 PH) are endothelin receptor antagonists (ERA), phosphodiesterase-5 inhibitors (PDEi), and prostacyclins.[2,27] Although it may be tempting to consider using targeted pulmonary vasodilator therapy approved for PAH in patients with Group 2 PH, doing so is generally of limited efficacy and more importantly may be associated with increased harm. These agents may be associated with fluid retention, hepatotoxicity, or systemic hypotension. In addition, pulmonary vasodilator therapy has at least the theoretical risk of increasing pulmonary venous return to a non-compliant left heart with already elevated filling pressures, thereby increasing the risk of pulmonary edema. These agents can also worsen ventilation-perfusion mismatch and subsequent hypoxia.[6–8,40]

For the main drug classes of pulmonary vasodilator therapy, several studies including randomized, controlled trials have evaluated their safety and efficacy in treating Group 2 PH (Table 26.2).[8,40–43] For ERA agents, the Endothelin Antagonist Bosentan for Lowering Cardiac Events in Heart Failure (ENABLE) trial and the Heart Failure ET(A) Receptor Blocker Trial (HEAT) have shown *worsening* HF symptoms and a trend toward *increased* mortality.[8,40,42–44] Moreover, the Macitentan in Subjects with Combined Pre- and Post-Capillary Pulmonary Hypertension due to Left Ventricular Dysfunction (MELODY-1) trial has evaluated patients specifically with the Cpc-PH form of Group 2 PH, and found that the treatment group exhibited *worsening* HF, manifest by fluid retention, and *worsening* functional class.[8,45] Similarly, for prostacyclin therapy, the Flolan International Randomized Trial (FIRST) was discontinued early due to a strong trend toward *greater* proportions of deaths in the study group.[40,46] In addition, PDEi agents have been studied for Group 2 PH treatment with disappointing results. The Phosphodiesterase-5 Inhibition to Improve Clinical Status and Exercise Capacity in Heart Failure with Preserved Ejection Fraction (RELAX) study enrolled 216 patients with HFpEF, of whom many had Group 2 PH. The trial did not show any improvement in functional capacity, its primary endpoint, with sildenafil compared with placebo.[8,47] Furthermore, a sub-study of RELAX in HFpEF patients with Group 2 PH and RV dysfunction also showed no improvement in functional capacity or RV function in response to sildenafil.[48] Moreover, the Sildenafil for Improving Outcomes After Valvular Correction (SIOVAC) study randomized patients with Group 2 PH after undergoing valve surgery to either sildenafil or placebo. The sildenafil group had *worse* clinical outcomes,

TABLE 26.2: Example of Randomized Control Trials for Pulmonary Hypertension (PH) Medications in Group 2 PH; Overall, There Is No Significant Benefit and Possible Harm from Many of the Agents

Class	Trial	Patients	Drug	Outcomes and Results
Endothelin receptor antagonists (ERA)	ENABLE	1613 pts with NYHA IIIB–IV HF and LVEF <35%	Bosentan	Clinical composite: no change Fluid retention: ↑
	HEAT	157 pts with NYHA III HF	Darusentan	Cardiac index: ↑ HF, mortality: ↑ (trend)
	MELODY-1	63 pts with NYHA II–III HF, LVEF ≥30%, and Cpc-PH	Macitentan	Fluid retention: ↑ (trend) Functional class: ↓ (trend)
Prostacyclin	FIRST	471 pts with NYHA IIIB–IV HF and LVEF <25%	Epoprostenol	Mortality: ↑ (trend, trial terminated early)
Phosphodiesterase inhibitor (PDEi)	RELAX	216 pts with NYHA II–IV HF with LVEF ≥50%	Sildenafil	Peak O_2 consumption: no change Functional capacity: no change
	SIOVAC	200 pts with mPAP ≥30 mmHg and VHD with repair/replacement >1 year prior	Sildenafil	Clinical composite: ↑ HF hospitalizations: ↑

Abbreviations: NYHA: New York Heart Association, HF: heart failure, Cpc-PH: combined pre- and postcapillary pulmonary hypertension, VHD: valvular heart disease.
Sources: Adapted from Franco (2018); Guazzi and Labate (2016); Packer et al. (2017); Packer et al. (2005); Luscher et al. (2002).

based on a composite of death, HF hospitalizations, change in functional class, and patient global self-assessment that was primarily driven by worsening HF. The sildenafil group also had worsening LV and RV dilation.[8,49] Based on these trials, PDEis are unlikely to be helpful to Group 2 PH patients and may even be harmful.[2,6]

Among the few studies to suggest a possible use for sildenafil in treating HFrEF and HFpEF patients with Group 2 PH are typically single-center trials with limited sample sizes and concern for selection bias. Interestingly, most of those studies that have described a potential benefit were from studies enrolling patients with predominantly the Cpc-PH form of Group 2 PH.[11,40,50–52] Thus, in carefully selected patients, it is conceivable that PDEi agents may play a selective role in Cpc-PH via pulmonary vasodilation and RV unloading without significant systemic hypotension in appropriately selected patients.[6,40,53] However, larger-scale trials are required before such agents can be recommended, even in this Group 2 PH subset of patients.

Overall, the mainstay of pharmacotherapy for treating Group 2 PH remains aggressive treatment of left heart disease. Though pulmonary vasodilators including ERA, prostacyclins, and PDEi have been evaluated, none has been demonstrated to be beneficial, and some may be harmful to patients. Furthermore, other novel therapies, including guanylate cyclase stimulators and inorganic nitrates/nitrites, are in the early stages of investigation but enthusiasm for these agents in treating Group 2 PH is modest at best.[8,40] For most patients with Group 2 PH, particularly those with HFrEF, when conventional therapies to treat left heart disease have been exhausted, the patient should be evaluated for advanced HF therapies.

Left Ventricular Assist Devices and Heart Transplantation

In the setting of advanced or stage D HF with severe Group 2 PH, proceeding directly with heart transplantation is a relative contraindication, given the increased risk of RV failure and increased mortality post-transplant.[25,26,31,33] In this scenario, the use of durable mechanical circulatory support has revolutionized the field as a bridge-to-transplant strategy.[3,6,54–56] Several observational studies have shown that patients with Ipc-PH or Cpc-PH have significant improvements in PA pressures, PVR, and TPG. Furthermore, LVAD therapy has been shown to be superior to medical therapy in improving these hemodynamics in patients with Group 2 PH (Figure 26.4).[57] The findings suggest that the chronic unloading provided by the LVAD allows for improvement in filling pressures as well as possibly for reverse remodeling of the pulmonary vasculature.[54–61] In most of these studies, at least 70% of patients with significantly elevated PVR prior to LVAD have improvement in PVR (to usually <3 WU) that allow the patient to be listed for heart transplantation.[6,54,57,60,61] Of the LVAD patients that have improvements in hemodynamics, most occur within one month of implantation and nearly all improvements occur within the first three to six months.[31,33,60,61]

For those LVAD patients with residual PH and/or RV dysfunction with a normal pulmonary capillary wedge pressure, pulmonary vasodilator therapy can be considered.[2,6,40,55,56] The theoretical concerns about increased venous return to a noncompliant left ventricle with pulmonary vasodilator therapy may be somewhat mitigated by an LVAD. A study that evaluated sildenafil therapy in LVAD patients with refractory PH demonstrated a significant improvement in PA, PVR, and RV function without adverse effects on PCWP or cardiac output when compared with LVAD patients in the placebo group.[62] Thus, there may be a role for pulmonary vasodilator therapy for LVAD patients with refractory PH, though more robust data is needed and its role is likely to be restricted to a minority of patients.

Use of an LVAD in the setting of Group 2 PH does not appear to adversely affect short- or long-term outcomes following heart transplantation. For example, LVAD patients with Group 2 PH have been shown to have similar ten-year survival compared with LVAD patients without PH.[63] Moreover, LVAD patients with Cpc-PH have been shown to achieve similar post-transplant survival at three years when compared with age- and sex-matched transplant patients without PH or LVAD support.[3,59]

Conclusion

Group 2 PH and RV dysfunction is highly prevalent in left heart disease and is associated with significantly increased risk of mortality. Although TTE can be useful as a screening tool, the definitive diagnostic test to fully characterize PH is a right heart catheterization with possible vasodilator testing. The mainstay of treatment for Group 2 PH remains management of the underlying left heart disease without a role currently for use of pulmonary vasodilator therapy. In many cases of PH in end-stage HF, LVAD therapy will result in near resolution of the PH and may be an effective bridge to heart transplantation.

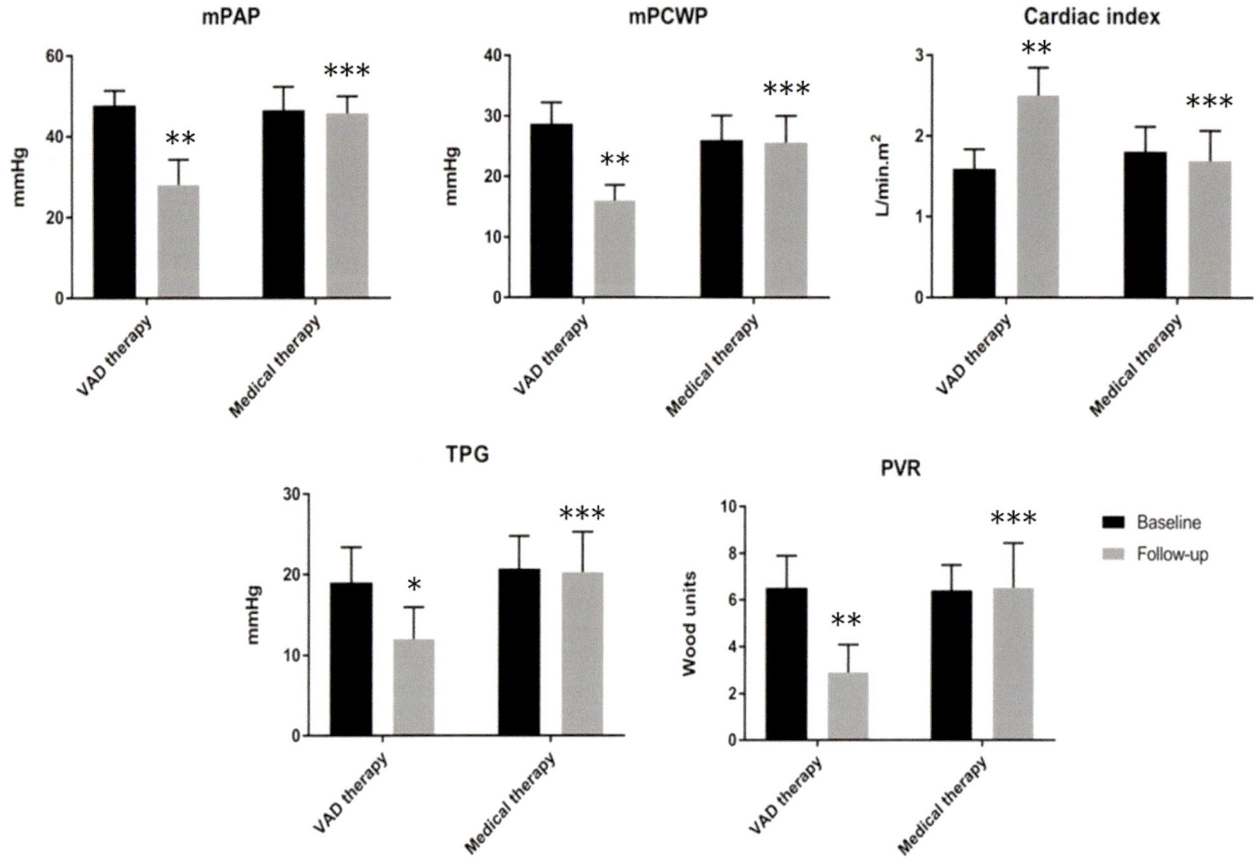

FIGURE 26.4 Comparison of left ventricular assist device (VAD) therapy *versus* medical therapy in patients with advanced heart failure (HF) and Group 2 pulmonary hypertension (PH) demonstrates superiority of LVAD therapy in achieving improvement of hemodynamic parameters at median follow-up of 5 months. *Abbreviations*: mPAP: mean pulmonary artery pressure, mPCWP: mean pulmonary capillary wedge pressure, TPG: transpulmonary gradient, PVR: pulmonary vascular resistance. *p<0.05 vs baseline. **p<0.01 vs baseline. ***p<0.01 vs LVAD group. (Reproduced with permission from Kumarasinghe et al., *ESC Heart Failure* 2018;5(4):695–702.)

References

1. Simonneau G, Montani D, Celermajer DS, et al. Haemodynamic definitions and updated clinical classification of pulmonary hypertension. *Eur Respir J.* 2019;53(1):1801913. doi:10.1183/13993003.01913-2018
2. Galiè N, Humbert M, Vachiery JL, et al. 2015 ESC/ERS guidelines for the diagnosis and treatment of pulmonary hypertension. *Eur Heart J.* 2016;37(1):67–119. doi:10.1093/eurheartj/ehv317
3. Fang JC, Demarco T, Givertz M, et al. World Health Organization Pulmonary Hypertension Group 2: pulmonary hypertension due to left heart disease in the adult - a summary statement from the Pulmonary Hypertension Council of the International Society for Heart and Lung Transplantation. *J Hear Lung Transplant.* 2012;31(9):913–33. doi:10.1016/j.healun.2012.06.002
4. Guha A, Amione-Guerra J, Park MH. Epidemiology of pulmonary hypertension in left heart disease. *Prog Cardiovasc Dis.* 2016;59(1):3–10. doi:10.1016/j.pcad.2016.07.001
5. Galiè N, McLaughlin V., Rubin LJ, Simonneau G. An overview of the 6th World Symposium on Pulmonary Hypertension. *Eur Respir J.* 2019;53(1):1802148. doi:10.1183/13993003.02148-2018
6. Berthelot E, Bauer F, Eicher JC, et al. Pulmonary hypertension in chronic heart failure: definitions, advances, and unanswered issues. *ESC Hear Fail.* 2018;5(5):755–63. doi:10.1002/ehf2.12316
7. Guazzi M, Naeije R. Pulmonary hypertension in heart failure: pathophysiology, pathobiology, and emerging clinical perspectives. *J Am Coll Cardiol.* 2017;69(13):1718–34. doi:10.1016/j.jacc.2017.01.051
8. Franco V. Management of pulmonary hypertension: associated with left heart disease. *Heart Fail Clin.* 2018;14(4):545–51. doi:10.1016/j.hfc.2018.06.009
9. Clark CB, Horn EM. Group 2 pulmonary hypertension: pulmonary venous hypertension: epidemiology and pathophysiology. *Cardiol Clin.* 2016;34(3):401–11. doi:10.1016/j.ccl.2016.04.010
10. Melenovsky V, Hwang SJ, Redfield M, Zakeri R, Lin G, Borlaug BA. Left atrial remodeling and function in advanced heart failure with preserved or reduced ejection fraction. *Circ Hear Fail.* 2015;8(2):295–303. doi:10.1161/CIRCHEARTFAILURE.114.001667
11. Guazzi M, Borlaug BA. Pulmonary hypertension due to left heart disease. *Circulation.* 2012;126(8):975–90. doi:10.1161/CIRCULATIONAHA.111.085761
12. Huang W, Kingsbury MP, Turner MA, Donnelly JL, Flores NA, Sheridan DJ. Capillary filtration is reduced in lungs adapted to chronic heart failure: morphological and haemodynamic correlates. *Cardiovasc Res.* 2001;49(1):207–17. doi:10.1016/S0008-6363(00)00223-6
13. Austin ED, Loyd JE. The genetics of pulmonary arterial hypertension. *Circ Res.* 2014;115(1):189–200. doi:10.1161/CIRCRESAHA.115.303404
14. Ma L, Chung WK. The role of genetics in pulmonary arterial hypertension. *J Pathol.* 2017;241(2):273–80. doi:10.1002/path.4833
15. Yin C, Li K, Yu Y, et al. Genome-wide association study identifies loci and candidate genes for non-idiopathic pulmonary hypertension in Eastern Chinese Han population. *BMC Pulm Med.* 2018;18(1):158. doi:10.1186/s12890-018-0719-0
16. Harjola VP, Mebazaa A, Čelutkiene J, et al. Contemporary management of acute right ventricular failure: a statement from the Heart Failure Association and the Working Group on Pulmonary Circulation and Right Ventricular Function of the European Society of Cardiology. *Eur J Heart Fail.* 2016;18(3):226–41. doi:10.1002/ejhf.478
17. Tedford RJ, Hassoun PM, Mathai SC, et al. Pulmonary capillary wedge pressure augments right ventricular pulsatile loading. *Circulation.* 2012;125(2):289–97. doi:10.1161/CIRCULATIONAHA.111.051540
18. Gerges M, Gerges C, Pistritto AM, et al. Pulmonary hypertension in heart failure epidemiology, right ventricular function, and survival. *Am J Respir Crit Care Med.* 2015;192(10):1234–46. doi:10.1164/rccm.201503-0529OC
19. Gerges C, Gerges M, Lang MB, et al. Diastolic pulmonary vascular pressure gradient: a predictor of prognosis in "out-of-proportion" pulmonary hypertension. *Chest.* 2013;143(3):758–66. doi:10.1378/chest.12-1653

20. Palazzini M, Dardi F, Manes A, et al. Pulmonary hypertension due to left heart disease: analysis of survival according to the haemodynamic classification of the 2015 ESC/ERS guidelines and insights for future changes. *Eur J Heart Fail.* 2018;20(2):248–55. doi:10.1002/ejhf.860
21. Ghio S, Gavazzi A, Campana C, et al. Independent and additive prognostic value of right ventricular systolic function and pulmonary artery pressure in patients with chronic heart failure. *J Am Coll Cardiol.* 2001;37(1):183–8. doi:10.1016/S0735-1097(00)01102-5
22. Kjaergaard J, Akkan D, Iversen K, et al. Prognostic importance of pulmonary hypertension in patients with heart failure. *Am J Cardiol.* 2007;99(8):1146–1150. doi:10.1016/j.amjcard.2006.11.052
23. Kalogeropoulos AP, Siwamogsatham S, Hayek S, et al. Echocardiographic assessment of pulmonary artery systolic pressure and outcomes in ambulatory heart failure patients. *J Am Heart Assoc.* 2014;3(1):e000363. doi:10.1161/JAHA.113.000363
24. Miller WL, Grill DE, Borlaug BA. Clinical features, hemodynamics, and outcomes of pulmonary hypertension due to chronic heart failure with reduced ejection fraction: pulmonary hypertension and heart failure. *JACC Hear Fail.* 2013;1(4):290–9. doi:10.1016/j.jchf.2013.05.001
25. Kirklin JKJK, Naftel DCDC, McGiffin DC, et al. Analysis of morbid events and risk factors for death after cardiac transplantation. *J Am Coll Cardiol.* 1988;11(5):917–24. doi:10.1016/S0735-1097(98)90045-6
26. Costard-Jäckle A, Fowler MB. Influence of preoperative pulmonary artery pressure on mortality after heart transplantation: testing of potential reversibility of pulmonary hypertension with nitroprusside is useful in defining a high risk group. *J Am Coll Cardiol.* 1992;19(1):48–54. doi:10.1016/0735-1097(92)90050-W
27. McLaughlin V V., Archer SL, Badesch DB, et al. ACCF/AHA 2009 expert consensus document on pulmonary hypertension. A report of the American College of Cardiology Foundation Task Force on Expert Consensus Documents and the American Heart Association Developed in Collaboration with the American College of Chest Physicians, American Thoracic Society, Inc., and the Pulmonary Hypertension Association. *J Am Coll Cardiol.* 2009;53(17):1573–619. doi:10.1016/j.jacc.2009.01.004
28. Rich JD, Shah SJ, Swamy RS, Kamp A, Rich S. Inaccuracy of doppler echocardiographic estimates of pulmonary artery pressures in patients with pulmonary hypertension: implications for clinical practice. *Chest.* 2011;139(5):988–93. doi:10.1378/chest.10-1269
29. Fisher MR, Forfia PR, Chamera E, et al. Accuracy of doppler echocardiography in the hemodynamic assessment of pulmonary hypertension. *Am J Respir Crit Care Med.* 2009;179(7):615–21. doi:10.1164/rccm.200811-1691OC
30. Rich JD. Counterpoint: can Doppler echocardiography estimates of pulmonary artery systolic pressures be relied upon to accurately make the diagnosis of pulmonary hypertension? No. *Chest.* 2013;143(6):1536–9. doi:10.1378/chest.13-0297
31. Mehra MR, Kobashigawa J, Starling R, et al. Listing criteria for heart transplantation: International Society for heart and lung transplantation guidelines for the care of cardiac transplant candidates-2006. *J Hear Lung Transplant.* 2006;25(9):1024–42. doi:10.1016/j.healun.2006.06.008
32. Schwartzenberg S, Redfield MM, From AM, Sorajja P, Nishimura RA, Borlaug BA. Effects of vasodilation in heart failure with preserved or reduced ejection fraction: implications of distinct pathophysiologies on response to therapy. *J Am Coll Cardiol.* 2012;59(5):442–51. doi:10.1016/j.jacc.2011.09.062
33. Mehra MRMR, Canter CECE, Hannan MMM, et al. The 2016 International Society for Heart Lung Transplantation listing criteria for heart transplantation: a 10-year update. *J Hear Lung Transplant.* 2016;35(1):1–23. doi:10.1016/j.healun.2015.10.023
34. Givertz MM, Hare JM, Loh E, Gauthier DF, Colucci WS. Effect of bolus milrinone on hemodynamic variables and pulmonary vascular resistance in patients with severe left ventricular dysfunction: a rapid test for reversibility of pulmonary hypertension. *J Am Coll Cardiol.* 1997;28(7):1775–80. doi:10.1016/S0735-1097(96)00399-3
35. Mehra MR. Guidelines for listing candidates for heart transplant: a 10-year update. *JAMA Cardiol.* 2017;2(1):98–99. doi:10.1001/jamacardio.2016.3756
36. Tampakakis E, Leary PJ, Selby VN, et al. The diastolic pulmonary gradient does not predict survival in patients with pulmonary hypertension due to left heart disease. *JACC Hear Fail.* 2015;3(1):9–16. doi:10.1016/j.jchf.2014.07.010
37. Mehra MR. Guidelines for listing candidates for heart transplant: a 10-year update. *JAMA Cardiol.* Published online 2016. doi:10.1001/jamacardio.2016.3756
38. Costard-Jackle A, Fowler MB. Influence of preoperative pulmonary artery pressure on mortality after heart transplantation: testing of potential reversibility of pulmonary hypertension with nitroprusside is useful in defining a high risk group. *J Am Coll Cardiol.* 1992;19(1):48–54.
39. Tampakakis E, Leary PJ, Selby VN, et al. The diastolic pulmonary gradient does not predict survival in patients with pulmonary hypertension due to left heart disease. *JACC Hear Fail.* 2015;3(1):9–16. doi:10.1016/J.JCHF.2014.07.010
40. Guazzi M, Labate V. Group 2 PH: medical therapy. *Prog Cardiovasc Dis.* 2016;59(1):71–7. doi:10.1016/j.pcad.2016.06.003
41. Packer M, McMurray JJ V, Krum H, et al. Long-term effect of endothelin receptor antagonism with bosentan on the morbidity and mortality of patients with severe chronic heart failure: primary results of the ENABLE trials. *JACC Hear Fail.* 2017;5(5):317–26. doi:10.1016/j.jchf.2017.02.021
42. Packer M, McMurray J, Massie BM, et al. Clinical effects of endothelin receptor antagonism with bosentan in patients with severe chronic heart failure: results of a pilot study. *J Card Fail.* 2005;11(1):12–20. doi:10.1016/j.cardfail.2004.05.006
43. Luscher TF, Enseleit F, Pacher R, et al. Hemodynamic and neurohumoral effects of selective endothelin A (ETA) receptor blockade in chronic heart failure: the heart failure ETA receptor blockade trial (HEAT). *Circulation.* 2002;106(21):2666–72. doi:10.1161/01.CIR.0000038497.80095.E1
44. Packer M, McMurray JJV, Krum H, et al. Long-term effect of endothelin receptor antagonism with bosentan on the morbidity and mortality of patients with severe chronic heart failure: primary results of the ENABLE trials. *JACC Hear Fail.* 2017;5(5):317–26. doi:10.1016/j.jchf.2017.02.021
45. Vachiéry JL, Delcroix M, Al-Hiti H, et al. Macitentan in pulmonary hypertension due to left ventricular dysfunction. *Eur Respir J.* 2018;51(2):1701886. doi:10.1183/13993003.01886-2017
46. Califf RM, Adams KF, McKenna WJ, et al. A randomized controlled trial of epoprostenol therapy for severe congestive heart failure: the Flolan International Randomized Survival Trial (FIRST). *Am Heart J.* 1997;134(1):44–54. doi:10.1016/S0002-8703(97)70105-4
47. Redfield MM, Chen HH, Borlaug BA, et al. Effect of phosphodiesterase-5 inhibition on exercise capacity and clinical status in heart failure with preserved ejection fraction: a randomized clinical trial. *JAMA.* 2013;309(12):1268–77. doi:10.1001/jama.2013.2024
48. Hussain I, Mohammed SF, Forfia PR, et al. Impaired right ventricular-pulmonary arterial coupling and effect of sildenafil in heart failure with preserved ejection fraction. *Circ Hear Fail.* 2016;9(4):e002729. doi:10.1161/CIRCHEARTFAILURE.115.002729
49. Bermejo J, Yotti R, García-Orta R, et al. Sildenafil for improving outcomes in patients with corrected valvular heart disease and persistent pulmonary hypertension: a multicenter, double-blind, randomized clinical trial. *Eur Heart J.* 2018;39(15):1255–64. doi:10.1093/eurheartj/ehx700
50. Guazzi M, Vicenzi M, Arena R, Guazzi M. Pulmonary hypertension in heart failure with preserved ejection fraction: a target of phosphodiesterase-5 inhibition in a 1-year study. *Circulation.* 2011;124(2):164–74. doi:10.1161/CIRCULATIONAHA.110.983866
51. Lewis GD, Shah R, Shahzad K, et al. Sildenafil improves exercise capacity and quality of life in patients with systolic heart failure and secondary pulmonary hypertension. *Circulation.* 2007;116(14):1555–62. doi:10.1161/CIRCULATIONAHA.107.716373
52. Guazzi M, Samaja M, Arena R, Vicenzi M, Guazzi MD. Long-term use of sildenafil in the therapeutic management of heart failure. *J Am Coll Cardiol.* 2007;50(22):2136–44. doi:10.1016/j.jacc.2007.07.078
53. Guazzi M, Gomberg-Maitland M, Arena R. Pulmonary hypertension in heart failure with preserved ejection fraction. *J Hear Lung Transplant.* 2015;34(3):273–81. doi:10.1016/j.healun.2014.11.003
54. Krishnamurthy Y, Cooper LB, Parikh KS, et al. Pulmonary hypertension in the era of mechanical circulatory support. *ASAIO J.* 2016;62(5):505–12. doi:10.1097/MAT.0000000000000408
55. Rao SD, Menachem JN, Birati EY, Mazurek JA. Pulmonary hypertension in advanced heart failure: assessment and management of the failing RV and LV. *Curr Heart Fail Rep.* 2019;16(5):119–29. doi:10.1007/s11897-019-00431-4
56. Sparrow CT, LaRue SJ, Schilling JD. Intersection of pulmonary hypertension and right ventricular dysfunction in patients on left ventricular assist device support: is there a role for pulmonary vasodilators? *Circ Heart Fail.* 2018;11(1):e004255. doi:10.1161/CIRCHEARTFAILURE.117.004255
57. Kumarasinghe G, Jain P, Jabbour A, et al. Comparison of continuous-flow ventricular assist device therapy with intensive medical therapy in fixed pulmonary hypertension secondary to advanced left heart failure. *ESC Hear Fail.* 2018;5(4):695–702. doi:10.1002/ehf2.12284
58. John R, Liao K, Kamdar F, Eckman P, Boyle A, Colvin-Adams M. Effects on pre- and posttransplant pulmonary hemodynamics in patients with continuous-flow left ventricular assist devices. *J Thorac Cardiovasc Surg.* 2010;140(2):447–52. doi:10.1016/j.jtcvs.2010.03.006
59. Zimpfer D, Zrunek P, Sandner S, et al. Post-transplant survival after lowering fixed pulmonary hypertension using left ventricular assist devices. *Eur J Cardio-thoracic Surg.* 2007;31(4):698–702. doi:10.1016/j.ejcts.2006.12.036
60. Etz CD, Welp HA, Tjan TD, et al. Medically refractory pulmonary hypertension: treatment with nonpulsatile left ventricular assist devices. *Ann Thorac Surg.* 2007;83(5):1697–705. doi:10.1016/j.athoracsur.2007.01.019

61. Mikus E, Stepanenko A, Krabatsch T, et al. Reversibility of fixed pulmonary hypertension in left ventricular assist device support recipients. *Eur J Cardio-thoracic Surg.* 2011;40(4):971–7. doi:10.1016/j.ejcts.2011.01.019
62. Tedford RJ, Hemnes AR, Russell SD, et al. PDE5A inhibitor treatment of persistent pulmonary hypertension after mechanical circulatory support. *Circ Heart Fail.* 2008;1(4):213–9. doi:10.1161/CIRCHEARTFAILURE.108.796789
63. Moayedifar R, Zuckermann A, Aliabadi-Zuckermann A, et al. Long-term heart transplant outcomes after lowering fixed pulmonary hypertension using left ventricular assist devices. *Eur J Cardio-thoracic Surg.* 2018;54(6):1116–21. doi:10.1093/ejcts/ezy214

Chapter 27
THE PATIENT WITH NON-GROUP 2 PULMONARY HYPERTENSION

Sophia Anastasia Mouratoglou and George Giannakoulas

Definitions, Epidemiology, and Outcomes

Pulmonary hypertension (PH) is a pathophysiological disorder involving multiple clinical conditions and potentially complicating most cardiovascular and respiratory diseases. PH is defined as mean pulmonary artery pressure (MPAP) ≥20 mmHg at rest as assessed by right heart catheterization.[1] PH is classified into five different groups (Figure 27.1). Although classification is driven by underlying pathophysiological changes and despite the fact that these clinical groups are characterized by comparable hemodynamic changes, the underlying mechanisms, diagnostic approaches, prognostic, and therapeutic implications are completely different. "Precapillary" PH describes a group of patients suffering from different clinical conditions characterized by MPAP ≥20 mmHg and pulmonary artery wedge pressure (PCWP) ≤15 mmHg (Figure 27.2) and encompasses all groups of PH with the exception of group 2 PH (secondary to left heart disease), which is characterized by postcapillary PH (PCWP >15 mmHg) and is reviewed in Chapter 26.[1,2] Right heart failure is the final result of PH and is characterized by impaired right ventricular function that leads to insufficient blood flow to the pulmonary circulation and/or elevated filling pressures at rest or during physiologically demanding conditions.

Certain clinical conditions, e.g., connective tissue disorders (especially scleroderma), congenital heart disease, portal hypertension, and infections (human immunodeficiency virus and schistosomiasis), are strongly associated with the development of Group 1 PH or pulmonary arterial hypertension (PAH) and patients suffering from these conditions are at risk of PAH. Drugs and other substances (e.g., anorexigens, rapeseed oil adulterated by aniline ("toxic oil syndrome," etc.) may also lead to PAH.

Although Group 2 PH is the most common form, precapillary PH characterizes almost 25% of patients with PH. Registries report considerable changes in disease phenotype over the past decades. These include substantial changes in age, sex, comorbidities, and survival since the early 1980s, when the mean age of PAH diagnosis was 36±15 years.[3] Current registries raise the age of PAH diagnosis to the 6th decade of life.[4] PAH is estimated to affect 15–60 cases per million of the adult population, with 5–10 new cases per million being reported yearly. Of these, most are characterized as idiopathic, heritable, or drug-induced, with connective tissue diseases remaining the second most frequent cause of PAH. Regardless of its clinical heterogeneity, PAH remains a disease with poor clinical outcome and severe prognosis. Despite recent advances in therapy and increased awareness of the disease, it remains incurable with reduced survival ranging from 2.8 years when left untreated to 7 years in the current PAH targeted treatment era,[5,6] rates which underscore the need for a better transfer of novel scientific knowledge into health care interventions.

PH is relatively common in patients with parenchymal lung disease (Group 3 PH) and its prevalence varies widely depending on the diagnostic method, the definition of PH used, and the patient population studied, ranging from 16% to 36% in patients with end-stage chronic lung disease.[7,8] Mild elevations of MPAP are seen in patients with severe chronic obstructive pulmonary disease, whereas combined emphysema/fibrosis syndrome is more commonly associated with more severe PH. Patients with chronic lung disease-associated PH have a significantly worse prognosis compared with patients with lung disease but without PH.[8,9]

Group 4 PH includes patients with obstructions of the pulmonary artery and the incidence of this disease is 0.9 new cases per million per year. Although the prevalence of chronic thromboembolic PH (CTEPH) is lower than that of PAH, reported to be 3.2 cases per million, the prevalence of the disease among patients surviving an acute pulmonary embolism is said to be much higher, ranging from 0.5% to 3.8% in registries.[10] Clinical conditions, such as thrombophilic disorders, splenectomy, ventriculoarterial (VA) shunt, and infected pacemakers, are associated with higher incidence of the disease.[11,12]

Basic Pathophysiology of Pulmonary Arterial Hypertension and Right Heart Failure

Precapillary PH is characterized by complex pathological changes in the setting of small pulmonary arterioles, which amongst others include accumulation of different vascular cells in the pulmonary arterial wall (pulmonary artery smooth muscle cells, endothelial cells, fibroblasts, myofibroblasts, and pericytes), loss of precapillary arteries, and an exaggerated perivascular infiltration of inflammatory cells (B- and T-lymphocytes, mast cells, dendritic cells, macrophages, etc.).[13–16] These changes result in severe loss and obstructive remodeling of the pulmonary vascular bed, resulting in a rise in pulmonary arterial pressure and in pulmonary vascular resistance.

In normal hearts, RV is thinner, smaller, and has a more crescent-like shape compared with the thicker and elliptically shaped left ventricle. To understand the continuum of ventricular adaptation to PH, the term "coupling" has been used to describe the energy transfer of right ventricular to arterial load. Coupling is being described by systolic and arterial elastance, (Ees/Ea) whose derivation is based on the pressure–volume loop. A well-adapted RV has preserved ventriculoarterial coupling, in contrast to a maladapted one that has different degrees of altered ventriculoarterial coupling (Figure 27.3). Adaptive remodeling is characterized by concentric patterns (higher mass-to-volume ratio) and preserved stroke volume, systolic function, and normal filling pressures (e.g., right ventricular remodeling of patients with Eisenmenger syndrome). Several mechanisms contribute to maladaptive remodeling of the pressure-overloaded right ventricle. These include neurohormonal activation, oxidative and nitrosative stress, inflammation, and activation of myocardial apoptotic pathways.[17] Decreased cardiac output leads to a reduction of tissue perfusion that finally

DOI: 10.1201/9780429244544-33

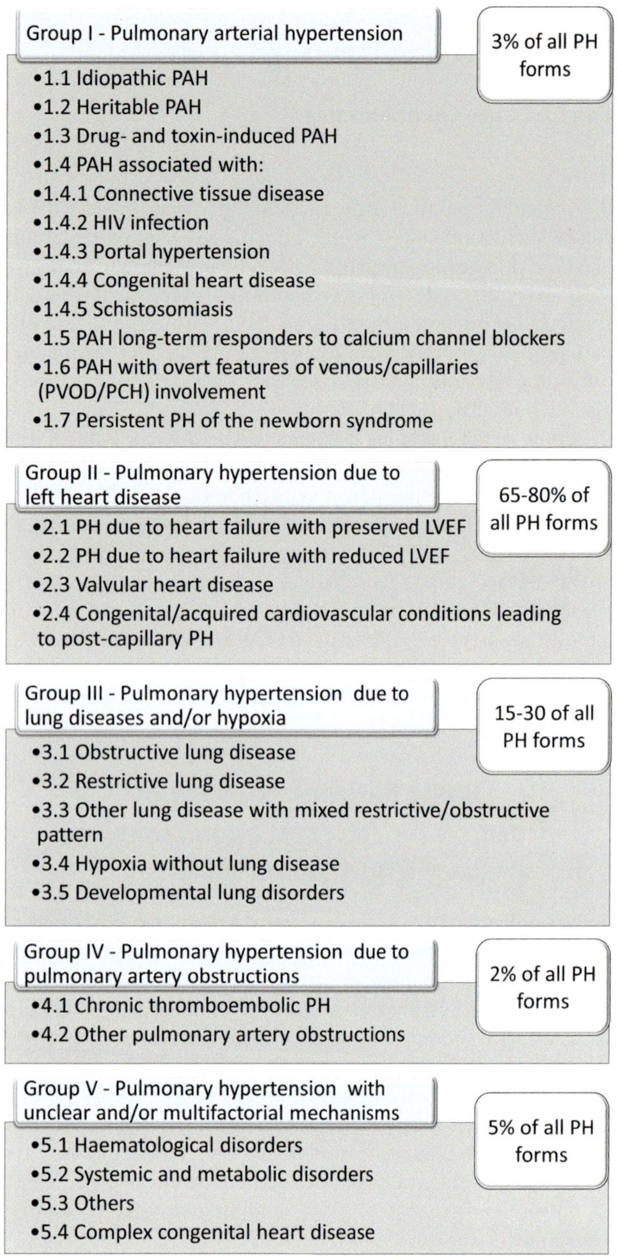

FIGURE 27.1 Updated clinical classification of pulmonary hypertension.

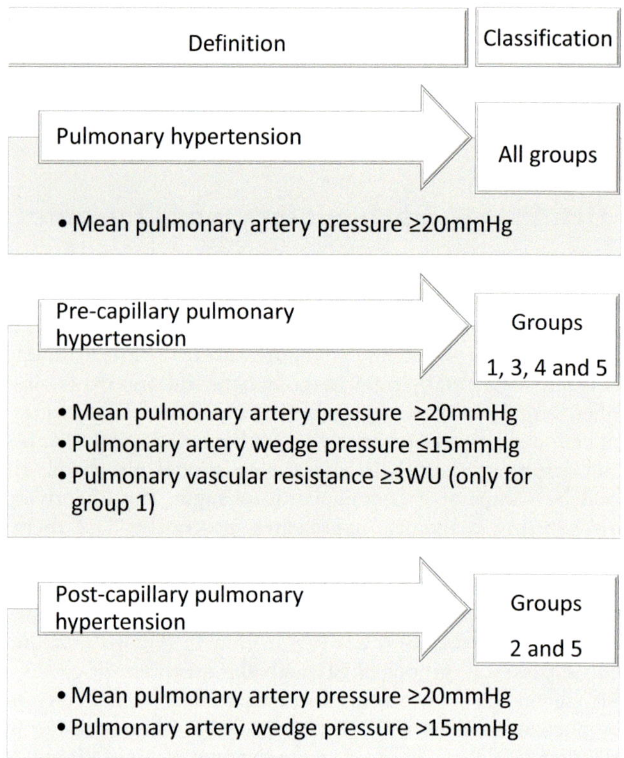

FIGURE 27.2 Hemodynamic definition and clinical classification of pulmonary hypertension.

results in activation of neurohormonal pathways. The latter, although beneficial at first (maintenance of blood pressure and renal perfusion), eventually further impairs cardiac function.[17] Right heart failure is associated with activation of the endothelin system, which is linked to more severe ventricular dysfunction and reduced exercise capacity.[18] Modulation of the endothelin system with endothelin receptor antagonists in PAH may lead to a decrease in pulmonary vascular resistance, better ventricular remodeling, and improved functional status.[19] Unfortunately, RV cannot sustain long-term pressure overload, reacting with global dilatation. This leads to a vicious circle, as RV dilatation leads to increased wall tension that subsequently increases myocardial oxygen demand, while simultaneously decreasing RV perfusion, conditions resulting in worse contractility translated into reduced stroke volume, impaired systolic function, and increased filling pressures.[20]

The left ventricle is involved in PH also, since both ventricles share the interventricular septum, are encircled with common myocardial fibers, and are enclosed by the pericardium.[21] This ventricular interdependence is expressed as rapid leftward septal bowing as a consequence of myocardial stretch during late right ventricular ejection,[22] as well as of interventricular relaxation dyssynchrony caused by the prolonged contraction of the RV free wall relative to the septum and the left ventricular free wall.[23,24] The characteristic septal curvature seen in PH is presented in Figure 27.4 and has been found to cause mechanical inefficiency that contributes to left ventricular underfilling[23] and atrophy,[25] while its duration is a prognostic factor in PH.[26]

Basic Pathophysiology of Chronic Lung Disease-Induced and Thromboembolic Pulmonary Hypertension

In patients with chronic parenchymal lung disease, the increase in pulmonary vascular resistance is the result of a complex interaction between mechanical factors, reflexive hypoxic pulmonary vasoconstriction, and pulmonary vascular remodeling. The process of pulmonary vascular remodeling involves mainly the small pulmonary arteries and is characterized by neovascularization, intimal thickening, and medial hypertrophy.[27] The pathophysiology behind this includes chronic hypoxia, airway and vascular wall inflammation, and cigarette smoking injury.[28,29] All these factors lead to vascular endothelial damage and subsequent structural changes within the vascular wall. There is also evidence supporting the involvement of the postcapillary pulmonary venous vasculature in all PH groups with varying degrees of intensity. In chronic respiratory disease, postcapillary involvement is likely

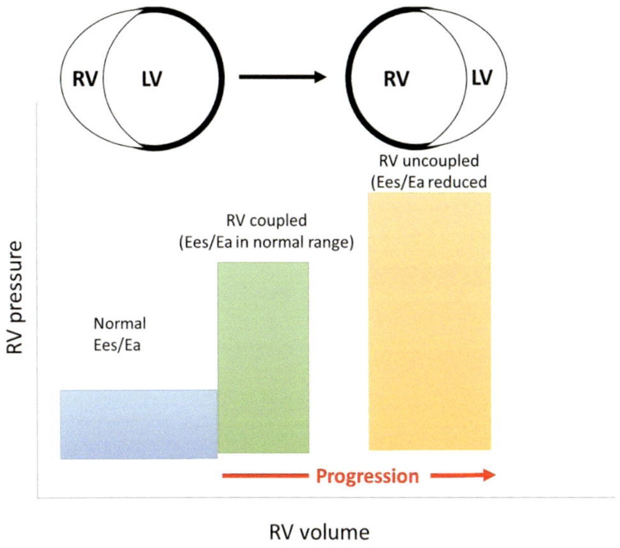

FIGURE 27.3 Pressure–volume loops of patients with and without pulmonary hypertension. Upper part: Right ventricle under normal conditions and in pulmonary hypertension. Increased pressure overload leads to increased right ventricular wall stress and subsequently to hypertrophy and dilatation. Lower part: Pressure–volume loops in normal controls and patients with pulmonary hypertension with maintained coupling and with increased RV volume. In controls and in patients with maintained ventriculoarterial coupling, the Ees/Ea ratio remains within the normal range. In patients with decreased coupling, the Ees/Ea ratio is also decreased, and wall stress is increased. Ees is the slope of the end-systolic pressure/volume relationship and is used as a measure of RV contractility, and Ea is a measure of the arterial load. (Modified from Vonk Noordegraaf et al. *J Am Coll Cardiol* 2013;62:22–33.)

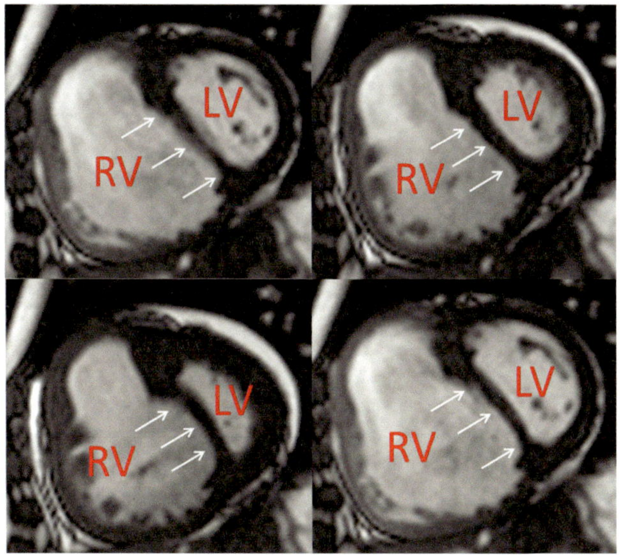

FIGURE 27.4 Leftward septal bowing in a patient with pulmonary arterial hypertension. Right ventricular pressure overload results in interventricular septal bowing towards left ventricle, resulting in impaired left ventricular filling and function. (Modified from Mouratoglou et al. *J Cardiovasc Magn Reson*. 2014;16:P240.)

to be explained, at least in part, by parenchymal destruction and inflammation in patients with lung fibrosis and emphysema. In patients with idiopathic pulmonary fibrosis, the pulmonary vasculopathy in areas of fibrosis is similar to that of patients with chronic obstructive lung disease with the addition of intimal fibrosis with resulting vascular lumen obliteration. The fibrotic areas also demonstrate vascular regression, whereas the non-fibrotic areas have increased growth of structurally abnormal vasculature that may contribute to increased vascular resistance.[30]

Although linked with pulmonary embolism, the pathophysiologic development of CTEPH extends beyond thrombosis. Recently, the role of small vessel abnormalities in the lungs of patients with CTEPH has received a major update, as the scope of small vessel involvement of CTEPH is found to extend beyond the precapillary small arteries. Histopathologic changes in the pulmonary venous and capillary systems, similar to that seen in pulmonary veno-occlusive disease and pulmonary capillary hemangiomatosis, as well as systemic to pulmonary anastomoses and hypertrophied bronchial collaterals, have been reported in lungs of CTEPH patients.[14]

RV adaptation to pressure overload in CTEPH may be different compared with other forms of PH. The primary location of vascular resistance in the pulmonary circulation appears to affect the RV afterload in a different way. Dissimilarities in RV afterload between proximal vs distal obstruction of the pulmonary arterial bed have been reported. This may have implications for the target of various therapies for CTEPH. For example, the RV in CTEPH may have different recovery or response, depending on whether an intervention relieves the proximal mechanical disease or its microvascular component.[31,32] These observations are important reminders that CTEPH is not just chronic thrombus with varying degrees of precapillary changes, similar to idiopathic PAH, but rather, a more complex disease with heterogeneous and less predictable involvement of the entire pulmonary circulation and associated collateral vasculature.

Diagnostic Evaluation and Diagnostic Tools

The diagnosis of PH requires clinical suspicion based on symptoms and physical examination as well as on a comprehensive set of diagnostic tests to confirm whether hemodynamic criteria for PH are met and to describe the etiology and the severity of the disease. The diagnosis of PH requires the involvement of a multidisciplinary team, for the identification of underlying causes of PH and the management of patients, especially with respect to those who may have more than one causes of PH (Figure 27.2). An algorithm for the diagnosis of PH has been proposed in current guidelines and recently updated after the 6th World Symposium of PH (Figure 27.5). The symptoms of the disease remain non-specific and are characterized by but not limited to exertional dyspnea, fatigue, weakness, chest pain, syncope, etc. Later, symptoms of right heart failure may be present, mainly congestion. The severity of heart failure is often sub-categorized according to World Health Organization (WHO) Functional Class and by the degree of congestion.[1,2] Clinical examination reveals non-specific signs [e.g., augmented second heart sound (P2 component), right ventricular lift, jugular venous distension, hepatojugular reflux, ascites, hepatomegaly and/or splenomegaly, edema, tricuspid regurgitation or pulmonary regurgitation cardiac murmurs, and S3 gallop], but has great importance in clinical

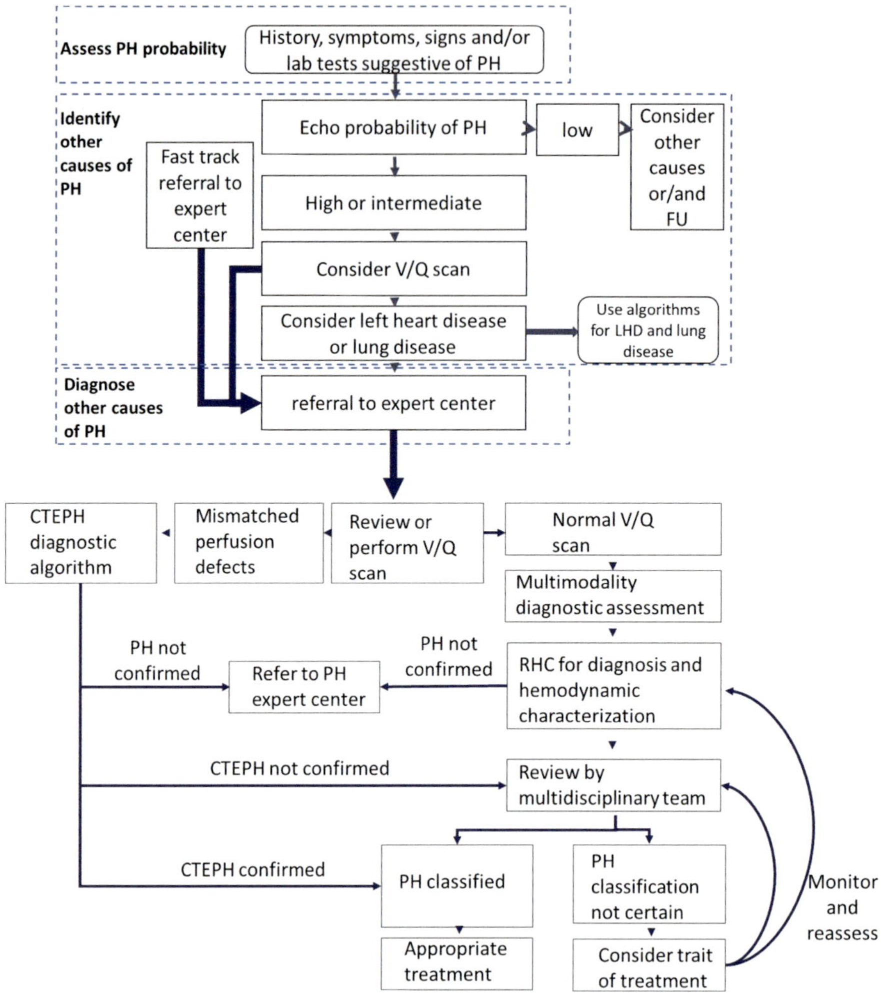

FIGURE 27.5 Diagnostic algorithm of pulmonary hypertension. (Modified from Galie et al. *Eur Heart J* 2015;37:67–119 and Frost et al. *Eur Respir J* 2019;53:1801904.)

evaluation of the disease severity and on patients' evaluation during follow-up.

ECG may demonstrate right axis deviation, right bundle branch block, signs of RV hypertrophy or strain, p-pulmonale (right atrial abnormality), or even QTc prolongation. These are more prominent in later stages of the disease and are associated with a poorer prognosis,[33] although a normal ECG does not exclude the diagnosis of PH.[2] Blood tests, although not useful in diagnosing PH, may identify the etiology of some forms of PH and detect end-organ damage. Routine biochemistry, hematology, and thyroid function tests are required in all patients, as well as several other specific blood tests, such as serological testing to detect underlying connective tissue disease, hepatitis, and human immunodeficiency virus (HIV), as well as thrombophilia screening in patients with CTEPH. Liver function tests may be abnormal because of elevated hepatic venous pressure due to congestion, primary liver disease and/or endothelin receptor antagonist (ERA) therapy. Thyroid disease is common in PAH and may develop during the disease. This should always be considered in cases of abrupt clinical deterioration.[1,2] Serum natriuretic peptide levels may be elevated in patients with PH, are an independent risk predictor,[34] and serial measurements are recommended.[2]

Patients with sporadic or familial PAH should be advised on genetic testing and counseling because of the strong possibility that they may carry a disease-causing mutation and a BMPR2 mutation screening should be offered. When no BMPR2 mutations are identified, screening for other, rarer mutations may be considered (ACVRL1 and mutations in *ENG, KCNK3, CAV1* genes, etc.). Patients with sporadic or familial pulmonary veno-occlusive disease/ pulmonary capillary hemangiomatosis (PVOD/PCH) should be tested for EIF2AK4 mutations as the presence of a bi-allelic EIF2AK4 mutation is sufficient to confirm PVOD/PCH without lung biopsy.[1,2]

To facilitate the differential diagnosis of PH and to provide significant information on its clinical classification, lung function tests may differentiate PH associated with chronic lung disease from other forms of PH, in which mild to moderate reduction of lung volumes may be seen, usually in the later stages of the disease, and the reduction is related to disease severity.[35]

Role of Imaging and Right Heart Catheterization

Chest X-Ray

Chest X-ray is not pathognomonic of PAH. Although abnormal in most patients at the time of diagnosis, a normal chest X-ray may not exclude the diagnosis of PAH. Most common findings may include central pulmonary arterial dilatation and loss of the peripheral blood vessels (peripheral pruning) or right atrial and RV enlargement (elevation of cardiac apex) in more advanced cases. The importance of chest X-ray lies not in the information the examination provides but in the differential diagnosis of the underlying condition causing PH (parenchymal lung disease or pulmonary venous congestion due to left heart disease, etc.).

Echocardiography

Echocardiography is the first-line non-invasive examination performed for the evaluation of suspicion of PH.[2] It is important to note that echocardiography by itself may not confirm the diagnosis of PH or lead to treatment decisions, but may trigger the need for further evaluation. Echocardiographic probability of PH may be high, intermediate, or low. Estimated peak tricuspid regurgitation velocity >3.4 m/s (or >2.9 m/s in symptomatic high-risk patients) is a sign of the high probability of PH and may indicate the need for right heart catheterization. Other echocardiographic signs that provide assessment of right ventricular size and pressure overload, the pattern of blood flow velocity towards the pulmonary artery, the diameter of the pulmonary artery, and an estimate of right atrial pressure are indicative of PH and presented in detail in Figure 27.6.

In addition to diagnosis, echocardiography is a valuable tool in differentiating the underlying cause of PH, by identifying congenital heart disease or left heart disease. Last, but not least, echocardiography provides valuable information on the disease severity and numerous parameters assessing right atrial and ventricular size, function, and hemodynamics have been found to be affected by advanced treatment[36] and offer prognostic significance in PH.[37,38] Indeed, presence of pericardial effusion, increased right atrial size, and impaired right ventricular function are included in the risk stratification algorithm of current guidelines.[2]

Ventilation/Perfusion (V/Q) Scan

Ventilation/perfusion scan is the method of choice for the diagnosis of chronic thromboembolic PH as a normal- or low-probability V/Q scan can effectively exclude CTEPH. However, an abnormal V/Q scan can also be seen in PAH as small peripheral unmatched and non-segmental defects in perfusion may be present.

Computer Tomography

Computer tomography (CT) imaging, and in particular high-resolution CT, contrast enhanced CT, and pulmonary angiography, is a valuable tool for the differential diagnosis of PH, providing information on vascular, parenchymal, and mediastinal pulmonary stroma and identifying the cause of the disease (e.g., CTEPH or lung disease—interstitial lung disease and emphysema—PVOD, pulmonary capillary hemangiomatosis, or esophageal dilation in systematic scleroderma, or congenital cardiac lesions such as anomalous pulmonary venous drainage). CT pulmonary angiography may provide evidence of surgically accessible CTEPH and identify the typical angiographic findings of CTEPH, such as total obstruction, bands, webs, and intimal irregularities, although traditional invasive pulmonary angiography is still required for the evaluation of CTEPH for assessing the need for surgical or percutaneous treatment.[39]

Cardiac Magnetic Resonance Imaging

The role of cardiac magnetic resonance (CMR) imaging in the diagnosis and management of PH, although important,

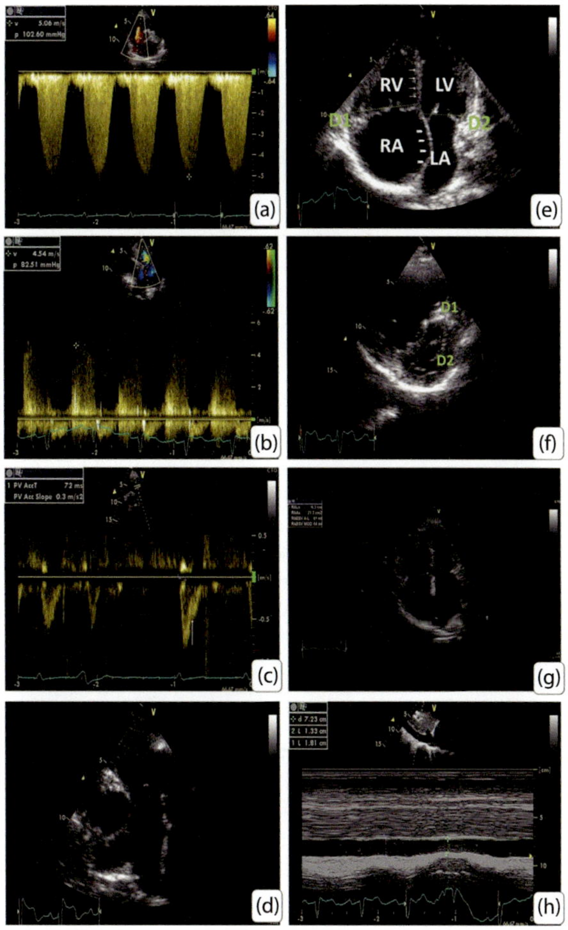

Peak tricuspid regurgitation velocity (m/s)	Presence of other echocardiographic signs of PH	Echocardiographic probability of PH
≤2.8 or not measurable	No	Low
≤2.8 or not measurable	Yes	Intermediate
2.9-3.4	No	
2.9-3.4	Yes	High
>3.4	Not required	

FIGURE 27.6 Echocardiographic signs suggestive of pulmonary hypertension. Tricuspid regurgitant velocity >3.4 m/s requires no supportive signs for classifying the probability of pulmonary hypertension as "high" (a). In tricuspid regurgitant velocity values <3.4 m/s, the presence of echocardiographic signs of pulmonary hypertension from at least two different categories should be present to alter the level of echocardiographic probability of pulmonary hypertension: 1. The pulmonary artery: Doppler findings suggestive of high pulmonary artery pressures (early diastolic pulmonary regurgitant velocity >2.2 m/s) (b), high pulmonary artery resistance (right ventricular outflow track Doppler acceleration time <105 ms and/or mid-systolic notching) (c), dilated pulmonary artery >25 mm (d). 2. The ventricles: Signs of interventricular interaction: right ventricular enlargement (right ventricle/left ventricle basal diameter ratio >1) (e), interventricular septal displacement towards left ventricle (left ventricular eccentricity index >1.1 in systole or/and in diastole) (f). 3. Inferior vena cava and right atrium: Signs of venous congestion: right atrial end-systolic area >18 cm^2 (g) or inferior cava diameter >21 mm with decreased inspiratory collapse (<50% with a sniff or <20% with quiet inspiration) (h).

remains relatively limited by its high cost and the need for specialized facilities not widely available at every center. It can nevertheless provide valuable, accurate, and highly reproducible information on the size, morphology, and function of the right heart, while data originating from CMR studies indicate their value in the prognosis of the disease, with the dimensions of the right ventricle expressed by its mass and volume, as well as its systolic function being recognized as determinants of prognosis.[40,41]

Right Heart Catheterization

Right heart catheterization (RHC) is the method of choice for the diagnosis (Figure 27.1) and treatment decisions in PH and, according to current guidelines, should follow all other investigations to achieve two goals: to avoid unnecessary examinations and targeted treatments in patients with alternative diagnosis (e.g., left heart disease) and to establish the correct diagnosis in patients with suspicion of PAH (Figure 27.5). Despite being an invasive examination, RHC has minimal risks of increased morbidity and mortality when performed in expert centers. During RHC, the following measurements should be performed: right atrial pressure, right ventricular systolic and end-diastolic pressure, systolic/diastolic and mean pulmonary artery pressure, pulmonary artery wedge pressure, pulmonary artery oxygen saturation, and cardiac output. Of these, surrogate markers, such as transpulmonary pressure gradient (mean pulmonary artery pressure minus pulmonary artery wedge pressure), pulmonary vascular resistance (transpulmonary pressure gradient/cardiac output), and cardiac index (cardiac output/body surface area) can be calculated. Pits and pitfalls that usually need to be overcome are:

- The correct level of zero (should be at the mid-thoracic line in a supine patient).
- The determination of all measurements at end-expiration and the recording of pulmonary artery wedge pressure as the mean of three measurements.
- The correct oximetry including samples from inferior and superior vena cava and pulmonary artery to suspect cardiac shunts.
- The determination of cardiac output by thermodilution or a direct Fick method (the latter in patients with congenital shunts)

In patients with idiopathic, hereditary, or drug-induced PAH, a pulmonary vasoreactivity test should also be performed to identify those few patients that could benefit from treatment with a calcium channel blocker. Inhaled nitric oxide (NO) at 10–20 parts per million (ppm) is the standard for vasoreactivity testing, but IV epoprostenol, IV adenosine, or inhaled iloprost can also be used. A positive acute response is defined as a reduction of mean PAP by ≥10 mmHg to reach an absolute value of mean PAP ≤40 mmHg with an increased or unchanged cardiac output.[2]

In addition to routinely performed measurements, in patients with high suspicion of left heart disease and pulmonary artery wedge pressure <15 mmHg, an acute volume challenge on left heart filling pressures should be considered. A fluid bolus of 500 mL appears to be safe and may discriminate between patients with PAH and those with left ventricular diastolic dysfunction.[2] In patients with pulmonary artery wedge pressure between 12 and 15 mmHg, an increase ≥18 mmHg after fluid challenge is considered abnormal and may be indicative of heart failure with preserved ejection fraction.

Pharmacotherapy

Despite advances in the pharmacotherapy of PAH in recent decades, the disease remains non-curable and retains remarkably high rates of morbidity and mortality. There are three well-known pathways that contribute to the pathogenesis of PAH: the endothelin, nitric oxide, and prostacyclin pathways (Figure 27.7). Treatments targeting these pathways are well established in clinical practice, such as endothelin receptor antagonists (ERAs), phosphodiesterase-5 (PDE-5) inhibitors, soluble guanylate cyclase stimulators (sGCs), and prostanoids.

Endothelin Receptor Antagonists

Endothelin 1 is a potent vasoconstrictor which effects its biologic actions through activation of two distinct receptor isoforms: the endothelin A (ETA) and endothelin B (ETB) receptors. Binding of endothelin 1 to ETA and ETB on pulmonary smooth muscle cells promotes vasoconstriction, whereas activation of ETB receptors on endothelial cells causes vasodilation through increased prostacyclin and nitric oxide levels.

Bosentan is an endothelin 1 antagonist that blocks both ETA and ETB receptors by binding to them. Bosentan treatment is initiated at a dose of 62.5 mg twice daily for four weeks and then the dose is increased to the approved maintenance dose of 125 mg twice daily. In the BREATH-1 trial, patients in the bosentan arm showed a significant improvement in the 6-minute walk test distance and WHO functional class compared with the placebo arm[42] In mildly symptomatic PAH, improvements in pulmonary vascular resistance and delayed time to clinical worsening vs placebo were observed in the EARLY study.[43] Bosentan was also evaluated with respect to response of other forms of PAH, such as Eisenmenger syndrome (BREATH-5 study),[44,45] in pediatric patients,[46] HIV-related PAH,[47] and in those with porto-pulmonary hypertension.[48] Monitoring of liver transaminases is required in patients treated with bosentan as elevated aspartate aminotransferase or alanine aminotransferase levels more than three times the upper limit of normal subject are not uncommon during therapy and may necessitate dose reduction or treatment discontinuation.

Ambrisentan is a selective ETA receptor antagonist administered once daily in a dose of 5 mg or 10 mg. As no significant increase in liver enzymes was observed in clinical trials, no liver function monitoring is deemed necessary. Ambrisentan showed a favorable result in 6-minute walk distance and in WHO functional class and a decrease in B-type natriuretic peptide (BNP) serum levels, as well as a delay in time to clinical worsening compared with placebo in two randomized, controlled clinical trials (ARIES 1 and ARIES 2),[49] with a maintained result in functional capacity after two years of drug administration (ARIES E).[50]

Macitentan is a tissue-targeting endothelin receptor antagonist characterized by high lipophilicity. The safety and efficacy of macitentan were examined in the SERAPHIN trial, the first event-driven randomized, controlled trial in PAH.[51] Macitentan 10 mg administered once daily achieved reduction of the primary composite endpoint of death, atrial septostomy,

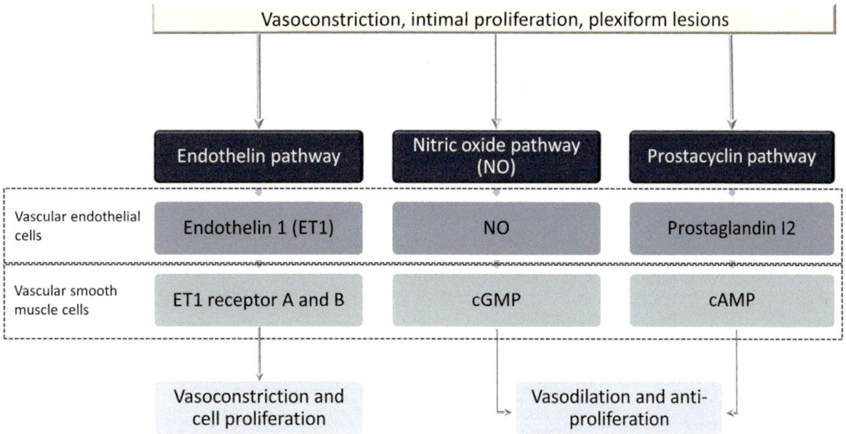

FIGURE 27.7 Different pathways of endothelial dysfunction that are targeted in the treatment of pulmonary rterial hypertension. *Abbreviations*: cAMP: cyclic adenosine monophosphate, cGMP: cyclic guanosine monophosphate.

lung transplantation, initiation of treatment with IV or subcutaneous prostanoids, or worsening of PAH. The favorable effects were also seen in patients under sequential combination therapy, to whom macitentan was added on their previous PAH treatment (mainly PDE-5 inhibitor).[51]

PDE-5 Inhibitors

PDE-5 inhibitors act on the NO pathway, by inhibiting cGMP metabolism, thereby maintaining the beneficial vasodilatory effects of NO. The safety and efficacy of sildenafil, a PDE-5 inhibitor, were tested in a short term (12-week) randomized, trial that showed improvement in 6-minute walk distance and WHO functional class when compared with controls (SUPER-1 study),[52] and these results were maintained after one and three years of treatment (SUPER-3 study).[53] The recommended dose of sildenafil is 20 mg three times daily.

Tadalafil is another PDE-5 inhibitor, administered in a single daily dose of 40 mg, that showed favorable effects on 6-minute walk test distance, hemodynamics, and time to clinical worsening when compared with placebo both in treatment-naïve patients and in patients under background advanced treatment for PAH, in a randomized, controlled, clinical trial.[54]

Soluble Guanylate Cyclase Stimulators (sGCs)

Riociguat is a novel agent, which also targets the NO pathway but by enhancing cGMP production. The target dose is 2.5 mg three times daily, and titration is driven by blood pressure. The favorable effects of riociguat on exercise capacity, hemodynamics, WHO functional class, and time to clinical worsening vs placebo were demonstrated in a clinical trial, in which almost half of the patients were already on background advanced treatment for PAH.[55] In the REPLACE trial, which examined the effect of switching to riociguat in patients with inadequate response to PDE-5 inhibitors, clinical improvement was achieved in 41% of the 111 patients in the riociguat group and 20% of the 113 patients in the PDE-5 inhibitor group (OR 2.78; 95% CI 1.53–5.06; P=0.0007).[56] Riociguat is also the only agent approved for inoperable or recurrent chronic thromboembolic PH after pulmonary endarterectomy.[57]

Prostacyclin Analogues

Epoprostenol is a synthetic analogue of the naturally occurring prostacyclin and is a potent pulmonary vasodilator. However, its short half-life (3 to 6 min) necessitates continuous IV infusion by a portable pump through a permanent catheter. The drug should be initiated and carefully up-titrated in the hospital in experienced centers. Infusion rates vary, determined by patient tolerance of side effects (e.g., jaw pain, headache, diarrhea, pain in extremities, nausea, and vomiting). The usual starting dose is 2 ng/kg/min. Various up-titration schemes have been proposed.[58] Epoprostenol was the first drug used for the treatment of PAH. In randomized, controlled trials, epoprostenol improved exercise capacity and hemodynamics and reduced mortality (over a period of 12 weeks and 3 years), compared with placebo.[59–61] To date, this is the only approved treatment for PAH that reduces mortality. These results were confirmed by observational studies[62,63] and by the French registry,[64,65] in which survival benefit was greatest in treatment-naïve patients who received upfront combination therapy with epoprostenol and oral medications. Epoprostenol use is limited by the need for strict adherence to protocols for sterile drug preparation and IV administration, as serious complications (e.g., catheter-related infection, cellulitis, pneumothorax, and thrombosis) have been observed. Caution should be paid to avoid abruptly stopping the continuous infusion, as this may lead to rebound PH with grave consequences, which may even lead to death.

Iloprost is a prostanoid analogue administered either IV or by inhalation. The latter is usually well tolerated, and the starting dose is 15 μg/day up-titrated to the target of 30 μg/day, divided into six equal doses. Iloprost has improved WHO functional class combined by improvement of 6-min walk distance, as well as hemodynamics and quality of life when compared with placebo in a randomized, controlled clinical trial.[66] Although syncope occurred with similar frequency in the two groups, this side effect was more frequently rated as serious in the Iloprost group. However, syncope was not associated with clinical deterioration in that trial.[66] The use of iloprost is associated with jaw pain, flushing, and cough, sometimes limiting patient adherence.

Treprostinil is a synthetic prostanoid that can be administered IV, subcutaneously (sc), or inhaled. It is stable at room temperature and has a half-life of four hours, characteristics that allow for continuous sc infusion. Treprostinil is also produced in formulations that allow oral use. The treatment with subcutaneous treprostinil is initiated at a dose of 1–2 ng/kg/min, up-titrated by 2 ng/kg/min, with the optimal dose determined by patient tolerability and the development of side effects, such as headache, jaw pain, myalgia, and flushing. Neuropathic pain at the site of sc infusion is the most severe side effect, affecting adherence. SC treprostinil improves exercise capacity and hemodynamics in patients with PAH,[67] and also has favorable effects in patients with PAH related to congenital heart disease[68] and chronic thromboembolic PH.[69] Intravenous treprostinil had favorable results on functional capacity in a randomized, double-blind, placebo-control, clinical trial prematurely discontinued due to ethical issues.[70] Inhaled treprostinil also generated promising results on 6-minute walk distance, quality of life, and NT-proBNP level when used as an add-on therapy on patients already on background advanced treatment with bosentan or sildenafil,[71] although oral treprostinil has yielded mixed results in clinical trials, ranging from no improvement on functional capacity to reduction of the risk of clinical worsening when administered soon after the initiation of background advanced PH therapy.[72–75]

Selexipag is a selective prostacyclin IP receptor agonist available for oral administration at a starting dose of 200 μg twice daily, gradually up-titrated to the target dose of 1600 μg twice daily. The most common side effects are similar to those seen by other prostanoids. Selexipag reduced the composite of death, hospitalization for PAH worsening, disease progression, and listing for transplantation in a large, event-driven, randomized, trial, in which 80% of patients were on background oral PAH advanced treatment.[76,77]

Ralinepag, a selective, non-prostanoid prostacyclin receptor agonist with a 24-h terminal half-life was found to reduce pulmonary vascular resistance in PAH patients already under advanced treatment, in a phase 2 study.[78] The safety and efficacy of ralinepag is currently being investigated in a multicenter, randomized, double-blind, placebo-controlled study implementing hard clinical end points such as PAH related death or hospitalization.[79]

Currently, scientific interest is focused on novel therapeutic pathways, such as the bone morphogenetic protein pathway, where signaling is associated with both hereditary and idiopathic subtypes of PH. Sotatercept, a fusion protein that binds activins and growth differentiation factors in an attempt to restore balance between growth-promoting and growth-inhibiting signaling pathways, was found to reduce pulmonary vascular resistance in a cohort of PAH patients already on background advanced PAH treatment.[80]

Goals of Therapy and Novel Therapeutic Targets

Treatment goals in PAH have been modified over time. Currently, a goal-oriented strategy that uses known prognostic indicators as treatment targets is supported by data from clinical trials and registries and embraced by current guidelines[2] Patients who are stabilized or who improve slightly can still receive additional therapy if treatment goals are not met. Risk assessment remains the gold standard in the evaluation and decision making concerning patients with PAH and regular assessments at tailored intervals are recommended. The comprehensive assessment should address the possibility of clinical deterioration, the determination of its cause (PAH or other cause), right ventricular function, and risk assessment. Currently, there are several risk assessment calculators, namely the French Pulmonary Hypertension Network (FPHN) registry risk equation,[81] the PH connection equation,[82] the Scottish composite score[83] the US Registry to Evaluate Early and Long-term PAH Disease Management (REVEAL) risk score,[84,85] and the 2015 ESC/ERS PH guidelines risk table.[2] All scores use multiple parameters, including clinical (presence of symptoms, functional class, 6-min walk test distance), hemodynamics (right atrial pressure, cardiac index), neurohormonal (natriuretic peptides), and echocardiographic markers (right atrial size, presence of pericardial effusion). Based on these scores, patients are then categorized as low, intermediate, or high risk.

Therapeutic Approaches and Options

The first step is referral to a center of PH expertise, as PH therapy requires an individualized approach. Patients are expected to perform lifestyle modifications, to achieve a better clinical status, and are thus encouraged to join patient support groups or ask for psychosocial support. Physical activity is adapted to avoid symptoms. Supervised exercise rehabilitation is useful, although excessive physical activity leading to symptoms is discouraged. Pregnancy should also be discouraged as it carries a high maternal risk. Air travel is not prohibited, but supplementary oxygen may be indicated in some patients. Genetic counseling should be offered to selected patients.

Supportive measures are also proposed, including diuretics in patients with signs of right heart failure and congestion, and ambulatory O_2 administration in patients with hypoxemia and correction of anemia. Digoxin may be used in patients with atrial tachyarrhythmias to slow the ventricular rate. Standard treatment of left heart failure such as angiotensin-converting enzyme inhibitors, angiotensin-2 receptor antagonists, beta-blockers, and ivabradine should be saved only for the treatment of comorbidities and is discouraged in patients with PAH[2,86] Calcium channel blockers (CCBs) are reserved for patients with idiopathic, heritable, or anorexigen-induced PAH who have positive acute vasoreactivity testing.[2] The most commonly used CCBs for PAH are nifedipine, diltiazem, and amlodipine, starting on a low dose and slowly titrating to the maximum tolerated dose. Target daily doses that have shown efficacy in idiopathic PAH are 60 to 240 mg for nifedipine, 240 to 720 mg for diltiazem, and 20 mg for amlodipine. Common adverse effects include systemic hypotension and lower extremity edema. Patients started on CCBs should be continuously re-assessed to identify clinical and hemodynamic improvements and continuing response; lack of response should prompt addition of PAH-targeted therapies.

Table 27.1 provides a brief overview of currently available advanced treatment options for pulmonary arterial hypertension, their standard dosage, and most common side effects. The updated treatment algorithm for PAH is described in Figure 27.8. To attain a low risk profile, a more aggressive approach is currently proposed, and combination therapy is strongly encouraged in expert centers, whereas monotherapy is reserved for specific categories of PAH (Table 27.2). Combination therapy to target multiple pathways is now

TABLE 27.1: Currently Available Advanced Treatment Options for Pulmonary Arterial Hypertension

Targeted Pathway	Type	Drug	Dosage	Side Effects
Oral Therapies				
Nitric oxide pathway	PDE-5i	Sildenafil	20 mg TiD	Headaches, flushing, diarrhea, non-arteritic anterior ischemic optic neuropathy, priapism
		Tadalafil	40 mg OD	Headache, nasopharyngitis, optic neuropathy, priapism
	sGCs	Riociguat	2.5 mg TiD	Headaches, dyspepsia, peripheral edema
Endothelin- 1 pathway	ERAs	Bosentan	125 mg BiD	Hepatotoxicity (8–12%), peripheral edema, anemia, sinusitis, headaches
		Ambrisentan	10 mg OD	Peripheral edema, headaches, anemia, nasal congestion
		Macitentan	10 mg OD	Headache, nasopharyngitis, anemia
Prostacyclin pathway	Prostanoids	Treprostinil	3 mg TiD (or greater)	Headaches, diarrhea, nausea, jaw pain
	Prostacyclin agonist	Selexipag	200 mcg BiD. to 1600 mcg BiD	Headache, diarrhea, jaw pain, vomiting, pain in extremities, hyperthyroidism
Inhaled Therapies				
Prostacyclin pathway	Prostanoids	Treprostinil	18–54 mg Q8H to Q3H	Cough, throat irritation, syncope
		Iloprost	2.5 or 5.0 mg, Q6H to Q4H	Syncope, cough, flushing, jaw pain
		Epoprostenol	10–50 ng/kg/min	Thrombocytopenia, rebound pulmonary hypertension
Nitric oxide pathway		Nitric oxide	5–40 ppm	Methemoglobinemia at high doses (>40 ppm)
Parenteral Therapies				
Prostacyclin pathway	Prostanoids	Treprostinil sc Treprostinil IV	1.25 ng/kg/min initial to goal 20–80 ng/kg/min (or higher)	Headache, diarrhea, thrombocytopenia, hypotension, jaw pain, hyperthyroidism
		Epoprostenol IV	2 ng/kg/min initial to goal 20–40 ng/kg/min (or higher)	Thrombocytopenia, headache, jaw pain, diarrhea, flushing, hyperthyroidism

Abbreviations: PDE-5i: phosphodiesterase-5 inhibitors, sGCs: soluble guanile cyclase stimulator, ERA: endothelin receptor antagonist, BiD: two times daily, TiD: three times daily, OD: once daily, Q3H: every three hours, Q4H: every four hours, Q6H: every six hours, Q8H every eight hours.

considered the standard of care in PAH based on strong evidence,[87,88] supporting the role of both initial and sequential combination therapy.[2,86] The latter, although the most widely utilized strategy for years, has now been replaced by initial combination strategy. However, in the light of recent clinical trials[89–91] using robust endpoints, such as hospitalization and mortality, initial combination with more than one class of PAH-specific drugs, e.g., using an ERA and a PDE-5 inhibitor, or/and IV epoprostenol in selected high-risk patients, is highly encouraged.[2,86]

Pulmonary Endarterectomy and Balloon Pulmonary Angioplasty

CTEPH is the only category of PH that can be fully treated with resolution of symptoms, either by surgical treatment with pulmonary endarterectomy (PEA) or, more recently, by percutaneous intervention with balloon pulmonary angioplasty (BPA). PEA is the preferred therapeutic option in CTEPH, offering significant improvement in hemodynamic profile, clinical status, and mortality in patients with operable lesions, compared with those treated with medical therapy alone (90% three-year[92] and 72% ten-year survival,[93] compared with 70% three-year survival of non-operated CTEPH patients). Therefore, patients with CTEPH should be evaluated for potential interventions by multidisciplinary teams in centers with surgical expertise. Although the definition of operability remains elusive, patients with prior history of venous thromboembolism, no signs of right heart failure, no comorbidities, and in retained functional class (WHO functional class II or III), as well as patients with more clear radiological disease, especially when located in lower lobes, and those with lower PVR (<1000 dyn.sec.cm^{-5}) have better long-term prognosis after PEA.[94]

Percutaneous balloon pulmonary angioplasty is a treatment option in selected patients with inoperable CTEPH or residual PH after PEA. The technique attracts interest as an alternative to PEA as it offers an option to improve hemodynamics and functional status at limited cost and with few complications when performed in expert centers.[2]

Conclusion

Although pulmonary hypertension as a clinical entity and fatal disease has been known since the 1960s, therapeutic options until recently were limited to non-specific drugs and were ineffective. Research in the field has evolved and advanced therapies have been introduced, changing the course of the disease. Clinical trials using soft clinical endpoints, such as 6-min walk test distance, have now been replaced by multicenter clinical trials with "harder" endpoints. Novel pathways are being explored, expanding the possible therapeutic targets, including genetic mutations (e.g., BMPR2 mutations, etc.), epigenetic modifications (e.g., histone deacetylase inhibition, etc.), growth factors (e.g., platelet-derived growth factor receptor-α and -β inhibition by tyrosine kinase receptor inhibitors), inflammation

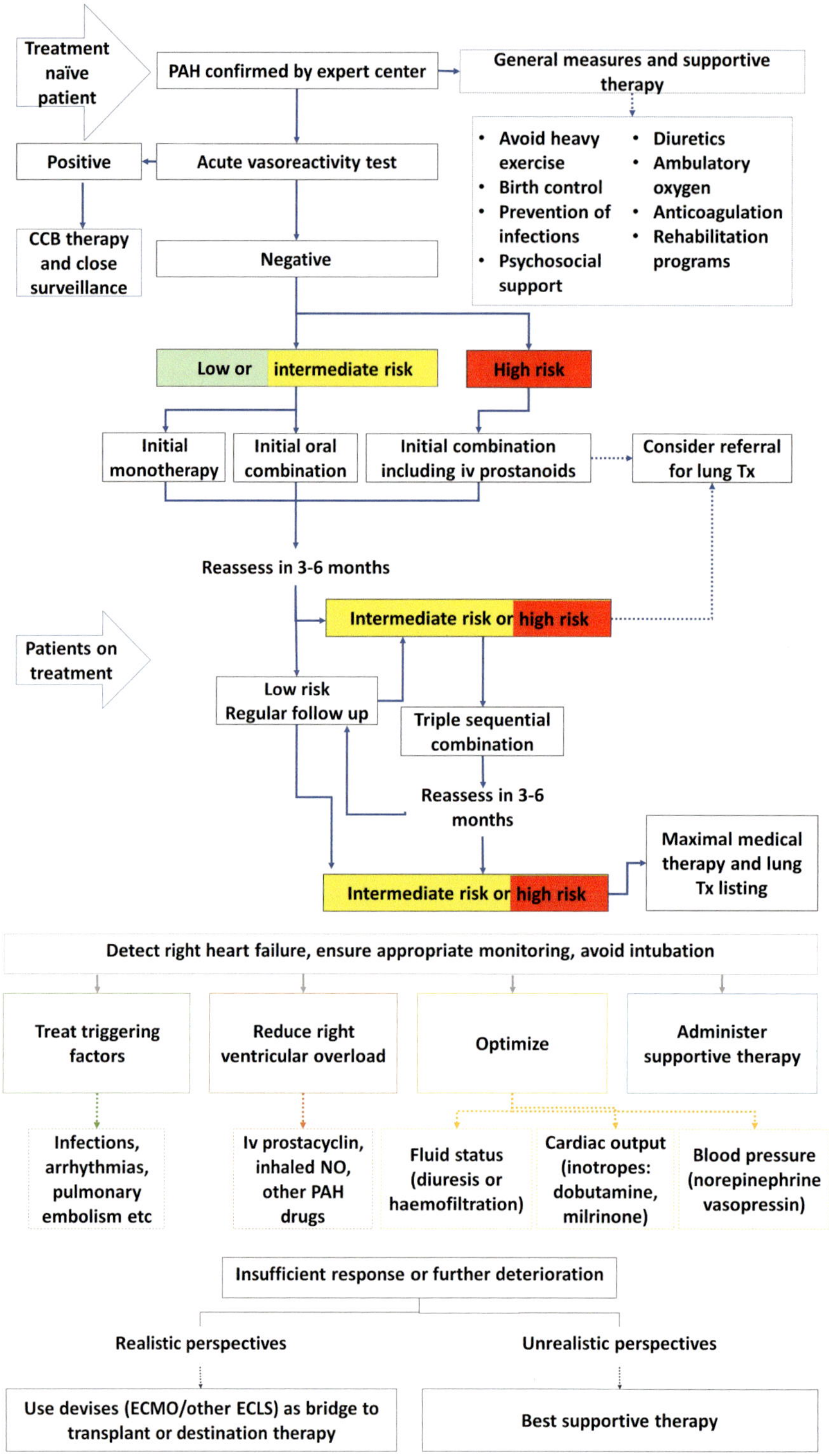

FIGURE 27.8 Proposed treatment algorithm in patients with pulmonary arterial hypertension. In patients with negative vasoreactivity test supportive and advanced pulmonary arterial hypertension, treatment is started with either monotherapy or initial combination therapy, according to patient's risk assessment. Triple or double combination therapy including parenteral prostanoids is saved for patients in the high-risk category, for which listing for lung transplantation should also be explored as a therapeutic target. The reduction of risk and the re-classification of the patient to the low-risk status is followed by a structured follow-up, in which evaluation of risk status is performed. Failure of the initial therapeutic approach to result in a low-risk status may highlight the need for treatment escalation with triple therapy (or sequential double therapy in the case of initial monotherapy) or with the addition of parenteral prostanoids and referral for lung transplantation in case risk status is determined as "high." In any case, the failure to achieve low-risk status should be followed by treatment up-titration and patients in high-risk status should be considered for lung transplantation. Severe right heart failure should also be treated by eliminating possible triggering factors, reducing right ventricular overload with the use of vasodilators and by optimizing body fluid status and cardiac function. The use of extracorporeal life support devices is encouraged in expert centers but saved only for patients with realistic life perspectives.

TABLE 27.2: Possible Indications of Monotherapy in Pulmonary Arterial Hypertension

- Idiopathic, heritable, and drug-induced pulmonary arterial hypertension patient responders to acute vasoreactivity tests and with WHO FC I/II and sustained hemodynamic improvement (same or better than achieved in the acute test) after at least one year on calcium channel blocker therapy only
- Long-term-treated historical pulmonary arterial hypertension patients with monotherapy (>5–10 years) stable with low risk profile
- Idiopathic pulmonary arterial hypertension patients>75 years old with multiple risk factors for heart failure with preserved ejection fraction (e.g., arterial hypertension, diabetes mellitus, coronary artery disease, atrial fibrillation, obesity)
- Pulmonary arterial hypertension patients with suspicion or high probability of pulmonary veno-occlusive disease or pulmonary capillary hemangiomatosis
- Patients with pulmonary arterial hypertension associated with HIV infection or portal hypertension or uncorrected congenital heart disease (e.g., Eisenmenger syndrome), as they were not included in RCTs of initial combination therapy
- Pulmonary arterial hypertension patients with very mild disease (e.g., WHO FC I, mPAP <30 mmHg, PVR <5 WU, normal right ventricle at echocardiography), who might be detected early with screening programs
- Combination therapy unavailable or contraindicated (e.g., severe liver disease)

Abbreviations: FC: Functional Class, mPAP: mean pulmonary arterial pressure, PAP: pulmonary arterial pressure, PVR: pulmonary vascular resistance, RCT: randomized controlled trial, WHO: World Health Organization, WU: Wood Units.
Sources: Modified from Galie et al. *Eur Respir J* 2019;53:1801889 and Galie et al. *Eur Heart J* 2015;37:67–119.

(monoclonal antibodies, pro-apoptotic agents, interleukin receptor antagonists, etc.), estrogen signaling, oxidative stress, and serotonin modulation, or even stem cell therapy and interventional techniques such as pulmonary artery denervation. Despite these advances, PAH currently remains incurable and carries a severe prognosis, necessitating further research.

References

1. Frost A, Badesch D, Gibbs JSR, et al. Diagnosis of pulmonary hypertension. *Eur Respir J.* 2019;53(1):1801904.
2. Galie N, Humbert M, Vachiery J-L, et al. 2015 ESC/ERS guidelines for the diagnosis and treatment of pulmonary hypertension. *Eur Heart J.* 2015;37(1):67–119.
3. Rich S, Dantzker DR, Ayres SM, et al. Primary pulmonary hypertension: a national prospective study. *Ann Intern Med.* 1987;107(2):216–23.
4. Hoeper MM, Huscher D, Ghofrani HA, et al. Elderly patients diagnosed with idiopathic pulmonary arterial hypertension: results from the COMPERA registry. *Int J Cardiol.* 2013;168(2):871–80.
5. Benza RL, Miller DP, Barst RJ, Badesch DB, Frost AE, McGoon MD. An evaluation of long-term survival from time of diagnosis in pulmonary arterial hypertension from the REVEAL registry. *CHEST.* 2012;142(2):448–56.
6. D'Alonzo GE, Barst RJ, Ayres SM, et al. Survival in patients with primary pulmonary hypertension: results from a national prospective registry. *Ann Intern Med.* 1991;115(5):343–9
7. Andersen CU, Mellemkjær S, Nielsen-Kudsk JE, et al. Echocardiographic screening for pulmonary hypertension in stable COPD out-patients and NT-proBNP as a rule-out test. *COPD.* 2012;9(5):505–12.
8. Andersen KH, Iversen M, Kjaergaard J, et al. Prevalence, predictors, and survival in pulmonary hypertension related to end-stage chronic obstructive pulmonary disease. *J Heart Lung Transplant.* 2012;31(4):373–80.
9. Nadrous HF, Pellikka PA, Krowka MJ, et al. Pulmonary hypertension in patients with idiopathic pulmonary fibrosis. *CHEST.* 2005;128(4): 2393–9.
10. Ende-Verhaar YM, Cannegieter SC, Vonk Noordegraaf A, et al. Incidence of chronic thromboembolic pulmonary hypertension after acute pulmonary embolism: a contemporary view of the published literature. *Eur Respir J.* 2017;49(2):1601792.
11. Kim NH. Group 4 pulmonary hypertension: chronic thromboembolic pulmonary hypertension: epidemiology, pathophysiology, and treatment. *Cardiol Clin.* 2016;34(3):435–41.
12. Bonderman D, Wilkens H, Wakounig S, et al. Risk factors for chronic thromboembolic pulmonary hypertension. *Eur Respir J.* 2009;33(2):325.
13. Fayyaz AU, Edwards WD, Maleszewski JJ, et al. Global pulmonary vascular remodeling in pulmonary hypertension associated with heart failure and preserved or reduced ejection fraction. *Circulation.* 2018;137(17):1796–810.
14. Dorfmüller P, Günther S, Ghigna M-R, et al. Microvascular disease in chronic thromboembolic pulmonary hypertension: a role for pulmonary veins and systemic vasculature. *Eur Respir J.* 2014;44(5):1275.
15. Huertas A, Guignabert C, Barberà JA, et al. Pulmonary vascular endothelium: the orchestra conductor in respiratory diseases. *Eur Respir J.* 2018;51(4):1700745.
16. Mouratoglou SA, Giannakoulas G, Deftereos S, et al. Intra- and intercellular calcium handling in pulmonary arterial hypertension. *Med Chem.* 2016;12(2):162–9.
17. Bogaard HJ, Abe K, Vonk Noordegraaf A, Voelkel NF. The right ventricle under oressure: cellular and molecular mechanisms of right-heart failure in pulmonary hypertension. *Chest.* 2009;135(3):794–804.
18. Nagaya N, Nishikimi T, Uematsu M, et al. Plasma brain natriuretic peptide as a prognostic indicator in patients with primary pulmonary hypertension. *Circulation.* 2000;102(8):865–70.
19. Channick RN, Sitbon O, Barst RJ, Manes A, Rubin LJ. Endothelin receptor antagonists in pulmonary arterial hypertension. *J Am Coll Cardiol.* 2004;43(12) Supplement S:62–67.
20. Vonk Noordegraaf A, Chin KM, Haddad F, et al. Pathophysiology of the right ventricle and of the pulmonary circulation in pulmonary hypertension: an update. *Eur Respir J.* 2019;53(1):1801900.
21. Naeije R. The overloaded right heart and ventricular interdependence. *Cardiovasc Res.* 2017;113:1474–85.
22. Lumens J, Arts T, Marcus JT, Vonk-Noordegraaf A, Delhaas T. Early-diastolic left ventricular lengthening implies pulmonary hypertension-induced right ventricular decompensation. *Cardiovasc Res.* 2012;96(2):286–95.
23. Marcus JT, Gan CT-J, Zwanenburg JJM, et al. Interventricular mechanical asynchrony in pulmonary arterial hypertension: left-to-right delay in peak shortening is related to right ventricular overload and left ventricular underfilling. *J Am Coll Cardiol.* 2008;51(7):750–7.
24. Vonk-Noordegraaf A, Haddad F, Chin KM, et al. Right heart adaptation to pulmonary arterial hypertension: physiology and pathobiology. *J Am Coll Cardiol.* 2013;62(25) Supplement:22–33.
25. Manders E, Bogaard H-J, Handoko ML, et al. Contractile dysfunction of left ventricular cardiomyocytes in patients with pulmonary arterial hypertension. *J Am Coll Cardiol.* 2014;64(1):28–37.
26. Mouratoglou SA, Kallifatidis A, Pitsiou G, et al. Duration of interventricular septal shift toward the left ventricle is associated with poor clinical outcome in precapillary pulmonary hypertension: a cardiac magnetic resonance study. *Hellenic J Cardiol.* 2020;61(2):112–7.
27. Peinado VI, Pizarro S, Barberà JA. Pulmonary vascular involvement in COPD. *CHEST.* 2008;134(4):808–14.
28. Peinado VI, Barberà JA, Ramírez J, et al. Endothelial dysfunction in pulmonary arteries of patients with mild COPD. *Am J Physiol* 1998;274(6):908–13.
29. Barberà JA, Peinado VI, Santos S, Ramirez J, Roca J, Robert R-R Reduced expression of endothelial nitric oxide synthase in pulmonary arteries of smokers. *Am J Respir Crit Care Med.* 2001;164(4):709–13.
30. Farkas L, Gauldie J, Voelkel NF, Kolb M. Pulmonary hypertension and idiopathic pulmonary fibrosis: a tale of angiogenesis, apoptosis, and growth factors. *Am J Respir Cell Mol Biol* 2011;45(1):1–15.
31. MacKenzie Ross RV, Toshner MR, Soon E, Naeije R, Pepke-Zaba J. Decreased time constant of the pulmonary circulation in chronic thromboembolic pulmonary hypertension. *Am J Physiol Heart Circ Physiol.* 2013;305(2):259–64.
32. Giusca S, Popa E, Amzulescu MS, et al. Is right ventricular remodeling in pulmonary hypertension dependent on etiology? An echocardiographic study. *Echocardiography.* 2016;33(4):546–54.

33. Bossone E, Paciocco G, Iarussi D, et al. The prognostic role of the ECG in primary pulmonary hypertension. *CHEST.* 2002;121(2):513–8.
34. Giannakoulas G, Mouratoglou S-A, Gatzoulis MA, Karvounis H. Blood biomarkers and their potential role in pulmonary arterial hypertension associated with congenital heart disease. A systematic review. *Int J Cardiol.* 2014;174(3):618–23.
35. Sun X-G, Hansen JE, Oudiz RJ, Wasserman K. Pulmonary function in primary pulmonary hypertension. *J Am Coll Cardiol.* 2003;41(6):1028–35.
36. Wright LM, Dwyer N, Celermajer D, Kritharides L, Marwick TH. Follow-up of pulmonary hypertension with echocardiography. *JACC Cardiovasc Imaging.* 2016;9(6):733–46.
37. Baggen VJM, Driessen MMP, Post MC, et al. Echocardiographic findings associated with mortality or transplant in patients with pulmonary arterial hypertension: a systematic review and meta-analysis. *Neth Heart J.* 2016;24(6):374–89.
38. Mouratoglou SA, Dimopoulos K, Kamperidis V, et al. Right atrial function predicts clinical outcome in patients with precapillary pulmonary hypertension. *J Am Soc Echocardiogr.* 2018;31(10):1137–45.
39. Reichelt A, Hoeper MM, Galanski M, Keberle M Chronic thromboembolic pulmonary hypertension: evaluation with 64-detector row CT versus digital substraction angiography. *Eur J Radiol.* 2008;(1):7149–54.
40. van Wolferen SA, Marcus JT, Boonstra A, Marques KM, Bronzwaer JG, Spreeuwenberg MD. Prognostic value of right ventricular mass, volume, and function in idiopathic pulmonary arterial hypertension. *Eur Heart J.* 2007;28(10):1250–7.
41. van de Veerdonk MC, Kind T, Marcus JT, et al. Progressive right ventricular dysfunction in patients with pulmonary arterial hypertension responding to therapy. *J Am Coll Cardiol.* 2011;58(24):2511–9.
42. Rubin LJ, Badesch DB, Barst RJ, et al. Bosentan therapy for pulmonary arterial hypertension. *N Engl J Med.* 2002;346(12):896–903.
43. Galie N, Rubin LJ, Hoeper MM, et al. Treatment of patients with mildly symptomatic pulmonary arterial hypertension with bosentan (EARLY study): a double-blind, randomised controlled trial. *Lancet.* 2008;371(9630):2093–100.
44. Berger RMF, Beghetti M, Galie N, et al. Atrial septal defects versus ventricular septal defects in BREATHE-5, a placebo-controlled study of pulmonary arterial hypertension related to Eisenmenger's syndrome: a subgroup analysis. *Int J Cardiol* 2011;144(3):373–8.
45. Gatzoulis MA, Beghetti M, Galie N, et al. Longer-term bosentan therapy improves functional capacity in Eisenmenger syndrome: results of the BREATHE-5 open-label extension study. *Int J Cardiol.* 2008;127(1):27–32.
46. Rosenzweig EB, Ivy DD, Widlitz A, et al. Effects of long-term bosentan in children with pulmonary arterial hypertension. *J Am Coll Card.* 2005;46(4):697–704.
47. Sitbon O, Gressin V, Speich R, et al. Bosentan for the treatment of human immunodeficiency virus–associated pulmonary arterial hypertension. *Am J Resp Crit Care Med.* 2004;170(11):1212–7.
48. Hoeper MM, Halank M, Marx C, et al. Bosentan therapy for portopulmonary hypertension. *Eur Resp J.* 2005;25(3):502.
49. Galie N, Olschewski H, Oudiz RJ, et al. Ambrisentan for the treatment of pulmonary arterial hypertension. Results of the ambrisentan in pulmonary arterial hypertension, randomized, doubleblind, placebo-controlled, multicenter, efficacy (ARIES) study 1 and 2. *Circulation.* 2008;117(23):3010–3019.
50. Oudiz RJ, Galiè N, Olschewski H, et al. Long-term ambrisentan therapy for the treatment of pulmonary arterial hypertension. *J Am Coll Card.* 2009;54(21):1971–81.
51. Pulido T, Adzerikho I, Channick RN, et al. Macitentan and morbidity and mortality in pulmonary arterial hypertension. *N Engl J Med.* 2013;369(9):809–18.
52. Galie N, Ghofrani HA, Torbicki A, et al. Sildenafil citrate therapy for pulmonary arterial hypertension. *N Engl J Med* 2005;353(20):2148–57.
53. Rubin LJ, Badesch DB, Fleming TR, et al. Long-term treatment with sildenafil citrate in pulmonary arterial hypertension: the SUPER-2 study. *Chest.* 2011;140(5):1274–83.
54. Galie N, Brundage BH, Ghofrani HA, et al. Tadalafil therapy for pulmonary arterial hypertension. *Circulation.* 2009;119(22):2894–903.
55. Ghofrani H-A, Galie N, Grimminger F, et al. Riociguat for the treatment of pulmonary arterial hypertension. *N Engl J Med* 2013;369(4):330–40.
56. Hoeper MM, Al-Hiti H, Benza RL, et al. Switching to riociguat versus maintenance therapy with phosphodiesterase-5 inhibitors in patients with pulmonary arterial hypertension (REPLACE): a multicentre, open-label, randomised controlled trial. *Lancet Respir Med.* 2021;9(6):573–84.
57. Ghofrani H-A, D'Armini AM, Grimminger F, et al. Riociguat for the treatment of chronic thromboembolic pulmonary hypertension. *N Engl J Med* 2013;369(4):319–29.
58. Sitbon O, Vonk Noordegraaf A. Epoprostenol and pulmonary arterial hypertension: 20years of clinical experience. *Eur Resp J.* 2017;26(143):160055.
59. Sitbon O, Delcroix M, Bergot E, et al. EPITOME-2: an open-label study assessing the transition to a new formulation of intravenous epoprostenol in patients with pulmonary arterial hypertension. *Am Heart J.* 2014;167(2):210–7.
60. Barst RJ, Rubin LJ, Long WA, et al. A comparison of continuous intravenous epoprostenol (prostacyclin) with conventional therapy for primary pulmonary hypertension. *N Engl J Med.* 1996;334(5):296–301.
61. Badesch DB, Tapson VF, McGoon MD, et al. Continuous intravenous epoprostenol for pulmonary hypertension due to the scleroderma spectrum of disease: a randomized, controlled trial. *Ann Intern Med.* 2000;132(6):425–34.
62. McLaughlin VV, Shillington A, Rich S. Survival in primary pulmonary hypertension: the impact of epoprostenol therapy. *Circulation.* 2002;106(12):1477–82.
63. Badesch DB, McGoon MD, Barst RJ, et al. Longterm survival among patients with ccleroderma-associated pulmonary arterial hypertension treated with intravenouseEpoprostenol. *J Reumatol.* 2009;36(10):2244.
64. Sitbon O, Humbert M, Nunes H, et al. Long-term intravenous epoprostenol infusion in primary pulmonary hypertension: prognostic factors and survival. *J Am Coll Cardiol.* 2002;40(4):780–8.
65. Bergot E, Sitbon O, Cottin V, et al. Current epoprostenol use in patients with severe idiopathic, heritable or anorexigen-associated pulmonary arterial hypertension: data from the French pulmonary hypertension registry. *Int J Cardiol.* 2014;172(3):561–7.
66. Olschewski H, Simonneau G, Galie N, et al. Inhaled iloprost for severe pulmonary hypertension. *N Engl J Med* 2002;347(5):322–9.
67. Lang I, Gomez-Sanchez M, Kneussl M, et al. Efficacy of long-term subcutaneous treprostinil sodium therapy in pulmonary hypertension. *Chest.* 2006;129(6):1636–43.
68. Skoro-Sajer N, Gerges C, Balint OH, et al. Subcutaneous treprostinil in congenital heart disease-related pulmonary arterial hypertension. *Heart.* 2018;104(14):1195–9.
69. Sadushi-Kolici R, Jansa P, Kopec G, et al. Subcutaneous treprostinil for the treatment of severe non-operable chronic thromboembolic pulmonary hypertension (CTREPH): a double-blind, phase 3, randomised controlled trial. *Lancet Respir Med.* 2019;7(3):239–48.
70. Tapson VF, Gomberg-Maitland M, McLaughlin VV, et al. Safety and efficacy of IV treprostinil for pulmonary arterial hypertension: a prospective, multicenter, open-label, 12-week trial. *Chest.* 2006;129(3):683–8.
71. McLaughlin VV, Benza RL, Rubin LJ, et al. Addition of inhaled treprostinil to oral therapy for pulmonary arterial hypertension: a randomized controlled clinical trial. *J Am Coll Cardiol.* 2010;55(18):1915–22.
72. Jing Z-C, Parikh K, Pulido T, et al. Efficacy and safety of oral treprostinil monotherapy for the treatment of pulmonary arterial hypertension: a randomized, controlled trial. *Circulation.* 2013;127(5):624–33.
73. Tapson VF, Torres F, Kermeen F, et al. Oral treprostinil for the treatment of pulmonary arterial hypertension in patients on background endothelin receptor antagonist and/or phosphodiesterase type 5 inhibitor therapy (the FREEDOM-C Study): a randomised controlled trial. *Chest.* 2012;142(6):1383–90.
74. Tapson VF, Sanchez Diaz CJ, Bohns Meyer GM, et al. Treatment with oral treprostinil delays time to clinical worsening in patients with pulmonary arterial hypertension – results from FREEDOM-EV. *J Heart Lung Transplant.* 2019;38(4):S94–5.
75. White RJ, Jerjes-Sanchez C, Bohns Meyer GM, et al. Combination therapy with oral treprostinil for pulmonary arterial hypertension. A double-blind placebo-controlled clinical trial. *Am J Respir Crit Care Med.* 2019;201(6):707–17.
76. Sitbon O, Channick R, Chin KM, et al. Selexipag for the treatment of pulmonary arterial hypertension. *N Engl J Med.* 2015;373(26):2522–33.
77. Simonneau Gr, Torbicki A, Hoeper MM, et al. Selexipag: an oral, selective prostacyclin receptor agonist for the treatment of pulmonary arterial hypertension. *Eur Respir J.* 2012;40(4):874.
78. Torres F, Farber H, Ristic A, et al. Efficacy and safety of ralinepag, a novel oral IP agonist, in PAH patients on mono or dual background therapy: results from a phase 2 randomised, parallel group, placebo-controlled trial. *Eur Respir J.* 2019;54(4):1901030.
79. (U.S.) NloM. A study evaluating the efficacy and safety of ralinepag to improve treatment outcomes in PAH patients. August 13, 2018;NCT03626688. https://clinicaltrials.gov/ct2/show/NCT03626688.
80. Humbert M, McLaughlin V, Gibbs JSR, et al. Sotatercept for the treatment of pulmonary arterial hypertension. *NEJM.* 2021;384(13):1204–15.
81. Humbert M, Sitbon O, Chaouat A, et al. Survival in patients with idiopathic, familial, and anorexigen-associated pulmonary arterial hypertension in the modern management era. *Circulation.* 2010;122(2):156–63.
82. Thenappan T, Glassner C, Gomberg-Maitland M. Validation of the pulmonary hypertension connection equation for survival prediction in pulmonary arterial hypertension. *Chest.* 2012;141(3):642–50.

83. Lee W-TN, Ling Y, Sheares KK, Pepke-Zaba J, Peacock AJ, Johnson MK. Predicting survival in pulmonary arterial hypertension in the UK. *Eur Resp J.* 2012;40(3):604.
84. Benza RL, Miller DP, Gomberg-Maitland M, et al. Predicting survival in pulmonary arterial hypertension. *Circulation.* 2010;122(2):164–72.
85. Benza RL, Miller DP, Foreman AJ, et al. Prognostic implications of serial risk score assessments in patients with pulmonary arterial hypertension: a Registry to Evaluate Early and Long-Term Pulmonary Arterial Hypertension Disease Management (REVEAL) analysis. *J Heart Lung Transplant.* 2015;34(3):356–61.
86. Galiè N, Channick RN, Frantz RP, et al. Risk stratification and medical therapy of pulmonary arterial hypertension. *Eur Respir J.* 2019;53(1):1801889.
87. Sitbon O, Gaine S Beyond a single pathway: combination therapy in pulmonary arterial hypertension. *Eur Respir Rev.* 2016(25):408–17.
88. Burks M, Stickel S, Galiè N. Pulmonary arterial hypertension: combination therapy in practice. *Am J Cardiovasc Drugs.* 2018;18(4):249–57.
89. Humbert M, Barst RJ, Robbins IM, et al. Combination of bosentan with epoprostenol in pulmonary arterial hypertension: BREATHE-2. *Eur Respir J.* 2004;24(3):353–9.
90. Kemp K, Savale L, O'Callaghan DS, et al. Usefulness of first-line combination therapy with epoprostenol and bosentan in pulmonary arterial hypertension: an observational study. *J Heart Lung Transplant.* 2012;31(0):150–8.
91. Galie N, Barbera JA, Frost AE, et al. Initial use of ambrisentan plus tadalafil in pulmonary arterial hypertension. *N Engl J Med* 2015;373(9):834–44.
92. Delcroix M, Lang I, Pepke-Zaba J, et al. Long-term outcome of patients with chronic thromboembolic pulmonary hypertension. *Circulation.* 2016;133(9):859–71.
93. Cannon John E, Su L, Kiely David G, et al. Dynamic risk stratification of patient long-term outcome after pulmonary endarterectomy. *Circulation.* 2016;133(18):1761–71.
94. Kim NH, Delcroix M, Jais X, et al. Chronic thromboembolic pulmonary hypertension. *Eur Resp J.* 2019;53(1):1801915.

Section VII
Special Cases of Heart Failure

DOI: 10.1201/9780429244544-34

Chapter 28
HEART FAILURE IN ADULT CONGENITAL HEART DISEASE

Andrew Constantine, Ana Barradas-Pires, Isma Rafiq, Justyna Rybicka, Michael A. Gatzoulis, and Konstantinos Dimopoulos

Introduction

Congenital heart disease (CHD) is the most common inborn malformation, with an estimated prevalence of 5–10 per 1000 live births.[1,2] Building on the triumph of the cardio-pulmonary bypass circuit over half a century ago, the success of CHD surgery, along with improved diagnostic, medical, and peri-operative care, have created a growing population of adults with CHD (ACHD). Current estimates put the ACHD population of the United States at 1.4 million[3] with an increasing prevalence of ACHD of great complexity.[4] Accordingly, the mortality burden has shifted significantly towards adulthood.[5] It is now well recognized that CHD, far from being cured, is associated with life-long morbidity portended by arrhythmias, residual hemodynamic lesions, pulmonary vascular disease (PVD), repeated interventions, and myocardial scarring. Heart failure (HF) is the final common pathway of many of these entities, with a lifetime prevalence of > 30% in patients with complex CHD and is the leading cause of death in ACHD patients over the age of 40 (Figure 28.1).[6,7]

Despite this, international HF guidelines do not provide any guidance on the treatment of CHD-related HF.[8] There are, indeed, major differences between acquired vs CHD-related HF: in the latter, the development of HF may indicate a changing hemodynamic milieu requiring reoperation or intervention, which can reverse or delay the progression of HF by decades. Hence, significant expertise and a multidisciplinary approach are required to manage ACHD patients with HF effectively.

In this chapter, we describe the CHD conditions with the highest likelihood of developing HF and examine the diagnosis and management, including the role of pharmacological, device and interventional therapies, in these groups.

Epidemiology of Heart Failure in ACHD

Compared to the pandemic of HF secondary to acquired heart disease, the burden of ACHD-related HF is much lower, although it represents a new, rapidly growing population of increasing complexity. Accurate estimation of the incidence and prevalence of HF in ACHD is challenging, not least because of the difficulty in exporting a universally applicable definition of HF from the acquired population. According to American College of Cardiology/American Heart Association guidelines, patients with structural heart disease, hence all CHD patients, are at risk of HF and are given HF status (stage B HF). Other definitions, such as HF as a "clinical syndrome caused by an abnormality of the heart and recognized by a characteristic pattern of hemodynamic, renal, neural, and hormonal responses,"[9] may better capture ACHD patients suffering from HF. Estimates of the prevalence of HF in the ACHD population have used various definitions and few are based on HF-related hospital admissions. Over the past three decades, mortality in ACHD patients has shifted from peri-operative causes to long-term complications, mainly HF. Population-based studies looking at contemporary cohorts consistently place HF as the first or second most common cause of death, accounting for 25–30% of all deaths and 45% of deaths from cardiovascular causes.[10,11] In our own cohort of over 7,000 patients, chronic HF was the leading cause of death in 42.5% of patients overall, and in two-thirds of patients with a systemic right ventricle (RV).[6]

The incidence of HF varies greatly depending on the underlying CHD. Patients with single ventricles or systemic RVs are at increased risk of HF from early life. By adulthood, HF is present in up to 40% of patients with a Fontan circulation and 20% of patients following an atrial switch (Mustard or Senning) procedure for transposition of the great arteries (TGA).[12] In the Dutch national registry, chronic HF accounted for over one-third of deaths in those with congenitally corrected transposition of the great arteries (ccTGA), univentricular hearts, and tetralogy of Fallot (ToF).[13]

Unlike in HF from acquired heart disease, HF is encountered in young patients with CHD, affecting 6.5% of all patients by 42 years of age, and 14.8% in complex CHD.[14] As in acquired disease, however, advancing age remains a strong predictor of HF in ACHD and the condition is likely to become even more prevalent as more patients with complex disease become older.

An analysis of US hospital admissions of ACHD patients in 2007 identified HF as the cause for 20% of cases, and was associated with increased mortality (hazard ratio 3.3, 95% confidence intervals 2.6–4.1).[15] European data reported an incidence of first HF admission of 1.2 per 100 patient-years, with certain diagnoses (univentricular heart, TGA, atrioventricular septal defects) associated with a higher risk.

The epidemiology of HF in ACHD has seen remarkable changes over the past few decades. The future impact of HF in this population will be determined by the downstream effects of better surgical techniques and introduction of interventional strategies allowing for earlier and more physiological correction and "migration" of pharmacological and device-related strategies from the wider HF population to an aging ACHD population with more complex disease.

Mechanisms of Heart Failure in ACHD

ACHD is an extremely heterogeneous group of anatomic phenotypes, each with its own specific clinical nuances and concerns. Mechanisms causing HF in CHD stem from a combination of the underlying defect and hemodynamic lesion causing volume or pressure overload, systemic arterial, venous or pulmonary hypertension (PH), cyanosis, coronary artery disease, arrhythmias, dyssynchrony, and chronotropic incompetence. Surgical and percutaneous repair creates a new substrate for late post-operative sequelae (e.g., surgical scars, post-operative coronary abnormalities, conduit stenoses). There is also a contribution from genetic factors affecting sarcomeric structure and function, including an association between some forms of CHD and cardiomyopathy,[16,17] although the genes and pathways involved have not been completely elucidated. CHD

DOI: 10.1201/9780429244544-35

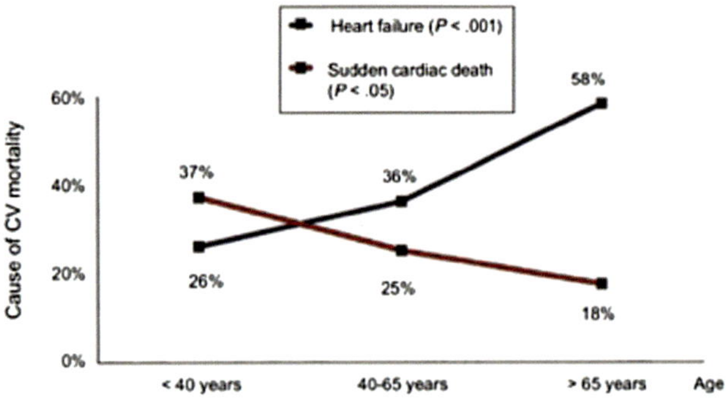

FIGURE 28.1 Mortality from heart failure and sudden cardiac death by age in patients with adult congenital heart disease. (Reproduced with permission from Oliver et al. *Int J Cardiol.* 2017;245:119–24.)

is compounded by acquired disease, including systemic hypertension, obesity, and atherosclerotic coronary artery disease, which can accrue with age. Concurrently, there is evidence of marked activation of the endothelin, sympathoadrenergic, and renin-aldosterone systems in adults with CHD.[18] The final common pathway involves systolic and diastolic ventricular dysfunction, with further neurohormonal activation, myocardial fibrosis, negative remodeling, and the possibility of systemic complications.

Exercise intolerance is commonly the main clinical feature of HF in ACHD. Non-cardiac factors contribute to exercise intolerance, including parenchymal pulmonary disease or kyphoscoliosis (commonly associated with CHD) and systemic effects of chronic HF (e.g., skeletal muscle abnormalities).[19] Cardiopulmonary exercise testing (CPET) is particularly helpful for elucidating the severity and mechanisms of exercise intolerance and is a core part of the assessment of the ACHD patient.

Patients presenting with new-onset or decompensated HF should be assessed to identify modifiable causes. Hemodynamic lesions should be assessed for surgery or transcatheter intervention in a multidisciplinary approach. In most CHD patients, HF is the result of hemodynamic burden caused by the CHD, combined with associated lesions, comorbidity, and sequelae, e.g., arrhythmias, myocardial dysfunction, scarring related to prior surgery, and concurrent lung disease. Therefore, management of HF in ACHD relies on identifying the mechanisms behind the onset and progression of HF.

Lesion-Specific Considerations and Therapeutic Options

Most ACHD patients presenting with HF belong to one of four anatomic types: repaired ToF, univentricular heart (mostly Fontan-type circulation), systemic RVs (TGA or ccTGA), or PH.

Right Heart Failure in Tetralogy of Fallot

ToF is the most common cyanotic CHD, accounting for 7–10% of all cardiac malformations.[20] The anterocephalad deviation of the "outlet" portion of the septum accounts for all the four associated lesions: ventricular septal defect (VSD), right ventricular outflow obstruction (RVOTO), aorta overriding the RV, and RV hypertrophy. The RVOTO often includes a sub-infundibular component related to RV hypertrophied septoparietal trabeculations.[21] Up to 20% of patients can also have coronary anomalies.

ToF includes a spectrum of anatomies based on the severity of RVOT obstruction, ranging from mild pulmonary stenosis (PS) to pulmonary atresia. In the latter, the pulmonary circulation is completely dependent on the ductus arteriosus or major aortopulmonary collaterals and the pulmonary arteries can be hypoplastic or absent, making repair difficult.

Surgical repair of ToF consists of closing the VSD and achieving relief of the RVOTO. Early techniques, using a ventriculotomy and transannular patch, disrupted the pulmonary annulus integrity and have gradually been replaced by transatrial or transpulmonary approaches, valve-sparing techniques, and smaller RVOT patches. These reflect an effort to avoid significant pulmonary regurgitation (PR). ToF repair has significantly changed the prognosis of these patients.

Despite this, the majority of patients reaching adulthood do have some form of sequela, mainly significant PR. Severe PR leads to significant dilatation of the RV, RV impairment, risk of ventricular arrhythmias, and impaired exercise capacity.[22] Therefore, timely intervention for significant PR is important. As a rule, patients with severe PR, symptoms, or severe RV dilatation should be offered pulmonary valve replacement to avoid further irreversible dilatation and dysfunction.[23]

Unfortunately, RV dysfunction is not uncommon in ToF patients, even after addressing hemodynamic lesions, and its management remains unclear. Standard HF therapy, such as beta-blockers, has not been shown to provide significant benefits.[24] A small, randomized trial in the UK only showed an improvement in RV long axis function with ramipril in patients with ToF and significant PR, but no improvement in the overall RV function or exercise capacity.[25]

Left ventricular (LV) dysfunction is present in up to 21% of ToF patients, mainly attributed to an abnormal ventricular interdependence: the volume-loaded RV (in the setting of severe PR) shifts the ventricular septum towards the left, affecting LV function. LV impairment is more frequent in patients after late ToF repair, performed in earlier surgical eras.[19] Coronary abnormalities should also be excluded in the presence of LV impairment. Many expert centers manage LV impairment in the setting of ToF as per the European Society of Cardiology HF Guidelines, similar to non-CHD patients, even though caution is necessary when extrapolating from non-CHD HF.

The Systemic Right Ventricle

Patients with a systemic RV are those in whom the RV is in the subaortic position and include:

- Univentricular circulations, in which the dominant ventricle is morphologically right.
- Biventricular circulations, in which there is either:
  - Atrioventricular (AV) and ventriculoarterial (VA) discordance: ccTGA, also known as levo- or L-transposition or double discordance (Figure 28.2a and b).
  - AV concordance and VA discordance (i.e., TGA or D-transposition) following an atrial switch procedure (Figure 28.2c, d, and e).

Many other complex anatomical arrangements exist and are beyond the scope of this chapter.

Conditions involving a systemic RV are rare in the general population (global prevalence up to 0.67 cases per 1000 live births),[26] but in ACHD cohorts they account for 10–12% of cases.[27] Additionally, the progressive nature of this condition,

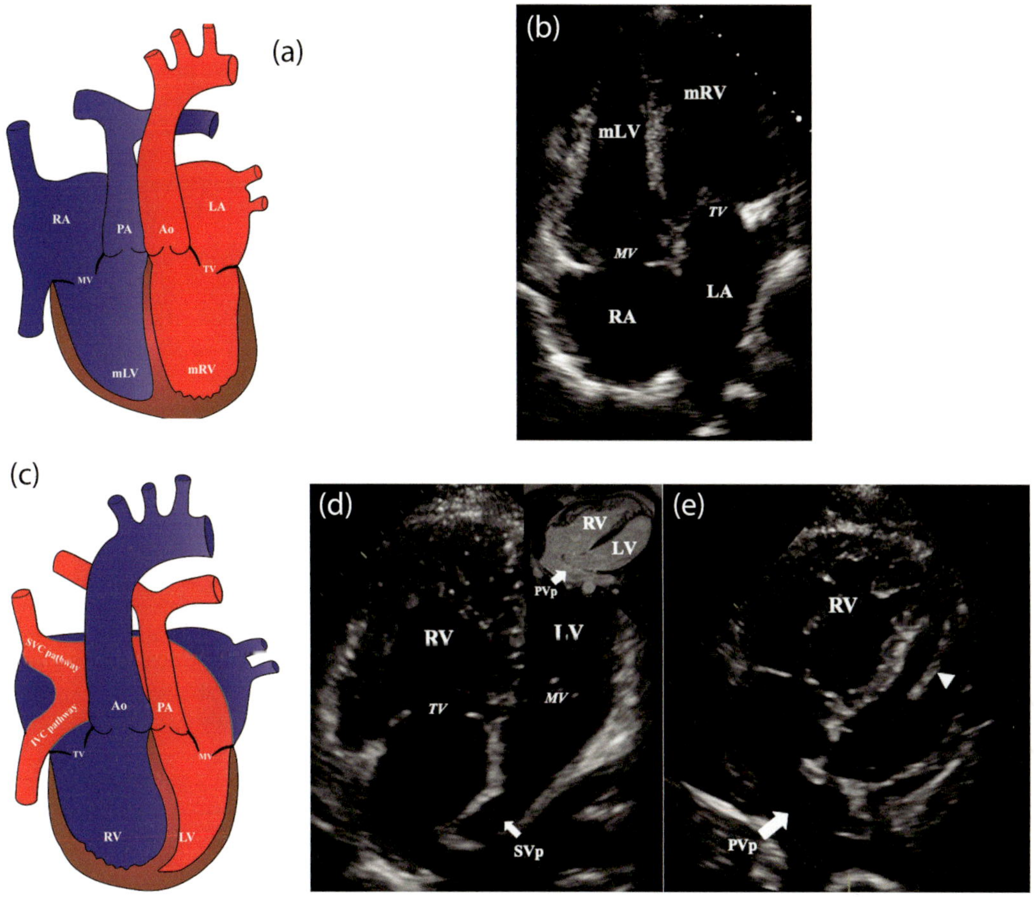

FIGURE 28.2 Panels (a) and (b) show the anatomy in congenitally corrected transposition of the great arteries (ccTGA), with systemic venous inflow passing from the right atrium (RA) to the morphologic left ventricle (mLV) through the mitral valve (MV), and into the pulmonary artery (PA). The morphologic right ventricle (mRV) is in the subaortic position (systemic) and receives blood from the pulmonary circulation via the left atrium (LA). Panels (c), (d), and (e) display TGA following an atrial switch operation. In the unoperated patient, blood moves from the RA to the RV and is pumped out of the heart into the aorta (Ao). The pulmonary venous return into LA then passes into the LV and into the PA. These parallel circulations are reliant on flow through the foramen ovale or an atrial septal defect at the atrial level, or through a patent ductus arteriosus at the level of the great vessels. The situation quickly becomes critical after birth. In the atrial switch operation, atrial baffles made from atrial tissue (Senning) or pericardial/synthetic material (Mustard) are formed to create pathways from the superior and inferior vena cavae to direct the systemic venous inflow to the mitral valve and the LV. In the Mustard patient (d, inset in d), the systemic RV is typically hypertrophied and dilated. The systemic venous (SVp) and pulmonary venous (PVp) pathways are shown. The development of systemic ventricular dysfunction and HF is accompanied by further RV dilatation and a small, crescent-shaped LV (e). A pacemaker lead is visualized in the subpulmonary LV (arrowhead).

resulting in a high incidence of HF and associated morbidity, means that they are overrepresented in terms of patient contact and resource utilization in ACHD services.

The RV develops embryologically from the secondary heart field and is inherently different from the LV, from cellular function through to geometry. It is designed to function in the subpulmonary position and can cope with large changes in preload, providing there is a low, relatively constant afterload. The RV has a more triangular shape compared to the near-conical shape of the LV and curves over the LV. This arrangement, with a shared interventricular septum, contributes to significant ventricular interdependence; the LV contributes 20–40% of the RV systolic pressure and resulting output. The thick-walled LV consists of a layer of circular myofibers sandwiched between subepicardial oblique and subendocardial longitudinal myofibers. In the thin-walled RV, this layered pattern is missing,[28] although RV hypertrophy in the setting of CHD can alter this architecture to resemble the pattern seen in the LV.[29] When in the systemic position, gross adaptive changes occur, including significant RV hypertrophy and increased ventricular mass, to amplify wall stress and maintain cardiac output in the face of a high (systemic) afterload.

TGA Following Atrial Switch Procedure (Mustard/Senning Procedure)

The atrial switch procedure was a pioneering operation that allowed the survival of those born with TGA beyond infancy and early childhood. This was the surgery of choice for TGA until it was superseded, in the 1980s and early 1990s, by the arterial switch operation. The atrial switch operation was aimed at redirecting flow through the heart ("physiologic correction") but maintained the RV as the systemic ventricle (Figure 28.2). Medium-term survival following a Mustard or Senning repair has been excellent, with most patients remaining asymptomatic or minimally symptomatic until adulthood.[30] However, the systemic RV is a substrate for late sequelae, including RV dysfunction,[31] pulmonary hypertension, impaired exercise tolerance,[32] arrhythmias, and premature death.[33] Subendocardial ischemia related to RV hypertrophy and inadequate myocardial perfusion is thought to account for the long-term decline in RV function.[34] In systemic RVs, the systemic AV valve is a tricuspid valve and is often regurgitant.

The systemic and pulmonary venous pathways created within the atria during the Mustard and Senning procedures present an additional challenge. Ventricular preload depends on adequate pathway function and atrial compliance, which is limited, impacting on stroke volume especially at increased heart rates.[35] Indeed, supraventricular arrhythmias are common after extensive surgery and scarring at atrial level. Sinus node dysfunction[36] and chronotropic incompetence, progressive cyanosis due to baffle leaks, PS, and/or pulmonary hypertension (typically postcapillary but occasionally precapillary or combined) contribute to the significant exercise intolerance observed in this cohort. Moreover, right-to-left shunting can predispose patients with a systemic RV to paradoxical embolic events.[37]

Congenitally Corrected TGA

The anatomic arrangement in ccTGA is shown in Figure 28.2 and in practice consists of a systemic RV and subpulmonary LV: deoxygenated blood reaches the lungs via the LV, while oxygenated blood is delivered to the periphery by the RV. The clinical presentation is variable, although most patients develop clinically manifest HF with moderate-to-severe RV dysfunction by the third or fourth decades of life.[38] The natural history and age at presentation are driven by the systemic RV and tricuspid valve function, as well as associated lesions: VSD in 70–88%,[39,40] PS in 50–70%, atrial septal defect in 55%, and patent ductus arteriosus (PDA) in 33%, among others. Primary tricuspid valve abnormalities are present in 30–70%, often with an Ebstein-like apical displacement of the septal and posterior tricuspid valve leaflets.

The coronary circulation is typically "anomalous" in ccTGA and a reduced coronary reserve has been described, even in the absence of ischemic symptoms.[41] The conduction system in ccTGA is also abnormal, with anterior displacement of the atrioventricular (AV) node and the His bundles, and a higher incidence of AV block and chronotropic incompetence. This limits the role of beta-blocker therapy.

The Management of HF in Patients with a Systemic RV

To date, there is little evidence to guide the management of HF in patients with a systemic RV. Expert assessment is crucial to understanding the mechanisms responsible for the development of HF, and to address reversible causes, such as severe tricuspid regurgitation, pathway obstruction, chronotropic incompetence, arrhythmias, etc. Many expert centers manage patients with a failing systemic RV similar to a failing systemic LV, following non-CHD HF evidence and guidelines, even though extrapolating from other cohorts carries risks. Small, randomized-controlled trials (RCTs) have been performed but suffer from notable limitations. In an RCT of valsartan involving ccTGA and atrial switch patients, there was a significant effect on RV ejection fraction in the subgroup with symptoms, although the primary end-point was negative.[42] Observational data on beta-blockers has suggested a reduction in symptoms and perhaps the risk of SCD,[43] although little evidence exists on mineralocorticoid receptor antagonists.[44] All patients with advanced HF should be assessed for heart transplantation, after careful assessment of invasive hemodynamics to exclude precapillary PH. Unfortunately, TGA patients often have associated significant allosensitization. Few patients with a systemic RV have been offered mechanical assist devices, even though there are challenges relating to the anatomic features of the RV and associated cardiovascular lesions.

Univentricular Circulation and the Fontan Palliation

Univentricular hearts include those with tricuspid or mitral atresia and double inlet LV or RV, in which a biventricular repair cannot be achieved as one of the ventricles is hypoplastic or the atrioventricular valve is straddling. Management in early life is aimed at ensuring adequate pulmonary blood flow (limiting cyanosis), whilst avoiding excessive pulmonary blood flow (that can trigger PVD or overload the systemic ventricle, causing progressive ventricular dysfunction). Infants born with a univentricular heart have a high mortality, with a five-year survival rate ranging from 13% to 60%.[45]

The Fontan circulation has been one of the great successes of CHD surgery. This procedure connects the systemic venous return to the pulmonary arteries without the interposition of a subpulmonary ventricle,[46] abolishing cyanosis and chronic volume overload. It is typically a staged procedure, completed by between two and four years of age,[47] with a ten-year postoperative survival of 91% in one large, retrospective cohort study. However, the Fontan circulation lacks a subpulmonary ventricle and depends on passive blood flow through the pulmonary vascular bed, maintained by the pressure gradient between the systemic veins and the pulmonary circulation.[48] This creates a state of chronic systemic venous hypertension and cardiac output that is dependent on systemic ventricular preload. Specialist care is important in addressing the complications and long-term needs of patients with a Fontan circulation (Table 28.1).

The term "Fontan failure" has been adopted by ACHD specialists to describe the complications resulting from mounting inefficiencies in the Fontan circulation, along with the multisystem results of chronic systemic venous hypertension and low cardiac output. It encompasses clinical entities, including impaired exercise capacity, recurrent atrial arrhythmias, thromboembolism, Fontan-associated liver disease, protein-losing enteropathy, plastic bronchitis (almost exclusively seen in children), chronic ascites, and peripheral edema.[49–51] Clinically manifest HF affects at least 40% of the adult Fontan population, with numbers expected to increase as this population ages.[12]

Effective management of such patients relies on optimizing the efficiency of the Fontan circuit, as well as efficiently and safely troubleshooting any complications. Thus, specialist-driven care with regular assessment is necessary. Management strategies for reducing systemic venous pressure and treating ascites, pleural effusions, and peripheral edema involve the careful use of diuretics. Low resistance through the Fontan circuit may be achieved by optimizing surgical techniques to reduce distortions and turbulence in the Fontan pathway, addressing Fontan pathway or branch pulmonary artery stenoses, and the use of pulmonary vasodilators. Even though Fontan patients are unlikely to reach a mean pulmonary pressure of 25 mmHg, an increased PVR has been reported, relating to microemboli, the absence of pulsatile flow, and endothelial dysfunction. Pulmonary vasodilators have been assessed in

TABLE 28.1: Variables Associated with Worse Survival in the ACHD Population

Modality	Clinical Variable Associated with Worse Survival
Bedside tests	Lower resting oxygen saturations
Exercise capacity	Shorter 6MWT distance, lower peak VO_2
Chest radiography (postero-anterior)	Raised cardiothoracic ratio
Echocardiography	RA/RV dilatation, reduced TAPSE, reduced RV FAC, greater degree of TR, presence of pericardial effusion
	Composite echo score: TAPSE <15 mm, increased RV S:D duration ratio ≥1.5, RA area ≥25 cm², RA:LA area ratio ≥1.5
Blood testing	Renal dysfunction
	Hyponatremia
	Elevated BNP
	Elevated high-sensitivity troponin T
	Elevated C-reactive protein
	Hypoalbuminemia

Abbreviations: 6MWT = 6-minute walk test; BNP = B-type natriuretic peptide; FAC = fractional area contraction; LA = left atrium; RA = right atrium; RV = right ventricle; S:D = ratio of right ventricular effective systolic to diastolic duration; TAPSE = tricuspid annular plane systolic excursion; TR = tricuspid regurgitation; VO_2 = oxygen uptake.

several small studies, including prospective, randomized trials,[52–54] with small improvements in exercise capacity and hemodynamics. Lacking definitive evidence, further studies are needed before therapeutic recommendations can be made.

A fenestration (a small communication between the Fontan pathway and the systemic atrium) is often created during Fontan surgery to allow decompression of the Fontan pathway in the immediate post-operative period. This fenestration can be closed percutaneously to abolish cyanosis. Other sources of cyanosis include veno-venous collaterals or arteriovenous collaterals in the lungs. The latter are common when no hepatic venous blood reaches the lungs.

Atrial pacing in Fontan patients with bradycardia may enhance cardiac output,[55] but there is little evidence on the efficacy of resynchronization therapy. Generally, surgical implantation of epicardial leads is required. Arrhythmias are common in Fontan patients, especially those with the older atriopulmonary Fontan circulation, in which severe dilatation of the right atrium is nearly universal and can cause HF decompensation. Prompt, direct, current cardioversion is recommended for all Fontan patients, and ablation can be attempted when the arrhythmia is persistent or recurrent. However, access to the atria depends on the anatomy, and retrograde access (through the aorta) using magnetic navigation and advanced electrophysiological mapping techniques in tertiary ACHD centers is recommended.[56]

The role of conventional HF therapies is less clear in the management of Fontan patients. Afterload reduction, though theoretically of benefit in improving cardiac output, could cause hypotension and reduced preload. There is no evidence to support the use of low-dose ACE-inhibition in patients with a failing single ventricle.[57,58]

Eisenmenger Syndrome and Other PH Related to CHD

PH, defined as a mean pulmonary arterial pressure of ≥25 mmHg at rest, is encountered in many types of CHD. Hemodynamically, PH can be distinguished by mean pulmonary wedge or left atrial pressure ≤15 mmHg in precapillary vs >15 mmHg in postcapillary PH. The latter is typically the result of "left-sided" heart disease, which, in CHD, may be related to systemic RV or LV dysfunction, left ventricular outflow tract obstruction, left AV valve disease, or pulmonary venous stenosis.

Pulmonary arterial hypertension in CHD (PAH-CHD) is precapillary PH, with a raised PVR >3 Wood Units (WU), and develops in 5–10% of patients.[59,60] It is classified into four groups: Eisenmenger syndrome, PAH associated with a prevalent systemic-to-pulmonary shunt, PAH with a small or coincidental shunt, and PAH after corrective cardiac surgery.[61]

Eisenmenger syndrome occurs in the context of a large systemic-to-pulmonary shunt, usually a post-tricuspid defect such as a VSD or PDA. Over time, this causes pressure and volume overload of the pulmonary circulation and results in PVD. The progressive rise in PVR is accompanied by a reduction in the degree of systemic-to-pulmonary shunting. Once the pressures in the ventricles become equal, the shunt becomes bi-directional and cyanosis occurs at rest and is exacerbated on exertion. Since Paul Wood's seminal work on the condition in 1958,[62,63] it has been acknowledged that PVD develops earlier in patients with large post-tricuspid than in pre-tricuspid shunts (e.g., ASDs).

An understanding of Eisenmenger syndrome pathophysiology is integral for differentiating this condition from idiopathic PAH and building an appropriate management strategy for these patients. RV adaptation can differ significantly between idiopathic PAH and Eisenmenger. Unlike patients with idiopathic PAH, where heterometric adaptation predominates and the untreated prognosis is guarded, the RV in Eisenmenger syndrome adapts well despite, or because of, a lifetime of systemic-level PH. Many adult patients with Eisenmenger syndrome have RV hypertrophy with little or no dilatation and good contractility (mainly homeomeric adaptation).[64] These benefits are not afforded to patients with pre-tricuspid defects, in whom the phenotype more closely resembles idiopathic disease.[65]

Despite the apparent advantages of the Eisenmenger phenotype compared to other forms of PAH, adult Eisenmenger patients are significantly impaired and have a reduced survival compared with other groups of CHD patients,[6] with a 10-year survival of 69% in treatment-naïve patients.[66] The transition from a compensated state to progressive RV failure usually occurs in the third or fourth decade. HF is a leading cause of death in this population and has become more common in recent decades.[67] There are numerous published markers of an increased mortality in Eisenmenger syndrome, which have been summarized in the multicenter study by Kempny et al. [68]

Chronic cyanosis itself is responsible for many of the clinical manifestations of Eisenmenger syndrome, including exercise intolerance, secondary erythrocytosis, hyperviscosity symptoms (rare), thrombocytopenia, and coagulopathy, which predispose patients to both bleeding and thrombosis.[69,70] Iron deficiency is commonly encountered and supplementation can improve exercise capacity and quality of life.[71] Extracardiac complications like cerebrovascular disease, cerebral abscess,[72] gout,[73] and renal impairment[74] may impact quality of life and survival.

The management of Eisenmenger patients should take place in a center specializing in the care of PAH-CHD. The greatest change in the management of Eisenmenger patients has occurred over the past 15 years with the advent of PAH-specific therapies, which act on the endothelin, nitric oxide, and prostacyclin pathways. In contemporary practice, PAH therapies are started in the majority of Eisenmenger patients in the developed world, in order to improve quality of life, exercise tolerance, and survival.[75,76]

Diagnostic Toolkit

HF remains primarily a clinical syndrome. Clinical, biochemical, functional, and imaging metrics are used to improve diagnostic accuracy and risk stratification. Most of these variables are interdependent and are best employed as part of a complete patient evaluation. Additionally, HF is a dynamic state, and these markers need to be interpreted as such, and in a manner specific to the underlying CHD. Frequent reassessment by a physician with expertise in CHD is necessary.

Symptoms

Symptoms of HF in ACHD are similar to non-CHD HF and depend on the underlying anatomy. Patients with right-sided lesions typically present with predominantly "right-sided" HF, i.e., with peripheral congestion, ascites, and signs of raised central venous pressure. Multiorgan (e.g., renal and hepatic) involvement is common in more advanced disease and can significantly complicate management. Syncope is a red-flag symptom that deserves special consideration in ACHD, especially in younger patients. Idiosyncratic presentations may occur: worsening of cyanosis in those with large shunts and changing pulmonary and systemic vascular resistances or patients with a Fontan circulation and persistent fenestration; or a variety of presentations in patients with chronic severe elevation of systemic venous pressure, e.g., protein losing enteropathy and lymphatic dysfunction in Fontan patients. Arrhythmias, both ventricular and supraventricular, are also common and are often a marker of deteriorating cardiac function.[77]

Electrocardiography (ECG)

ECGs in CHD must be interpreted with respect to the underlying defect, surgical history, and the patient's usual pattern. Supraventricular arrhythmias, commonly macroreentrant "atrial tachycardias," may not be easy to identify on a 12-lead ECG, when p waves are "hidden" within the QRS complex.

Imaging

Chest Radiography

The plain chest radiograph provides information about the heart and surrounding structures, including visceral and atrial situs, the position of the heart, signs of prior thoracic surgery, and the position of radio-opaque devices. Knowledge of the cardiac silhouette allows quick assessment of chamber enlargement, aortic anatomy, and venous drainage. The pattern of pulmonary vascular markings can alert the physician to the presence of pulmonary venous or arterial hypertension, as well as to pulmonary plethora or oligemia. In the acute setting, assessing signs of congestive HF, pulmonary edema, consolidation, and assessment of line and tube positioning are an essential part of daily practice.

Echocardiography

Echocardiography is fundamental to the assessment of any ACHD patient. Specialist training and accreditation are required for effective performance and interpretation of echocardiography in complex CHD. A full study often involves modified, oblique views and non-standard windows. New technologies, including two-dimensional speckle-tracking, three-dimensional chamber quantification, and anatomical assessment, can provide additional information. In the echocardiographic assessment of a patient with ACHD, the following should be provided:

- Sequential, segmental anatomical diagnosis
- Associated and residual lesions
- Ventricular systolic and diastolic function
- Hemodynamics (valves, shunts, estimate of central venous pressure), including presence and severity of PH
- Evidence of endocarditis
- Pericardial or pleural effusion

Cardiovascular Magnetic Resonance (CMR) and Computed Tomography (CT)

CMR is an indispensable part of the ACHD diagnostic toolkit. It has an unparalleled ability to quantify chamber volumes, evaluate the right ventricular outflow tract, conduits, and branch pulmonary arteries, and provide a non-invasive estimate of fibrosis burden and shunt fraction. Hybrid CMR fluoroscopic-guided cardiac catheterization procedures are used, especially in the pediatric population, for accurate assessment of PVR [78,79] and to guide cardiac interventions.[80] They can also be used to assess regional ischemia and viability.

CT remains the modality of choice for imaging the coronary arteries and is exceptional in the assessment of venous connections and collaterals, and the arterial tree. It is also invaluable in patients who have a contraindication to CMR scanning, including those with a non-conditional pacemaker or implantable cardioverter defibrillator (ICD).

Biomarkers

Laboratory testing is useful in the assessment of the ACHD patient with HF for the identification of:

- Conditions masking or masquerading as HF (e.g., anemia, iron deficiency, thyroid dysfunction)
- Markers indicative of the presence and severity of HF (BNP or NT-proBNP)
- Infection (acute phase reactants including C-reactive protein, blood cultures)
- End-organ dysfunction (renal and liver function)

Elevated levels of BNP[81] and NT-proBNP[82] are strong predictors of mortality in ACHD patients, and normal levels of NT-proBNP ($\leq$14 pmol/L) can reliably predict a low risk of death and HF. The value of measuring natriuretic peptides at regular intervals and lesion-specific cut-offs requires further study.

Cardiac Catheterization

Invasive hemodynamic assessment is usually undertaken following non-invasive evaluation and may be performed as a stand-alone diagnostic procedure or as the first part of a percutaneous intervention. Indications include confirmation of non-invasive gradients, including across the outflow tracts, conduits, and pathways (following an atrial switch operation), assessment of coronary anatomy, diastolic function, constrictive pericarditis, and measurement of the transhepatic gradient. Accurate measurement of PVR with assessment of reversibility is performed in patients with PH and those undergoing transplant assessment. General anesthesia may be required, and the risks should be weighed against the benefits.

Exercise Testing

CPET is helpful for elucidating the degree and mechanisms of exercise intolerance and can help distinguish between cardiac and respiratory causes of limitation. Lesion-specific ranges of normal should be considered in the interpretation of the data.[83] Peak oxygen uptake (VO_2) is an independent prognostic indicator in ACHD, and a lower value predicts a higher risk of hospitalization or death.[84] The quotient of the minute ventilation and CO_2 production (VE/VCO_2 slope) is a relatively effort-independent indicator of ventilatory efficiency and is a marker of pulmonary perfusion and physiological dead space. Finally, chronotropic incompetence (failure to achieve ≥80% of peak predicted heart rate) is common in ACHD and is strongly correlated to an adverse prognosis.[85]

Special Therapeutic Considerations in ACHD

Heart Failure Prevention and Lifestyle Considerations

Patients followed in specialist CHD centers receive lifestyle advice from childhood onward. Transition services, preparing CHD patients for adult life and the transfer from pediatric to ACHD services, educate patients on the merits of a healthy lifestyle and physical activity. Exercise recommendations should be individualized, based on underlying anatomy and physiology, and the results of cardiopulmonary exercise testing.

Pharmacological Therapy for Chronic HF in ACHD

The aims of pharmacological therapy in ACHD patients presenting with HF are to relieve symptoms and improve cardiac function and prognosis. However, to date, there is very little evidence to guide treatment in specific ACHD cohorts. In our practice:

Diuretics are commonly used in patients presenting with congestive heart failure, including intravenous diuretics in patients with severe congestion, refractory to oral diuretics, with or without the synergistic use of a thiazide diuretic (e.g., metolazone or bendroflumethiazide). Spironolactone or eplerenone can be used, especially in patients with "right-sided" congestion and/or hypokalemia.

ACE inhibitors or angiotensin receptor blockers are often used in patients with systemic ventricular dysfunction, including those with a systemic RV. They are avoided, however, in patients with significant left ventricular tract obstruction, and caution is required in Fontan patients to avoid a drastic reduction in systemic venous pressures and ventricular preload.

Beta-blockers are frequently used in patients with severe systemic ventricular dysfunction, or in the presence of arrhythmias. Caution is required in patients with RV dysfunction and conduction abnormalities.

In cases of refractory congestive HF, inotropes such as dobutamine, dopamine, or milrinone are routinely used. In the operative setting, vasopressors are often initiated prior to the induction of anesthesia, often with the concurrent use of inotropic agents with pulmonary vasodilator properties, such as milrinone. There is also growing experience of the peri-operative use of levosimendan, a calcium sensitizer with inotropic and vasodilating properties, to improve hemodynamics.[86,87] Its elimination half-life of 70–80 hours means it could be used for outpatient management of ACHD patients with HF, but studies are lacking.[88]

Percutaneous and Surgical Interventions

All ACHD patients presenting with HF should be thoroughly assessed for the presence of reversible causes, including lesions that can be addressed surgically or percutaneously. ACHD patients may benefit from the repair of a shunt, valve dysfunction, or obstructive lesion (e.g., aortic coarctation) to the point where HF is reversed. As HF progresses, the risks of intervention increase and the benefits may not be as clear-cut; eventually, a number of these patients are deemed inoperable and are referred for transplantation or palliative care.

Arrhythmias, Electrophysiology, and Device Therapy in ACHD

Arrhythmias are common in the ACHD population[10] and are closely interlinked with HF.[89] Directed antiarrhythmic therapy, electrophysiological studies, and catheter ablation procedures for both atrial and ventricular arrhythmias are frequently used in the treatment of ACHD patients with HF. Expert care is required, including careful planning of access routes, 3D anatomical mapping, and other novel technologies, such as magnetic navigation.[90]

Sudden cardiac death (SCD) remains common in ACHD patients under 40 years of age,[7] with a greater prevalence in patients late after repair for ToF,[91,92] and those with a previously aborted SCD or ventricular tachycardia (VT). Indications for ICD therapy for secondary prevention of SCD are similar to those for the non-CHD population. However, selection of patients who would benefit from primary prevention is more difficult (see section on ToF). Additional technical considerations in the CHD population include routes of access to the atria or subpulmonary ventricle,[93] and the risk of systemic thromboembolism in those with large shunts or single ventricle physiology. Placement of epicardial systems provides an alternative strategy, with good long-term outcomes.[94]

Cardiac resynchronization therapy (CRT) is recommended for patients with acquired HF on optimal medical therapy, based on symptoms, systemic ventricular function, evidence of electrical dyssynchrony, and the absence of atrial fibrillation.[95] In this population, there is mounting evidence of improvements in exercise capacity, quality of life, ventricular function, and survival.[96,97] CRT placement, particularly when an ICD is being planned, may provide additional benefit to some ACHD patients, but strong evidence is lacking. Access to the coronary sinus or one of its ventricular branches may be hampered or precluded by anomalous position of the coronary sinus, or previous surgery.

The ACHD Patient in Intensive Care

Care of the ACHD patient in this setting requires forward planning and a multidisciplinary approach from specialists in CHD, intensive care, and anesthetics, along with availability of CHD interventionalists, surgeons, and the advanced HF team.

Advanced decision making is key, with involvement of the patient and their relatives, taking into account the presence of treatable, reversible causes vs the progression of the underlying CHD and overall prognosis.

RV Failure

The management of acute LV failure in ACHD often follows the principles for the non-CHD population. RV failure is more common in ACHD patients and can be difficult to manage. It is observed in patients with right-sided lesions (e.g., Ebstein anomaly, late repair of ToF) (Figure 28.3) and those with PH, both precapillary (PVD) or postcapillary (long-standing left-sided lesions). Moreover, ACHD patients with acute or decompensated HF often present with RV dysfunction related to previous or ongoing hemodynamic lesions or repeat bypass surgery.[98] Support for the RV includes:

- Avoidance of hypoxia[99] or anemia.[100]
- Avoidance of intubation, if possible. If mechanical ventilation is necessary, avoid acidosis or hypercarbia, minimizing the use of positive end-expiratory pressure.
- Maintenance of AV synchrony.
- Optimization of preload, contractility, and afterload through careful fluid balance, with meticulous monitoring of central venous pressure, central venous saturations, fluid balance charts, daily weights, and renal function.
- Ensure adequate coronary arterial perfusion and an optimal metabolic state. Vasopressors are useful to maintain an adequate perfusion pressure by raising the systemic mean arterial pressure to above RV pressure.

Short-Term Mechanical Circulatory Support (MCS)

In patients who are failing medical HF therapy, the use of short-term MCS should be considered, most commonly in the form of extra-corporeal membrane oxygenation (ECMO). The use of veno-arterial (V-A) ECMO provides cardiac support, unloading the RV while maintaining oxygenation. This should be implanted by a CHD surgeon with an intimate understanding of the patient's anatomy, as variation of the normal cannula positions may be required. In a contemporary US cohort of ACHD patients undergoing cardiac surgery in pediatric centers, ECMO was utilized in 1.1% of patients, with a significant 67% mortality rate.[101] Complications are common, but the use of ECMO as a bridge to long-term MCS or transplantation can be lifesaving as long as careful patient selection and planning takes place.

Advanced Heart Failure Therapy in ACHD

When no suitable targets for conventional surgical or interventional therapy are present and HF becomes refractory to medical therapy, patients should be considered for transplantation or MCS.[6] Despite the increasing demand for transplant, only 3% of heart transplants worldwide were performed in ACHD patients between 2009 and 2017.[102] The number of organs transplanted in CHD patients is forecast to increase only modestly over the coming decade,[103] mainly limited by the number of available organs. Moreover, the higher peri-operative mortality in the ACHD vs non-CHD cohorts may contribute to the low numbers transplanted. Transplant programs focusing on ACHD patients, including surgeons and physicians with ACHD expertise, have been shown to improve transplant outcomes considerably.[104] Survival after one year from transplant is better in ACHD than in matched non-CHD transplant recipients.[102,105]

Patients should be referred early, as multiorgan failure is common in the advanced stages of HF and may preclude transplantation or require multiple organ transplantation. ACHD patients are generally younger and may adapt better to abnormal physiologic states for prolonged periods, behaving unlike non-CHD HF patients. This carries the risk of underestimating the degree of limitation in young ACHD patients. CHD-specific transplantation listing criteria are urgently needed to account for these differences in pathophysiology and presentation.[106,107] A multidisciplinary approach is, therefore, required (Figure 28.4)[108] using criteria that are both generic and ACHD specific (Table 28.2).[8]

Barriers to transplantation for ACHD patients include:

- Higher allosensitization rate (preformed antibodies to human leukocyte antigens) due to prior blood product transfusions, pregnancies, prior surgery with the use of homograft or allograft tissues, and MCS.
- Anatomical complexity and prior cardiac surgery, with reconstruction of several structures at heart

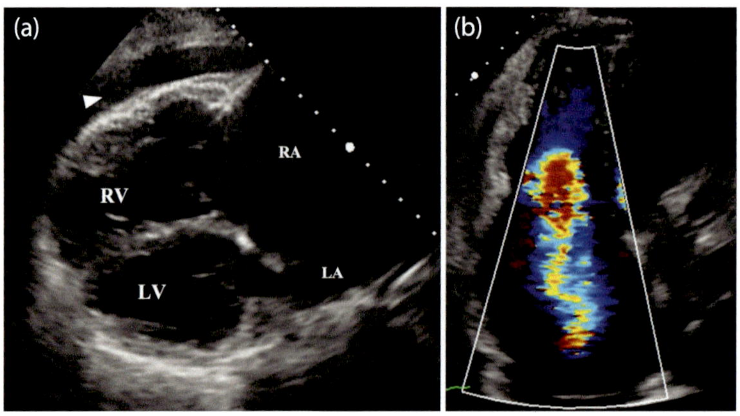

FIGURE 28.3 Congenital dysplasia of the tricuspid valve (a) with apical displacement of the annulus and pericardial effusion (arrowhead), resulting in low cardiac output and HF. Note the massive enlargement of the right atrium (RA). (b) Color flow Doppler from the same patient demonstrating a broad regurgitant jet that originates from the mid-cavity of the right ventricle (RV). *Abbreviations*: LA=left atrium; LV=left ventricle.

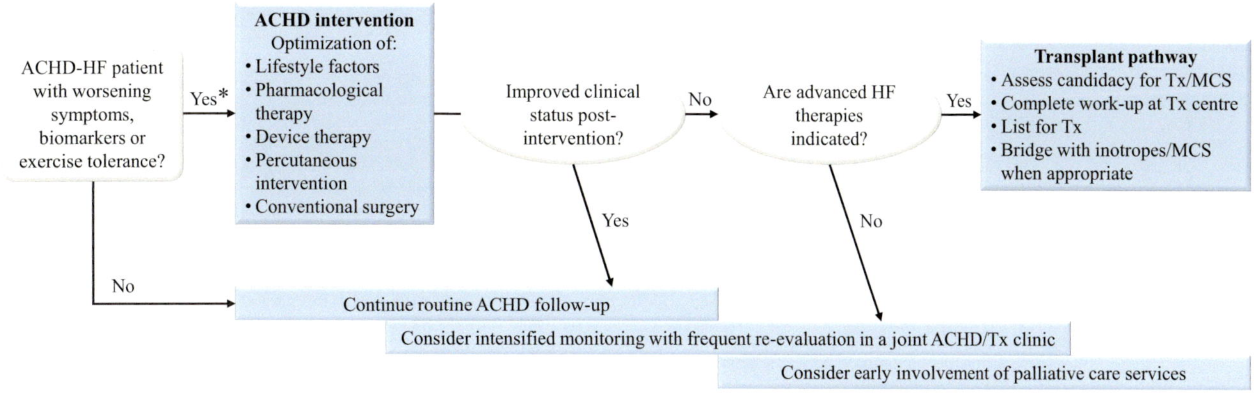

FIGURE 28.4 Proposed treatment algorithm for a patient with heart failure related to congenital heart disease, with the adult congenital heart disease and advanced heart failure multidisciplinary team at the center of the evaluation process. *Abbreviations*: (A)CHD = (adult) congenital heart disease; HF = heart failure; MCS = mechanical circulatory support; MDT = multidisciplinary team; Tx = transplant. (Modified from Ross et al. *Circulation*. 2016;133(8):802–20.)

TABLE 28.2: Clinical Features of Advanced Heart Failure Which May Act as Triggers for Transplant Assessment

Repeated (≥2) hospitalizations for heart failure in the past year
Progressive deterioration in renal function
Unexplained weight loss (i.e., cardiac cachexia)
Intolerance of ACE inhibitors or beta-blockers due to worsening heart failure or hypotension
Frequent hypotension (systolic blood pressure <90 mmHg)
Recent escalation of diuretics to maintain volume status (e.g., requiring a daily furosemide equivalent dose >160 mg/day and/or the concurrent use of thiazide diuretic therapy with metolazone or bendroflumethiazide)
Progressive hyponatremia
Frequent ICD therapy
Additional High-Risk Clinical Features in ACHD
Patients with CHD and the above symptoms who will not benefit from conventional surgical, interventional, or electrophysiological intervention
Patients with CHD and aborted-sudden cardiac death or life-threatening arrhythmias refractory to therapy
Atrial tachyarrhythmias in patients with CHD of great complexity (especially those with a Fontan circulation or atrial switch procedure for transposition of the great arteries)
Persistent protein-losing enteropathy despite optimal therapy in Fontan patients
Symptomatic cyanosis not considered amenable to surgical correction
Patients with PAH-CHD starting triple combination PAH therapy
Recurrent severe hemoptysis
Conventional surgery is too high risk or expected results are suboptimal/short-lasting

Abbreviations: ACE = angiotensin-converting enzyme; (A)CHD = (adult) congenital heart disease; ICD = implantable cardioverter defibrillator; PAH = pulmonary arterial hypertension; PAH-CHD = pulmonary arterial hypertension related to congenital heart disease.

transplantation, requiring congenital surgical expertise, extra donor tissue, and longer ischemic times.

- Liver disease, particularly in Fontan patients from long-standing systemic venous hypertension, which requires input from liver specialists.
- Higher rate of associated genetic syndromes, with associated extra-cardiac comorbidities and learning difficulties.

Policy changes in the United States and the United Kingdom have somewhat disadvantaged ACHD patients, with an increase in the proportion of organs going to "super-urgent" (status 1A) and "urgent" (status 1B) listed candidates, whereas patients with CHD are more commonly listed as "routine" (status 2).[105] This has led to proposals to change the current organ allocation system to better reflect the relative waiting list mortality rate and the needs of special populations,[109] or to hold separate criteria for organ allocation for CHD patients. On being listed, ACHD patients are less likely to receive a transplant or MCS, and are more likely to die or be delisted for clinical worsening while awaiting transplantation.[110,111]

Long-term MCS, as a bridge-to-transplant or destination therapy, has similar short-term results to heart transplantation, and technological advances and investment in this area are improving medium- and long-term outcomes. MCS is underutilized in the ACHD population and is of major potential benefit in improving the reversible component of PVD and improving extra-cardiac organ function through delivery of a reliable cardiac output. Unfortunately, ACHD patients experience an excess early mortality following MCS, and patients requiring a biventricular assist device or total artificial heart have a poor outcome.[112] MCS using devices require adaptation for use in systemic RVs and for the Fontan circulation.

Conclusion

As the ACHD population expands and ages, an increasing number of patients will be presenting in specialist and non-specialist centers with HF. All cardiologists should have a working understanding of the principles underlying the diagnosis and management of HF in ACHD, providing safe triage and initial management, while seeking advice from specialists in the field.

References

1. Hoffman JIE, Kaplan S. The incidence of congenital heart disease. *J Am Coll Cardiol.* 2002;39(12):1890–900. doi:10.1016/S0735-1097(02)01886-7
2. Marelli AJ, Mackie AS, Ionescu-Ittu R, Rahme E, Pilote L. Congenital heart disease in the general population: changing prevalence and age distribution. *Circulation.* 2007;115(2):163–72. doi:10.1161/CIRCULATIONAHA.106.627224
3. Gilboa SM, Devine OJ, Kucik JE, et al. Congenital heart defects in the United States: estimating the magnitude of the affected population in 2010. *Circulation.* 2016;134(2):101–9. doi:10.1161/CIRCULATIONAHA.115.019307
4. Marelli AJ, Ionescu-Ittu R, Mackie AS, Guo L, Dendukuri N, Kaouache M. Lifetime prevalence of congenital heart disease in the general population from 2000 to 2010. *Circulation.* 2014;130(9):749–56. doi:10.1161/CIRCULATIONAHA.113.008396
5. Khairy P, Ionescu-Ittu R, Mackie AS, Abrahamowicz M, Pilote L, Marelli AJ. Changing mortality in congenital heart disease. *J Am Coll Cardiol.* 2010;56(14):1149–57. doi:10.1016/j.jacc.2010.03.085
6. Diller G-P, Kempny A, Alonso-Gonzalez R, et al. Survival prospects and circumstances of death in contemporary adult congenital heart disease patients under follow-up at a large tertiary centre. *Circulation.* 2015;132(22):2118–25. doi:10.1161/CIRCULATIONAHA.115.017202
7. Oliver JM, Gallego P, Gonzalez AE, et al. Impact of age and sex on survival and causes of death in adults with congenital heart disease. *Int J Cardiol.* 2017;245:119–24. doi:10.1016/j.ijcard.2017.06.060
8. Yancy CW, Jessup M, Bozkurt B, et al. 2013 ACCF/AHA guideline for the management of heart failure: a report of the American College of Cardiology Foundation/American Heart Association Task Force on Practice Guidelines. *J Am Coll Cardiol.* 2013;62(16):e147–239. doi:10.1016/j.jacc.2013.05.019
9. Poole-Wilson PA, Buller NP. Causes of symptoms in chronic congestive heart failure and implications for treatment. *Am J Cardiol.* 1988;62(2):31A–34A. doi:10.1016/S0002-9149(88)80082-1
10. Zomer AC, Vaartjes I, Uiterwaal CSPM, et al. Circumstances of death in adult congenital heart disease. *Int J Cardiol.* 2012;154(2):168–72. doi:10.1016/j.ijcard.2010.09.015
11. Engelings CC, Helm PC, Abdul-Khaliq H, et al. Cause of death in adults with congenital heart disease — an analysis of the German National Register for Congenital Heart Defects. *Int J Cardiol.* 2016;211:31–6. doi:10.1016/j.ijcard.2016.02.133
12. Norozi K, Wessel A, Alpers V, et al. Incidence and risk distribution of heart failure in adolescents and adults with congenital heart disease after cardiac surgery. *Am J Cardiol.* 2006;97(8):1238–43. doi:10.1016/j.amjcard.2005.10.065
13. Verheugt CL, Uiterwaal CSPM, van der Velde ET, et al. Mortality in adult congenital heart disease. *Eur Heart J.* 2010;31(10):1220–9. doi:10.1093/eurheartj/ehq032
14. Gilljam T, Mandalenakis Z, Dellborg M, et al. Development of heart failure in young patients with congenital heart disease: a nation-wide cohort study. *Open Heart.* 2019;6(1):e000858. doi:10.1136/openhrt-2018-000858
15. Rodriguez FH, Moodie DS, Parekh DR, et al. Outcomes of heart failure-related hospitalization in adults with congenital heart disease in the United States. *Congenit Heart Dis.* 2013;8(6):513–9. doi:10.1111/chd.12019
16. Wessels MW, Willems PJ. Mutations in sarcomeric protein genes not only lead to cardiomyopathy but also to congenital cardiovascular malformations. *Clin Genet.* 2008;74(1):16–9. doi:10.1111/j.1399-0004.2008.00985.x
17. Kelle AM, Bentley SJ, Rohena LO, Cabalka AK, Olson TM. Ebstein anomaly, left ventricular non-compaction, and early onset heart failure associated with a de novo α-tropomyosin gene mutation. *Am J Med Genet A.* 2016;170(8):2186–90. doi:10.1002/ajmg.a.37745
18. Bolger AP, Sharma R, Li W, et al. Neurohormonal activation and the chronic heart failure syndrome in adults with congenital heart disease. *Circulation.* 2002;106(1):92–9. doi:10.1161/01.cir.0000020009.30736.3f
19. Stout KK, Broberg CS, Book WM, et al. Chronic heart failure in congenital heart disease: a scientific statement from the American Heart Association. *Circulation.* 2016;133(8):770–801. doi:10.1161/CIR.0000000000000352
20. Babu-Narayan SV, Gatzoulis MA. 47 — Tetralogy of Fallot. In: Gatzoulis MA, Webb GD, Daubeney PEF, eds. *Diagnosis and management of adult congenital heart disease (3rd edition).* Elsevier; 2018:474–88. doi:10.1016/B978-0-7020-6929-1.00047-2
21. Bailliard F, Anderson RH. Tetralogy of Fallot. *Orphanet J Rare Dis.* 2009;4(1):2. doi:10.1186/1750-1172-4-2
22. Bouzas B, Kilner PJ, Gatzoulis MA. Pulmonary regurgitation: not a benign lesion. *Eur Heart J.* 2005;26(5):433–9. doi:10.1093/eurheartj/ehi091
23. Stout KK, Daniels CJ, Aboulhosn JA, et al. 2018 AHA/ACC guideline for the management of adults with congenital heart disease: a report of the American College of Cardiology/American Heart Association Task Force on Clinical Practice Guidelines. *Circulation.* 2019;139(14):e698–800. doi:10.1161/CIR.0000000000000603
24. Norozi K, Bahlmann J, Raab B, et al. A prospective, randomized, double-blind, placebo controlled trial of beta-blockade in patients who have undergone surgical correction of tetralogy of Fallot. *Cardiol Young.* 2007;17(4):372–9. doi:10.1017/S1047951107000844
25. Babu-Narayan SV, Uebing A, Davlouros PA, et al. Randomised trial of ramipril in repaired tetralogy of Fallot and pulmonary regurgitation: the APPROPRIATE study (ACE inhibitors for Potential PRevention Of the deleterious effects of Pulmonary Regurgitation In Adults with repaired TEtralogy of Fallot). *Int J Cardiol.* 2012;154(3):299–305. doi:10.1016/j.ijcard.2010.09.057
26. Liu Y, Chen S, Zühlke L, et al. Global birth prevalence of congenital heart defects 1970–2017: updated systematic review and meta-analysis of 260 studies. *Int J Epidemiol.* Published online February 19, 2019. doi:10.1093/ije/dyz009
27. Pfitzer C, Helm PC, Ferentzi H, et al. Changing prevalence of severe congenital heart disease: results from the National Register for Congenital Heart Defects in Germany. *Congenital Heart Disease.* 2017;12(6):787–93. doi:10.1111/chd.12515
28. Ho SY, Nihoyannopoulos P. Anatomy, echocardiography, and normal right ventricular dimensions. *Heart.* 2006;92(Suppl 1):i2–i13. doi:10.1136/hrt.2005.077875
29. Sanchez-Quintana D, Anderson RH, Ho SY. Ventricular myoarchitecture in tetralogy of Fallot. *Heart.* 1996;76(3):280–6. doi:10.1136/hrt.76.3.280
30. Roos-Hesselink JW, Meijboom FJ, Spitaels SEC, et al. Decline in ventricular function and clinical condition after Mustard repair for transposition of the great arteries (a prospective study of 22–29 years). *Eur Heart J.* 2004;25(14):1264–70. doi:10.1016/j.ehj.2004.03.009
31. Cuypers JAAE, Eindhoven JA, Slager MA, et al. The natural and unnatural history of the Mustard procedure: long-term outcome up to 40 years. *Eur Heart J.* 2014;35(25):1666–74. doi:10.1093/eurheartj/ehu102
32. Winter MM, van der Bom T, de Vries LCS, et al. Exercise training improves exercise capacity in adult patients with a systemic right ventricle: a randomized clinical trial. *Eur Heart J.* 2012;33(11):1378–85. doi:10.1093/eurheartj/ehr396
33. Schwerzmann M, Salehian O, Harris L, et al. Ventricular arrhythmias and sudden death in adults after a Mustard operation for transposition of the great arteries. *Eur Heart J.* 2009;30(15):1873–9. doi:10.1093/eurheartj/ehp179
34. Hauser M, Meierhofer C, Schwaiger M, Vogt M, Kaemmerer H, Kuehn A. Myocardial blood flow in patients with transposition of the great arteries – risk factor for dysfunction of the morphologic systemic right ventricle late after atrial repair. *Circ J.* 2015;79(2):425–31. doi:10.1253/circj.CJ-14-0716
35. Winter MM, van der Plas MN, Bouma BJ, Groenink M, Bresser P, Mulder BJM. Mechanisms for cardiac output augmentation in patients with a systemic right ventricle. *Int J Cardiol.* 2010;143(2):141–6. doi:10.1016/j.ijcard.2009.01.065
36. Vetter VL, Tanner CS, Horowitz LN. Electrophysiologic consequences of the Mustard repair of d-transposition of the great arteries. *J Am Coll Cardiol.* 1987;10(6):1265–73.
37. De Pasquale G, Bonassin Tempesta F, Lopes BS, et al. High prevalence of baffle leaks in adults after atrial switch operations for transposition of the great arteries. *Eur Heart J Cardiovasc Imaging.* 2017;18(5):531–5. doi:10.1093/ehjci/jew276
38. Graham TP, Bernard YD, Mellen BG, et al. Long-term outcome in congenitally corrected transposition of the great arteries: a multi-institutional study. *J Am Coll Cardiol.* 2000;36(1):255–61.
39. Connelly MS, Liu PP, Williams WG, Webb GD, Robertson P, McLaughlin PR. Congenitally corrected transposition of the great arteries in the adult: functional status and complications. *J Am Coll Cardiol.* 1996;27(5):1238–43. doi:10.1016/0735-1097(95)00567-6
40. Hraska V, Duncan BW, Mayer JE, Freed M, del Nido PJ, Jonas RA. Long-term outcome of surgically treated patients with corrected transposition of the great arteries. *J Thorac Cardiovasc Surg.* 2005;129(1):182–91. doi:10.1016/j.jtcvs.2004.02.046
41. Hauser M, Bengel FM, Hager A, et al. Impaired myocardial blood flow and coronary flow reserve of the anatomical right systemic ventricle in patients with congenitally corrected transposition of the great arteries. *Heart.* 2003;89(10):1231–5. doi:10.1136/heart.89.10.1231
42. van der Bom Teun, Winter Michiel M., Bouma Berto J., et al. Effect of valsartan on systemic right ventricular function. *Circulation.* 2013;127(3):322–30. doi:10.1161/CIRCULATIONAHA.112.135392
43. Khairy P, Harris L, Landzberg MJ, et al. Sudden death and defibrillators in transposition of the great arteries with intra-atrial baffles: a multi-center study. *Circ Arrhythm Electrophysiol.* 2008;1(4):250–7. doi:10.1161/CIRCEP.108.776120

44. Dos L, Pujadas S, Estruch M, et al. Eplerenone in systemic right ventricle: double blind randomized clinical trial. The Evedes Study. *Int J Cardiol.* 2013;168(6):5167–73. doi:10.1016/j.ijcard.2013.07.163
45. Best KE, Rankin J. Long-term survival of individuals born with congenital heart disease: a systematic review and meta-analysis. *J Am Heart Assoc.* 2016;5(6). doi:10.1161/JAHA.115.002846
46. Fontan F, Baudet E. Surgical repair of tricuspid atresia. *Thorax.* 1971;26(3):240–248.
47. Kaulitz R. Current treatment and prognosis in children with functionally univentricular hearts. *Archiv Dis Child.* 2005;90(7):757–62. doi:10.1136/adc.2003.034090
48. Gewillig M, Brown SC. The Fontan circulation after 45 years: update in physiology. *Heart.* 2016;102(14):1081–6. doi:10.1136/heartjnl-2015-307467
49. Rychik J. Protein-losing enteropathy after Fontan operation. *Congenit Heart Dis.* 2007;2(5):288–300. doi:10.1111/j.1747-0803.2007.00116.x
50. Kiesewetter CH, Sheron N, Vettukattill JJ, et al. Hepatic changes in the failing Fontan circulation. *Heart.* 2007;93(5):579–84. doi:10.1136/hrt.2006.094516
51. Hebert A, Jensen AS, Mikkelsen UR, et al. Hemodynamic causes of exercise intolerance in Fontan patients. *Int J Cardiol.* 2014;175(3):478–83. doi:10.1016/j.ijcard.2014.06.015
52. Hebert A, Mikkelsen UR, Thilen U, et al. Bosentan improves exercise capacity in adolescents and adults after Fontan operation: the TEMPO (Treatment with Endothelin Receptor Antagonist in Fontan Patients, a Randomized, Placebo-Controlled, Double-Blind Study Measuring Peak Oxygen Consumption) study. *Circulation.* 2014;130(23):2021–30. doi:10.1161/CIRCULATIONAHA.113.008441
53. Cedars AM, Saef J, Peterson LR, et al. Effect of ambrisentan on exercise capacity in adult patients after the Fontan procedure. *Am J Cardiol.* 2016;117(9):1524–32. doi:10.1016/j.amjcard.2016.02.024
54. Giardini A, Balducci A, Specchia S, Gargiulo G, Bonvicini M, Picchio FM. Effect of sildenafil on haemodynamic response to exercise and exercise capacity in Fontan patients. *Eur Heart J.* 2008;29(13):1681–7. doi:10.1093/eurheartj/ehn215
55. Cohen MI, Rhodes LA, Wernovsky G, Gaynor JW, Spray TL, Rychik J. Atrial pacing: an alternative treatment for protein-losing enteropathy after the Fontan operation. *J Thorac Cardiovasc Surg.* 2001;121(3):582–3. doi:10.1067/mtc.2001.110681
56. Ueda A, Suman-Horduna I, Mantziari L, et al. Contemporary outcomes of supraventricular tachycardia ablation in congenital heart disease: a single-center experience in 116 patients. *Circ Arrhythm Electrophysiol.* 2013;6(3):606–13. doi:10.1161/CIRCEP.113.000415
57. Kouatli AA, Garcia JA, Zellers TM, Weinstein EM, Mahony L. Enalapril does not enhance exercise capacity in patients after Fontan procedure. *Circulation.* 1997;96(5):1507–12.
58. Hsu DT, Zak V, Mahony L, et al. Enalapril in infants with single ventricle: results of a multicenter randomized trial. *Circulation.* 2010;122(4):333–40. doi:10.1161/CIRCULATIONAHA.109.927988
59. Duffels MGJ, Engelfriet PM, Berger RMF, et al. Pulmonary arterial hypertension in congenital heart disease: an epidemiologic perspective from a Dutch registry. *Int J Cardiol.* 2007;120(2):198–204. doi:10.1016/j.ijcard.2006.09.017
60. van Riel ACMJ, Schuuring MJ, van Hessen ID, et al. Contemporary prevalence of pulmonary arterial hypertension in adult congenital heart disease following the updated clinical classification. *Int J Cardiol.* 2014;174(2):299–305. doi:10.1016/j.ijcard.2014.04.072
61. Galiè N, Humbert M, Vachiery J-L, et al. 2015 ESC/ERS guidelines for the diagnosis and treatment of pulmonary hypertension: the joint task force for the diagnosis and treatment of pulmonary hypertension of the European Society of Cardiology (ESC) and the European Respiratory Society (ERS) Endorsed by: Association for European Paediatric and Congenital Cardiology (AEPC), International Society for Heart and Lung Transplantation (ISHLT). *Eur Resp J.* 2015;46(4):903–75. doi:10.1183/13993003.01032-2015
62. Wood P. The Eisenmenger syndrome or pulmonary hypertension with reversed central shunt. I. *Br Med J.* 1958;2(5098):701–9. doi:10.1136/bmj.2.5098.701
63. Wood P. The Eisenmenger syndrome or pulmonary hypertension with reversed central shunt. *Br Med J.* 1958;2(5099):755–62. doi:10.1136/bmj.2.5099.755
64. Hopkins WE. The remarkable right ventricle of patients with Eisenmenger syndrome. *Coron Artery Dis.* 2005;16(1):19–25.
65. Moceri P, Kempny A, Liodakis E, et al. Physiological differences between various types of Eisenmenger syndrome and relation to outcome. *Int J Cardiol.* 2015;179:455–60. doi:10.1016/j.ijcard.2014.11.100
66. Diller G-P, Kempny A, Inuzuka R, et al. Survival prospects of treatment naïve patients with Eisenmenger: a systematic review of the literature and report of own experience. *Heart.* 2014;100(17):1366–72. doi:10.1136/heartjnl-2014-305690
67. Hjortshøj CMS, Kempny A, Jensen AS, et al. Past and current cause-specific mortality in Eisenmenger syndrome. *Eur Heart J.* 2017;38(26):2060–7. doi:10.1093/eurheartj/ehx201
68. Kempny A, Hjortshøj CS, Gu H, et al. Predictors of death in contemporary adult patients with Eisenmenger syndrome: a multicenter study. *Circulation.* 2017;135(15):1432–40. doi:10.1161/CIRCULATIONAHA.116.023033
69. Silversides CK, Granton JT, Konen E, Hart MA, Webb GD, Therrien J. Pulmonary thrombosis in adults with Eisenmenger syndrome. *J Am Coll Cardiol.* 2003;42(11):1982–7.
70. Broberg CS, Ujita M, Prasad S, et al. Pulmonary arterial thrombosis in Eisenmenger syndrome is associated with biventricular dysfunction and decreased pulmonary flow velocity. *J Am Coll Cardiol.* 2007;50(7):634–42. doi:10.1016/j.jacc.2007.04.056
71. Tay ELW, Peset A, Papaphylactou M, et al. Replacement therapy for iron deficiency improves exercise capacity and quality of life in patients with cyanotic congenital heart disease and/or the Eisenmenger syndrome. *Int J Cardiol.* 2011;151(3):307–12. doi:10.1016/j.ijcard.2010.05.066
72. Baumgartner EA, Abbott ME. Interventricular septal defect with dextroposition of aorta and dilatation of the pulmonary artery ("Eisenmenger complex") terminating by cerebral abscess. *Am J Med Sci.* 1929;177:639–47. doi:10.1097/00000441-192905000-00003
73. Oya H, Nagaya N, Satoh T, et al. Haemodynamic correlates and prognostic significance of serum uric acid in adult patients with Eisenmenger syndrome. *Heart.* 2000;84(1):53–8. doi:10.1136/heart.84.1.53
74. Dimopoulos K, Diller G-P, Koltsida E, et al. Prevalence, predictors, and prognostic value of renal dysfunction in adults with congenital heart disease. *Circulation.* 2008;117(18):2320–8. doi:10.1161/CIRCULATIONAHA.107.734921
75. Galiè N, Beghetti M, Gatzoulis MA, et al. Bosentan therapy in patients with Eisenmenger syndrome: a multicenter, double-blind, randomized, placebo-controlled study. *Circulation.* 2006;114(1):48–54. doi:10.1161/CIRCULATIONAHA.106.630715
76. Dimopoulos K, Inuzuka R, Goletto S, et al. Improved survival among patients with Eisenmenger syndrome receiving advanced therapy for pulmonary arterial hypertension. *Circulation.* 2010;121(1):20–5. doi:10.1161/circulationaha.109.883876
77. Drakopoulou M, Nashat H, Kempny A, et al. Arrhythmias in adult patients with congenital heart disease and pulmonary arterial hypertension. *Heart.* 2018;104(23):1963–9. doi:10.1136/heartjnl-2017-312881
78. Razavi R, Hill DLG, Keevil SF, et al. Cardiac catheterisation guided by MRI in children and adults with congenital heart disease. *Lancet.* 2003;362(9399):1877–82. doi:10.1016/S0140-6736(03)14956-2
79. Kuehne T, Yilmaz S, Schulze-Neick I, et al. Magnetic resonance imaging guided catheterisation for assessment of pulmonary vascular resistance: in vivo validation and clinical application in patients with pulmonary hypertension. *Heart.* 2005;91(8):1064–9. doi:10.1136/hrt.2004.038265
80. Tzifa Aphrodite, Krombach Gabriele A., Krämer Nils, et al. Magnetic resonance–guided cardiac interventions using magnetic resonance–compatible devices. *Circulation.* 2010;3(6):585–92. doi:10.1161/CIRCINTERVENTIONS.110.957209
81. Giannakoulas G, Dimopoulos K, Bolger AP, et al. Usefulness of natriuretic peptide levels to predict mortality in adults with congenital heart disease. *Am J Cardiol.* 2010;105(6):869–73. doi:10.1016/j.amjcard.2009.11.041
82. Baggen VJM, van den Bosch AE, Eindhoven JA, et al. Prognostic value of N-terminal Pro-B-type natriuretic peptide, troponin-T, and growth-differentiation factor 15 in Adult congenital heart disease. *Circulation.* 2017;135(3):264–79. doi:10.1161/CIRCULATIONAHA.116.023255
83. Diller G-P, Dimopoulos K, Okonko D, et al. Exercise intolerance in adult congenital heart disease: comparative severity, correlates, and prognostic implication. *Circulation.* 2005;112(6):828–35. doi:10.1161/CIRCULATIONAHA.104.529800
84. Inuzuka R, Diller G-P, Borgia F, et al. Comprehensive use of cardiopulmonary exercise testing identifies adults with congenital heart disease at increased mortality risk in the medium term. *Circulation.* 2012;125(2):250–9. doi:10.1161/CIRCULATIONAHA.111.058719
85. Diller G-P, Dimopoulos K, Okonko D, et al. Heart rate response during exercise predicts survival in adults with congenital heart disease. *J Am Coll Cardiol.* 2006;48(6):1250–6. doi:10.1016/j.jacc.2006.05.051
86. Ebade AA, Khalil MA, Mohamed AK. Levosimendan is superior to dobutamine as an inodilator in the treatment of pulmonary hypertension for children undergoing cardiac surgery. *J Anesth.* 2013;27(3):334–9. doi:10.1007/s00540-012-1537-9
87. Ricci Z, Garisto C, Favia I, Vitale V, Di Chiara L, Cogo PE. Levosimendan infusion in newborns after corrective surgery for congenital heart disease: randomized controlled trial. *Intensive Care Med.* 2012;38(7):1198–204. doi:10.1007/s00134-012-2564-6
88. Rafiq I, Freeman LJ. Pulsed levosimendan therapy in the management of chronic end stage cardiac failure in "adult congenital heart disease." *Int J Cardiol.* 2015;195:283–4. doi:10.1016/j.ijcard.2015.03.426
89. Ho SY, Anderson RH. Conduction tissue in congenital heart surgery. *World J Surg.* 1985;9(4):550–67. doi:10.1007/BF01656057

90. Harrison JL, Jensen HK, Peel SA, et al. Cardiac magnetic resonance and electroanatomical mapping of acute and chronic atrial ablation injury: a histological validation study. *Eur Heart J.* 2014;35(22):1486–95. doi:10.1093/eurheartj/eht560
91. Murphy JG, Gersh BJ, Mair DD, et al. Long-term outcome in patients undergoing surgical repair of tetralogy of Fallot. *N Engl J Med.* 1993;329(9):593–9. doi:10.1056/NEJM199308263290901
92. Silka MJ, Hardy BG, Menashe VD, Morris CD. A population-based prospective evaluation of risk of sudden cardiac death after operation for common congenital heart defects. *J Am Coll Cardiol.* 1998;32(1):245–51.
93. Hansky B, Blanz U, Peuster M, et al. Endocardial pacing after Fontan-type procedures. *Pacing Clin Electrophysiol.* 2005;28(2):140–8. doi:10.1111/j.1540-8159.2005.04006.x
94. Paech C, Kostelka M, Dähnert I, Flosdorff P, Riede FT, Gebauer RA. Performance of steroid eluting bipolar epicardial leads in pediatric and congenital heart disease patients: 15 years of single center experience. *J Cardiothorac Surg.* 2014;9:84. doi:10.1186/1749-8090-9-84
95. Normand C, Linde C, Singh J, Dickstein K. Indications for cardiac resynchronization therapy: a comparison of the major international guidelines. *JACC: Heart Failure.* 2018;6(4):308–16. doi:10.1016/j.jchf.2018.01.022
96. Cleland JGF, Daubert J-C, Erdmann E, et al. The effect of cardiac resynchronization on morbidity and mortality in heart failure. *N Engl J Med.* 2005;352(15):1539–49. doi:10.1056/NEJMoa050496
97. Moss AJ, Hall WJ, Cannom DS, et al. Cardiac-resynchronization therapy for the prevention of heart-failure events. *N Engl J Med.* 2009;361(14):1329–38. doi:10.1056/NEJMoa0906431
98. Bando K, Turrentine MW, Sharp TG, et al. Pulmonary hypertension after operations for congenital heart disease: analysis of risk factors and management. *J Thorac Cardiovasc Surg.* 1996;112(6):1600–7; discussion 1607–9. doi:10.1016/S0022-5223(96)70019-3
99. Zamanian RT, Haddad F, Doyle RL, Weinacker AB. Management strategies for patients with pulmonary hypertension in the intensive care unit. *Crit Care Med.* 2007;35(9):2037–50.
100. Kempny A, Dimopoulos K, Fraisse A, et al. Blood viscosity and its relevance to the diagnosis and management of pulmonary hypertension. *J Am Coll Cardiol.* 2019;73(20):2636–42.
101. Dolgner SJ, Krieger EV, Wilkes J, et al. Predictors of extracorporeal membrane oxygenation support after surgery for adult congenital heart disease in children's hospitals. *Congenit Heart Dis.* Published online March 5, 2019. doi:10.1111/chd.12758
102. Khush KK, Cherikh WS, Chambers DC, et al. The International Thoracic Organ Transplant Registry of the International Society for Heart and Lung Transplantation: thirty-fifth adult heart transplantation report-2018; focus theme: multiorgan transplantation. *J Heart Lung Transplant.* 2018;37(10):1155–68. doi:10.1016/j.healun.2018.07.022
103. Dimopoulos K, Muthiah K, Alonso-Gonzalez R, et al. Heart or heart-lung transplantation for patients with congenital heart disease in England. *Heart.* 2019;105(8):596–602. doi:10.1136/heartjnl-2018-313984
104. Menachem JN, Golbus JR, Molina M, et al. Successful cardiac transplantation outcomes in patients with adult congenital heart disease. *Heart.* 2017;103(18):1449–54. doi:10.1136/heartjnl-2016-310933
105. Gelow JM, Song HK, Weiss JB, Mudd JO, Broberg CS. Organ allocation in adults with congenital heart disease listed for heart transplant: impact of ventricular assist devices. *The Journal of Heart and Lung Transplantation.* 2013;32(11):1059–64. doi:10.1016/j.healun.2013.06.024
106. Alonso-Gonzalez R. Advanced heart failure in congenital heart disease: role of heart transplant and ventricular assist devices. *Rev Esp Cardiol (Engl Ed).* 2019;72(4):285–7. doi:10.1016/j.rec.2018.09.018
107. Jansen K, Constantine A, Condliffe R, Tulloh R, Clift P, Moledina S, Wort SJ, Dimopoulos K. Pulmonary arterial hypertension in adults with congenital heart disease: markers of disease severity, management of advanced heart failure and transplantation. *Expert Rev Cardiovasc Ther.* 2021;19(9):837–55.
108. Ross HJ, Law Y, Book WM, et al. Transplantation and mechanical circulatory support in congenital heart disease: a scientific statement from the American Heart Association. *Circulation.* 2016;133(8):802–20. doi:10.1161/CIR.0000000000000353
109. OPTN/UNOS Thoracic Organ Transplantation Committee. Proposal to modify the adult heart allocation system. Published online January 25, 2016. Accessed June 12, 2019. https://optn.transplant.hrsa.gov/media/1244/08_adult_heart_allocation_part1.pdf
110. Davies RR, Russo MJ, Yang J, Quaegebeur JM, Mosca RS, Chen JM. Listing and transplanting adults with congenital heart disease. *Circulation.* 2011;123(7):759–67. doi:10.1161/CIRCULATIONAHA.110.960260
111. Alshawabkeh LI, Hu N, Carter KD, et al. Wait-list outcomes for adults with congenital heart disease listed for heart transplantation in the U.S. *J Am Coll Cardiol.* 2016;68(9):908–17. doi:10.1016/j.jacc.2016.05.082
112. Poh CL, Chiletti R, Zannino D, et al. Ventricular assist device support in patients with single ventricles: the Melbourne experience. *Interact Cardiovasc Thorac Surg.* 2017;25(2):310–6. doi:10.1093/icvts/ivx066

Chapter 29
CANCER THERAPIES AND CARDIAC DYSFUNCTION

Victoria Shklar, Katherine Godfrey, and Michelle E. Bloom

Introduction

Translational medicine has vastly improved our understanding of cancer development and progression and has allowed for the rapid development of new chemotherapy and alternative therapeutic regimens, improving the quality of life and rates of survival in patients with cancer. Early detection and treatment have in many cases transformed cancer from a fatal disease to a chronic condition. Improved cancer survival implicitly uncovers a wide spectrum of toxicities attributable to novel cancer therapies, including those of a cardiac nature. Multidisciplinary care is critical, as cancer outcomes can be influenced by cardiovascular health. In turn, cardiovascular health can influence cancer treatment selection, and cardiac toxicity can impact cancer treatment. Cardiovascular disease (CVD) due to cancer treatment can ultimately alter cancer survivorship.

Cancer therapies, including cytotoxic chemotherapy, molecular targeted therapies, immunotherapy, and mediastinal irradiation, have been linked to a wide spectrum of cardiac toxicities, including cardiomyopathy, ischemia, hypertension, arrhythmias, myocarditis, myocardial fibrosis, and others. These toxicities may limit a patient's ability to complete effective cancer therapy and have been associated with significant morbidity and mortality. In many cases, the risk of death from CVD exceeds that from cancer itself or tumor recurrence[1] For example, CVD has been shown to be the main cause of death in older female breast cancer survivors.[2]

The aging population of cancer patients lends itself to a higher burden of cardiovascular risk factors, comorbidities, and poor cardiac reserve. Insufficient evidence regarding long-term consequences of cancer treatment-related CVD (CTRCD) might lead to ineffective prevention of adverse events and possible inappropriate interruption of life-saving therapies. Current research is aimed at identifying the best surveillance and prevention strategies to identify those at risk of early cardiac toxicity. Many cardiologists and oncologists still regard the left ventricular ejection fraction (LVEF) as the determining factor for cardiac toxicity. Unfortunately, by the point of LVEF decline, many patients have already presented with clinical heart failure (HF). Because the field of cardio-oncology and the topic of cardiac toxicity related to cancer therapy is vast and diverse, this chapter will focus on cancer treatment-related cardiomyopathy and HF.

Definitions and Classification

While several guideline and consensus documents have been published, there is currently no universal definition or standardized approach to surveillance and management of "cardiac toxicity" related to cancer therapy.[3] In a broader sense, cardiotoxicity, or CTRCD, refers to any cardiac injury (functional or structural) related to cancer treatment.[3] Understanding the pathophysiology of CTRCD is important for predicting, treating, and preventing these side effects. A previous classification system attempted to distinguish between drugs that cause irreversible damage (myocyte death, e.g., anthracyclines) vs reversible damage (myocyte dysfunction, e.g., trastuzumab).[4] However, more recent understanding suggests a spectrum, rather than distinct categories, with trastuzumab possibly causing permanent damage (particularly when cardiac comorbidities preexist) and anthracycline cardiomyopathy potentially reversing with early therapy.[5–7] Re-challenging with the offending "reversible" drug is usually well tolerated, especially after initiating cardiac protective therapy.[8,9]

Definitions of subclinical cardiac toxicity vary but have previously been proposed to include a reduction in LVEF by >10% to an absolute value <50% (Table 29.1).[10–13] The American Society of Echocardiography and the European Association of Cardiovascular Imaging define toxicity as a >5% decrease in LVEF from the baseline in symptomatic and >10% in asymptomatic patients to an absolute value of <53%, reflecting the more widespread acceptance that LVEF 53–73% is considered to be normal.[3] Further definition includes >15% in global longitudinal strain (GLS) on echocardiography from baseline.[1]

Risk Factors and Epidemiology

Cardiac disease and cancer are the first and second leading causes of mortality in North America, accounting for >50% of total deaths,[14] and share underlying biological mechanisms and risk profiles. With the aging population, there are growing numbers of patients living with or at risk of developing both diseases.[15] As cancer death rates fall, the number of patients living with and surviving cancer is growing, leading to a higher prevalence of non-cancer related deaths. For example, older women with breast cancer are more likely to die of a disease other than their cancer, and CVD has been shown to be the most frequent cause.[1,16] In older, postmenopausal women, CVD mortality is higher in breast cancer survivors than in women without a history of breast cancer[17] Overall, heart disease accounts for >10% of non-cancer causes of death in cancer patients.[18] However, only about half of patients with cancer and CVD are referred to cardiology.[19] Among different cancer types, HF ranges in incidence from 3.5% in breast cancer to 11.8% in lung cancer.[19]

Cardiac risk factor identification, albeit challenging and poorly defined, is paramount to cancer and cardiac therapeutic decisions. Patients felt to be at highest risk of cardiovascular compromise related to cancer therapy may benefit from heightened and more frequent surveillance and earlier interventions. The pathophysiology of cardiac toxicity is complex and multifaceted, involving traditional cardiovascular risk of the patient coupled with intrinsic risk of the cancer therapy itself. Early referral for cardiac evaluation should be considered in higher-risk patients.[20] Identifying at-risk patients is challenging, but several factors have been identified and risk scores developed.[21,22] Table 29.2 summarizes commonly used risk assessment models, which should include clinical history and examination, screening for CV risk factors, calculation of ASCVD risk score, and baseline measurement of cardiac function including cardiac biomarkers, electrocardiogram, and echocardiogram.[3,15,23,24]

DOI: 10.1201/9780429244544-36

TABLE 29.1: Definitions of Cardiotoxicity

Reference	Definition
Schwartz et al.[11]	Decline in LVEF >10% to final LVEF <50%
Cardiac Review and Evaluation Committee[10]	(1) Cardiomyopathy characterized by a decrease in LVEF, either global or more severe in the septum (2) Symptoms of HF (3) Associated signs of HF, including but not limited to S3 gallop, tachycardia, or both (4) Decline in LVEF of at least 5% to <55% with signs or symptoms of HF, or a decline in LVEF of at least 10% to below 55% without signs or symptoms of HF
American Society of Echocardiography and European Association of Cardiovascular Imaging[1]	>5% decrease in LVEF in symptomatic patients, or >10% decrease in LVEF from baseline in asymptomatic patients to an absolute value <53%, or >15% in GLS on echocardiography from baseline
Food and Drug Administration[12]	>20% decrease in LVEF, or >10% decrease to below lower limit of normal or absolute LVEF of 45% (anthracycline toxicity)
Breast Cancer International Research Group[13]	>10% reduction from baseline LVEF (asymptomatic left ventricular dysfunction)
National Cancer Institute[14]	Grade 1: Asymptomatic with elevations in biomarkers or abnormalities on imaging Grade 2: Symptoms with moderate activity or exertion Grade 3: Symptoms at rest or with minimal activity or exertion; hospitalization; new onset of symptoms Grade 4: Severe, life-threatening symptoms requiring urgent intervention, such as hemodynamic support Grade 5: Death

Abbreviations: GLS: global longitudinal strain, HF: heart failure, LVEF: left ventricular ejection fraction.

TABLE 29.2: Overview of Risk-Prediction Models

Reference	Population	Description	Risk Factors Included
Ezaz et al.[21]	Older women with early-stage breast cancer who received adjuvant trastuzumab therapy	Seven-point risk score for three-year HF risk which stratifies patients into low, medium, or high risk	Age, adjuvant chemotherapy, coronary artery disease, atrial fibrillation or flutter, diabetes mellitus, hypertension, renal failure
Romond et al.[28]	Women with HER2+ breast cancer without distant metastatic disease who underwent surgery	Statistical model for estimating cardiac risk associated with addition of trastuzumab to paclitaxel after AC	Age, baseline LVEF
Dranitsaris et al.[27]	Women with metastatic breast cancer receiving doxorubicin	Designed to estimate absolute risk with each cycle of doxorubicin-based chemotherapy	Age, weight, previous anthracycline exposure, performance status, number of cycles
Herrmann et al.[9]	Patients undergoing chemotherapy	Risk score calculated based on drug-related risk category plus patient-related risk factors, stratifying patients into very low-, low-, intermediate-, high-, or very high-risk groups	Age, female gender, hypertension, CAD or CAD equivalent, cardiomyopathy or heart failure, diabetes mellitus, prior or current anthracycline, prior or current chest radiation

Abbreviations: AC: doxorubicin/cyclophosphamide, CAD: coronary artery disease, HF: heart failure, LVEF: left ventricular ejection fraction.

Cancer and cardiac disease share multiple modifiable risk factors. These include tobacco use, alcohol consumption, obesity, physical inactivity, hypertension, hyperlipidemia, diabetes mellitus, and chronic inflammation.[15] Initial evaluation should include assessment for traditional cardiovascular risk factors including hypertension, diabetes mellitus, smoking, obesity, previous left ventricular dysfunction or HF, coronary artery disease, arrhythmias, valvular dysfunction, older age, female gender, and postmenopausal status. Cancer therapy-related factors for CTRCD include lifetime cumulative dose for certain agents, e.g., anthracyclines, combination of multiple agents with potential for cardiotoxicity, infusion regimen, rate of administration, schedule of administration, and electrolyte imbalances. Some single nucleotide polymorphisms (SNPs) have been implicated, suggesting that genetic variation may modulate risk. Heavy alcohol intake (at least eight drinks per week) may portend higher risk of cardiotoxicity.[25,26] Although there is no universally accepted validated risk score to definitively categorize patients, several have been proposed yet not validated in prospective studies (Table 29.2).[9,21,27,28]

Anthracyclines

Anthracyclines are a class of chemotherapeutics used in the management of many solid and hematologic cancers, most prominently for breast cancer. These drugs, including doxorubicin, daunorubicin, epirubicin, and idarubicin, are responsible for the earliest described form of chemotherapy-induced cardiotoxicity and as such are the most well studied. Anthracyclines rapidly localize to the nucleus where they integrate with DNA, thus disrupting RNA production and DNA metabolism (Figure 29.1). Their cytotoxicity is primarily due to inhibition of topoisomerase II, which then prevents DNA repair and results in apoptosis.[29] There are two isozymes of topoisomerase, Top IIa, which is expressed in rapidly dividing cells, and Top IIb, which is expressed in quiescent cells like cardiac myocytes.[30] The non-selective nature of anthracyclines

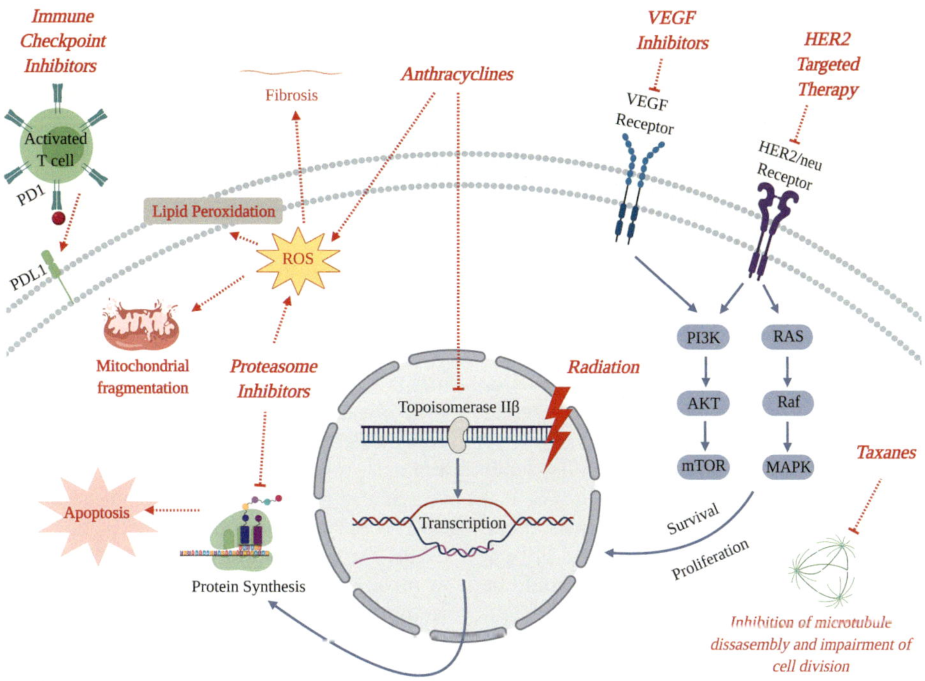

FIGURE 29.1 Cardiac myocyte with illustrated mechanisms of cardiotoxicity due to cancer therapy. Anthracyclines inhibit topoisomerase II, which prevents DNA repair and results in apoptosis. Anthracyclines also cause oxidative stress through the production of ROS, leading to fibrosis and lipid peroxidation of cardiac membranes. Inhibition of HER2 activation and signaling by drugs like trastuzumab and pertuzumab compromise proliferation and pro-survival pathways. ICIs prevent T cell deactivation by activating negative regulatory pathways. Taxanes interfere with microtubule function required for cell mitosis by polymerizing tubulin. Alkylating agents interfere with DNA base pairing, leading to strand breakage and impairment of cross-linking needed for DNA replication. Inhibition of the VEGF signaling cascade leads to inhibition of survival pathways. Proteasome inhibitors increase ubiquitylated proteins, resulting in mitochondrial dysfunction, ROS production, and ultrastructural changes that result in apoptosis. (Image adapted from Bloom et al. Cancer therapy-related cardiac dysfunction and heart failure: Part 1: Definitions, pathophysiology, risk factors, and imaging. *Circ Heart Fail.* 2016;9(1):e002661. Created with BioRender.com.)

results in binding of these agents to Top IIb, resulting in myocyte death.[31] Anthracyclines also cause oxidative stress through the formation of reactive oxygen species (ROS), which result in fibrosis and lipid peroxidation of cardiac membranes,[32] and may directly impair proliferation of cardiac progenitor cells, thus impairing recovery from stressors and inhibiting pro-survival signaling.[33,34]

Anthracycline-induced cardiotoxicity can be acute, early-onset, chronic, progressive, or late-onset chronic progressive.[23,32,35] Acute toxicity is rare (<1% of cases), and usually manifests as transient, generally reversible decline in myocardial contractility immediately after infusion.[23] The early-onset, chronic, progressive form occurs during treatment or within one year in 1.6–2.1% of patients. The late-onset, chronic, progressive form represents most cases and occurs over one year after treatment completion, sometimes decades later, in 1.6–5% of patients. Both chronic forms are marked by dilated cardiomyopathy and are usually irreversible.[23] Anthracycline toxicity has been shown to be dose dependent and related to the lifetime cumulative dose.[36,37] Incidence of HF due to doxorubicin is 1–2% with a cumulative dose of 300 mg/m^2, 3–5% with a cumulative dose of 400 mg/m^2, 15.7% at 500 mg/m^2, and 48% at 650 mg/m^2.[38] These estimates do not take into account pre-existing cardiac dysfunction. The recommended maximum lifetime cumulative dose is therefore set at 500 mg/m^2.[38] Risk factors, such as prior cardiac insult and existing CVD, age, female gender, and use of concomitant agents known to have cardiotoxicity, predispose to anthracycline-induced cardiotoxicity.[23,39,40] Intravenous bolus administration, and higher single doses increase risk.[23] Liposomal formulations may be less harmful and cardioprotective agents may be co-administered to help reduce the harmful effects.[11–43]

HER2 Targeted Therapies

The blockade of the human epidermal growth factor receptor 2 (HER2) signaling pathway alters cancer progression in multiple malignancies, but particularly in breast tumors which frequently overexpress HER2.[44,45] HER2, a tyrosine kinase transmembrane receptor encoded by the *ErbB2* gene, is expressed in various tissues, including the heart.[46] HER2 is a key regulator of cardiomyocyte growth and proliferation and plays a key role in cardiac response to oxygenic stress.[47–49] Trastuzumab and pertuzumab are recombinant humanized monoclonal antibodies that target different subdomains of HER2. They inhibit HER2 activation and signaling in the heart, thereby compromising cardioprotective mechanisms (Figure 29.1). Combination of anthracyclines with trastuzumab therapy induces a "two-hit" phenomenon in which anthracyclines are a "first hit" causing oxidative stress, and trastuzumab lowers cardiac protective mechanisms.[50]

HER2-targeted therapies are associated with the development of left ventricular (LV) systolic dysfunction and HF.[45,51] In general, cardiac dysfunction resulting from trastuzumab occurs early, has variable severity, is dose independent, and is usually reversible without ultrastructural changes.[8,52] The incidence of trastuzumab cardiac toxicity varies, but overall portends a relative risk of 5.1 when compared with non-trastuzumab-containing breast cancer chemotherapy regimens[53] Combination therapy with trastuzumab and pertuzumab is sometimes used due to mechanistic synergy, and, despite initial concerns for the potential of additive toxicity, the incidence of HF with dual HER-2 blockade appears to be comparable to single-agent therapy.[54,55] High rates of toxicity are seen in patients that receive HER2 therapies and concurrent or prior treatment with anthracyclines, with the time between the two correlating inversely with risk.[56,57] Other risk factors for HF are not unique to HER2 therapy, and include age, low baseline LVEF, obesity, coronary artery disease, hypertension, valvular disease, smoking, and renal failure.[21,32]

The FDA recommends holding trastuzumab for at least four weeks if LVEF drops[3] ≥16% from pretreatment values or if it falls below normal and[3] >10% from pretreatment values. It can be resumed if, within 4–8 weeks, the LVEF returns to normal and the absolute decrease from baseline is ≤15%. It should be discontinued permanently if there is a persistent (over eight weeks) LVEF decline or if cessation is required on more than three occasions for cardiomyopathy.[58]

Immune Therapy

Immune checkpoint inhibitors (ICI) have changed the landscape of cancer therapeutics. Tumor cells modulate regulatory immune system processes of T cell response by activating two negative regulatory pathways—the programmed cell death 1 (PD-1) and PD-1 ligand (PD-L1) pathway, and the cytotoxic T-lymphocyte associated antigen 4 (CTLA4)/B7 pathway. As a broad class, these agents are designed to reverse the immune system inhibition induced by cancer cells.[32] This class includes monoclonal antibodies targeting CTLA-4 (ipilimumab), PD-1 (nivolumab and pembrolizumab), and PD-L1 (atezolizumab, avelumab, durvalumab). Although ICIs are promising for several advanced malignancies and are well tolerated, they can lead to unintended autoimmunity against native tissues via phenomena referred to as immune-related adverse events (IRAEs). As ICIs directly attack malignant cells by preventing T cell deactivation (Figure 29.1), unintended targets prevent down-regulation of auto-reactive T cells and, as such, often lead to immune dysregulation that manifests as symptoms clinically resembling autoimmune disease. Almost every organ can be affected, including the skin, liver, eyes, kidneys, bowel, endocrine tissues, and central nervous system. Anti-CTLA4 therapy inhibits the immune pathway further upstream in the cascade whereas anti-PD-1 therapy acts more on peripheral tissues, lending the former to more severe IRAEs. These therapies are felt to lead to more adverse events when combined.[32]

Cardiac complications of ICIs, namely myocarditis, are currently reported as rare but severe and sometimes fatal. The incidence is likely underestimated owing to the lack of routine cardiac monitoring during clinical trials with these agents.[59] Combination of anti-CTLA4 and PD-1 therapy is the biggest risk factor.[59–61] In a safety database of ~20,000 patients, 18 cases (0.09%) of severe myocarditis were reported with single-agent PD-1 inhibitor but the incidence was higher with combined therapy (0.27%).[61] In a single-center experience, a rate of 1.14% has been reported for all ICIs, with 0.5% on PD-1 monotherapy and 2.4% with combination CTLA4 and PD-1.[59] In a multicenter study of 752 patients with melanoma treated with ipilimumab, one case of myocardial fibrosis was reported.[62] There has also been one case of LV dysfunction and one case of Takotsubo cardiomyopathy reported.[63,64] Myocarditis appears to occur early in the course of therapy and presentation can include atrial and ventricular arrhythmias, conduction abnormalities, or progressive HF persisting beyond the discontinuation of therapy.[59,61] Many cases present with another autoimmune event, such as rash, hepatitis, or myositis.[32,61] There have been no studies thus far to assess late-onset chronic cardiotoxicity after completion of therapy.

Diagnostic imaging and laboratory evaluation appears largely similar to myocarditis of other etiologies, including elevation in brain natriuretic peptide (BNP) and troponin levels, and abnormal EKG, though interestingly roughly 50% of patients present with preserved systolic function.[59] Histological analysis has demonstrated infiltration of the myocardium by lymphocytes and macrophages, as well as infiltration of the sinus and atrioventricular nodes. It is thought that immune-mediated myocarditis occurs from immune activation of cardiac and tumor tissue. The activated T cells may target an antigen that is shared by myocytes and tumor cells. Also, PD-L1 is highly expressed on injured cardiomyocytes and on infiltrating CD8+ T cells. It appears that PD-L1 is protective, and its inhibition contributes to cardiomyocyte vulnerability to injury.[65]

The American Society of Clinical Oncology (ASCO) recommends baseline EKG for all patients, and consideration of troponin, especially with combination therapy.[66] For patients with high clinical suspicion of cardiac toxicity, cardiology consultation and additional cardiac testing are recommended, including cardiac magnetic resonance imaging (MRI), cardiac catheterization, and endomyocardial biopsy, when appropriate. Treatment includes permanent discontinuation of ICI therapy, hospital admission, and high-dose steroids (methylprednisolone 1 g/day × 3 days), with the potential addition of other immune-modulating therapies, such as mycophenolic acid, infliximab, or anti-thymocyte globulin.[66]

Microtubule Inhibitors

Taxanes, such as paclitaxel, docetaxel, and cabazitaxel, work by interfering with microtubule function required for cell mitosis by polymerizing tubulin (Figure 29.1). These agents are used to treat a variety of cancers, including breast and ovarian. Up to 8% of patients treated with taxanes develop cardiotoxicity, mostly in combination with an anthracycline.[67] Taxanes are suspected to increase plasma levels of anthracyclines, thereby increasing anthracycline uptake into the heart.[68] Thus, it is generally recommended to separate their administration by at least 4–6 hours to decrease the risk of cardiotoxicity.[69] However, HF incidence with these agents is reportedly low.

Alkylating Agents

Alkylating agents interfere with DNA base pairing, leading to strand breaks and impairment of cross-linking needed for DNA replication (Figure 29.1). Acute LV dysfunction has been reported in 7–28% of patients receiving cyclophosphamide.[23] This cardiotoxicity appears to be dose related (≥150 mg/kg and 1.5 g/m²/day) and generally occurs within one to ten days after the first dose.[23,70] Currently, it is encountered less frequently due to lower and fractioned administrations, unrelated to cumulative dose. The mechanism behind this life-threatening, yet reversible, complication is unclear, but inactivation of glutathione redox cycling has been suggested. Ifosfamide can induce HF as well, with a dose-response trend (doses ≥12.5 g/m²) and can also be reversible.[71] Other alkylating agents have been reported to cause cardiotoxicity in combination with other drugs.[49,72]

VEGF Receptor Inhibitors and Tyrosine Kinase Inhibitors

Vascular endothelial growth factor (VEGF) promotes the growth and development of blood vessels supplying malignant tumors by stimulating tyrosine kinase receptors on the cell surface. VEGF has multiple isoforms and binds to three tyrosine kinase receptors. Different modes of inhibiting the VEGF signaling cascade have been developed to inhibit angiogenesis, including monoclonal antibodies against extracellular components and inhibitors of the intracellular ATP-binding domain of specific tyrosine kinases. The latter approach is not as specific and often leads to diverse inhibition of additional kinases, thus producing unwanted effects (Figure 29.1).[73] Drugs that inhibit VEGF-mediated angiogenesis have been linked to hypertension, ischemia, LV dysfunction, and HF. Hypertension is a class effect of VEGF-TKI, occurring in up to 80% of patients, often leading to HF.[35,74] The LV dysfunction associated with these drugs is at least partially reversible.[75,76] Incidence of LV dysfunction and HF is poorly defined and likely underestimated. VEGF inhibitors have been reported to cause asymptomatic LVEF decline in a quarter of patients, and symptomatic HF in 4–8%.[35,75] Some meta-analyses have estimated the incidence of combined LV dysfunction and HF with VEGF inhibitors or TKIs at approximately 3.6%.[77]

Bevacizumab, a monoclonal antibody, can lead to a decrement in LVEF of 10%³ in over one-quarter of patients, while almost one-half of patients develop hypertension.[78] Sunitinib can lead to HF in up to 8% of patients, while up to 28% develop a drop in LVEF of ≥10%, and 47% suffer from hypertension.[75,76] Sorafenib causes hypertension in 17–43% of patients.[79,80] Bevacizumab, when combined with taxanes, significantly increases the risk of HF.[81] Several BCR-ABL TKIs have been developed and are used for chronic myeloid leukemia, including imatinib, dasatinib, nilotinib, bosutinib, and ponatinib. These agents are used for long-term therapy. Imatinib has been associated with a low incidence of ventricular dysfunction (0.5–1.7%).[82]

Proteasome Inhibitors

Proteasome inhibitors, such as carfilzomib, bortezomib, and ixazomib, are well known for their therapeutic roles in multiple myeloma, cardiac amyloidosis, and certain lymphomas. Compared with other tissues, proteasome activity is increased in the heart; thus, disruption of protein homeostasis in cardiac myocytes results in cardiotoxicity, including HF. These drugs create an intracellular imbalance with an increase in ubiquitylated proteins and activation of pathways that lead to myocardial hypertrophy. They also result in mitochondrial dysfunction, ROS production, and ultrastructural changes that result in cardiac myocyte apoptosis, necrosis, and release of troponin (Figure 29.1).[83,84] Of note, many patients have advanced disease and have been exposed to other cardiotoxic agents and have higher background cardiovascular risk (e.g., amyloid). Thus, the characterization and understanding of cardiovascular events in this population is complex.

Bortezomib is a reversible proteasome inhibitor which is overall felt to be relatively safe, with low rates of LV dysfunction and HF in over a decade of clinical use.[85] The incidence of HF from bortezomib is in the range 2–5%. Meta-analysis rate of high-grade cardiac toxicity, including HF and sudden cardiac death, is estimated at 2.3%.[86] Carfilzomib is an irreversible proteasome inhibitor used in reversed/relapsed multiple myeloma, with more potent activity than bortezomib. According to a pooled analysis of phase II studies on carfilzomib, 22% of patients experienced cardiac side effects, of which 7.2% exhibited HF and 2% developed cardiomyopathy. Among 60 myeloma patients treated with carfilzomib-based regimens, 12% experienced reversible LVEF reduction by 20%³ at 15 months.[87] There was no dose-response association between carfilzomib and incidence of cardiac events. Carfilzomib toxicity is often reversible after drug cessation.[87] In a trial of refractory multiple myeloma, there was a trend toward grade 3 or higher HF in the carfilzomib versus bortezemib arm, with grading defined by the Medical Dictionary for Regulatory Activities preferred terms.[88]

Radiation Therapy

Radiation therapy is an effective treatment for a wide range of malignancies and is used on about 35% of cancer patients within one year of diagnosis.[89] Radiation exposure on the thorax is mainly used as an adjunctive therapy for breast, lung, or esophageal cancer, as well as for lymphoma. Irradiation of the heart can result in a wide range of cardiac toxicities, including atherosclerosis, valvular injury, fibrosis, pericardial disease, and myocarditis, with an estimated incidence of 10–30%.[90] LV dysfunction and HF occur rarely as a result of acute radiation myocarditis or more commonly as a long-term consequence of fibrosis.[91] Radiation myocarditis often presents with signs of constrictive pericardial disease and an enlarged cardiac silhouette on imaging, while tissue sections often show fibrosis in the anterior wall of the heart.[91] This results in ineffective contraction by myocytes, with decreased systolic function. Subclinical cardiac changes can occur weeks, months, or years after radiation therapy, but clinical toxicity usually manifests itself years after exposure.[92,93] Interestingly, over one-half of the patients that develop HF from radiation therapy have HFpEF or only a mild reduction in LVEF.[91,93] Risk factors include cumulative radiation doses >30 Gy, radiation fraction doses >2 Gy/day, longer intervals from time of radiation, concomitant chemotherapy (especially anthracyclines), location of radiation (anterior, left sided, mediastinal, mantle), younger age at irradiation, and coexisting cardiovascular risk factors.[94–96]

Prevention and Surveillance

Biomarkers

Biomarkers are useful in the early identification, risk stratification, and monitoring of CTRCD, as well as for assessment of cardioprotective effectiveness.[3,97,98] Biomarkers are minimally invasive, cheaper than imaging, and reproducible.[99] The high negative predictive value of some biomarkers allows for identification of low-risk patients, who can then avoid intensive, long-term cardiac monitoring.[23,100] Most biomarker data involve troponins and natriuretic peptides, although other markers have been studied.[99,101] There are currently no standards for use of biomarkers, though many centers incorporate biomarkers in surveillance and management.[3,102]

Elevations in both troponin I and T have been observed to precede detectable reductions in LVEF,[98,103] leading some to recommend the measurement of troponin immediately before and after each cycle of cancer therapy.[23] In patients receiving anthracyclines, increases in troponin level may predict poor response to cardiac therapy,[104] lack of LVEF recovery after treatment, and benefit from preventive therapy.[100] Absence of troponin elevation has a high negative predictive value in patients receiving high-dose chemotherapy,[100,105] while an early increase predicts diastolic dysfunction in up to 34% of patients.[101,106] Its elevation at the completion of treatment predicts subsequent reduction in LVEF and cardiac events.[107] Troponin has been proposed as a biomarker in the high-sensitivity detection of ICI-related myocarditis.[59,97]

Natriuretic peptides have shown mixed results for detection of cardiotoxicity. Natriuretic peptide levels may be more useful for their negative predictive value.[3] Although there is no evidence to guide cancer therapy according to these levels, increases in N-terminal-proBNP (NT-proBNP) are associated with abnormal LV thickness-to-dimension ratios,[108] suggestive of LV remodeling. The European Society of Cardiology (ESC) does recommend the use of natriuretic peptides to detect early cardiac injury and during follow-up.[23] Further study is needed to better characterize the role of NT-proBNP in the cancer population. Other biomarkers, though not as well studied, have shown promise, as summarized in Table 29.3.

Role of Imaging

It is generally considered standard of care to assess LV function by some imaging modality prior to initiating potentially cardiotoxic therapy, but surveillance frequency during and following therapy is not well defined.[109] ASCO recommends that patients with concerning clinical signs or symptoms should have an echocardiogram for diagnostic work-up (or MRI or nuclear, if echo is unavailable or not feasible).[109] Asymptomatic patients at high risk of CTRCD should have an echocardiogram between 6 and 12 months after completion of cancer therapy. Those with abnormal testing should be referred to a cardiologist; there are no recommendations for those with normal testing. A report from the American Society of Echocardiography and the European Association of Cardiovascular Imaging recommends a baseline LVEF and follow-up echocardiography every three months for all patients specifically receiving trastuzumab, followed by repeat imaging six months after therapy completion.[3] According to the European Society for Medical Oncology guidelines, patients receiving anthracyclines or trastuzumab should have serial monitoring to assess cardiac function at baseline, three, six, and nine months during treatment, and then at 12 and 18 months after initiation.[23] In the absence of symptoms, infrequent monitoring thereafter is appropriate in those with metastatic disease, where oncologic mortality risk outweighs cardiovascular risk.[23]

The simplest and most used method to assess LVEF is 2-dimensional echocardiography (2DE). The American Society of Echocardiography suggests the addition of contrast to two-dimensional echocardiography 2DE for better definition of endocardial borders in patients with breast implants or mastectomy.[110] However, 2DE may be unable to detect small (<10%) changes in LVEF, which may have important implications. Newer approaches, e.g., 3D echocardiography and strain imaging with speckle tracking or tissue doppler imaging (TDI), have gained traction. These techniques are dependent on image quality and operator experience and may not be widely available, but they do provide a more accurate determination of LVEF. As a result, they may allow for earlier detection of subtle changes. Global longitudinal strain (GLS) reduction has been shown to precede gross LV dysfunction in patients who later develop HF, and abnormal strain can be seen early, despite preserved LVEF.[107,111] A change in GLS >11% was the strongest predictor of cardiotoxicity in a study of patients receiving trastuzumab with or without anthracyclines.[112] Others have suggested a similar cut-off of >10% from baseline after three months. Subclinical LV dysfunction as defined by GLS was found to have a sensitivity range of 65–86% and a specificity range of 73–95%.[11] A relative decrease of GLS >15% from baseline is considered indicative of subclinical LV dysfunction, a relative decrease <8% is consistent with no evidence of subclinical LV dysfunction, while 8–15% is a gray zone that requires closer follow-up, potentially including a repeat study two to three weeks after the initial study.[3]

In addition to LVEF, it is essential to monitor right ventricular (RV) function. Subclinical changes in RV systolic and diastolic parameters have been noted in multiple studies.[101] It is important during echocardiography to focus on chamber size, tricuspid annular plane systolic excursion, estimation of pulmonary artery systolic pressure, and RV diastolic parameters.[3]

Cardiac magnetic resonance imaging (MRI) is a gold standard for ventricular functional and structural components. However, MRI use is limited by cost, lack of availability, processing times, and patient factors, e.g., pacemakers and claustrophobia. LV mass index independently predicts major adverse cardiac events in patients with cardiomyopathy from anthracyclines.[113] Myocardial fibrosis is a marker of LV remodeling and can be associated with worse prognosis.[99] MRI is generally reserved for cases with poor echocardiographic windows or inconclusive results, particularly when discontinuation of cancer therapy is being considered.[3,11,101,109]

Multi-gated acquisition (MUGA) scan, once a common modality for cardiac functional assessments due to its high reproducibility and availability, has now largely been replaced by echocardiography.[114] In addition to providing limited information on cardiac structure and function, MUGA has the added risk of secondary cancer due to radiation exposure (7.8 mSv/study).[114,115]

Cardioprotective Agents and Therapies for Prevention

Cardioprotective therapy studies investigating the role of angiotensin-converting enzyme inhibitors (ACEIis), angiotensin-receptor blockers (ARBs), and beta-blockers for prophylaxis have shown wide variation in the prevention of CTRCD (Tables 29.4 and 29.5). Both beta-blockers and ACEis are thought to help prevent HF by reducing afterload.[116] The OVERCOME trial demonstrated that enalapril and carvedilol in patients with hematological malignancies may prevent LV systolic dysfunction, but did not decrease incidence of diastolic dysfunction.[42] The PRADA trial assigned early-stage breast cancer patients with adjuvant anthracycline regimens to candesartan, metoprolol succinate, or matching placebos.[117] No effect of metoprolol on LVEF was observed, but candesartan was found to provide protection against early decline in LVEF. The MANTICORE trial showed a small attenuation of LVEF decline by both perindopril and bisoprolol in trastuzumab-treated breast cancer patients.[118] Most recently, CECCY, the largest trial for the primary prevention of anthracycline cardiotoxicity, showed carvedilol to have a neutral effect at six months follow-up.[119] However, carvedilol did decrease troponin levels and diastolic dysfunction.[119]

TABLE 29.3: **Prevention and Surveillance**

Mode	Purpose	Suggested Use	Considerations
Biomarkers			
Troponin I, T	Observed to precede reductions in LVEF and/or diastolic dysfunction; may predict poor response to cardiac therapy in those receiving anthracyclines; proposed to aid in detection of ICI-related myocarditis; may assist in distinguishing between reversible and irreversible cardiac injury by identifying myocardial cell necrosis	Consider measurement immediately before and after each cycle of cancer therapy	Low cost, minimally invasive, reproducible
Natriuretic peptides	Associated with LV remodeling	ESC recommends use for detection of early cardiac injury and during follow-up	Low cost, minimally invasive, reproducible
High-sensitivity C-reactive protein	Predictive of LVEF decline in breast cancer patients treated with trastuzumab in some studies; others showed no association		
Myeloperoxidase	Preliminary studies show levels rising early in treatment, persistent throughout course, and associated with cardiotoxicity		
Cytochrome C	Released when mitochondrial membrane disrupted by anthracyclines, increased levels observed in some pathological conditions like cardiac arrest and cardioplegia; studies ongoing to investigate possible role in predicting LVD in cancer patients		
Galectin-3, ST-2, growth differentiation factor 15	Studies have shown no association with cardiotoxicity		
Imaging		All patients prior to cardiotoxic therapy; recommendations for frequency during and following therapy varies	
2D Echo	LVEF, RV function	Varies, commonly done before therapy and every three months after	May be unable to detect smaller changes in LVEF
3D Echo (strain imaging w/ speckle tracking or tissue Doppler imaging)	LVEF, GLS, RV function	Varies, commonly done before therapy and every three months after	Techniques dependent on imaging quality and operative experience, may not be widely available, but provide more accurate determination of LVEF and earlier detection of changes
MRI	Ventricular functional and structural components	Reserve for cases with poor echo windows or inconclusive results	Expensive, lack of availability, long processing time, patient factors
MUGA scan	Ventricular functional and structural components	Mostly replaced with echo	High reproducibility and availability, but provides limited information on structure and function; risk of secondary cancer due to radiation exposure

Abbreviations: Echo: echocardiogram, ESC: European Society of Cardiology, GLS: global longitudinal strain, ICI: immune checkpoint inhibitor, LV: left ventricle, LVD: left ventricular dysfunction, LVEF: left ventricular ejection fraction, MRI: magnetic resonance imaging, MUGA: multi-gated acquisition scan, RV: right ventricle.

Statins have been shown to be protective against CTRCD, significantly lowering the risk of HF in cancer patients,[116,120] potentially through anti-inflammatory and anti-fibrotic properties and interfering with two of the main mechanisms of anthracycline cardiotoxicity, namely ROS generation and topoisomerase II inhibition.[121] A recent study demonstrated that statins are at least as potent as dexrazoxane, beta-blockers, or angiotensin antagonists in the prevention of anthracycline-induced cardiotoxicity.[116] However, most studies have been retrospective; only a handful of small-scale prospective studies are available, focused on anthracycline-based regimens.[121]

Dexrazoxane, an iron-chelating agent, is an FDA-approved drug for the prevention of anthracycline-induced cardiotoxicity. Dexrazoxane competes for ATP-binding sites on topoisomerase IIb, leading to a configurational change that prevents complex formation with anthracyclines.[122] Dexrazoxane also decreases iron levels, which prevents the formation of anthracycline-iron complexes and subsequent ROS formation.[123, 124] In patients previously treated with anthracyclines, dexrazoxane has been shown to markedly reduce HF.[43,116] It also diminishes the increase in troponin levels after anthracycline use.[125] Dexrazoxane is recommended by the FDA for metastatic breast cancer patients who received a cumulative dose of $\geq$300 mg/m^2 doxorubicin and are continuing doxorubicin therapy.[126] ASCO supports the use of dexrazoxane in patients planned for high-dose anthracyclines (e.g., doxorubicin $\geq$250 mg/m^2, epirubicin $\geq$600 mg/m^2).[109] The European Medicines Agency has made similar recommendations, only allowing its use

TABLE 29.4: ACE Inhibitors and Beta-Blockers

Trial	Population	Results
OVERCOME[42]	Patients with hematological malignancies	Enalapril and carvedilol may prevent LV systolic dysfunction; did not decrease incidence of diastolic dysfunction
PRADA[117]	Early-stage breast cancer patients with adjuvant anthracycline regimens	Metoprolol had no effect on LVEF, while candesartan was protective
MANTICORE[118]	Trastuzumab-treated breast cancer patients	Small attenuation of LVEF decline by perindopril and bisoprolol
CECCY[119]	Anthracycline-treated patients	Carvedilol had a neutral effect at six-month follow-up, but decreased troponin levels and diastolic dysfunction

Abbreviations: ACE: angiotensin-converting enzyme, LV: left ventricle, LVEF: left ventricular ejection fraction.

TABLE 29.5: Proposed Cardioprotective Agents

Agent	Mechanism
ACEI, ARB	Afterload reduction
Beta-blockers	Afterload reduction
Statins	Anti-inflammatory and anti-fibrotic properties, interference with ROS generation, topoisomerase II inhibition
Dexrazoxane	Topoisomerase II inhibition, reduction of iron levels, decrease in ROS generation
Natural antioxidants	Reduction in ROS generation
Structured exercise therapy	Improvement in cardiorespiratory fitness

Abbreviations: ACEi: angiotensin-converting enzyme inhibitor, ARB: angiotensin II receptor blocker, ROS: reactive oxygen species.

for advanced or metastatic breast cancer patients who have received a cumulative dose of 300 mg/m^2 doxorubicin or 540 mg/m^2 epirubicin.[127] Dexrazoxane myocardial uptake is rapid, necessitating infusion within 30 min prior to anthracycline administration.[32,128] A 50% dose reduction is indicated for creatinine clearance <40 mL/min.[126] Dexrazoxane use is limited by concerns about impaired anthracycline effectiveness and increased risk of a secondary malignancy.

Natural antioxidants have been explored for their roles in cardioprotection.[129] Several agents have been suggested for their potential role in curbing the excessive production of ROS by cancer therapy. None of these are part of routine clinical use due to concerns that they may protect both normal and cancer cells against free radicals generated by most chemotherapeutics.

Structured exercise therapy is already a key component of comprehensive rehabilitation among various cardiac conditions, but cancer is not currently a qualifying condition for exercise rehabilitation.[130] Cardiorespiratory fitness declines 5–26% in response to exposure to certain cancer therapies[131,132] and may not recover after treatment cessation.[133,134] A recent comprehensive review of clinical trials yielded mixed results.[135] The analysis did conclude that overall exercise improves cardiorespiratory fitness after completion of cancer therapy. Various screening and evaluation approaches can be applied but must be individualized. Currently, there is no standardized exercise model that has been developed for these patients, but models will need to incorporate different training modalities, doses, and length of training programs.

Treatment

Strategies aimed at preventing LV dysfunction appear to be more effective than interventions aimed at counteracting existing damage. Although no clear guidelines for the treatment of CTRCD exist, routine clinical management remains the accepted standard of care for established asymptomatic LV dysfunction.[136] Prompt initiation of ACEi or ARB and beta-blockers is recommended after identification of LVEF impairment, with up-titration to the maximal tolerated dose.[10,137] LVEF recovers when therapy is initiated early (within one to two months), but improvement is unlikely after 12 months.[137] LVEF recovery is usually partial.[10] Enalapril and carvedilol are more effective in combination.[10,138] Both American and European Guidelines recommend combination treatment with an ACEi or ARB and a beta-blocker in patients with symptomatic HF, asymptomatic LV dysfunction, and those with LVEF decreases >10% to an absolute value below 50%.[136] There is no consensus on discontinuation of HF therapies in the event of full LVEF recovery, though in clinical practice these agents are most often continued if tolerated.[138,139]

Other therapies for chemotherapy-induced cardiomyopathy may be applicable, including implantable cardioverter defibrillators, chronic resynchronization therapy, LV assist devices, and orthotopic heart transplantation.[140] Practitioners should carefully consider the cancer prognosis and reversibility of LV dysfunction in such patients before proceeding with advanced therapies.

Dose alteration, interruption, or cessation of cancer therapy may be necessary in certain HF cases. These cases are often complicated and should be considered in the context of shared oncologic and cardiac risk. Patient care should be individualized and involve shared decision making between cardiologists and oncologists.

References

1. Chapman JA, Meng D, Shepherd L, et al. Competing causes of death from a randomized trial of extended adjuvant endocrine therapy for breast cancer. *J Natl Cancer Inst.* 2008;100:252–60.
2. Patnaik JL, Byers T, DiGuiseppi C, Dabelea D, Denberg TD. Cardiovascular disease competes with breast cancer as the leading cause of death for older females diagnosed with breast cancer: a retrospective cohort study. *Breast Cancer Res.* 2011;13:R64.
3. Plana JC, Galderisi M, Barac A, et al. Expert consensus for multimodality imaging evaluation of adult patients during and after cancer therapy: a report from the American Society of Echocardiography and the European Association of Cardiovascular Imaging. *Eur Heart J Cardiovasc Imaging.* 2014;15:1063–93.

4. Suter TM, Ewer MS. Cancer drugs and the heart: importance and management. *Eur Heart J.* 2013;34:1102–11.
5. Tanaka S, Ikari A, Nitta T, Horiuchi T. Long-term irreversible trastuzumab-induced cardiotoxicity for metastatic breast cancer in a patient without cardiac risk factors. *Oxf Med Case Reports.* 2017;2017:omx038.
6. ElZarrad MK, Mukhopadhyay P, Mohan N, et al. Trastuzumab alters the expression of genes essential for cardiac function and induces ultrastructural changes of cardiomyocytes in mice. *PLoS One.* 2013;8:e79543.
7. Wells QS, Lenihan DJ. Reversibility of left ventricular dysfunction resulting from chemotherapy: can this be expected? *Prog Cardiovasc Dis.* 2010;53:140–8.
8. Ewer MS, Vooletich MT, Durand JB, et al. Reversibility of trastuzumab-related cardiotoxicity: new insights based on clinical course and response to medical treatment. *J Clin Oncol.* 2005;23:7820–6.
9. Herrmann J, Lerman A, Sandhu NP, et al. Evaluation and management of patients with heart disease and cancer: cardio-oncology. *Mayo Clin Proc.* 2014;89:1287–306.
10. Cardinale D, Colombo A, Bacchiani G, et al. Early detection of anthracycline cardiotoxicity and improvement with heart failure therapy. *Circulation.* 2015;131:1981–8.
11. Thavendiranathan P, Poulin F, Lim KD, et al. Use of myocardial strain imaging by echocardiography for the early detection of cardiotoxicity in patients during and after cancer chemotherapy: a systematic review. *J Am Coll Cardiol.* 2014;63:2751–68.
12. Seidman A, Hudis C, Pierri MK, et al. Cardiac dysfunction in the trastuzumab clinical trials experience. *J Clin Oncol.* 2002;20:1215–21.
13. Schwartz RG, McKenzie WB, Alexander J, et al. Congestive heart failure and left ventricular dysfunction complicating doxorubicin therapy. Seven-year experience using serial radionuclide angiocardiography. *Am J Med.* 1987;82:1109–18.
14. Weir HK, Anderson RN, Coleman King SM, et al. Heart disease and cancer deaths - trends and projections in the United States, 1969–2020. *Prev Chronic Dis.* 2016;13:E157.
15. Vincent L, Leedy D, Masri SC, Cheng RK. Cardiovascular disease and cancer: is there increasing overlap? *Curr Oncol Rep.* 2019;21:47.
16. Hanrahan EO, Gonzalez-Angulo AM, Giordano SH, et al. Overall survival and cause-specific mortality of patients with stage T1a,bN0M0 breast carcinoma. *J Clin Oncol.* 2007;25:4952–60.
17. Mehta LS, Watson KE, Barac A, et al. Cardiovascular disease and breast cancer: where these entities intersect: a scientific statement from the American Heart Association. *Circulation.* 2018;137:e30–e66.
18. Zaorsky NG, Churilla TM, Egleston BL, et al. Causes of death among cancer patients. *Ann Oncol.* 2017;28:400–7.
19. Al-Kindi SG, Oliveira GH. Prevalence of preexisting cardiovascular disease in patients with different types of cancer: the unmet need for onco-cardiology. *Mayo Clin Proc.* 2016;91:81–3.
20. Klein R, Nadouri D, Osler E, et al. Diastolic dysfunction can precede systolic dysfunction on MUGA in cancer patients receiving trastuzumab-based therapy. *Nucl Med Commun.* 2019;40:22–9.
21. Ezaz G, Long JB, Gross CP, Chen J. Risk prediction model for heart failure and cardiomyopathy after adjuvant trastuzumab therapy for breast cancer. *J Am Heart Assoc.* 2014;3:e000472.
22. Bhave M, Shah AN, Akhter N, Rosen ST. An update on the risk prediction and prevention of anticancer therapy-induced cardiotoxicity. *Curr Opin Oncol.* 2014;26:590–9.
23. Curigliano G, Cardinale D, Suter T, et al. Cardiovascular toxicity induced by chemotherapy, targeted agents and radiotherapy: ESMO clinical practice guidelines. *Ann Oncol.* 2012;23 Suppl 7:vii155–66.
24. Tajiri K, Aonuma K, Sekine I. Cardio-oncology: a multidisciplinary approach for detection, prevention and management of cardiac dysfunction in cancer patients. *Jpn J Clin Oncol.* 2017;47:678–82.
25. Lemieux J, Diorio C, Cote MA, et al. Alcohol and HER2 polymorphisms as risk factor for cardiotoxicity in breast cancer treated with trastuzumab. *Anticancer Res.* 2013;33:2569–76.
26. Reinbolt RE, Patel R, Pan X, et al. Risk factors for anthracycline-associated cardiotoxicity. *Support Care Cancer.* 2016;24:2173–80.
27. Dranitsaris G, Rayson D, Vincent M, et al. The development of a predictive model to estimate cardiotoxic risk for patients with metastatic breast cancer receiving anthracyclines. *Breast Cancer Res Treat.* 2008;107:443–50.
28. Romond EH, Jeong JH, Rastogi P, et al. Seven-year follow-up assessment of cardiac function in NSABP B-31, a randomized trial comparing doxorubicin and cyclophosphamide followed by paclitaxel (ACP) with ACP plus trastuzumab as adjuvant therapy for patients with node-positive, human epidermal growth factor receptor 2-positive breast cancer. *J Clin Oncol.* 2012;30:3792–9.
29. Tewey KM, Rowe TC, Yang L, Halligan BD, Liu LF. Adriamycin-induced DNA damage mediated by mammalian DNA topoisomerase II. *Science.* 1984;226:466–8.
30. Vejpongsa P, Yeh ET. Topoisomerase 2beta: a promising molecular target for primary prevention of anthracycline-induced cardiotoxicity. *Clin Pharmacol Ther.* 2014;95:45–52.
31. Lyu YL, Kerrigan JE, Lin CP, et al. Topoisomerase IIbeta mediated DNA double-strand breaks: implications in doxorubicin cardiotoxicity and prevention by dexrazoxane. *Cancer Res.* 2007;67:8839–46.
32. Caspi O, Aronson D. Surviving cancer without a broken heart. *Rambam Maimonides Med J.* 2019;10:1–22.
33. De Angelis A, Piegari E, Cappetta D, et al. Anthracycline cardiomyopathy is mediated by depletion of the cardiac stem cell pool and is rescued by restoration of progenitor cell function. *Circulation.* 2010;121:276–92.
34. Huang C, Zhang X, Ramil JM, et al. Juvenile exposure to anthracyclines impairs cardiac progenitor cell function and vascularization resulting in greater susceptibility to stress-induced myocardial injury in adult mice. *Circulation.* 2010;121:675–83.
35. Markman TM, Markman M. Cardio-oncology: mechanisms of cardiovascular toxicity. *F1000Res.* 2018;7:113.
36. Von Hoff DD, Layard MW, Basa P, et al. Risk factors for doxorubicin-induced congestive heart failure. *Ann Intern Med.* 1979;91:710–7.
37. Alexander J, Dainiak N, Berger HJ, et al. Serial assessment of doxorubicin cardiotoxicity with quantitative radionuclide angiocardiography. *N Engl J Med.* 1979;300:278–83.
38. Swain SM, Whaley FS, Ewer MS. Congestive heart failure in patients treated with doxorubicin: a retrospective analysis of three trials. *Cancer.* 2003;97:2869–79.
39. Jones RL, Swanton C, Ewer MS. Anthracycline cardiotoxicity. *Expert Opin Drug Saf.* 2006;5:791–809.
40. Volkova M, Russell R, 3rd. Anthracycline cardiotoxicity: prevalence, pathogenesis and treatment. *Curr Cardiol Rev.* 2011;7:214–20.
41. Safra T. Cardiac safety of liposomal anthracyclines. *Oncologist.* 2003;8 Suppl 2:17–24.
42. Bosch X, Rovira M, Sitges M, et al. Enalapril and carvedilol for preventing chemotherapy-induced left ventricular systolic dysfunction in patients with malignant hemopathies: the OVERCOME trial (preventiOn of left Ventricular dysfunction with Enalapril and caRvedilol in patients submitted to intensive ChemOtherapy for the treatment of Malignant hEmopathies). *J Am Coll Cardiol.* 2013;61:2355–62.
43. van Dalen EC, Caron HN, Dickinson HO, Kremer LC. Cardioprotective interventions for cancer patients receiving anthracyclines. *Cochrane Database Syst Rev.* 2011:CD003917.
44. Slamon DJ, Clark GM, Wong SG, et al. Human breast cancer: correlation of relapse and survival with amplification of the HER-2/neu oncogene. *Science.* 1987;235:177–82.
45. Slamon DJ, Leyland-Jones B, Shak S, et al. Use of chemotherapy plus a monoclonal antibody against HER2 for metastatic breast cancer that overexpresses HER2. *N Engl J Med.* 2001;344:783–92.
46. The Human Protein Atlas. ERBB2. https://www.proteinatlas.org/ENSG00000141736-ERBB2/tissue. Accessed April 7, 2022.
47. Ozcelik C, Erdmann B, Pilz B, et al. Conditional mutation of the ErbB2 (HER2) receptor in cardiomyocytes leads to dilated cardiomyopathy. *Proc Natl Acad Sci U S A.* 2002;99:8880–5.
48. Pugatsch T, Abedat S, Lotan C, Beeri R. Anti-erbB2 treatment induces cardiotoxicity by interfering with cell survival pathways. *Breast Cancer Res.* 2006;8:R35.
49. Monsuez JJ, Charniot JC, Vignat N, Artigou JY. Cardiac side-effects of cancer chemotherapy. *Int J Cardiol.* 2010;144:3–15.
50. Zeglinski M, Ludke A, Jassal DS, Singal PK. Trastuzumab-induced cardiac dysfunction: a "dual-hit." *Exp Clin Cardiol.* 2011;16:70–4.
51. Bowles EJ, Wellman R, Feigelson HS, et al. Risk of heart failure in breast cancer patients after anthracycline and trastuzumab treatment: a retrospective cohort study. *J Natl Cancer Inst.* 2012;104:1293–305.
52. Ewer MS, Lippman SM. Type II chemotherapy-related cardiac dysfunction: time to recognize a new entity. *J Clin Oncol.* 2005;23:2900–2.
53. Moja L, Tagliabue L, Balduzzi S, et al. Trastuzumab containing regimens for early breast cancer. *Cochrane Database Syst Rev.* 2012:CD006243.
54. Valachis A, Nearchou A, Polyzos NP, Lind P. Cardiac toxicity in breast cancer patients treated with dual HER2 blockade. *Int J Cancer.* 2013;133:2245–52.
55. von Minckwitz G, Procter M, de Azambuja E, et al. Adjuvant pertuzumab and trastuzumab in early HER2-positive breast cancer. *N Engl J Med.* 2017;377:122–31.
56. Farolfi A, Melegari E, Aquilina M, et al. Trastuzumab-induced cardiotoxicity in early breast cancer patients: a retrospective study of possible risk and protective factors. *Heart.* 2013;99:634–9.
57. Ganz PA, Romond EH, Cecchini RS, et al. Long-term follow-up of cardiac function and quality of life for patients in NSABP protocol B-31/NRG oncology: a randomized trial comparing the safety and efficacy of doxorubicin and cyclophosphamide (AC) followed by paclitaxel with AC followed by paclitaxel and trastuzumab in patients with node-positive breast cancer with tumors overexpressing human epidermal growth factor receptor 2. *J Clin Oncol.* 2017;35:3942–8.
58. FDA Drug Label for Herceptin (trastuzumab). Available at: https://www.accessdata.fda.gov/drugsatfda_docs/label/2010/103792s5250lbl.pdf. Accessed June 19, 2019.
59. Mahmood SS, Fradley MG, Cohen JV, et al. Myocarditis in patients treated with immune checkpoint inhibitors. *J Am Coll Cardiol.* 2018;71:1755–64.

60. Jain V, Bahia J, Mohebtash M, Barac A. Cardiovascular complications associated with novel cancer immunotherapies. *Curr Treat Options Cardiovasc Med.* 2017;19:36.
61. Johnson DB, Balko JM, Compton ML, et al. Fulminant myocarditis with combination immune checkpoint blockade. *N Engl J Med.* 2016;375:1749–55.
62. Voskens CJ, Goldinger SM, Loquai C, et al. The price of tumor control: an analysis of rare side effects of anti-CTLA-4 therapy in metastatic melanoma from the ipilimumab network. *PLoS One.* 2013;8:e53745.
63. Roth ME, Muluneh B, Jensen BC, Madamanchi C, Lee CB. Left ventricular dysfunction after treatment with ipilimumab for metastatic melanoma. *Am J Ther.* 2016;23:e1925–8.
64. Geisler BP, Raad RA, Esaian D, Sharon E, Schwartz DR. Apical ballooning and cardiomyopathy in a melanoma patient treated with ipilimumab: a case of takotsubo-like syndrome. *J Immunother Cancer.* 2015;3:4.
65. Tarrio ML, Grabie N, Bu DX, Sharpe AH, Lichtman AH. PD-1 protects against inflammation and myocyte damage in T cell-mediated myocarditis. *J Immunol.* 2012;188:4876–84.
66. Brahmer JR, Lacchetti C, Schneider BJ, et al. Management of immune-related adverse events in patients treated with immune checkpoint inhibitor therapy: American Society of Clinical Oncology Clinical Practice Guideline. *J Clin Oncol.* 2018;36:1714–68.
67. Gharib MI, Burnett AK. Chemotherapy-induced cardiotoxicity: current practice and prospects of prophylaxis. *Eur J Heart Fail.* 2002;4: 235–42.
68. Minotti G, Menna P, Salvatorelli E, Cairo G, Gianni L. Anthracyclines: molecular advances and pharmacologic developments in antitumor activity and cardiotoxicity. *Pharmacol Rev.* 2004;56:185–229.
69. Martin M, Pienkowski T, Mackey J, et al. Adjuvant docetaxel for node-positive breast cancer. *N Engl J Med.* 2005;352:2302–13.
70. Gottdiener JS, Appelbaum FR, Ferrans VJ, Deisseroth A, Ziegler J. Cardiotoxicity associated with high-dose cyclophosphamide therapy. *Arch Intern Med.* 1981;141:758–63.
71. Quezado ZM, Wilson WH, Cunnion RE, et al. High-dose ifosfamide is associated with severe, reversible cardiac dysfunction. *Ann Intern Med.* 1993;118:31–6.
72. Nieto Y, Cagnoni PJ, Bearman SI, et al. Cardiac toxicity following high-dose cyclophosphamide, cisplatin, and BCNU (STAMP-I) for breast cancer. *Biol Blood Marrow Transplant.* 2000;6:198–203.
73. Uitdehaag JC, de Roos JA, van Doornmalen AM, et al. Comparison of the cancer gene targeting and biochemical selectivities of all targeted kinase inhibitors approved for clinical use. *PLoS One.* 2014;9:e92146.
74. Small HY, Montezano AC, Rios FJ, Savoia C, Touyz RM. Hypertension due to antiangiogenic cancer therapy with vascular endothelial growth factor inhibitors: understanding and managing a new syndrome. *Can J Cardiol.* 2014;30:534–43.
75. Chu TF, Rupnick MA, Kerkela R, et al. Cardiotoxicity associated with tyrosine kinase inhibitor sunitinib. *Lancet.* 2007;370:2011–9.
76. Eschenhagen T, Force T, Ewer MS, et al. Cardiovascular side effects of cancer therapies: a position statement from the Heart Failure Association of the European Society of Cardiology. *Eur J Heart Fail.* 2011;13:1–10.
77. Dobbin SJH, Cameron AC, Petrie MC, et al. Toxicity of cancer therapy: what the cardiologist needs to know about angiogenesis inhibitors. *Heart.* 2018;104:1995–2002.
78. Qi WX, Fu S, Zhang Q, Guo XM. Bevacizumab increases the risk of severe congestive heart failure in cancer patients: an up-to-date meta-analysis with a focus on different subgroups. *Clin Drug Investig.* 2014;34:681–90.
79. Kane RC, Farrell AT, Saber H, et al. Sorafenib for the treatment of advanced renal cell carcinoma. *Clin Cancer Res.* 2006;12:7271–8.
80. Wu S, Chen JJ, Kudelka A, Lu J, Zhu X. Incidence and risk of hypertension with sorafenib in patients with cancer: a systematic review and meta-analysis. *Lancet Oncol.* 2008;9:117–23.
81. Fanous I, Dillon P. Cancer treatment-related cardiac toxicity: prevention, assessment and management. *Med Oncol.* 2016;33:84.
82. Kerkela R, Grazette L, Yacobi R, et al. Cardiotoxicity of the cancer therapeutic agent imatinib mesylate. *Nat Med.* 2006;12:908–16.
83. Meiners S, Dreger H, Fechner M, et al. Suppression of cardiomyocyte hypertrophy by inhibition of the ubiquitin-proteasome system. *Hypertension.* 2008;51:302–8.
84. Nowis D, Maczewski M, Mackiewicz U, et al. Cardiotoxicity of the anticancer therapeutic agent bortezomib. *Am J Pathol.* 2010;176: 2658–68.
85. Koulaouzidis G, Lyon AR. Proteasome inhibitors as a potential cause of heart failure. *Heart Fail Clin.* 2017;13:289–95.
86. Xiao Y, Yin J, Wei J, Shang Z. Incidence and risk of cardiotoxicity associated with bortezomib in the treatment of cancer: a systematic review and meta-analysis. *PLoS One.* 2014;9:e87671.
87. Dimopoulos MA, Roussou M, Gavriatopoulou M, et al. Cardiac and renal complications of carfilzomib in patients with multiple myeloma. *Blood Adv.* 2017;1:449–54.
88. Dimopoulos MA, Moreau P, Palumbo A, et al. Carfilzomib and dexamethasone versus bortezomib and dexamethasone for patients with relapsed or refractory multiple myeloma (ENDEAVOR): a randomised, phase 3, open-label, multicentre study. *Lancet Oncol.* 2016;17:27–38.
89. McLaughlin PY, Kong W, de Metz C, et al. Do radiation oncology outreach clinics affect the use of radiotherapy? *Radiother Oncol.* 2018;127:143–9.
90. Carver JR, Shapiro CL, Ng A, et al. American Society of Clinical Oncology clinical evidence review on the ongoing care of adult cancer survivors: cardiac and pulmonary late effects. *J Clin Oncol.* 2007;25:3991–4008.
91. Filopei J, Frishman W. Radiation-induced heart disease. *Cardiol Rev.* 2012;20:184–8.
92. Jacob S, Pathak A, Franck D, et al. Early detection and prediction of cardiotoxicity after radiation therapy for breast cancer: the BACCARAT prospective cohort study. *Radiat Oncol.* 2016;11:54.
93. Saiki H, Petersen IA, Scott CG, et al. Risk of heart failure with preserved ejection fraction in older women after contemporary radiotherapy for breast cancer. *Circulation.* 2017;135:1388–96.
94. McGale P, Darby SC, Hall P, et al. Incidence of heart disease in 35,000 women treated with radiotherapy for breast cancer in Denmark and Sweden. *Radiother Oncol.* 2011;100:167–75.
95. Lancellotti P, Nkomo VT, Badano LP, et al. Expert consensus for multi-modality imaging evaluation of cardiovascular complications of radiotherapy in adults: a report from the European Association of Cardiovascular Imaging and the American Society of Echocardiography. *J Am Soc Echocardiogr.* 2013;26:1013–32.
96. Rehammar JC, Jensen MB, McGale P, et al. Risk of heart disease in relation to radiotherapy and chemotherapy with anthracyclines among 19,464 breast cancer patients in Denmark, 1977–2005. *Radiother Oncol.* 2017;123:299–305.
97. Michel L, Rassaf T, Totzeck M. Biomarkers for the detection of apparent and subclinical cancer therapy-related cardiotoxicity. *J Thorac Dis.* 2018;10:S4282–95.
98. Christenson ES, James T, Agrawal V, Park BH. Use of biomarkers for the assessment of chemotherapy-induced cardiac toxicity. *Clin Biochem.* 2015;48:223–35.
99. Biasillo G, Cipolla CM, Cardinale D. Cardio-oncology: gaps in knowledge, goals, advances, and educational efforts. *Curr Oncol Rep.* 2017;19:55.
100. Cardinale D, Sandri MT, Colombo A, et al. Prognostic value of troponin I in cardiac risk stratification of cancer patients undergoing high-dose chemotherapy. *Circulation.* 2004;109:2749–54.
101. Bloom MW, Hamo CE, Cardinale D, et al. Cancer therapy-related cardiac dysfunction and heart failure: part 1: definitions, pathophysiology, risk factors, and imaging. *Circ Heart Fail.* 2016;9:e002661.
102. Tan LL, Lyon AR. Role of biomarkers in prediction of cardiotoxicity during cancer treatment. *Curr Treat Options Cardiovasc Med.* 2018;20:55.
103. Colombo A, Sandri MT, Salvatici M, Cipolla CM, Cardinale D. Cardiac complications of chemotherapy: role of biomarkers. *Curr Treat Options Cardiovasc Med.* 2014;16:313.
104. Cardinale D, Colombo A, Torrisi R, et al. Trastuzumab-induced cardiotoxicity: clinical and prognostic implications of troponin I evaluation. *J Clin Oncol.* 2010;28:3910–6.
105. Larsen CM, Mulvagh SL. Cardio-oncology: what you need to know now for clinical practice and echocardiography. *Echo Res Pract.* 2017;4:R33–R41.
106. Cardinale D, Bacchiani G, Beggiato M, Colombo A, Cipolla CM. Strategies to prevent and treat cardiovascular risk in cancer patients. *Semin Oncol.* 2013;40:186–98.
107. Sawaya H, Sebag IA, Plana JC, et al. Assessment of echocardiography and biomarkers for the extended prediction of cardiotoxicity in patients treated with anthracyclines, taxanes, and trastuzumab. *Circ Cardiovasc Imaging.* 2012;5:596–603.
108. Lipshultz SE, Miller TL, Scully RE, et al. Changes in cardiac biomarkers during doxorubicin treatment of pediatric patients with high-risk acute lymphoblastic leukemia: associations with long-term echocardiographic outcomes. *J Clin Oncol.* 2012;30:1042–9.
109. Armenian SH, Lacchetti C, Barac A, et al. Prevention and monitoring of cardiac dysfunction in survivors of adult cancers: American Society of Clinical Oncology Clinical Practice Guideline. *J Clin Oncol.* 2017;35:893–911.
110. Mulvagh SL, Rakowski H, Vannan MA, et al. American Society of Echocardiography consensus statement on the clinical applications of ultrasonic contrast agents in echocardiography. *J Am Soc Echocardiogr.* 2008;21:1179–201; quiz 1281.
111. Trivedi SJ, Choudhary P, Lo Q, et al. Persistent reduction in global longitudinal strain in the longer term after radiation therapy in patients with breast cancer. *Radiother Oncol.* 2019;132:148–54.
112. Negishi K, Negishi T, Hare JL, et al. Independent and incremental value of deformation indices for prediction of trastuzumab-induced cardiotoxicity. *J Am Soc Echocardiogr.* 2013;26:493–8.

113. Neilan TG, Coelho-Filho OR, Pena-Herrera D, et al. Left ventricular mass in patients with a cardiomyopathy after treatment with anthracyclines. *Am J Cardiol.* 2012;110:1679–86.
114. Kolla BC, Roy SS, Duval S, et al. Cardiac imaging methods for chemotherapy-related cardiotoxicity screening and related radiation exposure: current practice and trends. *Anticancer Res.* 2017;37:2445–9.
115. Mettler FA, Jr., Huda W, Yoshizumi TT, Mahesh M. Effective doses in radiology and diagnostic nuclear medicine: a catalog. *Radiology.* 2008;248:254–63.
116. Kalam K, Marwick TH. Role of cardioprotective therapy for prevention of cardiotoxicity with chemotherapy: a systematic review and meta-analysis. *Eur J Cancer.* 2013;49:2900–9.
117. Gulati G, Heck SL, Ree AH, et al. Prevention of cardiac dysfunction during adjuvant breast cancer therapy (PRADA): a 2 x 2 factorial, randomized, placebo-controlled, double-blind clinical trial of candesartan and metoprolol. *Eur Heart J.* 2016;37:1671–80.
118. Pituskin E, Mackey JR, Koshman S, et al. Multidisciplinary approach to novel therapies in cardio-oncology research (MANTICORE 101-breast): a randomized trial for the prevention of trastuzumab-associated cardiotoxicity. *J Clin Oncol.* 2017;35:870–7.
119. Avila MS, Ayub-Ferreira SM, de Barros Wanderley MR, Jr., et al. Carvedilol for prevention of chemotherapy-related cardiotoxicity: the CECCY trial. *J Am Coll Cardiol.* 2018;71:2281–90.
120. Seicean S, Seicean A, Plana JC, Budd GT, Marwick TH. Effect of statin therapy on the risk for incident heart failure in patients with breast cancer receiving anthracycline chemotherapy: an observational clinical cohort study. *J Am Coll Cardiol.* 2012;60:2384–90.
121. Henninger C, Fritz G. Statins in anthracycline-induced cardiotoxicity: Rac and Rho, and the heartbreakers. *Cell Death Dis.* 2017;8:e2564.
122. Classen S, Olland S, Berger JM. Structure of the topoisomerase II ATPase region and its mechanism of inhibition by the chemotherapeutic agent ICRF-187. *Proc Natl Acad Sci U S A.* 2003;100:10629–34.
123. Ichikawa Y, Ghanefar M, Bayeva M, et al. Cardiotoxicity of doxorubicin is mediated through mitochondrial iron accumulation. *J Clin Invest.* 2014;124:617–30.
124. Hasinoff BB. The interaction of the cardioprotective agent ICRF-187 [+)-1,2-bis(3,5-dioxopiperazinyl-1-yL)propane); its hydrolysis product (ICRF-198); and other chelating agents with the Fe(III) and Cu(II) complexes of adriamycin. *Agents Actions.* 1989;26:378–85.
125. Lipshultz SE, Scully RE, Lipsitz SR, et al. Assessment of dexrazoxane as a cardioprotectant in doxorubicin-treated children with high-risk acute lymphoblastic leukaemia: long-term follow-up of a prospective, randomised, multicentre trial. *Lancet Oncol.* 2010;11:950–61.
126. Pfizer. Zinecard (dexrazoxane) [package insert]. U.S. Food and Drug Administration. 2014. https://www.accessdata.fda.gov/drugsatfda_docs/label/2014/020212s017lbl.pdf. Accessed 6/19/19.
127. European Medicines Agency website. Cardioxane. 2017. Available at: https://www.ema.europa.eu/en/medicines/human/referrals/cardioxane (Accessed June 19, 2019).
128. Sepe DM, Ginsberg JP, Balis FM. Dexrazoxane as a cardioprotectant in children receiving anthracyclines. *Oncologist.* 2010;15:1220–6.
129. Zhang J, Cui X, Yan Y, et al. Research progress of cardioprotective agents for prevention of anthracycline cardiotoxicity. *Am J Transl Res.* 2016;8:2862–75.
130. Lakoski SG, Eves ND, Douglas PS, Jones LW. Exercise rehabilitation in patients with cancer. *Nat Rev Clin Oncol.* 2012;9:288–96.
131. Hurria A, Jones L, Muss HB. Cancer treatment as an accelerated aging process: assessment, biomarkers, and interventions. *Am Soc Clin Oncol Educ Book.* 2016;35:e516–22.
132. Jarden M, Hovgaard D, Boesen E, Quist M, Adamsen L. Pilot study of a multimodal intervention: mixed-type exercise and psychoeducation in patients undergoing allogeneic stem cell transplantation. *Bone Marrow Transplant.* 2007;40:793–800.
133. Jones LW, Courneya KS, Mackey JR, et al. Cardiopulmonary function and age-related decline across the breast cancer survivorship continuum. *J Clin Oncol.* 2012;30:2530–7.
134. Adams MJ, Lipsitz SR, Colan SD, et al. Cardiovascular status in long-term survivors of Hodgkin's disease treated with chest radiotherapy. *J Clin Oncol.* 2004;22:3139–48.
135. Scott JM, Nilsen TS, Gupta D, Jones LW. Exercise therapy and cardiovascular toxicity in cancer. *Circulation.* 2018;137:1176–91.
136. Zamorano JL, Lancellotti P, Rodriguez Munoz D, et al. 2016 ESC position paper on cancer treatments and cardiovascular toxicity developed under the auspices of the ESC Committee for practice guidelines: the task force for cancer treatments and cardiovascular toxicity of the European Society of Cardiology (ESC). *Eur Heart J.* 2016;37:2768–801.
137. Cardinale D, Colombo A, Lamantia G, et al. Anthracycline-induced cardiomyopathy: clinical relevance and response to pharmacologic therapy. *J Am Coll Cardiol.* 2010;55:213–20.
138. Ponikowski P, Voors AA, Anker SD, et al. 2016 ESC guidelines for the diagnosis and treatment of acute and chronic heart failure: the task force for the diagnosis and treatment of acute and chronic heart failure of the European Society of Cardiology (ESC). Developed with the special contribution of the Heart Failure Association (HFA) of the ESC. *Eur J Heart Fail.* 2016;18:891–975.
139. Yancy CW, Jessup M, Bozkurt B, et al. 2017 ACC/AHA/HFSA focused update of the 2013 ACCF/AHA guideline for the management of heart failure: a report of the American College of Cardiology/American Heart Association Task Force on Clinical Practice Guidelines and the Heart Failure Society of America. *J Card Fail.* 2017;23:628–51.
140. Hamo CE, Bloom MW, Cardinale D, et al. Cancer therapy-related cardiac dysfunction and heart failure: part 2: prevention, treatment, guidelines, and future directions. *Circ Heart Fail.* 2016;9:e002843.

Chapter 30
PERIPARTUM CARDIOMYOPATHY AND HEART FAILURE IN PREGNANCY

Anita Saraf and Fred H. Rodriguez III

Introduction

In the United States, cardiac disease is the leading cause of mortality in pregnancy, contributing to 25.9% of pregnancy-related deaths annually, as reported by the Pregnancy Mortality Surveillance System in the period 2011–2015.[1] The incidence of heart failure (HF) in pregnancy continues to rise, partly through improved recognition of the disease but also due to a change in demographics of the obstetric population. Average maternal age at childbirth is increasing, as is the proportion of high-risk pregnancies through assisted reproductive techniques. Although scientific advances have allowed many women to carry pregnancies successfully, the cardiovascular burden imparted by the hemodynamic and hormonal changes of pregnancy and long-term consequences on women's health are not yet fully appreciated. Pregnancy-related HF either develops *de novo*, in which case it is referred to as peripartum cardiomyopathy (PPCM), or is exacerbated during pregnancy because of preexisting structural heart disease, including congenital heart disease. In either case, HF symptoms are confounded by normal signs and symptoms of pregnancy, such as peripheral edema, shortness of breath, and fatigue. Delay in HF diagnosis in pregnant women, by even as little as a week, can be catastrophic for the woman and her baby.[2] Hence, continued education about pregnancy-related HF amongst health care providers and increased vigilance for signs of HF are essential in establishing standards of care and decreasing mortality.

Cardiovascular Physiology during Pregnancy

During pregnancy, the cardiovascular system undergoes hemodynamic and structural changes, including a decrease in systemic vascular resistance and an increase in cardiac output (CO), to accommodate the demands of a growing fetus and other organ systems (Table 30.1).[3] Plasma volume increases by 50% by week 34 of gestation.[4] However, cardiovascular demands increase as early as week 8 of gestation, when there is an increase in CO by 20%. This increased flow state is accommodated primarily by a decrease in systemic vascular resistance but also through an increase in stroke volume and heart rate. Echocardiographic and magnetic resonance imaging studies have shown an increase in left ventricular (LV) end-diastolic volume, an increase in LV mass, and an increase in CO during pregnancy.[5] Furthermore, CO increases by an additional 15% in twin pregnancies as compared to singleton pregnancies and is associated with a greater increase in cardiac chamber dimensions.[6] Though multiple cardiac parameters are altered during pregnancy,[7] myocardial contractility,[8] and left and right ventricular ejection fractions do not change in pregnancy.[5] Labor and delivery, by far, impose the most hemodynamic stress on the heart. CO increases by 60–80% at the onset of labor.[7] This is attributed to multiple acute changes, including increasing heart rate, increased preload from autotransfusion from the uterus into the systemic circulation as well as an increase in catecholamine response.[9] In addition to associated hemodynamic changes, the body of the expectant mother undergoes significant hormonal changes as well.

Clinical Signs and Physical Examination Findings

A comprehensive history and a thorough physical exam are essential in distinguishing signs of HF from normal signs and symptoms of pregnancy (Table 30.2). While fatigue, decreased exercise capacity, abdominal discomfort, mild pedal edema, and heart palpitations may normally occur as pregnancy progresses, a persistent cough or similar respiratory symptoms, new onset of nausea and food aversion in the 2nd and 3rd trimester of pregnancy, paroxysmal nocturnal dyspnea, orthopnea, significant pitting edema, or persistent tachycardia should alert the health care provider to seek additional tests to exclude HF. Physical examination reflective of elevated jugular venous pressure, persistent sinus tachycardia, or new murmurs indicating mitral regurgitation may indicate the presence of HF (Table 30.3). However, a third heart sound (S3) and systolic flow murmurs are findings of a normal pregnancy as well. An electrocardiogram can quantify the severity of tachycardia and identify changes in QRS as well as ST-T wave morphology. Holter monitoring can quantify arrhythmia burden. Echocardiography is a cornerstone in evaluating cardiac function and diagnosing new-onset HF in pregnancy. However, in cases where HF precedes pregnancy or there is known structural heart disease, changes in echocardiographic findings may be more subtle. Even with a normal pregnancy, there is a mild increase in the volume of cardiac cambers.[10] In these cases, serial monitoring of biomarkers such as B-type natriuretic peptide (BNP) throughout pregnancy may provide insights into the progression of HF.[11,12] BNP <100 pg/mL has been shown to have a negative predictive value of 100% for identifying cardiac events during pregnancy.[11] Additional imaging techniques, such as magnetic resonance imaging (MRI), have also been used during pregnancy but are limited to identifying fibrosis and presence of scar tissue due to contraindication of gadolinium use during pregnancy.

Peripartum Cardiomyopathy

The definition of peripartum cardiomyopathy (PPCM) in the United States was established in 1997 by the participants of the National Heart Lung Blood Institute (NHLBI) workshop[13] and is defined as the onset of HF between one month before delivery up to five months postpartum. The European Society of Cardiology guidelines are less stringent and their definition states PPCM as "HF secondary to LV systolic dysfunction towards the end of pregnancy and in the months following delivery, with the majority diagnosed post-partum."[14] In addition to the clinical signs of HF, the definition

DOI: 10.1201/9780429244544-37

TABLE 30.1: Hemodynamic Changes during Pregnancy, Labor, and Delivery, and the Postpartum Period

Hemodynamic Parameter	Change during Normal Pregnancy	Change during Labor and Delivery	Change during Postpartum
Blood volume	↑ 50%	↑	↓
Heart rate	↑ 10–15 beats/min	↑	↓
Cardiac output	↑ 50% (by third trimester)	↑	↓
Systolic blood pressure	↓ 10–20 mmHg	↑	↓
Stroke volume	↑ First and second trimesters	↑	↓
Systemic vascular resistance	↓	↑	↓
Basal oxygen consumption	↑	↑	↓

Source: Reprinted from Hebson, Saraf, and Book. Risk assessment and management of the mother with cardiovascular disease. *Clin Perinatol.* 2016;43(1):1–22.

TABLE 30.2: Normal and Abnormal Signs in Pregnancy

Normal Signs and Symptoms in Pregnancy	Abnormal Signs in Pregnancy
Increase in heart rate by 10–20 bpm	Persistent tachycardia > 100 bpm
Occasional brief palpitations, premature ventricular, and atrial complexes	Paroxysmal nocturnal dyspnea
Fatigue	Orthopnea
Shortness of breath on exertion	Persistent cough
S3	4th Heart sound
Soft systolic or flow murmurs	Diastolic murmurs
Mild peripheral edema	Jugular venous distention
Abdominal discomfort	Persistent nausea and vomiting in 2nd or 3rd trimester

TABLE 30.3: Diagnostic Work-Up for HF in Pregnancy and Peripartum Cardiomyopathy

Physical examination	Tachycardia, elevated jugular venous pulsation, 3rd heart sound, holosystolic murmur of tricuspid or mitral regurgitation. Displaced apical impulse. Pulmonary edema with crackles or peripheral edema.
Clinical signs	Dyspnea, orthopnea, paroxysmal nocturnal dyspnea, cough, chest pain, abdominal pain
EKG	Sinus tachycardia Non-specific ST-T wave changes
Laboratory results	Elevated BNP or N-terminal proBNP
Echocardiogram	Global left ventricular (LV) systolic dysfunction with varying degrees of LV dilation. Right ventricular dilation Bi-atrial dilation Atrio-ventricular valve regurgitation. Women with PPCM with full myocardial recovery have decreased contractile reserve as measured by dobutamine stress echo.
MRI findings	Used for diagnosis of LV thrombus and wall motion abnormalities. Gadolinium should be avoided during pregnancy.

requires absence of identifiable causes of HF, absence of recognizable heart disease prior to the last month of pregnancy, and LV systolic dysfunction by echocardiography with an ejection fraction <45% or a fractional shortening <30% (Table 30.4).[15] Determining the incidence of PPCM is limited by variability in reporting standards across the world.[16] In the United States, incidence is estimated at 1 in 968 live births,[17] whereas in Asia and South Africa its incidence is 1 in 1,000 live births.[18] United Kingdom and Japan have much lower incidence of 1 in 5,000–10,000 live births[16] and 1 in 6,000 live births, respectively.[19] Similarly, PPCM-associated mortality shows regional variability; six-month outcomes have shown 2% mortality in Germany,[20] 12.6% mortality in South Africa,[21] and 24% mortality in Turkey.[22] In a multi-center trial within the United States, Investigations of Pregnancy-Associated Cardiomyopathy (IPAC), 13% of patients had major events or severe cardiomyopathy at one year.[23]

Risk Factors for PPCM

As compared to the worldwide population, incidence of PPCM is up to 16-fold higher in women in Haitian or South African populations.[13] Older age, a history of hypertension, increased parity, and twin pregnancies increase the risk of PPCM. Most women in the United States are diagnosed between 27–33 years of age and >60% of women are older than 30 years at diagnosis. History of hypertension, including chronic hypertension and pregnancy-induced hypertension (onset after 18 weeks of gestation), and preeclampsia, increase the risk of PPCM. Multiparity has previously been identified as a risk factor; however, recent studies have shown that PPCM occurs during first and second pregnancies as well. PPCM has been reported in 24–37% of primigravidae women.[24] Adverse outcomes are associated with an initial LVEF of <30%, LV dilation with LV end-diastolic diameter of ≥6.0 cm, and right ventricular (RV) involvement[14]

TABLE 30.4: Criteria for Diagnosing Peripartum Cardiomyopathy

Criteria for Diagnosing PPCM
NHLB (United States) definition: Onset of heart failure one month prior and up to five months after delivery
European Society of Cardiology definition: Heart failure secondary to LV systolic dysfunction towards the end of pregnancy and in the months following delivery, with the majority diagnosed postpartum
Additional criteria:
• Absence of identifiable causes of heart failure
• Absence of recognizable heart disease prior to last month of pregnancy
• LV systolic dysfunction by echocardiography with an LV ejection fraction of <45% or fractional shortening of <30%

Pathophysiology of PPCM

Thus far, a single unifying hypothesis defining the origin of PPCM has not been identified. Multiple mechanisms have been suggested as possible driving factors in inducing PPCM and have been described comprehensively by Lindley et al[25] and others.[2,12,16,26–33] Given regional and familial clustering of PPCM, there is a clear genetic predisposition. Furthermore, there is a significant overlap between PPCM and idiopathic, dilated cardiomyopathy within family clusters, and, in these cases, mutations causing premature truncation of protein titin may be responsible.[34] Other implicated mutations have involved proteins associated with titin, suggesting that functional disruption of titin within the cardiomyocyte may be central to the development of PPCM.[35] However, titin-associated cardiomyopathies constitute only a small percentage of PPCM.[34]

Other pathophysiologic mechanisms have suggested an angiogenic imbalance during late pregnancy.[30,33,36] In late gestation, the placenta secretes numerous anti-angiogenic factors, e.g., soluble fms-like tyrosine kinase 1,[33] that are disproportionately upregulated in preeclampsia and PPCM.[31] This exaggerated anti-angiogenic response by the placenta causes endothelial dysfunction, microvascular ischemia, and cardiomyocyte death.[34] With multiple gestations, these antiangiogenic factors are further upregulated, thereby increasing the risk of PPCM in these pregnancies. Additionally, pregnancy-related hypertension and preeclampsia are being increasingly recognized as precursors to vascular dysfunction, and the association between pregnancy-related hypertension and both preeclampsia and PPCM further supports this hypothesis.[37]

Dysregulation of the maternal immune system has been implicated in PPCM as well, and multiple hypotheses that implicate autoimmune response to the myocardium have been studied. To allow fetal tolerance, adaptive immunity is suppressed during pregnancy.[38] As a result, natural killer (NK) cells) decline during pregnancy, whereas granulocytes and monocytes that are part of innate immunity increase. In an IPAC sub-study, which investigated the role of immune cells in PPCM, women with PPCM showed a significantly reduced level of NK cells and these levels remained suppressed for longer periods postpartum. NK cells are implicated in reducing cardiac eosinophilic infiltration and countering cardiac viral infection. PPCM cardiac tissue demonstrates increased eosinophilic infiltration and inflammatory findings associated with viral infections.[27] These findings support the hypothesis that decreased numbers of circulating NK cells facilitate an exaggerated eosinophilic infiltration and inflammatory response after external, noxious stimuli such as a viral infection.[32] Additionally, an inflammatory response toward migrating fetal cells that settle in the heart has also been implicated in PPCM. High titers of antibodies toward cardiac myosin heavy chains have been identified in the sera of patients with PPCM.[26]

Prognosis in PPCM

PPCM carries a significant burden of morbidity in the form of arrhythmias, cardiogenic shock, cardiac arrest, and death (Table 30.5). Multiple studies have investigated the prognosis of PPCM in women and their ability to successfully carry future pregnancies. The results vary based on region and ethnicity and are tied to early identification of PPCM and intervention. Whereas some studies had no reported mortality[39] globally reported mortality ranges from 7% and 50% in association with PPCM at 12 months.[24] A compilation of findings from various studies shows that factors associated with lack of cardiac recovery were LV end-diastolic dimension of >5.6 cm[39] to >6.1 cm[40] (based on parameters of the study), presence of LV thrombus[39] and African American race.[39] A delay of as little as one week in diagnosing PPCM has been tied to adverse outcomes in 48% of PPCM patients[2]. Women who recover their systolic function mainly do so within six months of onset,[15] although delayed recovery up to 19 months on average has been reported in some studies.[22] The greatest risk with future pregnancies is associated with women who have not recovered their LV ejection fraction (LVEF) to >50%. However, even in women with recovered LVEF, one study[41] showed that 21% had significant reduction of LVEF (>20% from baseline) in the first subsequent pregnancy, 21% developed symptoms of HF, and 14% had a decreased LVEF at last follow-up. Other studies have reproduced these results with similar findings,[42] suggesting that recovery of LV systolic function does not preclude worsening cardiac function with subsequent pregnancies. Hence, women should be counseled accordingly.

Differential Diagnosis for HF during Pregnancy

Dilated Cardiomyopathy

Although PPCM presents as a dilated cardiomyopathy (DCM) phenotype, other causes for DCM, including viral myocarditis, hypertensive heart disease, ischemic heart disease, familial cardiomyopathy, and drug-induced cardiomyopathy, should be considered. A comprehensive work-up to rule out these etiologies of LV systolic dysfunction is essential to treat reversible causes of cardiomyopathy in pregnancy. Work-up can include a myocardial biopsy, coronary angiography, and a thorough history of drug and alcohol use. Distinguishing PPCM from DCM is essential, as these two conditions have different rates of cardiac functional recovery and relapse with subsequent pregnancies. Full recovery of cardiac function is more likely in PPCM. The IPAC study showed a full recovery in over 65% of patients with PPCM in the United States.[23] PPCM occurs mostly during the peripartum and postpartum period, whereas DCM usually manifests in the second trimester.[43] PPCM can also occur recurrently during pregnancy whereas

TABLE 30.5: Adverse Outcomes Associated with Peripartum Cardiomyopathy

Outcome	Incidence
Severe heart failure requiring transplant	0.5% per year–10% in 43 months
Thromboembolism	6.6% per year–17% in 43 months
Cardiogenic shock	2.6% per year
Cardiac arrest	2.2% per year
Mechanical circulatory support	1.5% per year
Arrhythmias	18.7%[60] in hospitalized patients with PPCM
Death	2% during a 6-month follow-up–24% during a 30-month follow-up based on population
Recurrence of PPCM with pregnancy	21% when EF has recovered 25% when EF was <36%[12]

Sources: Kolte, Khera, Aronow, et al. Temporal trends in incidence and outcomes of peripartum cardiomyopathy in the United States: a nationwide population-based study. *J Am Heart Assoc.* 2014;3(3):e001056. Haghikia, Podewski, Libhaber, et al. Phenotyping and outcome on contemporary management in a German cohort of patients with peripartum cardiomyopathy. *Basic Res Cardiol.* 2013;108(4):366. Libhaber, Sliwa, Bachelier, et al. Low systolic blood pressure and high resting heart rate as predictors of outcome in patients with peripartum cardiomyopathy. *Int J Cardiol.* 2015;190:376–82. Biteker, Ilhan, Biteker, et al. Delayed recovery in peripartum cardiomyopathy: an indication for long-term follow-up and sustained therapy. *Eur J Heart Fail.* 2012;14(8):895–901. Amos, Jaber, Russell. Improved outcomes in peripartum cardiomyopathy with contemporary. *Am Heart J.* 2006;152(3):509–13. Elkayam, Tummala, Rao, et al. Maternal and fetal outcomes of subsequent pregnancies in women with peripartum cardiomyopathy. *N Engl J Med.* 2001;344(21):1567–1571. Elkayam Risk of subsequent pregnancy in women with a history of peripartum cardiomyopathy. *J Am Coll Cardiol.* 2014;64(15):1629–36. Mallikethi-Reddy, Akintoye, Trehan, et al. Burden of arrhythmias in peripartum cardiomyopathy: Analysis of 9841 hospitalizations. *Int J Cardiol.* 2017;235:114–17.

DCM does not have this predisposition,[43] thereby influencing counseling for subsequent pregnancies. Additionally, PPCM can lead to rapid clinical worsening in some cases, associated with high mortality.[44]

Hypertrophic Cardiomyopathy

Hypertrophic cardiomyopathy (HCM) is a clinical condition associated with LV hypertrophy and presents differently from DCM on clinical examination (dynamic murmur associated with the LV outflow tract obstruction) and echocardiographic findings (LV wall thickness of 15 mm or more). HCM can develop at different stages in life and can go undiagnosed until the pregnant mother seeks medical assistance. Given that pregnancy is a hypervolemic state, HCM is tolerated well in asymptomatic pregnant women. However, during the third trimester and peripartum period, with maternal increase in heart rate, symptoms of dynamic outflow obstruction and HF can become more prominent. Although systolic dysfunction in HCM is rare, increase in LV hypertrophy during pregnancy contributes to increase in diastolic dysfunction and this can clinically present as decompensated HF. In both these cases, judicious use of beta-blockers to reduce heart rate and increase diastolic filling can alleviate symptoms. Amongst beta-blockers, atenolol should be avoided since it is pregnancy class D agent (see also below). In patients with symptomatic HCM and severe LV hypertrophy, aggressive monitoring for arrhythmias and evaluation for sudden cardiac death should be considered.

Congenital Heart Disease

While *de novo* diagnosis of congenital heart disease (CHD) in pregnancy is rare, there is concern for HF exacerbation due to valvular dysfunction and intrinsic myocardial dysfunction. Ideally, pre-pregnancy counseling and intervention should prevent adverse cardiac events in these patients. However, given that >50% of pregnancies are unplanned, HF in patients with CHD is widely observed and consequential to the outcomes for both the mother and baby. For additional details on management of HF in CHD, including pregnancy, please see Chapter 31.

Medical Management of Heart Failure during Pregnancy

The management of a pregnant woman in HF should prioritize hemodynamic stabilization of the mother, followed by reduction of HF symptoms and improving long-term outcomes. An important consideration in pregnant and nursing women with HF is the selection of agents that are safe for the baby. Table 30.6 summarizes the current classification of drugs used to treat HF in pregnancy.

The Hemodynamically Unstable Patient

Management of a hemodynamically unstable pregnant woman requires immediate stabilization by providing cardiovascular and respiratory support. Respiratory support may involve invasive or non-invasive ventilation with a positive end-expiratory pressure with the goal of minimizing pulmonary edema. Cardiovascular support may require inotropic agents, such as dobutamine or milrinone, to increase CO, both of which are relatively safe during pregnancy. Nitroglycerine can reduce preload and afterload. If pregnancy is continued, nitroprusside should be used cautiously due to the risk of fetal thiocyanate toxicity.[45] Diuretics should be titrated to minimize dehydration that can lead to placental-utero insufficiency. Systolic blood pressure of 90–100 mmHg or mean arterial pressure >70 mmHg[46] and PaO_2>70 mmHg or SaO_2>95%[47] are essential for maintaining good perfusion of the fetus. Monitoring end-organ perfusion is integral in improving outcomes in cases where pregnancy is continued. Thus, invasive hemodynamic monitoring is essential to titrating medications and determining the extent of circulatory support. This can be accomplished through an intra-arterial line for monitoring

TABLE 30.6: Medication Safety Classification during Pregnancy and Breastfeeding

Medication	Use	Major Effects	Pregnancy	Lactation
Antiarrhythmic				
Adenosine	Arrhythmia (SVT)	None reported	✓	✓
Digoxin	Arrhythmia, CHF	Low birth weight, prematurity	✓	∼
Lidocaine	Arrhythmia, anesthesia	Neonatal CNS depression	✓	✓
Procainamide	Arrhythmia	None reported	∼	∼
Sotalol	Arrhythmia	Placental and fetal growth retardation	✓	✗
Antihypertensive				
BBs	Hypertension; Heart failure; Cardiomyopathy	Bradycardia IUGR (atenolol); Transient hypoglycemia	✓ Except Atenolol.	✓
ACEis	Hypertension; Heart failure; Cardiomyopathy	Teratogenicity	✗	✗
Calcium channel blockers	Hypertension; Arrhythmia	None reported; Nifedipine is preferred	✓	✓
Aldomet (methyldopa)	Hypertension	None reported	✓	✓
Hydralazine	Hypertension; Heart failure	Fetal distress with maternal hypotension	✓	✓
Clonidine	Hypertension	Maternal rebound tachycardia None to fetus	✓	✗
Nitrates	Hypertension	Fetal distress with maternal hypotension Can cause fetal/infant hypotension	∼	∼
Entresto	Heart failure	Teratogenicity	✗	✗
Diuretics				
Loop diuretics	Diuretic	Intravascular volume depletion; impairs placental perfusion	✓	✓
Thiazide diuretics	Diuretic	Intravascular volume depletion; impairs placental perfusion May reduce milk production	✓	✓
Anticoagulants				
Warfarin	Mechanical valve, hypercoagulable state, DVT, AF, Eisenmenger syndrome	Teratogenicity restricted to first trimester and at doses >5 mg/d. Crosses placenta, should not be used near time of delivery	✗	✓
Low-molecular-weight heparin	Mechanical valve, hypercoagulable state, DVT, AF, Eisenmenger syndrome	Hemorrhage, unclear effects on maternal bone mineral density	✓	✓
Unfractionated heparin	Mechanical valve, hypercoagulable state, DVT, AF, Eisenmenger syndrome	Maternal osteoporosis, hemorrhage, thrombocytopenia, thrombosis	✓	✓
Direct-acting anticoagulants	Thromboembolism	No current data on safety in pregnancy. Drugs can cross placenta	✗	✗
Fondaparinux	HIT in pregnancy	None reported	✓	✓

(*Continued*)

TABLE 30.6 (Continued): Medication Safety Classification during Pregnancy and Breastfeeding

Medication	Use	Major Effects	Pregnancy	Lactation
Antiplatelets				
Aspirin	Antiplatelet	<100 mg during pregnancy Risk of Reye syndrome at higher doses with lactation	Safe < 100 mg	Safe
Clopidogrel	Antiplatelet for MI, TIA	None reported	Safe	Safe
Glycoprotein IIB/IIIA inhibitors	Antiplatelet	Limited data, none reported	Safe	No data

Safe *Use with caution* *Not safe*

Abbreviations: AF, atrial fibrillation; CNS, central nervous system; DVT, deep vein thrombosis; HIT, heparin-induced thrombocytopenia; IUGR, intrauterine growth retardation; MI, myocardial infarction; SVT, supraventricular tachycardia; TIA, transient ischemic attack.

blood pressure. A central venous catheter for monitoring pulmonary and LV filling pressures can be used to titrate diuretics and inotropic support. Diuresis is obtained through intravenous loop diuretics in combination with thiazides, if necessary. Urgent fetal delivery through cesarian section is indicated in cases of hemodynamic instability when the patient is critically ill, irrespective of gestational age. Mechanical support for medically refractory HF can involve balloon pump or extracorporeal membrane oxygenation. Since recovery of myocardial function is not unreasonable in PPCM, use of long-term ventricular support devices or assessment for transplant needs to be considered on a case-by-case basis. Furthermore, given that pregnancy causes increased burden of panel-reactive antibodies, candidacy for transplant as well as long-term survival of the transplanted organ are challenges that need to be considered while listing these patients for transplantation.

The Hemodynamically Stable Patient

In hemodynamically stable pregnant women with volume overload, every effort should be made to continue pregnancy for as long as possible or until at least 37 weeks of gestation, when the baby reaches term. Diuretics are used judiciously to reduce symptoms of volume overload, such as shortness of breath and pedal edema, while avoiding dehydration. Beta-blockers (excluding atenolol) improve cardiovascular remodeling and minimize arrhythmias and are recommended for at least six months after myocardial recovery.[48] Careful monitoring for fetal bradycardia is recommended during pregnancy when on a beta-blocker. While angiotensin-converting enzyme inhibitors (ACEis) and angiotensin-receptor blockers (ARBs) are standard medications in HF management and facilitate afterload reduction, these agents are contraindicated in pregnancy due to fetal toxicity. However, benazepril, captopril, and enalapril have been tested in nursing women and are safe for babies.[49] Hydralazine and nitrates, however, can be used for afterload reduction in pregnant women. Spironolactone and other mineralocorticoid receptor antagonists are contraindicated in pregnancy. Digoxin has a good safety profile during pregnancy and can be used to improve LV contraction, as well as to reduce arrhythmias and tachycardia.

In a hemodynamically stable euvolemic patient with PPCM, in addition to continuing beta-blockers and optimal dose diuretics, salt and fluid restriction are recommended to maintain euvolemic state. In patients with an LVEF <35%, anticoagulation with warfarin or low-molecular-weight heparin is recommended to prevent LV thrombus formation at least during pregnancy and the first two months postpartum.[18,50] Vaginal delivery[51] of the baby with second-stage assistance[52] is recommended in stable patients with HF who are not on anticoagulants. Uterine to systemic autotransfusion after delivery can cause volume overload in a patient and can be managed with intravenous diuretics after delivery. Therefore, close monitoring after delivery is essential.

Future Directions and Unanswered Questions

While great strides have been made in increasing awareness of PPCM and establishing guidelines for care, there continues to be scope for progress in further understanding and treating the disease. Although there are multiple possible mechanisms that cause PPCM, the triggers for the disease are unknown. Hypertension-associated diseases in pregnancy such as preeclampsia, eclampsia, and gestational hypertension, are present in 65% of patients who develop PPCM[53] and the association between hypertension and PPCM continues to be studied. There is great interest in identifying biomarkers over the course of pregnancy to determine onset and severity of PPCM. These include inflammatory biomarkers, such as high-sensitivity C-reactive protein, interferon-γ, interleukin-6, tumor necrosis factor (TNF), and transforming growth factor-β.[28,29,54,55] Additional biomarkers, including those involved in angiogenic imbalance, such as soluble fms-like tyrosine kinase-1,[33] microRNA-146a,[56] asymmetric dimethylarginine,[20] cathepsin D,[57] and apoptosis signaling molecules, such as Fas/Apo1,[58] are being investigated. Novel treatments for PPCM continue to be studied. Based on initial results suggesting that PPCM is exacerbated by cardiotoxic prolactin metabolites, bromocriptine was added to beta-blockers, ACEi, and ARB in a prospective registry in Germany.[20] This study showed a non-significant difference in full LVEF recovery in PPCM patients receiving bromocriptine, although recovery was less frequent in patients with very low baseline LVEF.[20] In another trial, 63 patients with PPCM and LVEF ≤35% were randomized to receive standard HF treatment with either one-week or eight-week bromocriptine treatment.[59] No significant differences were observed between the two groups in terms of LVEF recovery by six months (from 28±10% to 49±12% in the one-week arm vs 27±10% to 51±10% in the 8-week arm; P=0.38) or in HF hospitalization rates, thereby suggesting that a one-week addition of bromocriptine is sufficient. A higher full recovery rate was reported in this study than in

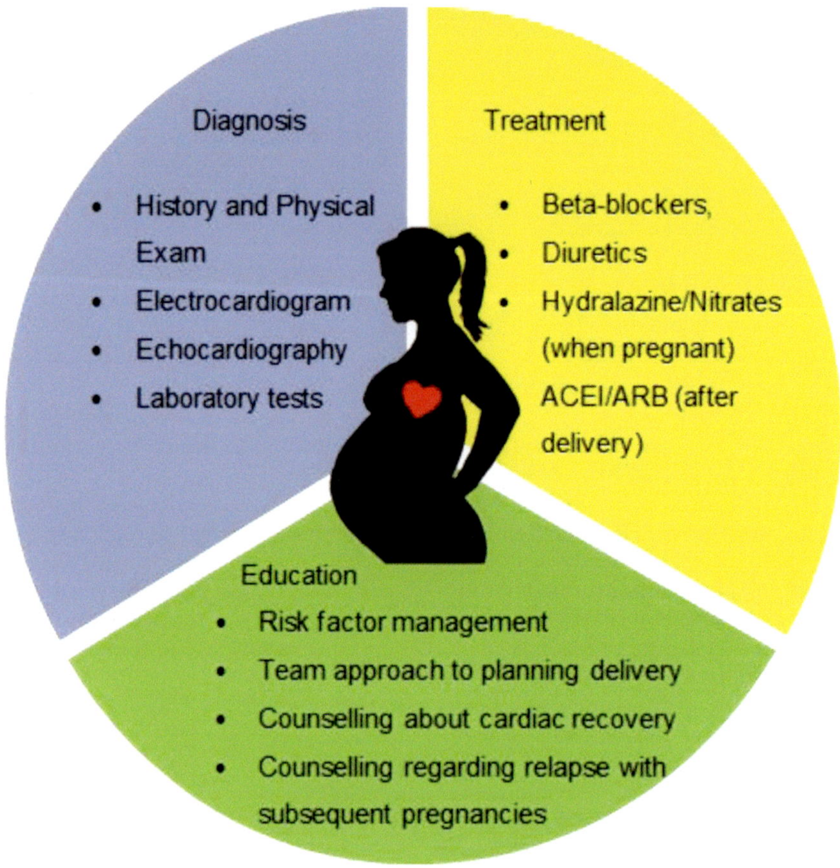

FIGURE 30.1 Approach to PPCM in a pregnant woman.

other studies of PPCM, suggesting a benefit to bromocriptine therapy.[59] A limitation of that study was that all patients but one were of Caucasian race. The inotrope levosimendan has been explored for use in PPCM patients. A randomized study of 24 women showed that the addition of the drug to a standard HF regimen did not improve outcomes in PPCM patients.[60] Interestingly, in another small study of patients with cardiogenic shock, response to levosimendan was more pronounced among patients with PPCM-related vs other causes of shock, as evident by improved hemodynamics 48 hours after treatment. This seems to warrant further investigation on the use of levosimendan for this subset of patients.[61] Pentoxifylline, an inhibitor of TNF, appeared to have a beneficial effect on LVEF in patients from South Africa[62] but showed no benefit in a Haitian population.[28] Identifying molecular targets and treatments for these targets continues to be an active area of interest in PPCM.

Conclusion

A comprehensive approach involving diagnosis, treatment, and patient education is essential in improving outcomes in women with PPCM (Figure 30.1). As awareness of PPCM increases in the community, early recognition and treatment will help improve outcomes for the mother and the baby. An increased understanding of the pathophysiological mechanisms that trigger PPCM is essential in discovering novel methods to monitor and treat this disease. Current guidelines recommend the use of beta-blockers throughout and ACEI/ARB after delivery to improve LV systolic function. Of note, PPCM carries a risk of recurrence with additional pregnancies, albeit at low incidence. Hence, counseling and educating the patient regarding recurrence and long-term outcomes is integral to providing comprehensive care to the patient.

References

1. Petersen EE, Davis NL, Goodman D, et al. Vital signs: pregnancy-related deaths, United States, 2011–2015, and strategies for prevention, 13 states, 2013–2017. *MMWR Morb Mortal Wkly Rep.* 2019;68:423–9.
2. Goland S, Modi K, Bitar F, et al. Clinical profile and predictors of complications in peripartum cardiomyopathy. *J Card Fail.* 2009;15:645–50.
3. Hebson C, Saraf A, Book WM. Risk assessment and management of the mother with cardiovascular disease. *Clin Perinatol.* 2016;43:1–22.
4. Soma-Pillay P, Nelson-Piercy C, Tolppanen H, Mebazaa A. Physiological changes in pregnancy. *Cardiovasc J Afr.* 2016;27:89–94.
5. Ducas RA, Elliott JE, Melnyk SF, et al. Cardiovascular magnetic resonance in pregnancy: insights from the cardiac hemodynamic imaging and remodeling in pregnancy (CHIRP) study. *J Cardiovasc Magn Reson.* 2014;16:1.
6. Hunter S, Robson SC. Adaptation of the maternal heart in pregnancy. *Br Heart J.* 1992;68:540–3.
7. Sanghavi M, Rutherford JD. Cardiovascular physiology of pregnancy. *Circulation.* 2014;130:1003–8.
8. Poppas A, Shroff SG, Korcarz CE, et al. Serial assessment of the cardiovascular system in normal pregnancy. Role of arterial compliance and pulsatile arterial load. *Circulation.* 1997;95:2407–15.
9. Jones CM, 3rd, Greiss FC, Jr. The effect of labor on maternal and fetal circulating catecholamines. *Am J Obstet Gynecol.* 1982;144:149–53.
10. Cong J, Fan T, Yang X, et al. Structural and functional changes in maternal left ventricle during pregnancy: a three-dimensional speckle-tracking echocardiography study. *Cardiovasc Ultrasound.* 2015;13:6.
11. Tanous D, Siu SC, Mason J, et al. B-type natriuretic peptide in pregnant women with heart disease. *J Am Coll Cardiol.* 2010;56:1247–53.
12. Forster O, Hilfiker-Kleiner D, Ansari AA, et al. Reversal of IFN-gamma, oxLDL and prolactin serum levels correlate with clinical improvement in patients with peripartum cardiomyopathy. *Eur J Heart Fail.* 2008;10:861–8.

13. Pearson GD, Veille JC, Rahimtoola S, et al. Peripartum cardiomyopathy: National Heart, Lung, and Blood Institute and Office of Rare Diseases (National Institutes of Health) workshop recommendations and review. *JAMA*. 2000;283:1183–8.
14. Regitz-Zagrosek V, Roos-Hesselink JW, Bauersachs J, et al. 2018 ESC guidelines for the management of cardiovascular diseases during pregnancy. *Eur Heart J*. 2018;39:3165–241.
15. Hibbard JU, Lindheimer M, Lang RM. A modified definition for peripartum cardiomyopathy and prognosis based on echocardiography. *Obstet Gynecol*. 1999;94:311–6.
16. Patel PA, Roy A, Javid R, Dalton JA. A contemporary review of peripartum cardiomyopathy. *Clin Med (Lond)*. 2017;17:316–321.
17. Kolte D, Khera S, Aronow WS, et al. Temporal trends in incidence and outcomes of peripartum cardiomyopathy in the United States: a nationwide population-based study. *J Am Heart Assoc*. 2014;3:e001056.
18. Arany Z, Elkayam U. Peripartum cardiomyopathy. *Circulation*. 2016;133:1397–409.
19. Lok SI, Kirkels JH, Klopping C, Doevendans PA, de Jonge N. Peripartum cardiomyopathy: the need for a national database. *Neth Heart J*. 2011;19:126–33.
20. Haghikia A, Podewski E, Libhaber E, et al. Phenotyping and outcome on contemporary management in a German cohort of patients with peripartum cardiomyopathy. *Basic Res Cardiol*. 2013;108:366.
21. Libhaber E, Sliwa K, Bachelier K, Lamont K, Bohm M. Low systolic blood pressure and high resting heart rate as predictors of outcome in patients with peripartum cardiomyopathy. *Int J Cardiol*. 2015;190:376–82.
22. Biteker M, Ilhan E, Biteker G, Duman D, Bozkurt B. Delayed recovery in peripartum cardiomyopathy: an indication for long-term follow-up and sustained therapy. *Eur J Heart Fail*. 2012;14:895–901.
23. McNamara DM, Elkayam U, Alharethi R, et al. Clinical outcomes for peripartum cardiomyopathy in North America: results of the IPAC study (Investigations of Pregnancy-Associated Cardiomyopathy). *J Am Coll Cardiol*. 2015;66:905–14.
24. Okeke T, Ezenyeaku C, Ikeako L. Peripartum cardiomyopathy. *Ann Med Health Sci Res*. 2013;3:313–9.
25. Lindley KJ, Verma AK, Blauwet LA. Peripartum cardiomyopathy: progress in understanding the etiology, management, and prognosis. *Heart Fail Clin*. 2019;15:29–39.
26. Ansari AA, Fett JD, Carraway RE, et al. Autoimmune mechanisms as the basis for human peripartum cardiomyopathy. *Clin Rev Allergy Immunol*. 2002;23:301–24.
27. Borczuk AC, van Hoeven KH, Factor SM. Review and hypothesis: the eosinophil and peripartum heart disease (myocarditis and coronary artery dissection)--coincidence or pathogenetic significance? *Cardiovasc Res*. 1997;33:527–32.
28. Fett JD. Peripartum cardiomyopathy: a puzzle closer to solution. *World J Cardiol*. 2014;6:87–99.
29. Fett JD, Ansari AA. Inflammatory markers and cytokines in peripartum cardiomyopathy: a delicate balance. *Expert Opin Ther Targets*. 2010;14:895–8.
30. Goland S, Weinstein JM, Zalik A, et al. Angiogenic imbalance and residual myocardial injury in recovered peripartum cardiomyopathy patients. *Circ Heart Fail*. 2016;9:e003349.
31. Llurba E, Crispi F, Verlohren S. Update on the pathophysiological implications and clinical role of angiogenic factors in pregnancy. *Fetal Diagn Ther*. 2015;37:81–92.
32. McTiernan CF, Morel P, Cooper LT, et al. Circulating T-cell subsets, monocytes, and natural killer cells in peripartum cardiomyopathy: results from the multicenter IPAC study. *J Card Fail*. 2018;24:33–42.
33. Patten IS, Rana S, Shahul S, et al. Cardiac angiogenic imbalance leads to peripartum cardiomyopathy. *Nature*. 2012;485:333–8.
34. Ware JS, Li J, Mazaika E, et al. Shared genetic predisposition in peripartum and dilated cardiomyopathies. *N Engl J Med*. 2016;374:233–41.
35. van Spaendonck-Zwarts KY, Posafalvi A, van den Berg MP, et al. Titin gene mutations are common in families with both peripartum cardiomyopathy and dilated cardiomyopathy. *Eur Heart J*. 2014;35:2165–73.
36. Bello NA, Arany Z. Molecular mechanisms of peripartum cardiomyopathy: A vascular/hormonal hypothesis. *Trends Cardiovasc Med*. 2015;25:499–504.
37. Brennan LJ, Morton JS, Davidge ST. Vascular dysfunction in preeclampsia. *Microcirculation*. 2014;21:4–14.
38. Sacks G, Sargent I, Redman C. An innate view of human pregnancy. *Immunol Today*. 1999;20:114–8.
39. Amos AM, Jaber WA, Russell SD. Improved outcomes in peripartum cardiomyopathy with contemporary. *Am Heart J*. 2006;152:509–13.
40. Witlin AG, Mabie WC, Sibai BM. Peripartum cardiomyopathy: a longitudinal echocardiographic study. *Am J Obstet Gynecol*. 1997;177:1129–32.
41. Elkayam U, Tummala PP, Rao K, et al. Maternal and fetal outcomes of subsequent pregnancies in women with peripartum cardiomyopathy. *N Engl J Med*. 2001;344:1567–71.
42. Elkayam U. Risk of subsequent pregnancy in women with a history of peripartum cardiomyopathy. *J Am Coll Cardiol*. 2014;64:1629–36.
43. Bhakta P, Biswas BK, Banerjee B. Peripartum cardiomyopathy: review of the literature. *Yonsei Med J*. 2007;48:731–47.
44. van Hoeven KH, Kitsis RN, Katz SD, Factor SM. Peripartum versus idiopathic dilated cardiomyopathy in young women--a comparison of clinical, pathologic and prognostic features. *Int J Cardiol*. 1993;40:57–65.
45. Brown CM, Garovic VD. Drug treatment of hypertension in pregnancy. *Drugs*. 2014;74:283–96.
46. Arnold JM, Howlett JG, Dorian P, et al. Canadian Cardiovascular Society Consensus Conference recommendations on heart failure update 2007: prevention, management during intercurrent illness or acute decompensation, and use of biomarkers. *Can J Cardiol*. 2007;23:21–45.
47. Bhatia PK, Biyani G, Mohammed S, Sethi P, Bihani P. Acute respiratory failure and mechanical ventilation in pregnant patient: a narrative review of literature. *J Anaesthesiol Clin Pharmacol*. 2016;32:431–9.
48. Hilfiker-Kleiner D, Haghikia A, Nonhoff J, Bauersachs J. Peripartum cardiomyopathy: current management and future perspectives. *Eur Heart J*. 2015;36:1090–7.
49. Beardmore KS, Morris JM, Gallery ED. Excretion of antihypertensive medication into human breast milk: a systematic review. *Hypertens Pregnancy*. 2002;21:85–95.
50. Regitz-Zagrosek V, Roos-Hesselink JW, Bauersachs J, et al. 2018 ESC guidelines for the management of cardiovascular diseases during pregnancy. *Kardiol Pol*. 2019;77:245–326.
51. European Society of G, Association for European Paediatric C, German Society for Gender M, et al. ESC guidelines on the management of cardiovascular diseases during pregnancy: the Task Force on the Management of Cardiovascular Diseases during Pregnancy of the European Society of Cardiology (ESC). Eur Heart J. 2011;32:3147–97.
52. Cauldwell M, Von Klemperer K, Uebing A, et al. The management of the second stage of labour in women with cardiac: A mixed methods study. *Int J Cardiol*. 2016;222:732–6.
53. Harper MA, Meyer RE, Berg CJ. Peripartum cardiomyopathy: population-based birth prevalence and 7-year mortality. *Obstet Gynecol*. 2012;120:1013–9.
54. Fett JD, Sannon H, Thelisma E, Sprunger T, Suresh V. Recovery from severe heart failure following peripartum cardiomyopathy. *Int J Gynaecol Obstet*. 2009;104:125–7.
55. Sarojini A, Sai Ravi Shanker A, Anitha M. Inflammatory markers-serum level of C-reactive protein, tumor necrotic factor-alpha, and interleukin-6 as predictors of outcome for peripartum cardiomyopathy. *J Obstet Gynaecol India*. 2013;63:234–9.
56. Halkein J, Tabruyn SP, Ricke-Hoch M, et al. MicroRNA-146a is a therapeutic target and biomarker for peripartum cardiomyopathy. *J Clin Invest*. 2013;123:2143–54.
57. Hilfiker-Kleiner D, Kaminski K, Podewski E, et al. A cathepsin D-cleaved 16 kDa form of prolactin mediates postpartum cardiomyopathy. *Cell*. 2007;128:589–600.
58. Sliwa K, Skudicky D, Bergemann A, et al. Peripartum cardiomyopathy: analysis of clinical outcome, left ventricular function, plasma levels of cytokines and Fas/APO-1. *J Am Coll Cardiol*. 2000;35:701–5.
59. Hilfiker-Kleiner D, Haghikia A, Berliner D, et al. Bromocriptine for the treatment of peripartum cardiomyopathy: a multicentre randomized study. *Eur Heart J*. 2017;38:2671–2679.
60. Biteker M, Duran NE, Kaya H, et al. Effect of levosimendan and predictors of recovery in patients with peripartum cardiomyopathy, a randomized clinical trial. *Clin Res Cardiol*. 2011;100:571–7.
61. Labbene I, Arrigo M, Tavares M, et al. Decongestive effects of levosimendan in cardiogenic shock induced by postpartum cardiomyopathy. *Anaesth Crit Care Pain Med*. 2017;36:39–42.
62. Sliwa K, Skudicky D, Candy G, et al. The addition of pentoxifylline to conventional therapy improves outcome in patients with peripartum cardiomyopathy. *Eur J Heart Fail*. 2002;4:305–9.

Chapter 31
DILATED CARDIOMYOPATHY

Marco Merlo, Alessia Paldino, Giulia De Angelis, and Gianfranco Sinagra

Definition and Classification

Dilated cardiomyopathy (DCM) is a heart muscle disease that is morphologically and functionally characterized by left ventricular (LV) or biventricular progressive dilation and systolic dysfunction in the absence of abnormal loading conditions (i.e., pressure or volume overload) or coronary artery disease severe enough to justify the dysfunction.[1,2] However, there is no universal classification for DCM.[3]

A pathogenic gene mutation is detectable in almost 50% of DCM cases.[4] Currently, DCM is viewed as a complex interaction between environmental triggers (such as tachyarrhythmias, alcohol, chemotherapy, inflammation) and a highly heterogeneous mix of genes and mutations.[5–7] A better understanding of the genotype-phenotype relationship would lead to improvements in management of DCM patients, from an earlier diagnosis to better prognostic stratification and targeted therapy.[5]

DCM may be subcategorized as sporadic, or isolated, when a single member of a family is affected, and familial, when occurring in two or more related family members or in the presence of a relative with sudden cardiac death (SCD) before the age of 35. A relative prevalence of 30–50% for familial DCM is reported in the current guidelines, with 40% having an identifiable gene mutation.[8,9] The identification of non-proband patients at an early stage of DCM by a complete family screening gives the chance to start an optimal medical therapy earlier and to improve prognosis.[10,11]

The Global Burden of DCM

Recent studies suggest that DCM is fairly common, affecting approximately up to 1 in 250 people in the general population.[12] The disease affects typically young patients in their 3rd to 5th decade of life, with a male-to-female ratio of 3:1. Patients are often scarcely symptomatic at the onset, with a long duration of LV dysfunction, low rate of comorbidities and, consequently, a low rate of cardiovascular events.[13] Therefore, DCM represents a special case of heart failure (HF) with reduced left ventricular ejection fraction (LVEF).

Etiological Definition

Etiological characterization is the cornerstone of management of DCM (Table 31.1). However, DCM is a heterogeneous and complex disease and etiologic assessment is challenging. For patients with non-ischemic DCM, clinicians should consider potentially reversible causes of LV dysfunction, which are likely to improve with specific therapeutic interventions. In cases of severe LV dysfunction and HF of recent onset, differentiating between genetically determined vs post-myocarditis DCM vs acute myocarditis has important prognostic implications. Approximately 50% of patients with active myocarditis presenting with HF experience significant improvement in the first 6 to 12 months under standard or specific therapy. On the other hand, recent reports suggest that a number of genetically determined structural modifications are associated with acute myocarditis and the development of post-myocarditis DCM, by favoring the persistence and progression of inflammation.[14]

Other non-genetically determined DCMs are tachycardia-induced, catecholamine-induced, or toxic (alcohol, chemotherapy, or cocaine), secondary to systemic inflammatory disorders (e.g., Churg-Strauss syndrome, sarcoidosis), or associated with significant arterial hypertension. These forms are characterized by a high propensity for LV reverse remodeling when the initial trigger is removed.[15,16]

When all the above causes are excluded, a familial or genetically determined DCM may be hypothesized. Whenever a direct cause leading to the phenotype of DCM cannot be determined, the term “idiopathic” DCM is used, which mostly reflects our inability to identify an underlying etiology. These forms represent currently about 20–30% of non-ischemic DCM in clinical practice. An unknown genetic or inflammatory background could be thought of as the major determinant of idiopathic DCM.

Genetics and Pathophysiology

The proportion of DCM cases with a genetic basis has long been underestimated due to variable clinical presentation, incomplete penetrance (not all gene carriers manifest the disease), and the lack of distinguishing phenotypic features in most cases. The main mode of inheritance is autosomal dominant, but X-linked recessive, autosomal recessive, and mitochondrial transmission are also recognized as isolated cardiac diseases or in the context of multiorgan syndromes.[17] Currently, the landscape of DCM genetics is rapidly extending with the advent of comprehensive molecular genetic analysis facilitated by the high-quality next-generation sequencing extended panels.[7,18]

More than 50 genes encoding a wide variety of proteins of the sarcomere, cytoskeleton, nuclear envelope, sarcolemma, ion channels, and intercellular junctions have been associated with DCM and many more will soon be recognized.[4,5] Specific mutations of these genes alter various pathways and cellular structures and negatively affect muscle contraction, function of ion channels and sensitivity to electrolytes, calcium homeostasis, and generation-transmission of mechanical force in the myocardium. The fact that this genetic heterogeneity results in a common phenotype has been explained by Bowles and Towbin with the “final common pathway” hypothesis: different mutations alter various proteins involved in a common pathway, the disruption of which leads to DCM.[19]

Genetic testing should be considered in patients with a diagnosis of DCM in order to identify possible pathogenic variants and facilitate future clinical management and family screening.[11] The presence of certain diagnostic “red flags” and a family history of the disease suggest genetic forms of DCM.[17] In these cases, genetic testing should be recommended. Moreover, genotype-phenotype correlation is fundamental for thorough risk

DOI: 10.1201/9780429244544-38

TABLE 31.1: Etiological Characterization of Dilated Cardiomyopathy (DCM)

Genetic	Inflammatory Causes	Medications
• **Isolated DCM** • TTN predictors • LMNA predictors • Cytoskeletal and Z-disk genes • Sarcomeric genes • Desmosomal genes • Ion channels • Other • **DCM in the context of neuromuscular disorders** • Duchenne and Becker muscular dystrophies • Emery-Dreifuss muscular dystrophy • Limb-Girdle muscular dystrophy • Myotonic dystrophy • Myofibrillar myopathies • **DCM in the context of syndromic diseases** • Mitochondrial diseases • Barth syndrome • Alström syndrome	• **Infectious diseases** • Viral • Bacterial • Fungal • Parasitic • Protozoal (Chagas disease) • **Autoimmune systemic disorders** • Systemic lupus erythematosus • Rheumatoid arthritis • Scleroderma • Dermatomyositis • Vasculitis • **Sarcoidosis**	• **Chemotherapeutic agents** • Anthracyclines • Cyclophosphamide • Trastuzumab • **Antiretroviral drugs** • Zidovudine • Didanosine • Zalcitabine • **Other** • Chloroquine • Clozapine • Phenothiazines
Toxins	**Endocrinologic Disorders**	**Other**
• Ethanol • Cocaine • Amphetamines	• Hyper- or hypo thyroidism • Growth hormone excess or deficiency • Pheochromocytoma • Diabetes mellitus • Cushing's disease	• Peripartum cardiomyopathy • Tachycardiomyopathy • DCM secondary to hemochromatosis

stratification and choice of therapy.[5] The principal genotype-phenotype correlations in DCM are reported in Table 31.2.

Titin-TTN

Titin (*TTN*) codes for titin, the largest sarcomeric protein of the heart muscle. Truncating mutations of *TTN* represent the most common known genetic cause of DCM, being discovered in 19–25% of familial DCM and 11–18% of sporadic cases.[20] The A-band is a critical portion of *TTN* because of its biomechanical sensing and signaling functions, involved in a causative mutation leading to the disease.[21] However, *TTN* truncating variants can be detected in 2–3% of subjects without overt cardiomyopathy.[22] *TTN* truncating mutations have been associated with mild and treatable DCM with mortality rates similar to that of the general DCM population.[20] However, an arrhythmogenic phenotype with higher interstitial fibrosis and reduced ventricular hypertrophy has been reported.[23]

Lamin-LMNA

Mutations in lamin (*LMNA*) gene, which encodes the nuclear proteins lamin A and C, have been shown to cause various phenotypes associated with DCM, including those with limb-girdle or Emery-Dreifuss muscular dystrophy. *LMNA* mutations are present in ~8% of patients with DCM, with an autosomal dominant inheritance pattern. *LMNA*-related DCM typically involves cardiac conduction abnormalities and skeletal muscle involvement with high creatinine kinase levels. These patients are at high risk of malignant ventricular arrhythmias and SCD, independent of LVEF. Indeed, *LMNA* pathogenic variants are currently considered to be an indicator for implantable cardioverter-defibrillators (ICD) for primary prevention, regardless of LVEF.[24]

Filamin-FLNC

Filamin C (FLNC) has recently been included in genetic screening for cardiomyopathy. *FLNC* encodes filamin C, a large, intermediate filament involved in sarcomeric and Z-disk stability.[25] Truncated variants in *FLNC* account for about 4% of DCM cases and 3% of arrhythmogenic DCM cases.[26,27] Indeed, *FLNC* truncating mutations seem to be a cause of an overlapping phenotype of dilated and left dominant arrhythmogenic cardiomyopathy, characterized by increased deposition of fibrotic tissue between cardiomyocytes, represented by subepicardial-transmural fibrosis in inferolateral LV wall, and complicated by malignant ventricular arrhythmias and SCD.[27] Recently, *FLNC* variants have been added to the indications for primary ICD implantation, next to *LMNA* and phospholamban (*PLN*) variants.[28] Moreover, almost 5% of carriers for these *FLNC* variants have a right ventricular involvement or hypertrophic/restrictive phenotype.

Other Genes

Many other genes can lead to different heterogeneous phenotypes, including DCM, but also other forms of cardiomyopathies.

- In addition to the Brugada and long QT type 3 syndromes, mutations in genes encoding sodium ion channels (i.e., sodium channel protein type 5 subunit alpha: *SCN5A* gene) have been linked to DCM. In particular, the Arg222Gln mutation has been detected in familial DCM characterized by frequent ventricular arrhythmias, cardiac conduction disease, and atrial fibrillation.[29]
- Missense mutations of the ryanodine receptor 2-encoding gene (*RYR2*), coding for one of the components of the sarcoplasmic reticulum calcium channel, are known to result in catecholaminergic polymorphic ventricular tachycardia (CPVT). However, a different variant has been found in two families with an overlap syndrome of CPVT and DCM in some members.[30]
- Mutations in desmosomal genes have been typically shown to cause arrhythmogenic right ventricular cardiomyopathy (ARVC)[31] but have now been linked to isolated DCM and

TABLE 31.2: Principal Genotype-Phenotype Correlations in Dilated Cardiomyopathy

Gene	Phenotype	Guideline Recommendations
LMNA	• AV-blocks, intraventricular conduction delays, supraventricular and ventricular arrhythmias, SCD • Skeletal muscle involvement and high CPK levels • Limb-girdle or Emery-Dreifuss muscular dystrophy	Class IIa level of evidence B for ICD implantation in presence of risk factors (NSVT during ambulatory electrocardiogram monitoring, LVEF <45% at first evaluation, male sex, and non-missense mutations).
FLNC	• Ventricular arrhythmias and SCD • LV inferolateral subepicardial/transmural fibrosis • Right ventricular involvement • Hypertrophic/restrictive phenotype • Lower rate of LVRR • Myofibrillar myopathy	Class IIa level of evidence B for ICD implantation in presence of LVEF <45% or NSVT.
PLN	• Early progressive HF and heart transplantation • Ventricular arrhythmias	Class IIa level of evidence C for ICD implantation in presence of ACM and an LVEF <45%.
TTN	• LVRR rate ≥ 50% • Ventricular arrhythmias • Cardiac fibrosis • Reduced hypertrophy	N/A
SCN5A	• Brugada syndrome and long QT type 3 • Ventricular and supraventricular arrhythmias (particularly AF) • AV-block	N/A
RYR2	• CPVT	N/A
DSP	• Ventricular arrhythmias • Right ventricular involvement • LV fibrosis	N/A
DES	• Conduction system disease (various degree AV-block) • Ventricular arrhythmias and SCD • Probably LV fibrosis • Myofibrillar myopathy	N/A

Abbreviations: ACM: arrhythmogenic cardiomyopathy; AV: atrioventricular; CPK: creatine-phosphokinase; CPVT: catecholaminergic polymorphic ventricular tachycardia; DES: desmin; DSP: desmoplakin; FLNC: filamin C; HF: heart failure; ICD: implantable cardioverter defibrillator; LMNA: laminA/C; LVEF: left ventricular ejection fraction; LVRR: left ventricular reverse remodeling; NSVT: non-sustained ventricular tachycardia; PLN: phospholamban; RYR2: ryanodine receptor 2; SCD: sudden cardiac death; SCN5A: sodium channel protein type 5 subunit alpha; TTN: titin.

overlap syndromes. For example, frameshift and nonsense mutations in *DSP*, encoding for desmoplakin, can induce LV fibrosis and dysfunction associated with increased arrhythmic burden, with or without involvement of the right ventricle.[32] Carvajal syndrome (woolly hair, keratoderma, DCM) is an autosomal recessive cardiocutaneus disease caused by homozygous *DSP* mutants.

- Mutations in *DES*, the gene encoding for desmin, an intermediate filament of the cytoskeleton, can cause skeletal myopathy, mixed skeletal-cardiac disease ("desmin-related myopathy"), and cardiomyopathy (DCM as well as hypertrophic or restrictive). *DES* accounts for only 1–2% of DCM-related mutations,[33] but truncated variants seem to be associated with early-onset and more severe forms of DCM with atrioventricular blocks[34] and diffuse LV fibrosis (unpublished data from Heart Muscle Disease Registry of Trieste [HMDR]).
- Sarcomeric genes, encoding proteins such as β myosin heavy chain (*MYH7*), cardiac troponin T (*TNNT2*) and tropomyosin (*TPM1*), are also frequently mutated in DCM, with a prevalence of 5–10%.[35] This group of genes is characterized by significant overlap of phenotypes, with different phenotypes in the same family, and has been associated in some reports with adverse prognosis.[36,37]
- Some rare mutations have been associated with worse prognosis. Arg9Cys and Arg14del, two mutations of the *PLN* gene (encoding phospholamban, an inhibitor of the sarcoplasmic reticulum calcium-transporting ATPase), have been associated with progressive HF and malignant ventricular arrhythmias, respectively, in a selected population in the Netherlands.[38,39] Also PLN has recently become an indication for early ICD implantation.[28] A small number of studies have reported a malignant phenotype of DCM with severe HF, arrhythmias, and a need for cardiac transplantation in carriers of mutations in *RBM20*, a gene encoding a nuclear RNA-binding protein with the function of regulating splicing of the transcript of genes involved in cardiac development.[40,41]

Clinical Spectrum of DCM

DCM may present with a wide and heterogeneous range of clinical scenarios. The most frequent presentation is systolic HF.[12] However, improvement of diagnostic techniques and broader familial screening allowed earlier diagnosis and revealed intermediate and preclinical phenotypes of DCM.[10]

Some cases of DCM are characterized by severe LV dysfunction in the absence of dilation or with mild dilation, also known as hypokinetic non-dilated cardiomyopathy[1] or mildly dilated cardiomyopathy[42] (Figure 31.1). Mildly dilated cardiomyopathy is often the initial manifestation of subsequent overt DCM; however, it may also be the phenotypic expression of atypical genotypes, such as *DES* or *LMNA* variants, often characterized by restrictive filling pattern and ventricular arrhythmias.

Malignant arrhythmias or SCD may be the first sign of either an underlying genetic disease (i.e., *LMNA* mutations, neuromuscular disorders), or a distinct arrhythmogenic phenotype

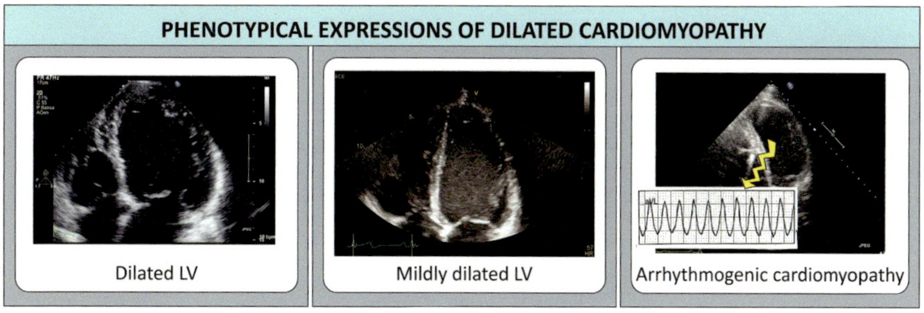

FIGURE 31.1 Phenotypic expression of DCM. Different phenotypic manifestations of DCM are possible; in particular, dilated cardiomyopathy, non- or mildly dilated cardiomyopathy, or arrhythmogenic cardiomyopathy may be the representation of the same disease at different stages or may reflect the etiological heterogeneity of DCM.

of DCM, which affects approximately one-third of DCM patients.[43] The arrhythmogenic DCM should be differentiated from the left dominant phenotype of ARVC.[31,44] Some features of arrhythmogenic DCM have been recently described: unexplained syncope (likely due to ventricular tachyarrhythmia); rapid non-sustained ventricular tachycardia, defined as five or more consecutive ventricular beats lasting <30 s with a rate ≥150/min on 24-hour Holter monitoring; ≥1,000 premature ventricular contractions, or ≥50 couplets, in 24 hours.[43] Currently, arrhythmogenic DCM, ARVC, and left dominant ARVC seem to represent manifestations of the same spectrum, currently known as arrhythmogenic cardiomyopathy.[45] Arrhythmogenic cardiomyopathy carries a heterogeneous genetic background (desmosomal genes, *DES*, *LMNA*, *FLNC*, *SCN5A*, *PLN*, *RBM20*) and similar phenotypes, which can be explained by the "final common pathway" hypothesis.[19,28] Moreover, a family history of arrhythmogenic cardiomyopathy is detectible in ~60% of cases.[45]

Finally, patients should always be evaluated for cardiac signs and symptoms related to multisystem disease.

Diagnosis

Improvement of diagnostic techniques, along with systematic family screening, have allowed for earlier identification of subclinical forms of DCM with prognostic benefit.[13] The most important tools are summarized below. These tools should be used in an integrated way to reach a definite diagnosis (Figure 31.2).[17] For family screening, please refer to "Therapy and Clinical Management of DCM – Early Diagnosis."

Laboratory Tests

B-type natriuretic peptide (BNP) or N-terminal-proBNP should be assessed at initial evaluation and regularly during follow-up.[46] Galectin-3 and ST2 could be useful prognostic markers in stable DCM.[47] Serum creatine phosphokinase should be measured in all patients, since elevated levels are typical of specific phenotypes, including laminopathies, dystrophin-related disorders, or desminopathies.[48]

Electrocardiography (ECG)

Although DCM is not typically characterized by specific ECG findings, a careful analysis can provide several clues about the etiology as well as the duration of the disease. For example, dystrophin-related DCM is generally characterized by a "posterolateral pseudonecrosis" aspect, atrioventricular blocks can suggest a mutation in *LMNA*, and myotonic dystrophy and Emery Dreifuss disease can be associated with sinus bradycardia and atrial standstill.[17] Left atrial enlargement is frequent in DCM and is usually an expression of a long-standing disease.[48] Left bundle-branch block is usually a marker of long-standing disease with prognostic and therapeutic implications.[49,50] In general, the ECG is important prognostically. Antero-lateral T-wave inversion, low QRS voltages, and fragmented QRS have been reported as independent predictors of death, heart transplantation, SCD, and malignant ventricular arrhythmias in a cohort of 414 patient with DCM.[51,52]

Echocardiography

Two-dimensional Doppler echocardiography is still the most important tool in the assessment of DCM.[53] In addition to LV systolic function and size, a complete evaluation is warranted. The presence and severity of functional mitral regurgitation provide important information for management and prognosis.[54] Left ventricular diastolic function should be systematically assessed for estimation of left ventricular filling pressures and identification of restrictive filling pattern.[55,56] The right ventricle, along with estimation of pulmonary arterial pressure, is also essential in risk stratification in DCM.[57]

Myocardial deformation imaging (e.g., speckle-tracking echocardiography-derived strain) offers greater sensitivity than LVEF for identifying subtle abnormalities of systolic function and may assume a role in the early detection of disease, especially for unaffected gene mutation carriers.[58] Furthermore, baseline evaluation of global longitudinal strain (GLS) seems to predict recovery of LVEF in patients with non-ischemic cardiomyopathy.[59] Also, re-evaluation of GLS during follow-up could predict future deterioration of LV function in HF patients with a recovered LVEF.[60]

Cardiac Magnetic Resonance (CMR)

CMR is considered the gold standard for assessment of ventricular volumes and ejection fraction, enabling confident diagnosis of DCM in borderline cases and improving the characterization of phenotype severity.[61] Moreover, tissue characterization can be useful in differentiating the various etiologies of DCM. The detection of myocardial edema (e.g., active myocarditis or sarcoidosis) and the presence and distribution of late gadolinium enhancement (LGE) (e.g., myocarditis, Chagas disease, sarcoidosis, etc.) are essential in the definition of the etiology of DCM.[62]

Recently, mounting evidence suggests an important prognostic role for LGE in DCM patients. The presence and, less clearly, the extent and location of LGE could be useful in predicting the response to optimal medical therapy[63] or cardiac resynchronization therapy, such as LV reverse remodeling (LVRR), and the risk of SCD or major ventricular arrhythmia independently from LVEF.[62,64,65]

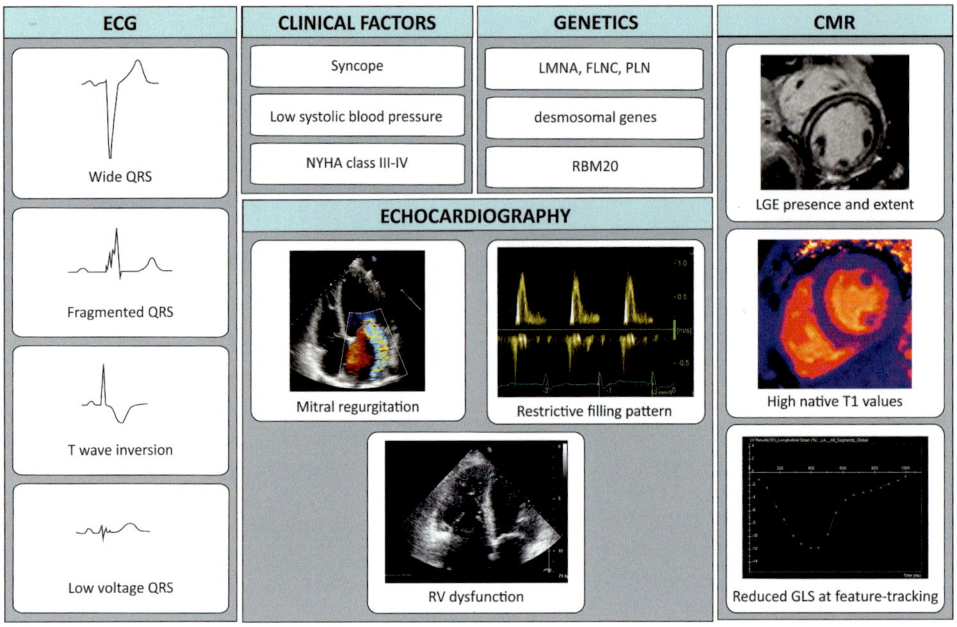

FIGURE 31.2 Prognostic stratification in DCM patients. Risk stratification of DCM patients should rely on multiparametric models based on both clinical and instrumental features and should be performed both at baseline and during follow-up. Here, we summarize the most important parameters that have proven to be associated with worse outcomes in DCM patients. ECG features are wide QRS, especially left bundle branch block, fragmented or low-voltage QRS, or T wave inversion. At echocardiography, the presence of moderate to severe functional mitral regurgitation, right ventricular dysfunction, or a restrictive filling pattern are linked to higher mortality. Late gadolinium enhancement (LGE) at cardiac magnetic resonance (CMR) is an independent and powerful predictor of both arrhythmic risk and heart failure risk. T1-mapping and global longitudinal strain (GLS) are also emerging as predictors of poor outcome. Mutations in many genes have been clearly associated with higher arrhythmic risk, in particular *LMNA*, *FLNC*, and *PLN*, but more recently also *RBM20* and desmosomal genes.

Moreover, new techniques, such as T1 mapping, can quantify extracellular inflammation and fibrosis and assess prognosis in myocarditis, infiltrative disease, and DCM.[62] GLS by feature-tracking CMR has been shown to be a powerful predictor of mortality in non-ischemic cardiomyopathy, proving prognostic information incremental to risk factors such as LVEF and LGE extent.[66] Combined with other CMR parameters, feature-tracking seems to improve the prediction of LVRR in patients with recently diagnosed non-ischemic cardiomyopathy receiving evidence-based treatment.[67]

Left and Right Heart Catheterization

In the diagnostic assessment of a depressed LVEF of unknown origin, coronary angiography is always required to rule out coronary artery disease. Cardiac computed tomography can be considered as an alternative, particularly when the probability of ischemic disease is low. Right heart catheterization should be reserved for select cases, e.g., in patients with advanced disease who are candidates for long-term mechanical circulatory support or cardiac transplantation.[68]

Endomyocardial Biopsy

The role of endomyocardial biopsy in the etiological characterization of DCM is largely controversial. Modern immunohistochemical methods improve sensitivity compared with the traditional histopathological Dallas criteria. Although broader use has been proposed with the goal of detecting myocarditis,[69] biopsy should be generally reserved for select cases of newly diagnosed non-ischemic LV dysfunction with a high degree of suspicion of acute myocarditis. Patients with severe HF, non-response to treatment, hemodynamic impairment, or life-threatening arrhythmias, where immunosuppression or antiviral therapy are considered,[70,71] appear to be the best candidates for endomyocardial biopsy.

Therapy and Clinical Management of DCM

DCM is a common cause of HF and the treatment reflects the management of chronic HF with reduced LVEF recommended by international guidelines.[24,72] In clinical practice, every effort should be taken towards an individualized identification of the cause of LV dysfunction.[24] Precise diagnosis of underlying etiology is a critical step towards personalized medicine for these patients and seems to be the best prospect in the treatment of DCM.[73]

History, physical examination, and a comprehensive differential analysis are necessary. Patients with these disorders often have medical management needs beyond their cardiac care needs and thus precise diagnosis of underlying etiology is critical to optimize treatment.

Current data show an eight-year survival of ~87%.[13] Interestingly, the annual incidence of major cardiovascular adverse events (death or heart transplant) is around 2% and the occurrence of SCD has dropped to 0.5%/year.[13,74] Cornerstones of this survival improvement are early diagnosis and LVRR achieved with evidence-based therapies.

Early Diagnosis

Screening of family members has led to an improved early diagnosis in DCM with an accompanying improvement in prognosis of DCM in recent decades.[13] Therefore, all family members should be screened systematically when approaching a patient with newly diagnosed DCM. A complete screening is recommended for proband's first-degree relatives.[11] A family history of three or more generations and a complete pedigree analysis are mandatory, with attention to family occurrence of HF before the age of 60, SCD, pacemaker implantation early in life, and skeletal myopathies (e.g., Duchenne or Becker disease) or presence of sensorineural hearing loss (congenital or occurring after the second decade of life) as suggestion of syndromic disease.[75] Periodic clinical, ECG, and echocardiographic screening is recommended for genotype-positive relatives.[11] According to guidelines, genetic testing of first-degree relatives is recommended, starting from the age of 10 to 12, when a specific mutation (pathogenic or likely pathogenic) is identified in the proband, although earlier testing can be considered for laminopathies.[11]

Reverse Remodeling: The Importance of Follow-Up

DCM has long been considered to be an irreversible condition. The cumulative experience derived from referral centers suggests that ~40% of patients could experience significant LVRR[76,77] with evidence-based pharmacological and device therapy.[24]

Evidence suggests that LVRR concludes after 12 up to 24 months of optimal treatment; LVRR provides strong incremental prognostic information over baseline evaluation.[76] Importantly, LVRR seems to be preceded by early (three to six months) improvement of echocardiographic markers, such as functional mitral regurgitation and right ventricular dysfunction,[78] which represent early therapeutic markers and useful prognostic tools. Baseline smaller LV dimensions, less hemodynamic impairment, absence of left bundle branch block, and no LGE on CMR are important predictors of LVRR.[74,77] Further identification of predictors of LVRR appears to be an important target for future research.

The genetic background of LVRR has been recently explored. Mutations in genes encoding cytoskeleton Z-disk (*DES*, *FLNC*, and *DMD*), obscurin-like 1 (*OBSL1*), nexilin F-actin binding protein (*NEXN*), myopalladin (*MYPN*), nebulette (*NEBL*), and LIM domain binding 3 (*LDB3*) have been associated with a lower rate of LVRR compared with *TTN* genotype in a study population of 152 DCM patients.[79]

Also, cardiac resynchronization therapy (CRT) has been proven to positively influence LVRR specifically in DCM.[73,80] Indeed, a higher percentage of "super-responders" to CRT has been reported for patients with DCM compared with other cardiomyopathies.[81] However, a possible diagnosis of reversible "left bundle branch block-induced cardiomyopathy," a pathological condition not well defined yet, should be considered as the cause of LV dysfunction in some of these cases.[81]

The natural history of DCM is generally characterized by initial improvement of ventricular involvement (in some cases, normalization of LV size and systolic function), usually within two years from optimization of therapy, followed by a subsequent period of stability.[82] Finally, from the 6th to 8th year of follow-up, new disease progression has been described.[82] Therefore, at the current state of knowledge, treatment should be continued lifelong, as well as in improved DCM patients. Patients with DCM should be re-evaluated continuously.[17] In some cases, new coronary artery disease or acute myocarditis can explain the worsening of LV systolic function or ventricular arrhythmic burden.[17] Therefore, comorbidities should be systematically ruled out during follow-up of patients with DCM.[17] These issues underline the importance not only of an accurate and complete initial diagnosis, but also of a continuous, individualized, long-term follow-up evaluation in DCM.

Open Issues in the Clinical Management of DCM

Despite the significant improvement in overall survival, the clinical management of DCM is still challenging, and DCM continues to represent an important indication for heart transplantation. Areas of uncertainty, reported below, require future research to further improve prognosis of DCM.

Genetic Testing in DCM

Almost 50% of DCM cases have a genetic origin; however, not all responsible genes are known.[12]

Although the genetic analysis of DCM is important because it allows for early diagnosis in family members, it has less of an impact for the patients themselves, as examples of "genetic treatment" are still few and not widely accessible. The current exceptions concern patients who carry the *LMNA* gene mutation:

- Class IIa indication by international guidelines for ICD implantation early during follow-up, in the presence of certain additional risk factors and independently of LV disfunction severity.[24]
- A new molecule, ARRY-797, is currently being tested in a phase III clinical trial, after showing promising results in phase II. The small molecule acts by inhibiting the p38-MAPK pathway, which appears to be up-regulated in the deficit of *LMNA*.

In a recent international consensus statement, a new recommendation for ICD implantation in patients with arrhythmogenic cardiomyopathy and a gene mutation of *LMNA*, *PLN*, or *FLNC*, also in the absence of severe LV dysfunction, has been suggested.[28] The detection of pro-arrhythmic gene mutations will be useful in the near future for a more precise prognostic stratification and targeted therapy in patients with DCM.[5]

Arrhythmic Stratification

The risk stratification for SCD in patients with DCM is still an open discussion. Recent studies show that only 31% of patients still meet the criteria for ICD implantation after six months of optimal medical therapy.[83] Accordingly, before deciding on an ICD implant, at least three to six months of optimal medical therapy are necessary.[24] However, ~2% of patients with DCM die suddenly after diagnosis.[78] Thus, how to select early candidates for ICD in primary prevention or for wearable ICD is still an open question. However, LV dilatation, wider QRS complex, and poor tolerance to β-blocker up-titration, more than LVEF, have been identified at baseline as early predictors of SCD and major ventricular arrhythmia in a large population of patients with DCM.[78]

On the other hand, ICD implantation is still debated for prevention of overall mortality in non-ischemic DCM. Recently, the DANISH trial has showed a similar overall mortality with or without ICD, but a benefit on overall mortality, other than SCD, was demonstrated in younger patients.[84] Therefore, the selection of patients with non-ischemic DCM for ICD implantation on the basis of LVEF and NYHA class, the only parameters validated and reported by guidelines, appears to be inadequate and further investigation is needed to refine patient selection.[85]

In the future, we should aim to evaluate each individual patient with DCM using multi-parametric models. Dynamic models (i.e., including different parameters at different time-points) during the natural history of the disease are proposed, due to the possible long-term and complex evolution of DCM. Those models should be comprehensive. An accurate etiological definition—followed by ECG, Holter monitoring, echocardiography (beyond LVEF, including speckle tracking evaluation), CMR (including quantification of late gadolinium enhancement, new techniques such as T1 mapping or GLS assessed by feature tracking), and cardiopulmonary exercise testing—and genetic data at the baseline should be systematically considered. Finally, periodic risk re-assessment of the patient's global and arrhythmic risk should be planned.[73]

References

1. Pinto YM, Elliott PM, Arbustini E, et al. Proposal for a revised definition of dilated cardiomyopathy, hypokinetic non-dilated cardiomyopathy, and its implications for clinical practice: a position statement of the ESC working group on myocardial and pericardial diseases. *Eur Heart J.* 2016;37:1850–8.
2. Elliott P, Andersson B, Arbustini E, et al. Classification of the cardiomyopathies: a position statement from ESC. *Eur Heart J.* 2008;29:270–6.
3. Arbustini E, Narula N, Dec GW, et al. The MOGE(S) classification for a phenotype–genotype nomenclature of cardiomyopathy. *J Am Coll Cardiol.* 2013;62:2046–72.
4. Mestroni L, Brun F, Spezzacatene A, et al. GENETIC CAUSES OF DILATED CARDIOMYOPATHY. *Prog Pediatr Cardiol.* 2014;37:13–18.
5. Paldino A, De Angelis G, Merlo M, et al. Genetics of dilated cardiomyopathy: clinical implications. *Curr Cardiol Rep.* 2018;20:83.
6. Hazebroek MR, Moors S, Dennert R, et al. Prognostic pelevance of gene-environment interactions in patients with dilated cardiomyopathy applying the MOGE(S) classification. *J Am Coll Cardiol.* 2015;66:1313–23.
7. Haas J, Frese KS, Peil B, et al. Atlas of the clinical genetics of human dilated cardiomyopathy. *Eur Heart J.* 2015;36:1123–35.
8. Ganesh SK, Arnett DK, Assimes TL, et al. Genetics and genomics for the prevention and treatment of cardiovascular disease: update. *Circulation.* 2013;128:2813–51.
9. Taylor MRG, Carniel E, Mestroni L. Cardiomyopathy, familial dilated. *Orphanet J Rare Dis.* 2006;1:27.
10. Moretti M, Merlo M, Barbati G, et al. Prognostic impact of familial screening in dilated cardiomyopathy. *Eur J Heart Fail.* 2010;12: 922–7.
11. Hershberger RE, Givertz MM, Ho CY, et al. Genetic evaluation of cardiomyopathy—A Heart Failure Society of America Practice Guideline. *J Card Fail.* 2018;24:281–302.
12. Hershberger RE, Hedges DJ, Morales A. Dilated cardiomyopathy: the complexity of a diverse genetic architecture. *Nat Rev Cardiol.* 2013;10:531–47.
13. Merlo M, Pivetta A, Pinamonti B, et al. Long-term prognostic impact of therapeutic strategies in patients with idiopathic dilated cardiomyopathy: changing mortality over the last 30 years. *Eur J Heart Fail.* 2014;16:317–24.
14. Belkaya S, Kontorovich AR, Byun M, et al. Autosomal recessive cardiomyopathy presenting as acute myocarditis. *J Am Coll Cardiol.* 2017;69:1653–65.
15. Maisch B. Alcoholic cardiomyopathy: the result of dosage and individual predisposition. *Herz.* 2016;41:484–93.
16. Dandamudi G, Rampurwala AY, Mahenthiran J, et al. Persistent left ventricular dilatation in tachycardia-induced cardiomyopathy patients after appropriate treatment and normalization of ejection fraction. *Hear Rhythm.* 2008;5:1111–4.
17. Merlo M, Cannatà A, Gobbo M, et al. Evolving concepts in dilated cardiomyopathy. *Eur J Heart Fail.* 2018;20:228–39.
18. McNally EM, Mestroni L. Dilated cardiomyopathy: genetic determinants and mechanisms. *Circ Res.* 2017;121:731–48.
19. Bowles NE, Bowles KR, Towbin JA. The "final common pathway" hypothesis and inherited cardiovascular disease. *Herz.* 2000;25:168–75.
20. Herman DS, Lam L, Taylor MRG, et al. Truncations of titin causing dilated cardiomyopathy. *N Engl J Med.* 2012;366:619–28.
21. Akinrinade O, Alastalo T-P, Koskenvuo JW. Relevance of truncating titin mutations in dilated cardiomyopathy. *Clin Genet.* 2016;90:49–54.
22. Akinrinade O, Koskenvuo JW, Alastalo TP. Prevalence of titin truncating variants in general population. *PLoS One.* 2015;10:e0145284.
23. Verdonschot JAJ, Hazebroek MR, Derks KWJ, et al. Titin cardiomyopathy leads to altered mitochondrial energetics, increased fibrosis and long-term life-threatening arrhythmias. *Eur Heart J.* 2018;39:864–73.
24. Ponikowski P, Voors AA, Anker SD, et al. 2016 ESC guidelines for the diagnosis and treatment of acute and chronic heart failure. *Eur Heart J.* 2016;37:2129–200.
25. Stossel TP, Condeelis J, Cooley L, et al. Filamins as integrators of cell mechanics and signalling. *Nat Rev Mol Cell Biol.* 2001;2:138–45.
26. Begay RL, Graw SL, Sinagra G, et al. Filamin C truncation mutations are associated with arrhythmogenic dilated cardiomyopathy and changes in the cell–cell adhesion structures. *JACC Clin Electrophysiol.* 2018;4:504–14.
27. Ortiz-Genga MF, Cuenca S, Dal Ferro M, et al. Truncating FLNC mutations are associated with high-risk dilated and arrhythmogenic cardiomyopathies. *J Am Coll Cardiol.* 2016;68:2440–51.
28. Towbin JA, McKenna WJ, Abrams DJ, et al. 2019 HRS expert consensus statement on evaluation, risk stratification, and management of arrhythmogenic cardiomyopathy. *Hear Rhythm.* 2019;16:e373–e407.
29. McNair WP, Sinagra G, Taylor MRG, et al. SCN5A mutations associate with arrhythmic dilated cardiomyopathy and commonly localize to the voltage-sensing mechanism. *J Am Coll Cardiol.* 2011;57:2160–8.
30. Marjamaa A, Laitinen-Forsblom P, Lahtinen AM, et al. Search for cardiac calcium cycling gene mutations in familial ventricular arrhythmias resembling catecholaminergic polymorphic ventricular tachycardia. *BMC Med Genet.* 2009;10:12.
31. Corrado D, Basso C, Judge DP. Arrhythmogenic cardiomyopathy. *Circ Res.* 2017;121:784–802.
32. Garcia-Pavia P, Syrris P, Salas C, et al. Desmosomal protein gene mutations in patients with idiopathic dilated cardiomyopathy undergoing cardiac transplantation: a clinicopathological study. *Heart.* 2011;97:1744–52.
33. Taylor MRG, Slavov D, Ku L, et al. Prevalence of desmin mutations in dilated cardiomyopathy. *Circulation.* 2007;115:1244–51.
34. Capetanaki Y, Papathanasiou S, Diokmetzidou A, et al. Desmin related disease: a matter of cell survival failure. *Curr Opin Cell Biol.* 2015;32:113–20.
35. Kamisago M, Sharma SD, DePalma SR, et al. Mutations in sarcomere protein genes as a cause of dilated cardiomyopathy. *N Engl J Med.* 2000;343:1688–96.
36. Hershberger RE, Hedges DJ, Morales A. Dilated cardiomyopathy: the complexity of a diverse genetic architecture. *Nat Rev Cardiol.* 2013;10:531–47.
37. Merlo M, Sinagra G, Carniel E, et al. Poor prognosis of rare sarcomeric gene variants in patients with dilated cardiomyopathy. *Clin Transl Sci.* 2013;6:424–8.
38. Fish M, Shaboodien G, Kraus S, et al. Mutation analysis of the phospholamban gene in 315 South Africans with dilated, hypertrophic, peripartum and arrhythmogenic right ventricular cardiomyopathies. *Sci Rep.* 2016;6:22235.
39. van der Zwaag PA, van Rijsingen IAW, Asimaki A, et al. Phospholamban R14del mutation in patients diagnosed with dilated cardiomyopathy or arrhythmogenic right ventricular cardiomyopathy: evidence supporting the concept of arrhythmogenic cardiomyopathy. *Eur J Heart Fail.* 2012;14:1199–207.
40. Maatz H, Jens M, Liss M, et al. RNA-binding protein RBM20 represses splicing to orchestrate cardiac pre-mRNA processing. *J Clin Invest.* 2014;124:3419–30.
41. Brauch KM, Karst ML, Herron KJ, et al. Mutations in ribonucleic acid binding protein gene cause familial dilated cardiomyopathy. *J Am Coll Cardiol.* 2009;54:930–41.
42. Gigli M, Stolfo D, Merlo M, et al. Insights into mildly dilated cardiomyopathy: temporal evolution and long-term prognosis. *Eur J Heart Fail.* 2017;19:531–9.
43. Spezzacatene A, Sinagra G, Merlo M, et al. Arrhythmogenic phenotype in dilated cardiomyopathy: natural history and predictors of life-threatening arrhythmias. *J Am Heart Assoc.* 2015;4:e002149.
44. Mestroni L, Sbaizero O. Arrhythmogenic cardiomyopathy. *Circulation.* 2018;137:1611–3.
45. Protonotarios A, Elliott PM. Arrhythmogenic cardiomyopathies (ACs): diagnosis, risk stratification and management. *Heart.* 2019; heartjnl-2017-311160.
46. Amorim S, Campelo M, Moura B, et al. The role of biomarkers in dilated cardiomyopathy: assessment of clinical severity and reverse remodeling. *Rev Port Cardiol.* 2017;36:709–16.
47. Wojciechowska C, Romuk E, Nowalany-Kozielska E, et al. Serum Galectin-3 and ST2 as predictors of unfavorable outcome in stable dilated cardiomyopathy patients. *Hell J Cardiol.* 2017;58:350–9.
48. Rapezzi C, Arbustini E, Caforio ALP, et al. Diagnostic work-up in cardiomyopathies: bridging the gap between clinical phenotypes and final diagnosis. A position statement from the ESC Working Group on Myocardial and Pericardial Diseases. *Eur Heart J.* 2013;34:1448–58.
49. Aleksova A, Carriere C, Zecchin M, et al. New-onset left bundle branch block independently predicts long-term mortality in patients with idiopathic dilated cardiomyopathy: data from the Trieste Heart Muscle Disease Registry. *Europace.* 2014;16:1450–9.

50. Gentile P, Paldino A, Cannatà A, et al. Left bundle branch block in dilated cardiomyopathy with intermediate left ventricular dysfunction: clinical phenotyping and outcome correlates. *Int J Cardiol.* 2019;278:180–5.
51. Merlo M, Zaffalon D, Stolfo D, et al. ECG in dilated cardiomyopathy. *J Cardiovasc Med.* 2019;120:450–8.
52. Goldberger JJ, Subačius H, Patel T, et al. Sudden cardiac death risk stratification in patients with nonischemic dilated cardiomyopathy. *J Am Coll Cardiol.* 2014;63:1879–89.
53. Lang RM, Badano LP, Mor-Avi V, et al. Recommendations for cardiac chamber quantification by echocardiography in adults: an update from the American Society of Echocardiography and the European Association of Cardiovascular Imaging. *Eur Hear J – Cardiovasc Imaging.* 2015;16:233–71.
54. Rossi A, Dini FL, Faggiano P, et al. Independent prognostic value of functional mitral regurgitation in patients with heart failure. A quantitative analysis of 1256 patients with ischaemic and non-ischaemic dilated cardiomyopathy. *Heart.* 2011;97:1675–80.
55. Pinamonti B, Zecchin M, Di Lenarda A, et al. Persistence of restrictive left ventricular filling pattern in dilated cardiomyopathy: an ominous prognostic sign. *J Am Coll Cardiol.* 1997;29:604–12.
56. Pinamonti B, Di Lenarda A, Sinagra G, et al. Restrictive left ventricular filling pattern in dilated cardiomyopathy assessed by Doppler echocardiography: clinical, echocardiographic and hemodynamic correlations and prognostic implications. Heart Muscle Disease Study Group. *J Am Coll Cardiol.* 1993;22:808–15.
57. Merlo M, Gobbo M, Stolfo D, et al. The prognostic impact of the evolution of RV function in idiopathic DCM. *JACC Cardiovasc Imaging.* 2016;9:1034–42.
58. Yu Y, Yu S, Tang X, et al. Evaluation of left ventricular strain in patients with dilated cardiomyopathy. *J Int Med Res.* 2017;45:2092–100.
59. Swat SA, Cohen D, Shah SJ, et al. Baseline longitudinal strain predicts recovery of left ventricular ejection fraction in hospitalized patients with nonischemic cardiomyopathy. *J Am Heart Assoc.* 2018;7:e09841.
60. Adamo L, Perry A, Novak E, et al. Abnormal global longitudinal strain predicts future deterioration of left ventricular function in heart failure patients with a recovered left ventricular ejection fraction. *Circ Hear Fail.* 2017;10:e003788.
61. Strohm O, Schulz-Menger J, Pilz B, et al. Measurement of left ventricular dimensions and function in patients with dilated cardiomyopathy. *J Magn Reson Imaging.* 2001;13:367–71.
62. Porcari A, De Angelis G, Romani S, et al. Current diagnostic strategies for dilated cardiomyopathy: a comparison of imaging techniques. *Expert Rev Cardiovasc Ther.* 2019;17:53–63.
63. Halliday BP, Baksi AJ, Gulati A, et al. Outcome in dilated cardiomyopathy related to the extent, location, and pattern of late gadolinium enhancement. *JACC Cardiovasc Imaging.* 2019;12:1645–55.
64. Leong DP, Chakrabarty A, Shipp N, et al. Effects of myocardial fibrosis and ventricular dyssynchrony on response to therapy in new-presentation idiopathic dilated cardiomyopathy: insights from cardiovascular magnetic resonance and echocardiography. *Eur Heart J.* 2012;33:640–8.
65. Di Marco A, Anguera I, Schmitt M, et al. Late gadolinium enhancement and the risk for ventricular arrhythmias or sudden death in dilated cardiomyopathy. *JACC Hear Fail.* 2017;5:28–38
66. Romano S, Judd RM, Kim RJ, et al. Feature-tracking global longitudinal strain predicts death in a multicenter population of patients with ischemic and nonischemic dilated cardiomyopathy incremental to ejection fraction and late gadolinium enhancement. *JACC Cardiovasc Imaging.* 2018;11:1419–29.
67. Merlo M, Masè M, Vitrella G, et al. Usefulness of addition of magnetic resonance imaging to echocardiographic imaging to predict left ventricular reverse remodeling in patients with nonischemic cardiomyopathy. *Am J Cardiol.* 2018;122:490–7.
68. Mehra MR. Guidelines for listing candidates for heart transplant. *JAMA Cardiol.* 2017;2:98.
69. Caforio ALP, Pankuweit S, Arbustini E, et al. Current state of knowledge on aetiology, diagnosis, management, and therapy of myocarditis: a position statement of the European Society of Cardiology Working Group on Myocardial and Pericardial Diseases. *Eur Heart J.* 2013;34:2636–48.
70. Sinagra G, Anzini M, Pereira NL, et al. Myocarditis in clinical practice. *Mayo Clin Proc.* 2016;91:1256–66.
71. Pollack A, Kontorovich AR, Fuster V, et al. Viral myocarditis—diagnosis, treatment options, and current controversies. *Nat Rev Cardiol.* 2015;12:670–80.
72. Yancy CW, Jessup M, Bozkurt B, et al. 2017 ACC/AHA/HFSA focused update of the 2013 ACCF/AHA guideline for the management of heart failure: a report of the American College of Cardiology/American Heart Association Task Force on Clinical Practice Guidelines and the Heart Failure Society of America. *Circulation.* 2017;136:e137–61.
73. Merlo M, Caiffa T, Gobbo M, et al. Reverse remodeling in dilated cardiomyopathy: insights and future perspectives. *IJC Hear Vasc.* 2018;18:52–57.
74. Castelli G, Fornaro A, Ciaccheri M, et al. Improving survival rates of patients with idiopathic dilated cardiomyopathy in tuscany over 3 decades. *Circ Hear Fail.* 2013;6:913–21.
75. Burkett EL, Hershberger RE. Clinical and genetic issues in familial dilated cardiomyopathy. *J Am Coll Cardiol.* 2005;45:969–81.
76. Merlo M, Pyxaras SA, Pinamonti B, et al. Prevalence and prognostic significance of left ventricular reverse remodeling in dilated cardiomyopathy receiving tailored medical treatment. *J Am Coll Cardiol.* 2011;57:1468–76.
77. Matsumura Y, Hoshikawa-Nagai E, Kubo T, et al. Left ventricular reverse remodeling in long-term (12 years) survivors with idiopathic dilated cardiomyopathy. *Am J Cardiol.* 2013;111:106–10.
78. Losurdo P, Stolfo D, Merlo M, et al. Early arrhythmic events in idiopathic dilated cardiomyopathy. *JACC Clin Electrophysiol.* 2016;2:535–43.
79. Dal Ferro M, Stolfo D, Altinier A, et al. Association between mutation status and left ventricular reverse remodelling in dilated cardiomyopathy. *Heart.* 2017;103:1704–10.
80. Serdoz LV, Daleffe E, Merlo M, et al. Predictors for restoration of normal left ventricular function in response to cardiac resynchronization therapy measured at time of implantation. *Am J Cardiol.* 2011;108:75–80.
81. Zecchin M, Proclemer A, Magnani S, et al. Long-term outcome of "super-responder" patients to cardiac resynchronization therapy. *Europace.* 2014;16:363–71.
82. Merlo M, Stolfo D, Anzini M, et al. Persistent recovery of normal left ventricular function and dimension in idiopathic dilated cardiomyopathy during long-term follow-up: does real healing exist? *J Am Heart Assoc.* 2015;4:e001504.
83. Zecchin M, Merlo M, Pivetta A, et al. How can optimization of medical treatment avoid unnecessary implantable cardioverter-defibrillator implantations in patients with idiopathic dilated cardiomyopathy presenting with "SCD-HeFT criteria?" *Am J Cardiol.* 2012;109:729–35.
84. Køber L, Thune JJ, Nielsen JC, et al. Defibrillator implantation in patients with nonischemic systolic heart failure. *N Engl J Med.* 2016;375:1221–30.
85. Stolfo D, Ceschia N, Zecchin M, et al. Arrhythmic risk stratification in patients with idiopathic dilated cardiomyopathy. *Am J Cardiol.* 2018;121:1601–9.

Chapter 32
STRESS CARDIOMYOPATHY (TAKOTSUBO SYNDROME)

Marco Giuseppe Del Buono, Juan Guido Chiabrando, Krishna Ravindra, and Antonio Abbate

Introduction

Stress cardiomyopathy (SCMP) or Takotsubo syndrome, also known as broken heart syndrome or apical ballooning syndrome, is an acute and reversible form of myocardial stunning often precipitated by an emotional or physical stress, not explained by an obstruction of an epicardial coronary artery as in acute coronary syndrome (ACS). It is often encountered in women, especially of post-menopausal age.[1]

The first case of acute and transient myocardial dysfunction was described in a patient with pheochromocytoma by Iga et al., although the authors did not use the term "takotsubo."[2] Two years later in 1991, "takotsubo," the Japanese name for the octopus pot, was introduced by Sato et al. to describe the shape of left ventriculogram in a patient with suspected ACS.[3] Despite the efforts made to understand this syndrome, the pathophysiology is still largely unknown. Enhanced sympathetic activity and excessive catecholamine release seem to play a key role in determining myocardial dysfunction in stress cardiomyopathy.[1,4,5] Due to the self-limiting nature of the syndrome, SCMP was initially believed to be a benign disorder associated with a good prognosis; however, over time, it has become clear that SCMP is associated with a non-negligible risk of complications, long-term increase in mortality rate, and recurrence [1,6–8]

Definition and Diagnosis

SCMP is an acute and reversible (<21 days) form of left ventricular (LV) systolic dysfunction, in the absence of an occluded culprit epicardial coronary artery, often following an intense emotionally or physically stressful event.[1,4,6] As such, LV regional wall motion abnormalities typically extend beyond the territory supplied by a single epicardial coronary artery, with a circumferential (non-coronary) pattern. The classically described anatomical variant is "apical ballooning," which is characterized by apical hypokinesia or akinesia accompanied by basal compensatory hyperkinesia.[6] Clinical presentation and electrocardiographic findings are similar to those of patients presenting with ACS.[1,6] Suspicion of SCMP should be based on clinical context (emotional or physical trigger in the preceding days); the characteristic disproportionately mild elevation of plasma cardiac troponin and creatine kinase myocardial band (CK-MB) levels in comparison with the significant elevation in natriuretic peptide levels (B-type natriuretic peptide [BNP] or N-terminal-pro-BNP [NT-proBNP]), and the suggestive non-invasive cardiovascular imaging findings.[1,9–11] However, the aforementioned non-invasive tools are typically inconclusive, making coronary angiography usually necessary in order to exclude an acute obstruction of an epicardial coronary artery.

Different diagnostic criteria for SCMP have been proposed over the years. The most commonly used is the Revised Mayo Clinic Criteria.[12] In addition, new diagnostic criteria have been recently proposed in the last consensus paper from the European Society of Cardiology, referred to as the International Takotsubo Diagnostic Criteria (InterTAK Diagnostic Criteria), summarized in Table 32.1.[13] Neurologic disorders (e.g., subarachnoid hemorrhage, stroke, or seizures) and pheochromocytoma have now been listed among potential triggers. Furthermore, the presence of significant coronary artery disease is no longer considered an absolute exclusion criterion for the diagnosis.[13]

Epidemiology

Since its first description in Japan in 1991, SCMP has been increasingly recognized across the world. It now represents approximately 1–2% of patients presenting at emergency departments with troponin-positive suspected ACS,[14] with an overall incidence of approximately 15 to 30 cases per 100,000 per year.[7] It occurs more commonly in women, and predominantly in those of older age[6] The largest registry in the word, the International Takotsubo Registry, reported a relative prevalence of 89.9% women, with a mean age of 66.4 years. SCMP in males is less frequent, but it is more often precipitated by a physical event. The recurrence rate for all patients is estimated to be 1.8% per patient year.[6]

Pathophysiology

The pathophysiology of SCMP is still largely unknown, and several pathophysiological mechanisms have been proposed. A pivotal study by Wittstein et al. showed extremely high levels of plasma catecholamines and stress-related neuropeptides in patients with SCMP, compared with Killip class III ACS patients, suggesting a direct causal link between plasma catecholamines and stress cardiomyopathy.[4] However, these findings were not confirmed in subsequent studies, in which plasma levels of catecholamines were found to be normal or only slightly elevated.[15] This heterogenicity may be at least in part explained by the differences in techniques and in cut-off thresholds used between laboratories.[15] Recalculation of the plasma epinephrine in Wittstein's study, according to published values, revealed only a modest increase of plasma epinephrine.[15] Only recently, using a neuroimaging approach, is the key role of a brain-heart connection in SCMP becoming clear. In the acute phases, an increase in cerebral blood flow to the hippocampus, brainstem, and basal ganglia has been documented, with a progressive normalization in the recovery phase.[16–19] The complex neocortical and limbic integration following the interpretation of a threatening stimulus activates the neuro-hormonal stress response in the hypothalamus, resulting in the activation of brainstem and spinal cord noradrenergic neurons and sympathetic adrenomedullary circuits.[16–18] Hypoconnectivity of central brain regions associated with autonomic functions and regulation of the limbic system in patients with SCMP suggest that functional alterations at the level of the central nervous system may result in the onset of the syndrome in response to

DOI: 10.1201/9780429244544-39

TABLE 32.1: Diagnostic Criteria for Stress Cardiomyopathy (Takotsubo Syndrome)

International Takotsubo Diagnostic Criteria (InterTAK Diagnostic Criteria)

1. Patients show transient left ventricular dysfunction (hypokinesia, akinesia, or dyskinesia), presenting as apical ballooning or midventricular, basal, or focal wall motion abnormalities. Right ventricular involvement can be present. Besides these regional wall motion patterns, transitions between all types can exist. The regional wall motion abnormality usually extends beyond a single epicardial vascular distribution; however, rare cases can exist where the regional wall motion abnormality is present in the subtended myocardial territory of a single coronary artery (focal Takotsubo syndrome).[a]
2. An emotional, physical, or combined trigger can precede the Takotsubo syndrome event, but this is not obligatory.
3. Neurologic disorders (e.g., subarachnoid hemorrhage, stroke/transient ischemic attack, or seizures) as well as pheochromocytoma may serve as triggers for Takotsubo syndrome.
4. New-onset ECG abnormalities are present (ST-segment elevation, ST-segment depression, T-wave inversion, and QTc prolongation); however, rare cases exist without any ECG changes.
5. Serum levels of cardiac biomarkers (troponin and creatine kinase) are moderately elevated in most cases; significant elevation of brain natriuretic peptides is common.
6. Significant coronary artery disease is not a contraindication in Takotsubo syndrome.
7. Patients have no evidence of infectious myocarditis.[b]
8. Postmenopausal women are predominantly affected.

Revised Mayo Clinic Criteria

1. Transient hypokinesis, akinesis, or dyskinesis of the left ventricular midsegments with or without apical involvement; the regional wall motion abnormalities extend beyond a single epicardial vascular distribution; a stressful trigger is often, but not always present.[c]
2. Absence of obstructive coronary disease or angiographic evidence of acute plaque rupture.[d]
3. New electrocardiographic abnormalities (either ST-segment elevation and/or T-wave inversion) or modest elevation in cardiac troponin level.
4. Absence of pheochromocytoma or myocarditis. In either of these situations, the diagnosis of SCMP should be made with caution, and a clear stressful precipitating trigger must be sought.

[a] Wall motion abnormalities may remain for a prolonged period of time or documentation of recovery may not be possible, for example, as a result of death before evidence of recovery is captured.
[b] Cardiac magnetic resonance imaging is recommended to exclude infectious myocarditis and diagnose confirmation of Takotsubo syndrome.
[c] There are rare exceptions to these criteria such as those patients in whom the regional wall motion abnormality is limited to a single coronary territory.
[d] It is possible that a patient with obstructive coronary atherosclerosis may also develop stress cardiomyopathy. However, this is very rare in our experience and in the published literature, perhaps because such cases are misdiagnosed as an acute coronary syndrome.

a stressful trigger.[18] Sympathetic nervous system overactivity following an emotional or physical stress may lead to a local myocardial spillover of catecholamines and neuropeptides (e.g., neuropeptide Y [NPY]), resulting in direct myocardial toxicity and/or an acute microvascular dysfunction resulting in a supply-demand mismatch and myocardial stunning.[1] Elevated norepinephrine levels in the coronary sinus have been found in patients with stress cardiomyopathy, suggesting an increase in the local release of myocardial catecholamines.[20] As LV β-adrenergic receptor density has an apical-basal gradient, the apex presents with the highest receptor density and lower sympathetic innervation; thus, the apex is more sensitive to high levels of catecholamines.[21] However, cases of recurrent SCMP with variant forms challenge this idea and support a homogeneous ventricular adrenoceptor density.

Why SCMP occurs only in a small portion of individuals after a stressful event is still unclear. An individual predisposition to an increased sympathetic drive and presynaptic concentration of norepinephrine/NPY granules, as well as conditions associated with chronic endothelial and microvascular dysfunction (i.e., diabetes mellitus, postmenopausal state, asthma/chronic obstructive lung diseases, underlying myocardial diseases), may predispose to an acute microvascular and myocardial dysfunction following sympathetic activation (Figure 32.1).[1,5,22–28] The high prevalence in postmenopausal women may be explained by the increased central sympathetic drive, NPY concentration, endothelial dysfunction, and oxidative stress levels (predisposing to microvascular dysfunction).[1,25,26] Patients with psychiatric disorders (e.g., anxiety, depression) or on antidepressants (e.g., selective norepinephrine reuptake inhibitors) may have exaggerated sympathetic adrenergic response to emotional stress.[27] Asthma exacerbation is another trigger of TS. Patients with history of asthma show higher NPY levels, and during acute asthma attacks may have an increased release of NPY at the myocardial level.[1,24] Furthermore, the use of β_2 adrenergic receptor agonists, epinephrine, and mast-cell degranulation (containing tumor necrosis factor-α and interleukin-1) may contribute to the catecholaminergic cardiac dysfunction.[1,24] Insights into pathophysiology also come from case series describing the occurrence of SCMP during cancer treatment as a result of cancer-related stress or treatment-related coronary microvascular dysfunction (i.e., vascular endothelial growth factor inhibitors) predisposing to SCMP after a stressful trigger.[29,30] The mechanism of SCMP is similar to "neurogenic stunning myocardium" described in the past during intracerebral hemorrhage, ischemic stroke, seizures, and brain trauma, that have now been listed among the neurological triggers for stress cardiomyopathy.[1,13,31]

Triggers

SCMP is often triggered by an emotional or physical stress; however, about one-third of patients have no evidence of an identifiable preceding stressful event.[6] Emotional triggers often include the death of a loved one, natural disasters, financial troubles, and sexual abuse. Interestingly, SCMP-like episodes may also follow pleasant events, a phenomenon known as "happy heart syndrome."[6,32] Physical triggers are more common than emotional stress factors and include a plethora of medical conditions such as, but not limited to, acute respiratory failure, surgery, central nervous system conditions, infection/sepsis, and trauma.[1,6] Physical stressful events are more often identified as triggers in male patients, whereas emotional triggers more frequently precede SCMP in women (Table 32.2).

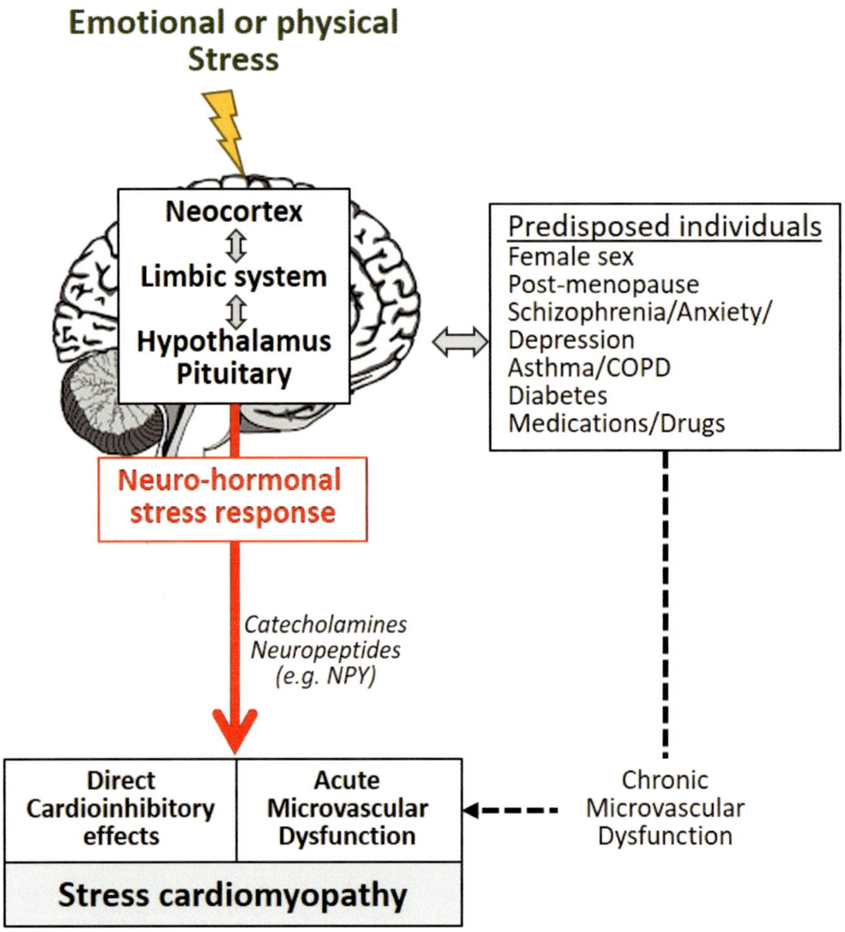

FIGURE 32.1 Schematic representation of the pathophysiology of stress cardiomyopathy.

Anatomical Variants

Since the initial description of the classical (typical) apical ballooning pattern, accounting for 75–80% of all variants, several variants of LV involvement have been described over time (Figure 32.2).[1,6] The mid-ventricular pattern is the second most frequent variant, present in up to 15% of cases and is characterized by the akinesis or hypokinesis of the middle part of the LV with hypercontractile apical and basal segments. Reverse (inverted) or basal pattern is characterized by basal and mid-ventricular akinesis or hypokinesis with apical sparing. Rarely, focal types have been described and are characterized by wall motion abnormalities limited to isolated segment(s). Other rare variants include biventricular dysfunction and isolated right ventricular impairment, usually associated with severe hemodynamic compromise, and global dysfunction. The latter is more often encountered in SCMP triggered by pheochromocytoma or acute neurological disorders.[1,6] As previously discussed, the pathophysiological explanation for different anatomical variants is still largely debated given the fact that (1) the apical-basal β-adrenoceptor density gradient has never been confirmed in humans, and (2) it may only account for the apical ballooning variant.

Clinical Presentation

The clinical presentation of patients with SCMP is non-specific. The most common presenting symptoms are chest pain and dyspnea.[1,6] Syncope, acute heart failure, and arrhythmias are less frequent.[1,6,33] The non-specific presentation makes the diagnosis challenging for clinicians. Furthermore, coexisting or precipitating acute illnesses (e.g., acute respiratory failure, sepsis, cerebrovascular accident) can mask the classical symptoms of chest pain and dyspnea leading to an under- or mis-diagnosis.

Differential Diagnosis

Besides ACS, clinicians should be aware of other causes of cardiac and non-cardiac chest pain, especially when concomitant with electrocardiography (ECG) abnormalities. Table 32.3 summarizes the principal conditions to consider in the differential diagnosis of patients presenting to emergency departments with chest pain and ECG abnormalities.

Diagnostic Work-Up

Pre-Test Probability

Because clinical presentation, ECG abnormalities, and cardiac biomarkers on admission are commonly indistinguishable from classical ACS, to facilitate initial evaluation in the emergency department, the InterTAK Diagnostic score has recently been proposed.[34] This score encompasses seven clinical, anamnestic, and ECG variables that can be easily obtained. Each is assigned a score value (Table 32.4, https://www.takotsubo-registry.com/takotsubo-score.html), providing a pre-test probability for SCMP versus ACS.

TABLE 32.2: Triggers Associated with Stress Cardiomyopathy

Emotional Stress[14,46,47]
Tragic events involving a beloved one, receiving bad news (legal, medical, social, or financial), interpersonal arguments, assault, public speaking, car accident, natural disasters (e.g., earthquakes), after adulterous intercourse.

Physical Stress
Surgical or non-surgical procedures: e.g., cholecystectomy, hysterectomy, cesarean section, radiotherapy, colonoscopy.
Cardiac procedures: e.g., arrhythmia ablation, pacemaker implantation, electrical cardioversion.
Medical conditions: e.g., respiratory exacerbation of asthma or chronic obstructive pulmonary disease, pneumothorax, pulmonary embolism, acute cholecystitis, pheochromocytoma, seizures, limbic encephalitis, spinal cord injury, ischemic/hemorrhagic stroke, global amnesia, head trauma, Guillain-Barré syndrome, posterior reversible encephalopathy syndrome, subarachnoid hemorrhage, advanced amyotrophic lateral sclerosis.
Medications and illicit drugs: e.g., cocaine, marijuana, Adderall, nortriptyline overdose, venlafaxine overdose, albuterol, metoprolol withdrawal, epinephrine, 5-fluorouracil, duloxetine, opiate and alcohol withdrawal, methamphetamines and cancer treatment (e.g., bevacizumab), abuse of energy drinks.

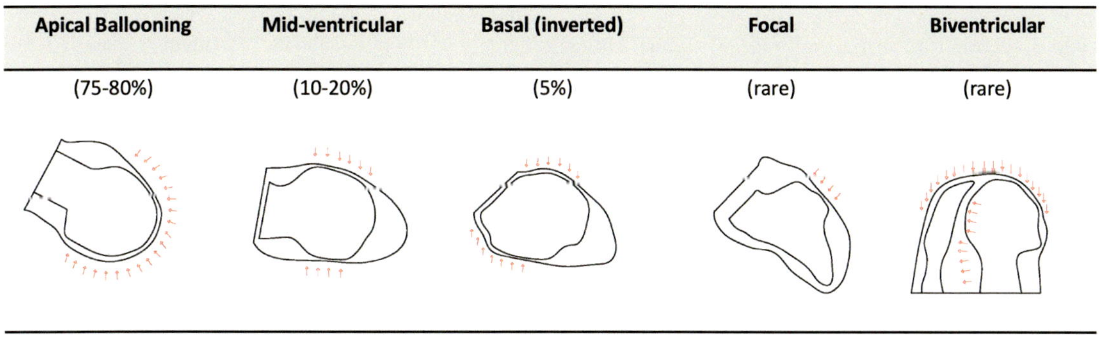

FIGURE 32.2 Anatomical variants of stress cardiomyopathy.

TABLE 32.3: Conditions to Consider in the Differential Diagnosis of Stress Cardiomyopathy Presenting with Chest Pain and ECG Abnormalities

- Myocardial infarction with obstructive CAD
- Myocardial infarction with no obstructive CAD (MINOCA)
- Acute pulmonary embolism
- Acute myopericarditis
- Pheochromocytoma or exogenous catecholamine excess (cocaine, methamphetamines)*
- Hypertrophic cardiomyopathy
- Others (e.g., aortic dissection, myocardial contusion)

* Pheochromocytoma may represent a robust and durable substrate for stress cardiomyopathy, precipitating an acute event following a stressful trigger. Cocaine and methamphetamines may cause coronary vasospasm as well as direct myocardial toxicity.

Cardiac Biomarkers

Serum troponin and CK-MB levels are generally only mildly elevated in patients with SCMP. Their increase is usually disproportionately low compared with the extent of wall motion abnormalities and with the increase in BNP and NT-proBNP plasma levels. The BNP-to-troponin and BNP-to-CK-MB ratios may help to differentiate between SCMP and ACS with a good specificity; however, sensitivity is low (Table 32.5).[9,10]

Electrocardiographic Abnormalities

T-wave inversion and QTc prolongation are the most common ECG abnormalities at diagnosis of SCMP. The "classic" evolution of ECG changes, represented by a transient ST-segment elevation, followed by negative T waves and transient T-wave reversion with the development of deep, inverted T waves, has been debunked by subsequent studies (Figure 32.3).[35–37] ST-segment depression is less frequent (<10%) than in ACS. Several criteria have been proposed to differentiate between ACS and SCMP with regard to ECG abnormalities.[38] However, due to the high heterogenicity of ECG findings (as a result of variable patterns of wall motion abnormalities, triggers, time from symptom onset, racial differences, etc.), ECG is often not of great help when trying to differentiate between SCMP and ACS (Table 32.5).[36,37]

Echocardiography

Transthoracic echocardiography is the simplest method to detect global and segmental LV systolic function, the presence of complications (mitral regurgitation in the setting of dynamic LV outflow tract obstruction (LVOTO), papillary muscle dysfunction, apical thrombus formation, or myocardial wall rupture), and is fundamental in hemodynamic monitoring and management guidance.[1] The key characteristic of SCMP, differentiating it from other causes of myocardial damage, is that wall motion abnormalities typically extend beyond the territory supplied by a single epicardial coronary. New echocardiographic techniques, such as speckle tracking with multidirectional assessment of LV deformation, increase the

TABLE 32.4: InterTAK Diagnostic Score

Criterion	Points
Female sex	25
Emotional trigger	24
Physical trigger	13
Absence of ST-segment depression	12
Psychiatric disorders	11
Neurologic disorders	9
QTc prolongation	6
Diagnosis (cut-off value [range 0–100])	
≥50	**≤31**
Takotsubo syndrome (Specificity 95%)	Acute coronary syndrome (Specificity 95%)

sensitivity in detecting myocardial wall motion abnormalities (Table 32.5).[39]

Coronary Angiography, Ventriculography, and Coronary Intravascular Imaging

Because of the striking resemblance of SCMP to ACS, coronary angiography is usually performed to rule out an acute thrombotic occlusion of the coronary arteries in SCMP. Most of the patients with SCMP have normal or near-normal epicardial coronary arteries at coronary angiography (Figure 32.4). However, because of the high prevalence of coronary artery disease (CAD) in patients of older age, patients with SCMP may also have obstructive CAD (bystander finding) and therefore its presence should not a priori exclude the diagnosis of SCMP.[40] In patients without a culprit coronary lesion, ventriculography is performed to detect and differentiate the anatomical variants. In select cases, where coronary angiography shows normal or near-normal coronary arteries and ventriculography remains inconclusive, intravascular imaging with intravascular ultrasound and optical coherence tomography, as well as intracoronary provocative tests (with acetylcholine or ergonovine), may help elucidate the underlying cause of myocardial infarction with non-obstructive coronary artery lesions (Table 32.5).[41]

Cardiac Computed Tomography Scan

In patients at very low risk of CAD (recent cardiac catheterization, young age with a low-risk profile), at high risk of complications (active bleeding, frail patients), or in those with a prior episode of SCMP and suspicion of recurrence, a less invasive procedure, such as cardiac computed tomography scan, may help in confirming the presence or absence of significant coronary stenotic lesions.

Cardiac Magnetic Resonance

Cardiac magnetic resonance (CMR) is the first-line modality for a detailed non-invasive assessment of left and right ventricular systolic function and early detection of structural myocardial complications (e.g., pericardial effusion, mitral regurgitation, LVOTO, and myocardial wall rupture).[11] It also plays a unique role in the differential diagnosis. The presence of transmural edema in SCMP, typically with a circumferential extension, matches with the areas of wall motion abnormalities displaying a non-coronary distribution.[11] Myocardial edema is a transient phenomenon, normally resolving between three and six months. A characteristic feature of SCMP on CMR is the absence of late gadolinium enhancement (LGE), and its distribution within the myocardial wall can help differentiate SCMP from myocardial infarction, in which LGE is subendocardial or transmural with an epicardial coronary artery distribution (Figure 32.5). Furthermore, LGE can help differentiate SCMP from myocarditis, in which LGE is typically focal and "patchy," with a subepicardial or midventricular non-coronary distribution (Table 32.5).[1,11]

Management

Acute Treatment

In the absence of randomized, controlled trials, to date the management of SCMP is based solely on clinical experience. Because SCMP is clinically difficult to distinguish from ACS, patients are usually treated with antithrombotic drugs until a final diagnosis is made. In patients with heart failure without signs of cardiogenic shock, treatment is usually similar as for patients with heart failure and reduced ejection fraction (i.e., beta-blockers, angiotensin-converting enzyme [ACE] inhibitors, or angiotensin II receptor blockers [ARBs]), except that diuretics and vasodilators should be used with caution on account of the risk of developing LVOTO. In patients with cardiogenic shock, appropriate management depends upon whether significant LVOTO is present or not. Patients without significant LVOTO may require temporary inotropic therapy (e.g., milrinone, dobutamine, or dopamine), and, if needed, temporary mechanical support (with, e.g., Impella or intra-aortic balloon pump). Continuous echocardiographic assessment is required as inotropic agents may worsen LVOTO by increasing basal hypercontractility. In patients with cardiogenic shock and LVOTO, inotropes are not indicated. Intravenous fluids and low doses of short-acting β-blockers (e.g., esmolol, metoprolol) may improve LVOTO; however, these measures may be poorly tolerated from a hemodynamic standpoint. Peripherally acting vasopressors (e.g., phenylephrine or vasopressin) may be considered to increase blood pressure without further worsening LVOTO. If medical therapy fails to improve hemodynamics, temporary mechanical circulatory support with, e.g., Impella or extra-corporeal membrane oxygenation, is recommended.[1,42,43]

Long-Term Management

As in the acute setting, there are no randomized trials data regarding the choice and the long-term duration of medical therapy. Observational data showed that use of ACE inhibitors or ARBs were associated with improved survival at one year;[6] such survival benefit has not been observed with β-blockers.[6] Likewise, there is no evidence to support the use of antiplatelet medications after a final diagnosis of SCMP.

Complications

Despite the reversibility of the syndrome, SCMP is associated with a significant risk of in-hospital complications and mortality.[6,7] These include acute heart failure and cardiogenic shock (due to acute pump failure, LVOTO, functional mitral regurgitation, or myocardial wall rupture), supraventricular or ventricular arrhythmias (especially in the context of prolonged QTc interval), advanced atrioventricular block, thromboembolic events, pericarditis, intramyocardial hemorrhage, or cardiac rupture (free wall rupture or ventricular septum defect).[1,6] Cardiac arrest may occur at presentation or during the subacute phase with a reported incidence of 5.9%, and is associated

TABLE 32.5: **Differential Diagnosis of Patients with Stress Cardiomyopathy (Takotsubo Syndrome)**

Clinical Presentation	Electrocardiography	Echocardiography	Angiographic Findings	CMR	Cardiac Biomarkers
Stress Cardiomyopathy					
Usually in post-menopausal female. Emotional or physical trigger Chest pain, dyspnea, arrhythmias, heart failure/cardiogenic shock, cardiac arrest	ST-segment elevation, T wave inversion, QTc prolongation. ST-segment depression is less common.	Apical, mid-ventricular, basal, or focal hypo/akinesia.*	Absence of a culprit obstructive coronary artery lesion in angiography and/or intravascular imaging. Ventriculography identifies the anatomical variant.	Edema: Transmural ventricular edema in the areas of ventricular dysfunction Cine-CMR: Regional wall motion abnormalities according to the anatomical patterns LGE: Generally absent (cut-off>5 SD)	NT-proBNP and BNP ↑↑ Troponin and CK-MB ↑
Myocardial Infarction					
High pre-test probability of coronary artery disease Chest pain, dyspnea, arrhythmias, heart failure/cardiogenic shock, cardiac arrest	ST-segment elevation, ST-segment depression, and/or T-wave inversion.	Regional wall motion abnormalities according with epicardial coronary artery distribution.	Coronary artery disease with acute plaque rupture and thrombus formation.	Edema: Subendocardial or transmural at sites of wall motion abnormalities Cine-CMR: Regional wall motion abnormalities according to epicardial coronary artery distribution LGE: Bright LGE, typically subendocardial or transmural in an epicardial coronary artery distribution	Troponin and CK-MB levels ↑↑ BNP and NT-proBNP ↑
Myocarditis					
Middle-age population Often preceded by an upper respiratory infection or enteritis Chest pain, dyspnea, acute heart failure, syncope, palpitations, cardiac arrest	Non-specific ST- and/or T-wave changes (diffuse ST-segment elevation is usually seen in myopericarditis).	Global or segmental systolic dysfunction. Pericardial effusion may be also present.	Absence of obstructive coronary artery disease or angiographic evidence of acute plaque destabilization.	Edema: Typically subepicardial, basal and lateral Cine-CMR: Global, or regional contractile dysfunction LGE: Low intensity, focal, "patchy," subepicardial or midventricular with a non-coronary distribution	Troponin and CK-MB ↑ BNP and NT-proBNP ↑

Abbreviations: BNP: B-type natriuretic peptide; CK-MB: creatine kinase myocardial band; CMR: cardiac magnetic resonance; LGE: late gadolinium enhancement; NT-proBNP: N-terminal pro-B-type natriuretic peptide.

with worse short- and long-term mortality.[33,44] These patients are more likely to be younger and male, and have atrial fibrillation, neurologic comorbidities, physical triggers, longer QT interval, atypical forms of SCMP and lower LV ejection fraction on admission. Due to the increased risk of arrhythmias, ECG monitoring is therefore recommended in the acute phase and wherever possible until ECG, QTc and LV ejection fraction recover.

Secondary Prevention

Prevention of Arrhythmias

Beta-blockers are frequently used in stable patients based on the assumption of an increased sympathetic drive in patients with SCMP. However, β-blockers should be used with caution in patients with prolonged QTc due to the risk of *Torsade de pointes* and ventricular arrhythmias. Furthermore, β-blockers have failed to improve one-year survival.[6] Due to the self-limiting course of the disease, an implantable cardioverter defibrillator in patients experiencing malignant ventricular arrhythmias or cardiac arrest is generally not recommended. However, due to the risk of recurrence, a wearable defibrillator (LifeVest) or a subcutaneous implantable cardioverter defibrillator may be considered case by case.[44]

Prevention of Thromboembolism

In patients with typical SCMP, the increase in blood stasis in the akinetic apical segments of the LV predisposes to thrombus formation. Prophylactic anticoagulation is recommended if large areas of akinesis are present and should be continued until LV function recovers. For patients with thrombus formation, treatment is recommended for three months, as for patients with ACS.[1]

Prevention of Recurrence

Stress cardiomyopathy is associated with a 2% risk per year of recurrence and can be precipitated by different triggers and with a different anatomical pattern over the patient's entire lifespan.[6] Observational data suggest that ACE inhibitors and ARBs are associated with lower risk of recurrence, whereas β-blockers unexpectedly failed to prevent recurrence despite their potential effects on mitigating increased sympathetic

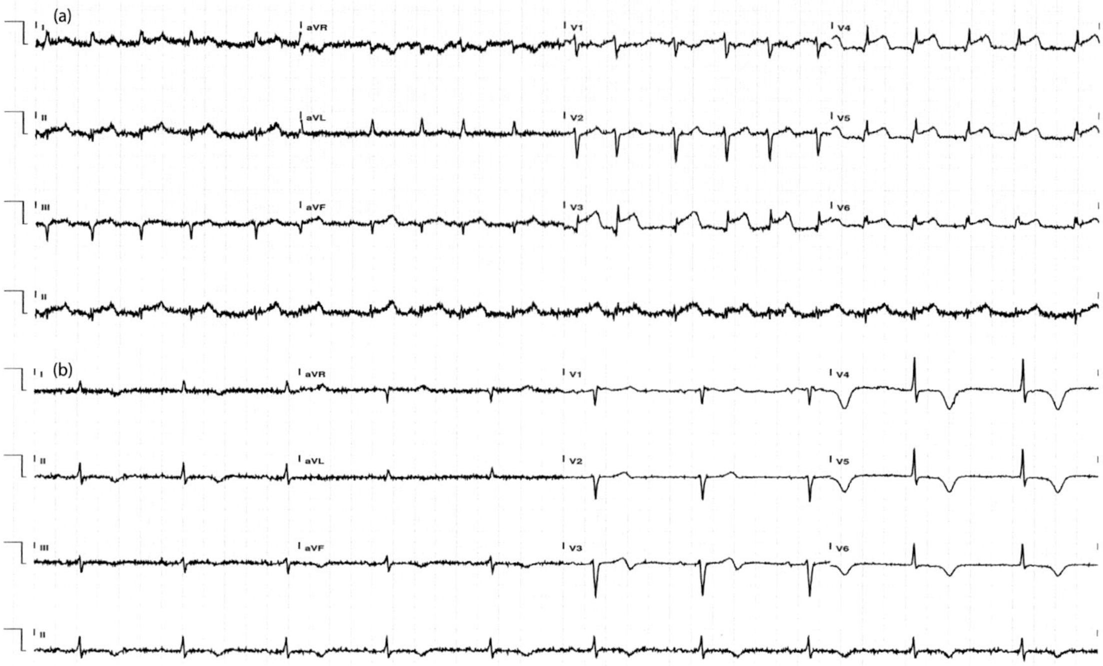

FIGURE 32.3 ECG changes in stress cardiomyopathy. ST-segment elevation is usually seen in anterior leads in the acute phase (a), leading to deep T-wave inversion (b) and QTc prolongation (in the same leads) in the subacute phase.

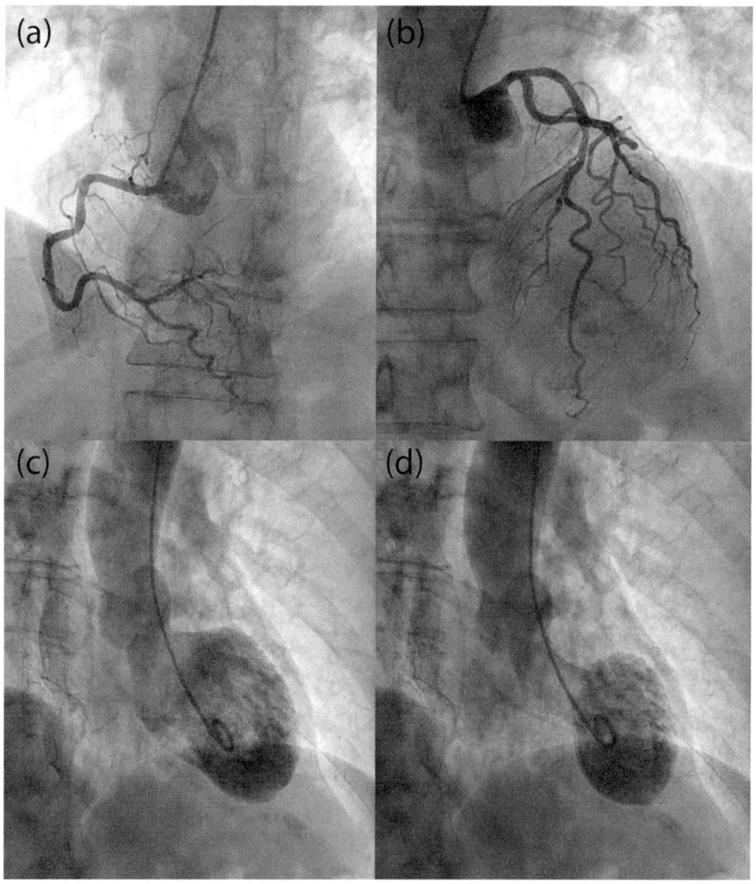

FIGURE 32.4 Angiographic findings. Absence of obstructive coronary artery lesions at coronary angiography (a) Right coronary artery; (b) left coronary artery. Ventriculography shows the typical wall motion abnormalities with apical ballooning and basal hypercontractility. (c) Late diastole; (d) late systole.

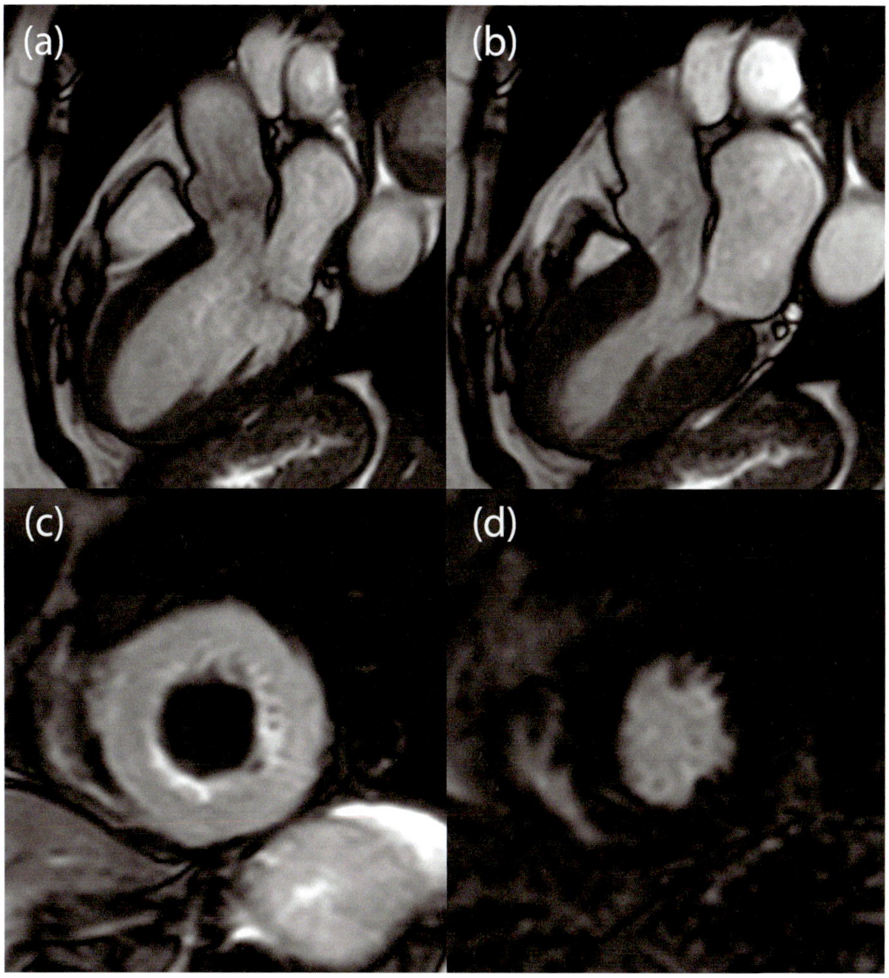

FIGURE 32.5 Cardiac magnetic resonance findings. CMR performed in the subacute phase of SCMP. Cine-CMR 2-chamber view showing the typical wall motion abnormalities with apical ballooning and basal sparing. (a) Late diastole; (b) late systole. T2-weighted short axis sequences showing circumferential transmural edema in the apical segments (c) matching the dysfunctional ventricular contraction areas observed with cine CMR sequences. CMR short-axis view depicting absence of late gadolinium enhancement (d).

tone, anxiety, and microvascular dysfunction.[6] Notably, given the high frequency of untreated, underlying psychiatric illness, a special attention to and an integrated assessment of psychiatric comorbidities is required.

Prognosis

Due to the significant short- and long-term mortality risks, comparable with those in patients diagnosed with ACS, SCMP is no longer considered a benign syndrome. In the International Takotsubo Registry, which included 1,750 patients, in-hospital mortality was 4.1%, with a 7.1% risk of major adverse cardiac and cerebrovascular events (including death, stroke, or transient ischemic attack) during the first 30 days after admission.[6] During long-term follow-up, the rates of all-cause mortality and major adverse cardiac and cerebrovascular events were 5.6% and 9.9% per patient-year, respectively.[6] Notably, SCMP triggered by emotional stress had a favorable short- and long-term prognosis compared with the prognosis in those patients where SCMP was triggered by a physical stress (with the worst short-term prognosis associated with neurological triggers).[8] However, the poor prognosis of these patients is likely largely attributable to the underlying, catastrophic, physical condition (e.g., intracranial hemorrhage).[8] Additionally, the long-term prognosis may be affected by persistent structural and functional myocardial abnormalities. Scally et al. showed that patients with a prior (>12 months) episode of SCMP experienced persistent symptoms of heart failure and reduced cardiorespiratory fitness compared with age-matched healthy controls, despite a recovered ejection fraction.[45] Using speckle-tracking echocardiography and CMR (with T1 mapping and 31P magnetic resonance spectroscopy), these investigators revealed several abnormalities of LV performance, including impaired cardiac deformation (reduced apical circumferential and global longitudinal strain), increased native T1 values (suggesting presence of microscopic fibrosis), and impaired cardiac energetic status.[45] Taken together, these data suggest that the prognosis of SCMP is multifactorial and depends on patient characteristics (e.g., age, underlying comorbidities, trigger) and the long-term structural and metabolic alterations in their myocardium.

Conclusion

Stress cardiomyopathy is an acute and reversible form of acute heart failure associated with a significant risk of complications and mortality. A prompt diagnosis is necessary to guide the optimal management. Future research efforts should be directed to understanding the pathophysiology of this syndrome in order to implement specific treatment options and improve prognosis.

References

1. Medina de Chazal H, Del Buono MG, Keyser-Marcus L, Ma L, Moeller FG, Berrocal D, Abbate A. Stress cardiomyopathy diagnosis and treatment: JACC state-of-the-art review. *J Am Coll Cardiol.* 2018;72:1955–71.
2. Iga K, Gen H, Tomonaga G, Matsumura T, Hori K. Reversible left ventricular wall motion impairment caused by pheochromocytoma--a case report. *Jpn Circ J.* 1989;53:813–8.
3. Kurisu S, Sato H, Kawagoe T, et al. Takotsubo-like left ventricular dysfunction with ST-segment elevation: a novel cardiac syndrome mimicking acute myocardial infarction. *Am Heart J.* 2002;143:448–55.
4. Wittstein IS, Thiemann DR, Lima JAC, et al. Neurohumoral features of myocardial stunning due to sudden emotional stress. *N Engl J Med.* 2005;352:539–48.
5. Pelliccia F, Kaski JC, Crea F, Camici PG. Pathophysiology of Takotsubo Syndrome. *Circulation.* 2017;135:2426–41.
6. Templin C, Ghadri JR, Diekmann J, et al. Clinical features and outcomes of Takotsubo (stress) cardiomyopathy. *N Engl J Med.* 2015;373:929–38.
7. Brinjikji W, El-Sayed AM, Salka S. In-hospital mortality among patients with takotsubo cardiomyopathy: a study of the National inpatient sample 2008 to 2009. *Am Heart J.* 2012;164:215–21.
8. Ghadri JR, Kato K, Cammann VL, et al. Long-term prognosis of patients with Takotsubo syndrome. *J Am Coll Cardiol.* 2018;72:874–82.
9. Madhavan M, Borlaug BA, Lerman A, Rihal CS, Prasad A. Stress hormone and circulating biomarker profile of apical ballooning syndrome (Takotsubo cardiomyopathy): insights into the clinical significance of B-type natriuretic peptide and troponin levels. *Heart.* 2009;95:1436–41.
10. Randhawa MS, Dhillon AS, Taylor HC, Sun Z, Desai MY. Diagnostic utility of cardiac biomarkers in discriminating takotsubo cardiomyopathy from acute myocardial infarction. *J Card Fail.* 2014;20:2–8.
11. Abbas A, Sonnex E, Pereira RS, Coulden RA. Cardiac magnetic resonance assessment of takotsubo cardiomyopathy. *Clin Radiol.* 2016;71:e110–9.
12. Bybee KA, Kara T, Prasad A, et al. Systematic review: transient left ventricular apical ballooning: a syndrome that mimics ST-segment elevation myocardial infarction. *Ann Intern Med.* 2004;141:858–65.
13. Ghadri J-R, Wittstein IS, Prasad A, et al. International expert consensus document on takotsubo syndrome (part I): clinical characteristics, diagnostic criteria, and pathophysiology. *Eur Heart J.* 2018;39:2032–46.
14. Gianni M, Dentali F, Grandi AM, et al. Apical ballooning syndrome or takotsubo cardiomyopathy: a systematic review. *Eur Heart J.* 2006;27:1523–9.
15. Y-Hassan S. Plasma epinephrine levels and its causal link to takotsubo syndrome revisited: critical review with a diverse conclusion. *Cardiovasc Revascularization Med.* 2019;20:907–14.
16. Suzuki H, Matsumoto Y, Kaneta T, et al. Evidence for brain activation in patients with takotsubo cardiomyopathy. *Circ J.* 2014;78:256–8.
17. Klein C, Hiestand T, Ghadri J-R, et al. Takotsubo syndrome – predictable from brain imaging data. *Sci Rep.* 2017;7:5434.
18. Templin C, Hänggi J, Klein C, et al. Altered limbic and autonomic processing supports brain-heart axis in Takotsubo syndrome. *Eur Heart J.* 2019;40:1183–7.
19. Sonnino C, Van Tassell BW, Toldo S, et al. Lack of soluble circulating cardiodepressant factors in takotsubo cardiomyopathy. *Auton Neurosci.* 2017;208:170–2.
20. Kume T, Kawamoto T, Okura H, et al. Local release of catecholamines from the hearts of patients with tako-tsubo-like left ventricular dysfunction. *Circ J.* 2008;72:106–8.
21. Lyon AR, Rees PS, Prasad S, Poole-Wilson PA, Harding SE. Stress (Takotsubo) cardiomyopathy—a novel pathophysiological hypothesis to explain catecholamine-induced acute myocardial stunning. *Nat Clin Pract Cardiovasc Med.* 2008;5:22–9.
22. Stiermaier T, Santoro F, El-Battrawy I, et al. Prevalence and prognostic impact of diabetes in Takotsubo syndrome: insights from the international, multicenter GEIST registry. *Diabetes Care.* 2018;41:1084–8.
23. Del Buono MG, Carbone S, Abbate A. Comment on Stiermaier et al. Prevalence and prognostic impact of diabetes in Takotsubo syndrome: insights from the international, multicenter GEIST registry. *Diabetes Care.* 2018;41:1084–8. *Diabetes Care.* 2018;41:e121–e121.
24. Pontillo D, Patruno N, Stefanoni R. The tako-tsubo syndrome and bronchial asthma: the chicken or the egg dilemma. *J Cardiovasc Med.* 2011;12:149.
25. Vitale C, Mendelsohn ME, Rosano GMC. Gender differences in the cardiovascular effect of sex hormones. *Nat Rev Cardiol.* 2009;6:532–42.
26. Escobar CM, Krajewski SJ, Sandoval-Guzmán T, Voytko M Lou, Rance NE. Neuropeptide Y gene expression is increased in the hypothalamus of older women. *J Clin Endocrinol Metab.* 2004;89:2338–43.
27. Grippo AJ, Johnson AK. Stress, depression and cardiovascular dysregulation: a review of neurobiological mechanisms and the integration of research from preclinical disease models. *Stress.* 2009;12:1–21.
28. Del Buono MG, Montone RA, Camilli M, et al. Takotsubo syndrome and left ventricular non-compaction cardiomyopathy: casualty or causality? *Auton Neurosci Basic Clin.* 2019;218:64–7.
29. Franco TH, Khan A, Joshi V, Thomas B. Takotsubo cardiomyopathy in two men receiving bevacizumab for metastatic cancer. *Ther Clin Risk Manag.* 2008;4:1367–70.
30. Coen M, Rigamonti F, Roth A, Koessler T. Chemotherapy-induced Takotsubo cardiomyopathy, a case report and review of the literature. *BMC Cancer.* 2017;17:394.
31. Biso S, Wongrakpanich S, Agrawal A, et al. A review of neurogenic stunned myocardium. *Cardiovasc Psychiatry Neurol.* 2017;2017: 5842182.
32. Ghadri JR, Sarcon A, Diekmann J, et al. Happy heart syndrome: role of positive emotional stress in takotsubo syndrome. *Eur Heart J.* 2016;37:2823–9.
33. Del Buono MG, O'Quinn MP, Garcia P, et al. Cardiac arrest due to ventricular fibrillation in a 23-year-old woman with broken heart syndrome. *Cardiovasc Pathol.* 2017;30:78–81.
34. Ghadri JR, Cammann VL, Jurisic S, et al. A novel clinical score (InterTAK Diagnostic Score) to differentiate takotsubo syndrome from acute coronary syndrome: results from the International Takotsubo registry. *Eur J Heart Fail.* 2017;19:1036–42.
35. Akashi YJ, Goldstein DS, Barbaro G, Ueyama T. Takotsubo cardiomyopathy: a new form of acute, reversible heart failure. *Circulation.* 2008;118:2754–62.
36. Mitsuma W, Kodama M, Ito M, et al. Serial electrocardiographic findings in women with Takotsubo cardiomyopathy. *Am J Cardiol.* 2007;100:106–9.
37. Guerra F, Giannini I, Capucci A. The ECG in the differential diagnosis between takotsubo cardiomyopathy and acute coronary syndrome. *Expert Rev Cardiovasc Ther.* 2017;15:137–44.
38. Frangieh AH, Obeid S, Ghadri J, et al. ECG criteria to differentiate between Takotsubo (stress) cardiomyopathy and myocardial infarction. *J Am Heart Assoc.* 2016;5:e003418.
39. Dias A, Franco E, Rubio M, et al. Usefulness of left ventricular strain analysis in patients with takotsubo syndrome during acute phase. *Echocardiography.* 2018;35:179–83.
40. Kurisu S, Inoue I, Kawagoe T, et al. Prevalence of incidental coronary artery disease in tako-tsubo cardiomyopathy. *Coron Artery Dis.* 2009;20:214–8.
41. Tamis-Holland JE, Jneid H, Reynolds HR, et al. Contemporary diagnosis and management of patients with myocardial infarction in the absence of obstructive coronary artery disease: a scientific statement from the American Heart Association. *Circulation.* 2019;139:e891–908.
42. Aalberts JJJ, Klinkenberg TJ, Mariani MA, van der Harst P. Mechanical circulatory support for refractory cardiogenic shock in Takotsubo syndrome: a case report and review of the literature. *Eur Hear J – Case Reports.* 2017;1:ytx005.
43. Beneduce A, Fausta Bertoldi L, Melillo F, et al. Mechanical circulatory support with impella percutaneous ventricular assist device as a bridge to recovery in Takotsubo syndrome complicated by cardiogenic shock and left ventricular outflow tract obstruction. *JACC Cardiovasc Interv.* 2019;12:e31–2.
44. Gili S, Cammann VL, Schlossbauer SA, et al. Cardiac arrest in takotsubo syndrome: results from the InterTAK Registry. *Eur Heart J.* 2019;40:2142–51.
45. Scally C, Rudd A, Mezincescu A, et al. Persistent long-term structural, functional, and metabolic changes after stress-induced (Takotsubo) cardiomyopathy. *Circulation.* 2018;137:1039–48.
46. Bybee KAa, Kara T, Prasad A, et al. Review systematic review: transient left ventricular apical ballooning. *Ann Intern Med.* 2004;141:858–65.
47. Tsuchihashi K, Ueshima K, Uchida T, et al. Transient left ventricular apical ballooning without coronary artery stenosis: a novel heart syndrome mimicking acute myocardial infarction. *J Am Coll Cardiol.* 2001;38:11–8.

Chapter 33
HYPERTROPHIC CARDIOMYOPATHY

Ahmad Masri and Stephen B. Heitner

Introduction

Hypertrophic cardiomyopathy (HCM) is a heterogeneous, autosomal dominant, genetic disorder caused by sarcomeric mutations that result in myocardial hypercontractility, reduced compliance, myofibrillar disarray, hypertrophy of the left ventricle (LV), and fibrosis.[1,2] It is the most common inherited cardiac condition, affecting 1 out of 500 individuals with conservative estimates, and one of the leading causes of sudden cardiac death in the young.[3] Reduced exercise capacity and symptoms of exertional dyspnea and chest pain result from impaired relaxation and reduced compliance of the LV, left ventricular outflow tract (LVOT) obstruction, and mitral regurgitation (MR). In addition to septal hypertrophy, abnormalities of the mitral valve (MV) and subvalvular apparatus contribute to systolic anterior motion (SAM) and LVOT obstruction, the characteristic features of obstructive HCM.

Since the initial clinical description in the 1950s,[4] HCM has evolved from what was thought to be a rare and fatal condition to a relatively common disease with complex phenotypic manifestations. Nowadays, patients with HCM generally have an excellent overall prognosis,[5] but many remain with significant disease-related morbidity.[6] HCM is a progressive condition, and as such, inadequately treated patients can suffer. Conversely, patients treated aggressively and according to contemporary standards often enjoy an excellent overall quality of life.[7–11] As such, a careful history, physical examination, and evaluation of imaging, exercise, and biomarker data are crucial.

Clinical Evaluation

History and Physical Examination

Patients with HCM may present with a wide range of symptoms, including chest pain, dyspnea, dizziness, fatigue, syncope, or sudden death. It is important to recognize that some patients have minimal or no symptoms. In one HCM cohort study, 70% of patients had mild or no symptoms, and 20% of patients achieved estimated life expectancy of ≥70 years.[9] On physical examination, a systolic murmur may be heard best at the left lower sternal border, which is augmented by maneuvers that decrease preload ("Valsalva" or "squat-to-stand") and diminished by maneuvers that increase afterload (isometric hand-grip and squatting). Displaced apical impulse is often noted, the carotid upstroke may be bifid, and an S4 heart sound may be present.

Electrocardiogram (EKG)

A 12-lead EKG is recommended during initial evaluation, which may show findings of left ventricular hypertrophy (LVH) based on voltage criteria (Sokolov-Lyon criteria being most commonly used, i.e., S-wave depth in lead V1 + tallest R wave height in lead V5–V6 > 35 mm) and widespread Q waves.[12] These abnormalities, however, do not correlate with severity or pattern of hypertrophy. The exception is with apical variant HCM, where LVH and deep inverted T waves can be seen in lead V2-V6 (Yamaguchi pattern, Figure 33.1).[13] EKG can be normal in 5%–10% of patients with HCM, and, therefore, EKG alone cannot be used to rule out HCM.[14]

Transthoracic Echocardiogram (TTE)

Echocardiography is the primary modality for evaluating and monitoring patients with suspected or confirmed HCM. Traditionally, morphologic diagnosis is based on presence of hypertrophy (≥15 mm) in the absence of other potential systemic causes of hypertrophy, such as long-standing hypertension or athlete's heart.[3] Milder hypertrophy (≥13 mm) is sometimes considered diagnostic in patients with positive family history or other features of HCM.[15] Classically, the basal anteroseptum is involved, but various patterns, as well as diffuse hypertrophy, have been described.[16] A focused apical view may identify localized hypertrophy ("apical variant HCM"), which may be associated with apical aneurysm (Figure 33.2a). If present, this can lead to thrombus formation and predisposition to thromboembolic events or stroke (Figure 33.2b).

Often, LV function is hyperdynamic, and systolic dysfunction—the so-called "end-stage" or "burned out" HCM—is uncommon.[17] Importantly, increased left atrial (LA) size is common and associated with more frequent cardiovascular events.[10] Increased LA size correlates with decreased exercise capacity in non-obstructive HCM.[18] Approximately one-third of HCM cases are non-obstructive and seem to follow a relatively benign course.[19]

In obstructive HCM, SAM of the MV leaflets is characteristic, resulting in dynamic LVOT obstruction and posteriorly directed MR in the absence of organic MV pathology (Figure 33.3a, b, and c). Significant obstruction at rest (≥30 mmHg), with provocation, or exercise (≥50 mmHg), is present in up to 70% of patients with HCM.[19] Obstruction results from a variety of mechanisms, including LVOT narrowing from septal hypertrophy, papillary muscle displacement, and elongated MV leaflets.[20,21] Septal-SAM contact results in a pressure gradient between the LV and the aorta at the sub-valvular level, and was the very first physiological abnormality described in the 1950s, resulting in the initial term "idiopathic hypertrophic subaortic stenosis."[22] Presently, it is known that obstruction may occur in the mid-cavity or apical regions depending on the location of the hypertrophy. In the United States, the apical variant is uncommon (1–2% of HCM cases); however, in Japan and other Asian countries, it is more common.[23,24]

Tissue Doppler imaging (TDI) is a useful technique for differentiating HCM from athlete's heart. The latter tends to show normal or super-normal values, whereas there is evidence of abnormal myocardial mechanics in HCM.[25] Evaluation of mechanics using myocardial deformation imaging (strain) suggests that patients with HCM have reduced longitudinal but increased circumferential strain.[26] Left ventricular opacification with echo-contrast is important for detecting the presence of apical variant HCM, LV aneurysms, and LV thrombus (Figure 33.4). Additionally, echo-contrast is used intra-procedurally for the delineation of the perfusion territory of isolated septal perforator arteries prior to alcohol septal

DOI: 10.1201/9780429244544-40

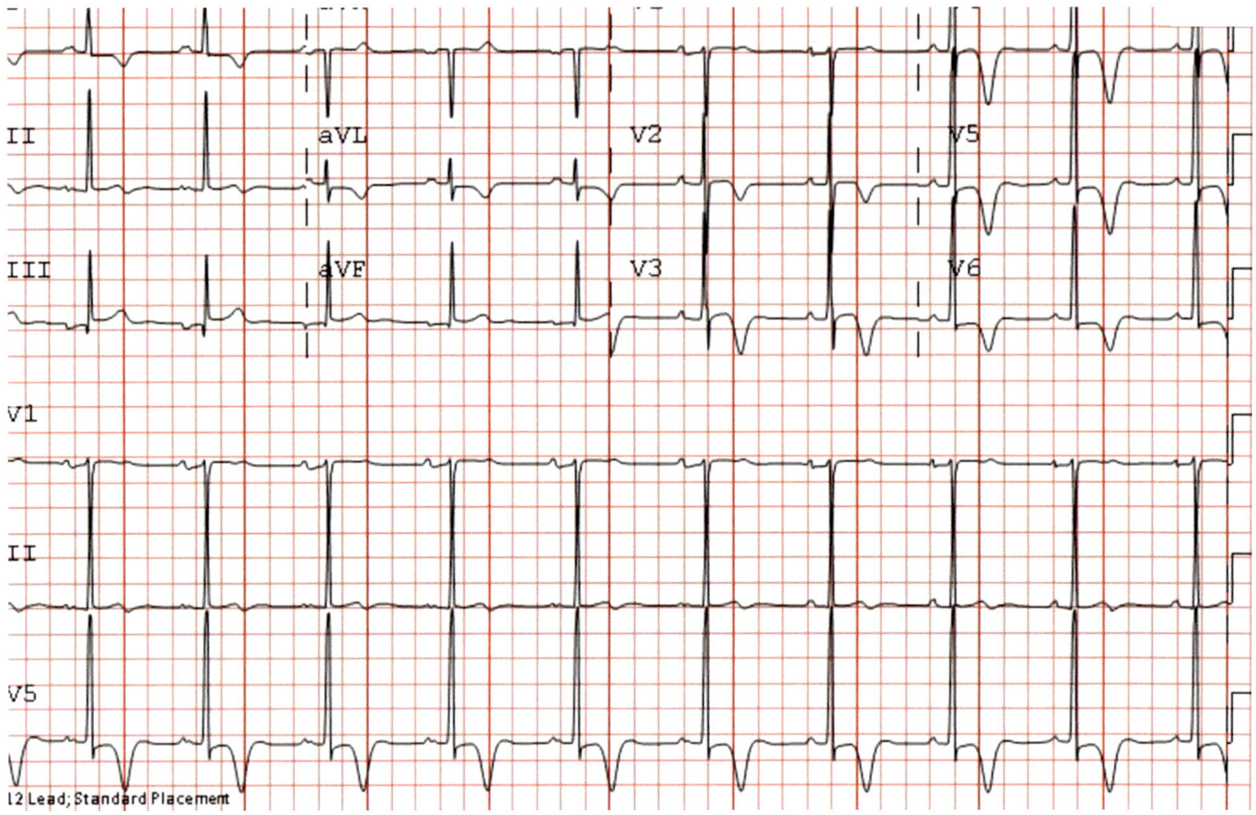

FIGURE 33.1 Classic electrocardiographic finding in a patient with apical HCM, showing giant T-wave inversion in precordial leads (Yamaguchi syndrome).

ablation (ASA).[27] Tissue characterization using myocardial contrast echocardiography is an area of active research.

Stress Echocardiogram

Obstruction of the LVOT is dynamic, in response to volume status, afterload, and preload. Although pharmacologic provocation of LVOT obstruction is feasible with amyl nitrite, isoproterenol, or dobutamine, physiologic exercise is always preferable. Exercise stress testing provides data regarding functional capacity, occult symptoms, and prognosis.[28] Moreover, post-prandial exercise evaluation has been shown to unmask occult LVOT obstruction as a result of splanchnic vasodilation and decreasing afterload in a subset of patients.[29] The hemodynamic response to exercise has implications for the risk of sudden cardiac death and may sway the provider to recommend placement of an implantable cardiac defibrillation (ICD).[30] A resting LVOT gradient of ≥30 mmHg or provoked gradient of ≥50 mmHg are considered significant, and in the presence of symptoms there is potential to gain both improved quality of life as well as increased longevity through appropriately chosen septal reduction therapies or disopyramide use.[31–33] Although not performed routinely in all patients, metabolic parameters, such as anaerobic threshold and peak oxygen consumption, can be measured by cardiopulmonary exercise stress test, which provides comprehensive assessment of functional capacity and can add to the prognostic information on individual patients.[34]

Transesophageal Echocardiogram (TEE)

TEE can be valuable in selected patients with poor acoustic windows. TEE can be used for more complete evaluation of the mitral sub-valvular apparatus and help exclude subaortic or supra-aortic membrane. All patients undergoing myectomy benefit from careful surgical planning with multimodality imaging. In many instances, revision of the MV and sub-valvular structures is necessary for complete relief of LVOT obstruction, and intraoperative TEE is a key tool in the hands of a skilled operator.[35]

Cardiac Magnetic Resonance Imaging (CMR)

CMR has emerged as a vital tool in contemporary management of HCM patients. Highly resolved images provide precise localization of hypertrophy, evaluation of the MV apparatus, papillary muscle morphology, and prognostic information from quantification of myocardial fibrosis (Figure 33.5a).[36–38] CMR has been useful for differentiation of HCM from phenocopies, such as hypertensive heart disease, athlete's heart, and infiltrative and metabolic cardiomyopathies (Figure 33.5b). CMR is vital for operative planning and has been used for 3D printing in order to facilitate this.[39]

Familial Screening and Genetic Testing

Cascade screening of relatives of patients with HCM is essential. First-degree relatives of the proband should undergo serial intermittent EKG and echocardiography in the absence of a known disease-causing genetic mutation.[30] Phenotypic screening frequency depends on the age of the relative, with children aged 7–18 years old requiring screening every 12–18 months, with relatives >18 years old tested only every 3–5 years. Genetic analysis is useful to confirm the genetic etiology and to differentiate isolated HCM from other syndromic conditions associated with it (such as Danon disease, Fabry disease, amyloidosis, and mitochondrial cardiomyopathy).

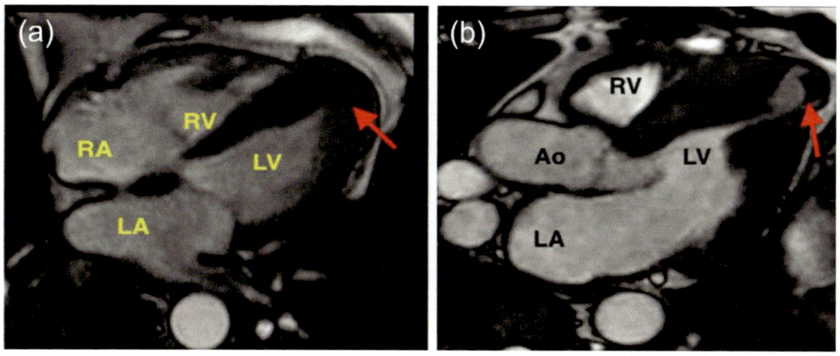

FIGURE 33.2 CMR steady-state free-precision sequences of (a) four-chamber view showing extensive apical thickening in a 62-year-old man with apical variant HCM and (b) three-chamber view showing thrombus in the LV apical region (arrow).

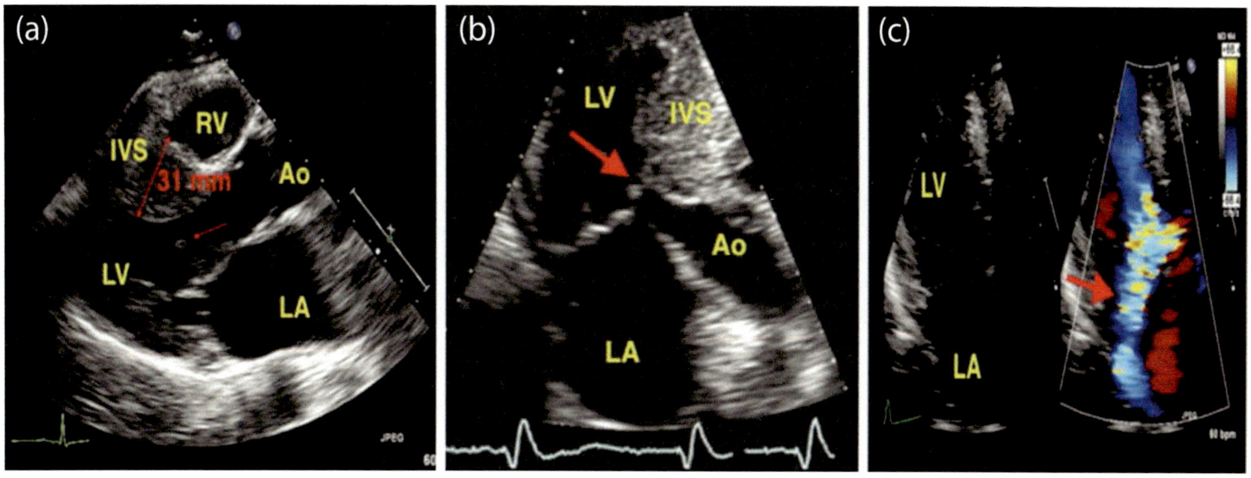

FIGURE 33.3 Echocardiographic findings in HCM. (a) Parasternal long-axis view of a 40-year-old man showing septal thickness of 31 mm and systolic anterior motion (SAM) of mitral valve (arrow). (b) Three-chamber apical view showing SAM septal contact (arrow). (c) Three-chamber apical view showing posteriorly directed mitral regurgitation jet (arrow).

A significant portion of HCM can also be attributed to *de novo* variants, compound variants, or pathogenic variants in multiple genes; each of these scenarios conveys a different risk to a proband's relatives.[40] Whereas genotyping is a useful tool for familial risk stratification, there are serious pitfalls and implications, especially on young individuals, that mandate thorough professional genetic counseling and understanding of the limitations of the technique.

Management of Hypertrophic Cardiomyopathy

Figure 33.6 summarizes our institutional approach to the management of HCM.

Pharmacotherapies

Figure 33.7 summarizes the available medications for the pharmacologic management of HCM. Symptoms are the primary driver for initiation of pharmacotherapy. Currently, there is no evidence that the currently available therapies could prevent the development of progression of HCM phenotypes. In pediatric patients, where symptoms may not be reliable, pharmacotherapy use can be based on physical examination and echocardiographic findings. Patients with non-obstructive HCM and heart failure with preserved ejection fraction are managed with diuretics for symptom control. Those who develop systolic dysfunction and heart failure with reduced ejection fraction should be treated according to current evidence-based medical therapy for heart failure. Several medications have been evaluated in clinical trials for symptom alleviation and improvement of exertional capacity (losartan,[41] spironolactone,[42] ranolazine,[43] eleclazine,[44] and perhexiline) but none have succeeded. Currently, there are ongoing studies evaluating valsartan[45] mavacamten[46] and CK-274[47] in treating the various phenotypes and stages of HCM.

β-Blockers

Non-vasodilating β-blockers (propranolol, metoprolol, atenolol) were the first class of drugs shown to be effective in obstructive HCM.[48] β-blockers are usually the first-line drugs to treat symptoms in obstructive HCM and have been shown to alleviate some symptoms and potentially improve exercise tolerance.[49,50] Central nervous system side effects (fatigue, depression, erectile dysfunction) continue to be problematic, especially in the young HCM population.

In general, long-acting formulations are preferred in the treatment of LVOT obstruction, with propranolol and metoprolol being the best-studied β-blockers. Despite limited evidence, agents with alpha-blocking activity (carvedilol,

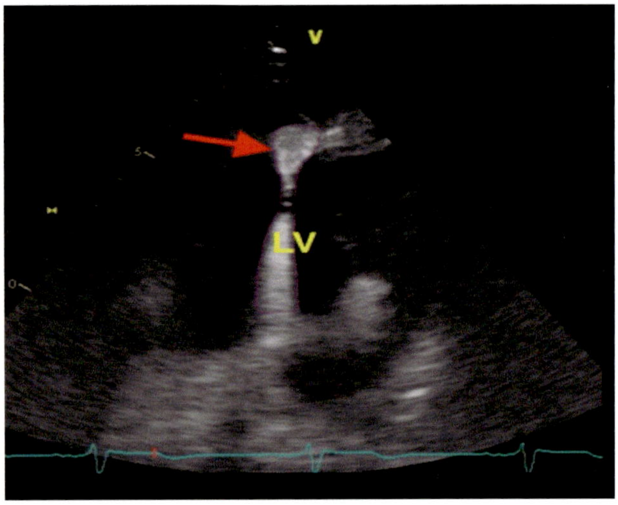

FIGURE 33.4 Echocardiogram with contrast-enhancing agent, revealing apical aneurysm in a 52-year-old man with apical variant HCM.

labetalol, bisoprolol) are thought to aggravate LVOT obstruction and, in general, are avoided in obstructive HCM, with the exception being patients with coexistent systemic hypertension. We have had success with careful institution of carvedilol when concomitant control of both obstructive HCM symptoms and hypertension was warranted. Nebivolol is a unique β-blocker which also produces an endothelium-derived nitric oxide-dependent vasodilation, resulting in reduction of blood pressure, and theoretically should be avoided in patients with obstructive HCM.

Calcium Channel Blockers (CCBs)

Traditionally, β-blockers are trialed initially and, if ineffective or not well tolerated, a non-dihydropyridine CCB (verapamil or diltiazem) is initiated. Recently, based on analysis of claims data, CCBs were associated with fewer adverse events than patients treated with β-blockers.[51] CCBs in general are associated with fewer side effects in younger patients than β-blockers. Similar to β-blockers, CCBs primarily ameliorate provocable, as opposed to resting, gradients. A strategy of using CCB first in young patients is appealing but is not yet supported by guidelines.[19]

Disopyramide

Disopyramide is a class I antiarrhythmic drug with negative inotropic properties which was found to be helpful in alleviating symptoms of obstructive HCM.[31,52–54] Disopyramide can reduce both resting and provocable LVOT obstruction. Disopyramide can successfully ameliorate symptoms of exertional shortness of breath, angina, pre-syncope, and syncope in up to two-thirds of patients with obstructive HCM.[55] Although generally well tolerated, disopyramide's anticholinergic side effects can limit its tolerability in a subset of patients. For the side effects of dry mouth and dry eyes, patients should be advised to drink more fluids, use saliva stimulants, such as lime water, and use artificial tears, if needed. Blurred vision and urinary retention are more troubling and typically require discontinuation of therapy. One can consider the addition of pyridostigmine for side effect control. Disopyramide can enhance conduction through the AV node, resulting in high ventricular response rates, and even ventricular fibrillation, in the setting of AF, and should always be prescribed with atrioventricular nodal blocking agents (β-blockers or CCBs). Disopyramide has the potential to be proarrhythmic and has QT-prolonging properties and traditionally has been started as an in-patient medication, with dose titration and regular evaluation of the QTc. Our practice is to introduce disopyramide on an out-patient basis and have routine monitoring of the EKG for QTc prolongation. A recent study showed the safety of this approach.[56] It is difficult to predict response to disopyramide and its tolerability. The onset of the drug effect is short, and most responders report alleviation of symptoms within 24–48 hours. Emergence of side effects could take longer. One observational study suggests that this agent is safe, effective, and may be associated with a survival advantage.[31]

Ranolazine

Ranolazine is an FDA-approved antianginal agent that acts through inhibition of the late sodium current ($I_{Na}L$). Ranolazine is safe in treatment of HCM and is a very useful adjunct for angina that is refractory to β-blockers or CCBs.[57] Although an open-label study in nonobstructive HCM (RHYME, NCT01721967) demonstrated improvement in patient-reported measures with ranolazine,[57] a phase II trial (RESTYLE-HCM) failed to demonstrate a significant effect on objective measures (peak VO_2, natriuretic peptides, diastolic function), although there was a reduction in PVC burden.[43] Additionally, the more potent $I_{Na}L$-inhibitor eleclazine, was ineffective in a large (n = 180), placebo-controlled trial (LIBERTY-HCM, NCT02291237).[58]

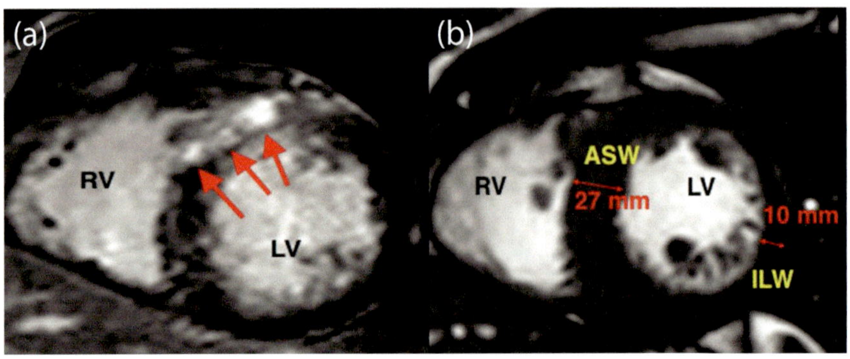

FIGURE 33.5 CMR short-axis acquisitions at the level of papillary muscles. (a) Post-gadolinium phase-sensitive inversion recovery sequence showing non-transmural late gadolinium enhancement (arrows) in a 53-year-old woman with known history of non-sustained ventricular tachycardia and HCM. (b) Steady-state free-precision sequence showing asymmetric thickening with anteroseptal wall (ASW) and inferolateral wall (ILW) measuring 27 mm and 10 mm, respectively.

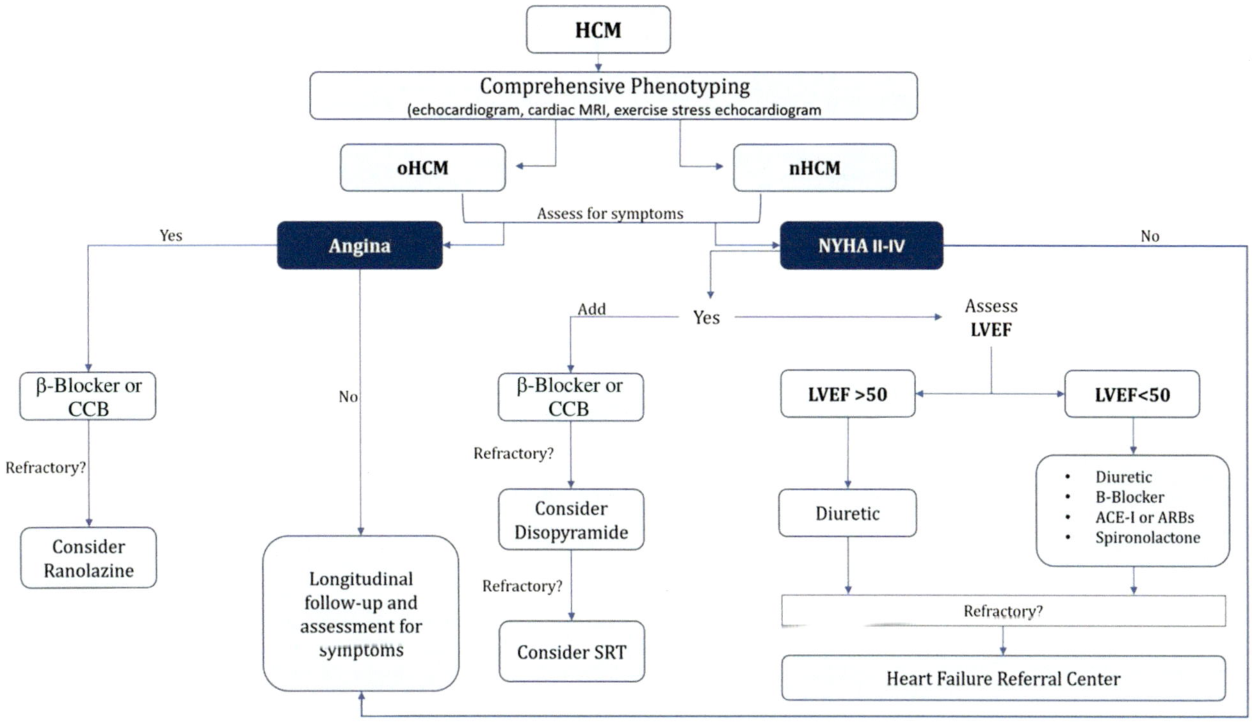

FIGURE 33.6 Overview of the pharmacotherapeutic approaches to patients with HCM. *Abbreviations*: oHCM: obstructive HCM; nHCM: non-obstructive HCM; MRI: magnetic resonance imaging; NYHA FC: New York Heart Association functional class; β-blocker: beta-blocker; CCB: calcium channel blocker; SRT: septal reduction therapy; LVEF: left ventricular ejection fraction; ACE-I: angiotensin-converting enzyme inhibitor; ARB: angiotensin receptor blocker.

Drug		Class	Effect on LVOTO	Effect on Angina	Dose Range	Common Side Effects
Beta Blockers	Metoprolol tartrate or Metoprolol succinate	Cardio-selective β-blocker	↓↓	↓↓↓	25-200 mg bid or 400 mg daily	Fatigue, depression, erectile dysfunction, bradycardia, hypotension, asthma exacerbation
	Propranolol or Propranolol ER	Non-selective β-blocker	↓↓	↓↓↓	20-40 mg tid/qid or 80-160 mg daily	
Calcium Channel Blockers	Verapamil or Verapamil ER	Non-dihydropyridine CCB	↓↓	↓↓	40-160 mg tid or 120-480 mg daily	Constipation, bradycardia, hypotension
	Diltiazem or Diltiazem ER	Non-dihydropyridine CCB	↓↓	↓↓	30-90 mg qid or 120-480 mg daily	
Disopyramide or Disopyramide ER		Class 1A antiarrhythmic	↓↓↓	↓↓↓	100-200 mg tid/qid or 100-300 mg bid	Dry eyes, dry mouth, constipation, urinary retention, blurred vision, QTc prolongation
Ranolazine		Late-sodium channel blocker	-	↓↓↓	500 - 1000mg bid	Dizziness, confusion, constipation, blurred vision, QTc prolongation

FIGURE 33.7 Common pharmacotherapies in symptomatic HCM. *Abbreviations*: LVOTO: left ventricular outflow tract obstruction; ER: extended release; CCB: calcium channel blocker; bid: twice daily; tid: three times daily; qid: four times daily.

Septal Reduction Therapies and Other Surgical Procedures

Septal reduction therapies should be considered in patients with HCM and symptoms attributed to LVOT obstruction. Both ASA and septal myectomy have similar short- and long-term hemodynamic and functional outcomes based on non-randomized studies. In general, surgical myectomy with appropriate MV revision is the treatment of choice in patients able to undergo sternotomy and the associated recovery time. ASA is an important therapy for older patients and those deemed to be at higher risk.[59] Important limitations for ASA include the technical feasibility based on anatomic limitations, the inability to address abnormalities related to the MV, and higher risk for development of complete heart block.[60,61] Newer techniques for septal reduction therapies are being developed, including radiofrequency ablation and high-intensity focused ultrasound, which remain in the early phases of development and beyond the scope of this chapter.

Abnormalities of the MV and related apparatus are common in HCM, leading to MR and worsening LVOT obstruction with SAM.[20,21] Mitral valve repair and sub-valvular revision is preferred over replacement. Techniques aimed at addressing MV and subvalvular abnormalities include anterior MV plication, papillary muscle realignment, chordal transposition, synthetic chord placement, or very occasional annuloplasty rings, if the patient has intrinsic MV disease. More recently, patients with SAM-septal contact and symptomatic LVOT obstruction have been successfully treated percutaneously using a MitraClip device.[62,63] Our center, as well as others, have reported encouraging results.[64]

Only rarely is MV replacement required, and, should this be a consideration, our experience is that mechanical valves are more appropriate. Sub-valvular protrusion of the bioprosthetic valve may result in a neo-LVOT and fixed LVOT obstruction, particularly in patients with small LV cavities. Thus, careful preoperative planning and an experienced surgeon to modify the valve orientation are paramount.

In selected cases where medical therapies fail, and septal reduction is contraindicated, preferential right ventricular pacing may reduce LVOT obstruction and relieve symptoms.[65,66] This strategy should not be routinely used as chronic and persistent right ventricular pacing has also been associated with reduced LV ejection fraction.[67]

Arrhythmias in HCM

Atrial fibrillation and atrial flutter (AF) are common in HCM, particularly as patients age. It is often symptomatic and poorly tolerated. Stroke risk is much higher when compared with standard non-valvular AF, and, as such, thromboembolic risk scores ($CHADS_2$, CHA_2DS_2-VASc, etc.) are not applicable in HCM.[68–71] In general, anticoagulation is recommended unless specifically contraindicated. Given the hemodynamic effects of loss of atrial contraction, a rhythm control strategy is preferred. Electrical cardioversion, antiarrhythmic medications, pulmonary vein isolation, surgical maze procedure, or left atrial appendage ligation at the time of surgical myectomy are useful treatment options. When considering antiarrhythmics, disopyramide is a good option in patients with concomitant LVOT obstruction, although it is a weak antiarrhythmic. These patients need an adequate dose of an AV nodal blocking agent in addition to disopyramide to avoid paradoxical shortened conduction and rapid ventricular rates. Amiodarone is also effective, but the dose- and duration-dependent likelihood of drug toxicity is a concern. Rate control with β-blockers or CCBs can be tried if rhythm control fails, but generally it is not a good strategy. Importantly, digoxin should be avoided due to the positive inotropic effect and the risk of worsening LVOT obstruction. Rarely, in refractory symptomatic AF, AV node ablation and placement of a pacemaker can be employed.

Sudden cardiac death (SCD) is the most dreaded manifestation of HCM and is most frequently a result of ventricular fibrillation. Although overall it is rare (<1% per year), it is more frequent in younger patients. Because SCD is attributable to ventricular arrhythmias, it is preventable by appropriate use of ICDs. Subcutaneous ICDs can be used to reduce the intravascular hardware burden in selected patients.[72] Currently, there is no evidence supporting a pharmacological treatment to prevent SCD in HCM. Antiarrhythmics are controversial in non-sustained ventricular tachycardia. Identifying patients at higher risk of SCD is a major challenge in HCM, since ICD implantation, especially in young patients, is by no means without consequence. Importantly, SCD risk re-stratification is necessary on an annual basis. Traditional risk factors include: (a) history of SCD or ventricular tachyarrhythmia (ventricular fibrillation, sustained ventricular tachycardia), (b) non-sustained ventricular tachycardia (>3 beats at >120 bpm on a Holter monitor); (c) massive hypertrophy (≥30 mm); (d) recent unexplained syncope; (e) first-degree relative with sudden unexplained death; and (f) a hypotensive/flat hemodynamic response to exercise.[30] Despite these being well-proven and life-saving markers, many patients undergo unnecessary ICD placement. Refinement of SCD risk assessment has been a subject of intense research and has resulted in several evolving markers. Among these are the amount of fibrosis on CMR,[37,73] LVOT gradient ≥30 mmHg,[74] apical aneurysm,[24] double or compound pathogenic sarcomeric gene variants, systolic dysfunction, and impaired coronary flow (myocardial ischemia).[30,75] O'Mahoney et al. have published a risk calculator that utilizes established risk markers and age to calculate risk. This calculator is endorsed by the European Society of Cardiology,[76] has been externally validated, especially for the extremes of risk,[77] and is helpful when discussing risk with patients and family members.[78] A shared decision model between the patient and the physician, taking into account the individual philosophy and risk tolerance, is essential.

Novel Pharmacotherapies

The previously discussed mainstay of treatment of obstructive HCM (β-blockers, CCBs, disopyramide) shares a negative inotropic effect, resulting in reduction of SAM-septal contact and LVOT obstruction. Despite their utility, current guideline-directed pharmacotherapies were never designed for the treatment of HCM and the supporting evidence is quite limited. In fact, there have been no randomized trials that demonstrate the efficacy of any agent to treat HCM,[79] and currently the only FDA-approved drug is propranolol based on a study of 13 patients published in 1966.[48] Moreover, non-obstructive HCM, which represents ~30% of patients, remains poorly addressed with no disease-modifying therapies to date. With greater understanding of the molecular underpinnings of HCM, several targeted therapies have recently been studied in clinical trials.

Myocardial Force Generation: Mavacamten and CK-274

The vast majority of mutations in HCM affect sarcomeric proteins, with ~70% involving genes encoding cardiac β-myosin heavy chain (*MYH7*) and myosin-binding protein C (*MYBPC*). Actin-myosin cross-bridging is an active process which results in muscle fiber shortening. Mutations in *MYH7* are known to affect the activity of the myosin ATPase unit, leading to increased myocardial force generation, whereas *MYBPC* plays a role in sarcomere organization and may serve as a brake on myofibril contraction.[80,81] Therefore, HCM mutations lead to a hypercontractile state with subsequent LV stiffening. Mavacamten, a first-in-class oral small molecule, targets this process by modulating cardiac β-myosin and causing reversible inhibition of actin-myosin cross-bridging.[82,83] In animal models, treatment with mavacamten reduced contractility, eliminated

SAM, relieved LVOT obstruction,[84] and improved the myocardial pressure-volume relationship.[85] Moreover, in a histologic study, treatment with mavacamten resulted in attenuation of the HCM phenotype with suppression of hypertrophy, cardiomyocyte disarray, and profibrotic gene expression.[86]

Mavacamten has been shown in phase II (PIONEER)[87] and phase III trials (EXPLORER)[88] to successfully decrease LVOT gradient, and improve peak VO_2, patient-reported outcomes, and New York Heart Association (NYHA) class, as well as decreasing N-terminal pro-B-type natriuretic peptide (NT-proBNP) levels. In EXPLORER, 251 patients were randomized to mavacamten vs placebo. Patients on mavacamten had greater reductions in post-exercise LVOT gradient (−36 mmHg, 95% confidence interval [CI] −43.2 to −28.1; p<0.0001), greater increases in peak VO_2 (+1.4 mL/kg per minute, 95% CI 0.6–2.1; p=0.0006), with 34% more patients in the mavacamten group having improvements by at least 1 NYHA class. Overall, mavacamten was safe and well tolerated, and all reductions in left ventricular ejection fraction were reversible.[88]

Multiple open-label extension studies (PIONEER-OLE, NCT03496168; MAVA-LTE, NCT03723655) are underway to examine long-term safety and effectiveness. Moreover, given that pre-clinical data suggest a beneficial effect on myocardial compliance, a phase-IIb placebo-controlled trial in non-obstructive HCM was conducted (MAVERICK-HCM, NCT03442764). Although overall the results from MAVERICK-HCM were neutral, an echo- and biomarker-based sub-group analysis showed promising results. Subsequent phase III trials in non-obstructive HCM are needed to confirm the hypotheses generated by MAVERICK-HCM.[89]

CK-274 is a next-generation cardiac myosin inhibitor that has shown safety and tolerability in a phase I clinical trial[47] and data from the phase II clinical trial (REDWOOD-HCM, NCT04219826) were presented in conference proceedings showing significant reduction in LVOT gradients. The phase III clinical trial (SEQUOIA-HCM, NCT05186818) is currently being conducted.[90]

Myocardial Energetics: Perhexiline and Trimetazidine

Sarcomeric mutations in HCM lead to inefficient ATP utilization, resulting in a depleted energy state and a compromise in important homeostatic functions.[91] HCM mutation carriers have impaired high-energy phosphate metabolism as evident by reduced phosphocreatine-to-ATP ratio.[92] As a compensatory mechanism, there is increased carbohydrate utilization relative to fatty acids (glucose being a more efficient energy source for ATP production)—akin to cardiomyocyte adaptation during ischemia.

Perhexiline is an oral inhibitor of carnitine palmitoyl transferase I (CPT-1) which reduces fatty acid uptake into mitochondria, resulting in greater cellular dependence on carbohydrates for ATP production.[93] Similar to diltiazem, perhexiline blocks the voltage-gated L-type calcium channels. Although a preclinical study[94] and an early phase clinical study (METAL-HCM, NCT00500552)[95] revealed favorable changes in the cardiac metabolome and improvement in exercise capacity compared to placebo, a multicenter phase-IIb clinical trial (NCT02862600) was terminated early due to lack of efficacy, and the drug has been abandoned as a potential therapy for nonobstructive HCM.

Similarly, trimetazidine, a metabolic modulator causing reversible inhibition of 3-ketoacyl-coenzyme A was recently shown to be ineffective for non-obstructive HCM (NCT01696370).[96]

Lifestyle Modification

Therapeutic interventions in HCM tend to target symptoms and prevention of complications. Although medications and septal reduction therapies are the mainstay treatment, lifestyle modification is an essential step in alleviating symptoms, and perhaps even altering the disease course. Physical inactivity, obesity, and psychological disturbances impact the livelihood and outcomes of patients with HCM.

Exercise type and frequency remain highly controversial disagreements in current expert consensus statements in the United States and Europe.[30,74,97] Current exercise guidelines focus on restricting physical activity of phenotype-positive HCM patients. Despite this intense controversy, there is no evidence showing detrimental effects of recreational or moderate-intensity exercise in patients with HCM. In fact, moderate-intensity personalized exercise programs have been shown to improve functional capacity and peak oxygen consumption (VO_2) without any evidence of disease progression, arrhythmias, or other adverse outcomes.[98] LIVE-HCM (Lifestyle and Exercise in HCM), a prospective observational study, will hopefully provide insight for developing exercise recommendations that can aid in patient-provider shared decision making.

Conclusion

Over the years, the heightened suspicion of HCM on imaging, establishment of centers of excellence, and the judicial use of ICDs have improved the outcomes of patients with HCM. The prevalence, diagnosis, risk stratification, and treatment of HCM continue to evolve. Although there have been no new medical treatments proven to be effective for HCM since the 1980s, the introduction of new agents which specifically target the underlying pathological pathways in HCM will change our overall approach to the disease, and potentially make invasive therapies obsolete.

References

1. Maron BJ. Clinical course and management of hypertrophic cardiomyopathy. *N Engl J Med.* 2018;379:655–68.
2. Spudich JA. Three perspectives on the molecular basis of hypercontractility caused by hypertrophic cardiomyopathy mutations. *Pflugers Arch.* 2019;471(5):707–17.
3. Maron BJ, Shirani J, Poliac LC. Sudden death in young competitive athletes. Clinical, demographic, and pathological profiles. *JAMA.* 1996;276:199–204.
4. Teare D. Asymmetrical hypertrophy of the heart in young adults. *Br Heart J.* 1958;20:1–8.
5. Maron BJ, Rowin EJ, Casey SA, et al. Hypertrophic cardiomyopathy in adulthood associated with low cardiovascular mortality with contemporary management strategies. *J Am Coll Cardiol.* 2015;65:1915–28.
6. Ho CY, Ashley EA, Michels M, Pereira AC, Jacoby D, Cirino AL, Fox JC, Lakdawala NK, Ware JS, Caleshu CA, Helms AS, Colan SD, Girolami F, Cecchi F, Seidman CE, Sajeev G, Signorovitch J, Green EM, Olivotto I. Genotype and lifetime burden of disease in hypertrophic cardiomyopathy: insights from the sarcomeric human cardiomyopathy registry (SHaRe). *Circulation.* 2018;138(14):1387–98.
7. Maron MS, Olivotto I, Betocchi S, et al. Effect of left ventricular outflow tract obstruction on clinical outcome in hypertrophic cardiomyopathy. *N Engl J Med.* 2003;348:295–303.
8. Maron BJ, Rowin EJ, Udelson JE, Maron MS. Clinical spectrum and management of heart failure in hypertrophic cardiomyopathy. *JACC Heart Fail.* 2018;6:353–63.
9. Maron BJ, Casey SA, Poliac LC, et al. Clinical course of hypertrophic cardiomyopathy in a regional United States cohort. *JAMA.* 1999;281:650–5.
10. Cecchi F, Olivotto I, Montereggi A, et al. Hypertrophic cardiomyopathy in Tuscany: clinical course and outcome in an unselected regional population. *J Am Coll Cardiol.* 1995;26:1529–36.
11. Spirito P, Chiarella F, Carratino L, et al. Clinical course and prognosis of hypertrophic cardiomyopathy in an outpatient population. *N Engl J Med.* 1989;320:749–55.

12. Gersh BJ, Maron BJ, Bonow RO, et al. 2011 ACCF/AHA guideline for the diagnosis and treatment of hypertrophic cardiomyopathy: a report of the American College of Cardiology Foundation/American Heart Association Task Force on Practice Guidelines. *J Am Coll Cardiol.* 2011;58(25):e212–60.
13. Yamaguchi H, Nishiyama S, Nakanishi S, Nishimura S. Electrocardiographic, echocardiographic and ventriculographic characterization of hypertrophic non-obstructive cardiomyopathy. *Eur Heart J.* 1983;4 Suppl F:105–19.
14. McLeod CJ, Ackerman MJ, Nishimura RA, Tajik AJ, Gersh BJ, Ommen SR. Outcome of patients with hypertrophic cardiomyopathy and a normal electrocardiogram. *J Am Coll Cardiol.* 2009;54(3):229–33.
15. Maron MS, Maron BJ, Harrigan C, et al. Hypertrophic cardiomyopathy phenotype revisited after 50 years with cardiovascular magnetic resonance. *J Am Coll Cardiol.* 2009;54(3):220–8.
16. Klues HG, Schiffers A, Maron BJ. Phenotypic spectrum and patterns of left ventricular hypertrophy in hypertrophic cardiomyopathy: morphologic observations and significance as assessed by two-dimensional echocardiography in 600 patients. *J Am Coll Cardiol.* 1995;26(7):1699–708.
17. Harris KM, Spirito P, Maron MS, et al. Prevalence, clinical profile, and significance of left ventricular remodeling in the end-stage phase of hypertrophic cardiomyopathy. *Circulation.* 2006;114(3):216–25.
18. Sachdev V, Shizukuda Y, Brenneman CL, et al. Left atrial volumetric remodeling is predictive of functional capacity in nonobstructive hypertrophic cardiomyopathy. *Am Heart J.* 2005;149(4):730–6.
19. Gersh BJ, Maron BJ, Bonow RO, et al. 2011 ACCF/AHA guideline for the diagnosis and treatment of hypertrophic cardiomyopathy: a report of the American College of Cardiology Foundation/American Heart Association Task Force on Practice Guidelines. *Circulation.* 2011;124:e783–831.
20. Kwon DH, Setser RM, Thamilarasan M, et al. Abnormal papillary muscle morphology is independently associated with increased left ventricular outflow tract obstruction in hypertrophic cardiomyopathy. *Heart.* 2008;94(10):1295–301.
21. Patel P, Dhillon A, Popovic ZB, et al. Left ventricular outflow tract obstruction in hypertrophic cardiomyopathy patients without severe septal hypertrophy: implications of mitral valve and papillary muscle abnormalities assessed using cardiac magnetic resonance and echocardiography. *Circ Cardiovasc Imaging.* 2015;8(7):e003132.
22. Braunwald E, Lambrew CT, Rockoff SD, et al. Idiopathic hypertrophic subaortic stenosis. I. A description of the disease based upon an analysis of 64 patients. *Circulation.* 1964;30(Suppl4):3–119.
23. Hughes RK, Knott KD, Malcolmson J, et al. Apical hypertrophic cardiomyopathy: the variant less known. *J Am Heart Assoc.* 2020;9(5):e015294.
24. Maron MS, Finley JJ, Bos JM, et al. Prevalence, clinical significance, and natural history of left ventricular apical aneurysms in hypertrophic cardiomyopathy. *Circulation.* 2008;118(15):1541–9.
25. Vinereanu D, Florescu N, Sculthorpe N, et al. Differentiation between pathologic and physiologic left ventricular hypertrophy by tissue Doppler assessment of long-axis function in patients with hypertrophic cardiomyopathy or systemic hypertension and in athletes. *Am J Cardiol.* 2001;88(1):53–8.
26. Carasso S, Yang H, Woo A, et al. Systolic myocardial mechanics in hypertrophic cardiomyopathy: novel concepts and implications for clinical status. *J Am Soc Echocardiogr.* 2008;21(6):675–83.
27. Faber L, Seggewiss H, Gleichmann U. Percutaneous transluminal septal myocardial ablation in hypertrophic obstructive cardiomyopathy: results with respect to intraprocedural myocardial contrast echocardiography. *Circulation.* 1998;98(22):2415–21.
28. Rowin EJ, Maron BJ, Olivotto I, Maron MS. Role of exercise testing in hypertrophic cardiomyopathy. *JACC Cardiovasc Imaging.* 2017;10(11):1374–86.
29. Feiner E, Arabadjian M, Winson G, et al. Post-prandial upright exercise echocardiography in hypertrophic cardiomyopathy. *J Am Coll Cardiol.* 2013;61(24):2487–8.
30. Gersh BJ, Maron BJ, Bonow RO, et al. 2011 ACCF/AHA guideline for the diagnosis and treatment of hypertrophic cardiomyopathy: executive summary: a report of the American College of Cardiology Foundation/American Heart Association Task Force on Practice Guidelines. *J Am Coll Cardiol.* 2011;58:2703–38.
31. Sherrid MV, Barac I, McKenna WJ, et al. Multicenter study of the efficacy and safety of disopyramide in obstructive hypertrophic cardiomyopathy. *J Am Coll Cardiol.* 2005;45:1251–8.
32. Rastegar H, Boll G, Rowin EJ, et al. Results of surgical septal myectomy for obstructive hypertrophic cardiomyopathy: the Tufts experience. *Ann Cardiothorac Surg.* 2017;6(4):353–63.
33. Ommen SR, Maron BJ, Olivotto I, et al. Long-term effects of surgical septal myectomy on survival in patients with obstructive hypertrophic cardiomyopathy. *J Am Coll Cardiol.* 2005;46(3):470–6.
34. Masri A, Pierson LM, Smedira NG, et al. Predictors of long-term outcomes in patients with hypertrophic cardiomyopathy undergoing cardiopulmonary stress testing and echocardiography. *Am Heart J.* 2015;169(5):684–692.e1.
35. Bonanno AM, Macfie R, Yadava M, et al. Use of intraoperative dobutamine stress echocardiography on outcomes of septal myectomy. *Semin Thorac Cardiovasc Surg.* 2021;33(4):1037–42.
36. Maron MS, Olivotto I, Harrigan C, et al. Mitral valve abnormalities identified by cardiovascular magnetic resonance represent a primary phenotypic expression of hypertrophic cardiomyopathy. *Circulation.* 2011;124(1):40–7.
37. Chan RH, Maron BJ, Olivotto I, et al. Prognostic value of quantitative contrast-enhanced cardiovascular magnetic resonance for the evaluation of sudden death risk in patients with hypertrophic cardiomyopathy. *Circulation.* 2014;130(6):484–95.
38. Adabag AS, Maron BJ, Appelbaum E, et al. Occurrence and frequency of arrhythmias in hypertrophic cardiomyopathy in relation to delayed enhancement on cardiovascular magnetic resonance. *J Am Coll Cardiol.* 2008;51(14):1369–74.
39. Farooqi KM, Cooper C, Chelliah A, et al. 3D Printing and heart failure: the present and the future. *JACC Heart Fail.* 2019;7(2):132–42.
40. Marian AJ, Braunwald E. Hypertrophic cardiomyopathy: genetics, pathogenesis, clinical manifestations, diagnosis, and therapy. *Circ Res.* 2017;121(7):749–70.
41. Axelsson A, Iversen K, Vejlstrup N, et al. Efficacy and safety of the angiotensin II receptor blocker losartan for hypertrophic cardiomyopathy: the INHERIT randomised, double-blind, placebo-controlled trial. *Lancet Diabetes Endocrinol.* 2015;3:123–31.
42. Maron MS, Chan RH, Kapur NK, et al. Effect of spironolactone on myocardial fibrosis and other clinical variables in patients with hypertrophic cardiomyopathy. *Am J Med.* 2018;131:837–41.
43. Olivotto I, Camici PG, Merlini PA, et al. Efficacy of ranolazine in patients with symptomatic hypertrophic cardiomyopathy: the RESTYLE-hcm randomized, double-blind, placebo-controlled study. *Circ Heart Fail.* 2018;11:e004124.
44. Elliott PM. Evolving story of clinical trials in hypertrophic cardiomyopathy. *Circ Heart Fail.* 2018;11:e004572.
45. Ho CY, McMurray JJV, Cirino AL, et al. The design of the valsartan for attenuating disease evolution in early sarcomeric hypertrophic cardiomyopathy (VANISH) trial. *Am Heart J.* 2017;187:145–155.
46. https://clinicaltrial.gov. A study to evaluate mavacamten in adults with symptomatic obstructive HCM who are eligible for septal reduction therapy (VALOR-HCM). (ClinicalTrials.gov Identifier: NCT04349072).
47. Laura A. Robertson DRA, E Robbie, Anna Osmukhina, Hanbin Li, Fady I. Malik, Scott D. Solomon. A first in human study of the selective cardiac myosin inhibitor, CK-3773274. *J Card Fail.* 25:S79–S80.
48. Cherian G, Brockington IF, Shah PM, Oakley CM, Goodwin JF. Beta-adrenergic blockade in hypertrophic obstructive cardiomyopathy. *Br Med J.* 1966;1:895–8.
49. Adelman AG, Shah PM, Gramiak R, Wigle ED. Long-term propranolol therapy in muscular subaortic stenosis. *Br Heart J.* 1970;32:804–11.
50. Flamm MD, Harrison DC, Hancock EW. Muscular subaortic stenosis. Prevention of outflow obstruction with propranolol. *Circulation.* 1968;38:846–58.
51. Gombar S, Moneghetti KJ, Callahan A, Jung K, Wheeler MT. Abstract 21307: beta-blockers inferior to calcium channel blockers in hypertrophic cardiomyopathy. *Circulation.* 2017;136:A21307.
52. Pollick C, Kimball B, Henderson M, Wigle ED. Disopyramide in hypertrophic cardiomyopathy. I. Hemodynamic assessment after intravenous administration. *Am J Cardiol.* 1988;62:1248–51.
53. Pollick C. Disopyramide in hypertrophic cardiomyopathy. II. Noninvasive assessment after oral administration. *Am J Cardiol.* 1988;62:1252–5.
54. Pollick C. Muscular subaortic stenosis: hemodynamic and clinical improvement after disopyramide. *N Engl J Med.* 1982;307:997–9.
55. Louie EK, Edwards LC, 3rd. Hypertrophic cardiomyopathy. *Prog Cardiovasc Dis.* 1994;36:275–308.
56. Adler A, Fourey D, Weissler-Snir A, et al. Safety of outpatient initiation of disopyramide for obstructive hypertrophic cardiomyopathy patients. *J Am Heart Assoc.* 2017;6(6):e005152.
57. Gentry JL, 3rd, Mentz RJ, Hurdle M, Wang A. Ranolazine for treatment of angina or dyspnea in hypertrophic cardiomyopathy patients (RHYME). *J Am Coll Cardiol.* 2016;68:1815–7.
58. Olivotto I, Hellawell JL, Farzaneh-Far R, et al. Novel approach targeting the complex pathophysiology of hypertrophic cardiomyopathy: the impact of late sodium current inhibition on exercise capacity in subjects with symptomatic hypertrophic cardiomyopathy (LIBERTY-HCM) trial. *Circ Heart Fail.* 2016;9:e002764.
59. Veselka J, Jensen MK, Liebregts M, et al. Long-term clinical outcome after alcohol septal ablation for obstructive hypertrophic cardiomyopathy: results from the Euro-ASA registry. *Eur Heart J.* 2016;37(19):1517–23.
60. Kwon DH, Smedira NG, Thamilarasan M, et al. Characteristics and surgical outcomes of symptomatic patients with hypertrophic cardiomyopathy with abnormal papillary muscle morphology undergoing papillary muscle reorientation. *J Thorac Cardiovasc Surg.* 2010;140(2):317–24.

61. El-Sabawi B, Nishimura RA, Barsness GW, et al. Temporal occurrence of arrhythmic complications after alcohol septal ablation. *Circulation: Cardiovascular Interventions*. 2020;13(2):e008540.
62. Schafer U, Kreidel F, Frerker C. MitraClip implantation as a new treatment strategy against systolic anterior motion-induced outflow tract obstruction in hypertrophic obstructive cardiomyopathy. *Heart Lung Circ*. 2014;23(5):e131–135.
63. Sorajja P, Pedersen WA, Bae R, et al. First experience with percutaneous mitral valve plication as primary therapy for symptomatic obstructive hypertrophic cardiomyopathy. *J Am Coll Cardiol*. 2016;67(24):2811–18.
64. Gupta S, Slater M, Heitner S, Wei K. Percutaneous mitral valve repair for management of systolic anterior motion and mitral regurgitation associated with hypertrophic cardiomyopathy. *J Am Coll Cardiol* 2016;68(18 Suppl):B327–B328.
65. Maron BJ, Nishimura RA, McKenna WJ, et al. Assessment of permanent dual-chamber pacing as a treatment for drug-refractory symptomatic patients with obstructive hypertrophic cardiomyopathy. A randomized, double-blind, crossover study (M-PATHY). *Circulation*. 1999;99(22):2927–33.
66. Kappenberger L, Linde C, Daubert C, et al. Pacing in hypertrophic obstructive cardiomyopathy. A randomized crossover study. PIC Study Group. *Eur Heart J*. 1997;18(8):1249–56.
67. Kiehl EL, Makki T, Kumar R, et al. Incidence and predictors of right ventricular pacing-induced cardiomyopathy in patients with complete atrioventricular block and preserved left ventricular systolic function. *Heart Rhythm*. 2016;13(12):2272–8.
68. Maron BJ, Olivotto I, Bellone P, et al. Clinical profile of stroke in 900 patients with hypertrophic cardiomyopathy. *J Am Coll Cardiol*. 2002;39(2):301–7
69. Lin TT, Sung YL, Ko TY, et al. Risk of ischemic stroke in patients with hypertrophic cardiomyopathy in the absence of atrial fibrillation – a nationwide cohort study. *Aging (Albany NY)*. 2019;11(23):11347–57.
70. Hirota T, Kubo T, Baba Y, et al. Clinical profile of thromboembolic events in patients with hypertrophic cardiomyopathy in a regional japanese cohort – results from Kochi RYOMA Study. *Circ J*. 2019;83(8):1747–54.
71. Jung H, Yang PS, Sung JH, et al. Hypertrophic cardiomyopathy in patients with atrial fibrillation: prevalence and associated stroke risks in a nationwide cohort study. *Thromb Haemost*. 2019;119(2):285–93.
72. Nazer B, Dale Z, Carrassa G, et al. Appropriate and inappropriate shocks in hypertrophic cardiomyopathy patients with subcutaneous implantable cardioverter-defibrillators: an international multicenter study. *Heart Rhythm*. 2020;17(7):1107–14.
73. Green JJ, Berger JS, Kramer CM, et al. Prognostic value of late gadolinium enhancement in clinical outcomes for hypertrophic cardiomyopathy. *JACC Cardiovasc Imaging*. 2012;5(4):370–7.
74. Elliott PM, Anastasakis A, Borger MA, et al. 2014 ESC guidelines on diagnosis and management of hypertrophic cardiomyopathy: the task force for the diagnosis and management of hypertrophic cardiomyopathy of the European Society of Cardiology (ESC). *Eur Heart J*. 2014;35:2733–79.
75. Marstrand P, Han L, Day SM, et al. Hypertrophic cardiomyopathy with left ventricular systolic dysfunction: insights from the SHaRe registry. *Circulation*. 2020;141:1371–83.
76. O'Mahony C, Jichi F, Pavlou M, et al. A novel clinical risk prediction model for sudden cardiac death in hypertrophic cardiomyopathy (HCM risk-SCD). *Eur Heart J*. 2014;35(30):2010–20.
77. O'Mahony C, Jichi F, Ommen SR, et al. International External Validation Study of the 2014 European Society of Cardiology Guidelines on Sudden Cardiac Death Prevention in Hypertrophic Cardiomyopathy (EVIDENCE-HCM). *Circulation*. 2018;137(10):1015–23.
78. O'Mahony C, Akhtar MM, Anastasiou Z, et al. Effectiveness of the 2014 European Society of Cardiology guideline on sudden cardiac death in hypertrophic cardiomyopathy: a systematic review and meta-analysis. *Heart*. 2019;105:623–31.
79. Spoladore R, Maron MS, D'Amato R, Camici PG, Olivotto I. Pharmacological treatment options for hypertrophic cardiomyopathy: high time for evidence. *Eur Heart J*. 2012;33:1724–33.
80. Frey N, Luedde M, Katus HA. Mechanisms of disease: hypertrophic cardiomyopathy. *Nat Rev Cardiol*. 2011;9:91–100.
81. Toepfer CN, Wakimoto H, Garfinkel AC, et al. Hypertrophic cardiomyopathy mutations in MYBPC3 dysregulate myosin. *Sci Transl Med*. 2019;11(476):eaat1199.
82. Kawas RF, Anderson RL, Ingle SRB, et al. A small-molecule modulator of cardiac myosin acts on multiple stages of the myosin chemomechanical cycle. *J Biol Chem*. 2017;292:16571–7.
83. Anderson RL, Trivedi DV, Sarkar SS, et al. Deciphering the super relaxed state of human beta-cardiac myosin and the mode of action of mavacamten from myosin molecules to muscle fibers. *Proc Natl Acad Sci U S A*. 2018;115:E8143–52.
84. Stern JA, Markova S, Ueda Y, et al. A small molecule inhibitor of sarcomere contractility acutely relieves left ventricular outflow tract obstruction in feline hypertrophic cardiomyopathy. *PLoS One*. 2016;11:e0168407.
85. del Rio C, Ueyama Y, Baker D, et al. Abstract 20593: in vivo cardiac effects of mavacamten (MYK-461): evidence for negative inotropy and improved compliance. *Circulation*. 2017;136:A20593.
86. Green EM, Wakimoto H, Anderson RL, et al. A small-molecule inhibitor of sarcomere contractility suppresses hypertrophic cardiomyopathy in mice. *Science*. 2016;351:617–21.
87. Heitner SB, Jacoby D, Lester SJ, et al. Mavacamten treatment for obstructive hypertrophic cardiomyopathy: a clinical trial. *Ann Intern Med*. 2019;170:741–8.
88. Olivotto I, Oreziak A, Barriales-Villa R, et al. Mavacamten for treatment of symptomatic obstructive hypertrophic cardiomyopathy (EXPLORER-HCM): a randomised, double-blind, placebo-controlled, phase 3 trial. *The Lancet*. 2020;396(10253):759–69.
89. Ho CY, Mealiffe ME, Bach RG, et al. Evaluation of mavacamten in symptomatic patients with nonobstructive hypertrophic cardiomyopathy. *J Am Coll Cardiol*. 2020;75:2649–60.
90. HFSA 2021. https://www.biospace.com/article/releases/cytokinetics-announces-results-from-redwood-hcm-and-galactic-hf-presented-in-late-breaking-clinical-trial-session-at-the-hfsa-annual-scientific-meeting/ Accessed March 25, 2022.
91. Ashrafian H, Redwood C, Blair E, Watkins H. Hypertrophic cardiomyopathy:a paradigm for myocardial energy depletion. *Trends in Genetics*. 2003;19:263–8.
92. Crilley JG, Boehm EA, Blair E, et al. Hypertrophic cardiomyopathy due to sarcomeric gene mutations is characterized by impaired energy metabolism irrespective of the degree of hypertrophy. *J Am Coll Cardiol*. 2003;41:1776–82.
93. Horowitz JD, Chirkov YY. Perhexiline and hypertrophic cardiomyopathy: a new horizon for metabolic modulation. *Circulation*. 2010;122:1547–9.
94. Gehmlich K, Dodd M, Allwood J, et al. Changes in the cardiac metabolome caused by perhexiline treatment in a mouse model of hypertrophic cardiomyopathy (Accepted Manuscript). *Molecular BioSystems*. 2015;11(2):564–73.
95. Abozguia K, Elliott P, McKenna W, et al. Metabolic modulator perhexiline corrects energy deficiency and improves exercise capacity in symptomatic hypertrophic cardiomyopathy. *Circulation*. 2010;122:1562–9.
96. Coats CJ, Pavlou M, Watkinson OT, et al. Effect of trimetazidine dihydrochloride therapy on exercise capacity in patients with nonobstructive hypertrophic cardiomyopathy: a randomized clinical trial. *JAMA Cardiol*. 2019;4(3):230–5.
97. Maron BJ, Chaitman BR, Ackerman MJ, et al. Recommendations for physical activity and recreational sports participation for young patients with genetic cardiovascular diseases. *Circulation*. 2004;109:2807–16.
98. Saberi S, Wheeler M, Bragg-Gresham J, et al. Effect of moderate-intensity exercise training on peak oxygen consumption in patients with hypertrophic cardiomyopathy: a randomized clinical trial. *JAMA*. 2017;317:1349–57.

Chapter 34
MYOCARDITIS

George Lazaros, Emilia Lazarou, and Dimitris Tousoulis

Introduction and Nomenclature

Myocarditis is defined as the acute inflammatory disorder of the heart resulting from a variety of infectious and noninfectious conditions, including systemic immune-mediated disorders, cardiotoxic agents, etc.[1,2] Myocarditis is diagnosed using established clinical, laboratory, imaging, histological, immunological, and immunohistochemical criteria, after other possible cardiovascular or extracardiac causes of acute myocardial dysfunction have been ruled out.[2]

In acute myocarditis with left ventricular dysfunction, the term "infective cardiomyopathy" is reserved for cases attributed to infection.[2–4] In this context, the term "viral cardiomyopathy" is used in cases of persistent cardiotropic viral genome in endomyocardial biopsy (EMB) samples, detected with polymerase chain reaction, and accompanied by inflammation. In contrast, the term "viral heart disease" denotes the presence of ongoing lytic viral infection without concurrent inflammation.[2–5] "Inflammatory cardiomyopathy" is used in cases of dilated cardiomyopathy due to biopsy-proven non-infectious myocarditis, demonstrated by the presence of inflammation in the absence of infectious microorganisms.[2–5] When neither viral genome nor inflammation is demonstrated in a patient with dilated cardiomyopathy, then the term "idiopathic dilated cardiomyopathy" is used in the absence of a pathogenic gene mutation (see Chapter 31).[5] This nomenclature is useful for clinical and research purposes and has contributed to overcoming the confusion created by different definitions in this setting.

Epidemiology and Etiology

Myocarditis is quite common, with an estimated annual incidence of approximately 22 cases per 100,000 subjects; in comparison, the incidence of acute pericarditis is 27.7 cases.[4,6] This estimate corresponds to 1.5 million cases of myocarditis worldwide.[4]

In addition to the acute mortality due either to sudden death (3% of all sudden death cases in a series)[7] or to fulminant myocarditis evolving into intractable cardiogenic shock,[8] another important concern with acute myocarditis is the potential for progression to dilated cardiomyopathy and heart failure (HF) in approximately 30% of cases.[3]

The etiology of myocarditis includes a wide range of infectious and noninfectious causes (Table 34.1). Viral infection is the most common, as evident from the detection of viral genome in endomyocardial biopsy (EMB) specimen.[9] Concerning the individual agents, a shift in epidemiology was recorded in recent years (as of 1990), with parvovirus B19 and human herpes virus 6 being the most commonly detected pathogens, as opposed to the predominance of enteroviruses (in particular Coxsackie B virus) and adenoviruses in earlier years.[5] However, in approximately 30% of patients, multiple agents are detected.[10] In these cases, a high mean viral load (genome equivalents per microgram of isolated nucleic acids) may discriminate between the causative agent and bystanders.[11,12] Apart from epidemiologic purposes, the identification of the viral agent may have clinical and prognostic implications. For instance, parvovirus infection has been linked with symptoms resembling mostly those of acute myocardial infarction, whereas human herpes virus myocarditis presents with acute HF symptoms and tends to evolve into dilated cardiomyopathy.[13]

With respect to non-infectious causes, the identification of the underlying cause is of paramount importance. In cases of an autoimmune disease or other systemic condition, every effort should be taken to treat the causative disorder. Similarly, in cases of toxic or hypersensitive myocarditis, withdrawal of the trigger may be sufficient to cause remission.

Pathogenesis and Progression to Dilated Cardiomyopathy

The pathogenesis of acute myocarditis in humans has not been fully elucidated even today. However, the availability of experimental models, mainly murine models, has contributed to a better understanding of the series of events linking viral infection, acute myocarditis, and progression to dilated cardiomyopathy and HF. In viral myocarditis, where most of the work has been done, the virus appears to enter the myocardial cells from the blood stream through specific myocardial receptors and coreceptors.[14,15] The role of receptors in myocarditis has been indirectly highlighted by the higher expression of CAR receptors in patients with viral cardiomyopathy as compared with those with healthy hearts or other heart diseases.[16] Viral replication within myocytes may lead to myocyte necrosis with exteriorization of antigens, such as cardiac myosin, and subsequent activation of the host's immune system, with mobilization and local confluence of macrophages and natural killers, which release cytokines.[14]

This series of events constitutes the first or acute phase of myocarditis, which lasts approximately four days. In this phase, EMB shows myocyte necrosis without inflammatory infiltrates. An extensive myocardial necrosis in this phase, depending on the balance between virus cardiotoxicity and intensity of host defensive mechanisms, may lead to fulminant myocarditis and intractable cardiogenic shock.[17]

The second or subacute phase of myocarditis is characterized by cellular cardiac infiltrates and may last anywhere from a few weeks to several months. In this phase, a series of autoimmune reactions occur, with the aim of viral clearance. Viral-specific T lymphocytes, macrophages, and cardiac dendritic cells release a variety of cytokines, including interleukins-1, -2, -4 to -6, and -17, tumor necrosis factor, and interferon-γ, targeting the infected myocytes. The released cytokines recruit antibody-producing B cells, which can insult damaged myocardial cells as well.[14]

In most cases, immune activation leads to virus clearance and restoration of normal left ventricular contractility. However, in some cases complete virus elimination is not achieved or the immune activation with persisting heart damage may continue

DOI: 10.1201/9780429244544-41

TABLE 34.1: **Most Common Etiologies in Acute Myocarditis**

		Most Common Etiologies in Acute Myocarditis
Infectious	Bacteria	*Streptococcus, Staphylococcus, Mycobacteria, Chlamydia, Gonococcus, Salmonella, Corynebacterium diphtheriae, Haemophilus influenzae, Pneumococcus, Meningococcus, Brucella, Mycoplasma pneumoniae, Legionella, Serratia*
	Viruses	Coxsackieviruses A and B, Echoviruses, Adenoviruses, Parvovirus B19, Human herpes virus 6, Human immunodeficiency virus, Hepatitis C virus, Epstein-Barr virus, Cytomegalovirus, Influenza A and B virus, Varicella-Zoster virus, herpes simplex virus, poliovirus, respiratory syncytial virus, rubella virus, measles virus, mumps virus, Arboviruses
	Protozoa	*Trypanosoma cruzi, Leishmania, Toxoplasma gondii*
	Parasites	*Echinococcus granulosus, Taenia solium, Trichinella spiralis*
	Fungi	*Candida, Actinomyces, Cryptococcus, Blastomyces, Histoplasma, Coccidioides*
	Spirochetes	*Borrelia, Leptospira*
	Rickettsiae	*Coxiella burnetti, Rickettsia ricketsii*
Immune-Mediated	Systemic lupus erythematosus, rheumatoid arthritis, Sjogren syndrome, sarcoidosis, Churg-Strauss syndrome, Takayasu arteritis, inflammatory bowel diseases, Wegener granulomatosis, rheumatic fever, giant cell myocarditis, necrotizing eosinophilic myocarditis, Kawasaki disease, allergens (such as vaccines and hypersensitivity reactions to various drugs, including, among others, penicillin, colchicine, furosemide, isoniazid, phenytoin, methyldopa, thiazide diuretics, amitriptyline, etc.)	
Toxic	Encompasses forms due to medications (anthracyclines, cocaine, cyclophosphamide, amphetamines, lithium, trastuzumab, clozapine, catecholamines, etc.), heavy metals, physical agents (electric shock, radiation, heat shock, hypothermia), ethanol	
Other	Snake, scorpion, spider, and insect stings, thyrotoxicosis, arsenic	

even in the absence of the viral genome. This may be due to antigenic or molecular mimicry, which consists of sustained immune activation due to the presence of common antigens between offending microorganism and cardiac structures. such as cardiac myosin (which has been exposed after myocardial injury) and human cell-surface protein laminin.[4,14,15,18] Thus, a third or chronic phase, lasting months to years, may occur even in the absence of symptoms.[14] This phase is characterized by persistent low-grade heart damage, fibrous replacement of the myocardium, and gradual transition to dilated cardiomyopathy and HF in up to 30% of cases.[1,4,14,15,19] The interplay between genetic and environmental factors is key for disease progression. Familial dilated cardiomyopathy has been described in up to 35% of affected patients (in the form of asymptomatic cardiac abnormalities), whereas sequencing studies have revealed causative mutations in up to 25% of affected patients.[3] Finally, autoimmune inflammation leading to fibrosis has been described in the absence of infections and has been attributed to heat shock proteins, immunogenic particles deriving from tissue injury, various drugs, and systemic autoimmune disorders.[4]

Additional mechanisms, independent of immune system activation, have been implicated in the progression of acute myocarditis to chronic dilated cardiomyopathy. Among others, protease 2A produced by enterovirus may lead to cardiomyopathy by proteolytic cleavage of dystrophin and other host proteins.[20] In the case of erythroviruses (including parvovirus), the infection and persistence in the endothelial cells, typical of this etiology, may lead to impaired nitric oxide (NO) production, altered coronary artery vasoreactivity (more prominent at the microcirculation level leading to myocardial injury), fibrosis, and heart dilatation.[21] The time course of viral myocarditis is summarized in Figure 34.1.

A major concern with respect to the link between myocarditis and chronic dilated cardiomyopathy is that current knowledge is based mainly on animal models. Whether these apply to human myocarditis should be explored in human studies.

Clinical Scenarios in Acute Myocarditis

Myocarditis involves a wide range of clinical manifestations, extending from asymptomatic (subclinical and incidentally revealed forms) to cases presenting with intractable cardiogenic shock or even sudden death as the first sign of the disease.[8] Myocarditis accounts for 3% of sudden death cases; in young athletes, the corresponding proportion is 5–12%.[7,22]

The most common symptoms of acute myocarditis include chest pain and dyspnea of variable intensity.[2] Symptoms usually appear within one to four weeks after a respiratory or gastrointestinal tract viral infection.[5] Physical examination usually yields non-specific findings and does not offer any specific clues. According to a position statement of the pertinent working group of the European Society of Cardiology (ESC), there are five possible scenarios in patients with biopsy-proven myocarditis (Table 34.2).[2]

The first scenario includes patients presenting with acute coronary syndrome-like symptoms, such as chest pain. Importantly, coronary artery disease or any possible cardiac or extracardiac condition accounting for these symptoms should be excluded (see also the subsection in this chapter on imaging features in the Diagnosis section). Patients may present with or without troponin elevation. In contrast to coronary syndromes, troponin has sustained release and prolonged plateau in myocarditis.[2] C-reactive protein may rise in any subtype of acute myocarditis; however, normal values do not rule out myocardial inflammation.[23]

The second clinical scenario encompasses myocarditis cases characterized by new onset HF of two weeks' to three months' duration, with dyspnea, fatigue, peripheral edema, ventricular arrhythmias, and heart block. Left and/or right ventricular systolic dysfunction is invariably present, whereas dilatation and/or increased thickness (due to edema) may be observed.[2] This is the typical scenario of fulminant myocarditis and includes giant cell myocarditis, necrotizing eosinophilic myocarditis, and toxic myocarditis, as well as other forms without a specific etiological diagnosis.

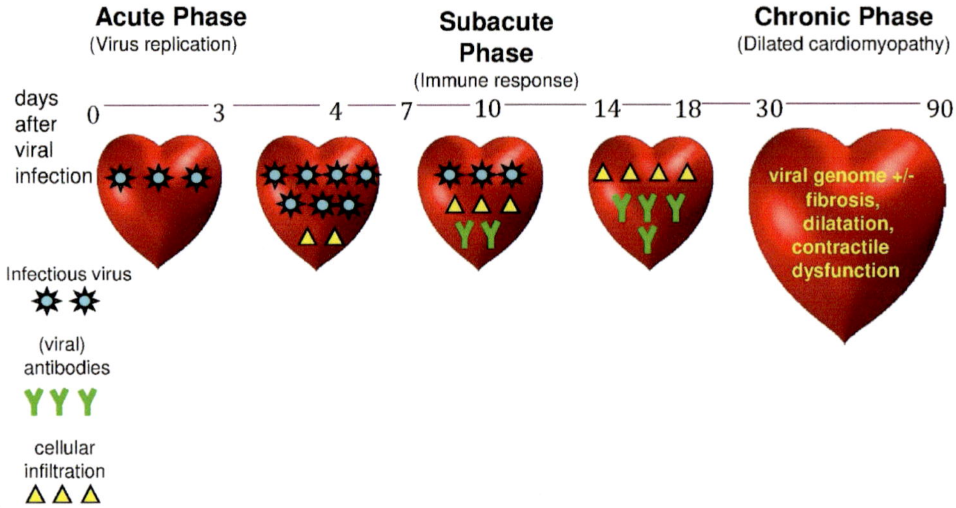

FIGURE 34.1 Time course of viral myocarditis. (Reproduced with permission from Kindermann et al. Update on myocarditis. *J Am Coll Cardiol*. 2012;59(9):779–92.)

TABLE 34.2: Diagnostic Criteria in Patients with Suspected Myocarditis

Clinical Scenarios	i. Infarct-like chest pain ii. New onset HF (less than three months) iii. Subacute or chronic heart failure (more than three months) iv. Unexplained arrhythmias or aborted sudden cardiac death v. Unexplained cardiogenic shock
Diagnostic Criteria	A. Electrocardiography, Holter, or stress test features* B. Troponin elevation C. Structural and functional abnormal findings with echocardiography, CMR, and coronary angiography* D. Edema and/or LGE distribution (namely tissue characterization parameters) compatible with myocarditis

Notes: Diagnosis is established in the presence of one or more clinical scenario along with one or more diagnostic criterion (e.g., i + D) provided that alternative diagnoses have been ruled out. In asymptomatic patients (not fitting any clinical scenario), two or more diagnostic criteria from different categories should be met.

* See relevant sections for details.

Abbreviations: CMR = cardiac magnetic resonance, LGE = late gadolinium enhancement.

The third clinical scenario includes patients with a profile similar to that described in the second scenario, but the duration of symptoms is >three months, sometimes with remissions and exacerbations. The imaging findings are consistent with dilated cardiomyopathy, with impaired contractility of the left and occasionally right ventricle, along with increased dimensions of left or both ventricles.

Finally, the fourth and fifth clinical scenarios include very sick patients presenting with aborted cardiac death or life-threatening ventricular arrhythmias (fourth scenario) and cardiogenic shock and poor left ventricular function (fifth scenario). As in all clinical scenarios, alternative cardiac and non-cardiac pathology should be excluded (e.g., coronary artery disease, valve or congenital heart disease, hyperthyroidism, etc.).[2]

In a subset of patients, estimated at 32–57% of myocarditis cases, pericardial involvement is observed with or without pericardial effusion.[24] However, non-steroidal anti-inflammatory drugs (NSAIDs), which constitute the cornerstone of the treatment for pericardial syndromes, should be used with caution in the setting of myocarditis, as in experimental models NSAIDs seem to enhance inflammation necrosis and worsen mortality.[14] These agents should be practically reserved for patients with prominently pericardial pain, and should be given at the lowest effective dose for pain control and for the shortest possible period, provided that left ventricular function is preserved.[6,8] Moreover, in contrast to "pure" pericarditis, colchicine is not recommended in myopericarditis, as there is no evidence to support its clinical benefit in this setting.[2]

Additional symptoms due to extracardiac involvement may accompany secondary myocarditis, such as immune-mediated diseases (including autoimmune disorders and auto-inflammatory diseases, where at least two organ systems are involved), human immunodeficiency virus (HIV) infection, etc.[1] In these cases, it is of utmost importance to suspect and diagnose any systemic condition underlying myocarditis, as treatment of the primary disorder should be the main target. Myocarditis in this context should be suspected in the presence of chest pain, dyspnea, HF, cardiogenic shock, and life-threatening arrhythmias with or without troponin elevation.[1] The diagnostic work-up should be individualized on the basis of clinical presentation and EMB can be a valuable tool in these cases.

Clinical Presentation According to Cause

Giant cell myocarditis is an uncommon but particularly severe form of myocarditis, with rapid progression to intractable HF and frequent need for heart transplantation.[4,25,26] Its incidence is estimated at 0.13 per 100,000 people annually and seems to increase over time; it is detected approximately in 3–5.6% of all myocarditis autopsies.[4,27–29] The mean age at onset is 43 and, in 19% of cases, an associated autoimmune disorder is reported.[4,29] Fulminant myocarditis is detected in 10% of patients undergoing EMB for recent-onset cardiomyopathy.[17] It is a distinct clinical entity with approximately 7% in-hospital mortality. However, patients who survive the acute event with aggressive hemodynamic support have excellent long-term prognosis with full recovery of cardiac function.[17] Finally, acute fulminant necrotizing myocarditis is a very uncommon and often fatal form of acute myocarditis presenting with rapidly progressing symptoms, leading to HF and shock. In contrast to other forms of eosinophilic myocarditis (such as hypersensitivity myocarditis), the exclusive target is the heart without concomitant multiorgan involvement.[30]

Myocardial involvement in sarcoidosis is particularly challenging. This condition often presents with conduction disturbances, ventricular arrhythmias, and occasionally sudden death, which is the major concern.[1] Sarcoidosis occurs usually between ages 20 and 50 and the histological hallmark of the disease is the detection of non-necrotizing granulomas in affected tissues.[1,31] Sarcoidosis manifestations include, among others, lymphadenopathy, pulmonary infiltrations, and skin and ocular lesions. Overt heart involvement is clinically apparent in up to 7% of cases, whereas autopsy series report cardiac involvement in up to 30% of cases.[1,31] Positron emission tomography imaging with fluorodeoxyglucose can detect active inflammation and scarring and is therefore a valuable tool for the diagnosis of sarcoidosis.[4]

Another cause of myocarditis associated with potentially reversible heart block is Lyme disease. Lyme borreliosis is the most common tick-borne disease in high-income countries.[32] Cardiac involvement has been described in up to 10% of untreated cases, with heart block being the most common feature.[3]

Chagas disease due to *Trypanosoma cruzi* is a major public health problem, especially in Latin America. Its clinical course includes an acute and a subsequent chronic phase. Severe acute disease including myocarditis occurs in <5% of cases after inoculation; the syndrome lasts one to two months and regresses spontaneously.[33] Untreated patients progress to chronic cardiac involvement at a rate of 1.4–5% per year with 14–45% showing cardiac involvement at some point.[33] Cardiac manifestations include heart block, complex ventricular arrhythmias, left ventricular dysfunction, eventually with apical aneurysm and frequent thrombus formation, dilated cardiomyopathy, and sudden death.[33]

Finally, another important cause of myocarditis, mainly due to the high prevalence of HIV infection worldwide, is HIV-related myocarditis and cardiomyopathy. In autopsy series, 52% of HIV-infected patients have findings compatible with myocarditis, and biventricular involvement is detected in 10% of cases.[34] Direct HIV-induced myocardial injury along with immune-mediated mechanisms and systemic inflammation have been implicated in the pathogenesis of HIV-related myocardial disease.[35] Accelerated myocardial fibrosis, as demonstrated by cardiac magnetic resonance (CMR) imaging, appears to play a key role in the development of cardiomyopathy and HF in HIV.[35] The prognosis of HIV-related cardiomyopathy is worse than in uninfected counterparts.[36] Effective treatment is important for the prevention of HIV cardiomyopathy, as poorly controlled infection has been associated with greater risk of HF.[35]

Diagnosis

Myocarditis is often difficult to diagnose, considering the clinical, laboratory, and imaging findings overlapping with other disorders. A high index of suspicion is required to plan a suitable work-up and obtain a correct diagnosis in a timely fashion.

Neither the ESC nor the American Heart Association or the American College of Cardiology has released formal guidelines on myocarditis to date. In the relevant position paper from the ESC, the diagnosis of myocarditis is established by the combination of one of the four possible clinical scenarios described above (in the absence of an alternative explanation) with at least one of (1) electrocardiographic, Holter monitoring, or stress test criteria; (2) elevated troponin (or other markers of myocardial necrosis); (3) imaging findings (echocardiography, CMR, angiography) showing functional or structural cardiac abnormalities; and (4) edema and typical late gadolinium enhancement (LGE) on CMR.[2] In asymptomatic patients, two or more criteria should be met to establish the diagnosis. The diagnostic criteria are summarized in Table 34.2.

Patients with acute myocarditis can present with a wide spectrum of clinical manifestations. Whether asymptomatic or oligosymptomatic patients (e.g., presenting with flu-like illness without prominent, cardiovascular symptoms) with mild troponin elevations should be admitted to the hospital is a matter of ongoing discussion. According to the ESC statement on myocarditis, these patients should be admitted and monitored until a final diagnosis is established, because, even in the absence of left ventricular dysfunction, the condition can rapidly evolve into a cardiovascular emergency.[2] Experts in the United States recommend a more conservative approach for patients with normal left ventricular systolic function, suggesting that out-patient management with reevaluation after 1–2 weeks to assess for troponin trend and HF symptoms and/or arrhythmias is reasonable.[2,37] A compromise between these two options would be a short-term in-hospital observation for initial work-up and subsequent discharge with outpatient follow-up in the absence of high-risk findings.

The work-up of patients presenting with suspected myocarditis includes a variety of tools, including electrocardiogram (ECG), biomarkers, imaging (mainly echocardiography and CMR), and invasive procedures, such as coronary angiography to exclude coronary artery disease and EMB. The diagnostic approach should be individualized depending on clinical presentation. Troponins should be trended in all patients, both for diagnostic purposes and to track disease activity.[2] Natriuretic peptides can be useful, especially in patients presenting with HF.[38] Viral serology to identify the causative agent, either through circulating antibodies or by polymerase chain reaction, is not generally recommended, taking into consideration the lack of correlation between peripheral blood and EMB findings.[23] The presence of heart-specific antibodies is useful for distinguishing between autoimmune myocarditis (presence of autoantibodies in the absence of inflammation on EMB) and inflammatory myocarditis (absence of autoantibodies in the presence of inflammation on EMB).[39] Recently, there has been a growing interest in the role of microRNAs (miRNAs) in the pathogenesis, treatment, and early recognition of patients prone to short- and long-term complications. Most important, certain miRNAs, such as miR-155, may be selected as therapeutic targets in acute myocarditis, taking into consideration the inflammation-enhancing properties of the latter.[40] The diagnostic ability of the rest of the available screening tools is briefly reported below.

Electrocardiogram (ECG)

An ECG should be obtained in all suspected cases of myocarditis. Although a non-specific tool, the ECG shows pathologic findings in most patients with acute myocarditis.[14,15] Most patients present with non-specific repolarization abnormalities. ST-segment elevation may raise differential diagnostic issues with acute myocardial infarction.[14] Newly appearing Q waves, abnormal QRS axis, and prolongation beyond 120 ms, a QTc greater than 440 ms, and ventricular ectopy have been associated with adverse outcome and a need for transplantation.[41]

Echocardiography

Echocardiography is of paramount importance in the overall management of myocarditis, both for initial assessment and for long-term follow-up. Although echocardiography does not provide specific clues with respect to myocarditis, it is useful in the differential diagnosis of alternative underlying disorders, including valvular disease, cardiomyopathies, congenital heart disease, etc.[2] An unusual finding specific to fulminant myocarditis is normal-sized chambers with severely impaired contractility and increased wall thickness due to myocardial edema, which resolves in the long term (Figure 34.2).[2,14] Transthoracic echocardiography should be offered to all suspected cases to assess chamber size, wall thickness, systolic and diastolic function, and the presence of pericardial effusion and intracavitary thrombi. Repeat studies are recommended in cases of clinical worsening and/or hemodynamic instability. Regional wall motion abnormalities are observed in up to 64% of myocarditis cases and therefore do not help to discriminate between myocarditis and coronary artery disease.[42] Systolic dysfunction of any degree is observed in 69% of cases, whereas diastolic dysfunction is recorded in most patients.[40] Echocardiography may additionally provide prognostic clues. Impaired left ventricular ejection fraction (LVEF), pulmonary hypertension, elevated left ventricular filling pressures, and right ventricular dysfunction (observed in approximately 23% of patients) have all been associated with adverse prognosis.[2,14,42] Global longitudinal strain may provide incremental information, revealing subtle systolic dysfunction, myocardial inflammation and fibrosis, and clues differentiating myocarditis from chronic, dilated cardiomyopathy.[5]

Cardiac Magnetic Resonance (CMR)

Tissue characterization without the need for ionizing radiation and iodinated contrast are the main strengths of CMR. Moreover, CMR can be used for EMB guidance, considering the patchy involvement of the myocardium. Potential limitations include contraindications in patients with advanced chronic renal disease or non-compatible electronic devices, the time-consuming nature of the procedure, and the inability of bedside evaluation. CMR should be performed early in the course of the disease, ideally towards the end of the first week. A follow-up CMR at least one month later is useful to detect persistent inflammation, which is predictive of adverse outcomes.[24] The CMR diagnostic criteria for myocarditis are based on the Lake Louise criteria following consensus of CMR experts.[24] These criteria include three different CMR techniques: (1) T2-weighted short-tau inversion recovery images which detect tissue edema; (2) T1-weighted sequences which reveal hyperemia and capillary leak (myocardial early gadolinium enhancement); and (3) T1-weighted inversion recovery sequences 10–15 min after administration of the paramagnetic agent to detect subepicardial and/or midmyocardial LGE, a marker of necrosis and fibrosis (Figure 34.3).[2,5,24] In the presence of two out of three of these criteria, the diagnostic accuracy of the Lake Louise criteria is 78%.[24] Quantitative techniques, such as native T1 mapping, T2 mapping, and extracellular volume mapping, have recently emerged as useful tools for confirming (or excluding) myocarditis.[43] Compared with Lake Louise criteria, only T1 mapping had a greater sensitivity, although each technique seems to offer distinct advantages.[44,45] The combination of T1 mapping plus LGE increases the diagnostic accuracy of CMR for myocarditis to 96% (range: 82–97%).[43]

Endomyocardial Biopsy

EMB is still considered the gold standard for the definite diagnosis of myocarditis and may additionally provide prognostic information. EMB is the final step in the diagnostic algorithm in patients with suspected myocarditis in the relevant ESC position statement. According to this algorithm, suspected cases should be hospitalized; coronary artery disease should be excluded (by conventional or computed tomography angiography), and then EMB should be offered.[2] Nevertheless, this practice has not been endorsed by all experts, as EMB is an invasive procedure with potential complications, and myocarditis is a self-limited condition in most cases. In this context, the joint American and European scientific statement on EMB

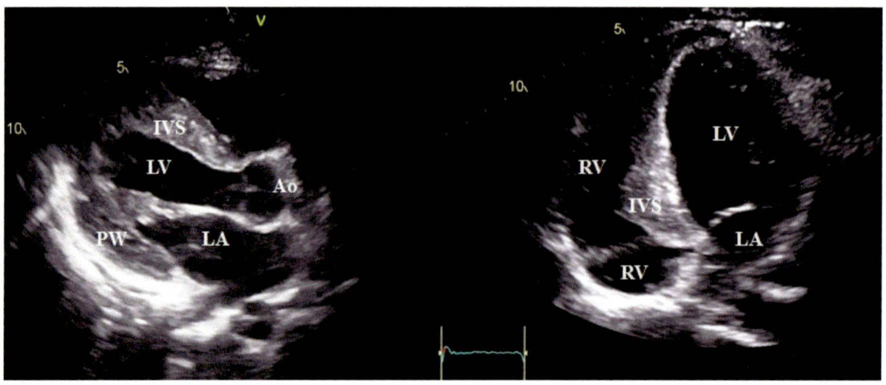

FIGURE 34.2 Increased septal thickness in a patient with acute myocarditis. Septal thickness normalized in the following four weeks. *Abbreviations*: IVS = interventricular septum, Ao = aorta, PW = left ventricular posterior wall, LA = left atrium, RA = right atrium, LV = left ventricle, RV = right ventricle.

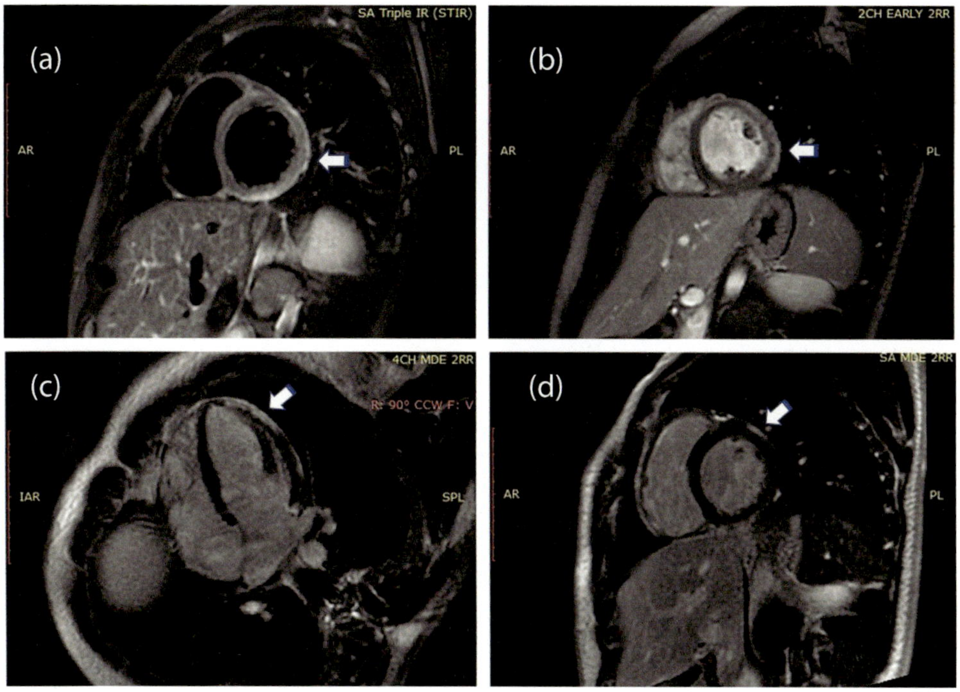

FIGURE 34.3 CMR in a patient with acute viral myocarditis. (a) Short-axis view, T2-weighted short-tau inversion recovery (*STIR*) image, depicting increased signal intensity due to edema in the inferolateral wall (arrow). (b) Early gadolinium enhancement with increased signal intensity in the mid lateral wall secondary to local hyperemia-inflammation (arrow). (c and d) Late gadolinium enhancement in the horizontal long-axis and short- axis views, respectively, showing increased signal in the subepicardial and midmyocardial region of the medial and apical lateral wall (arrows). (Courtesy of Dr. D. Klettas.)

recommends (class I) EMB for patients meeting these two clinical scenarios:[46] (1) new-onset (two weeks or shorter duration) HF with normal-sized or dilated left ventricle and hemodynamic compromise (which corresponds to fulminant myocarditis); or (2) HF of two weeks' to three months' duration, left ventricular dilatation, ventricular arrhythmias, or advanced heart block, unresponsive to conventional care within two weeks. Apart from cases presenting with overt hemodynamic impairment, progressive left or right HF symptoms despite optimal treatment and prolonged troponin release constitute additional indications for EMB.[2]

EMB specimens can be taken from either ventricle, and CMR may be helpful for a targeted biopsy.[2] At least three specimens should be obtained.[2] The complication rate is ~6%, and fatal complications have been observed in <0.5% of EMB cases.[46]

The Dallas histopathologic criteria were the first criteria used for the diagnostic and prognostic evaluation of myocarditis and included a qualitative assessment of the intensity of inflammation and (non-ischemic) necrosis.[47] In the absence of necrosis, myocarditis is considered borderline. The main drawback of the Dallas criteria was the low sensitivity and high inter-observer variability. The use of quantitative immunohistochemical criteria has overcome these limitations, with inflammation defined as ≥14 leucocytes/mm^2.[2,9] Immunochemistry can further distinguish between B cells (CD20+) and T cells (CD3+), as well as various T cell subpopulations.[5] In cases of dilated cardiomyopathy, ongoing inflammation is observed in 30% of EMBs.[48]

EMB may detect viral genomes and quantify viral load and replication by molecular analysis techniques.[2] However, a concurrent systemic viral infection should be excluded by parallel tests in the peripheral blood.[49] Viral persistence in EMB carries important therapeutic and prognostic value. Enterovirus persistence has been linked to increased mortality, whereas parvovirus B19 and human herpes virus 6 non-clearance is of uncertain significance.[5]

EMB is of paramount importance in suspected myocarditis, to reveal the underlying cause. In particular, the identification of certain etiologies, such as sarcoidosis, giant cell myocarditis, and eosinophilic myocarditis has important implications concerning treatment (both in the acute phase and in the long term) and prognosis[2] Cardiac sarcoidosis and rheumatoid arthritis are characterized by granulomas on EMB in the absence of viral genomes.[2] In cardiac sarcoidosis, giant cells may be detected but only within the non-caseous granulomas. The hallmark of giant cell myocarditis is the omnipresence of multinucleated giant cells in association with myocyte necrosis.[2,5,27]

Treatment

The treatment algorithm of acute myocarditis is summarized in Figure 34.4. Treatment strategy should consider several parameters, including etiology and clinical presentation, as well as imaging and EMB findings.

Upon myocarditis diagnosis, exercise restriction is recommended until LVEF recovers and arrhythmias do not occur. Since acute myocarditis resolves in most instances within two to four weeks, a return to everyday activities, always on an individualized basis, seems reasonable after this time period.[2] Participation in competitive sports is allowed after six months following a thorough reevaluation.[2] We summarize below the most appropriate treatment course in the individual patient according to the best available evidence.

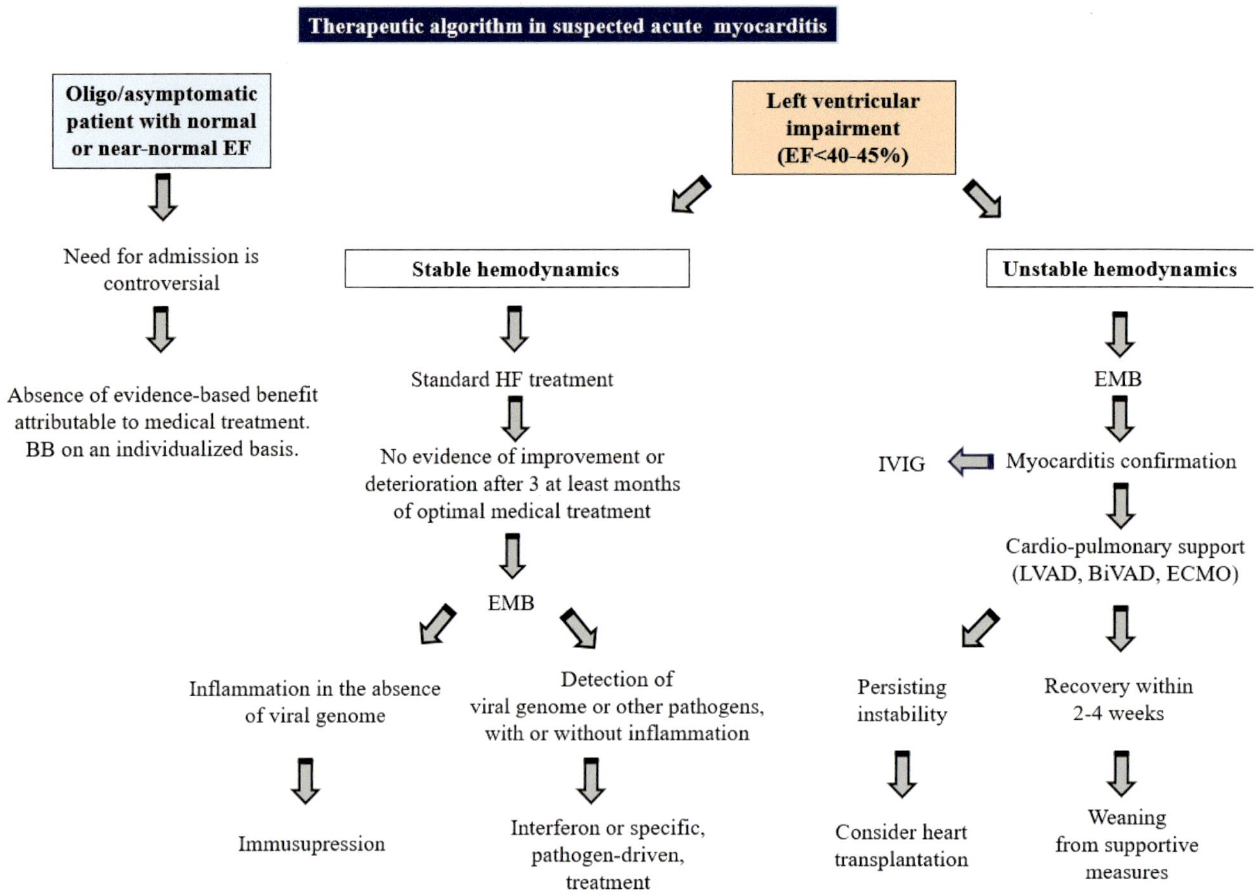

FIGURE 34.4 Proposed treatment algorithm in cases of acute myocarditis. *Abbreviations*: EF = ejection fraction, BB = beta-blockers, HF = heart failure, EMB = endomyocardial biopsy, ECMO = extra-corporeal membrane oxygenation, LVAD = left ventricular assist device, BiVAD = biventricular assist device.

Treatment of Patients with Normal or Near-Normal LVEF

This subgroup of patients is the least explored one, as evidence is scarce and treatment is largely empiric, with only small, non-randomized studies available. In a study of 44 patients with mean LVEF >50%, those receiving beta-blockers (BB) showed significant increases in LVEF at the six-month follow-up, whereas those receiving angiotensin-converting enzyme inhibitors (ACEis) did not.[8,50] In our institutional practice, BB are empirically administered to patients with pronounced sinus tachycardia, or in the presence of arrhythmias.

Treatment of Stable Patients with Impaired LVEF

In patients with reduced LVEF (<50%), treatment should follow HF guidelines.[51] However, most available evidence is an extrapolation from HF studies to patients with myocarditis.

Regarding individual medications in the context of myocarditis, BBs should be used with caution in severely ill patients with marginal hemodynamics, as BBs can precipitate cardiogenic shock. In non-decompensated patients, BBs appear to improve left ventricular function and survival and decrease rehospitalizations.[8] Experimental studies suggest that not all BBs share the same cardioprotective effects, with carvedilol demonstrating a better profile than other BBs, which may exert neutral or even detrimental effects in this context.[8,52]

ACEis and angiotensin II receptor blockers have been associated with reduced inflammatory burden, less necrosis and fibrosis, and reduced oxidative stress, all of which appear to be class effects.[8,14] These effects translate into favorable remodeling and improved LVEF. Most importantly, detrimental effects have not been reported for ACEis.[8,14] In models of viral myocarditis, mineralocorticoid receptor antagonists have been shown to decrease fibrosis and improve survival, reproducing the disease-modifying properties shown in HF.[53]

Concerning other medication classes, digoxin has been shown to increase the release of proinflammatory cytokines in animal studies, with detrimental effects on left ventricular function and mortality.[8,14] Among diuretics, used to relieve congestion, torasemide appears to reduce progression from myocarditis to dilated cardiomyopathy independently of its diuretic properties.[54]

An important question in patients with HF phenotype at presentation is the duration of HF treatment in cases where LVEF and cardiac dimensions are restored or near-normalized at follow-up. In a recent randomized pilot trial in patients who have seemingly recovered from dilated cardiomyopathy, treatment withdrawal was associated with relapse. In this line, until more robust clinical data are available, HF treatment should be offered on a long-term basis (probably indefinitely).[55] Antiarrhythmics should be administered on an individual basis and arrhythmia management should in general follow the guidelines for treatment of ventricular arrhythmias and prevention of sudden death.[56] For primary prevention of sudden cardiac death, an implantable cardioverter defibrillator should be offered to patients with NYHA class ≥2 and LVEF ≤35% after three or more months of optimal medical treatment, provided that life expectancy exceeds one year.[56] In cases deemed to be potentially reversible, LifeVests and temporary pacemakers (e.g., in reversible heart block in Lyme disease) are potential options.[2]

In myocarditis patients presenting with pericardial chest pain with or without effusion (perimyocarditis), NSAIDs should be given at the lowest effective dose and for the shortest possible time period.[2] Corticosteroids may offer an alternative in intolerant patients and those with contraindication to NSAIDs; the role of colchicine is unexplored[2] Of note, pericardial involvement (i.e., pericardial effusion or pericardial LGE) in acute myocarditis seems to be associated with worse prognosis.[57]

Treatment of Hemodynamically Unstable Patients

Cardiogenic shock is considered the most troublesome and fearful complication of acute myocarditis, second only to sudden cardiac death. The proposed management algorithm of these patients is depicted in Figure 34.4. Fulminant and giant cell myocarditis are the most common causes of cardiogenic shock. Patients with hemodynamic instability should be preferentially transferred to and managed in specialized centers with availability of heart catheterization, expertise in EMB, and cardiopulmonary support (extra-corporeal membrane oxygenation and ventricular assist devices). For patients unable to wean from advanced cardiac support, heart transplantation is an option. Although consideration for this option should not be delayed, the threshold should be high, as in some cases (especially fulminant myocarditis), full recovery may be observed.

Apart from supportive measures, data on medical treatment of fulminant myocarditis are sparse and controversial. Various treatment options, including immunosuppressive drugs, intravenous immunoglobulins, and corticosteroids, have been tested but the evidence is too weak to recommend any of these options.[17,58] In contrast, high doses of corticosteroids have proved beneficial in the subset of patients with necrotizing eosinophilic myocarditis.[30,46] Aggressive immunosuppression with two to four drugs (i.e., cyclosporine-based regimens with steroids, azathioprine, and muronomab CD-3 on an individual basis) is the recommended treatment in case of giant cell myocarditis.[4,8] With the combination of hemodynamic support and immunosuppression, clinical remission is achieved in approximately two-thirds of cases with a 42% transplant-free five-year survival.[26,28] Treatment discontinuation may lead to relapses.[8]

Patients with Persistent Symptoms and Left Ventricular Dysfunction

In this difficult-to-treat patient group, EMB findings are of paramount importance to guide immunomodulatory and antiviral therapeutic options. Patients with inflammatory cardiomyopathy, i.e., virus-negative, inflammation-positive patients with persistent HF symptoms and depressed LVEF (<45%), despite optimal treatment for at least six months, are candidates for immunosuppression.[8,14] Increased myocardial HLA expression and presence of circulating anti-heart antibodies further support immunosuppressive treatment.[8] To date, two major placebo-controlled trials (the Myocarditis Treatment Trial and the Tailored Immunosuppression in Inflammatory Cardiomyopathy [TIMIC]) trial have evaluated treatment with prednisolone and azathioprine combinations for six months in this setting.[59,60] The Myocarditis Treatment Trial was neutral,[59] but viral genome search was not performed. In TIMIC, which included viral-negative patients, immunosuppression was beneficial (improved LVEF and left ventricular dimensions).[60] Ongoing trials are expected to provide further data on this topic. In the context of immunomodulatory therapies, immunoadsorption is a procedure aiming at the removal of circulating antibodies. In myocarditis, autoantibodies appear to promote the progression of myocarditis to dilated cardiomyopathy. Initial experience from small studies showed a potential benefit with immunoadsorption; however, its role should be tested in larger studies.[8]

Cardiotropic viral genomes have been identified in up to 70% of patients with chronic dilated cardiomyopathy.[61] A critical question is whether the virus in question is a by-stander or if an active infection is ongoing. A high number of viral copies and evidence of replication indicate active infection and are important clues for the evaluation of virus activity, heralding possibly a higher success rate with antiviral agents, including immunoglobulins.[4] Among antiviral agents, treatment with interferon β-1b for six months in patients with symptomatic HF and EMB-proven enterovirus infection achieved virus clearance and improved NYHA class, quality of life, and patient global assessment.[62] On the other hand, elimination of other viruses, such as parvovirus B19 and human herpes virus 6, was incomplete in the same trial. Immunoglobulins have not been proved to be of benefit in dilated cardiomyopathy, although there are ongoing studies in certain subgroups of patients (including parvovirus myocarditis).[4,14] Preliminary data from specific antiviral treatments (virostatics), such as acyclovir, foscarnet, valaciclovir, or ganciclovir, according to the viral etiology, are encouraging.[63] On the other hand, antiretroviral therapy is the cornerstone of therapy in HIV-infected patients with cardiomyopathy.[35] The specific indications of immunosuppressive and antiviral treatment in myocarditis and/or dilated cardiomyopathy are summarized in Table 34.3.

Specific etiologies of myocarditis require pertinent therapies. Systemic autoimmune disorders (lupus, rheumatoid arthritis) will benefit from steroid or biological treatments. Corticosteroids in cardiac sarcoidosis prevent HF, although benefits have been reported even in advanced heart disease.[4] Most experts recommend a broader use of cardioverter defibrillators for primary prevention of sudden cardiac death in cardiac sarcoidosis.[64] Antiparasitic (benznidazole or nifurtimox) treatment for 60–90 days should be offered in Chagas disease and antibiotics in Lyme disease (oral amoxicillin or doxycycline for 14–21 days in mild-to-moderate disease and intravenous ceftriaxone, cefotaxime, or penicillin G in severe disease for 14 to 28 days).[32,33]

Prognosis

Myocarditis is a multifaceted disease with variable presentation, ranging from asymptomatic forms to forms presenting with sudden death or progressing to dilated cardiomyopathy and HF.[65] Survival among all-comers with acute myocarditis is estimated at 86% at three years and at 57% at five years.[39] In patients who develop dilated cardiomyopathy, five-year survival is <50%.[42] Underlying etiology, clinical features, and genetic factors are important prognostic elements. Of note, acute myocarditis is a self-limited disease in 50–57% of cases within two to four weeks of symptoms onset, which should always be

TABLE 34.3: Indications of Immunosuppressive and Antiviral Treatment in Myocarditis and Dilated Cardiomyopathy

Indications for Immunosuppression (Corticosteroids, Azathioprine, etc.) with One or More Agent, According to Underlying Etiology	• Absence of viral genome in EMB • No contraindications to immunosuppression • Symptomatic patients with dilated inflammatory cardiomyopathy and left ventricular ejection fraction <45% of at least six months' duration despite optimal HF treatment • Immune-mediated myocarditis, including autoimmune conditions (e.g., lupus), giant cell myocarditis, necrotizing eosinophilic myocarditis, sarcoidosis, etc. • Upregulation of HLA in EMB and circulating anti-heart and other organ-specific antibodies
Indications for Antiviral Treatment	• Interferon β-1b potentially beneficial in EMB-proven enteroviral infection and symptomatic HF (viral cardiomyopathy or viral heart disease) • Specific (pathogen-driven) antiviral treatment (virostatics) has shown encouraging results in patients with EMB-proven viral infection • Virus load quantification and determination of active replication should be taken into consideration for treatment decisions in patients with viral cardiomyopathy or viral heart disease
Intravenous Immunoglobulins	• Potentially beneficial in the treatment of fulminant cases along with supportive measures

Abbreviations: EMB = endomyocardial biopsy, HF = heart failure, HLA = human leucocyte antigen.

TABLE 34.4: Variables Associated with Worse Prognosis in Myocarditis

Clinical Presentation	Syncope, advanced NYHA class (either III or IV)
Electrocardiographic	QRS prolongation beyond 120 ms, presence of Q waves
Echocardiographic	Impaired left ventricular ejection fraction (<45%), biventricular involvement, elevated left ventricular filling pressures, pulmonary hypertension, pericardial involvement
CMR	Extension and septal localization of LGE, especially if persisting in follow-up studies, pericardial LGE
EMB	Intensity of necrosis and type of inflammation, giant cell myocarditis, necrotizing eosinophilic myocarditis, sarcoidosis, viral persistence in certain etiologies (e.g., enteroviral)
Others	Male sex (probably due to enhanced fibrotic response), virulence of offending virus, genetic substrate of the host

Abbreviations: CMR = cardiac magnetic resonance imaging, EMB = endomyocardial biopsy, LGE = late gadolinium enhancement, NYHA = New York Heart Association.

considered when planning treatment.[2,39] Partial recovery may be observed in approximately 25% of cases, whereas, in the remainder (~12–25%), left ventricular function may progressively deteriorate, leading to chronic dilated cardiomyopathy and HF.[2] In a recent Italian registry, low LVEF, low cardiac output, and complex ventricular arrhythmias conferred a high risk of serious adverse events, although risk was negligible in the absence of these features.[66] Patients presenting with prominent left ventricular dysfunction (EF <35% and end-diastolic dimension >6 cm) will recover spontaneously in 25% of cases, whereas the remainder will progress to either permanent left ventricular dysfunction (50%) or advanced HF and death.[42] In addition, pericardial involvement, either as pericardial effusion or pericardial LGE, and anteroseptal LGE, have recently emerged as independent prognostic factors.[57] Nevertheless, LVEF appears to be the most powerful prognostic factor on CMR.[67]

Even patients with an initially benign clinical course should be followed-up for at least two to three years, as cases with late clinical worsening have been occasionally recorded.[39,68] In addition, myocarditis may recur in approximately 10% of cases, even several years after the index episode, especially in genetically predisposed patients.[2,69,70] The most important prognostic factors are shown in Table 34.4.

Participation in sports after acute myocarditis is a challenging issue. Exercise restriction should be recommended to all patients for three to six months, a time which is considered sufficient for disease resolution. Return to full activities (including competitive sports) is allowed afterward, provided that LVEF is restored, and arrhythmias have not been detected with Holter monitoring and stress testing.[68] However, athletes with persisting LGE (and in particular those with septal enhancement, which may be linked to poor prognosis independently of LVEF) should remain under annual clinical surveillance.[68,71]

References

1. Caforio ALP, Adler Y, Agostini C, et al. Diagnosis and management of myocardial involvement in systemic immune-mediated diseases: a position statement of the European Society of Cardiology Working Group on Myocardial and Pericardial Disease. *Eur Heart J*. 2017;38(35):2649–62.
2. Caforio AL, Pankuweit S, Arbustini E, et al. Current state of knowledge on aetiology, diagnosis, management, and therapy of myocarditis: a position statement of the European Society of Cardiology Working Group on Myocardial and Pericardial Diseases. *Eur Heart J*. 2013;34(33):2636–48, 2648a–d.
3. Pinto YM, Elliott PM, Arbustini E, et al. Proposal for a revised definition of dilated cardiomyopathy, hypokinetic non-dilated cardiomyopathy, and its implications for clinical practice: a position statement of the ESC working group on myocardial and pericardial diseases. *Eur Heart J*. 2016;37(23):1850–8.
4. Heymans S, Eriksson U, Lehtonen J, Cooper LT, Jr. The quest for new approaches in myocarditis and inflammatory cardiomyopathy. *J Am Coll Cardiol*. 2016;68(21):2348–64.
5. Dominguez F, Kuhl U, Pieske B, Garcia-Pavia P, Tschope C. Update on myocarditis and inflammatory cardiomyopathy: reemergence of endomyocardial biopsy. *Rev Esp Cardiol (Engl Ed)*. 2016;69(2):178–87.
6. Adler Y, Charron P, Imazio M, et al. 2015 ESC guidelines for the diagnosis and management of pericardial diseases: the task force for the diagnosis and management of pericardial diseases of the European Society of Cardiology (ESC)Endorsed by: The European Association for Cardio-Thoracic Surgery (EACTS). *Eur Heart J*. 2015;36(42):2921–64.
7. Matoba R, Shikata I, Iwai K, et al. An epidemiologic and histopathological study of sudden cardiac death in Osaka Medical Examiner's Office. *Jpn Circ J*. 1989;53(12):1581–8.
8. Lazaros G, Oikonomou E, Tousoulis D. Established and novel treatment options in acute myocarditis, with or without heart failure. *Expert Rev Cardiovasc Ther*. 2017;15(1):25–34.
9. Schultheiss HP, Kuhl U, Cooper LT. The management of myocarditis. *Eur Heart J*. 2011;32(21):2616–25.
10. Kuhl U, Pauschinger M, Noutsias M, et al. High prevalence of viral genomes and multiple viral infections in the myocardium of adults with "idiopathic" left ventricular dysfunction. *Circulation*. 2005;111(7):887–93.
11. Nikolaou M, Lazaros G, Karavidas A, Hatzianastasiou S, Miliopoulos D, Adamopoulos S. Recurrent viral myocarditis: the emerging link toward dilated cardiomyopathy. *Hellenic J Cardiol*. 2018;59(1):60–3.

12. Bock CT, Klingel K, Kandolf R. Human parvovirus B19-associated myocarditis. *N Engl J Med.* 2010;362(13):1248–9.
13. Mahrholdt H, Wagner A, Deluigi CC, et al. Presentation, patterns of myocardial damage, and clinical course of viral myocarditis. *Circulation.* 2006;114(15):1581–90.
14. Kindermann I, Barth C, Mahfoud F, et al. Update on myocarditis. *J Am Coll Cardiol.* 2012;59(9):779–92.
15. Cooper LT, Jr. Myocarditis. *N Engl J Med.* 2009;360(15):1526–38.
16. Noutsias M, Fechner H, de Jonge H, et al. Human coxsackie-adenovirus receptor is colocalized with integrins alpha(v)beta(3) and alpha(v)beta(5) on the cardiomyocyte sarcolemma and upregulated in dilated cardiomyopathy: implications for cardiotropic viral infections. *Circulation.* 2001;104(3):275–80.
17. McCarthy RE, 3rd, Boehmer JP, Hruban RH, et al. Long-term outcome of fulminant myocarditis as compared with acute (nonfulminant) myocarditis. *N Engl J Med.* 2000;342(10):690–5.
18. Li Y, Heuser JS, Cunningham LC, Kosanke SD, Cunningham MW. Mimicry and antibody-mediated cell signaling in autoimmune myocarditis. *J Immunol.* 2006;177(11):8234–40.
19. Liu PP, Mason JW. Advances in the understanding of myocarditis. *Circulation.* 2001;104(9):1076–82.
20. Badorff C, Lee GH, Lamphear BJ, et al. Enteroviral protease 2A cleaves dystrophin: evidence of cytoskeletal disruption in an acquired cardiomyopathy. *Nat Med.* 1999;5(3):320–6.
21. Stewart GC, Lopez-Molina J, Gottumukkala RV, et al. Myocardial parvovirus B19 persistence: lack of association with clinicopathologic phenotype in adults with heart failure. *Circ Heart Fail.* 2011;4(1):71–8.
22. Maron BJ, Udelson JE, Bonow RO, et al. Eligibility and disqualification recommendations for competitive athletes with cardiovascular abnormalities: Task Force 3: hypertrophic cardiomyopathy, arrhythmogenic right ventricular cardiomyopathy and other cardiomyopathies, and myocarditis: a scientific statement from the American Heart Association and American College of Cardiology. *J Am Coll Cardiol.* 2015;66(21):2362–71.
23. Mahfoud F, Gartner B, Kindermann M, et al. Virus serology in patients with suspected myocarditis: utility or futility? *Eur Heart J.* 2011;32(7):897–903.
24. Friedrich MG, Sechtem U, Schulz-Menger J, et al. Cardiovascular magnetic resonance in myocarditis: A JACC white paper. *J Am Coll Cardiol.* 2009;53(17):1475–87.
25. Cooper LT, Jr., Berry GJ, Shabetai R. Idiopathic giant-cell myocarditis--natural history and treatment. Multicenter Giant Cell Myocarditis Study Group Investigators. *N Engl J Med.* 1997;336(26):1860–6.
26. Cooper LT, Jr., Hare JM, Tazelaar HD, et al. Usefulness of immunosuppression for giant cell myocarditis. *Am J Cardiol.* 2008;102(11):1535–9.
27. Kandolin R, Lehtonen J, Salmenkivi K, Raisanen-Sokolowski A, Lommi J, Kupari M. Diagnosis, treatment, and outcome of giant-cell myocarditis in the era of combined immunosuppression. *Circ Heart Fail.* 2013;6(1):15–22.
28. Ekstrom K, Lehtonen J, Kandolin R, Raisanen-Sokolowski A, Salmenkivi K, Kupari M. Long-term outcome and its predictors in giant cell myocarditis. *Eur J Heart Fail.* 2016;18(12):1452–8.
29. Kyto V, Saukko P, Lignitz E, et al. Diagnosis and presentation of fatal myocarditis. *Hum Pathol.* 2005;36(9):1003–7.
30. Callan PD, Baltabaeva A, Kamal M, et al. Acute fulminant necrotizing eosinophilic myocarditis: early diagnosis and treatment. *ESC Heart Fail.* 2017;4(4):660–4.
31. Hamzeh N, Steckman DA, Sauer WH, Judson MA. Pathophysiology and clinical management of cardiac sarcoidosis. *Nat Rev Cardiol.* 2015;12(5):278–88.
32. Kostic T, Momcilovic S, Perisic ZD, et al. Manifestations of Lyme carditis. *Int J Cardiol.* 2017;232:24–32.
33. Perez-Molina JA, Molina I. Chagas disease. *Lancet.* 2018;391(10115):82–94.
34. Anderson DW, Virmani R, Reilly JM, et al. Prevalent myocarditis at necropsy in the acquired immunodeficiency syndrome. *J Am Coll Cardiol.* 1988;11(4):792–9.
35. Savvoulidis P, Butler J, Kalogeropoulos A. Cardiomyopathy and heart failure in patients with HIV infection. *Can J Cardiol.* 2019;35(3):299–309.
36. Thienemann F, Sliwa K, Rockstroh JK. HIV and the heart: the impact of antiretroviral therapy: a global perspective. *Eur Heart J.* 2013;34(46):3538–46.
37. Sagar S, Liu PP, Cooper LT, Jr. Myocarditis. *Lancet.* 2012;379(9817):738–47.
38. Jensen J, Ma LP, Fu ML, Svaninger D, Lundberg PA, Hammarsten O. Inflammation increases NT-proBNP and the NT-proBNP/BNP ratio. *Clin Res Cardiol.* 2010;99(7):445–52.
39. Dennert R, Crijns HJ, Heymans S. Acute viral myocarditis. *Eur Heart J.* 2008;29(17):2073–82.
40. Corsten MF, Papageorgiou A, Verhesen W, et al. MicroRNA profiling identifies microRNA-155 as an adverse mediator of cardiac injury and dysfunction during acute viral myocarditis. *Circ Res.* 2012;111(4):415–25.
41. Ukena C, Mahfoud F, Kindermann I, Kandolf R, Kindermann M, Bohm M. Prognostic electrocardiographic parameters in patients with suspected myocarditis. *Eur J Heart Fail.* 2011;13(4):398–405.
42. Magnani JW, Dec GW. Myocarditis: current trends in diagnosis and treatment. *Circulation.* 2006;113(6):876–90.
43. Ferreira VM, Schulz-Menger J, Holmvang G, et al. Cardiovascular magnetic resonance in nonischemic myocardial inflammation: expert recommendations. *J Am Coll Cardiol.* 2018;72(24):3158–76.
44. Lurz P, Luecke C, Eitel I, et al. Comprehensive cardiac magnetic resonance imaging in patients with suspected myocarditis: the MyoRacer-trial. *J Am Coll Cardiol.* 2016;67(15):1800–11.
45. Pan JA, Lee YJ, Salerno M. Diagnostic performance of extracellular volume, native T1, and T2 mapping versus lake louise criteria by cardiac magnetic resonance for detection of acute myocarditis: a meta-analysis. *Circ Cardiovasc Imaging.* 2018;11(7):e007598.
46. Cooper LT, Baughman KL, Feldman AM, et al. The role of endomyocardial biopsy in the management of cardiovascular disease: a scientific statement from the American Heart Association, the American College of Cardiology, and the European Society of Cardiology. Endorsed by the Heart Failure Society of America and the Heart Failure Association of the European Society of Cardiology. *J Am Coll Cardiol.* 2007;50(19):1914–31.
47. Aretz HT. Myocarditis: the Dallas criteria. *Hum Pathol.* 1987;18(6):619–24.
48. Kuhl U, Schultheiss HP. Myocarditis: early biopsy allows for tailored regenerative treatment. *Dtsch Arztebl Int.* 2012;109(20):361–8.
49. Maisch B. Cardio-immunology of myocarditis: focus on immune mechanisms and treatment options. *Front Cardiovasc Med.* 2019;6:48.
50. Abstracts of the 17th Annual SCMR Scientific Sessions, 16–19 January 2014 New Orleans, LA, USA. *J Cardiovasc Magn Reson.* 2014;16(Suppl 1):M1-o8.
51. Ponikowski P, Voors AA, Anker SD, et al. 2016 ESC guidelines for the diagnosis and treatment of acute and chronic heart failure: the task force for the diagnosis and treatment of acute and chronic heart failure of the European Society of Cardiology (ESC)Developed with the special contribution of the Heart Failure Association (HFA) of the ESC. *Eur Heart J.* 2016;37(27):2129–200.
52. Yuan Z, Shioji K, Kihara Y, Takenaka H, Onozawa Y, Kishimoto C. Cardioprotective effects of carvedilol on acute autoimmune myocarditis: anti-inflammatory effects associated with antioxidant property. *Am J Physiol Heart Circ Physiol.* 2004;286(1):H83–90.
53. Xiao J, Shimada M, Liu W, Hu D, Matsumori A. Anti-inflammatory effects of eplerenone on viral myocarditis. *Eur J Heart Fail.* 2009;11(4):349–53.
54. Veeraveedu PT, Watanabe K, Ma M, et al. Torasemide, a long-acting loop diuretic, reduces the progression of myocarditis to dilated cardiomyopathy. *Eur J Pharmacol.* 2008;581(1–2):121–31.
55. Halliday BP, Wassall R, Lota AS, et al. Withdrawal of pharmacological treatment for heart failure in patients with recovered dilated cardiomyopathy (TRED-HF): an open-label, pilot, randomised trial. *Lancet.* 2019;393(10166):61–73.
56. Priori SG, Blomstrom-Lundqvist C, Mazzanti A, et al. 2015 ESC guidelines for the management of patients with ventricular arrhythmias and the prevention of sudden cardiac death: the task force for the management of patients with ventricular arrhythmias and the prevention of sudden cardiac death of the European Society of Cardiology (ESC). Endorsed by: Association for European Paediatric and Congenital Cardiology (AEPC). *Eur Heart J.* 2015;36(41):2793–867.
57. Di Bella G, Imazio M, Bogaert J, et al. Clinical value and prognostic impact of pericardial involvement in acute myocarditis. *Circ Cardiovasc Imaging.* 2019;12(2):e008504.
58. Gupta S, Markham DW, Drazner MH, Mammen PP. Fulminant myocarditis. *Nat Clin Pract Cardiovasc Med.* 2008;5(11):693–706.
59. Mason JW, O'Connell JB, Herskowitz A, et al. A clinical trial of immunosuppressive therapy for myocarditis. The myocarditis treatment trial investigators. *N Engl J Med.* 1995;333(5):269–75.
60. Frustaci A, Russo MA, Chimenti C. Randomized study on the efficacy of immunosuppressive therapy in patients with virus-negative inflammatory cardiomyopathy: the TIMIC study. *Eur Heart J.* 2009;30(16):1995–2002.
61. Hazebroek MR, Moors S, Dennert R, et al. Prognostic relevance of gene-environment interactions in patients with dilated cardiomyopathy: applying the MOGE(S) classification. *J Am Coll Cardiol.* 2015;66(12):1313–23.
62. Schultheiss HP, Piper C, Sowade O, et al. Betaferon in chronic viral cardiomyopathy (BICC) trial: effects of interferon-beta treatment in patients with chronic viral cardiomyopathy. *Clin Res Cardiol.* 2016;105(9):763–73.
63. Gkouziouta A, Lazaros G, Karavidas A, et al. Pathogen-driven treatment strategy in new onset dilated cardiomyopathy. Impact on ventricular function and clinical outcome. *Int J Cardiol.* 2016;209:15–16.

64. Birnie DH, Sauer WH, Bogun F, et al. HRS expert consensus statement on the diagnosis and management of arrhythmias associated with cardiac sarcoidosis. *Heart Rhythm.* 2014;11(7):1305–23.
65. Elliott P, Andersson B, Arbustini E, et al. Classification of the cardiomyopathies: a position statement from the European Society of Cardiology Working Group on Myocardial and Pericardial Diseases. *Eur Heart J.* 2008;29(2):270–6.
66. Ammirati E, Cipriani M, Moro C, et al. Clinical presentation and outcome in a contemporary cohort of patients with acute myocarditis. *Circulation.* 2018;138(11):1088–99.
67. Imazio M, Angelico G, Andriani M, et al. Prevalence and prognostic impact of septal late gadolinium enhancement in acute myocarditis with or without preserved left ventricular function. *Am J Cardiol.* 2018;122(11):1955–8.
68. Pelliccia A, Solberg EE, Papadakis M, et al. Recommendations for participation in competitive and leisure time sport in athletes with cardiomyopathies, myocarditis, and pericarditis: position statement of the Sport Cardiology Section of the European Association of Preventive Cardiology (EAPC). *Eur Heart J.* 2019;40(1):19–33.
69. Karavidas A, Lazaros G, Noutsias M, et al. Recurrent coxsackie B viral myocarditis leading to progressive impairment of left ventricular function over 8 years. *Int J Cardiol.* 2011;151(2):e65–67.
70. Kyto V, Sipila J, Rautava P. Rate and patient features associated with recurrence of acute myocarditis. *Eur J Intern Med.* 2014;25(10):946–50.
71. Aquaro GD, Perfetti M, Camastra G, et al. Cardiac MR with late gadolinium enhancement in acute myocarditis with preserved systolic function: ITAMY study. *J Am Coll Cardiol.* 2017;70(16):1977–87.

Chapter 35
INFILTRATIVE DISEASES
Amyloid

Melissa Lyle and Kunal Bhatt

Overview

Amyloidosis is a systemic disorder that results from the extracellular deposition of amyloid fibrils, insoluble structures comprised of misfolded proteins that self-assemble into aggregates of ß-pleated sheets. Amyloid fibrils can deposit in the heart, kidneys, liver, peripheral nerves, gastrointestinal tract, and other soft tissues. Amyloid nomenclature designates the amyloid fibril protein as protein A, followed by the abbreviated form of the precursor protein. For example, when amyloid fibrils are derived from immunoglobulin light chains the specific amyloid fibril protein is referred to as AL and the disease is AL amyloidosis.[1]

There are more than thirty amyloidogenic proteins, and the two proteins that most frequently infiltrate the heart are immunoglobulin light chains (AL) and transthyretin (ATTR).[2] At least eleven other proteins can misfold into amyloid fibrils that infiltrate the myocardium, including serum amyloid A (AA) protein, ß2-microglobulin (Aß2M), gelsolin (AGel), fibrinogen (AFib), and apolipoprotein A1 (AApoA1).[3] However, AL and ATTR amyloidosis remain the most common forms associated with cardiac manifestations and will be the focus of this chapter.

Epidemiology

Light chain (AL) amyloidosis remains rare, with an incidence of 10 cases per million individuals.[4] Transthyretin (ATTR) amyloidosis, however, is not rare, but often unrecognized. Transthyretin amyloid cardiomyopathy (ATTR-CM) is increasingly found to be a cause of heart failure (HF). ATTR amyloidosis can be hereditary, secondary to an inherited mutation (hATTR), or wild type (wtATTR), the latter often thought to be age related. Among autopsy studies of patients over age 75 with HF and preserved ejection fraction (HFpEF), 32% had amyloid deposits, highlighting the role of wtATTR in the pathophysiology of HFpEF.[5]

Clinical Assessment

Cardiac Manifestations

Cardiac amyloidosis specifically occurs when amyloid fibrils infiltrate the myocardium, and this extracellular deposition results in a restrictive cardiomyopathy. There are many mimickers of cardiac amyloidosis, including hypertrophic cardiomyopathy, hypertensive heart disease, athlete's heart, and lysosomal storage disorders. However, cardiac amyloidosis should be considered in the context of unexplained left ventricular hypertrophy.

The characteristic appearance of cardiac amyloidosis is increased biventricular wall thickness and severe diastolic dysfunction. Common symptoms associated with cardiac amyloidosis include fatigue and dyspnea, along with other non-specific findings of HF. Physical examination findings are often consistent with right-sided HF, including elevated jugular venous distention, abdominal ascites, and lower extremity edema.

Laboratory Evaluation

There is no specific laboratory test for cardiac amyloidosis, although serum free light chains and serum protein electrophoresis with immunofixation play a key role in the diagnosis of AL amyloidosis. Cardiac biomarkers, including N-terminal-pro brain natriuretic peptide (NT-proBNP) and troponin are frequently elevated in cardiac amyloidosis. Both NT-proBNP and troponin are prognostic markers included in various staging systems. The revised Mayo Clinic staging system for AL amyloid includes serum free light chains, troponin-T, and NT-proBNP,[6] and cardiac biomarkers are also utilized in the Mayo Clinic staging system for wtATTR amyloidosis.[7] Laboratory evaluation could also reveal abnormal liver function tests or elevated creatinine, depending on renal and liver involvement.

The serum concentration of transthyretin, previously called prealbumin, is typically within the range of 18–45 mg/dL, but can be affected by age, nutritional status, or increased inflammation. Previous studies have demonstrated that patients with wtATTR have lower serum transthyretin levels, with lower levels correlating with worse survival. Increasing transthyretin concentrations have also been documented with the use of the transthyretin stabilizer diflunisal, suggesting that serum transthyretin could be a potential marker for stabilization in addition to being a prognostic tool.[8]

Electrocardiography

As part of the initial clinical assessment for cardiac amyloidosis, an electrocardiogram (ECG) is usually performed. The amyloid fibril deposition in the myocardium will result in discrepancy between the QRS voltage on electrocardiography and the left ventricular hypertrophy visualized by echocardiography or magnetic resonance imaging, a low voltage-to-mass ratio.[9] Although low QRS voltage is often described as a classic finding in cardiac amyloidosis, it is not always present. Only 25–40% of ATTR-CM patients meet low voltage criteria,[10] whereas low QRS voltage may be seen in up to 60% of patients with AL amyloidosis.[11] A "pseudoinfarct pattern" with Q waves in two consecutive limb leads without prior myocardial infarction is another ECG finding in amyloidosis.

Both atrial and ventricular arrhythmias occur in cardiac amyloidosis. Amyloid fibrils can infiltrate the atria, resulting commonly in atrial arrhythmias such as atrial fibrillation and atrial flutter. The Transthyretin Amyloidosis Outcome Survey (THAOS), a global multicenter longitudinal registry of patients with ATTR amyloidosis, demonstrated that the prevalence of atrial fibrillation was 62.8% in wtATTR and 51.9% in hATTR, specifically with the Val122Ile mutation.[12] Bradyarrhythmias and progressive conduction abnormalities are also common

DOI: 10.1201/9780429244544-42

in cardiac amyloidosis. Permanent pacemaker implantation is needed in ~25% of patients with Val30Met hATTR, in 36% of Val122Ile ATTR patients, and in 43% of wtATTR patients, for conduction abnormalities or symptomatic bradycardia.[13]

Cardiac Imaging

Transthoracic echocardiography is one of the first diagnostic imaging tools in the evaluation of known or suspected cardiac amyloidosis (Table 35.1). However, it is important to note that the type of cardiac amyloidosis cannot be differentiated by echocardiography. Echocardiography typically illustrates biventricular wall thickness, usually with an interventricular wall thickness >12 mm being a diagnostic threshold, in addition to a thickened interatrial septum, atrioventricular valve thickening, bi-atrial enlargement, a "speckled" appearance of the myocardium, diastolic dysfunction, and often a small pericardial effusion (Figure 35.1). Global longitudinal strain (GLS) is often reduced with evidence of apical sparing, often referred to as the "cherry on top," given the bull's-eye plot of global longitudinal strain (Figure 35.1). The relative regional strain ratio (RRSR) is defined as the average apical longitudinal strain divided by the sum of the average mid and basal longitudinal strain, and a high RRSR is adversely prognostic in patients with cardiac amyloid[14] The biventricular wall thickness and reduction in contractility results in reduced stroke volume, and the stroke volume index is another independent echocardiographic prognostic marker, particularly in AL amyloidosis.[15]

Cardiac magnetic resonance imaging (MRI) can also be helpful for the diagnosis of cardiac amyloidosis. Non-specific findings include increased biventricular wall mass in addition to the more specific findings of diffuse non-ischemic pattern of late gadolinium enhancement and abnormal nulling of the myocardium.[16] Cardiac amyloidosis is associated with global subendocardial late gadolinium enhancement (LGE) in a non-coronary artery distribution pattern. Increased signal on native T1 mapping detects cardiac amyloidosis and is considered an early disease tracker.[17] Increased extracellular volume (ECV), a measurement of interstitial expansion, is elevated in cardiac amyloidosis secondary to interstitial amyloid deposition and another finding that aids in diagnosis.[18] Cardiac MRI helps to raise suspicion for the diagnosis of cardiac amyloidosis and even monitor disease progression; however, similar to echocardiography, MRI is unable to differentiate between AL and ATTR cardiac amyloidosis.

Nuclear bone scintigraphy using technetium-labeled bone radiotracer, either ^{99m}technetium pyrophosphate (PYP) in the United States or ^{99m}technetium 3,3-diphosphono-1,2-propanodicarboxylic acid in Europe, has been used to diagnose cardiac ATTR deposits (Figure 35.2). The affinity of TTR amyloid fibrils for these bone radiotracers is thought to be calcium related, but the exact mechanism remains unknown. Single-photon emission computed tomography (SPECT) can be utilized to ensure that the uptake is truly cardiac. A semi-quantitative score comparing cardiac tracer uptake to bone uptake of the rib is used with a range from grade 0, representing no uptake, to grade 3 demonstrating that cardiac uptake exceeds rib uptake. A quantitative heart-to-contralateral (H/CL) ratio exhibits high diagnostic accuracy for differentiating ATTR from AL when the ratio exceeds 1.5.[19] Grade 2 or 3 tracer uptake is associated with 100% specificity for ATTR-CM when performed in the absence of a monoclonal protein.[20] The caveat that nuclear scintigraphy is only interpretable in the absence of a monoclonal protein is important given that 27% of patients with AL amyloidosis actually had positive PYP scans.[20] Therefore, serum free light chains and serum and urine protein electrophoresis with immunofixation should always be obtained prior to nuclear scintigraphy. Even in the presence of grade 2 or 3 radiotracer uptake, if a concomitant monoclonal

TABLE 35.1: Imaging/Diagnostic Criteria for Cardiac Amyloid

Electrocardiographic Findings	Echocardiography	Cardiac MRI	Nuclear PYP
• Low voltage • Discordance between imaging findings and LVH on ECG • Pseudoinfarct pattern	• Biventricular wall thickening • Interatrial septal thickening • Valvular thickening • Diastolic dysfunction • Apical sparing on strain imaging	• Increased biventricular wall mass • Diffuse delayed gadolinium enhancement and abnormal nulling of myocardium • Increased signal on T1 mapping • Increased extracellular volume	• Quantitative heart-to-contralateral ratio exceeding 1.5

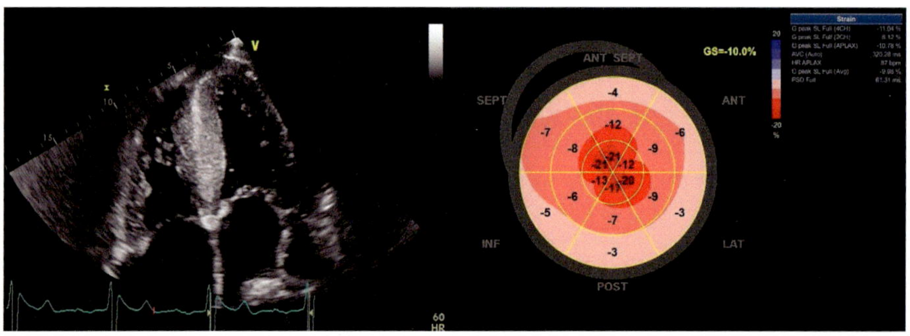

FIGURE 35.1 Four-chamber view of the heart by transthoracic echocardiography (left) illustrates biventricular wall thickening, with prominent thickening of the interventricular septum, and a "speckled" appearance of the myocardium. Bull's eye plot of global longitudinal strain (right) from the three apical left ventricular views demonstrates globally reduced strain with apical sparing ("cherry on top").

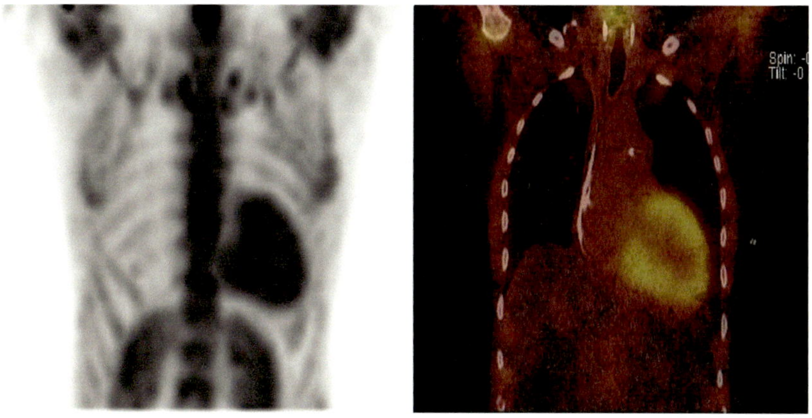

FIGURE 35.2 Planar and single-photon emission computerized tomography (SPECT) images with technetium-99m pyrophosphate (PYP) showing Perugini grade 3 uptake at three hours.

protein or abnormal free light chains ratio is present, an endomyocardial biopsy (EMB), in conjunction with a hematology consultation, may be warranted.

Endomyocardial Biopsy (EMB)

Tissue biopsy to illustrate amyloid deposits is necessary for the diagnosis of AL amyloid. EMB remains the gold standard for cardiac amyloidosis and is still utilized for ATTR-CM when nuclear scintigraphy cannot be interpreted. The ß-pleated sheet configuration of amyloid fibrils is clearly visualized by electron microscopy. Under light microscopy, when Congo red staining is utilized, amyloid deposits appear pink, whereas, under polarized light, they have a classic apple-green birefringence appearance.[21] Once Congo red-positive deposits are demonstrated and confirm the diagnosis of amyloidosis, it is vital to subtype the amyloid deposits either by immunohistochemistry or mass spectrometry. However, mass spectrometry-based proteomic analysis is currently the gold standard for fibril typing.[22]

Medical Management

In cardiac amyloidosis, both AL and ATTR, it is important to maintain euvolemia, therefore loop diuretics and aldosterone antagonists are frequently used in addition to salt restriction, but caution is needed to avoid hypotension. Most patients with cardiac amyloidosis cannot tolerate guideline-directed medical therapy, given hypotension, autonomic dysfunction, and low stroke volume; therefore, beta-blockers and vasodilators are not routinely recommended. Previously digoxin was considered to be contraindicated in AL amyloidosis, out of concerns that amyloid fibrils bind to digoxin with high affinity.[23] However, more recent studies demonstrated that digoxin for rate control in atrial fibrillation can be used cautiously in appropriately selected patients.[24] There is also potentially increased binding of calcium channel blockers (CCBs) to amyloid fibrils, increasing their effect. Therefore, non-dihydropyridine CCBs (diltiazem and verapamil) are not recommended in cardiac amyloidosis.

Patients with cardiac amyloidosis are at high risk of thromboembolism. El-Am et al. showed that patients with cardiac amyloidosis had a high cancellation rate of direct current cardioversion compared with controls, due to the presence of intracardiac thrombus despite appropriate anticoagulation. Given these findings, a transesophageal echocardiogram is recommended prior to cardioversion despite anticoagulation.[25] In a large autopsy study of patients with cardiac amyloidosis, 33% had an intracardiac thrombus identified, with AL amyloidosis being an independent risk factor for thromboembolism. Atrial thrombosis also occurred in normal sinus rhythm, most likely secondary to atrial mechanical dissociation.[26] Therefore, the decision for anticoagulation should be based on clinical context instead of just CHA2DS2-VASc score.

Diagnostic Approach

Although cardiac amyloidosis is increasingly recognized as a cause of HF, it is still under-diagnosed and often missed by internists and cardiologists. A survey of 533 patients with AL amyloidosis revealed that often the diagnosis was not established until one year or more after the onset of symptoms, and cardiologists made the correct diagnosis only 19% of the time.[27] It is important to be systematic in the diagnostic approach and have a high index of clinical suspicion, particularly with increased left ventricular wall thickness in the absence of a history of hypertension or in the setting of HF (Figure 35.3). Other clinical clues include discordance between left ventricular wall thickness and voltage on electrocardiography, elevated troponin in the absence of obstructive coronary disease, and extracardiac features, such as carpal tunnel syndrome or polyneuropathy (Table 35.2).

Once there is considerable suspicion of cardiac amyloidosis, laboratory evaluation is the first step of the diagnostic approach. Serum free light chains and serum and urine immunofixation must be obtained to rule out AL amyloidosis, given that this is a medical emergency. Troponin and NT-proBNP levels can also be obtained for staging purposes. If there is evidence of a monoclonal protein, a referral to hematology is necessary. The diagnosis of AL amyloidosis requires either a fat pad biopsy or a biopsy of a clinically involved organ. If there is no evidence of a monoclonal protein, nuclear scintigraphy can be used to screen for ATTR cardiac amyloidosis. If nuclear scintigraphy is positive, transthyretin gene sequencing must be obtained to differentiate between hATTR and wtATTR (Figure 35.3).

AL Amyloidosis

AL amyloidosis is secondary to extracellular deposition of immunoglobin light chains and is a clonal, non-proliferative plasma cell dyscrasia. These light chains can form amyloid fibrils that infiltrate the heart, in addition to a variety of other organs. Although AL amyloidosis can result in a restrictive

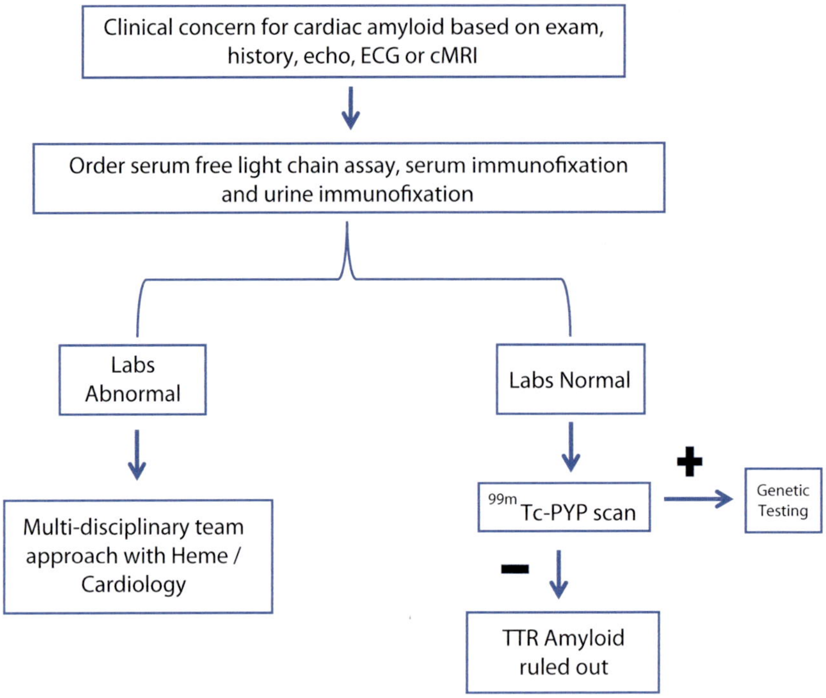

FIGURE 35.3 Diagnostic algorithm for transthyretin (TTR) cardiac amyloidosis.

TABLE 35.2: Clinical Features of Cardiac Amyloid and Red Flags

Clinical Features	Red Flags
Elevated jugular venous pressure	Elderly patients with heart failure with reduced ejection fraction (HFpEF)
Hepatomegaly	Elderly HFpEF patients with low flow-low gradient aortic stenosis
Ascites	New diagnosis of hypertrophic cardiomyopathy (HCM) after age 60
Peripheral edema	HFpEF patients with concomitant findings including:
Bilateral carpal tunnel syndrome	• Bilateral carpal tunnel syndrome
Spinal stenosis	• Spinal stenosis
Peripheral neuropathy of unclear etiology	• Spontaneous biceps tendon rupture "Popeye muscle"
Autonomic dysfunction	• Unexplained neuropathy
Spontaneous biceps tendon rupture	• Nephrotic range proteinuria
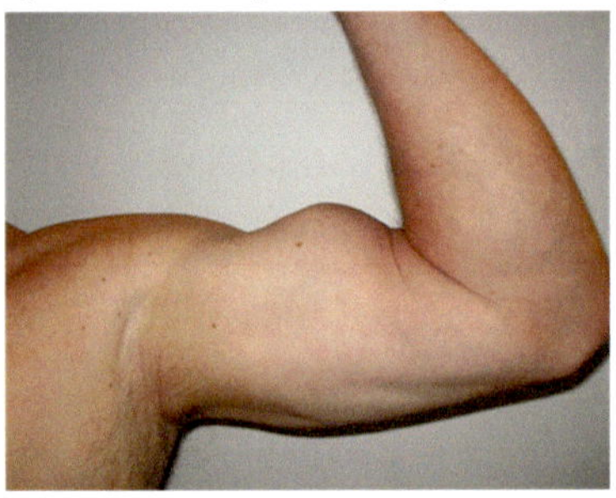	• Macroglossia/periorbital purpura • Orthostatic hypotension

cardiomyopathy, AL cardiac amyloidosis is also considered a "toxic-infiltrative cardiomyopathy,"[28] given that circulating light chains are directly toxic to cardiomyocytes, independent of fibril deposition. Light chains induce p38 mitogen-activated protein kinase (MAPK), eventually leading to oxidative stress, cellular dysfunction, and apoptosis.[29] Because of the direct cellular toxicity, there is a focus on lowering the amount of circulating pathologic light chains during therapeutic interventions.

Diagnosis

Cardiac AL amyloidosis may be considered if there is evidence of increased left ventricular wall thickness or diastolic dysfunction in addition to other organ findings, such as macroglossia, nephrotic syndrome, or gastrointestinal symptoms. Initial evaluation should include serum free light chains, serum protein electrophoresis with immunofixation, 24-hour urine protein electrophoresis with immunofixation, and troponin and NT-proBNP levels for staging purposes. The typical normal range for a $\kappa{:}\lambda$ ratio is 0.26–1.65 but can increase to 2.5 with renal dysfunction. A diagnosis of AL amyloidosis requires biopsy evidence of amyloid deposits.[30] An abdominal fat pad biopsy can be the first test, particularly given that there is higher yield in AL amyloid compared with ATTR. The sensitivity of an abdominal fat pad biopsy in AL amyloidosis is approximately 84%, although only 45% in hATTR and 15% in wtATTR.[31] If the abdominal fat pat biopsy does not reveal the diagnosis, then biopsy of the most clinically affected organ is recommended.

Prognosis

The overall prognosis for AL amyloidosis is poor, despite advances in therapies, with an estimated 42% overall survival after four years.[32] Cardiac involvement is the primary determinant of outcomes, with most patients dying from progressive HF or sudden cardiac death (SCD). The revised Mayo Clinic staging system ascribes one point for each of the following: free light chain difference ≥18 mg/dL, cardiac troponin T ≥0.025 ng/mL, and NT-proBNP ≥1800 pg/mL. Stages I to IV correspond to an estimated median survival of 7.8 years, 3.4 years, 1.2 years, and 0.5 years, respectively (Table 35.3).[6] A NT-proBNP >8,500 ng/L has been used to further stratify patients.[33] A more recent staging system was devised by Boston University and includes a troponin I cut-off of 0.1 ng/mL and a B-type natriuretic peptide (BNP) value of 81 pg/mL to divide patients into stages 1, 2, and 3, with stage 3b representing a higher-risk cohort of patients with a BNP value >700 pg/mL. Stages 1, 2, 3, and 3b correlate with a median survival of 10 years, 9.4 years, 4.3 years, and 1 year, respectively.[34] This improvement in survival is most likely reflective of new light chain suppressive therapies.

Management

There have been many advances in the treatment of AL amyloidosis. Prior to 1990, the first regimen for AL amyloidosis consisted of an alkylator, melphalan, and prednisone; although this regimen did improve outcomes, median survival was still only 18 months.[35] From 1990–2005, there was more focus on high- dose melphalan and autologous stem cell transplantation, with a median survival of 4.6 years at that time, with cardiac involvement serving as a prognostic indicator.[36] There has been substantial progress in light chain suppressive therapies. Currently, the most common chemotherapy regimen for patients with a new diagnosis of AL amyloidosis is a combination of the alkylator cyclophosphamide, the proteasome inhibitor bortezomib, and the steroid dexamethasone (CyBorD). Other proteasome inhibitors, such as carfilzomib, are utilized less often, given their potential cardiotoxicity. Immunomodulators, such as lenalidomide and pomalidomide, have also been used in AL amyloidosis treatment. The most recent new addition to the AL amyloidosis treatment arsenal is daratumumab, an antibody directed against CD38, with studies showing an overall hematologic response rate of 76% in patients with refractory AL amyloidosis.[37] The phase 3 ANDROMEDA clinical trial is currently investigating the role of up-front therapy with daratumumab plus traditional CyBorD therapy. Regardless of which regimen is utilized, the goal of these therapies is to reduce the amount of circulating light chains.

ATTR Amyloidosis

The transthyretin precursor protein is a carrier protein for thyroxine and holo-retinol binding protein and consists of four monomers that circulate as a tetramer. Transthyretin is mostly produced by the liver but can also be secreted by the choroid plexus and retinal pigmented epithelial cells. Destabilization of the tetramer can result in degradation into amyloidogenic monomers that misfold and self-aggregate to form ß-sheet-rich amyloid fibrils. ATTR amyloidosis is classified by the 127 amino acid sequence of the transthyretin gene, located on chromosome 18. If there is no mutation, then it is wild-type ATTR (wtATTR) amyloidosis, whereas hereditary ATTR (hATTR) is defined by the presence of a single amino acid mutation. Whereas the amino acid mutation accounts for the destabilization of the transthyretin tetramer, the instability of the wtATTR tetramer is attributed to the aging process.

Wild-Type ATTR

The prevalence of wtATTR is higher than previously thought, and wtATTR cardiomyopathy (wtATTR-CM) is now recognized as a relatively common cause of HF. Most of the registries illustrate a predominance of Caucasian men, although this could be related to referral bias. The average age of diagnosis is 75 years, with some rare patients diagnosed in their forties.[7] Extracardiac manifestations associated with wtATTR-CM include carpal tunnel syndrome in approximately 50% to 70% of patients, lumbar stenosis, spontaneous biceps tendon rupture in approximately 33% of patients, polyneuropathy in 10%, and autonomic dysfunction.[2,38] The exact prevalence of wtATTR remains unknown, but autopsy studies suggest a prevalence of 20 to 25% in octogenarians and approximately 37% in patients older than 95 years of age.[39] In hospitalized HFpEF patients who underwent nuclear scintigraphy, approximately 13% actually had wtATTR.[40] In patients with severe

TABLE 35.3: Stages of Cardiac Amyloidosis

	Model Stages	NT-proBNP (ng/L)	BNP (ng/L)	Cardiac Troponin T (mcg/L)	High-Sensitivity Cardiac Troponin T (ng/L)	Additional Risk Factors (RF)
AL Amyloidosis						
Mayo 2012 model	Stage 1 = no RF Stage II = 1 RF Stage III = 2RF Stage IV = 3RF	≥1800	≥400	≥0.025	≥40	dFLC ≥180 mgL^{-1}
ATTR Amyloidosis						
Mayo wtATTR	Stage I = no RF Stage II = 1 RF Stage III = 2RF	>3000	ND	>0.05	≥65	NA

Abbreviations: AL, light-chain amyloidosis; ATTR, transthyretin amyloidosis; BNP, brain natriuretic peptide; dFLC, difference between involved to uninvolved light chains; NA, not applicable; ND, no data; NT-proBNP, N-terminal pro B-type natriuretic peptide; RF, risk factor; wtATTR amyloidosis, wild-type transthyretin amyloidosis.

aortic stenosis referred for transcatheter aortic valve replacement, nuclear scintigraphy revealed that 16% overall and 22% of men had wtATTR-CM.[41] Amyloid fibrils deposit in the flexor retinaculum and tenosynovial tissue, resulting in carpal tunnel syndrome, often preceding ATTR-CM by five to ten years.[42] Of patients undergoing carpal tunnel syndrome release surgery, 10.2% were found to have amyloid deposits in samples of the tenosynovium.[43]

The THAOS registry reported worse survival outcomes in hATTR, particularly those cases with the Val122Ile mutation, compared with wtATTR amyloidosis.[12] The Mayo Clinic staging system for wtATTR-CM uses thresholds of troponin T greater than 0.05 ng/mL and NT-proBNP greater than 3,000 pg/mL to designate stage 1, 2, and 3 corresponding with both values below the threshold, one value above, or both above. The median survival was estimated at 66 months for stage 1, 40 months for stage 2, and 20 months for stage 3.[7]

Hereditary ATTR

Once ATTR amyloidosis is diagnosed, it is important to proceed with genetic testing to determine appropriate therapeutic options as well as to offer genetic counseling to family members. Hereditary ATTR amyloidosis (hATTR) has an autosomal dominant pattern of inheritance, but overall penetrance is unknown. The mechanism of amyloid fibril formation is similar regardless of the exact mutation. Over 120 mutations have been identified, the most common being Val30Met, Val122Ile, and Thr60Ala (Tables 35.4 and 35.5). The THAOS registry also identified the Leu111Met and Ile68Leu mutations as other causes of hATTR-CM (Table 35.1).[12] The Val30Met is the most common mutation worldwide; it is endemic in Portugal, Japan, and Sweden.[44,45] Although polyneuropathy is the most common manifestation, Val30Met can result in late-onset cardiomyopathy.

The Val122Ile mutation, which results from a valine-to-isoleucine substitution at position 122, is the most common hATTR variant in the United States. The Val122Ile mutation originated in western Africa and affects 3.4% of the African American population.[46] The Val122Ile is most frequently associated with cardiomyopathy, whether the allele is present in the heterozygous or homozygous state. Thr60Ala is the second most common mutation in the United States that results in cardiomyopathy.[2] It was originally identified in County Donegal in Ireland[47] and has an estimated population prevalence of 1% in northwest Ireland.[48] Although cardiomyopathy is frequent with Thr60Ala, there is also a high rate of neurologic involvement with autonomic dysfunction and peripheral neuropathy present in 75% and 54% of affected individuals, respectively.[49]

Treatment

Transthyretin Stabilization

In addition to symptomatic management of ATTR-CM with salt restriction, diuretics, and aldosterone antagonism, there have been advances in disease-specific interventions (Table 35.6). The rate-limiting step in amyloid fibril formation is the dissociation of the transthyretin tetramer, and stabilization of the tetramer has been a target for therapies. Diflunisal is a nonsteroidal anti-inflammatory agent (NSAID) that also binds and stabilizes TTR. Diflunisal was evaluated in patients with hereditary ATTR polyneuropathy, and improved quality of life and reduced neurologic impairment.[50] The true efficacy of diflunisal in ATTR-CM is not clear, but one study of 13 patients, including wtATTR and hATTR cardiac amyloidosis, demonstrated no significant change in left ventricular (LV) mass or function, a finding consistent with stabilization of the disease.[51] However, caution must be utilized with the administration of diflunisal given its potential for renal dysfunction, gastrointestinal bleeding, and heart failure exacerbations.

TABLE 35.4: TTR Mutations

Mutation	Endemic	Prevalence	Manifestations
Val122Ile	US and Western Africa	3.4% of African Americans; most common mutation in US	Mostly cardiac; 10% neuropathy
Thr60Ala	US (Appalachian region); northern part of Republic of Ireland	1% of northwest Ireland	Mix of cardiac and nerve involvement
Val30Met	Portugal, Sweden, Japan	Most common mutation worldwide	Polyneuropathy most common, but late-onset cardiomyopathy can occur
Leu111Met	Denmark	Rare	Earlier onset of cardiac involvement
Ile68Leu	Italy	Rare	Later onset of cardiac involvement (>55 years)

TABLE 35.5: Mutation-Dependent Phenotypes

Mostly Neurologic Phenotype	Mixed Neurologic and Cardiac Phenotype	Mostly Cardiac Phenotype
V30M (early onset)	**Neurologic > Cardiac**	T60A
F33L	R34T	L111M
C10R	G47A	I68L
S50R	A36P	V122I
	F64L	
	T49A	
	E89Q	
	V30M (late onset)	
	Cardiac > Neurologic	
	W41L	
	H88R	
	S23N	

TABLE 35.6: **Therapies for Transthyretin Amyloidosis**

Drug	Mechanism	Administration	Study Population	Tolerability	FDA Approval
Patisiran	siRNA (silencer)	Intravenous every 3 weeks	Neuropathy (~50% CM pts)	20% infusion reactions	Approved
Inotersen	ASO (silencer)	Weekly subcutaneous injection	Neuropathy (~60% CM pts)	Thrombocytopenia and glomerulonephritis	Approved
Tafamidis	Stabilizer	Oral, once daily	ATTR cardiomyopathy	GI upset and UTI (minimal)	Approved

Abbreviations: ASO: antisense oligonucleotide; ATTR: transthyretin amyloidosis; CM: cardiomyopathy; GI: gastrointestinal; siRNA: small interfering RNA; UTI: urinary tract infection.

Tafamidis is a novel compound that binds to the thyroxine-binding sites of TTR with high affinity, which inhibits tetramer dissociation into monomers. Previous trials illustrated that tafamidis slowed the progression of peripheral neuropathy in hATTR polyneuropathy, leading to its approval in other countries.[52] The phase 3 double-blind, placebo-controlled trial Transthyretin Amyloidosis Cardiomyopathy Clinical Trial (ATTR-ACT) assessed tafamidis (20 or 80 mg daily) in patients with wtATTR and hATTR. Tafamidis was associated with lower mortality compared with placebo, with a 13.4% absolute difference in mortality and a 32% relative risk reduction in cardiovascular hospitalizations. The estimated number needed to treat with 2.5 years of treatment is 7.5 to prevent one death. Tafamidis was well tolerated, with no significant adverse events.[53] Tafamidis achieved expedited approval by the US Food and Drug Administration (FDA). At a cost of $225,000 per patient per year, tafamidis is currently the most expensive cardiovascular drug, and cost continues to be a concern for future use of this medication.

Other agents that can stabilize TTR include epigallocatechin-3-gallate (EGCG) in green tea, which inhibits amyloid fibril formation, but further evidence is needed.[54] AG-10 is a compound that stabilizes wild-type TTR and TTR Val122Ile. A phase II study of 49 patients with ATTR-CM illustrated stabilization of TTR with AG-10,[55] and the phase III trial is currently ongoing. Tolcapone, a catechol-*O*-methyltransferase (COMT) inhibitor used as adjunctive therapy for Parkinson's disease, binds to TTR in human plasma, and stabilizes both wild-type and mutant TTR,[56] although studies are still pending.

TTR Gene Silencers

TTR gene silencing, either through RNA interference or antisense oligonucleotides, is another treatment strategy for ATTR amyloidosis. Small interfering RNAs (siRNAs) are delivered to hepatocytes and target gene expression leading to the degradation of TTR mRNA. Patisiran, a siRNA, resulted in a dose-dependent reduction of serum TTR levels in patients with hATTR polyneuropathy. The phase III APOLLO study included 225 patients with hATTR polyneuropathy randomized to receive either patisiran infusions or placebo, and patisiran resulted in improvement in the neuropathy impairment score (NIS) after 18 months of therapy.[57] In the pre-specified cardiac subgroup, consisting of patients with LV wall thickness ≥13 mm with no concomitant history of hypertension or valvular disease, patisiran resulted in an improvement in NT-proBNP, LV wall thickness, and global longitudinal strain.[58]

Antisense oligonucleotides (ASOs) are short, synthetic RNAs that inhibit the translation of mRNA. Inotersen is an ASO that inhibits hepatic expression of TTR, suppressing both wild-type and mutant TTR. The NEURO-TTR trial demonstrated that, in hATTR polyneuropathy, subcutaneous injections of inotersen resulted in improvement in symptoms related to polyneuropathy.[59] In a study of 22 patients with ATTR-CM, inotersen was associated with stabilization of the disease at 12 months, based on decreased left ventricular mass and improvement in 6-min walk test.[60] Side effects for TTR silencers include rare infusion reactions for patisiran and glomerulonephritis, and thrombocytopenia for inotersen. FDA approved both patisiran and inotersen for hATTR polyneuropathy, with the caveat that platelets and renal function should be monitored weekly with inotersen. TTR silencers are not currently being approved for hATTR-CM without neuropathy.

Fibril Degradation

Previously there was extensive investigation into TTR amyloid fibril disruption and removal of amyloid fibrils. The tetracycline antibiotic, doxycycline, in combination with tauro-ursodeoxycholic acid (TUDCA), an over-the-counter antioxidant and antiapoptotic, were administered to disrupt TTR fibrils. This combination was associated with no progression of cardiac or neurologic manifestations over the span of a year in patients with ATTR amyloidosis.[61] However, further investigations into fibril degradation have not been as promising. Antibodies targeted against monomeric amyloidogenic forms of TTR have been found to induce phagocytic uptake of the TTR aggregates to prevent amyloid fibril formation,[62] but further evaluation is warranted.

Advanced Therapy Option/Device Therapies

Defibrillators and Resynchronization Therapy

Historically, implantable cardioverter defibrillator (ICD) therapy was considered to be contraindicated in cardiac amyloidosis. However, this was from an era when ATTR amyloidosis was still considered rare and the median survival for patients with AL amyloidosis was less than one year. There was also concern that ICDs were not effective in patients with cardiac amyloidosis, particularly AL amyloid, given that SCD in this population was attributed to pulseless electrical activity (PEA) or electromechanical dissociation. However, ventricular arrhythmias have been found to be common in cardiac amyloidosis, particularly AL amyloidosis, with an estimated prevalence of 27%.[63] Several studies of cardiac amyloidosis patients have illustrated high rates of successful termination of ventricular arrhythmias by ICD. The Stanford Amyloid Center released their criteria for ICD implantation, which focuses on risk stratification for those cardiac amyloid patients with highest risk of SCD. No ICD implantation is recommended for NYHA IV or life expectancy less than one year. However, ICD is recommended for unexplained syncope, non-sustained ventricular tachycardia, or sustained ventricular tachycardia on outpatient telemetry, which should be performed every six months to one year.[64]

There is little evidence on the use of cardiac resynchronization therapy in cardiac amyloidosis. Typically, biventricular pacing is recommended if QRS>130 ms or there is concern for high right ventricular pacing burden. Donnellan et al. however did find that biventricular devices were associated with improvement in ejection fraction, mitral regurgitation severity, and NYHA functional class when clinically indicated in patients with cardiac amyloidosis.[65]

Mechanical Circulatory Support

Although left ventricular assist device (LVAD) implantation is technically feasible in patients with cardiac amyloidosis,[66,67] the smaller left ventricular size is often a contraindication, given the known increased mortality with LVAD implantation in a patient with a smaller left ventricular end-diastolic dimension.[67] The biventricular nature of cardiac amyloidosis also makes mechanical circulatory support (MCS) difficult. A study of 12 patients undergoing MCS as bridge-to-transplantation demonstrated that biventricular MCS, in the form of biventricular assist devices (or total artificial heart) are potential alternatives for durable MCS while awaiting transplantation.[68]

Transplantation

The aforementioned therapeutic agents for ATTR-CM have not been approved or studied in patients with NYHA IV or Stage D HF. In patients with advanced HF secondary to cardiac amyloidosis, orthotopic heart transplantation (OHT) offers a potential therapeutic option. Historically, there was a concern for poor post-transplantation survival outcomes in cardiac amyloidosis. An evaluation of the United Network for Organ Sharing registry from 1987 to 2002 found reduced one-year survival outcomes in patients with cardiac amyloidosis compared with non-amyloid patients undergoing OHT.[69] Grogan et al. reported a one-year post-transplant survival of 77% in patients with AL amyloidosis undergoing OHT, which was significantly lower than for patients undergoing OHT for other indications. More than half of the deaths were secondary to progressive amyloidosis.[70]

Recent reports demonstrate more promising outcomes for transplantation in cardiac amyloidosis. Rosenbaum et al. reported 100% three-year survival in patients with wtATTR-CM who underwent OHT.[71] With advances in new light chain therapies, outcomes for OHT in AL amyloidosis have also improved. Barrett et al. investigated 31 patients, 13 with AL and 18 with ATTR amyloidosis, who underwent OHT, and post-transplant mortality rates were similar compared with non-amyloid patients. Interestingly, outcomes were similar in patients with AL and ATTR amyloidosis.[72] Under the new UNOS allocation policy (October 2018), restrictive cardiomyopathy secondary to cardiac amyloidosis is designated status 4 in terms of urgency, which could potentially disadvantage this patient population, although further long-term follow-up is needed post-allocation policy change.

Conclusion

Amyloidosis is a systemic disease that results from misfolding of precursor proteins into amorphous aggregates that subsequently form insoluble fibrils that can deposit in the heart, liver, kidneys, gastrointestinal tract, peripheral nerves, and other soft tissues. Cardiac amyloidosis is an increasingly recognized cause of heart failure. The most common types of amyloid that result in cardiac amyloidosis are light chain (AL) and transthyretin (ATTR) amyloidosis. In the presence of a monoclonal protein, tissue biopsy is still necessary to differentiate between AL and ATTR amyloidosis, and a systematic approach is key to ensuring a correct diagnosis. There have been significant advances in light chain therapies for both AL amyloidosis- and ATTR-specific therapies, offering hope for both patient populations, particularly if early diagnosis is achieved.

References

1. Benson MD, Buxbaum JN, Eisenberg DS, et al. Amyloid nomenclature 2018: recommendations by the International Society of Amyloidosis (ISA) nomenclature committee. *Amyloid.* 2018;25(4):215–9.
2. Ruberg FL, Grogan M, Hanna M, Kelly JW, Maurer MS. Transthyretin amyloid cardiomyopathy: JACC state-of-the-art review. *J Am Coll Cardiol.* 2019;73(22):2872–91.
3. Gopal DM, Ruberg FL, Siddiqi OK. Impact of genetic testing in transthyretin (ATTR) cardiac amyloidosis. *Curr Heart Fail Rep.* 2019;16(5):180–8.
4. Kyle RA, Linos A, Beard CM, et al. Incidence and natural history of primary systemic amyloidosis in Olmsted County, Minnesota, 1950 through 1989. *Blood.* 1992;79(7):1817–22.
5. Mohammed SF, Mirzoyev SA, Edwards WD, et al. Left ventricular amyloid deposition in patients with heart failure and preserved ejection fraction. *JACC Heart Fail.* 2014;2(2):113–22.
6. Kumar S, Dispenzieri A, Lacy MQ, et al. Revised prognostic staging system for light chain amyloidosis incorporating cardiac biomarkers and serum free light chain measurements. *J Clin Oncol.* 2012;30(9):989–95.
7. Grogan M, Scott CG, Kyle RA, et al. Natural history of wild-type transthyretin cardiac amyloidosis and risk stratification using a novel staging system. *J Am Coll Cardiol.* 2016;68(10):1014–20.
8. Hanson JLS, Arvanitis M, Koch CM, et al. Use of serum transthyretin as a prognostic indicator and predictor of outcome in cardiac amyloid disease associated with wild-type transthyretin. *Circ Heart Fail.* 2018;11(2):e004000.
9. Sperry BW, Vranian MN, Hachamovitch R, et al. Are classic predictors of voltage valid in cardiac amyloidosis? A contemporary analysis of electrocardiographic findings. *Int J Cardiol.* 2016;214:477–81.
10. Rapezzi C, Merlini G, Quarta CC, et al. Systemic cardiac amyloidoses: disease profiles and clinical courses of the 3 main types. *Circulation.* 2009;120(13):1203–12.
11. Cyrille NB, Goldsmith J, Alvarez J, Maurer MS. Prevalence and prognostic significance of low QRS voltage among the three main types of cardiac amyloidosis. *Am J Cardiol.* 2014;114(7):1089–93.
12. Maurer MS, Hanna M, Grogan M, et al. Genotype and phenotype of transthyretin cardiac amyloidosis: THAOS (transthyretin amyloid outcome survey). *J Am Coll Cardiol.* 2016;68(2):161–72.
13. Okamoto S, Hornsten R, Obayashi K, Wijayatunga P, Suhr OB. Continuous development of arrhythmia is observed in Swedish transplant patients with familial amyloidotic polyneuropathy (amyloidogenic transthyretin Val30Met variant). *Liver Transpl.* 2011;17(2):122–8.
14. Senapati A, Sperry BW, Grodin JL, et al. Prognostic implication of relative regional strain ratio in cardiac amyloidosis. *Heart.* 2016;102(10):748–54.
15. Milani P, Dispenzieri A, Scott CG, et al. Independent prognostic value of stroke volume index in patients with immunoglobulin light chain amyloidosis. *Circ Cardiovasc Imaging.* 2018;11(5):e006588.
16. Syed IS, Glockner JF, Feng D, et al. Role of cardiac magnetic resonance imaging in the detection of cardiac amyloidosis. *JACC Cardiovasc Imaging.* 2010;3(2):155–64.
17. Fontana M, Banypersad SM, Treibel TA, et al. Native T1 mapping in transthyretin amyloidosis. *JACC Cardiovasc Imaging.* 2014;7(2):157–65.
18. Fontana M, Banypersad SM, Treibel TA, et al. Differential myocyte responses in patients with cardiac transthyretin amyloidosis and light-chain amyloidosis: a cardiac MR imaging study. *Radiology.* 2015;277(2):388–97.
19. Bokhari S, Castano A, Pozniakoff T, Deslisle S, Latif F, Maurer MS. (99m) Tc-pyrophosphate scintigraphy for differentiating light-chain cardiac amyloidosis from the transthyretin-related familial and senile cardiac amyloidoses. *Circ Cardiovasc Imaging.* 2013;6(2):195–201.
20. Gillmore JD, Maurer MS, Falk RH, et al. Nonbiopsy diagnosis of cardiac transthyretin amyloidosis. *Circulation.* 2016;133(24):2404–12.
21. Merlini G, Comenzo RL, Seldin DC, Wechalekar A, Gertz MA. Immunoglobulin light chain amyloidosis. *Expert Rev Hematol.* 2014;7(1):143–56.
22. Vrana JA, Gamez JD, Madden BJ, Theis JD, Bergen HR, 3rd, Dogan A. Classification of amyloidosis by laser microdissection and mass spectrometry-based proteomic analysis in clinical biopsy specimens. *Blood.* 2009;114(24):4957–9.
23. Rubinow A, Skinner M, Cohen AS. Digoxin sensitivity in amyloid cardiomyopathy. *Circulation.* 1981;63(6):1285–8.
24. Muchtar E, Gertz MA, Kumar SK, et al. Digoxin use in systemic light-chain (AL) amyloidosis: contra-indicated or cautious use? *Amyloid.* 2018;25(2):86–92.
25. El-Am EA, Dispenzieri A, Melduni RM, et al. Direct current cardioversion of atrial arrhythmias in adults with cardiac amyloidosis. *J Am Coll Cardiol.* 2019;73(5):589–97.

26. Feng D, Edwards WD, Oh JK, et al. Intracardiac thrombosis and embolism in patients with cardiac amyloidosis. *Circulation*. 2007;116(21):2420–6.
27. Lousada I, Comenzo RL, Landau H, Guthrie S, Merlini G. Light chain amyloidosis: patient experience survey from the amyloidosis research consortium. *Adv Ther*. 2015;32(10):920–8.
28. Falk RH, Alexander KM, Liao R, Dorbala S. AL (light-chain) cardiac amyloidosis: a review of diagnosis and therapy. *J Am Coll Cardiol*. 2016;68(12):1323–41.
29. Shi J, Guan J, Jiang B, et al. Amyloidogenic light chains induce cardiomyocyte contractile dysfunction and apoptosis via a non-canonical p38alpha MAPK pathway. *Proc Natl Acad Sci U S A*. 2010;107(9):4188–93.
30. Leung N, Nasr SH, Sethi S. How I treat amyloidosis: the importance of accurate diagnosis and amyloid typing. *Blood*. 2012;120(16):3206–13.
31. Quarta CC, Gonzalez-Lopez E, Gilbertson JA, et al. Diagnostic sensitivity of abdominal fat aspiration in cardiac amyloidosis. *Eur Heart J*. 2017;38(24):1905–8.
32. Kumar SK, Gertz MA, Lacy MQ, et al. Recent improvements in survival in primary systemic amyloidosis and the importance of an early mortality risk score. *Mayo Clin Proc*. 2011;86(1):12–8.
33. Palladini G, Sachchithanantham S, Milani P, et al. A European collaborative study of cyclophosphamide, bortezomib, and dexamethasone in upfront treatment of systemic AL amyloidosis. *Blood*. 2015;126(5):612–5.
34. Lilleness B, Ruberg FL, Mussinelli R, Doros G, Sanchorawala V. Development and validation of a survival staging system incorporating BNP in patients with light chain amyloidosis. *Blood*. 2019;133(3):215–23.
35. Kyle RA, Gertz MA, Greipp PR, et al. A trial of three regimens for primary amyloidosis: colchicine alone, melphalan and prednisone, and melphalan, prednisone, and colchicine. *N Engl J Med*. 1997;336(17):1202–7.
36. Skinner M, Anderson J, Simms R, et al. Treatment of 100 patients with primary amyloidosis: a randomized trial of melphalan, prednisone, and colchicine versus colchicine only. *Am J Med*. 1996;100(3):290–8.
37. Kaufman GP, Schrier SL, Lafayette RA, Arai S, Witteles RM, Liedtke M. Daratumumab yields rapid and deep hematologic responses in patients with heavily pretreated AL amyloidosis. *Blood*. 2017;130(7):900–2.
38. Connors LH, Sam F, Skinner M, et al. Heart failure resulting from age-related cardiac amyloid disease associated with wild-type transthyretin: a prospective, observational cohort study. *Circulation*. 2016;133(3):282–90.
39. Tanskanen M, Peuralinna T, Polvikoski T, et al. Senile systemic amyloidosis affects 25% of the very aged and associates with genetic variation in alpha2-macroglobulin and tau: a population-based autopsy study. *Ann Med*. 2008;40(3):232–9.
40. Gonzalez-Lopez E, Gallego-Delgado M, Guzzo-Merello G, et al. Wild-type transthyretin amyloidosis as a cause of heart failure with preserved ejection fraction. *Eur Heart J*. 2015;36(38):2585–94.
41. Castano A, Narotsky DL, Hamid N, et al. Unveiling transthyretin cardiac amyloidosis and its predictors among elderly patients with severe aortic stenosis undergoing transcatheter aortic valve replacement. *Eur Heart J*. 2017;38(38):2879–87.
42. Nakagawa M, Sekijima Y, Yazaki M, et al. Carpal tunnel syndrome: a common initial symptom of systemic wild-type ATTR (ATTRwt) amyloidosis. *Amyloid*. 2016;23(1):58–63.
43. Sperry BW, Reyes BA, Ikram A, et al. Tenosynovial and cardiac amyloidosis in patients undergoing carpal tunnel release. *J Am Coll Cardiol*. 2018;72(17):2040–50.
44. Andrade C. A peculiar form of peripheral neuropathy; familiar atypical generalized amyloidosis with special involvement of the peripheral nerves. *Brain*. 1952;75(3):408–27.
45. Sousa A, Coelho T, Barros J, Sequeiros J. Genetic epidemiology of familial amyloidotic polyneuropathy (FAP)-type I in Povoa do Varzim and Vila do Conde (north of Portugal). *Am J Med Genet*. 1995;60(6):512–21.
46. Buxbaum JN, Ruberg FL. Transthyretin V122I (pV142I)* cardiac amyloidosis: an age-dependent autosomal dominant cardiomyopathy too common to be overlooked as a cause of significant heart disease in elderly African Americans. *Genet Med*. 2017;19(7):733–42.
47. Wallace MR, Dwulet FE, Conneally PM, Benson MD. Biochemical and molecular genetic characterization of a new variant prealbumin associated with hereditary amyloidosis. *J Clin Invest*. 1986;78(1):6–12.
48. Reilly MM, Staunton H, Harding AE. Familial amyloid polyneuropathy (TTR ala 60) in north west Ireland: a clinical, genetic, and epidemiological study. *J Neurol Neurosurg Psychiatry*. 1995;59(1):45–9.
49. Sattianayagam PT, Hahn AF, Whelan CJ, et al. Cardiac phenotype and clinical outcome of familial amyloid polyneuropathy associated with transthyretin alanine 60 variant. *Eur Heart J*. 2012;33(9):1120–7.
50. Miller SR, Sekijima Y, Kelly JW. Native state stabilization by NSAIDs inhibits transthyretin amyloidogenesis from the most common familial disease variants. *Lab Invest*. 2004;84(5):545–52.
51. Castano A, Helmke S, Alvarez J, Delisle S, Maurer MS. Diflunisal for ATTR cardiac amyloidosis. *Congest Heart Fail*. 2012;18(6):315–9.
52. Coelho T, Maia LF, Martins da Silva A, et al. Tafamidis for transthyretin familial amyloid polyneuropathy: a randomized, controlled trial. *Neurology*. 2012;79(8):785–92.
53. Maurer MS, Schwartz JH, Gundapaneni B, et al. Tafamidis treatment for patients with transthyretin amyloid cardiomyopathy. *N Engl J Med*. 2018;379(11):1007–16.
54. Bieschke J, Russ J, Friedrich RP, et al. EGCG remodels mature alpha-synuclein and amyloid-beta fibrils and reduces cellular toxicity. *Proc Natl Acad Sci U S A*. 2010;107(17):7710–5.
55. Judge DP, Heitner SB, Falk RH, et al. Transthyretin stabilization by AG10 in symptomatic transthyretin amyloid cardiomyopathy. *J Am Coll Cardiol*. 2019;74(3):285–95.
56. Sant'Anna R, Gallego P, Robinson LZ, et al. Repositioning tolcapone as a potent inhibitor of transthyretin amyloidogenesis and associated cellular toxicity. *Nat Commun*. 2016;710787.
57. Adams D, Gonzalez-Duarte A, O'Riordan WD, et al. Patisiran, an RNAi therapeutic, for hereditary transthyretin amyloidosis. *N Engl J Med*. 2018;379(1):11–21.
58. Solomon SD, Adams D, Kristen A, et al. Effects of patisiran, an RNA interference therapeutic, on cardiac parameters in patients with hereditary transthyretin-mediated amyloidosis. *Circulation*. 2019;139(4):431–43.
59. Benson MD, Waddington-Cruz M, Berk JL, et al. Inotersen treatment for patients with hereditary transthyretin amyloidosis. *N Engl J Med*. 2018;379(1):22–31.
60. Benson MD, Dasgupta NR, Rissing SM, Smith J, Feigenbaum H. Safety and efficacy of a TTR specific antisense oligonucleotide in patients with transthyretin amyloid cardiomyopathy. *Amyloid*. 2017;24(4):219–25.
61. Obici L, Cortese A, Lozza A, et al. Doxycycline plus tauroursodeoxycholic acid for transthyretin amyloidosis: a phase II study. *Amyloid*. 2012;19 Suppl 134–6.
62. Hosoi A, Su Y, Torikai M, et al. Novel antibody for the treatment of transthyretin amyloidosis. *J Biol Chem*. 2016;291(48):25096–105.
63. Dubrey SW, Cha K, Anderson J, et al. The clinical features of immunoglobulin light-chain (AL) amyloidosis with heart involvement. *QJM*. 1998;91(2):141–57.
64. Varr BC, Zarafshar S, Coakley T, et al. Implantable cardioverter-defibrillator placement in patients with cardiac amyloidosis. *Heart Rhythm*. 2014;11(1):158–62.
65. Donnellan E, Wazni OM, Saliba WI, et al. Cardiac devices in patients with transthyretin amyloidosis: impact on functional class, left ventricular function, mitral regurgitation, and mortality. *J Cardiovasc Electrophysiol*. 2019;30(11):2427–32.
66. Swiecicki PL, Edwards BS, Kushwaha SS, Dispenzieri A, Park SJ, Gertz MA. Left ventricular device implantation for advanced cardiac amyloidosis. *J Heart Lung Transplant*. 2013;32(5):563–8.
67. Topilsky Y, Pereira NL, Shah DK, et al. Left ventricular assist device therapy in patients with restrictive and hypertrophic cardiomyopathy. *Circ Heart Fail*. 2011;4(3):266–75.
68. Kittleson MM, Cole RM, Patel J, et al. Mechanical circulatory support for cardiac amyloidosis. *Clin Transplant*. 2019;33(10):e13663.
69. Kpodonu J, Massad MG, Caines A, Geha AS. Outcome of heart transplantation in patients with amyloid cardiomyopathy. *J Heart Lung Transplant*. 2005;24(11):1763–5.
70. Grogan M, Gertz M, McCurdy A, et al. Long term outcomes of cardiac transplant for immunoglobulin light chain amyloidosis: The Mayo Clinic experience. *World J Transplant*. 2016;6(2):380–8.
71. Rosenbaum AN, Edwards BS. Current indications, strategies, and outcomes with cardiac transplantation for cardiac amyloidosis and sarcoidosis. *Curr Opin Organ Transplant*. 2015;20(5):584–92.
72. Barrett CD, Alexander KM, Zhao H, et al. Outcomes in patients with cardiac amyloidosis undergoing heart transplantation. *JACC Heart Fail*. 2020;8(6):461–8.

Chapter 36
INFILTRATIVE CARDIOMYOPATHIES
Fabry Disease and Iron-Overload Cardiomyopathy

Arthur Qi, Quynh Nguyen, Haran Yogasundaram, and Gavin Y. Oudit

Introduction

Infiltrative cardiomyopathy refers to a heterogeneous group of disorders which involves infiltration of the myocardium with various molecules and typically carries a poor prognosis.[1] Some infiltrative cardiomyopathies, such as Fabry disease, cause a hypertrophic phenotype with increased ventricular wall thickness, while others, such as iron-overload cardiomyopathy, cause a dilated phenotype with chamber enlargement and secondary wall thinning.[2] These conditions must be distinguished from similar conditions with true myocyte hypertrophy (e.g., hypertrophic cardiomyopathy, hypertensive heart disease) or dilatation (e.g., ischemic or dilated cardiomyopathy). Given the systemic nature of the infiltrative processes, assessment of non-cardiac involvement in infiltrative cardiomyopathies is paramount. In this chapter, we will highlight the cardiac manifestations of Fabry disease and iron-overload cardiomyopathy.

Fabry Disease

Etiology and Epidemiology

Fabry disease (FD), also known as Anderson-Fabry disease, is an X-linked recessive lysosomal storage disorder characterized by deficient α-galactosidase A (α-Gal A) enzymatic activity and gradual accumulation of glycosphingolipids, especially globotriaosylceramide (Gb3), within numerous cell types and tissues throughout the body. This progressive accumulation results in dermatological, gastrointestinal, ocular, neurological, cardiac, and renal manifestations.[3] Clinical presentation and progression is heterogeneous and is typically divided into two phenotypes, classic and variant. Over 585 pathogenic mutations have been identified in the α-Gal A (GLA) gene located on chromosome Xq.22.1 that result in variable levels of α-Gal A production and function, and, subsequently, clinical phenotypes.[4] Another consequence of the non-specific clinical picture of FD has been an underestimation of its prevalence and diagnosis; although the prevalence of FD is classically estimated at 1:40,000, newborn dried bloodspot screening indicates a prevalence of GLA mutations between 0.022% and 0.041%.[5,6]

Clinical Phenotypes and Pathogenesis

Patients with classic FD have severely diminished or absent α-Gal A activity. This phenotype affects hemizygous males, homozygous females, and some heterozygous females with skewed X-chromosome inactivation. The disease typically manifests in childhood or adolescence as acroparesthesias, diffuse angiokeratomas, corneal verticillata (Figure 36.1), heat intolerance, hypohidrosis, and abdominal pain crises.[3,7] In adulthood, patients develop cardiovascular, renal, and neurologic involvement that can progress to renal failure, cardiovascular disease, and cerebrovascular events. A critical feature of classic FD is accelerated glycosphingolipid deposition in the endothelium and smooth muscle of microvasculature, in addition to numerous organ systems, leading to progressive microvascular dysfunction, ischemia, and subsequent end-organ damage.[4,8] Clinical indices such as the Fabry International Prognostic Index and Mainz Severity Score Index have been used to assess disease activity, as well as to inform treatment and monitor disease progression.[9,10]

Variant FD is characterized by residual α-Gal A activity and affects males with less severe mutations and most heterozygous females. Variant FD typically affects either the heart or the kidneys alone and these pathogenic mutations are termed cardiac or renal variants. Patients with variant FD show little to no microvascular involvement and typically have a slower overall clinical progression.[3,7]

Cardiovascular Disease

Cardiovascular disease is the most significant cause of morbidity and mortality in FD.[4,7,11] Prominent cardiovascular manifestations include concentric left ventricular hypertrophy (LVH) and diastolic dysfunction with restrictive filling pattern resulting from Gb3-mediated infiltration and damage to microvasculature.[3,12] Accordingly, FD is an important differential diagnosis for infiltrative hypertrophic cardiomyopathy.[3] Interestingly, lysosomal Gb3 accumulation accounts for only 1–3% of mass in hypertrophic hearts.[13] Instead, Gb3 deposition activates pathologic signaling pathways, resulting in inflammation and oxidative stress, and leading to extracellular matrix and concentric myocardial remodeling that progresses to hypertrophy, necrosis, and fibrosis (Figure 36.2).[13,14] Microvascular damage also leads to reduced blood flow and resultant angina pectoris despite the absence of epicardial coronary artery stenosis (Figure 36.2).[3,13,14]

Minor valvular disease, specifically mild-to-moderate mitral and aortic regurgitation, is common in FD and results from infiltrative changes in valvular fibroblasts, leading to thickened and distorted valve leaflets and aortic root dilatation (Figure 36.2).[3,12–14] The greater impact on left-sided valves suggests a hemodynamic, pressure-mediated mechanism of valvular disease.[3,14]

Electrophysiological changes are common in FD. Early manifestations include shortened PR and prolonged QRS interval that can later progress to bundle branch and atrioventricular node blocks, atrial fibrillation, and sudden cardiac death (Figure 36.2).[3,13,14] Atrial fibrillation risk has been shown to be four times higher in FD patients than in the general population, which increases to 12 times in patients older than 50 years of age.[15] Age, left atrial size, LVH, and myocardial fibrosis have been identified as risk factors for greater arrhythmia burden.[16] In FD, traditional Holter monitoring has reported negative results in patients with a high number of clinically relevant supraventricular and ventricular arrhythmias, for which treatment was necessary to prevent stroke, syncope, and sudden cardiac death. Therefore, continuous monitoring devices, e.g., implantable loop recorders, may be useful in patients with FD due to their increased sensitivity.[11]

DOI: 10.1201/9780429244544-43

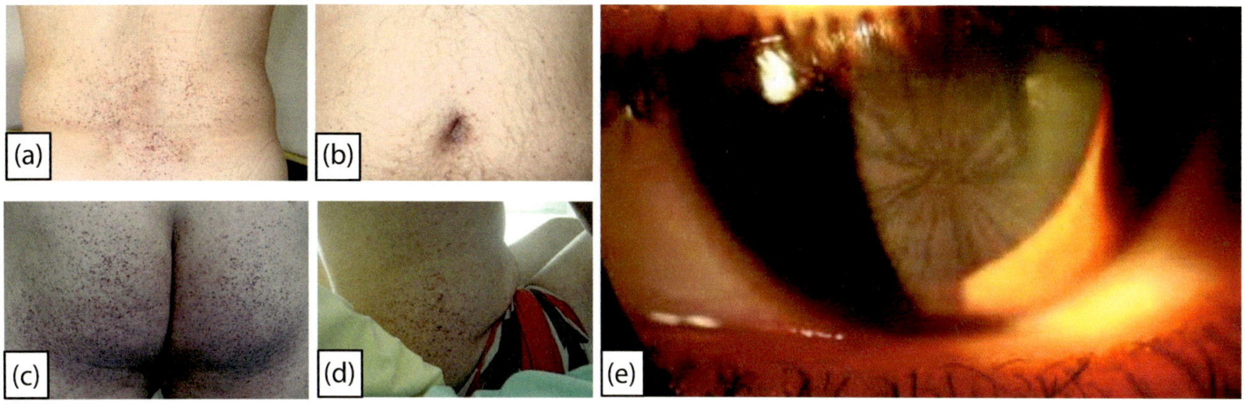

FIGURE 36.1 Diffuse angiokeratomas (tiny, painless papules), located on the lower back (a), umbilical (b), gluteal (c), and flank (d) regions, are characteristic dermatological manifestations of Fabry disease. (e) Cornea verticillata (bilateral whorl-like opacities located in the superficial corneal layers) are characteristic of Fabry disease.

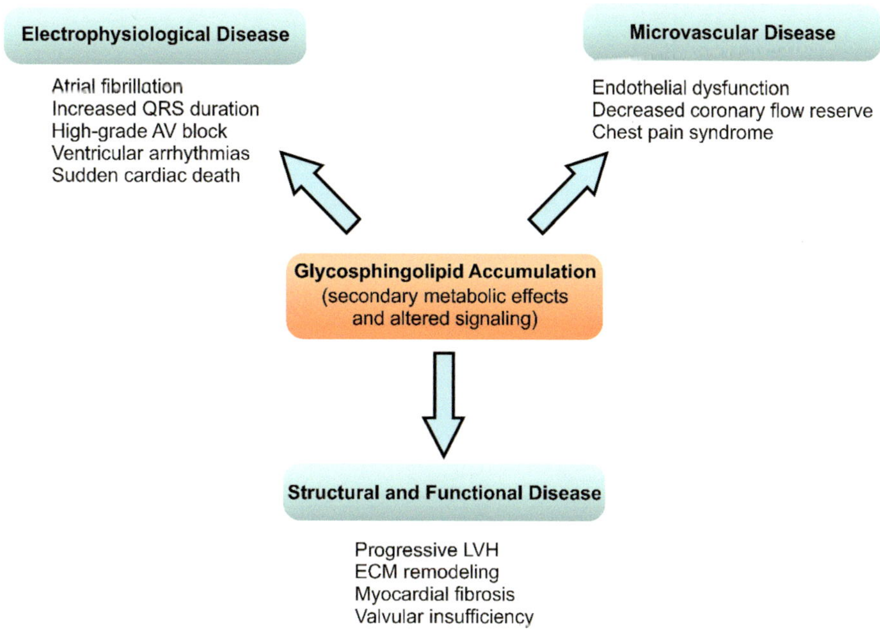

FIGURE 36.2 Pathophysiology and categorized cardiac manifestations in Fabry disease. *Abbreviations*: AV, atrioventricular; ECM, extracellular matrix; LVH, left ventricular hypertrophy. (Reproduced from Yogasundaram et al. *Can J Cardiol.* 2017;33(7):883–97 with permission from Elsevier.)

Other Manifestations

Progressive accumulation of lysosomal Gb3 in podocytes, mesangial cells, arteriolar endothelial, tubular epithelial, and interstitial renal cells results in microalbuminuria and reduced glomerular filtration rate, and progresses to irreversible ischemic changes in microvasculature that lead to renal failure. Additional manifestations include neurological events such as cryptogenic stroke, transient ischemic attack, sensorineural hearing loss, migraines, and neuropathic pain, with the latter being the most frequently reported symptom in FD patients (76% men and 64% women).[4,17] Gastrointestinal symptoms most commonly manifest as abdominal pain and diarrhea (27–55% men and 19–50% women), but can also include nausea, vomiting, and heartburn, and may relate to Gb3 deposition in enteric smooth muscle as well as nerves.[18–20]

Diagnostic Evaluation

The diagnosis of FD has historically been challenging due to non-specific presentation, leading to long delays between symptom onset and diagnosis, as well as misdiagnosis.[3] Diagnosis in males is initially based on the demonstration of deficient α-Gal A activity in plasma or leukocytes, with <5% of mean being highly suggestive of classic FD (Figure 36.3).[3,17] Enzyme activity in females and some males, however, can be highly variable, even with clinical disease. Therefore, genetic testing for GLA mutations is usually required to confirm diagnosis in males with non-diagnostic α-Gal A activity and females (Figure 36.3).[17,21] In indeterminate cases, biomarkers have some utility in the diagnosis of FD. Plasma Gb3 has been shown to be a poor plasma biomarker due to its variability in FD.[22,23] In contrast, plasma and urinary globotriaosylsphingosine (lyso-Gb3) is a sensitive and specific biomarker that is elevated in patients

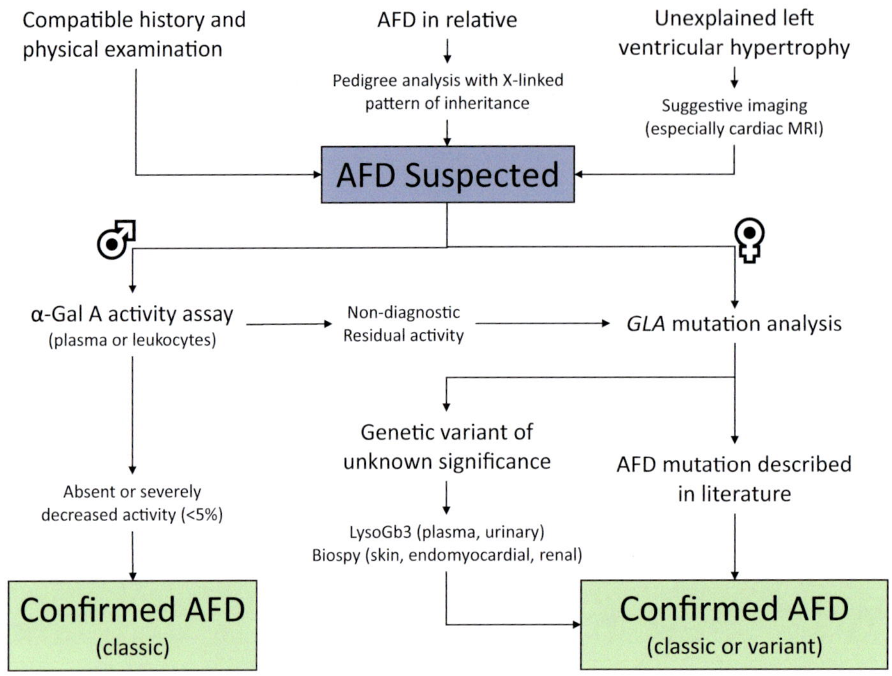

FIGURE 36.3 Proposed diagnostic algorithm for suspected Fabry disease. (Reproduced from Yogasundaram et al. *Can J Cardiol.* 2017;33(7):883–97 with permission from Elsevier.)

with FD and is especially useful in classifying genetic variants of unknown significance (Figure 36.3).[12,22,23]

Cardiac imaging offers a non-invasive method of assessing cardiovascular burden of FD. Echocardiography is useful for assessing LVH, valvular regurgitation, diastolic filling, and myocardial dysfunction. Strain and strain rate analysis is able to detect sub-clinical stages of impaired myocardial contractility in patients with diastolic dysfunction and myocardial fibrosis, while speckle tracking is useful for assessing left atrial function.[3,13] Cardiac magnetic resonance imaging (MRI) is the gold standard for assessing structural disease and myocardial fibrosis, and reliably discriminates FD-associated hypertrophy and fibrosis from other causes.[24,25] Specifically, late gadolinium enhancement discriminates FD from hypertrophic cardiomyopathy due to FD producing a distinct pattern of inferolateral basal and mid-wall distribution that spares the subendocardium.[24] In addition, non-contrast T1 mapping is capable of differentiating FD from other causes of concentric hypertrophy due to the uniquely shortened septal T1 time in FD.[25] Finally, cardiac nuclear perfusion imaging is necessary to evaluate microvascular dysfunction that leads to myocardial perfusion defects and fibrosis due to its unique ability to detect early cardiac inflammation in patients without any known cardiac involvement.[3]

Medical Management

Enzyme Replacement Therapy

Since its development in 2001, enzyme replacement therapy (ERT) has been the mainstay of treatment for FD. Two formulations of recombinant α-Gal A are currently approved: agalsidase α (0.2 mg/kg every two weeks) and agalsidase β (1 mg/kg every two weeks), both of which share the same amino acid structure as the native human enzyme but differ in originating cell lines. Both formulations are safe and effective in reducing glycosphingolipid levels in the plasma, heart, liver, and vasculature, leading to reductions in left ventricular (LV) mass, improved heart rate variability, stabilization of glomerular filtration, and improvement in gastrointestinal symptoms.[3,4,20] Therefore, ERT slows the progression of renal, cardiac, and central nervous system disease and in some instances partially reverses cardiomyopathy, especially in higher-risk elderly and male populations.[3,26,27] However, ERT should ideally be started early to slow or prevent irreversible changes, as its efficacy in advanced FD is limited.[4,28] Another challenge of ERT is the development of antibodies against the recombinant enzyme, which has been shown to occur in 20–56% participants across several studies.[29,30]

Pharmacological Chaperone Therapy

More recently, the iminosugar 1-deoxygalactonojirimycin (migalastat hydrochloride) has been approved for treatment of FD. It functions as a pharmacological chaperone and potent inhibitor of α-Gal A that binds the active site of the enzyme and improves its folding, stability, and lysosomal trafficking, after which it dissociates to allow an α-Gal A to catalyze the degradation of Gb3.[31–33] Migalastat has been shown to cause durable increase in α-Gal A activity and significant reduction in glycosphingolipid levels in lysates from the kidneys, heart, and liver.[31,32] Migalastat presents several advantages over ERT: its ability to cross the blood-brain barrier, oral rather than intravenous route of administration, and higher volume of distribution, which may enhance α-Gal A levels in multiple organs.[26,33] However, migalastat only improves the stability and activity of α-Gal A in patients with amenable missense mutations causing misfolding of α-Gal A, 78 of which have been identified to date.[31,32] Therefore, many nonsense and missense mutations resulting in both classic and variant phenotypes are not amenable to this treatment.

Substrate Reduction Therapy

Substrate reduction therapy, specifically eliglustat tartrate (Genz-112638), is an emerging treatment for FD, and represents an alternative approach to reducing glycosphingolipid levels that has proven effective in treating Gaucher disease, another glycosphingolipidosis.[34] Through inhibition of the glucosylceramide synthase enzyme that catalyzes the first step of glycosphingolipid synthesis, substrate reduction therapy reduces upstream production of glycosphingolipids.[23] In FD mouse models, substrate reduction therapy has been shown to reduce Gb3 and lyso-Gb3 levels in the kidneys, heart, and liver, with maximal effect when used in conjunction with ERT.[23,27] However, eliglustat was ineffective at lowering glycosphingolipid levels in the brain due to its poor ability to cross the blood-brain barrier.[35] A novel oral glucosylceramide synthase inhibitor, ibiglustat (Genz-682452), was designed to cross the blood brain barrier and has shown efficacy in lowering Gb3 and lyso-Gb3 levels in the brain, especially in conjunction with ERT.[34]

Gene Therapy

Gene therapy is a developing treatment for FD that offers a long-term treatment with minimal administration. Transduction of a functional GLA gene into FD mouse models via recombinant adeno-associated viral vectors with liver-specific promoters were shown to achieve supraphysiological levels of α-Gal A activity with simultaneous dramatic reduction in Gb3 levels in plasma, kidneys, heart, and liver for the duration of the study (14 weeks).[36] In addition, lentiviral α-Gal A transduction into FD patient CD34+ hematopoietic cells resulted in supraphysiological α-Gal A activity both ex vivo and when xenotransplanted into mouse FD models, where a reduction in splenic, hepatic, cardiac, and renal Gb3 levels was observed.[37] However, gene therapy has not yet been evaluated as a treatment modality for FD in humans.

Additional Considerations

In addition to disease-modifying FD therapy, patients should be monitored by a multidisciplinary team. Patients should undergo history, physical examination, as well as electrocardiography and echocardiography at baseline and annually if older than 35 years.[38] Lifestyle modification is also important in FD management due to its cardiovascular sequelae, including smoking cessation, a heart-healthy diet, and increased aerobic exercise.[3] Hypertension should preferably be treated using angiotensin-modulating agents due to their reno-protective effects.[3] Diabetes mellitus and simultaneous renal disease should be treated as per guidelines and statin therapy is indicated in patients with dyslipidemia. Low-dose aspirin is not recommended for primary stroke prevention in FD patients. Current guidelines recommend anticoagulation for stroke prevention in patients with atrial fibrillation and hypertrophic cardiomyopathy, regardless of risk stratification. In the absence of specific data, anticoagulation is indicated for patients with FD and atrial fibrillation.[39]

Conclusion

Fabry disease is a lysosomal storage disease with systemic sequelae that arise from diminished or absent α-Gal A enzyme activity, leading to serious cardiac, renal, and neurological disease. Cardiovascular disease is the number one cause of mortality in FD patients and manifests as LVH, diastolic dysfunction, microvascular dysfunction, and conduction disease. Diagnosis is based on α-Gal A activity and genetic testing in combination with clinical and biochemical disease markers. Traditional and novel biomarkers and cardiac imaging play crucial roles in following disease progression and response to therapy. The mainstays of treatment include aggressive conventional risk factor modification and ERT, with chaperone therapy, SRT, and gene therapy emerging as promising interventions.

Iron-Overload Cardiomyopathy (IOC)

Introduction

Iron is an essential component of cellular function and metabolism. As a transition metal, iron exists in either a ferrous (Fe^{2+}) or ferric (Fe^{3+}) ionic form and can readily undergo oxidation-reduction reactions between the two states.[40,41] Besides being a key component of hemoglobin and myoglobin, iron is an essential constituent of many proteins involved in the mitochondrial electron transport chain, such as cytochromes, NADPH dehydrogenases, and succinate dehydrogenases, as well as other enzymatic systems.[40,41] Iron homeostasis is therefore important for cellular function and, because of this, iron levels are tightly regulated under normal physiological conditions. Several regulatory proteins are involved in maintaining intracellular iron concentrations, via processes such as iron absorption, transport, and storage (Figure 36.4a).[42] Iron is mainly absorbed from the gastrointestinal tract or released from macrophages as Fe^{2+} via ferroportin. Iron release is in turn regulated by hepcidin, which inhibits iron transport by acting on ferroportin. Iron is converted from Fe^{2+} to Fe^{3+} by ceruloplasmin, transported within the circulation by transferrin, and stored in protein complexes such as ferritin. Iron metabolism is subject to numerous feedback mechanisms, and dysregulated iron homeostasis leads to hematologic, metabolic, and cardiovascular consequences.[43]

Primary and Acquired Iron Overload

Iron overload is defined as the accumulation of excessive iron in the body, which can be caused by both inherited and acquired etiologies.[43] Importantly, the human body lacks a physiologic mechanism for the excretion of excess iron. Primary hemochromatosis is a prototypical inherited cause of iron overload and is caused by mutations in genes involved in iron metabolism.[40] There are four types of hereditary hemochromatosis (Table 36.1). Type 1 is characterized by autosomal recessive mutations in the *HFE* gene which encodes a protein responsible for regulating hepcidin production. In type 1 hemochromatosis, increased iron absorption from the diet results in excessive iron accumulation in cells. A similar mechanism occurs in type 2 hemochromatosis, which is caused by autosomal recessive mutations in the *HJV* gene that codes for an iron regulatory protein named hemojuvelin. Defects in iron transporter proteins such as transferrin and ferroportin can give rise to autosomal recessive type 3 and autosomal dominant type 4 hemochromatosis, respectively.[40]

The most common causes of acquired iron overload are transfusion-dependent anemias, such as thalassemia and sickle cell disease (Table 36.1). Thalassemia is characterized by a deficiency in the synthesis of one or more globin chains of haemoglobin.[44] It is estimated that 1–5% of the world population are carriers of a mutant thalassemia allele; the disease is mostly prevalent in sub-Saharan Africa, the Mediterranean region, the Middle East, the Indian subcontinent, and East and Southeast Asia. Similarly, sickle cell disease, which results from mutations altering the β-globin chain of hemoglobin, is also known to be highly prevalent in Africa, India, the Mediterranean region, and the Middle East.[45] With migration, sickle cell disease has been introduced to areas

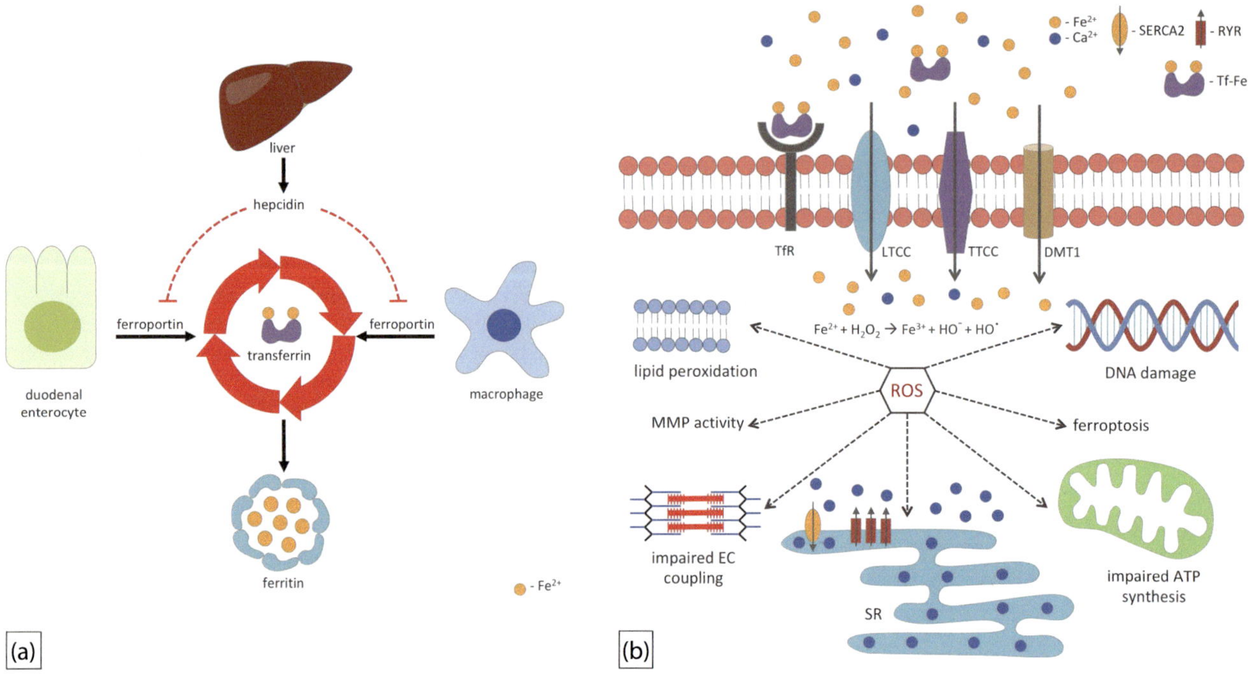

FIGURE 36.4 Overview of major proteins involved in iron homeostasis (a). Iron is absorbed from the gastrointestinal tract or released from macrophages through the action of ferroportin, which is inhibited by hepcidin. Iron is transported through the bloodstream via transferrin and is stored in complexes such as ferritin. Pathophysiology of iron-overload cardiomyopathy (c). Excessive iron accumulation in the cell generates ROS which activates numerous deleterious intracellular pathways. *Abbreviations*: TfR, transferrin receptor; Tf, transferrin; LTCC, L-type calcium channel; TTCC, T-type calcium channel; MMP, matrix metalloproteinase; EC, excitation-contraction; ROS, reactive oxygen species; RYR, ryanodine receptor; SR, sarcoplasmic reticulum; SERCA2, sarcoendoplasmic reticulum calcium ATPase 2.

TABLE 36.1: Primary and Secondary Causes of Iron-Overload Cardiomyopathy with Potential Inheritance Patterns

Conditions	Causes	Inheritance
Primary Hemochromatosis		
Type 1	*HFE* mutations	Autosomal recessive
Type 2	*HJV* mutations	Autosomal recessive
Type 3	*TfR2* mutations	Autosomal recessive
Type 4	*SLC40A1* mutations	Autosomal dominant
Secondary Iron Overload		
Thalassemia	Globin mutations	Autosomal recessive/dominant
Sickle cell anemia	*HBB* mutations	Autosomal recessive
Myelodysplastic syndrome	Multifactorial	—
Aplastic anemia	Multifactorial	—
Friedreich's ataxia	*FXN* mutations	Autosomal recessive
Chronic renal failure	Multifactorial	—
Increased iron intake	Diet, intravenous supplementation	—

in which it was not historically endemic, such as northern Europe and North America. In addition to thalassemia and sickle cell anemia, other hematological conditions, such as myelodysplastic syndrome, sideroblastic anemia, acute myeloid leukemia, and congenital dyserythropoietic anemia, are all associated with secondary iron overload resulting from frequent blood transfusion.[42,43] Additionally, iron overload has also been recognized in dialysis patients due to administration of erythropoiesis-stimulating agents and supplemental iron.[46]

Pathophysiology

In iron overload, excessive iron overwhelms the binding capacity of transferrin, leading to iron existing in a toxic, non-transferrin-bound, or labile state in the circulation.[47] Iron is transported into cardiomyocytes via multiple routes, including L-type and T-type calcium channels, bivalent metal transporter 1, and transferrin receptors.[48–50] Once in the cardiomyocyte, labile iron can damage various cellular structures and functions (Figure 36.4b). An important factor in iron-related cellular injury is the formation of reactive oxygen species.[42,43,51] Labile

Fe^{2+} can be converted to Fe^{3+} via the Haber-Weiss and Fenton reaction, which also generates reactive hydroxyl radicals.[49] Once the amount of reactive oxygen species produced exceeds the cell's antioxidant capacity, peroxidation of membrane lipids, cellular proteins, and nucleic acids result in intracellular oxidative damage.[43,51,52] Lipid peroxidation of mitochondrial membranes impairs oxidative phosphorylation and, subsequently, ATP production inside cardiomyocytes. In addition to cellular damage, excessive iron affects electrical conductivity via its deposition in the sinoatrial and atrioventricular nodes, and induces tissue fibrosis due to increased fibroblast activation and differentiation.[53] Increased Fe^{2+} transportation through L-type and T-type calcium channels interferes with intrinsic Ca^{2+} transportation in cardiomyocytes, resulting in impaired excitation-contraction coupling.[43,48,49,52] Elevated cytoplasmic Ca^{2+} concentrations due to reactive oxygen species-mediated suppression of SERCA2 damages cardiomyocyte contraction and relaxation. Iron-mediated cell death, matrix metalloproteinases, and tissue inhibitors of metalloproteinases may play a role in the pathogenesis of iron-overload cardiomyopathy (IOC).[54,55] There are key sex differences in iron-overload mediated effects on heart structure and function; females are markedly protected from IOC due to the protective effects of 17-beta estradiol.[56]

Clinical Presentation

In addition to IOC, iron overload is associated with several extracardiac manifestations, including hepatic dysfunction, pancreatic insufficiency leading to diabetes mellitus, pituitary and gonadal dysfunction, skin hyperpigmentation, and arthropathy often involving the second and third metacarpophalangeal joints. Early IOC manifests as diastolic dysfunction with restrictive filling and preserved left ventricle ejection fraction (LVEF) (Figure 36.5).[42,43,52] Stiff ventricles require higher filling pressures during diastole which leads to higher left atrial pressures and subsequent pulmonary hypertension. With prolonged pulmonary hypertension, patients can develop right ventricular (RV) remodeling, which eventually results in RV dilatation and right heart failure.

As the disease progresses, most patients will develop LV dilatation with reduced LVEF.[43] Cardiovascular MRI studies have demonstrated a strong inverse correlation between LVEF and myocardial iron deposition.[57] This inverse correlation was also observed in the RV. In late-stage iron overload, patients can develop dilated biventricular cardiomyopathy with reduced LVEF. Iron deposition in sinus and atrioventricular nodal cells, and myocardial fibrosis predispose IOC patients to conduction system disease.[58] Patients with iron overload may experience a variety of abnormal heart rhythms, such as atrioventricular block, conduction defects, bradyarrhythmias, tachyarrhythmias, and sudden cardiac death.[43]

Patients with IOC have pre-existing conditions that may complicate interpretation of clinical presentation. Transfusion-dependent patients almost invariably have anemia and vascular dysfunction. Therefore, diastolic and systolic dysfunction in these patients can be masked by an anemia-induced high output state.[59] Increased myocardial oxygen demand in the context of anemia and hypertrophic ventricles cause decreased myocardial perfusion and ischemia despite normal coronary arteries.[60] Myocardial perfusion is further compromised by unpredictable episodes of vasoocclusion due to polymerization of deoxygenated sickled hemoglobin in the case of sickle cell anemia.[61] This process, in combination with impaired coronary blood flow due to iron-mediated endothelial dysfunction, leads to higher risk of angina and myocardial infarction in patients with acquired IOC. Hemolytic anemia is another hallmark of sickle cell disease which results in chronic vasculopathy.[61] Free plasma hemoglobin depletes nitric oxide and generates reactive oxygen species while the released heme from hemoglobin activates the immune system, both of which lead to

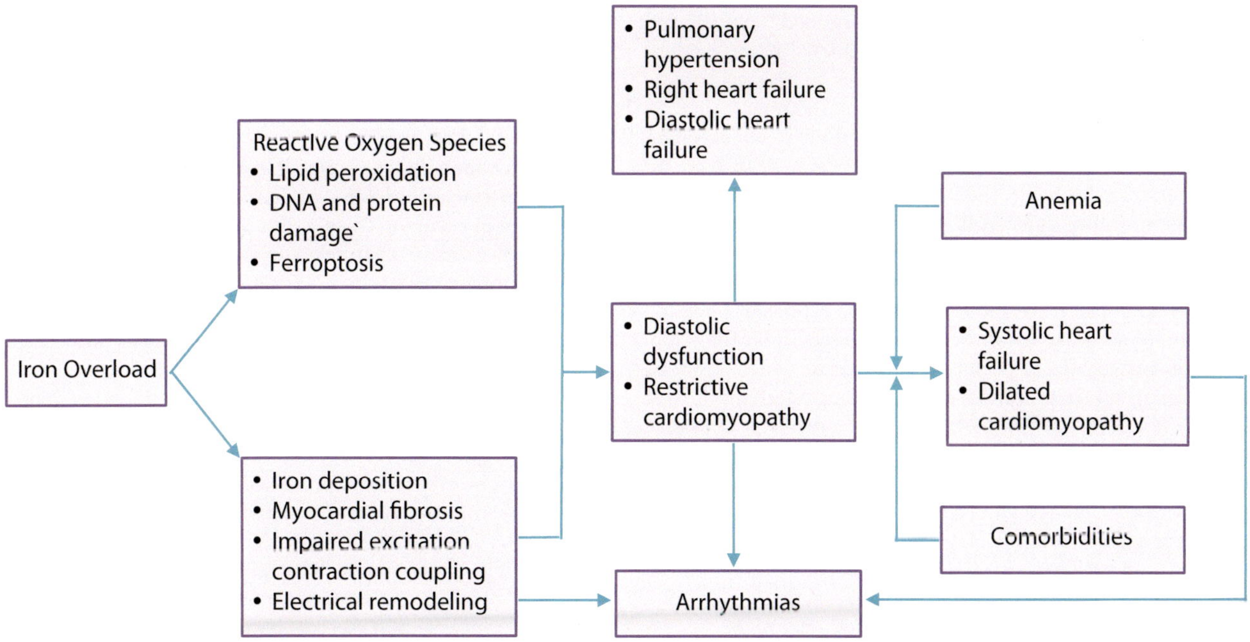

FIGURE 36.5 Pathophysiology of cardiac disease in iron-overload cardiomyopathy. Generation of reactive oxygen species and physical deposition of iron are two mechanisms by which iron-overload causes cardiac disease. Both systolic and diastolic heart failure are potential consequences of iron-overload cardiomyopathy. Comorbidities include liver disease, diabetes, endocrinopathies, and malnutrition.

endothelial dysfunction, vasoconstriction, and thromboembolism. Obstruction of small arterioles due to thromboembolism contributes to increased pulmonary vascular resistance, pulmonary hypertension, and eventually right heart failure in these patients.[62]

Diagnosis

A thorough history and physical examination may reveal signs and symptoms of heart failure as well as underlying causes or complication of IOC. For acquired IOC, the cumulative units of blood transfusion or intravenous iron that the patient has received are important information.[43]

Iron studies and genetic testing may be required when primary hemochromatosis is suspected. Serum ferritin is frequently elevated in patients with IOC. Even though serum ferritin is a non-specific marker that correlates poorly with myocardial iron deposition, elevated levels identify those at risk of developing IOC. Plasma B-type natriuretic peptide (BNP) is a useful prognostic marker, especially early in the course of the disease.[63] BNP might be elevated in heart failure patients with preserved LVEF before Doppler indices become abnormal.[64] Other biochemical tests, such as complete blood count, hemoglobin electrophoresis, and liver function or endocrine tests are helpful in identifying the underlying condition resulting in IOC, as well as evaluating the extent of iron-induced organ dysfunction.[42,43]

A standard electrocardiogram may identify conduction abnormalities.[42] Echocardiography can provide information on systolic and diastolic function, pericardial abnormalities, or valvular structure and function. Pseudo-normal or restrictive filling can be detected in early-stage IOC.[43] Later, echocardiography can reveal dilated phenotypes, characterized by ventricular dilatation and reduced LVEF, or restrictive phenotypes, characterized by dilatation of the left atrium and RV with preserved LVEF. However, conventional measures of systolic and diastolic function such as end-systolic volume, end-diastolic volume, EF, or fractional shortening are not sufficiently sensitive to detect early myocardial iron overload.[43] Strain and strain rate imaging allows for measurement of regional or global function of the myocardium and is more sensitive for evaluating subtle systolic and diastolic dysfunctions.[65]

Cardiac MRI-derived T2* relaxation time is an excellent non-invasive approach to quantify myocardial iron load. In an iron-overloaded heart, the iron paramagnetic effect creates local susceptibility-induced distortions on the magnetic field and shortens tissue relaxation time.[57] T2* allows measurement of magnetic field heterogeneity in regions of myocardial iron overload. Compared to traditional T1- or T2-based imaging, T2* is more sensitive for myocardial iron load quantification. Of note, myocardial T2* does not correlate with observed serum ferritin or liver iron levels[66] Low serum ferritin or liver iron are not predictive of lower IOC risk, since iron clearance is significantly slower in the heart than in other organs.[57] This becomes important when monitoring iron chelation therapy. T2* relaxation time is a good prognostic marker for heart failure and arrhythmias secondary to IOC. The reduction in mortality rates in patients with IOC can be partially attributed to the widespread use of T2* MRI in clinical practice.[67]

Finally, endomyocardial biopsy provides a definitive assessment of tissue iron levels. However, myocardial iron deposition is heterogeneous, which makes it challenging to evaluate global iron levels.[68,69] Endomyocardial biopsy is an invasive procedure with its own inherent risks; therefore, non-invasive approaches (e.g., cardiac MRI) are preferred in clinical practice.

Treatment

Therapy for iron overload differs depending on the underlying etiology, and typically involves either therapeutic phlebotomy or iron chelation therapy. The standard of care for primary hemochromatosis is phlebotomy to reduce total body iron and serum ferritin levels. When initiated early, phlebotomy is safe and effective for all four types of primary hemochromatosis.[42] Phlebotomy can prevent disease progression and improve survival in patients with IOC. Symptomatic patients or patients with elevated serum ferritin (>1,000 ng/mL) often require phlebotomy therapy. The goal of treatment is to reduce serum ferritin to <50 ng/mL and to maintain it at <100 ng/mL. Carriers of type I hemochromatosis mutations have increased risk of IOC and may require early intervention.[42,43,70]

The management of secondary IOC is largely through iron chelation therapy. Currently, there are three main iron chelators available: deferoxamine (parenteral), deferiprone (oral), and deferasirox (oral).[42,43] Iron removal iron chelation has proven effective in preventing the development of LV dysfunction, improving prognosis, and reducing mortality in patients with secondary IOC.[43] Combined chelation therapy using deferoxamine and deferiprone has been shown to reduce myocardial iron load and improve LVEF as well as endothelial function.[71] The dosing regimens depend on the total body iron level, the frequency of transfusions, and the severity of iron-induced damage in the heart and other organs. In this regard, T2* imaging is an excellent tool to evaluate myocardial iron deposition and monitor iron chelation therapy.[42,43]

Since iron-mediated oxidative stress significantly contributes to the pathophysiology of IOC, antioxidants may be beneficial in IOC. Combinational therapy consisting of iron chelators with antioxidants such as *N*-acetylcysteine or taurine reverse iron-induced damage in the brain and heart of a murine model with iron overload.[72,73] Dietary resveratrol supplementation ameliorated iron-induced oxidative stress, reduced myocardial fibrosis, and Ca^{2+} cycling defects, rescued advanced cardiomyopathy, and increased survival in iron-overloaded mice.[52,74] Antioxidants are a potential therapeutic intervention in the treatment of IOC; however, randomized, clinical trials remain to be performed before any of these drugs can be used in clinical practice.

Calcium channels are responsible for transporting iron into myocardial cells. Therefore, calcium channel blockers could be effective in reducing the severity of IOC.[48,49,75] Additionally, blockage of calcium channels can reduce iron-induced Ca^{2+} overload, improve diastolic function, and promote myocardial microvascular perfusion.[43] In randomized trials, dual therapy with the calcium channel blocker amlodipine and iron chelators reduced myocardial iron burden without serious adverse effects in patients with thalassemia.[76] Calcium channel blockers should be evaluated in larger clinical trials to establish their efficacy and safety profile in patients with IOC.

The only curative treatment for secondary IOC is bone marrow transplantation to correct the underlying hematologic defects. Other approaches, such as erythropoiesis modulation or stem cell gene therapy, are also under development. To date, there has been only one case report on reversing cardiomyopathy in a patient with IOC secondary to severe aplastic anemia, using stem cell transplantation.[77] Cardiac function could be normalized once iron overload from repetitive transfusions is stopped; therefore, these promising strategies offer potential alternatives for patients with secondary IOC. Patients with cardiac complications from iron overload, such as heart failure or conduction defects, are typically treated according to conventional guidelines. Management of comorbidities and risk factors for progression of cardiovascular disease are important in this patient population. Device therapy and advanced heart failure therapies, including heart transplantation, may be indicated for severe IOC.

Conclusion

Primary hemochromatosis and transfusion-dependent IOC are important causes of heart failure. Iron-induced cardiac dysfunction can manifest as restrictive cardiomyopathy or, more frequently, dilated cardiomyopathy, but these phenotypes can be complicated by pre-existing conditions. Besides traditional diagnostic tools, cardiac MRI with T2* imaging is an excellent non-invasive technique for quantifying iron deposition in myocardial cells. Current treatments directed at the underlying cause are limited to phlebotomy and iron chelation therapy. Promising approaches are under development and have the potential to facilitate treatment of IOC in the future.

References

1. Felker GM, Thompson RE, Hare JM, et al. Underlying causes and long-term survival in patients with initially unexplained cardiomyopathy. *N Engl J Med.* 2000;342(15):1077–84.
2. Seward JB, Casaclang-Verzosa G. Infiltrative cardiovascular diseases: cardiomyopathies that look alike. *J Am Coll Cardiol.* 2010;55(17):1769–79.
3. Yogasundaram H, Kim D, Oudit O, Thompson RB, Weidemann F, Oudit GY. Clinical features, diagnosis, and management of patients with Anderson-Fabry cardiomyopathy. *Can J Cardiol.* 2017;33(7):883–97.
4. El-Abassi R, Singhal D, England JD. Fabry's disease. *J Neurol Sci.* 2014;344(1–2):5–19.
5. Lin HY, Chong KW, Hsu JH, et al. High incidence of the cardiac variant of Fabry disease revealed by newborn screening in the Taiwan Chinese population. *Circ Cardiovasc Genet.* 2009;2(5):450–6.
6. Spada M, Pagliardini S, Yasuda M, et al. High incidence of later-onset Fabry disease revealed by newborn screening. *Am J Hum Genet.* 2006;79(1):31–40.
7. Adalsteinsdottir B, Palsson R, Desnick RJ, et al. Fabry disease in families with hypertrophic cardiomyopathy: clinical manifestations in the classic and later-onset phenotypes. *Circ Cardiovasc Genet.* 2017;10(4):e001639.
8. Desnick RJ, Brady R, Barranger J, et al. Fabry disease, an under-recognized multisystemic disorder: expert recommendations for diagnosis, management, and enzyme replacement therapy. *Ann Intern Med.* 2003;138(4):338–46.
9. Hughes DA, Malmenas M, Deegan PB, et al. Fabry international prognostic index: a predictive severity score for Anderson-Fabry disease. *J Med Genet.* 2012;49(3):212–20.
10. Whybra C, Kampmann C, Krummenauer F, et al. The Mainz Severity Score Index: a new instrument for quantifying the Anderson-Fabry disease phenotype, and the response of patients to enzyme replacement therapy. *Clin Genet.* 2004;65(4):299–307.
11. Weidemann F, Maier SK, Stork S, et al. Usefulness of an implantable loop recorder to detect clinically relevant arrhythmias in patients with advanced Fabry cardiomyopathy. *Am J Cardiol.* 2016;118(2):264–274.
12. Niemann M, Herrmann S, Hu K, et al. Differences in Fabry cardiomyopathy between female and male patients: consequences for diagnostic assessment. *JACC Cardiovasc Imaging.* 2011;4(6):592–601.
13. Putko BN, Wen K, Thompson RB, et al. Anderson-Fabry cardiomyopathy: prevalence, pathophysiology, diagnosis and treatment. *Heart Fail Rev.* 2015;20(2):179–91.
14. Linhart A, Elliott PM. The heart in Anderson-Fabry disease and other lysosomal storage disorders. *Heart.* 2007;93(4):528–35.
15. Shah JS, Hughes DA, Sachdev B, et al. Prevalence and clinical significance of cardiac arrhythmia in Anderson-Fabry disease. *Am J Cardiol.* 2005;96(6):842–6.
16. Thompson RB, Chow K, Khan A, et al. T(1) mapping with cardiovascular MRI is highly sensitive for Fabry disease independent of hypertrophy and sex. *Circ Cardiovasc Imaging.* 2013;6(5):637–45.
17. Desnick RJ. Fabry disease. In: Rosenberg RN, Pascual JM, eds. *Rosenberg's molecular and genetic basis of neurological and psychiatric disease.* Boston: Academic Press; 2015:419–30.
18. Spada M, Pagliardini S, Yasuda M, et al. High incidence of later-onset Fabry disease revealed by newborn screening. *Am J Hum Genet.* 2006;79(1):31–40.
19. Favalli V, Disabella E, Molinaro M, et al. Genetic screening of Anderson-Fabry disease in probands referred from multispecialty clinics. *J Am Coll Cardiol.* 2016;68(10):1037–50.
20. Wilcox WR, Feldt-Rasmussen U, Martins AM, et al. Improvement of Fabry disease-related gastrointestinal symptoms in a significant proportion of female patients treated with agalsidase beta: data from the Fabry registry. *JIMD Rep.* 2018;38:45–51.
21. Echevarria L, Benistan K, Toussaint A, et al. X-chromosome inactivation in female patients with Fabry disease. *Clin Genet.* 2016;89(1):44–54.
22. Rombach SM, Dekker N, Bouwman MG, et al. Plasma globotriaosylsphingosine: diagnostic value and relation to clinical manifestations of Fabry disease. *Biochim Biophys Acta.* 2010;1802(9):741–8.
23. Sakuraba H, Togawa T, Tsukimura T, Kato H. Plasma lyso-Gb3: a biomarker for monitoring fabry patients during enzyme replacement therapy. *Clin Exp Nephrol.* 2018;22(4):843–9.
24. De Cobelli F, Esposito A, Belloni E, et al. Delayed-enhanced cardiac MRI for differentiation of Fabry's disease from symmetric hypertrophic cardiomyopathy. *AJR Am J Roentgenol.* 2009;192(3):W97–102.
25. Sado DM, White SK, Piechnik SK, et al. Identification and assessment of Anderson-Fabry disease by cardiovascular magnetic resonance noncontrast myocardial T1 mapping. *Circ Cardiovasc Imaging.* 2013;6(3):392–8.
26. Del Pino M, Andres A, Bernabeu AA, et al. Fabry nephropathy: an evidence-based narrative review. *Kidney Blood Press Res.* 2018;43(2):406–21.
27. Ortiz A, Abiose A, Bichet DG, et al. Time to treatment benefit for adult patients with Fabry disease receiving agalsidase beta: data from the Fabry Registry. *J Med Genet.* 2016;53(7):495–502.
28. Simonetta I, Tuttolomondo A, Di Chiara T, et al. Genetics and gene therapy of Anderson-Fabry disease. *Curr Gene Ther.* 2018;18(2):96–106.
29. Deegan PB. Fabry disease, enzyme replacement therapy and the significance of antibody responses. *J Inherit Metab Dis.* 2012;35(2):227–43.
30. Schiffmann R, Kopp JB, Austin HA, 3rd, et al. Enzyme replacement therapy in Fabry disease: a randomized controlled trial. *JAMA.* 2001;285(21):2743–9.
31. Benjamin ER, Flanagan JJ, Schilling A, et al. The pharmacological chaperone 1-deoxygalactonojirimycin increases alpha-galactosidase A levels in Fabry patient cell lines. *J Inherit Metab Dis.* 2009;32(3):424–40.
32. Ishii S. Pharmacological chaperone therapy for Fabry disease. *Proc Jpn Acad Ser B Phys Biol Sci.* 2012;88(1):18–30.
33. Echevarria L, Benistan K, Toussaint A, et al. X-chromosome inactivation in female patients with Fabry disease. *Clin Genet.* 2016;89(1):44–54.
34. Ashe KM, Budman E, Bangari DS, et al. Efficacy of enzyme and substrate reduction therapy with a novel antagonist of glucosylceramide synthase for Fabry disease. *Mol Med.* 2015;21(1):389–99.
35. Marshall J, Ashe KM, Bangari D, et al. Substrate reduction augments the efficacy of enzyme therapy in a mouse model of Fabry disease. *PLoS One.* 2010;5(11):e15033.
36. Jeyakumar J, Kia A, McIntosh J, et al. Liver-directed gene therapy corrects Fabry disease in mice. *Mol Genet Metabol.* 2019;126(2):S80.
37. Huang J, Khan A, Au BC, et al. Lentivector iterations and pre-clinical scale-up/toxicity testing: targeting mobilized CD34(+) cells for correction of Fabry disease. *Mol Ther Methods Clin Dev.* 2017;5:241–58.
38. Eng CM, Germain DP, Banikazemi M, et al. Fabry disease: guidelines for the evaluation and management of multi-organ system involvement. *Genet Med.* 2006;8(9):539–48.
39. January CT, Wann LS, Alpert JS, et al. 2014 AHA/ACC/HRS guideline for the management of patients with atrial fibrillation: a report of the American College of Cardiology/American Heart Association Task Force on practice guidelines and the Heart Rhythm Society. *Circulation.* 2014;130(23):e199–267.
40. Andrews NC. Disorders of iron metabolism. *N Engl J Med.* 1999;341(26):1986–95.
41. Hentze MW, Muckenthaler MU, Andrews NC. Balancing acts: molecular control of mammalian iron metabolism. *Cell.* 2004;117(3):285–97.
42. Kremastinos DT, Farmakis D. Iron overload cardiomyopathy in clinical practice. *Circulation.* 2011;124(20):2253–63.
43. Murphy CJ, Oudit GY. Iron-overload cardiomyopathy: pathophysiology, diagnosis, and treatment. *J Card Fail.* 2010;16(11):888–900.
44. Taher AT, Weatherall DJ, Cappellini MD. Thalassaemia. *Lancet.* 2018;391(10116):155–67.
45. Gardner RV. Sickle cell disease: advances in treatment. *Ochsner J.* 2018;18(4):377–89.
46. Bailie GR, Larkina M, Goodkin DA, et al. Data from the dialysis outcomes and practice patterns study validate an association between high intravenous iron doses and mortality. *Kidney Int.* 2015;87(1):162–8.
47. Wood JC. Cardiac iron across different transfusion-dependent diseases. *Blood Rev.* 2008;22 Suppl 2S14–21.
48. Oudit GY, Sun H, Trivieri MG, et al. L-type Ca2+ channels provide a major pathway for iron entry into cardiomyocytes in iron-overload cardiomyopathy. *Nat Med.* 2003;9(9):1187–94.

49. Oudit GY, Trivieri MG, Khaper N, Liu PP, Backx PH. Role of L-type Ca2+ channels in iron transport and iron-overload cardiomyopathy. *J Mol Med (Berl).* 2006;84(5):349–64.
50. Kumfu S, Chattipakorn S, Srichairatanakool S, Settakorn J, Fucharoen S, Chattipakorn N. T-type calcium channel as a portal of iron uptake into cardiomyocytes of beta-thalassemic mice. *Eur J Haematol.* 2011;86(2):156–66.
51. Zhabyeyev P, Oudit GY. Hemochromatosis protein (HFE) knockout mice as a novel model of hemochromatosis: implications for study and management of iron-overload cardiomyopathy. *Can J Cardiol.* 2017;33(7):835–7.
52. Das SK, Wang W, Zhabyeyev P, et al. Iron-overload injury and cardiomyopathy in acquired and genetic models is attenuated by resveratrol therapy. *Sci Rep.* 2015;518132.
53. Rosenqvist M, Hultcrantz R. Prevalence of a haemochromatosis among men with clinically significant bradyarrhythmias. *Eur Heart J.* 1989;10(5):473–8.
54. Stockwell BR, Friedmann Angeli JP, Bayir H, et al. Ferroptosis: a regulated cell death nexus linking metabolism, redox biology, and disease. *Cell.* 2017;171(2):273–85.
55. Zhabyeyev P, Das SK, Basu R, et al. TIMP3 deficiency exacerbates iron overload-mediated cardiomyopathy and liver disease. *Am J Physiol Heart Circ Physiol.* 2018;314(5):H978–90.
56. Das SK, Patel VB, Basu R, et al. Females are protected from iron-overload cardiomyopathy independent of iron metabolism: key role of oxidative stress. *J Am Heart Assoc.* 2017;6(1):pii: e003456.
57. Anderson LJ, Holden S, Davis B, et al. Cardiovascular T2-star (T2*) magnetic resonance for the early diagnosis of myocardial iron overload. *Eur Heart J.* 2001;22(23):2171–9.
58. Pepe A, Positano V, Capra M, et al. Myocardial scarring by delayed enhancement cardiovascular magnetic resonance in thalassaemia major. *Heart.* 2009;95(20):1688–93.
59. Lau KC, Li AM, Hui PW, Yeung CY. Left ventricular function in beta thalassaemia major. *Arch Dis Child.* 1989;64(7):1046–51.
60. Alpert BS, Flood NL, Strong WB, Blair JR, Walpert JB, Levy AL. Responses to exercise in children with sickle cell trait. *Am J Dis Child.* 1982;136(11):1002–4.
61. Piccin A, Murphy C, Eakins E, et al. Insight into the complex pathophysiology of sickle cell anaemia and possible treatment. *Eur J Haematol.* 2019;102(4):319–30.
62. Hahalis G, Alexopoulos D, Kremastinos DT, Zoumbos NC. Heart failure in beta-thalassemia syndromes: a decade of progress. *Am J Med.* 2005;118(9):957–67.
63. Kremastinos DT, Hamodraka E, Parissis J, Tsiapras D, Dima K, Maisel A. Predictive value of B-type natriuretic peptides in detecting latent left ventricular diastolic dysfunction in beta-thalassemia major. *Am Heart J.* 2010;159(1):68–74.
64. Kremastinos DT, Tsiapras DP, Kostopoulou AG, Hamodraka ES, Chaidaroglou AS, Kapsali ED. NT-proBNP levels and diastolic dysfunction in beta-thalassaemia major patients. *Eur J Heart Fail.* 2007;9(5):531–6.
65. Gupta A, Kapoor A, Phadke S, et al. Use of strain, strain rate, tissue velocity imaging, and endothelial function for early detection of cardiovascular involvement in patients with beta-thalassemia. *Ann Pediatr Cardiol.* 2017;10(2):158–66.
66. Kletzmayr J, Horl WH. Iron overload and cardiovascular complications in dialysis patients. *Nephrol Dial Transplant.* 2002;17 Suppl 225–29.
67. Modell B, Khan M, Darlison M, Westwood MA, Ingram D, Pennell DJ. Improved survival of thalassaemia major in the UK and relation to T2* cardiovascular magnetic resonance. *J Cardiovasc Magn Reson.* 2008;10(1):42.
68. Olson LJ, Edwards WD, Holmes DR, Jr., Miller FA, Jr., Nordstrom LA, Baldus WP. Endomyocardial biopsy in hemochromatosis: clinicopathologic correlates in six cases. *J Am Coll Cardiol.* 1989;13(1):116–20.
69. Olson LJ, Edwards WD, McCall JT, Ilstrup DM, Gersh BJ. Cardiac iron deposition in idiopathic hemochromatosis: histologic and analytic assessment of 14 hearts from autopsy. *J Am Coll Cardiol.* 1987;10(6):1239–43.
70. Niederau C, Fischer R, Sonnenberg A, Stremmel W, Trampisch HJ, Strohmeyer G. Survival and causes of death in cirrhotic and in noncirrhotic patients with primary hemochromatosis. *N Engl J Med.* 1985;313(20):1256–62.
71. Tanner MA, Galanello R, Dessi C, et al. A randomized, placebo-controlled, double-blind trial of the effect of combined therapy with deferoxamine and deferiprone on myocardial iron in thalassemia major using cardiovascular magnetic resonance. *Circulation.* 2007;115(14):1876–84.
72. Oudit GY, Trivieri MG, Khaper N, et al. Taurine supplementation reduces oxidative stress and improves cardiovascular function in an iron-overload murine model. *Circulation.* 2004;109(15):1877–85.
73. Wongjaikam S, Kumfu S, Khamseekaew J, Chattipakorn SC, Chattipakorn N. Restoring the impaired cardiac calcium homeostasis and cardiac function in iron overload rats by the combined deferiprone and N-acetyl cysteine. *Sci Rep.* 2017;744460.
74. Das SK, Zhabyeyev P, Basu R, et al. Advanced iron-overload cardiomyopathy in a genetic murine model is rescued by resveratrol therapy. *Biosci Rep.* 2018;38(1):BSR20171302.
75. Oudit GY, Backx PH. Amlodipine therapy for iron-overload cardiomyopathy: the enduring value of translational research. *Can J Cardiol.* 2016;32(8):938–40.
76. Eghbali A, Kazemi H, Taherahmadi H, Ghandi Y, Rafiei M, Bagheri B. A randomized, controlled study evaluating effects of amlodipine addition to chelators to reduce iron loading in patients with thalassemia major. *Eur J Haematol.* 2017;99(6):577–81.
77. Nishio M, Endo T, Nakao S, Sato N, Koike T. Reversible cardiomyopathy due to secondary hemochromatosis with multitransfusions for severe aplastic anemia after successful non-myeloablative stem cell transplantation. *Int J Cardiol.* 2008;127(3):400–1.

INDEX

D

E

F

G

H

N

R

S